PART I FUNDAMENTALS OF STRUCTURE AND MOTION OF THE HUMAN BODY

PART II SKELETAL OSTEOLOGY (STUDY OF THE BONES)

PART III SKELETAL ARTHROLOGY (STUDY OF THE JOINTS)

PART IV MYOLOGY (STUDY OF THE MUSCULAR SYSTEM)

APPENDIX

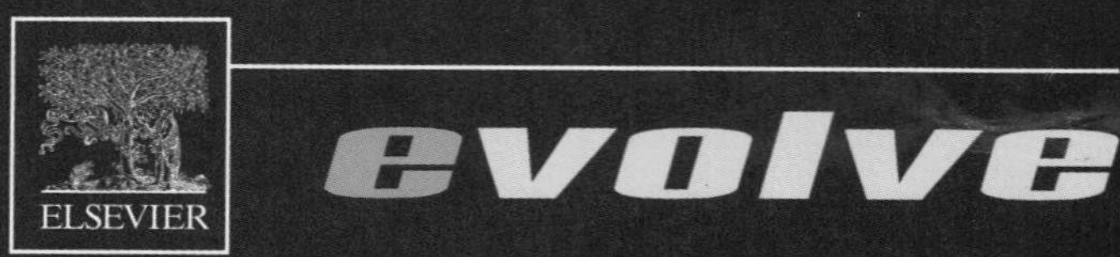

To access your Student Resources, visit:

http://evolve.elsevier.com/Muscolino/kinesiology/

Evolve® Student Learning Resources for **Muscolino: *Kinesiology: The Skeletal System and Muscle Function,*** offer the following features:

Student Resources

- **Answers to Review Questions in the Book**
  Look here to find answers to the review questions at the end of each chapter in the book!
- **Weblinks**
  Additional information is provided several via weblinks chosen by the author.
- **Drag and Drop Labeling Exercises**
  Enhance your review of the material by dragging and dropping labels into correct position on the 15 anatomic illustrations.
- **Crossword Puzzles**
  17 crossword puzzles (1 for each chapter) help you reinforce muscle names and terminology.
- **Glossary of Terms and Word Origins**
  All terms from the book are defined and explained, along with word origins, on the Evolve site.
- **Radiographs**
  Study these radiographs for realistic applications of material in the book.

http://evolve.elsevier.com/Muscolino/kinesiology/

KINESIOLOGY

The Skeletal System and Muscle Function

KINESIOLOGY

The Skeletal System and Muscle Function

JOSEPH E. MUSCOLINO, DC

Instructor, Connecticut Center for Massage Therapy
Westport, Connecticut
Owner, The Art and Science of Kinesiology, Redding, Connecticut

MOSBY

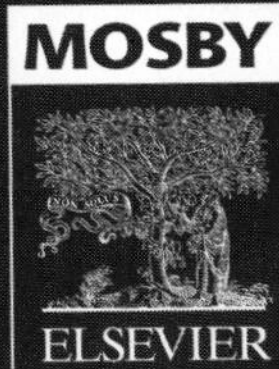

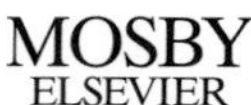

11830 Westline Industrial Drive
St. Louis, Missouri 63146

KINESIOLOGY: THE SKELETAL SYSTEM AND MUSCLE FUNCTION ISBN-13: 978-0-323-02524-9
ISBN-10: 0-323-02524-2

Copyright © 2006 by Mosby, Inc., an affiliate of Elsevier Inc.

All rights reserved. No part of this publication may be reproduced or transmitted in any form or by any means, electronic or mechanical, including photocopy, recording, or any information storage and retrieval system, without permission in writing from the publisher.

Permissions may be sought directly from Elsevier's Health Sciences Rights Department in Philadelphia, PA, USA: phone: (+1) 215 239 3804, fax: (+1) 215 239 3805, e-mail: healthpermissions@elsevier.com. You may also complete your request on-line via the Elsevier homepage (http://www.elsevier.com), by selecting 'Customer Support' and then 'Obtaining Permissions'.

Notice

Neither the Publisher nor the Author assume any responsibility for any loss or injury and/or damage to persons or property arising out of or related to any use of the material contained in this book. It is the responsibility of the treating practitioner, relying on independent expertise and knowledge of the patient, to determine the best treatment and method of application for the patient.

The Publisher

ISBN-13 978-0-323-02524-9

ISBN 0-323-02524-2

Publishing Director: *Linda Duncan*
Editor: *Kellie Fitzpatrick*
Developmental Editor: *Jennifer Watrous*
Editorial Assistant: *Elizabeth Clark*
Publishing Services Manager: *Julie Eddy*
Project Manager: *JoAnn Amore*
Designer: *Julia Dummitt*

Printed in The United States of America.

Last digit is the print number: 9 8 7 6 5 4 3 2 1

Working together to grow
libraries in developing countries
www.elsevier.com | www.bookaid.org | www.sabre.org
ELSEVIER BOOK AID International Sabre Foundation

This book is dedicated to my family.

To my parents, Carl and Vera,
who have given me everything of value,
most importantly love and support.
Thank you for teaching me to believe in myself.

To my big sister Diane and her family.
Diane, thank you for teaching me what true strength is.
Of everyone I know, you stand the tallest.

To my other big sister Dede and her family.
Dede, thank you for rescuing lost creatures
and for creating the center of our family.

And of course, to my wife, Simona,
and my two children, Randi and JC,
the centers of my life.

Forewords

Early in my career, I read a Zen proverb that said, "When the student is ready, the teacher will appear." Two years later, I not only found my first teacher on the subject of biomechanics, I also found my passion.

My first teacher was Tom Purvis, RPT, the founder of the Resistance Training Specialist Program. He gave me a strong foundation and taught me some important insights about learning. His profound statement still sticks with me: "Saying 'I've got it!' is the first sign that you don't! 'Getting it' is a lifelong process."

If biomechanics is an exact science, Dr. Joseph E. Muscolino has hit the nail on the head with his timely book entitled *Kinesiology: The Skeletal System and Muscle Function.* Joe makes "getting it" a much easier process! He told me that he has been working on this book for five years. But this book really represents a compilation of his experiences and perspectives throughout 20 years in a private chiropractic practice and more than 19 years as an instructor at the Connecticut Center for Massage Therapy.

I have worked as the Biomechanics Consultant for the Fitness Staff at ESPN, Canyon Ranch and the Greenbrier Healthy Living Spa. I have also taught biomechanics to many fitness professionals throughout New England. Frequently, colleagues will ask me to recommend a kinesiology book. I have often been at a loss. Now, I look forward to recommending Joe Muscolino's breakthrough book. Joe's superb blend of teaching experience and examples (light bulb boxes) will offer Athletic Trainers, Personal Trainers, Massage Therapists, Occupational Therapists, and Physical Therapists a remarkable resource that is visually appealing and put together in an accessible format.

It's not very often that a valuable resource like this comes along. Joe takes a very complex subject and makes it simple without being inaccurate...His insight on stressors and gait alone makes this book an asset to any library.

Rick C. Merriam, ACE, AFAA, LMT
F.I.T. First in-home personalized training
Canton, Connecticut

Massage therapy and bodywork are effective, beneficial approaches for enhancing wellness and treating soft-tissue disorders. Increasingly, massage and bodywork practitioners are sought after for treatment of a variety of pain complaints and injury conditions. The public's expectations place a high demand on the knowledge base of these practitioners. Consequently, the professional development of massage and bodywork therapists must accommodate the changing requirements of the profession. *Kinesiology: The Skeletal System and Muscle Function* meets the needs of emerging professionals and fills a critical gap in the resources available to schools and students.

Kinesiology is a critical component of the knowledge and skills necessary for today's soft-tissue therapist. By definition kinesiology is the study of anatomy (structure), neuromuscular physiology (function), and biomechanics (the mechanics of movement related to living systems). Competence in these principles is required even for those practitioners who work in an environment where massage or movement therapy is used only for relaxation or stress reduction. The need to understand proper movement can arise in the most basic soft-tissue treatment.

Take the instance of a client who initially states that she wants a relaxation treatment. Perhaps in the midst of the treatment she describes recurrent anterior knee pain and asks for attention to that area. Effective treatment requires addressing the tissues involved. In order to address the client's pain, the practitioner must ask the client which movements produce the pain, immediately applying the concepts of kinesiology in considering the client's discomfort. Suppose the client's pain is produced when squatting. The therapist should be able to identify knee flexion as the action that creates the pain. The practitioner could conclude that the hamstrings are the problematic tissue involved because this muscle group produces knee flexion by concentric action. However, the client specified anterior knee pain. Applying correct principles of kinesiology, the practitioner would then recognize the pain-producing action as an eccentric action of the quadriceps. Consequently, this minor amount of assessment would show that a musculotendinous disorder in the quadriceps or patellar tendon is a more likely cause of the client's pain.

The requirements for knowing the principles of kinesiology are even greater for those practitioners who actively choose to address soft-tissue pain and injury conditions. Treatment of any soft-tissue disorder begins with a comprehensive assessment of the problem. Accurate assessment is not possible without an understanding of how the body moves under normal circumstances. In the example above, adequate treatment would wholly depend on competent assessment of the condition. Treating the client's hamstrings would have proven ineffectual for what was truly a quadriceps or patellar tendon disorder. While the client might have benefited from the minor relief brought about by superficial overall massage, the specific pain complaint would not have been addressed.

Over the years of teaching orthopedic assessment and treatment to soft-tissue therapists, I have found many students deficient in their understanding of kinesiology. Similarly, students express frustration about understanding how to apply basic kinesiology principles in their practice. Although they receive some training in their initial coursework, traditional approaches to teaching kinesiology often provide little benefit to students. Overwhelmingly, basic courses in kinesiology prove to be insufficient and fail to connect the student with the skills necessary for professional success.

Learning muscle attachments and concentric actions tends to be the focus of most kinesiology curricula and is often turned into an exercise of rote memorization. Yet, there is significantly more to this important subject than these topics. Eccentric actions, force loads, angle of pull, axis of rotation, synergistic muscles, and other concepts are necessary for understanding human movement. These principles, in turn, are prerequisites for effective therapeutic treatment. An adequate understanding of kinesiology requires more than a curriculum plan that emphasizes memorization. A competent education in kinesiology requires a foundation in the functional application of its principles.

Including effective kinesiology training in the curriculum is a benefit for schools and their students. The success of a class or instructional program, however, is reliant on the instructional materials used. One of the key factors that limits a school's ability to develop quality kinesiology curricula is the lack of resources tailored specifically for the needs of massage therapists and bodyworkers. While there are numerous kinesiology texts published, *Kinesiology: The Skeletal System and Muscle Function* is the only text designed to be appropriate for the massage and movement therapist.

There are very few people capable of producing this badly needed resource. Joe Muscolino's scientific background and years of experience as an educator teaching anatomy, pathology, and kinesiology make him uniquely qualified for this project. His skill, talent, and demonstrated expertise are evidenced in this work and are of great benefit to the soft-tissue professions. During the years I've known Joe as a professional colleague, we have repeatedly engaged in animated discussions about how to raise the quality of training and improve educational resources available in the profession. With the publication of this book, he has hit the mark again and produced another outstanding contribution to our professional literature.

The structure of the text allows educators to easily incorporate the material into a beginning or advanced course. The organization and design of the subject matter makes the material easily accessible to students, as well. Review questions, learning objectives, key terms and concepts, and instructor support materials are designed to enhance high-order thinking skills instead of simple repetition of factual knowledge. In addition, the elaborate illustrations and user-friendly graphical layout make the book inviting and not intimidating to the reader. The instructor resources that accompany the book, including materials on CD and the web, demonstrate a genuine understanding of what is necessary for effective learning in kinesiology. Program directors and educators will significantly improve their training programs by using this profession-appropriate resource and the beneficial support materials provided.

One factor that represents the maturing of a profession is the development of supportive literature that addresses the unique needs of practicing professionals, educators, and students. This book has accomplished these goals and is destined to be a key resource for years to come. Muscolino's text excels in its ability to be both a comprehensive resource for the practicing professional and an excellent guide for students new to the field.

Whitney Lowe, LMT
Orthopedic Massage Education & Research Institute
Sisters, Oregon

Preface

Kinesiology: The Skeletal System and Muscle Function is unique in that it is the first kinesiology textbook written for the allied health fields of bodywork, movement therapies, and athletic training. The purpose of this book is to explain the concepts of kinesiology in a clear, simple, and straightforward manner, without dumbing down the material. Because this book is geared toward allied health fields, clinical applications are located throughout the text's narrative to explain relevant concepts.

The subject matter of this book is explained in a manner in which the reader or student is encouraged to think critically instead of memorize. This concept follows from a clear and orderly layout of the information. My belief is that no subject matter is difficult to learn if the *big picture* is first presented, and then the smaller pieces are presented in context to the big picture. An analogy to a jigsaw puzzle can be made wherein each piece of the puzzle represents a piece of information that must be learned. When all the pieces of the puzzle first come cascading out of the box, the idea of learning them and fitting them together can seem overwhelming; and indeed it is a daunting task if we do not first look at the big picture on the front of the box. However, if the big picture is first explained and understood, then our ability to learn and place into context all the small pieces is facilitated. This approach makes the job of being a student of kinesiology much easier!

The layout of information in this book is assisted by full-color illustrations that visually display the concepts that are being explained so that the student can *see* what is happening. Although good illustrations are always helpful, in a kinesiology textbook in which the subject matter is movement, they are especially important. Numerous resources are available for the reader or student, including learning outcomes, review questions, and the Evolve web site, which contains answers to the various questions, further in-depth readings, a comprehensive glossary of terms, and interactive exercises such as crossword puzzles, drag-and-drop exercises, and more.

For the instructor of kinesiology using this textbook for a class, the following resources are available: an image bank containing all illustrations found in the book, a test bank of over 1000 questions, and an instructor's resource manual. Furthermore, this book is designed as not only a reference textbook, but also as a source to be used within the classroom. Toward this end, it contains open bullets next to each piece of information that the student can easily check, which allows the instructor to assign clearly the material that the students are responsible to learn.

Finally, I would like to say that even though kinesiology can be viewed as the science of studying the biomechanics of body movement (and the human body certainly is a marvel of biomechanical engineering), kinesiology can also be seen as the study of an art form. Movement is more than simply lifting a glass or walking across a room; movement is the means by which we live our lives and express ourselves. Therefore science and art are part of the study of kinesiology. Whether you are just beginning the exploration of kinesiology, or you are an experienced student looking to expand your knowledge, I hope that *Kinesiology: The Skeletal System and Muscle Function* proves to be a helpful and friendly guide. Even more importantly, I hope that it also facilitates an enjoyment and excitement as you come to better understand and appreciate the wonder and beauty of human movement!

CONTENT

The term *kinesiology* literally means the study of motion. Because motion of the body is created by the forces of muscle contractions pulling on bones and moving body parts at joints, kinesiology involves the study of the musculoskeletal system. As such, bones, joints, and muscle are studied. This book covers these topics and is divided into four parts.

- ❑ Part I of this book covers essential terminology that is used in kinesiology. Terminology that is unambiguous is necessary to allow for clear communication, which is especially important when dealing with clients in the health, athletic training, and rehabilitation fields.
- ❑ Part II covers the skeletal system. This part explores the makeup of skeletal tissues and also contains a photographic atlas of all bones and bony landmarks, as well as joints, of the human body.
- ❑ Part III contains a detailed study of the joints of the body. The first two chapters explain the structure and function of joints in general. The next three chapters provide a thorough regional examination of all joints of the body.
- ❑ Part IV examines how muscles function. After covering the anatomy and physiology of muscle tissue, the larger kinesiologic concepts of muscle function are addressed. A big picture idea of what defines muscle contraction is explained. From this point, various topics such as types of muscle contractions, roles of muscles, types of joint motions, musculoskeletal assessment, control by the nervous system, posture, exercise, and the gait cycle are covered.

- ❑ At the end of the book, an appendix is provided containing a complete listing of all attachments and actions of the skeletal muscles of the body.

NOTE

This book has been written to stand on its own. However, it has also been written to complement and be used in conjunction with *The Muscular System Manual* (Mosby, 2005). *The Muscular System Manual* is a thorough and clearly presented atlas of the skeletal muscles of the human body. These two textbooks, along with the *Musculoskeletal Anatomy Coloring Book* (Mosby, 2004), the *Musculoskeletal Anatomy Flashcards* (Mosby, 2005), and *Flashcards for Bones, Joints, and Actions of the Human Body* (Mosby, 2006), give the student a complete set of resources to study and thoroughly learn all aspects of kinesiology.

Joseph E. Muscolino
December 2005

Acknowledgments

Usually only one name is listed on the front of a book, and that is the author's. This practice can give the reader the misconception that the author is the only person responsible for what lies in his or her hands. However, many people who work behind the scenes and are invisible to the reader have contributed to the effort. The *Acknowledgements* section of a book is the author's opportunity to both directly thank these people and acknowledge them to the readers.

First, I would like to thank William Courtland. William, now a fellow instructor at the Connecticut Center for Massage Therapy (C.C.M.T.), was the student who 5 years ago first recommended that I should write a kinesiology textbook. William, thanks for giving me the initial spark of inspiration to write. It took me 5 years to get this book done because I became waylaid with a few other books along the way, but here it finally is.

Because kinesiology is the study of movement, the illustrations in this book are just as important, if not more important than the written text. I am lucky to have had a brilliant team of five illustrators and two photographers. Jeannie Robertson illustrated the bulk of the figures in this book. Jeannie is able to portray three-dimensional movements of the body with sharp, accurate, simple, and clear full-colored illustrations. Tiziana Cipriani contributed a tremendous number of beautiful drawings to this book, including perhaps my two favorites, Figures 11-13*A* and *B*. Jean Luciano, my principle illustrator for *The Muscular System Manual,* also stepped in to help with a few beautiful illustrations, as did Nadine Sokol. Yanik Chauvin is the photographer who took the photos that appear in Chapters 7 through 9, as well as a few others. Yanik is extremely talented, as well as being one of the easiest people with whom to work. Frank Forney is an illustrator who came to this project via Electronic Publishing Services (EPS). Frank drew the computer drawings of the bones that were overlaid on Yanik's photos in Chapters 7 through 9. Frank proved to be an extremely able and invaluable asset to the artwork team. Last but not least is Dr. David Eliot of Touro University College of Osteopathic Medicine, who provided the bone photographs that are found in Chapter 4. Dr. Eliot is a PhD. anatomist whose knowledge of the musculoskeletal system is as vast as his photographs are beautiful. I was lucky to have him as a contributor to this book.

I would also like to thank the models for Yanik's photographs: Audrey Van Herck, Kiyoko Gotanda, Gamaliel Martinez Fonseca, Patrick Tremblay, and Simona Cipriani. The beauty and poise of their bodies was invaluable toward expressing the kinesiologic concepts of movement in the photographs for this book.

I must thank the authors of the other kinesiology textbooks that are presently in print. I like to think that we all stand on the shoulders of those who have come before us. Each kinesiology textbook is unique and has contributed to the field of kinesiology, as well as my knowledge base. I would particularly like to thank Donald Neumann, PT, PhD of Marquette University. His book, *Kinesiology of the Musculoskeletal System,* is, in my opinion, the best book ever written on joint mechanics. I once told Don Neumann that if I could have written just one book, I wish it would have been his.

Writing a book is not only the exercise of stating facts, but also the art of how to present these facts. In other words, a good writer should be a good teacher. Toward that end, I would like to thank all my present and past students at C.C.M.T. for helping me become a better teacher. I would also like to thank the entire staff and administration of C.C.M.T. for making working there such as pleasure.

For the act of actually turning this project into a book, I must thank the entire Mosby/Elsevier team in St. Louis who spent tremendous hours on this project, especially in the last few weeks of production, particularly Jennifer Watrous, Kellie Fitzpatrick, Elizabeth Clark, Ellen Kunkelmann, JoAnn Amore, Rich Barber, Linda McKinley, Julia Dummitt, and Julie Burchett. Thank you for making the birth of this book as painless as possible.

Finally, to echo my dedication, I would like to thank my entire family, who makes it all worthwhile!

About the Author

Dr. Joseph E. Muscolino has been teaching musculoskeletal and visceral anatomy and physiology, kinesiology, neurology, and pathology courses at the Connecticut Center For Massage Therapy (C.C.M.T.) for over 19 years. He has also been instrumental in course manual development and has assisted with curriculum development at C.C.M.T. He has published *The Muscular System Manual,* the *Musculoskeletal Anatomy Coloring Book,* and the *Musculoskeletal Anatomy Flashcards,* as well as articles in the *Massage Therapy Journal* and the *Journal of Bodywork and Movement Therapies. Flashcards for Bones, Joints, and Actions of the Human Body* will be published in 2006. Dr. Muscolino runs continuing education workshops on topics such as anatomy and physiology, kinesiology, deep-tissue massage, and joint mobilization, as well as cadaver workshops. He is approved by the National Certification Board for Therapeutic Massage and Bodywork (NCBTMB) as a provider of continuing education, and grants continuing education units (CEUs) for massage therapists toward certification renewal. In 2002, Dr. Muscolino participated on the NCBTMB Job Analysis Survey Task Force, as well as the Test Specification Meeting as a subject matter expert in anatomy, physiology, and kinesiology. He is also a member of both of the NCBTMB Continuing Education and Exam Committees and is a member of the Educational Review Operational Committee (EROC) of the *Massage Therapy Journal.*

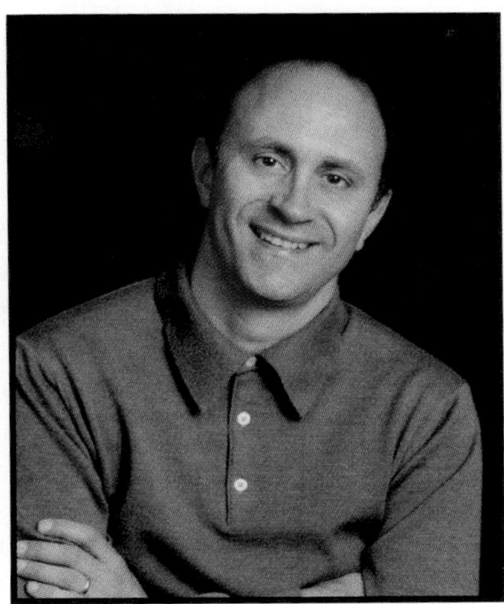

Dr. Muscolino holds a Bachelor of Arts degree in biology from the State University of New York at Binghamton, Harpur College. He attained his Doctor of Chiropractic degree from Western States Chiropractic College in Portland, Oregon, and is licensed in Connecticut, New York, and California. Dr. Muscolino has been in private practice in Connecticut for over 20 years and incorporates soft-tissue work into his chiropractic practice for all his patients.

If you would like further information regarding *Kinesiology: The Skeletal System and Muscle Function, The Muscular System Manual, Musculoskeletal Anatomy Coloring Book, Musculoskeletal Anatomy Flashcards,* or *Flashcards for Bones, Joints, and Actions of the Human Body,* or if you are an instructor and would like information regarding the many supportive materials such as *PowerPoint* slides, colored overhead transparency masters, test banks of questions, or instructor's manuals, please visit http://www.us.elsevierhealth.com. You can contact Dr. Muscolino directly at his web site: http://www.learnmuscles.com.

How to Use this Book

LAYOUT OF BOOK

This book has four major parts:

❑ Part I covers kinesiologic terminology
❑ Part II covers the bones of the body
❑ Part III covers the joints of the body
❑ Part IV covers the muscular system

Each of the major *parts* of this book contains a specific number of *chapters,* each of which covers a certain body of knowledge within the larger theme of the part. The chapters themselves are divided into compartmentalized *sections,* each containing a smaller body of knowledge within the theme of the chapter. In addition to the complete table of contents located at the beginning of the book, a separate outline is available for each chapter located at the beginning of the chapter. Each separate outline lists the sections of that chapter.

ORDER OF LAYOUT

Generally, the information within this book is laid out in the order that the musculoskeletal system is usually covered. Terminology is usually needed before bones can be discussed. Bones then need to be studied before the joints can be learned. Finally, once the terminology, bones, and joints have been learned, the muscular system can be explored. However, depending on the curriculum of your particular school, you might need to access the information in a different order and jump around within this book. The compartmentalized layout of the sections of this book easily allows for this freedom.*

STYLE OF LAYOUT

❑ The information within the text of this book is laid out in open-bulleted form: each piece of information follows an open square bullet. These open bullets act as check boxes that can be checked off as material is covered. This approach allows for an instructor to clearly alert the students to the material that they are responsible for learning. It also allows the reader or student to check off the material that he or she has read and learned.

❑ Scattered throughout the text of this book are lightbulb and spotlight icons. These icons alert the reader to additional information on the subject matter being presented. A contains an interesting fact or short amount of additional information; a contains a greater amount of information. In most cases, these illuminating boxes immediately follow the text statements that explain the concept. The box numbers are only cited within the text paragraph if the and boxes are slightly removed from the descriptive paragraph, such as on the following page. You have the choice of either going to the box that contains the additional information or simply bypassing it and reading on.

STUDY AIDS

This book contains numerous study aids:

❑ At the beginning of each chapter is a list of learning objectives. Refer to these objectives as you read each chapter of the book.

❑ After the objectives is an overview of the information of the chapter. I strongly suggest that you read this overview so that you have a big picture idea of what the chapter covers before delving into the details.

❑ Immediately after the overview is a list of key terms for the chapter, with the proper pronunciation included where necessary. These key terms are also in bold type when they first appear in the text. A complete glossary of all key terms from the book is located on the Evolve web site that accompanies this book.

❑ After the key terms is a list of word origins. These origins explore word roots (prefixes, suffixes, and so forth) that are commonly used in the field of kinesiology. Learning a word root once can enable you to make sense of tens or hundreds of other terms without having to look them up!

❑ At the end of each chapter is a list of review questions. Try to answer these without referring back to the text in the chapter. If you need additional help beyond what is written in the text, the answers to these questions are placed in the Evolve web site.

In addition to the previously mentioned aids, numerous other study tools are available on the Evolve web site, including crossword puzzles for mastering definitions, interactive drag-and-drop labeling exercises, additional readings on selected topics, and more. Access the Evolve web site by going to http://evolve.elsevier.com/Muscolino/kinesiology/.

---

*Note: This book covers the muscular system. However, beyond the listing of attachments, actions, and innervations of the skeletal muscles of the body, located in the appendix, its concentration is on the function of the muscular system; it is not an atlas of muscles. You may want to supplement your study of the musculoskeletal system with a separate atlas of muscles when first learning the attachments and actions of the skeletal muscles of the body. Although any good one can be used, this book was written to complement and be used in conjunction with *The Muscular System Manual,* second edition (Mosby, 2005).

Contents

PART I Fundamentals of Structure and Motion of the Human Body

Chapter 1

Parts of the Human Body

CHAPTER OUTLINE

CHAPTER OBJECTIVES

After completing this chapter, the student should be able to perform the following:

- ❑ List the major divisions of the body.
- ❑ List and locate the 11 major parts of the body.
- ❑ Describe the concept of and give an example of movement of a body part.
- ❑ List the aspects of and give an example of fully naming a movement of the body.
- ❑ Describe the concept and give an example of movement of smaller body parts located within larger (major) body parts.
- ❑ Explain the difference between and give an example of *true movement* of a body part compared with "going along for the ride."
- ❑ List and locate the major regions of the body.
- ❑ Define the key terms of this chapter.
- ❑ State the meanings of the word origins of this chapter.

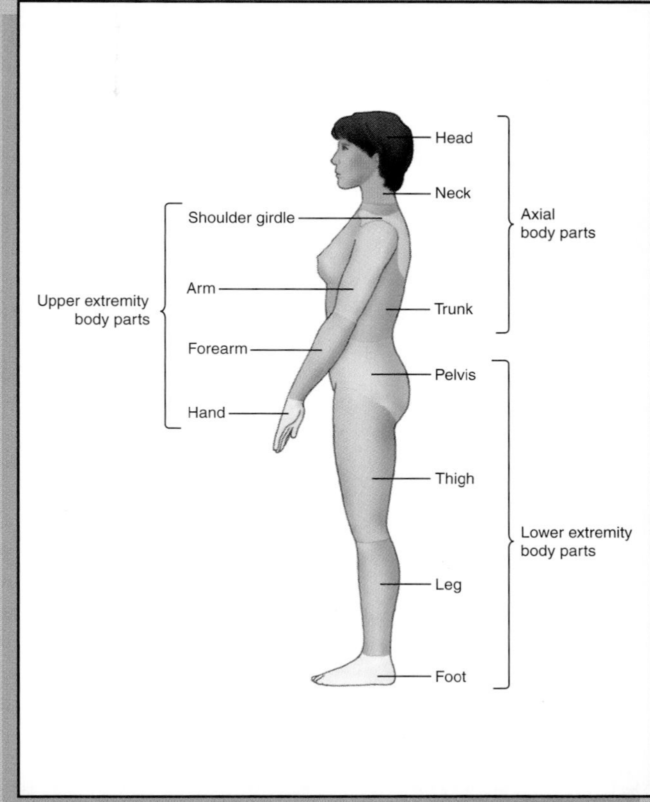

OVERVIEW

The human body is composed of 11 major parts that are located within the axial and appendicular portions of the body. Some of these major body parts have smaller body parts within them. Separating two adjacent body parts from each other is a joint. True movement of a body part involves movement of that body part relative to another body part at the joint that is located between them.

KEY TERMS

Abdominal (ab-DOM-i-nal)
Antebrachial (AN-tee-BRAKE-ee-al)
Antecubital (an-tee-KYU-bi-tal)
Anterior view (an-TEER-ee-or)
Appendicular (ap-en-DIK-u-lar)
Arm
Axial (AK-see-al)
Axillary (AK-sil-err-ee)
Body part
Brachial (BRAKE-ee-al)
Carpal (KAR-pal)
Cervical (SER-vi-kal)
Cranial (KRA-nee-al)
Crural (KROO-ral)
Cubital (KYU-bi-tal)
Digital (DIJ-i-tal)
Facial
Femoral (FEM-o-ral)
Foot
Forearm
Gluteal (GLOO-tee-al)
"Going along for the ride"
Hand
Head
Inguinal (ING-gwi-nal)
Interscapular (IN-ter-skap-u-lar)
Joint
Lateral view (LAT-er-al)
Leg
Lower extremity (eks-TREM-i-tee)
Lumbar (LUM-bar)
Mandibular (man-DIB-u-lar)
Neck
Palmar (PAL-mar)
Patellar (pa-TEL-ar)
Pectoral (PEK-to-ral)
Pelvis
Plantar (PLAN-tar)
Popliteal (pop-LIT-ee-al)
Posterior view (pos-TEER-ee-or)
Pubic (PYU-bik)
Sacral (SAY-kral)
Scapular (SKAP-u-lar)
Shoulder girdle
Supraclavicular (SUE-pra-kla-VIK-u-lar)
Sural (SOO-ral)
Thigh
Thoracic (tho-RAS-ik)
Trunk
Upper extremity (eks-TREM-i-tee)

WORD ORIGINS

- ❑ Ante—From Latin *ante,* meaning *before, in front of*
- ❑ Append—From Latin *appendo,* meaning *to hang something onto something*
- ❑ Ax—From Latin *axis,* meaning *a straight line*
- ❑ Fore—From Old English *fore,* meaning *before, in front of*
- ❑ Inter—From Latin *inter,* meaning *between*
- ❑ Lat—From Latin *latus,* meaning *side*
- ❑ Post—From Latin *post,* meaning *behind, in the rear, after*
- ❑ Supra—From Latin *supra,* meaning *on the upper side, above*

☐ 1.1 MAJOR DIVISIONS OF THE HUMAN BODY

- ❑ The human body can be divided into two major sections (Figure 1-1, Box 1-1):
  - ❑ The **axial** body
  - ❑ The **appendicular** body

Axial Body:

- ❑ The axial body is the central core axis of the body and contains the following body parts:
  - ❑ **Head**
  - ❑ **Neck**
  - ❑ **Trunk**

Appendicular Body:

- ❑ The appendicular body is made up of appendages that are "added onto" the axial body.
- ❑ The appendicular body can be divided into the right and left upper extremities and the right and left lower extremities.

BOX 1-1

When we learn how to name the location of a structure of the body or a point on the body (see Chapter 2), it will be crucial that we understand the difference between the axial body and the appendicular body.

- ❑ An **upper extremity** contains the following body parts:
  - ❑ **Shoulder girdle** (the scapula and clavicle)
  - ❑ **Arm**
  - ❑ **Forearm**
  - ❑ **Hand**
- ❑ A **lower extremity** contains the following body parts:
  - ❑ **Pelvis** (pelvic girdle) (Box 1-2)
  - ❑ **Thigh**
  - ❑ **Leg**
  - ❑ **Foot**

BOX 1-2

The pelvis is often considered to be part of the axial body. In actuality, it is a transitional body part that is part of both the axial body and the appendicular body. The pelvic girdle of the pelvis is composed of the bones of the pelvis. For symmetry, we will consider the pelvis to be part of the lower extremity (therefore the appendicular body), because the shoulder girdle is part of the upper extremity.

The word *girdle* is used because the pelvic and shoulder girdles resemble a girdle in that they encircle the body like a girdle does (actually, the shoulder girdle does not completely encircle the body because the two scapulae do not meet in back).

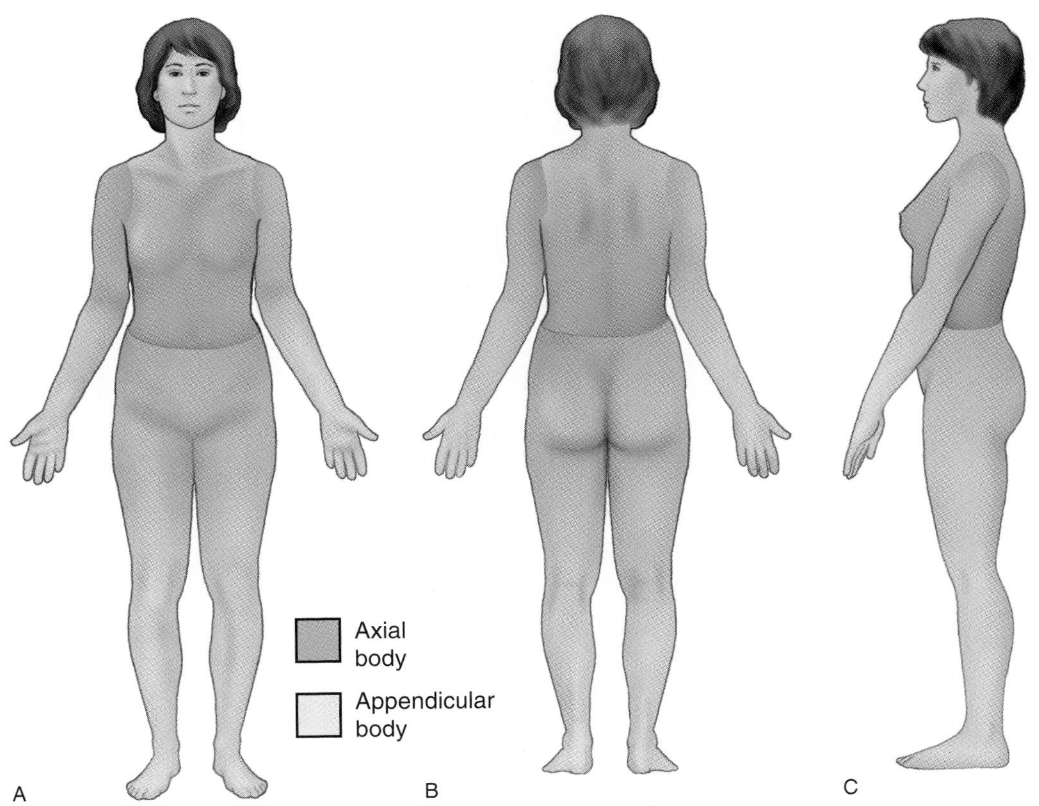

Figure 1-1 The major divisions of the human body: the axial body and the appendicular body. *A,* **Anterior view.** *B,* **Posterior view.** *C,* **Lateral view.**

1.2 MAJOR BODY PARTS

- A **body part** is a part of the body that can move independently of another body part that is next to it.
- Generally it is the presence of a bone (sometimes more than one bone) within a body part that defines the body part.
  - For example, the humerus defines the arm; the radius and ulna define the forearm.
- The human body has 11 major body parts (see Figure 1-2):
  - Axial body:
    - Head
    - Neck
    - Trunk
  - Appendicular body:
    - Lower extremity:
      - Pelvis
      - Thigh
      - Leg
      - Foot
    - Upper extremity:
      - Shoulder girdle
      - Arm
      - Forearm
      - Hand
- It is important to distinguish the thigh from the leg. The thigh is between the hip joint and the knee joint, whereas the leg is between the knee joint and the ankle joint.
- It is important to distinguish the arm from the forearm. The arm is between the shoulder joint and the elbow joint, whereas the forearm is between the elbow joint and the wrist joint.
- The shoulder girdle contains the scapulae and the clavicles.
  - Most sources include the sternum as part of the shoulder girdle.
  - The shoulder girdle is also known as the *pectoral girdle.*
- The pelvis as a body part includes the pelvic girdle of bones.
  - The pelvic girdle contains the two pelvic bones, the sacrum, and the coccyx.

BOX 1-3

The pelvis is a body part; the pelvic girdle is composed of the bones within the pelvis. Regarding the bones of the pelvic girdle, the sacrum and coccyx are technically bones of the spine and therefore bones of the axial body; the two pelvic bones are technically part of the lower extremities and therefore part of the appendicular body. For this reason, the pelvis is considered to be a transitional body part that is actually part of the axial body and the appendicular body.

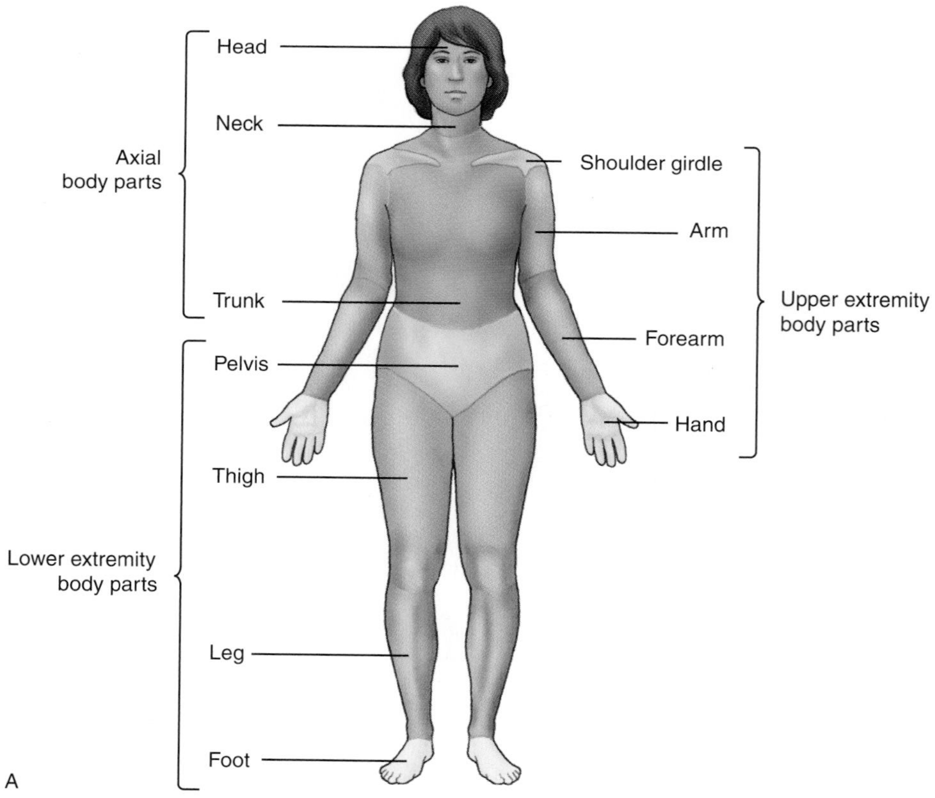

Figure 1-2 The 11 major parts of the human body. *A,* Anterior view. *B,* Posterior view. *C,* Lateral view.

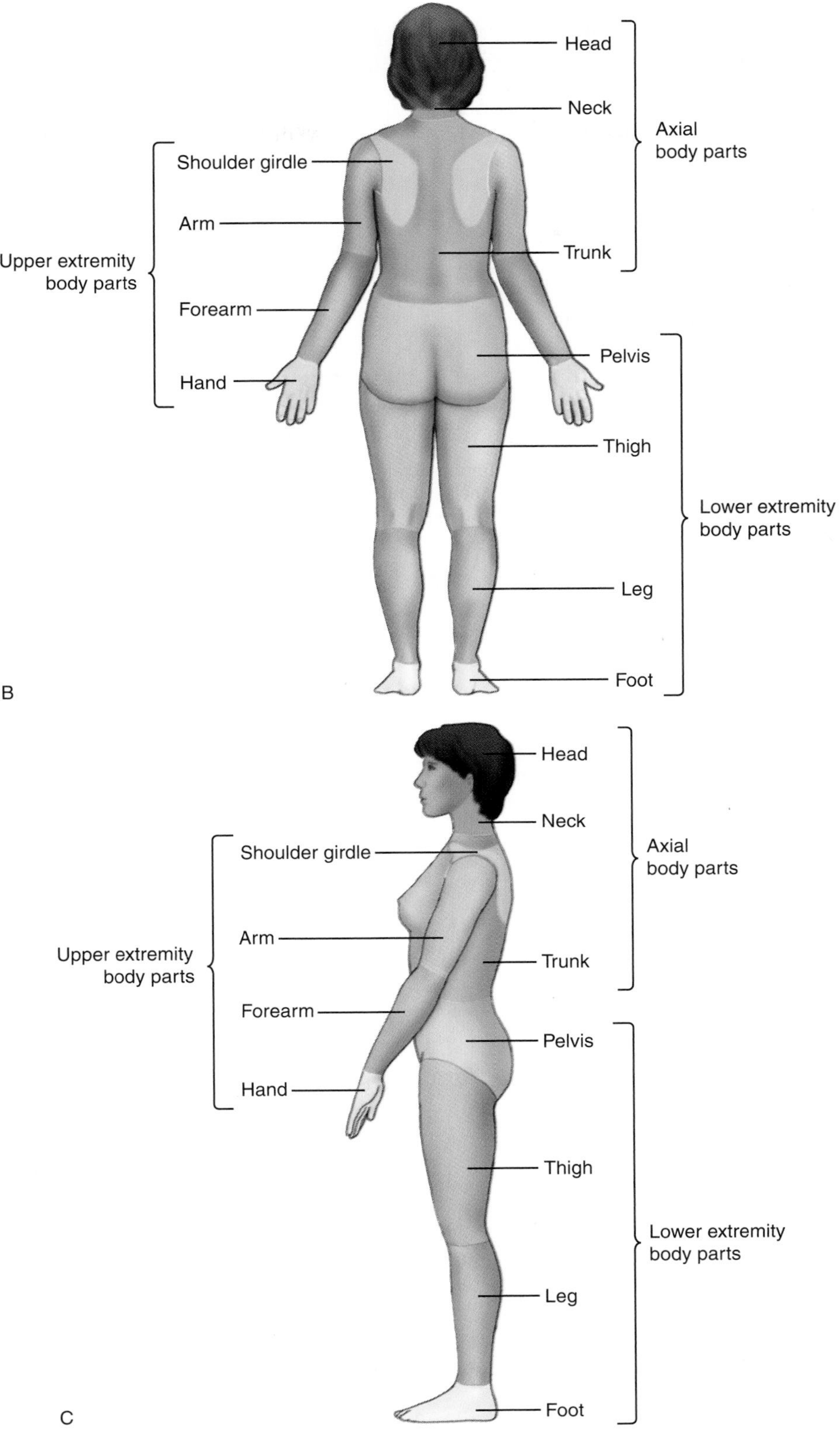

Figure 1-2, cont'd

☐ 1.3 JOINTS BETWEEN BODY PARTS

- What separates one body part from the body part next to it is the presence of a **joint** between the bones of the body parts. A joint is located between each two adjacent body parts (Figure 1-3).

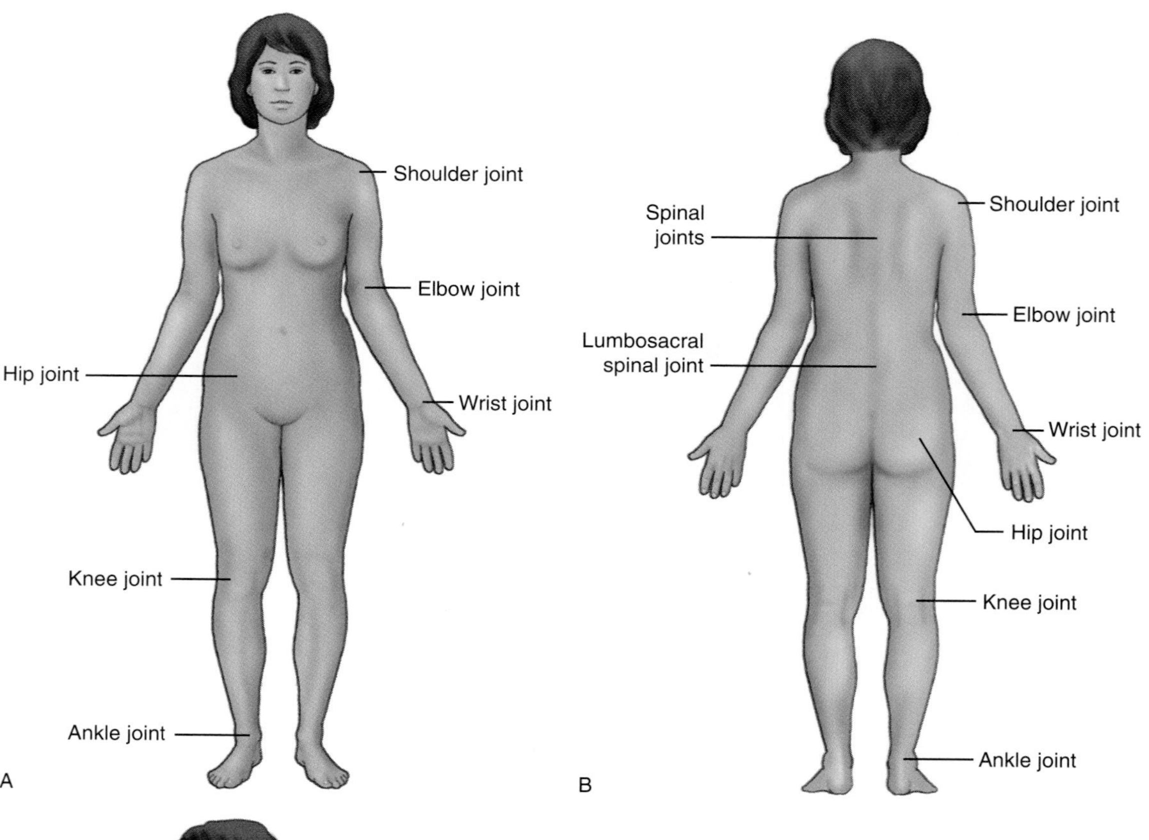

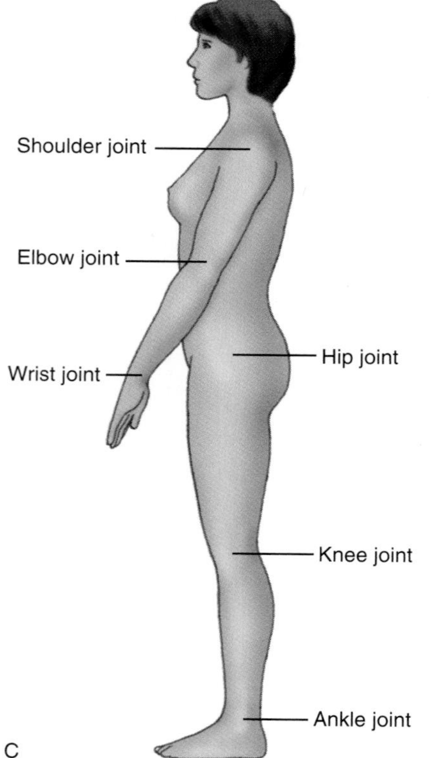

Figure 1-3 Illustration of the concept of a joint being located between two adjacent body parts. It is the presence of a joint that separates one body part from another body part. *A,* Anterior view. *B,* Posterior view. *C,* Lateral view.

- ❑ When we say that a body part moves, our general rule will be that the body part moves relative to another body part that is next to it.
- ❑ This movement occurs at the joint that is located between these two body parts (Figure 1-4).

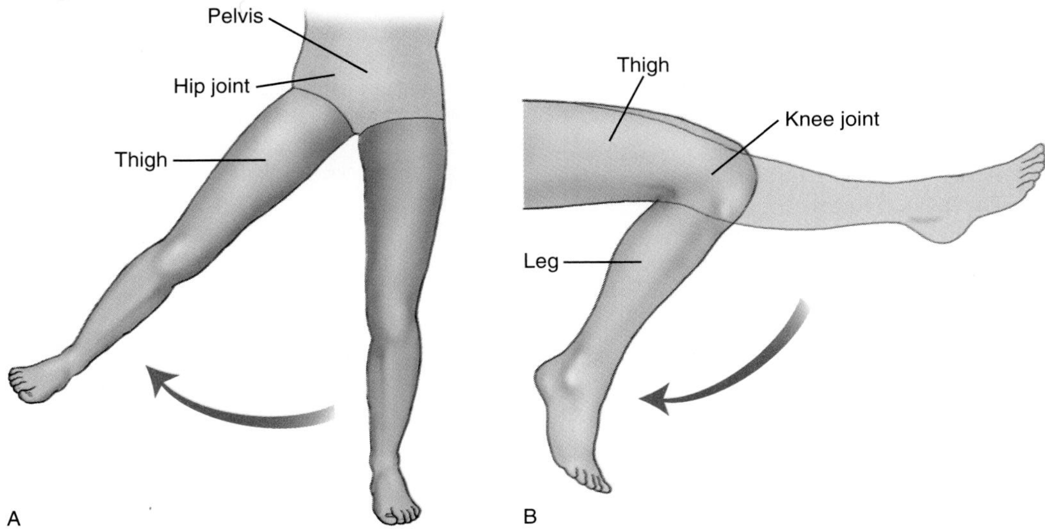

Figure 1-4 *A,* The thigh moving (abducting) relative to the pelvis. This motion is occurring at the hip joint, which is located between them. *B,* Leg moving (flexing) relative to the thigh. This motion is occurring at the knee joint, which is located between them.

☐ 1.4 MOVEMENT OF A BODY PART RELATIVE TO AN ADJACENT BODY PART

- ❑ When movement of our body occurs, we see the following:
  - ❑ It is a body part that is moving.
  - ❑ That movement is occurring at the joint that is located between that body part and the adjacent body part.
  - ❑ Therefore when a body part moves, it moves relative to an adjacent body part.
- ❑ To name this movement properly and fully, two things must be stated (Box 1-4):
  1. The name of the body part that is moving
  2. The joint where the movement is occurring

Figures 1-5, 1-6, and 1-7 show examples of movements of body parts relative to adjacent body parts.

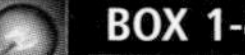

BOX 1-4

Most texts describe a movement of the body by stating only the body part that is moving or by stating only the joint where the motion is occurring. However, to be complete and fully describe and understand what is happening, both aspects should be stated. By doing this every time you describe a movement of the body, you will gain a better visual picture and understanding of the movement that is occurring.

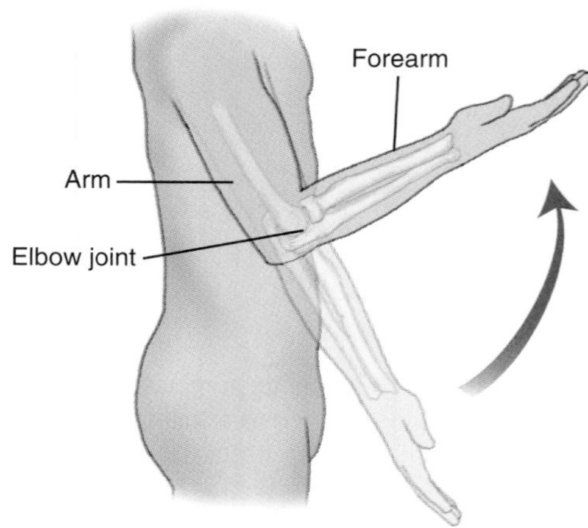

Figure 1-6 Illustration of a body movement. The body part that is moving is the forearm, and the joint where this movement is occurring is the elbow joint. We say that the forearm is moving (flexing) at the elbow joint. This motion of the forearm occurs relative to the body part that is next to the forearm (i.e., the arm).

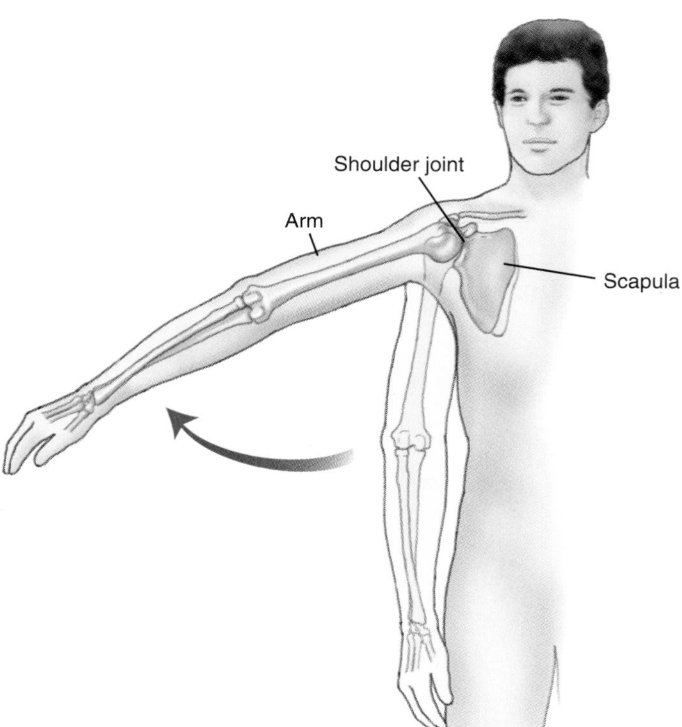

Figure 1-5 Illustration of a body movement. The body part that is moving is the arm, and the joint where this movement is occurring is the shoulder joint. We say that the arm is moving (abducting) at the shoulder joint. This motion of the arm occurs relative to the body part that is next to the arm (i.e., the shoulder girdle; more specifically, the scapula of the shoulder girdle).

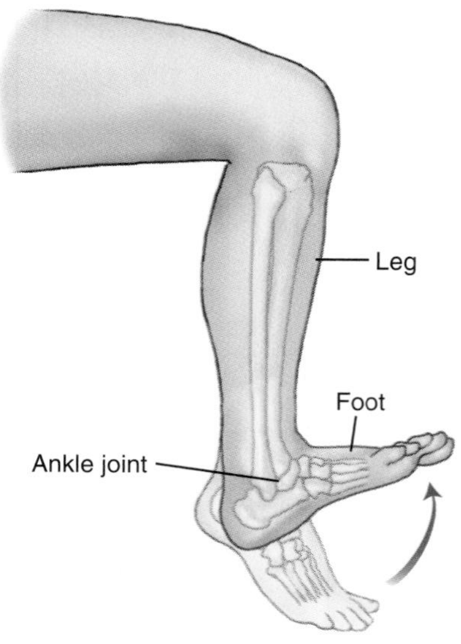

Figure 1-7 Illustration of a body movement. The body part that is moving is the foot, and the joint where this movement is occurring is the ankle joint. We say that the foot is moving (dorsiflexing) at the ankle joint. This motion of the foot occurs relative to the body part that is next to the foot (i.e., the leg).

1.5 MOVEMENT WITHIN A BODY PART

- We have seen that when a major body part moves, the movement occurs at the joint that is located between that body part and an adjacent body part.
- Because that joint is located between two different major body parts, when one body part moves relative to another body part, it can be said that the movement occurs *between* body parts.

- However, sometimes movement can occur *within* a major body part.
- This can occur whenever the major body part has two or more smaller body parts (i.e., bones) located within it. When this situation exists, movement can occur at the joint that is located between these smaller body parts (i.e., bones) within the major body part.
  - The simplest example of this is the hand. The hand is considered to be a major body part, and motion of the hand is described as occurring between it and the forearm at the wrist joint (Figure 1-8a). However, the hand has other body parts (i.e., the fingers) within it. Each finger is a body part in its own right, because a finger can move relative to the palm of the hand (Figure 1-8b). Further, each finger has three separate parts (i.e., bones) within it, and each of these parts can move independently as well (Figure 1-8c).
  - A second example is the forearm. The forearm is usually described as moving relative to the arm at the elbow joint (Figure 1-9a). However, the forearm has two bones within it, and joints are located between these two bones. Motion of one of these bones can occur relative to the other (Figure 1-9b). In this case each one of the two bones would be considered to be a separate smaller body part.

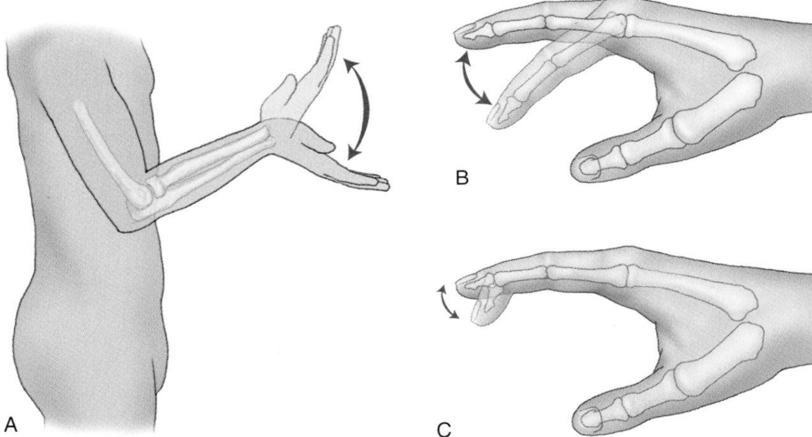

Figure 1-8 *A,* Lateral view showing the hand moving relative to the forearm at the wrist joint. *B,* Depiction of motion within the hand. This is a lateral view in which we see a finger moving relative to the palm of the hand at the joint that is located between them. *C,* Illustration of movement of one part of a finger relative to another part of the finger at the joint that is located between them. Note: *B* and *C* both illustrate the concept of movement occurring within a major body part because smaller body parts are within it.

- A third, more complicated example is the cervical spine. The cervical spine has seven vertebrae within it. The neck may be described as moving relative to the trunk that is beneath it (Figure 1-10a). However, each one of the seven vertebrae can move independently. Therefore motion can occur between vertebrae within the neck at the joints located between the vertebrae (Figure 1-10b).

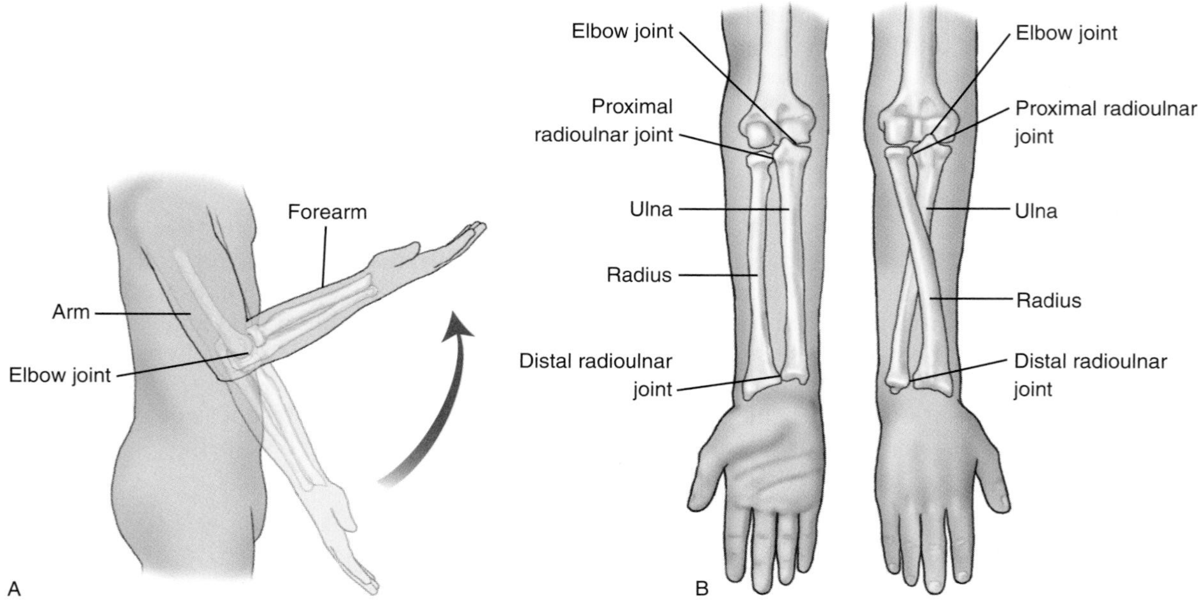

Figure 1-9 *A,* Lateral view showing the forearm moving (flexing) relative to the arm at the elbow joint. *B,* Movement of one of the bones (i.e., the radius) within the forearm, relative to the other bone (i.e., the ulna) of the forearm; this motion occurs at the radioulnar joints located between the two bones. The concept of movement occurring within a major body part is illustrated, because smaller body parts are within it.

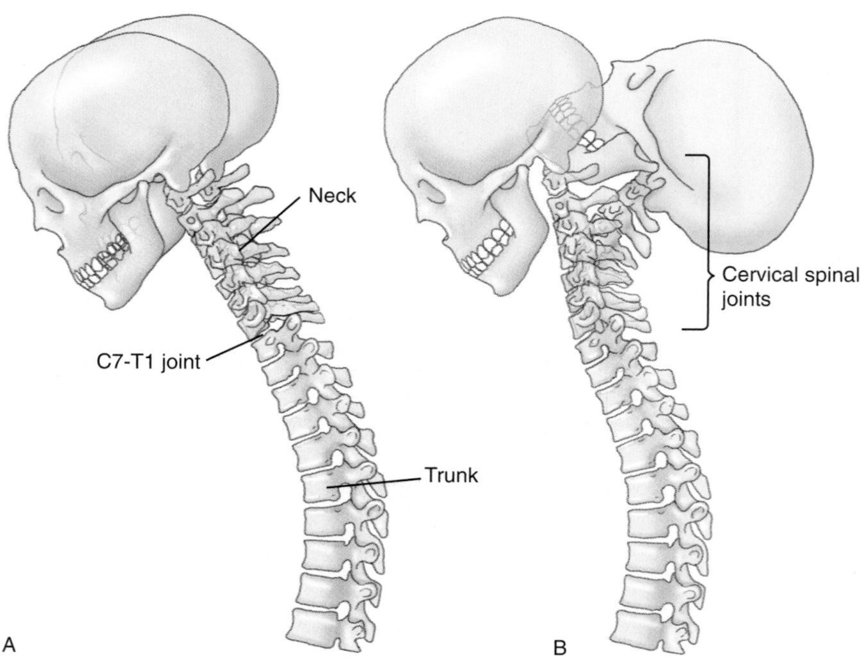

Figure 1-10 *A,* Lateral view of the neck showing the neck moving relative to the trunk at the spinal joint between them (C7-T1). *B,* Motion within the neck that is occurring between several individual vertebrae of the neck. This motion occurs at the spinal joints located between these bones. The concept of movement occurring within a major body part is illustrated, because smaller body parts are within it.

☐ 1.6 TRUE MOVEMENT OF A BODY PART VERSUS "GOING ALONG FOR THE RIDE"

- ❑ In lay terms, when we say that a body part has moved, it does not always mean true movement of that body part has occurred (according to the terminology that is used in the musculoskeletal field for describing joint movements).
- ❑ A distinction must be made between *true movement of a body part* and what we will call "going along for the ride."
- ❑ For true movement of a body part to occur, the body part must move relative to an adjacent body part (or the body part must have movement occur within it).
- ❑ For example, in Figure 1-11, we see that a person is moving the right upper extremity.
- ❑ In lay terms we might say that the person's right hand is moving because it is changing its position in space.
- ❑ However, in our terminology, the right hand is not moving because the position of the hand relative to the forearm is not changing (i.e., the right hand is not moving relative to the forearm [and motion is not occurring within the hand]).
- ❑ The movement that is occurring in Figure 1-11 is flexion of the forearm at the elbow joint. It is the forearm that is moving relative to the arm at the elbow joint.
- ❑ The hand is not moving in this scenario. We could say that the hand is merely "going along for the ride".

Figure 1-12 depicts true movement of the hand relative to the forearm.

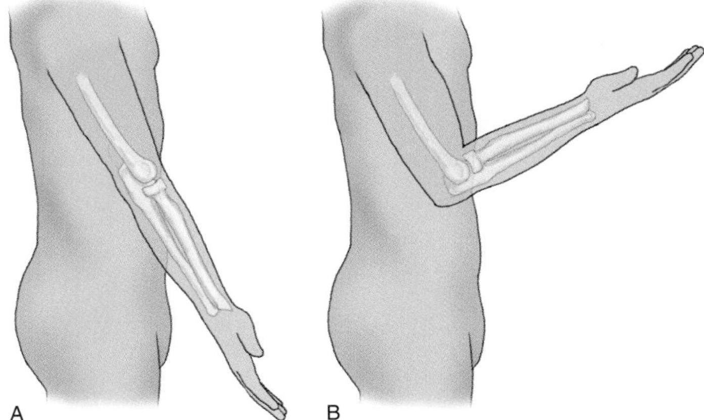

Figure 1-11 *A* and *B,* Illustration of the concept that the forearm is moving (because its position relative to the arm is changing). The motion that is occurring here is flexion of the forearm at the elbow joint. The hand is not moving, because its position relative to the forearm is not changing; the hand is merely "going along for the ride".

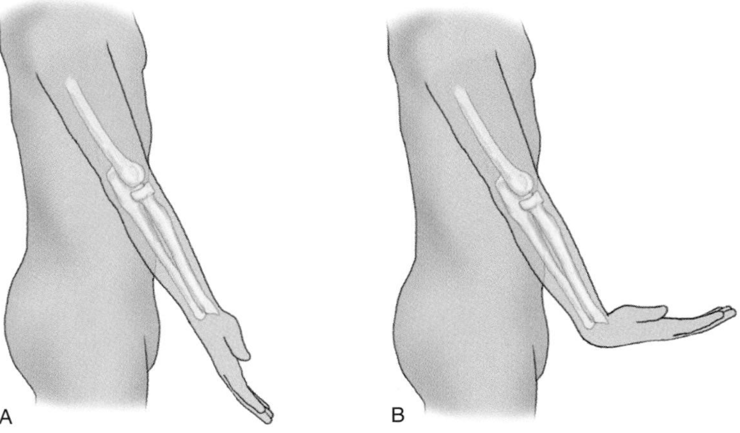

Figure 1-12 Illustration of true movement of the hand (because the position of the hand is changing relative to the forearm). This movement would be called *flexion* of the hand at the wrist joint.

1.7 REGIONS OF THE BODY

- Within the human body, areas or regions exist that are given names. Sometimes these regions are located within a body part; sometimes they are located across two or more body parts. Following are illustrations that show the various regions of the body (Figure 1-13).

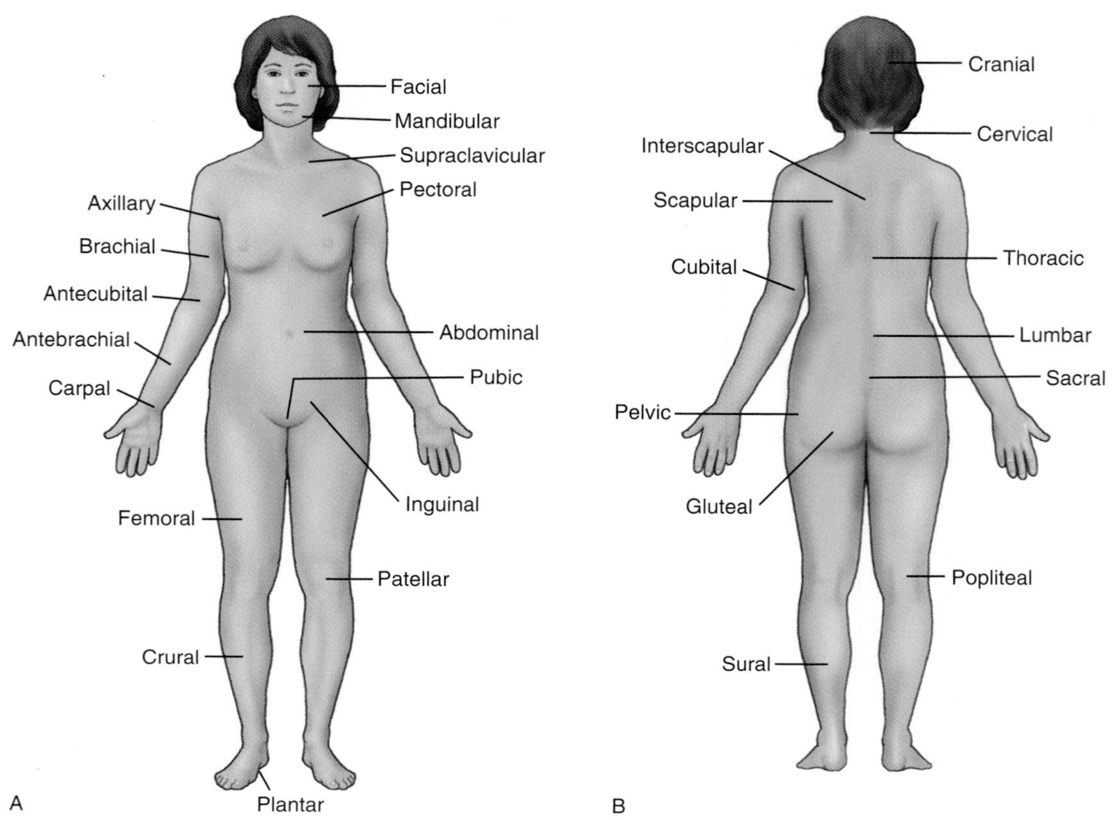

Figure 1-13 *A,* Anterior view of the body illustrating its major regions. *B,* Posterior view of the body illustrating its major regions.

REVIEW QUESTIONS

evolve Answers to the following review questions appear on the Evolve website accompanying this book.

1. What are the two major divisions of the human body?

2. What are the 11 major body parts of the human body?

3. What defines a body part?

4. What is the difference between the thigh and the leg?

5. What is the difference between the arm and the forearm?

6. What is the difference between the trunk and the pelvis?

7. What two things are stated to describe a movement of the body properly and fully?

8. How can movement occur within a body part?

9. What is the difference between *true movement* and "going along for the ride"?

10. Name five regions of the human body.

Chapter 2

Mapping the Human Body

CHAPTER OUTLINE

Section 2.1 Anatomic Position
Section 2.2 Location Terminology
Section 2.3 Anterior/Posterior
Section 2.4 Medial/Lateral
Section 2.5 Superior/Inferior and Proximal/Distal
Section 2.6 Superficial/Deep
Section 2.7 Location Terminology Illustration
Section 2.8 Planes
Section 2.9 Motion of the Human Body Within Planes
Section 2.10 Axes
Section 2.11 Planes and Their Corresponding Axes
Section 2.12 Visualizing the Axes—Door Hinge Pin Analogy
Section 2.13 Visualizing the Axes—Pinwheel Analogy

CHAPTER OBJECTIVES

After completing this chapter, the student should be able to perform the following:

- ❑ Describe and explain the importance of anatomic position.
- ❑ Explain how location terminology can be used to map the body.
- ❑ List and be able to apply the following pairs of terms that describe relative location on the human body: anterior/posterior, medial/lateral, superior/inferior, proximal/distal, and superficial/deep.
- ❑ List and be able to apply the following additional pairs of terms that describe relative location on the human body: ventral/dorsal, volar/dorsal, radial/ulnar, tibial/fibular, plantar/dorsal, and palmar/dorsal.
- ❑ List and describe the three cardinal planes.
- ❑ Explain the concept of an oblique plane.
- ❑ Explain how motion occurs within a plane and be able to give an example of motion occurring in each of the three cardinal planes and in an oblique plane.
- ❑ Define what an axis is and be able to explain how motion can occur relative to an axis.
- ❑ List the axes that correspond to each of the three cardinal planes.
- ❑ Be able to determine the axis for an oblique plane.
- ❑ Be able to give an example of motion occurring within each of the three cardinal planes and around each of the three cardinal axes.
- ❑ Be able to draw an analogy between the hinge pin of a door and the pin of a pinwheel to the axis of movement for each of the three cardinal planes.
- ❑ Define the key terms of this chapter.
- ❑ State the meanings of the word origins of this chapter.

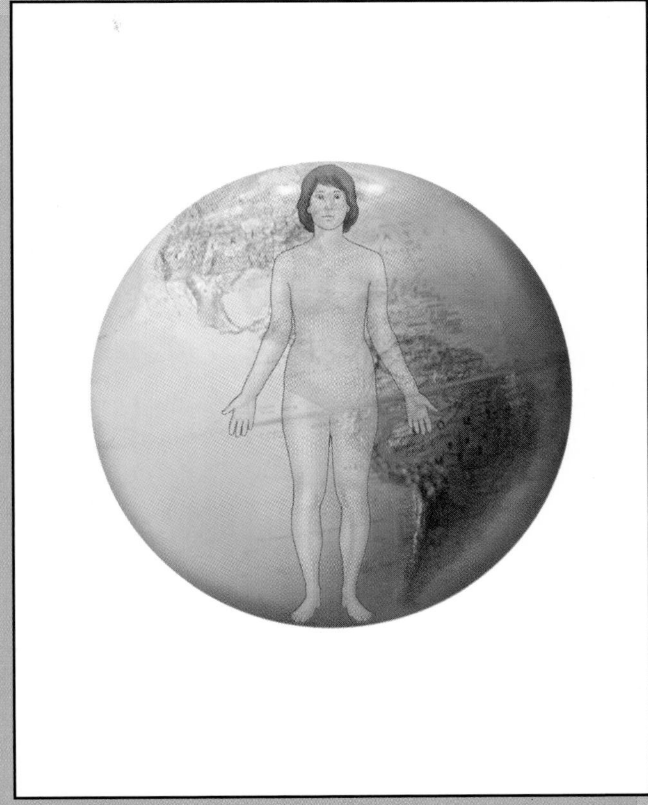

OVERVIEW

The field of kinesiology uses directional terms of relative location to describe and communicate the location of a structure of the body or a point on the body. These terms are similar to geographic directional terms such as *north* and *south*, *east* and *west*. However, instead of mapping the Earth, we use our terms to map the human body. We also need to map the space around the human body by describing the three dimensions or *planes* of space. Understanding the orientation of the planes is extremely important in the field of kinesiology because when the body moves, motion of body parts occurs within these planes. The concept of an axis is then explored, because most body movements are axial movements that occur within a plane and around an axis.

Putting the information that was learned in Chapter 1 together with the information that is presented in Chapter 2, the student will have a clear and fundamental understanding of body movement. That is, when motion of the human body occurs, a body part moves relative to an adjacent body part at the joint that is located between them; and if this motion is an axial movement, then it occurs within a plane and around an axis. After studying the bones in more detail in Chapters 3 and 4, the exact terms that are used to describe these movements of body parts are covered in Chapter 5.

KEY TERMS

Anatomic position (an-a-TOM-ik)
Angular movement
Anterior (an-TEER-ee-or)
Anteroposterior axis (an-TEER-o-pos-TEER-ee-or)
Axial movement (AK-see-al)
Axis, pl. axes (AK-sis, AK-seez)
Axis of rotation
Cardinal axis (KAR-di-nal)
Cardinal plane
Circular movement
Coronal plane (ko-RO-nal)
Deep
Distal
Dorsal (DOOR-sal)
Fibular (FIB-u-lar)
Frontal-horizontal axis
Frontal plane
Horizontal plane
Inferior (in-FEAR-ee-or)
Lateral
Mechanical axis
Medial (MEE-dee-al)
Mediolateral axis (MEE-dee-o-LAT-er-al)
Midsagittal plane (MID-SAJ-i-tal)
Oblique axis (o-BLEEK)
Oblique plane
Plane
Posterior (pos-TEER-ee-or)
Proximal (PROK-si-mal)
Radial (RAY-dee-al)
Rotary movement
Sagittal-horizontal axis (SAJ-i-tal)
Sagittal plane
Superficial
Superior (sue-PEER-ee-or)
Superoinferior axis (sue-PEER-o-in-FEER-ee-or)
Tibial (TI-bee-al)
Transverse plane
Ulnar (UL-nar)
Ventral (VEN-tral)
Vertical axis
Volar (VO-lar)

WORD ORIGINS

- ❑ Ana—From Latin *ana,* meaning *up*
- ❑ Dors—From Latin *dorsum,* meaning *the back*
- ❑ Infer—From Latin *inferus,* meaning *below, lower*
- ❑ Medial—From Latin *medialis,* meaning *middle*
- ❑ Oblique—From Latin *obliquus,* meaning *slanting*
- ❑ Rota—From Latin *rota,* meaning *wheel*
- ❑ Super—From Latin *superus,* meaning *higher, situated above*
- ❑ Tome—From Latin *tomus,* meaning *a cutting*
- ❑ Trans—From Latin *trans,* meaning *across, to the other side of*
- ❑ Ventr—From Latin *venter,* meaning *belly, stomach*

☐ 2.1 ANATOMIC POSITION

❏ Although the human body can assume an infinite number of positions, one position is used as the reference position for mapping the body. This position is used to name the location of body parts, structures, and points on the body and is called **anatomic position**. In anatomic position the person is standing erect, facing forward, with the arms at the sides, the palms facing forward, and the fingers and thumbs extended (Figure 2-1).

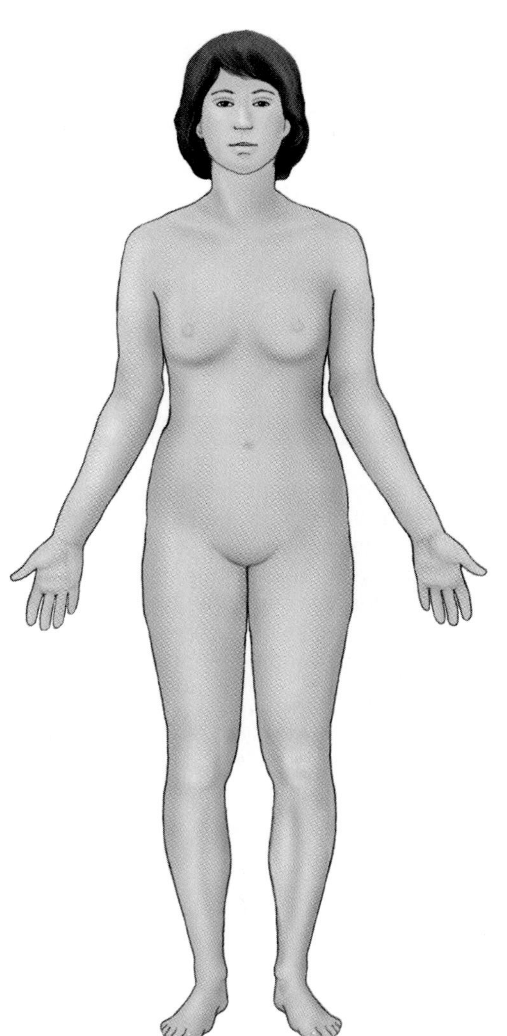

Figure 2-1 Anterior view of anatomic position. Anatomic position is the position assumed when a person stands erect, facing forward, with the arms at the sides, the palms facing forward, and the fingers and thumbs extended. Anatomic position is important because it is used as a reference position for naming locations on the human body.

2.2 LOCATION TERMINOLOGY

Naming Locations on the Human Body:

- Whenever we want to describe the location of a structure of the human body or the location of a specific point on the human body, we always do so in reference to anatomic position.
- Describing a location on the human body involves the use of specific directional terms that describe the location of one structure or point on the body relative to another structure or point on the body.
- The reason for specific terminologies like this to exist is that they help us to avoid the ambiguities of lay language. Therefore embracing and using these terms is extremely important in the health field where someone's health is dependent on clear communication.

BOX 2-1

An example of a lay term that is ambiguous and can create confusion and poor communication when describing a location on the human body is the word *under. Under* can mean *inferior,* or it can mean *deep*. Similarly, the word *above* can mean both *superior* and *superficial.*

- These terms always come in pairs; the terms of each pair are opposite to each other.
- These pairs of terms are similar to the terms *north/south, east/west,* and *up/down*. However, our terms specifically relate to relative directions on the human body.

BOX 2-2

It is important to emphasize that these are terms of *relative* anatomic location. A structure of the human body that is said to be *anterior* is so named because it is *anterior relative to another structure that is more posterior*. However, that same *anterior* structure may be *posterior to a third structure that is more anterior than it is*. For example, the sternum is anterior to the spine. However, the sternum is posterior to the skin that lies over it. Therefore depending on which structure we are comparing it to, the sternum may be described as *anterior* or *posterior.*

- In essence, we are mapping the human body and using specific terminology to describe points on this map. In the following sections are the pairs of directional terms for naming the relative location of structures or points on the human body.

BOX 2-3

Once these pairs of terms for relative location have been learned, they may be combined to describe a structure or point's location. For example, a point on the body may be both anterior and medial to another point. When these terms are combined, it is customary to drop the end of the first term, and combine the two terms together with the letter *o* (e.g., anterior and medial become *anteromedial*). It is also common practice for the terms *anterior* or *posterior* to come first.

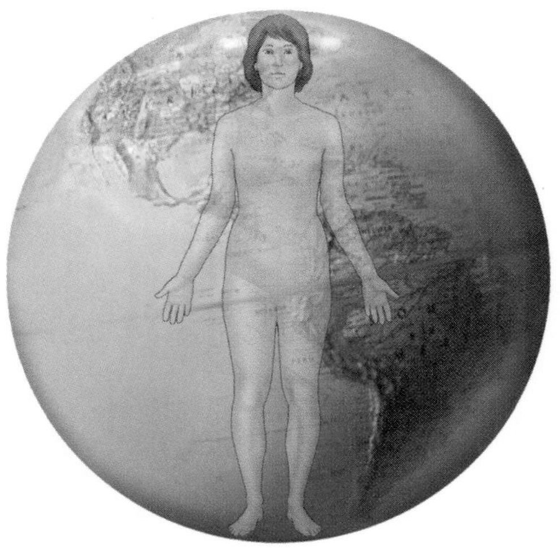

☐ 2.3 ANTERIOR/POSTERIOR

Anterior—Means *farther to the front*

Posterior—Means *farther to the back*

- The terms *anterior/posterior* can be used for the entire body (i.e., for the axial and the appendicular body parts).

  Examples: The sternum is anterior to the spine.
  The spine is posterior to the sternum (Figure 2-2).

  Examples: The patella is anterior to the femur.
  The femur is posterior to the patella (see Figure 2-2).

Notes:

- The terms *ventral/dorsal* are often used synonymously with anterior/posterior.
  - **Ventral** essentially means *anterior*.
  - **Dorsal** essentially means *posterior* (Box 2-4).
- The term **volar** is occasionally used in place of anterior for the hand region (*dorsal* is usually used as the opposite term in the pair).

BOX 2-4

Each body part has a soft, fleshy surface and a harder, firmer surface. The term *ventral* actually refers to the belly or the softer surface of a body part; the term *dorsal* refers to the back or the harder, firmer surface of a body part. The ventral surfaces of the entire upper extremity and axial body are located anteriorly; the ventral surface of the thigh is medial; the ventral surface of the leg is posterior; and the ventral surface of the foot is the inferior, plantar surface. The dorsal surfaces are on the opposite side of the ventral surfaces.

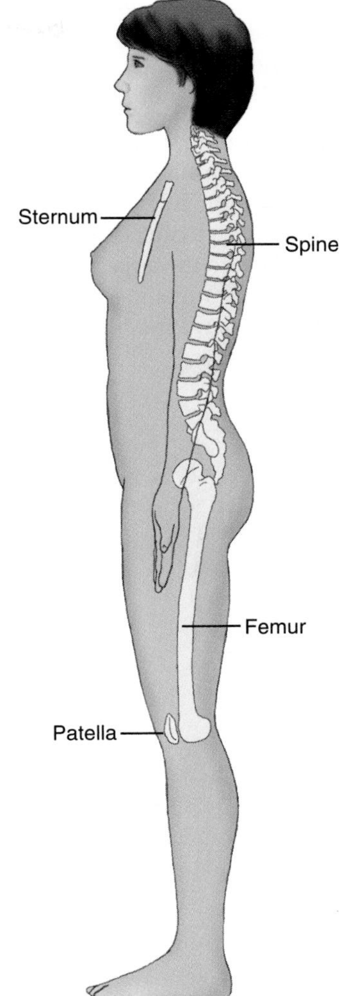

Figure 2-2 Lateral view of a person in anatomic position. The sternum is anterior to the spine; conversely, the spine is posterior to the sternum. The patella is anterior to the femur; conversely, the femur is posterior to the patella.

☐ 2.4 MEDIAL/LATERAL

- **Medial**—Means *closer to an imaginary line that divides the body into left and right halves* (Figure 2-3). (Note: This imaginary line that divides the body into left and right halves is the *midsagittal plane*; see Section 2.8.)
- **Lateral**—Means *farther from an imaginary line that divides the body into left and right halves* (i.e., more to the left side or the right side).
  - The terms *medial/lateral* can be used for the entire body (i.e., for the axial and the appendicular body parts).
  Example: The sternum is medial to the humerus. The humerus is lateral to the sternum (see Figure 2-3).
  Example: The little finger is medial to the thumb. The thumb is lateral to the little finger (see Figure 2-3).

Notes:

- In the forearm and the hand, the terms *ulnar/radial* can be used instead of *medial/lateral*. **Ulnar** means *closer to the ulna*, which is more medial. **Radial** means *closer to the radius*, which is more lateral.
- In the leg, the terms *tibial/fibular* can be used instead of medial/lateral. **Tibial** means *closer to the tibia*, which is more medial. **Fibular** means *closer to the fibula*, which is more lateral.

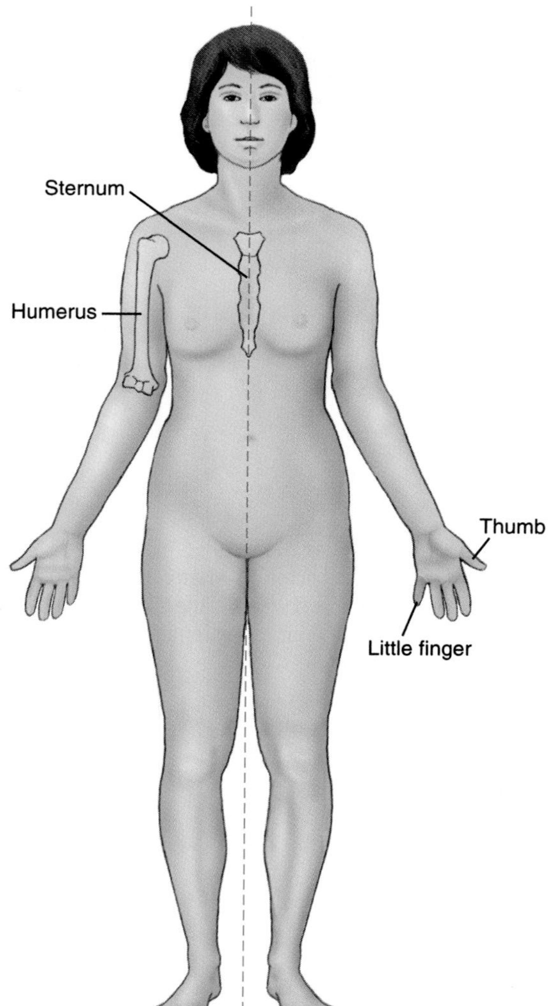

Figure 2-3 Anterior view of a person in anatomic position. The midline of the body, which is most medial in location, is represented by the vertical dashed line that divides the body into left and right halves. The sternum is medial to the humerus; conversely, the humerus is lateral to the sternum. The little finger is medial to the thumb; conversely, the thumb is lateral to the little finger.

☐ 2.5 SUPERIOR/INFERIOR AND PROXIMAL/DISTAL

- **Superior**—Means *above*
- **Inferior**—Means *below*

- The terms *superior/inferior* are used for the axial body parts only.
  Examples: The head is superior to the trunk.
  The trunk is inferior to the head (Figure 2-4a).
  Examples: The sternum is superior to the umbilicus.
  The umbilicus is inferior to the sternum (see Figure 2-4a).

Note:

- Although most sources apply these terms only to the axial body, some sources use these terms on the appendicular body as well.

- **Proximal**—Means *closer* (i.e., greater proximity) *to the axial body*
- **Distal**—Means *farther* (i.e., more distant) *from the axial body*
  - The terms *proximal/distal* are used for the appendicular body parts only.
    Examples: The arm is proximal to the forearm.
    The forearm is distal to the arm (Figure 2-4b).
    Examples: The thigh is proximal to the leg.
    The leg is distal to the thigh (see Figure 2-4b).

Note regarding the use of superior/inferior versus proximal/distal:

- Given that the terms *superior/inferior* are used on the axial body and are not used on the appendicular body, and the terms *proximal/distal* are used on the appendicular body and are not used on the axial body, a dilemma arises when we look to compare the relative location of a point that is on an extremity with a point that is on the axial body. For example, the psoas major muscle attaches from the trunk to the thigh. How would one describe its attachments? It is convention to use either one pair of terms or the other but not to mix between the two pairs of terms. In other words, you could describe the attachments of this muscle as being *superior and inferior*, or you could describe them as being *proximal and distal*. Do not mix these terms and describe the attachments as superior and distal (or proximal and inferior). Generally the terms *proximal/distal* are more commonly used.

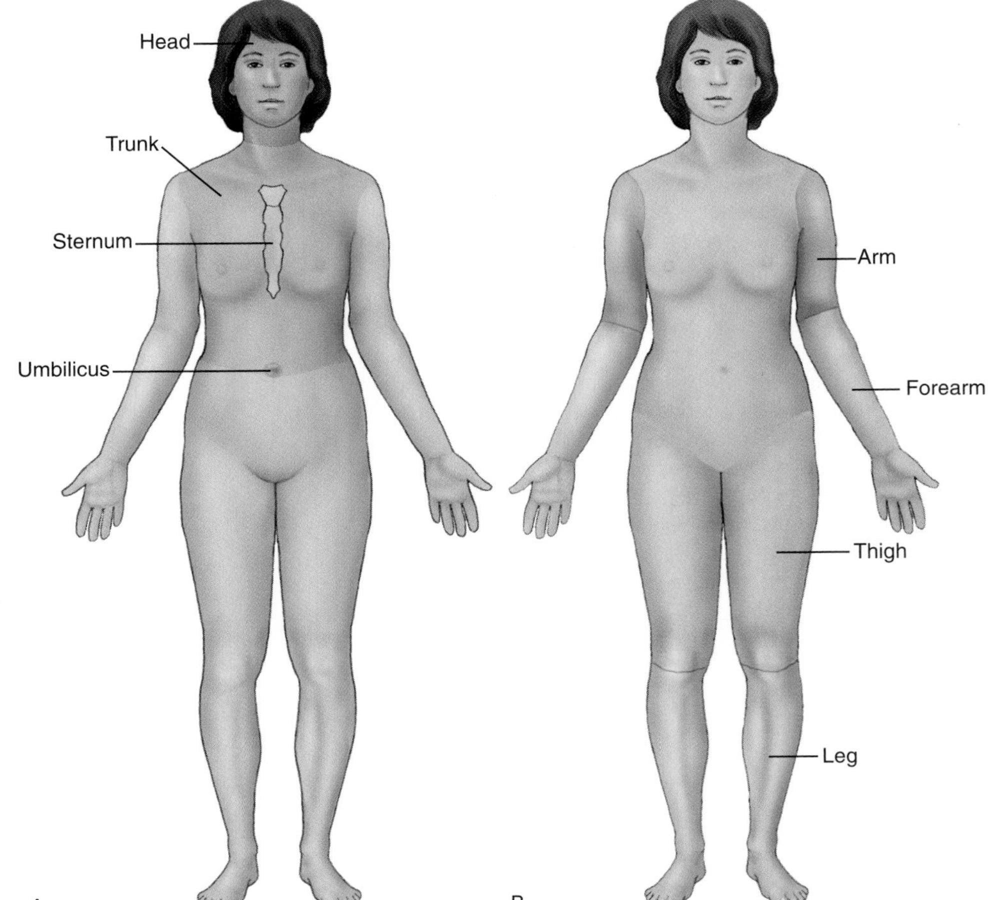

Figure 2-4 Anterior views of a person in anatomic position. *A,* The head is superior to the trunk; conversely, the trunk is inferior to the head. In addition, the sternum is superior to the umbilicus; conversely, the umbilicus is inferior to the sternum. *B,* The arm is proximal to the forearm; conversely, the forearm is distal to the arm. In addition, the thigh is proximal to the leg; conversely, the leg is distal to the thigh.

2.6 SUPERFICIAL/DEEP

- **Superficial**—Means *closer to the surface of the body*
- **Deep**—Means *farther from the surface of the body* (i.e., more internal or deep)
  - The terms *superficial/deep* can be used for the entire body (i.e., for the axial and the appendicular body parts).

    Example: The anterior abdominal wall muscles are superficial to the intestines.
    The intestines are deep to the anterior abdominal wall muscles (Figure 2-5).

    Example: The biceps brachii muscle is superficial to the humerus (arm bone).
    The humerus (arm bone) is deep to the biceps brachii muscle (see Figure 2-5).

Note:

- Whenever designating a structure of the human body as superficial or deep, it is important to state the perspective from which one is looking at the body. Furthermore, the deeper a structure is from one perspective of the body, the more superficial it is from the other perspective of the body.

BOX 2-5

When describing a structure as superficial or deep, it is important to specify the perspective from which one is looking at the body. This is important because one structure may be deep to another structure from one perspective but not deep to it from another perspective. An example is the brachialis muscle of the arm. The brachialis is usually thought of as deep to the biceps brachii muscle because from the anterior perspective the brachialis is deep to it. As a result, many bodyworkers do not realize that the brachialis is superficial (deep only to the skin) and easily accessible and palpable laterally and medially.

The deeper a structure is from one perspective of the body, the more superficial it is from the other perspective of the body. An example is the dorsal interossei pedis muscles of the feet. The dorsal interossei pedis muscles of the feet, are considered to be in the deepest plantar layer of musculature of the feet and viewed from the plantar perspective they are located deep to the plantar interossei muscles. However, from the dorsal perspective, the dorsal interossei pedis muscles are superficial to the plantar interossei muscles; and indeed, the dorsal interossei pedis muscles are more accessible and palpable from the dorsal side.

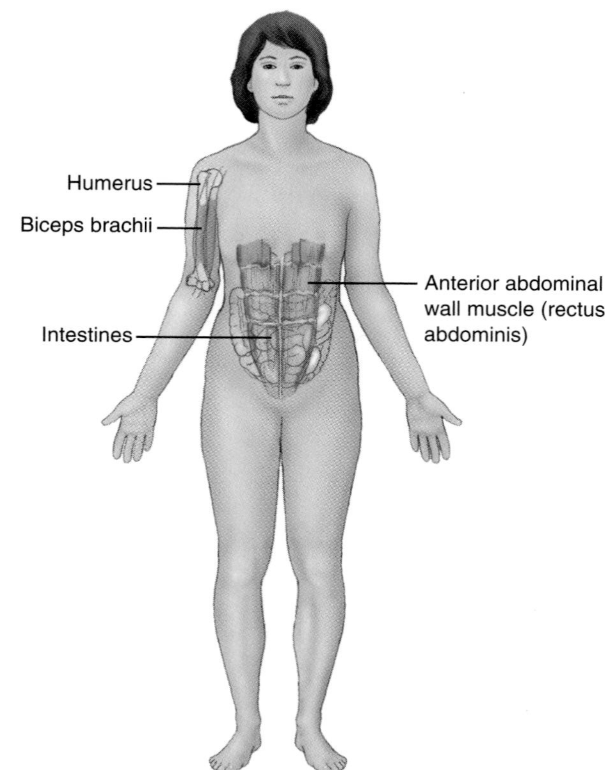

Figure 2-5 Anterior view of a person in anatomic position. The anterior perspective shows the rectus abdominis muscle of the anterior abdominal wall is superficial to the intestines (located within the abdominopelvic cavity); conversely, the intestines are deep to the rectus abdominis muscle. From the anterior perspective, the biceps brachii muscle is superficial to the humerus; conversely, the humerus is deep to the biceps brachii muscle.

☐ 2.7 LOCATION TERMINOLOGY ILLUSTRATION

Figure 2-6 is an anterior view of a person, illustrating the terms of relative location as they pertain to the body.

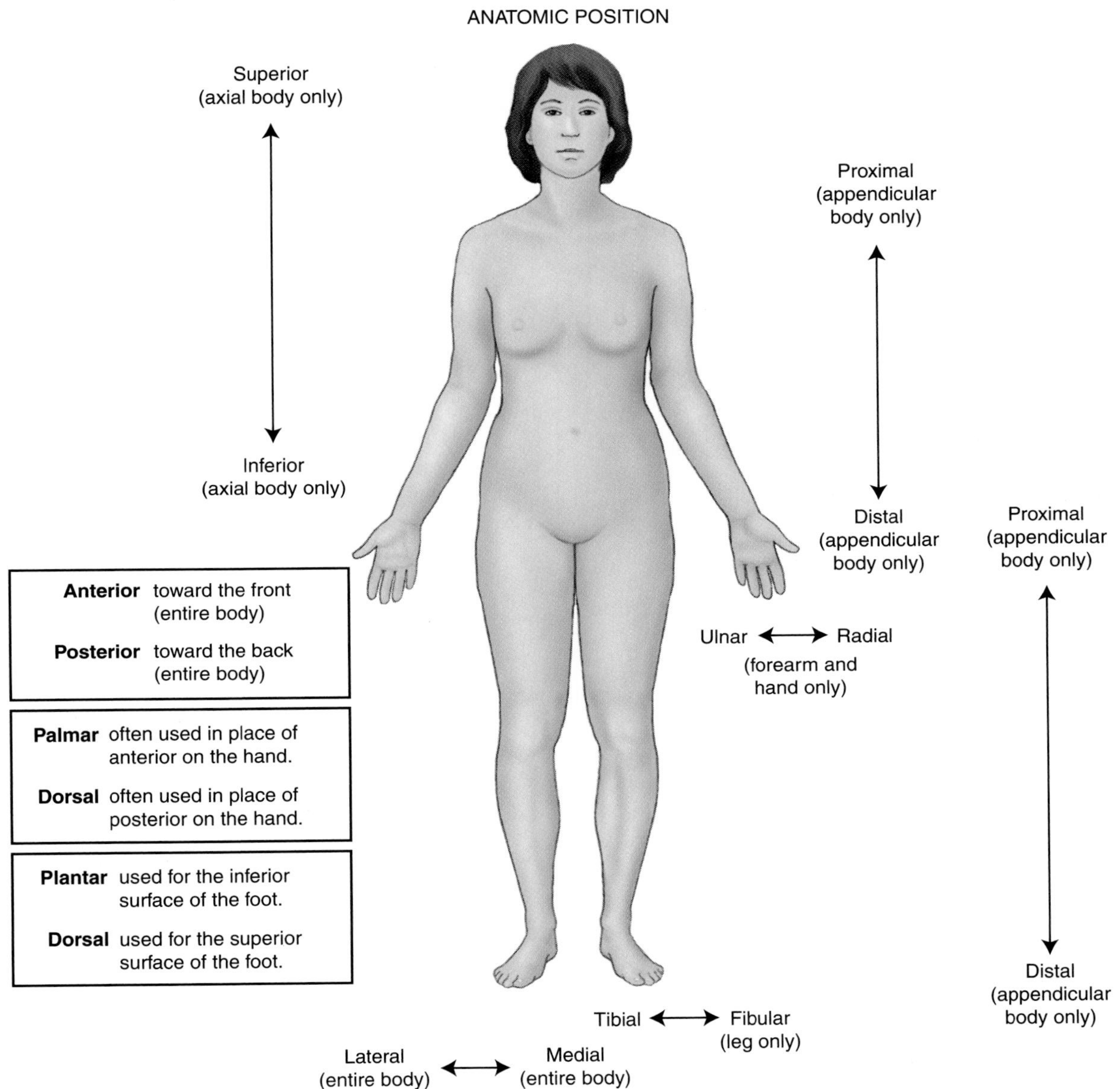

Figure 2-6 Various directional terms of location relative to anatomic position.

☐ 2.8 PLANES

All too often, planes are presented in textbooks with an illustration and a one-line definition for each one of them. Consequently, students often memorize them with a weak understanding of what they really are and their importance. Because a clear and thorough understanding of planes greatly facilitates learning and understanding the motions caused by muscular contractions, the following is presented.

- We have already mapped the human body to describe the location of structures and/or points of the body.
- However, when we want to describe motion of the human body, we need to describe or map the space through which motion occurs.
- As we all know, space is three-dimensional (3-D).
- Therefore to map space, we need to describe these three dimensions of space.
- We describe each one of these dimensions with a **plane**; because three dimensions exist, three types of planes exist.

BOX 2-6

The word *plane* actually means *a flat surface.* Each of the planes is a flat surface that cuts through space, describing a dimension of space.

- The three types of planes are called *sagittal, frontal,* and *transverse* (Figure 2-7).
- The human body or a part of the body can move in each of these three dimensions or planes:
  - A body part can move in an anterior to posterior (or posterior to anterior) direction. This direction describes the **sagittal plane**.
  - A body part can move in a left to right (or right to left) direction; this could also be described as a medial to lateral (or lateral to medial) direction of movement. This direction describes the **frontal plane**.
  - A body part can stay in place and spin (i.e., rotate). This direction describes the **transverse plane**.
- These three planes are called **cardinal planes** and are defined as follows:
  - A sagittal plane divides the body into left and right portions.

BOX 2-7

The sagittal plane that is located down the center of the body and divides the body wall into equal left and right halves is called the **midsagittal plane**.

  - A frontal plane divides the body into anterior and posterior portions.
  - A transverse plane divides the body into (upper) superior/proximal and (lower) inferior/distal portions.
- Please note the following:
  - These three cardinal planes are defined relative to anatomic position. (This is not to say that motion of the human body can only be initiated from anatomic position. It only means that these three cardinal planes were originally defined with the body parts in anatomic position.)
  - Any plane that is not purely sagittal, frontal, or transverse (i.e., has components of two or three of the cardinal planes) is called an **oblique plane**.
  - The sagittal and frontal planes are oriented vertically; the transverse plane is oriented horizontally.
  - An infinite number of sagittal, frontal, transverse, and oblique planes are possible.
- The frontal plane is also commonly called the **coronal plane**.
- The transverse plane is also commonly called the **horizontal plane**.

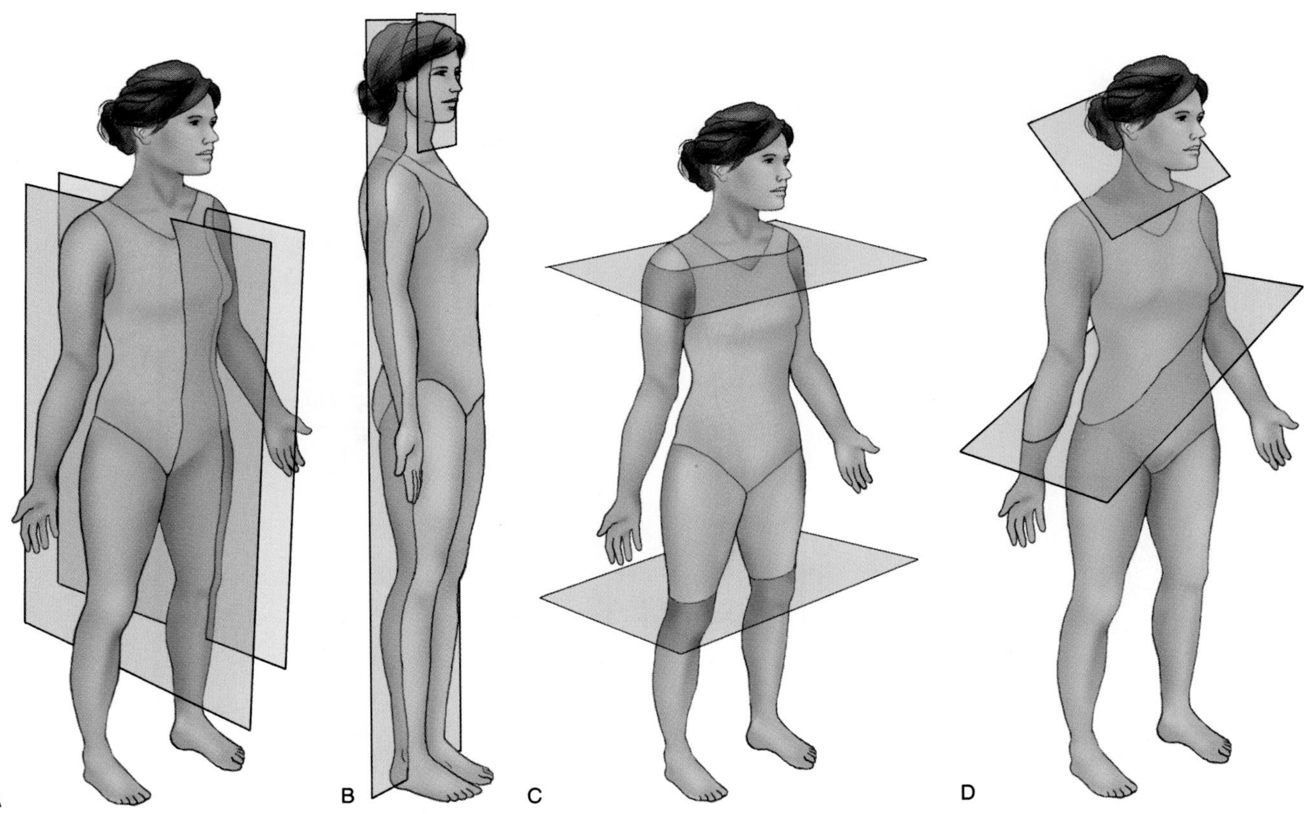

Figure 2-7 Anterolateral views of the body, illustrating the four types of planes: sagittal, frontal, transverse, and oblique. *A,* Two examples of sagittal planes; a sagittal plane divides the body into left and right portions. *B,* Two examples of frontal planes; a frontal plane divides the body into anterior and posterior portions. *C,* Two examples of transverse planes; a transverse plane divides the body into upper (superior and/or proximal) and lower (inferior and/or distal) portions. *D,* Two examples of oblique planes; an oblique plane is a plane that is not exactly sagittal, frontal, or transverse (i.e., it has components of two or three cardinal planes). The upper oblique plane has frontal and transverse components to it; the lower oblique plane has sagittal and transverse components to it.

2.9 MOTION OF THE HUMAN BODY WITHIN PLANES

- Because an understanding of the planes is an important part of understanding movements of the body, motion of the human body in each of the three planes should be examined. Figures 2-8a–d illustrate motion of the body in the sagittal, frontal, and transverse planes, as well as in an oblique plane, respectively. Figure 2-8e–h illustrates additional examples of motions within planes. (For a detailed discussion of the names of these motions, please see Chapter 5, Sections 5.11 through 5.25.)

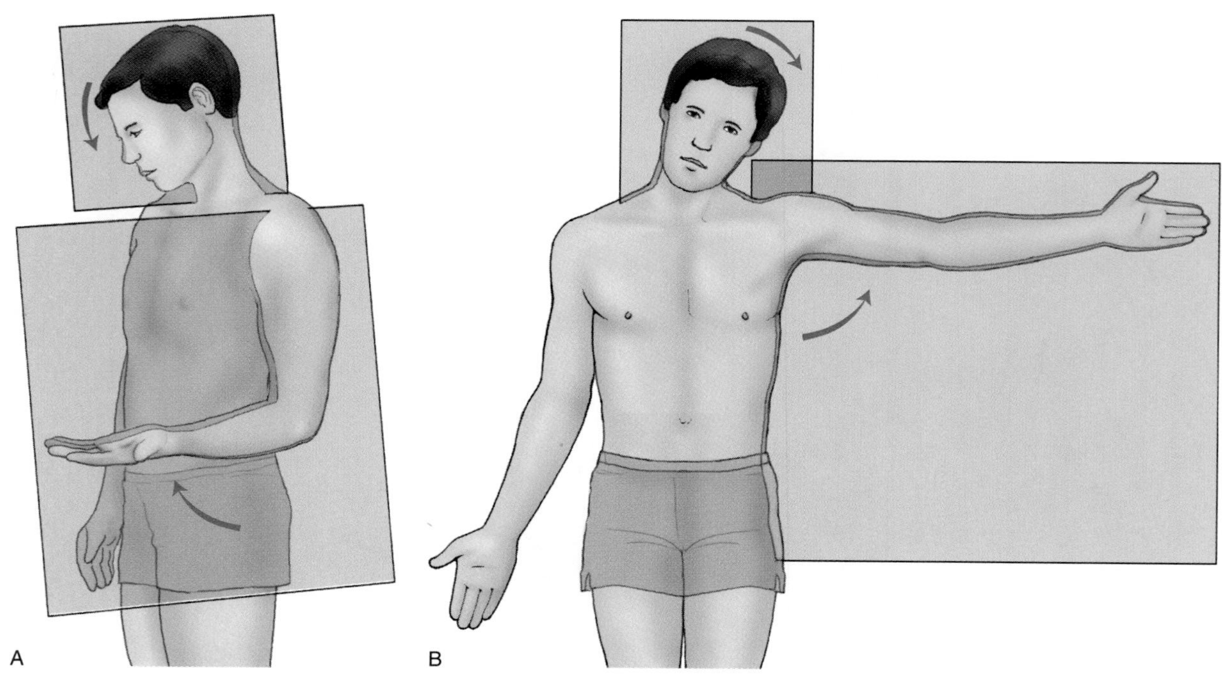

Figure 2-8 *A,* Anterolateral view illustrates two examples of the concept of motion of a body part within a sagittal plane. The head and neck are flexing (moving anteriorly) at the spinal joints; this motion is occurring within a sagittal plane. In addition, the left forearm is flexing (moving anteriorly) at the elbow joint; this motion is occurring within a sagittal plane. *B,* Anterior view illustrates two examples of the concept of motion of a body part within a frontal plane. The head and neck are left laterally flexing (bending to the left side) at the spinal joints; this motion is occurring within a frontal plane. In addition, the left arm is abducting (moving laterally away from the midline) at the shoulder joint; this motion is occurring within a frontal plane.

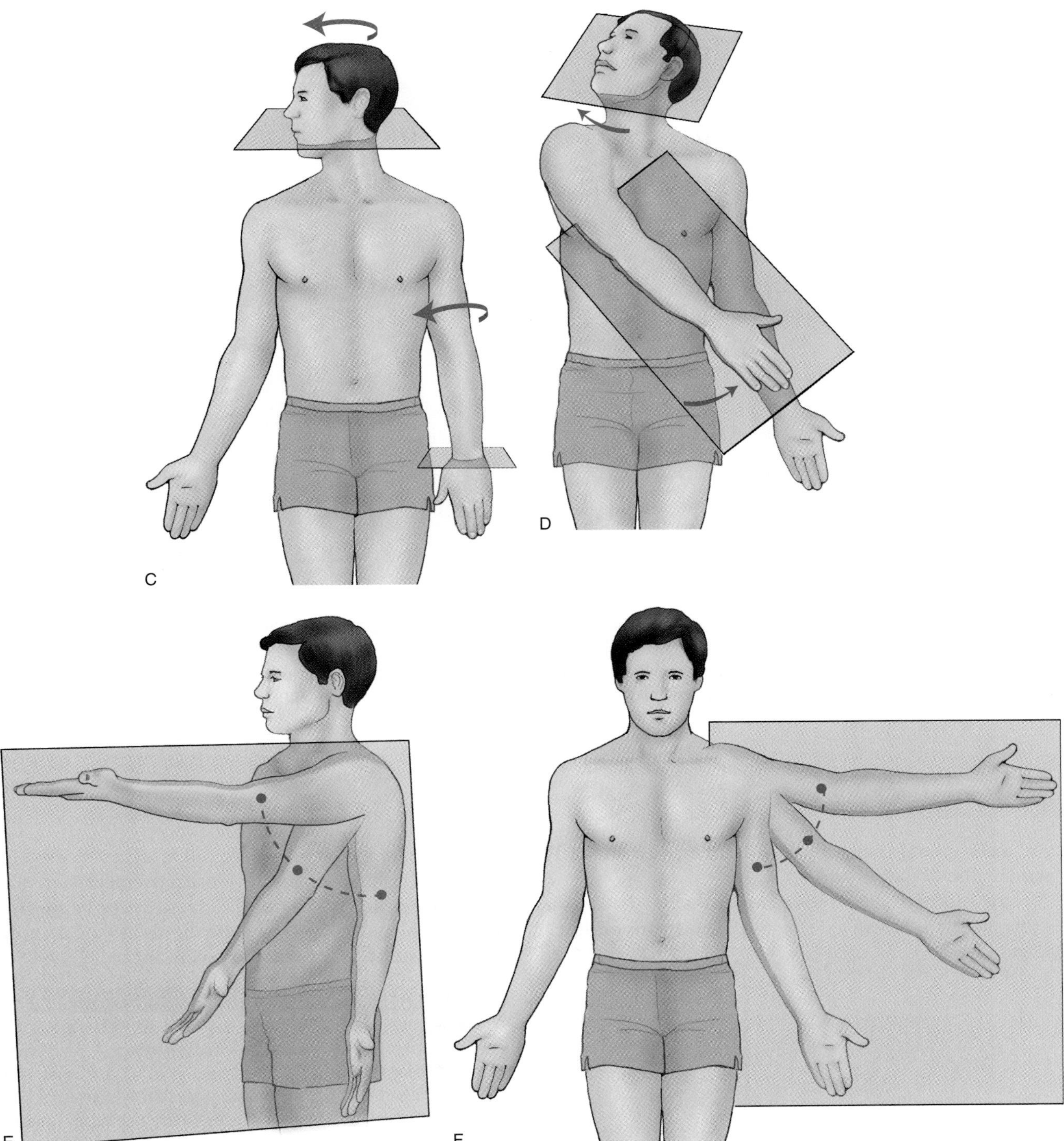

Figure 2-8, cont'd *C,* Anterior view illustrates two examples of the concept of motion of a body part within a transverse plane. The head and neck are rotating to the right (twisting/turning to the right) at the spinal joints; this motion is occurring within a transverse plane. In addition, the left arm is medially rotating (rotating toward the midline) at the shoulder joint; this motion is occurring within a transverse plane. *D,* Anterior view illustrates two examples of the concept of motion of a body part within an oblique plane (i.e., a plane that has components of two or three of the cardinal planes). The head and neck are doing a combination of sagittal, frontal, and transverse plane movements (at the spinal joints). These movements are extension (moving posteriorly) in the sagittal plane, left lateral flexion (bending to the left side) in the frontal plane, and right rotation (twisting/turning to the right) in the transverse plane. The right arm is also doing a combination of sagittal, frontal, and transverse plane movements (at the shoulder joint). These movements are flexion (moving anteriorly) in the sagittal plane, adduction (moving medially toward the midline) in the frontal plane, and medial rotation (rotating toward the midline) in the transverse plane. *E* to *H,* Motion of the arm at the shoulder joint within each of the three cardinal planes and an oblique plane. A point has been drawn on the arm; the arc that is created by the movement of this point has also been drawn in (in each case, the arc of motion of this point is within the plane of motion that the body part is moving within, illustrating that motion of a body part occurs within a plane). *E,* An anterolateral view illustrates the left arm flexing (moving anteriorly) at the shoulder joint within a sagittal plane. *F,* Anterior view illustrates the left arm abducting (moving laterally away from the midline) at the shoulder joint within a frontal plane.

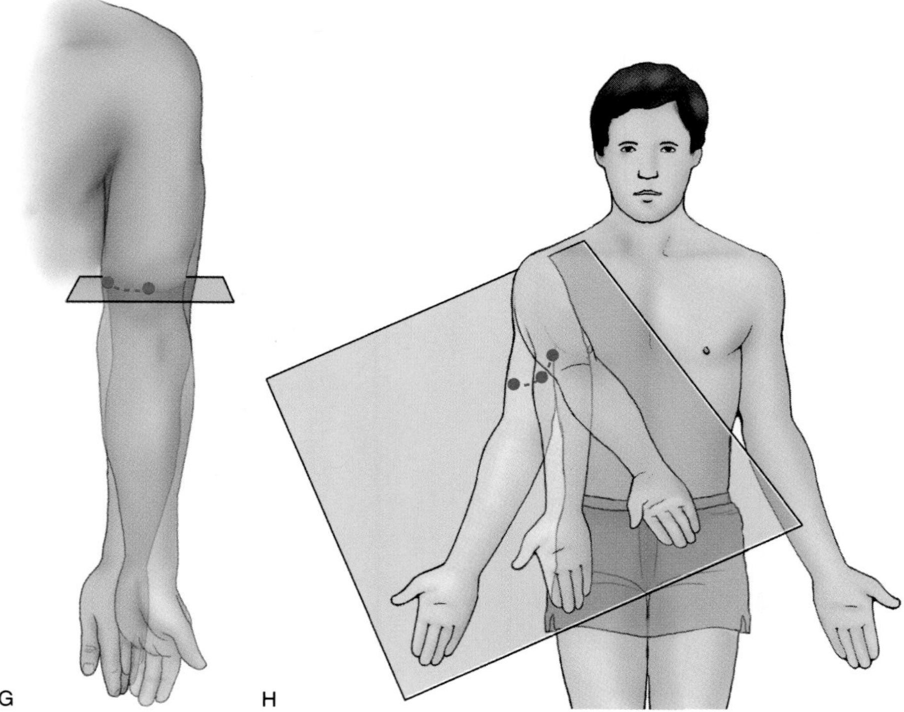

Figure 2-8, cont'd *G,* Anterior view illustrates the left arm laterally rotating (rotating away from the midline) at the shoulder joint within a transverse plane. *H,* Anterior view illustrates the right arm making a motion that is a combination of flexion (moving anteriorly) and adduction (moving toward the midline) at the shoulder joint within an oblique plane.

2.10 AXES

- An **axis** (plural: axes) is an imaginary line around which a body part moves.
- An axis is often called a **mechanical axis**.
- Movement around an axis is called **axial movement** (Figure 2-9).

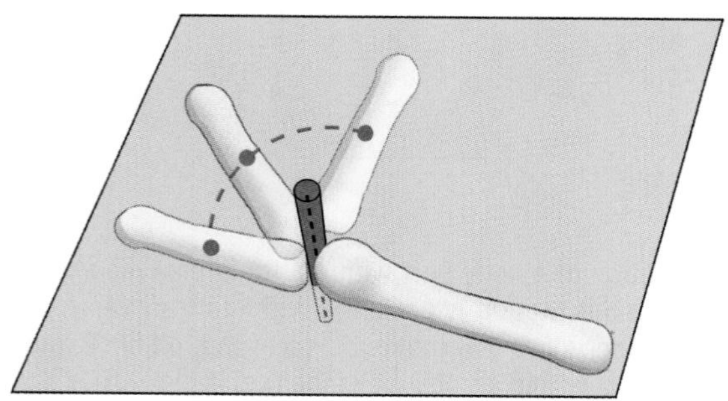

Figure 2-9 An axis is an imaginary line around which motion occurs. This figure illustrates the motion of a bone within a plane and around an axis; the axis is drawn in as a red tube. This type of movement is known as an *axial movement.* A point has been drawn on the bone, and the arc that is transcribed by the motion of this point can be seen to move in a circular path; for this reason, an axial movement is also known as a *circular movement.*

- When a body part moves around an axis, it does so in a circular fashion. For this reason, a movement that occurs around an axis is also called a **circular movement**.
- An axial movement can also be called an **angular movement** or a **rotary movement**.

BOX 2-8

Because a body part is often described as rotating around the axis, an axial movement can also be called a *rotary movement,* or even *rotation.* Indeed, an axis is often referred to as an ***axis of rotation.*** However, calling axial movements *rotary* or *rotation movements* is not recommended (at least not for the beginning kinesiology student), because one type of axial movement has the word *rotation* within its name (*spin* axial movements [e.g., right rotation, left rotation, lateral rotation, medial rotation]), whereas another type of axial movement (*roll* axial movements [e.g., flexion, extension, abduction, adduction]) does not have the word *rotation* within its name. Therefore it is easy to confuse these different types of axial movements with each other. Axial movements (and in particular spin and roll axial movements) are discussed in Chapter 5, Sections 5.7 and 5.8.

- The terms *axial movement, circular movement, angular movement,* and *rotary movement* are all synonyms. The concept of axial movement is visited again and covered in more detail in Chapter 5, Sections 5.5 through 5.7.

☐ 2.11 PLANES AND THEIR CORRESPONDING AXES

- When motion of a body part occurs, it can be described as occurring within a plane.
  - Depending on the type of motion that occurs, this motion within the plane can be further described as moving around an axis.
  - Therefore for each one of the three cardinal planes of the body, a corresponding **cardinal axis** exists; hence, three cardinal axes exist (Figure 2-10a–c).
  - For every motion that occurs within an oblique plane, a corresponding **oblique axis** exists (Figure 2-10d). Therefore an infinite number of oblique axes exist, one for each possible oblique plane.

- Naming an axis is straightforward; simply describe its orientation.
  - The three cardinal axes are the mediolateral, anteroposterior, and the superoinferior (vertical) axes (see Figures 2-10a–c).
- Please note that an axis about which motion occurs is always perpendicular to the plane in which the motion is occurring.
- An axial movement of a body part is one in which the body part moves within a plane and around an axis.

Mediolateral Axis:

- A **mediolateral axis** is a line that runs from medial to lateral (or lateral to medial [i.e., left to right or right to left]) in direction (see Figure 2-10a).
- Movements that occur in the sagittal plane move around a mediolateral axis.
- The mediolateral axis is also known as the **frontal-horizontal axis** because it runs horizontally and is located within the frontal plane.

Anteroposterior Axis:

- An **anteroposterior axis** is a line that runs anterior to posterior (or posterior to anterior) in direction (see Figure 2-10b).
- Movements that occur in the frontal plane move around an anteroposterior axis.
- The anteroposterior axis is also known as the **sagittal-horizontal** axis because it runs horizontally and is located within the sagittal plane.

Superoinferior Axis:

- A **superoinferior axis** is a line that runs from superior to inferior (or inferior to superior) in direction (see Figure 2-10c).
- Movements that occur in a transverse plane move around a superoinferior axis.
- The superoinferior axis is more commonly referred to as the **vertical axis** because it runs vertically. (This text will use the term *vertical axis* because it is an easier term for the reader/student to visualize.)

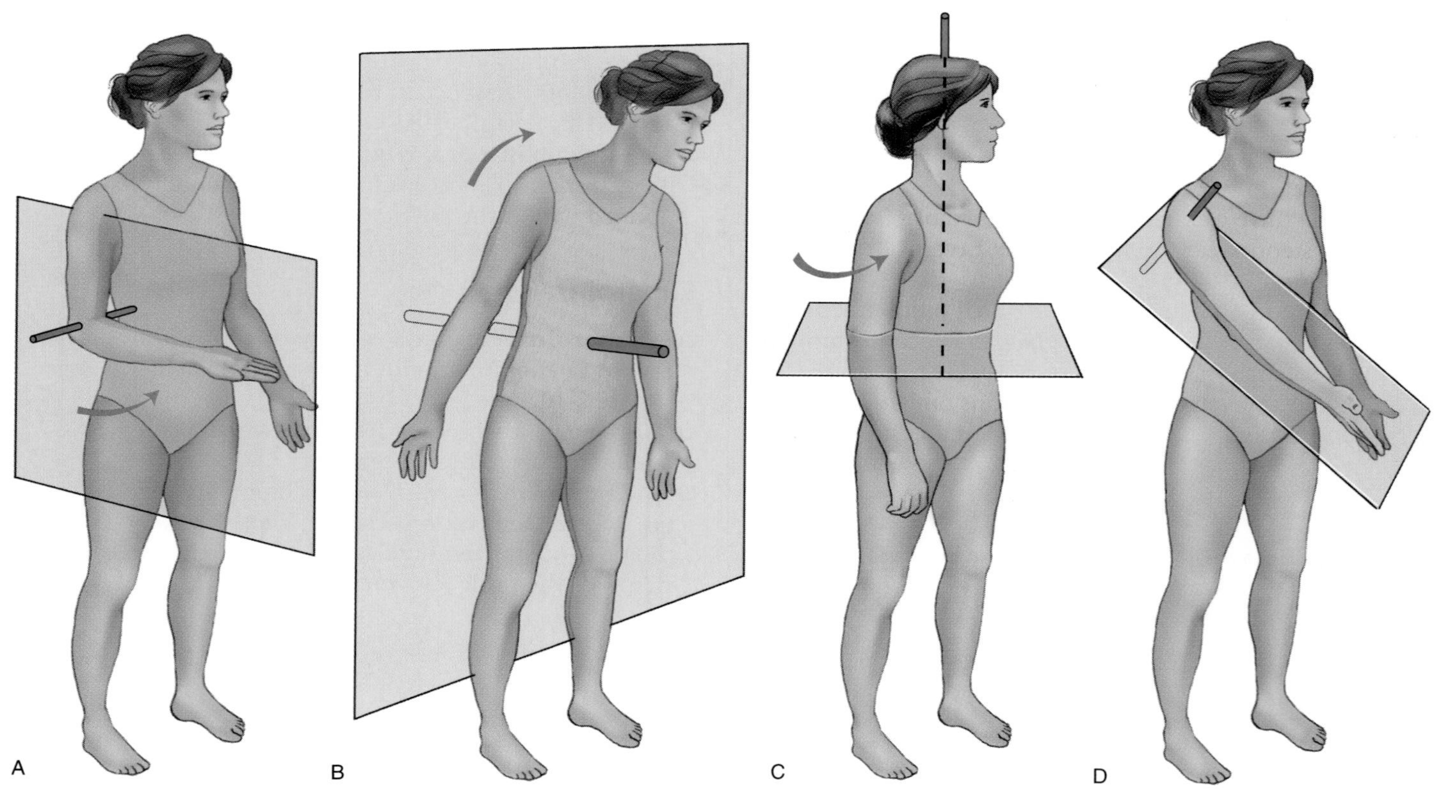

Figure 2-10 *A* to *D,* Anterolateral views that illustrate the corresponding axes for the three cardinal planes and an oblique plane; the axes are shown as red tubes. Note that an axis always runs perpendicular to the plane in which the motion is occurring. *A,* Motion occurring in the sagittal plane; because this motion is occurring around an axis that is running horizontally in a medial to lateral orientation, it is called the *mediolateral axis. B,* Motion occurring in the frontal plane; because this motion is occurring around an axis that is running horizontally in an anterior to posterior orientation, it is called the *anteroposterior axis. C,* Motion occurring in the transverse plane; because this motion is occurring around an axis that is running vertically in a superior to inferior orientation, it is called the *superoinferior axis,* or more simply, the *vertical axis. D,* Motion occurring in an oblique plane; this motion is occurring around an axis that is running perpendicular to that plane (i.e., it is the oblique axis for this oblique plane).

☐ 2.12 VISUALIZING THE AXES—DOOR HINGE PIN ANALOGY

- To help visualize an axis for motion, the following visual analogy may be helpful. An axis may be thought of as the hinge pin of a door. Just as a body part's motion occurs around its axis, a door's motion occurs around its hinge pin, which is its axis for motion (Figure 2-11).

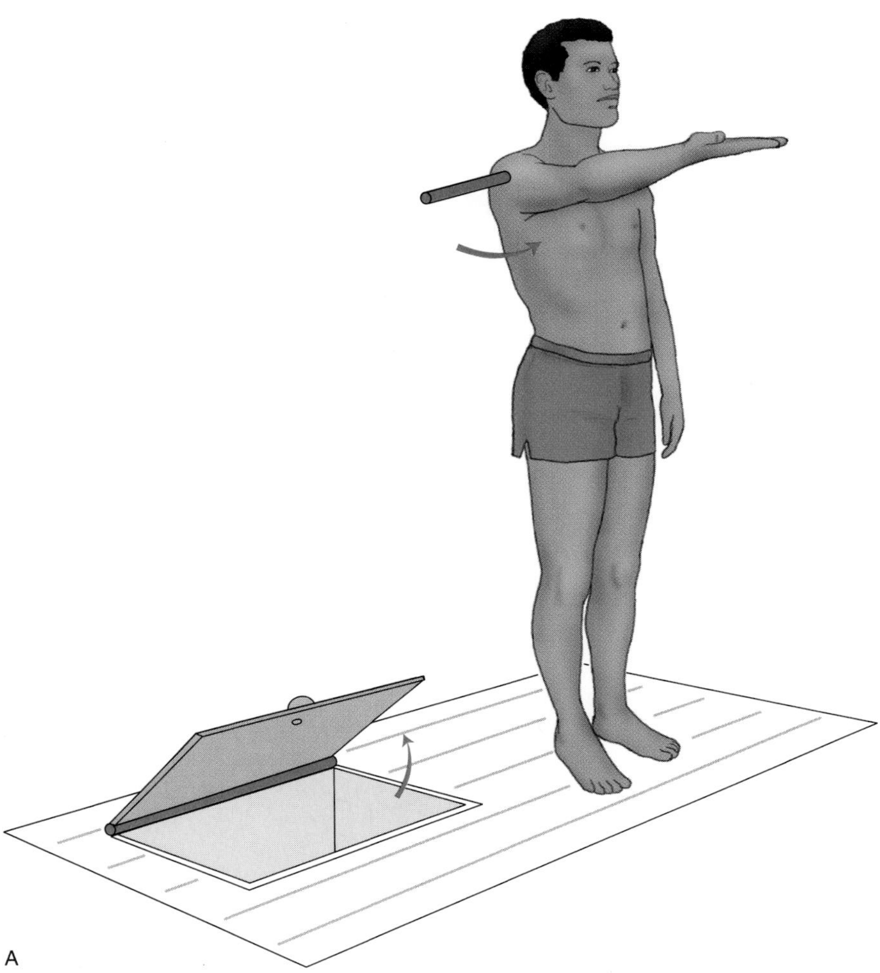

Figure 2-11 *A* to *C*, Anterolateral views that compare the axes of motion for movement of the arm to the axes of motion for a door that is moving (i.e., opening); the axes are drawn in as red tubes. *A*, A trap door in a floor that is moving (i.e., opening). The person standing next to the door is moving the arm in the same manner that the trap door is opening. These movements are occurring in the sagittal plane. If we look at the orientation of the hinge pin of the door, which is its axis of motion, we will see that it is medial to lateral in orientation. Note that the axis for the motion of the person's arm is also medial to lateral in orientation. Hence the axis for sagittal plane motion is mediolateral.

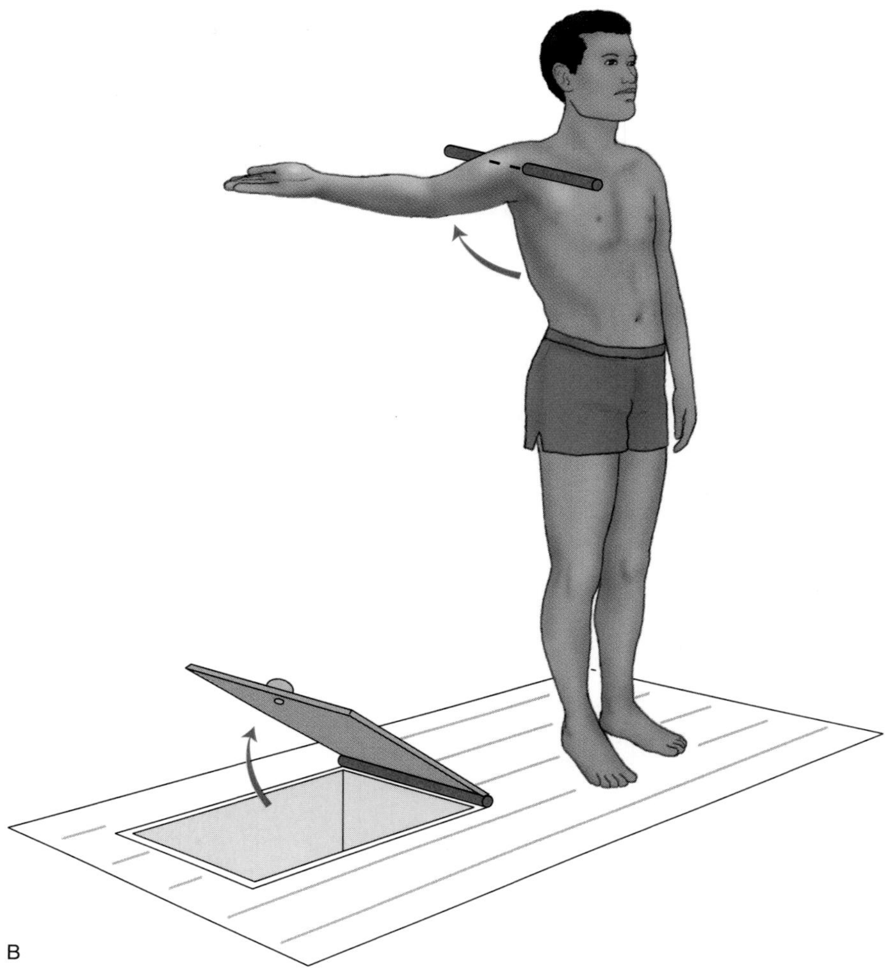

Figure 2-11, cont'd *B,* A trap door in a floor that is moving (i.e., opening). The person standing next to the door is moving the arm in the same manner that the trap door is opening. These movements are occurring in the frontal plane. If we look at the orientation of the hinge pin of the door, which is its axis of motion, we will see that it is anterior to posterior in orientation. Note that the axis for the motion of the person's arm is also anterior to posterior in orientation. Hence the axis for sagittal plane motion is anteroposterior.

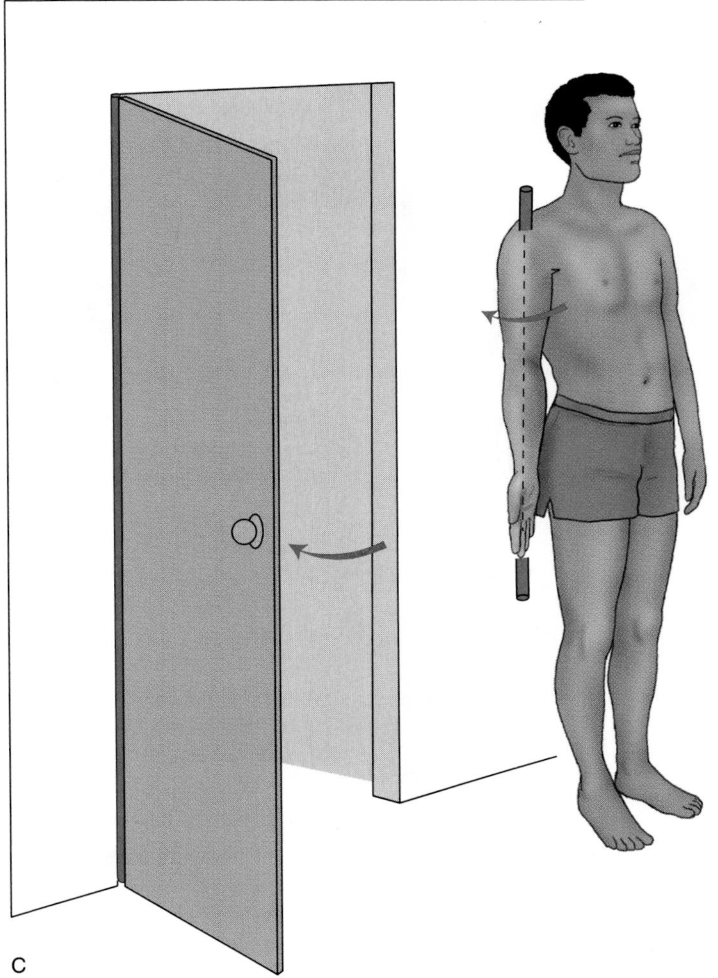

Figure 2-11, cont'd *C,* A door that is moving (i.e., opening). The person standing next to the door is moving the arm in the same manner that the door is opening. These movements are occurring in the transverse plane. If we look at the orientation of the hinge pin of the door, which is its axis of motion, we will see that it is superior to inferior in orientation (i.e., it is vertical). Note that the axis for the motion of the person's arm is also superior to inferior in orientation. Hence the axis for transverse plane motion is vertical.

☐ 2.13 VISUALIZING THE AXES—PINWHEEL ANALOGY

❑ Another visual analogy that may be helpful toward determining the axis of motion is a pinwheel. When a child blows on a pinwheel, the wheel of the pinwheel spins in a plane; the pin of the pinwheel is the axis about which the wheel spins. If you orient the motion of the wheel in any one of the three cardinal planes, then naming the orientation of the pin of the pinwheel will name the axis for that plane's motion (Figure 2-12a–c).

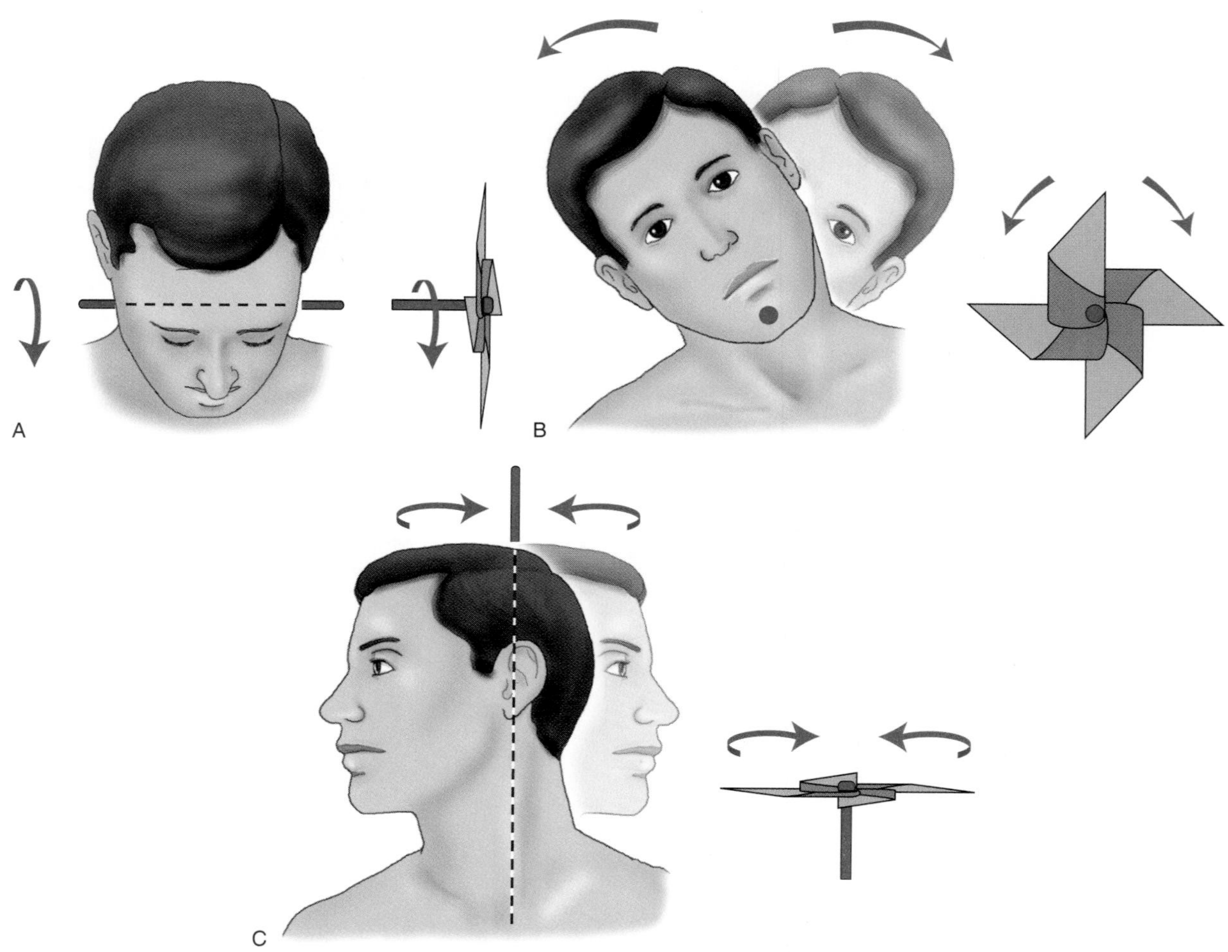

Figure 2-12 *A* to *C,* Anterior views that compare the axes of motion for movement of the head and neck to the axes of motion for the wheel of a pinwheel. The pin of the pinwheel represents the axis of motion of the pinwheel; the axes are drawn in as red tubes or a red dot. *A,* The motion of the person's head and neck and the motion of the wheel of the pinwheel are in the sagittal plane; the axis for sagittal plane motion is mediolateral. *B,* The motion of the person's head and neck and the motion of the wheel of the pinwheel are in the frontal plane; the axis for frontal plane motion is anteroposterior *(red dot). C,* The motion of the person's head and neck and the motion of the wheel of the pinwheel are in the transverse plane; the axis for transverse plane motion is vertical.

REVIEW QUESTIONS

evolve Answers to the following review questions appear on the Evolve website accompanying this book.

1. What is the position of the body when it is in anatomic position?

2. What is the importance of anatomic position?

3. What are the five major pairs of directional terms for naming the location of a structure of the body or a point on the body?

4. In what parts of the body can each of the pairs of directional terms of location be used?

5. If point *A* is located farther toward the front of the body than point *B* is, then how do we describe the location of point *A*? Point *B*?

6. If point *C* is located closer to the midline of the body than point *D* is, then how do we describe the location of point *C*? Point *D*?

7. If point *E* is located on the axial body closer to the top of the body than point *F* is, then how do we describe the location of point *E*? Point *F*?

8. If point *G* is located on the appendicular body closer to the axial body than point *H* is, then how do we describe the location of point *G*? Point *H*?

9. If point *I* is located both farther toward the front and farther toward the midline of the body than point *J* is, then how do we describe the location of point *I*? Point *J*?

10. If point *K* is located closer to the surface of the body than point *L* is, then how do we describe the location of point *K*? Point *L*?

11. What is a plane and what is the importance of understanding the concept of planes?

12. What are the four major types of planes?

13. What is an axis and what is the importance of understanding the concept of axes?

14. What are the corresponding axes for each of the three cardinal planes?

15. What is the relationship between axial motion and planes and axes?

16. How is the hinge pin of a door or the pin of a pinwheel analogous to the axis for an axial movement?

NOTES

Chapter 3

Skeletal Tissues

CHAPTER OUTLINE

CHAPTER OUTLINE

After completing this chapter, the student should be able to perform the following:

- ❑ List the four major classifications of bones by shape and give an example of each one.
- ❑ Place sesamoid bones into their major category of bones by shape and give an example of a sesamoid bone.
- ❑ Explain the concept of a supernumerary bone and give an example of a supernumerary bone.
- ❑ List and describe the major structural aspects of a long bone.
- ❑ List and describe the five major functions of bones.
- ❑ List and describe the components of bone as a connective tissue.
- ❑ Describe, compare, and contrast the structure of compact and spongy bone.
- ❑ Describe, compare, and contrast the two methods of bone development and growth: (1) endochondral ossification and (2) intramembranous ossification.
- ❑ Explain the purpose of the fontanels of the infant's skull.
- ❑ Name, locate, and state the closure time of the major fontanels of the infant's skull.
- ❑ Describe the steps by which a fractured bone heals.
- ❑ State and explain the meaning and importance of Wolff's law to the human skeleton and the fields of bodywork and exercise.
- ❑ Explain the relationship of the piezoelectric effect to Wolff's law.
- ❑ Explain the relationship between Wolff's law and degenerative joint disease (DJD) (also known as *osteoarthritis* [OA]).
- ❑ List and describe the components of cartilage as a connective tissue.
- ❑ Compare and contrast the three types of cartilage tissue.
- ❑ Compare and contrast the structure and function of tendons and ligaments.
- ❑ Explain why tendons and ligaments do not heal well when injured.
- ❑ Compare and contrast the structure and function of bursae and tendon sheaths.
- ❑ Compare and contrast the concepts of elasticity and plasticity.
- ❑ Relate the concepts of creep, thixotropy, and hysteresis to the fields of bodywork and exercise.

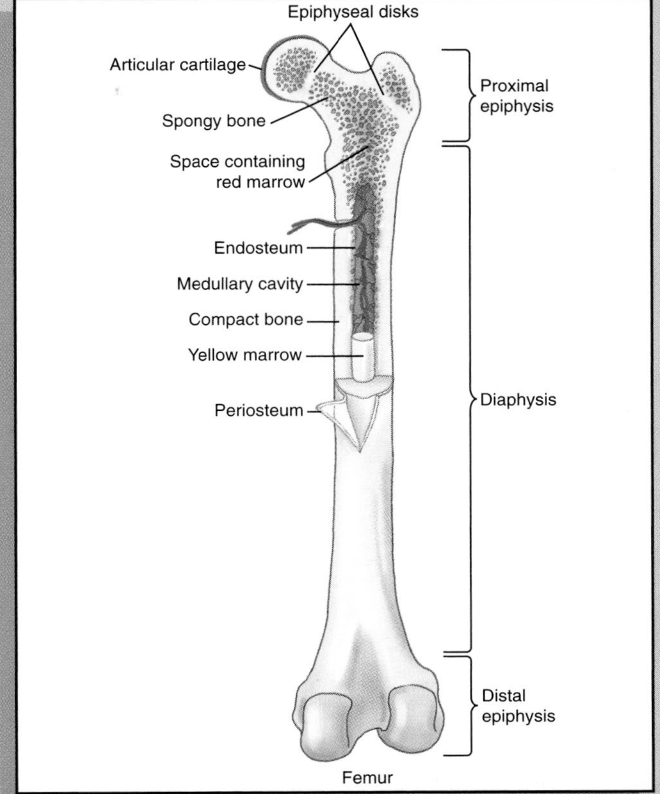

- ❑ Define the key terms of this chapter.
- ❑ State the meanings of the word origins of this chapter.

OVERVIEW

Many tissues contribute to the structure and function of the skeletal system, chief among them is bone tissue. The first sections of this chapter examine bone tissue macrostructure, microstructure, functions, and physiology. The later sections of this chapter then cover the other tissues that are necessary for skeletal system structure and function. These other tissues are cartilage, tendon, ligament, bursae, and tendon sheaths. The last section then covers the general properties that apply to all skeletal connective tissues.

KEY TERMS

Anterior fontanel (an-TEER-ee-or FON-ta-nel)
Anterolateral fontanel (AN-teer-o-LAT-er-al FON-ta-nel)
Aponeurosis, pl. aponeuroses (AP-o-noo-RO-sis, AP-o-noo-RO-seez)
Articular cartilage (ar-TIK-you-lar KAR-ti-lij)
Articular surface
Bone marrow
Bone spur
Bony callus
Bursa, pl. bursae (BER-sa, BER-see)
Bursitis (ber-SIGH-tis)
Calcitonin (KAL-si-TO-nin)
Callus
Canaliculus, pl. canaliculi (KAN-a-LIK-you-lus, KAN-a-LIK-you-lie)
Cancellous bone (KAN-se-lus)
Cartilage (KAR-ti-lij)
Chondroblast (KON-dro-blast)
Chondrocyte (KON-dro-site)
Chondroitin sulfate (kon-DROY-tin SUL-fate)
Collagen fibers (KOL-la-jen)
Compact bone
Connective tissue
Contractility
Cortex (KOR-teks)
Cortical surface (KOR-ti-kal)
Creep (KREEP)
Cytoplasmic processes (SI-to-PLAZ-mik)
Degenerative joint disease
Diaphysis, pl. diaphyses (die-AF-i-sis, die-AF-i-seez)
Elastic cartilage
Elasticity
Elastin fibers (ee-LAS-tin)
Endochondral ossification (en-do-KON-dral OS-si-fi-KAY-shun)
Endosteum (en-DOS-tee-um)
Epiphysial disc (e-PIF-i-zee-al)
Epiphysial line
Epiphysis, pl. epiphyses (e-PIF-i-sis, e-PIF-i-seez)
Fibroblast (FI-bro-blast)
Fibrocartilage (FI-bro-KAR-ti-lij)
Flat bones
Fontanel (FON-ta-NEL)
Frontal fontanel
Gel state (JEL)
Glucosamine (glue-KOS-a-meen)
Ground substance
Growth plate
Haversian canal (ha-VER-zhun)
Hematoma (HEEM-a-TOME-a)
Hematopoiesis (heem-AT-o-poy-E-sis)
Hyaline cartilage (HI-a-lin KAR-ti-lij)
Hydroxyapatite crystals (hi-DROK-see-AP-a-TIGHT)
Hysteresis (his-ter-E-sis)
Intramembranous ossification (in-tra-MEM-bran-us OS-si-fi-KAY-shun)
Irregular bones
Kinesiology (ki-NEE-see-OL-o-gee)
Lacuna, pl. lacunae (la-KOO-na, la-KOO-nee)
Lever
Ligament (LIG-a-ment)
Long bones
Mastoid fontanel (MAS-toyd FON-ta-NEL)
Matrix (MAY-triks)
Medullary cavity (MEJ-you-LAR-ree)
Membrane (MEM-brain)
OA
Occipital fontanel (ok-SIP-i-tal FON-ta-NEL)
Ossification center (OS-si-fi-KAY-shun)
Osteoarthritis (OS-tee-o-ar-THRI-tis)
Osteoblast (OS-tee-o-BLAST)
Osteoclast (OS-tee-o-KLAST)
Osteocyte (OS-tee-o-SITE)
Osteoid tissue (OS-tee-OYD)
Osteon (OS-tee-on)
Osteonic canal (OS-tee-ON-ik)
Parathyroid hormone (PAR-a-THI-royd)
Perichondrium (per-ee-KON-dree-um)
Periosteum (per-ee-OS-tee-um)
Periostitis (PER-ee-ost-EYE-tis)
Piezoelectric effect (PIE-zo-e-LEK-trik)
Plasticity (plas-TIS-i-tee)
Posterior fontanel (pos-TEER-ee-or FON-ta-nel)
Posterolateral fontanel (POS-teer-o-LAT-er-al FON-ta-nel)
Primary ossification center
Proteoglycans (PRO-tee-o-GLY-kans)
Radiograph (RAY-dee-o-graf)
Red bone marrow
Retinaculum, pl. retinacula (ret-i-NAK-you-lum, ret-i-NAK-you-la)
Round bones
Secondary ossification centers
Sesamoid bones (SES-a-moyd)
Short
Sol state (SOLE)
Sphenoid fontanel (SFEE-noyd FON-ta-NEL)
Spongy bone
Sprain
Strain
Stretch
Subchondral bone
Supernumerary bones (soo-per-NOO-mer-air-ee)
Synovial tendon sheath (si-NO-vee-al)
Tendinitis (ten-di-NI-tis)
Tendon

Tendon sheath
Tenosynovitis (TEN-o-sin-o-VI-tis)
Tensile strength (TEN-sile)
Thixotropy (thik-SOT-tro-pee)
Trabecula, pl. trabeculae (tra-BEK-you-la, tra-BEK-you-lee)
Viscoelasticity (VIS-ko-ee-las-TIS-i-tee)
Viscoplasticity (VIS-ko-plas-TIS-i-tee)
Volkmann's canal (FOK-mahns ka-NAL)
Weight bearing
Wolff's law (WOLF or VULF)
Wormian bones (WERM-ee-an)
Yellow bone marrow

WORD ORIGINS

- ❑ A (an)—From Latin *a,* meaning *not, without*
- ❑ Arthr—From Greek *arthron,* meaning *a joint*
- ❑ Articular—From Latin *articulus,* meaning *a joint*
- ❑ Blastic—From Greek *blastos,* meaning *to bud, to build, to grow*
- ❑ Chondr—From Greek *chondros,* meaning *cartilage*
- ❑ Clastic—From Greek *klastos,* meaning *to break up into pieces*
- ❑ Cortical—From Latin *cortex,* meaning *outer portion of an organ, bark of a tree*
- ❑ Cyte—From Greek *kyton,* meaning *a hollow, cell*
- ❑ Endo—From Greek *endon,* meaning *within, inner*
- ❑ Epi—From Greek *epi,* meaning *on, upon*
- ❑ Fibr, fibro—From Latin *fibra,* meaning *fiber*
- ❑ Graph—From Greek *grapho,* meaning *to write*
- ❑ Hem, hemato—From Greek *haima,* meaning *blood*
- ❑ Hyaline—From Greek *hyalos,* meaning *glass*
- ❑ Intra—From Latin *intra,* meaning *within, inner*
- ❑ Itis—From Greek *itis,* meaning *inflammation*
- ❑ Kines—From Greek *kinesis,* meaning *movement, motion*
- ❑ Medulla—From Latin *medulla,* meaning *inner portion, marrow*
- ❑ Num—From Latin *numerus,* meaning *number*
- ❑ Oid—From Greek *eidos,* meaning *resembling, appearance*
- ❑ Ology—From Greek *logos,* meaning *study of, discourse, word*
- ❑ Os, ossi—From Latin *os,* meaning *bone*
- ❑ Ost, osteo—From Greek *osteon,* meaning *bone*
- ❑ Peri—From Greek *peri,* meaning *around*
- ❑ Physi, physio—From Greek *physis,* meaning *body, nature*
- ❑ Piezo—From Greek *piesis,* meaning *pressure*
- ❑ Poiesis—From Greek *poiesis,* meaning *production, making*

3.1 CLASSIFICATION OF BONES BY SHAPE

- Structurally, bones can be divided into four major categories based upon their shape (Figure 3-1).
  - These four major classifications by shape are:
    - Long bones
    - Short bones
    - Flat bones
    - Irregular bones
  - These classifications can be useful when discussing the structure and function of bones. However, it should be kept in mind that all classification systems are at least somewhat arbitrary, and not every bone fits perfectly into one category; sometimes the classification of a bone may be difficult because it has attributes of two or more categories.
- **Long bones** are long (i.e., they have a longitudinal axis to them). This longitudinal axis is the shaft of the bone. At each end of the shaft of a long bone is an expanded portion that forms a joint (articulates) with another bone. (See Section 3.2 for the anatomy of a long bone in more detail.)
  - Examples of long bones are humerus, femur, radius, ulna, tibia, fibula, metacarpals, metatarsals, and phalanges.

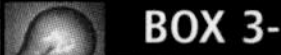

BOX 3-1

Even though some of the phalanges are quite short in length, they still have a longitudinal axis (i.e., a length to them) with expanded ends; therefore they qualify as long bones.

- **Short bones** are short (i.e., they are approximately as wide as they are long, and they are often described as being cube shaped).
  - Examples of short bones are the carpals of the wrist and the tarsals of the ankle.

BOX 3-2

Tarsal bones of the ankle region are considered to be short bones. An exception is the calcaneus of the tarsals (see Section 4.8, Figures 4-54 to 4-57), which is considered to be an irregular bone, not a short bone.

- **Flat bones** are flat; that is they are broad and thin, with either a flat or perhaps a curved surface.
  - Examples of flat bones are the ribs, sternum, cranial bones of the skull, and the scapula.

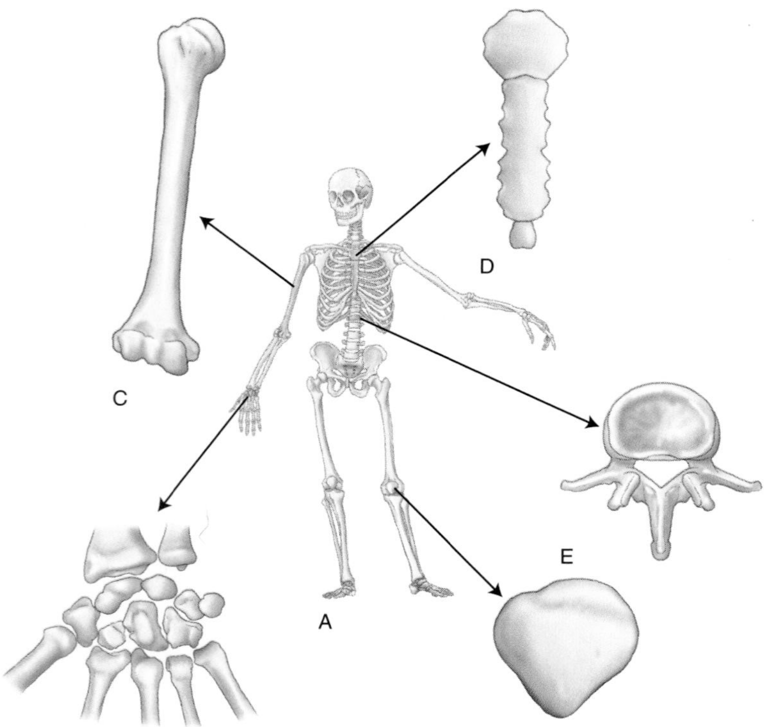

Figure 3-1 The four major classifications (shapes) of bones, as well as a sesamoid bone, which is a type of irregular bone. *A,* Anterior view of the full human skeleton. *B,* The carpals (wrist bones), which are examples of short bones. *C,* A humerus, which is an example of a long bone. *D,* A sternum, which is an example of a flat bone. *E,* A vertebra, which is an example of an irregular bone. *F,* A patella (i.e., kneecap), which is an example of a sesamoid bone; sesamoid bones are considered to be a type of irregular bone.

BOX 3-3

Given that the scapula has a spine, and acromion and coracoid processes, an argument could be made that it is an irregular bone. However, most sources place it as a flat bone.

- **Irregular bones** are irregular in shape (i.e., they do not neatly fall into any of the three preceding categories). They are neither clearly long, nor short, nor flat.
  - Examples of irregular bones are the vertebrae of the spine, the facial bones of the skull, and sesamoid bones.
    - **Sesamoid bones** are so named because they are shaped like a sesame seed (i.e., they are round).

BOX 3-4

Because sesamoid bones are round in shape, they are also known as **round bones**. Some sources consider sesamoid bones to be a separate 5th category of bones.

- The number of sesamoid bones in the human body varies from one individual to another. The only sesamoid bones that are consistently found in all people are the two patellae (kneecaps).

- Additional bones: The number of bones in the human skeleton is usually said to be 206. This number can vary slightly from individual to individual. Whenever a person has more than the usual number of 206 bones, these additional bones are called **supernumerary** bones. The following are examples of supernumerary bones:
  - Additional sesamoid bones (other than the two patellae), are considered to be supernumerary bones. In addition to the patellae, sesamoid bones are also usually present at the thumb and big toe.

BOX 3-5

Many individuals have additional sesamoids beyond the patellae and the sesamoids of the thumb and big toe; these additional sesamoids are usually located at other fingers.

  - **Wormian bones**, which are small bones that are sometimes found in the suture joints between cranial bones of the skull.
  - Note: Occasionally, individuals have additional anomalous bones such as a 6th lumbar vertebra or *cervical ribs*.

☐ 3.2 PARTS OF A LONG BONE

As Section 3.1 demonstrates, no one *typical* bone exists in the human skeleton; great differences in size and shape exist among bones. Even though differences exist among the various bones, it is valuable to examine the parts of a long bone (Figure 3-2) to gain a better understanding of the typical structure of bones in general.

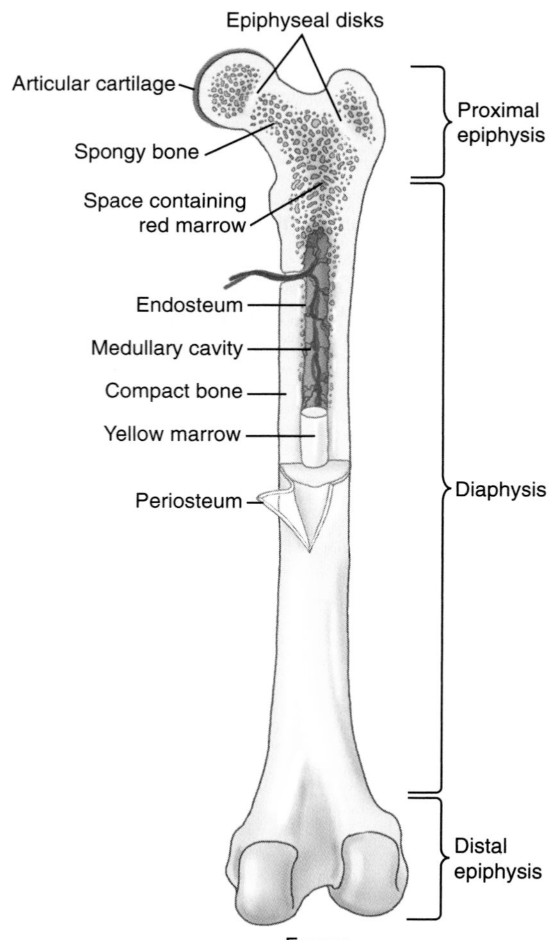

Figure 3-2 This is a view of a long bone (i.e., the femur) with the proximal portion opened up to expose the interior of the bone. The major structural components of a long bone are the diaphysis (i.e., the shaft) and the expanded ends (i.e., the epiphyses). Periosteum lines the entire outer surface of the bone, except the articular surfaces (i.e., joint surfaces), which are covered with articular cartilage. The inside of the diaphysis is primarily composed of compact bony tissue and also houses the medullary cavity, in which bone marrow is found. The epiphyses are primarily composed of spongy bone tissue.

Parts of a Long Bone:

Diaphysis:

- ❑ The **diaphysis** is the shaft of a long bone; its shape is that of a hollow cylindric tube.
- ❑ The purpose of the diaphysis is to be a rigid tube that can withstand strong forces without bending or breaking; it must accomplish this without excessive weight.
- ❑ The diaphysis is composed of compact bone tissue with a thin layer of spongy bone tissue lining its inside surface. For more information on compact and spongy bone tissue, see Section 3.5.
- ❑ Located within the diaphysis at its center is the medullary cavity, which contains bone marrow.

Epiphysis:

- ❑ An **epiphysis** (plural: epiphyses) is the expanded end of a long bone found at each end of the diaphysis. Hence, each long bone has two epiphyses.
- ❑ The purpose of an epiphysis is to articulate (form a joint) with another bone.
- ❑ By expanding, the epiphysis widens out, allowing for a larger joint surface, thus increasing the stability of the joint.
- ❑ The epiphysis is composed of spongy bone with a thin layer of compact bone tissue around the periphery.
- ❑ The spaces of spongy bone within the epiphysis contain red marrow.
- ❑ The articular surface of the epiphysis is covered with articular cartilage.

Articular Cartilage:

- ❑ **Articular cartilage** covers the **articular surfaces** (i.e., joint surfaces) of a bone.
- ❑ Being a softer tissue than bone, the purpose of articular cartilage is to provide cushioning and shock absorption for the joint.
- ❑ Articular cartilage is composed of hyaline cartilage. For more details on hyaline cartilage, see Section 3.10.
- ❑ It is worth noting that articular cartilage has a very poor blood supply; therefore it does not heal well after it has been damaged.

BOX 3-6

The process of degenerative joint disease (DJD) (or osteoarthritis **[OA]**) involves degeneration of the articular cartilage at a joint.

Periosteum:

- **Periosteum** surrounds the entire bone, except for the articular surfaces, which are covered with articular cartilage.
- Periosteum is a thin dense fibrous membrane.
- Periosteum has many purposes:
  - To provide a site of attachment for ligaments and the tendons of muscles

BOX 3-7

Fibers of ligaments and tendons literally interlace into the periosteal fibers of bone, thereby firmly anchoring the ligaments and tendons to the bone.

  - To house cells that are important in forming and repairing bone tissue
  - To house the blood vessels that provide vascular supply to the bone
- The periosteum of bone is highly innervated with nerve fibers and very pain sensitive when bruised.

BOX 3-8

The fact that periosteum is pain sensitive is clear to anyone who has ever banged the *shin* against a coffee table. The shin is the anterior shaft of the tibia where very little soft tissue exists between the skin and the bone to cushion the blow to the periosteum. Any trauma that causes inflammation of the periosteum is technically called **periostitis** but is often known in lay terms as a *bone bruise*.

Medullary Cavity:

- The **medullary cavity** is a tubelike cavity located within the diaphysis of a long bone.
- The medullary cavity houses a soft tissue known as **bone marrow** (red marrow and/or yellow bone marrow). For more details on bone marrow, see Section 3.3.

Endosteum:

- The **endosteum** is a thin membrane that lines the inner surface of the bone within the medullary cavity.
- The endosteum (like the periosteum) contains cells that are important in forming and repairing bone.

Other Components of a Bone:

- All bones are highly metabolic organs that require a rich blood supply. Therefore they are well supplied with arteries and veins.
- Bones are also well innervated with sensory and motor autonomic neurons (i.e., nerve cells). The periosteum of bones is particularly well innervated with sensory neurons.

☐ 3.3 FUNCTIONS OF BONES

- ❑ Bones serve many functions in our body; the five major functions of bones are listed following. Of these five major functions, the first two, structural support of the body and providing levers for body movements, are the two most important functions of bones for bodyworkers, trainers, and students of kinesiology.
  - ❑ Structural support of the body
  - ❑ Provide levers for body movements
  - ❑ Protection of underlying structures
  - ❑ Blood cell formation
  - ❑ Storage reservoir for calcium

Structural Support of the Body:

- ❑ The bones create a skeletal structure that provides a rigid framework for the body.
- ❑ By providing this framework, many tissues of the body literally attach to bones of the skeleton.
  - ❑ For example, the brain is attached by soft tissue (i.e., meninges) to the cranial bones, and the internal visceral organs of the abdominopelvic cavity are literally suspended from the spine by soft tissue ligaments (Figure 3-3).

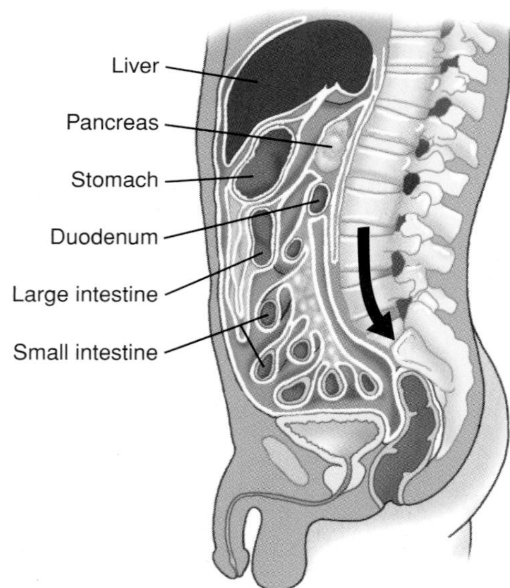

Figure 3-3 Bones create a skeletal structure that provides a rigid framework for the body. This rigid framework supports the internal organs as can be seen in this illustration in which the internal organs of the abdominopelvic cavity literally hang from, and are thereby supported by, the spine. Further, this rigid structure provides a weight-bearing structure through which the weight of the body parts that are located superiorly passes. The arrow drawn over the lower aspect of the spinal column represents the force of the weight of the body traveling through the spine.

- ❑ Further, the skeleton bears the weight of the tissues of the body and transfers this weight through the lower extremities to the ground.
- ❑ The study of posture is largely concerned with understanding the manner in which bones create an effective and healthy skeletal support structure for the tissues of the body. The topic of posture is covered in more detail in Chapter 17.

Provide Levers for Body Movements:

- ❑ The bones of the body are somewhat rigid elements that define the parts of the body.
- ❑ For example, the arm is defined by the presence of the humerus; the forearm is defined by the presence of the radius and ulna.
- ❑ By providing a rigid element within the body part, the bone of a body part provides a site to which muscles can attach. The force of a muscle contraction can then create movement of the bone and consequently movement of the body part within which the bone is located.
- ❑ In this manner, a bone is a **lever** for movement of a body part (Figure 3-4). (Note: Levers are covered in more detail in Sections 15.6 to 15.8.)

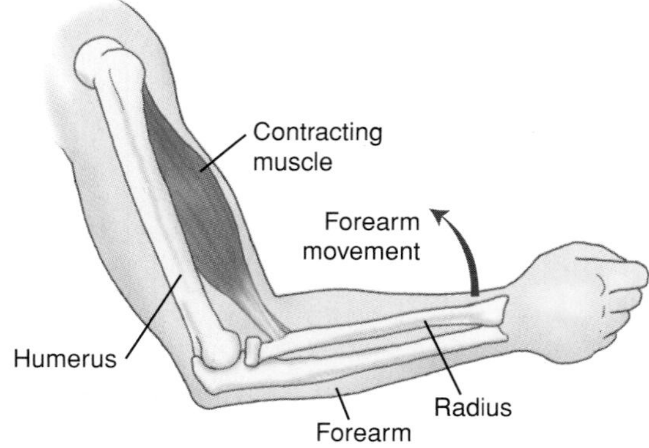

Figure 3-4 A bone provides a rigid lever by which a muscle can move a body part. The muscle pictured here attaches from the humerus of the arm to the radius of the forearm. This muscle is contracting, exerting an upward pull on the radius, causing the radius to move toward the humerus. Because the radius is rigid, when it moves the entire forearm moves. In this manner the radius acts as a rigid lever, and forces that act on it (in this case, the muscle pictured) move the body part that it is within. (Note: The muscle here does not represent an actual muscle in the human body. It is only drawn to illustrate the concept of how levers work.)

BOX 3-9

This function of bones providing levers for muscles to move parts of the body is key to the study of kinesiology. **Kinesiology** literally means the study of movement. Because movement occurs by the forces of muscle contractions acting on bony levers, kinesiology is the study of the function of the musculoskeletal system. (For more information on levers, see Sections 15.6 to 15.8.)

Protection of Underlying Structures:

- Physical damage to our body from traumas such as falls, motor vehicle accidents, and sports injuries is always a danger. Some tissues and organs of our body are particularly sensitive to trauma, critical to life, and need to be protected. Because bone tissue is rigid, it is ideal for providing protection to these underlying structures. For example:
  - The brain is safely encased within the cranial cavity, fully surrounded by the bones of the cranium (Figure 3-5a).
  - The spinal cord is located within the spinal canal, surrounded by the bony vertebrae.
  - The heart and lungs are located within the thoracic cavity, protected by the sternum and ribcage.

Blood Cell Formation:

- Bones house **red bone marrow** (also known as *red marrow*), the soft connective tissue that makes blood cells (Figure 3-5b).
- This process of blood cell production is called **hematopoiesis**.
- It is important to point out that red marrow produces all types of blood cells: red blood cells, white blood cells, and platelets.
- Red marrow is located within the medullary cavity of long bones and the spaces of spongy bones.
- As a child, red marrow is found in most every bone of the body. However, as a person ages, the red bone marrow is gradually replaced with **yellow bone marrow** (also known as *yellow marrow*); yellow marrow is essentially fat cells and therefore is not active in hematopoiesis.
- In an adult, red marrow is found primarily in the spongy bones of the axial skeleton (skull, sternum, ribs, clavicles, vertebrae, and pelvis) and in the medullary cavities of the humerus and femur.

Storage Reservoir for Calcium:

- Calcium is a mineral that is critical to the functioning of the human body.
  - Calcium is necessary for conduction of impulses in the nervous system, the contraction of muscles, and the clotting of blood.
- Because calcium is necessary for life, it is vital for the body to maintain proper levels of calcium in the bloodstream.
- When dietary intake of calcium is insufficient to meet the needs of the body, calcium can be taken from the bones to increase the blood level of calcium; when dietary intake of calcium exceeds the need by the body, calcium in the bloodstream can be deposited back into the bones.

BOX 3-10

The hormone **parathyroid hormone** (from the parathyroid glands) is responsible for withdrawing calcium from the bones; the hormone **calcitonin** (from the thyroid gland) is responsible for depositing calcium back into the bones.

- In this manner the bones act as a *reservoir* or *bank* from which calcium can be withdrawn and deposited, thereby maintaining proper blood levels of calcium for the body to function (see Figure 3-5c).

BOX 3-11

The type of bone cell that causes the release of calcium from the bones into the bloodstream is an osteoclast; the type of bone cell that causes the deposition of calcium from the bloodstream back into bones is an osteoblast. (For more information on bone cells, see Section 3.4.)

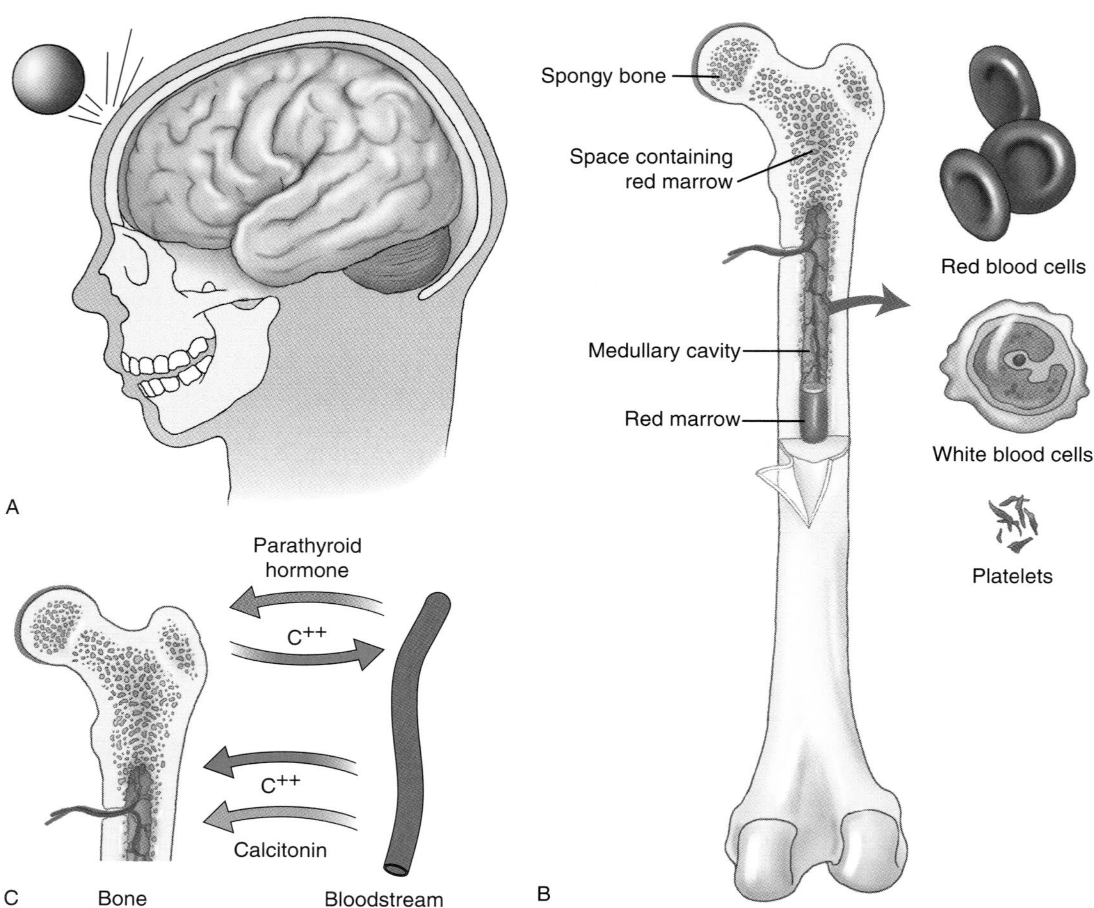

Figure 3-5 Three additional functions of bones. *A,* Bones protect underlying structures of the body. A hard object is seen hitting the head. The brain, located within the cranial cavity, is largely protected from the force of this blow by the bones of the skull. *B,* Hematopoiesis (i.e., the formation of blood cells). The red bone marrow seen in the medullary cavity of this long bone functions to create red blood cells, white blood cells, and platelets. *C,* Bones act as a reservoir or bank for blood levels of calcium. When the blood level of calcium is low, the body secretes parathyroid hormone, which causes the release of calcium from the bones into the bloodstream. When the blood level of calcium is high, the body secretes the hormone calcitonin, which causes excess calcium from the bloodstream to be deposited back into the bones.

☐ 3.4 BONE AS A CONNECTIVE TISSUE

❑ Bone is a type of **connective tissue**. As such, it is composed of bone cells and **matrix**.

> **BOX 3-12**
>
> Four major tissues exist in the human body: (1) nervous tissue (carries electrical impulses), (2) muscular tissue (contracts), (3) epithelial tissue (lines body surfaces open to a space or cavity), and (4) connective tissue (the most diverse of the four groups, generally considered to *connect* aspects of the body).
>
> The matrix of a connective tissue is defined as everything other than the cells and is often divided into the fiber component and the ground substance component. With regard to bone tissue, the fibers are collagen fibers and make up a portion of the organic matrix of bone; the remainder of the matrix (both organic and inorganic) would be the **ground substance**.

❑ The matrix of bone is often divided into its organic gel-like component and its inorganic rigid component.

Bone Cells:

❑ Three types of bone cells exist:
- ❑ **Osteoblasts**: Osteoblasts build up bone tissue by secreting matrix tissue of the bone.
- ❑ **Osteocytes**: Once osteoblasts are fully surrounded by the matrix of bone and lie within small chambers within the bony matrix, they are called *osteocytes*.
- ❑ These small chambers are called *lacunae* (singular: lacuna). (For more information on lacunae, see Section 3.5.)
- ❑ **Osteoclasts**: Osteoclasts break down bone tissue by breaking down the matrix tissue of the bone.

❑ It is important to realize that bone is a dynamic living tissue that has a balance of osteoblastic and osteoclastic activity occurring. This is true when a bone is growing, when it is repairing after an injury, and when calcium is being withdrawn and deposited into bone to maintain proper blood levels of calcium (which occurs throughout our entire life).

Organic Matrix:

❑ The gel-like organic matrix of bone adds to the resiliency of bone.

> **BOX 3-13**
>
> Certainly bones are more rigid than soft tissues of the body, but the organic gel-like component of bone matrix that is present in living bone gives it much more resiliency than the dried up fossilized bones that we see in a museum and often think of when we think of bones.

❑ The organic component of matrix is composed of collagen fibers and the gel-like osteoid tissue.

❑ This gel-like **osteoid tissue** contains large molecules called **proteoglycans**. Their major purpose is to trap fluid so that bone tissue does not become too dry and brittle.

> **BOX 3-14**
>
> Proteoglycans are protein/polysaccharide molecules that are composed primarily of glucosamine and chondroitin sulfate molecules. (For more information on proteoglycans, see Section 3.10.)
>
> The composition of a living healthy bone is approximately 25% water.

❑ Within this gel-like proteoglycan mix, collagen fibers are created and deposited by fibroblastic cells.

❑ **Collagen fibers** primarily add to a bone's tensile strength (its ability to withstand pulling forces).

> **BOX 3-15**
>
> Vitamin C is necessary for the production of collagen, and if its intake in the diet is insufficient, a condition called *scurvy* occurs. Hundreds of years ago, sailors at sea would often come down with this disease because of the lack of fresh foods containing vitamin C on long sea journeys. The British were the first to realize that if they took a certain fresh food on board their ships, their sailors would not get scurvy. The fresh food that they carried with them was limes. For this reason, people from Britain have long been known as *Limeys*.

Inorganic Matrix:

❑ The inorganic component of matrix is composed of the mineral content of bone (i.e., the calcium-phosphate salts of bone).

❑ These calcium-phosphate salts are also known as **hydroxyapatite crystals**.

❑ The calcium-phosphate salts give bone its rigidity.

☐ 3.5 COMPACT AND SPONGY BONE

The manner in which the components of bone tissue (cells and matrix) are organized can vary. Two different arrangements of bone tissue exist (Figure 3-6):

- ❑ **Compact bone** has a compact ordered arrangement of bone tissue.
- ❑ **Spongy bone** has an arrangement of bone tissue that is less compact, containing irregular spaces, that gives this tissue the appearance of a sponge.
  - ❑ Spongy bone is also known as **cancellous bone.**

Compact Bone:

- ❑ As stated, compact bone has a very ordered, tightly packed arrangement of the bony tissue (Figure 3-7).

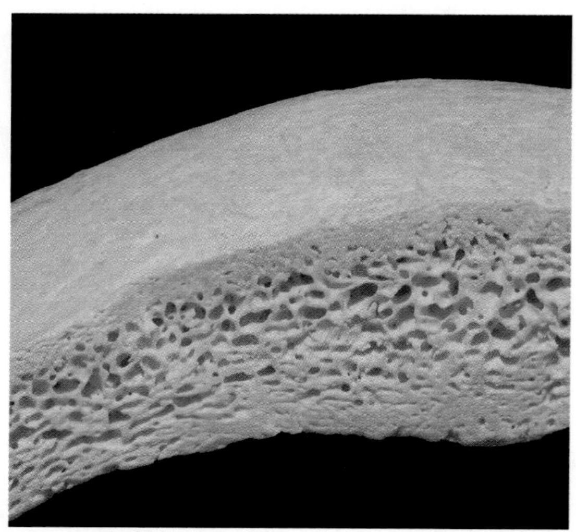

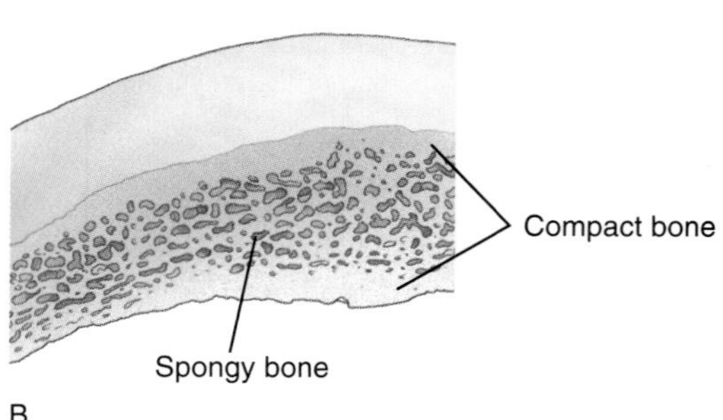

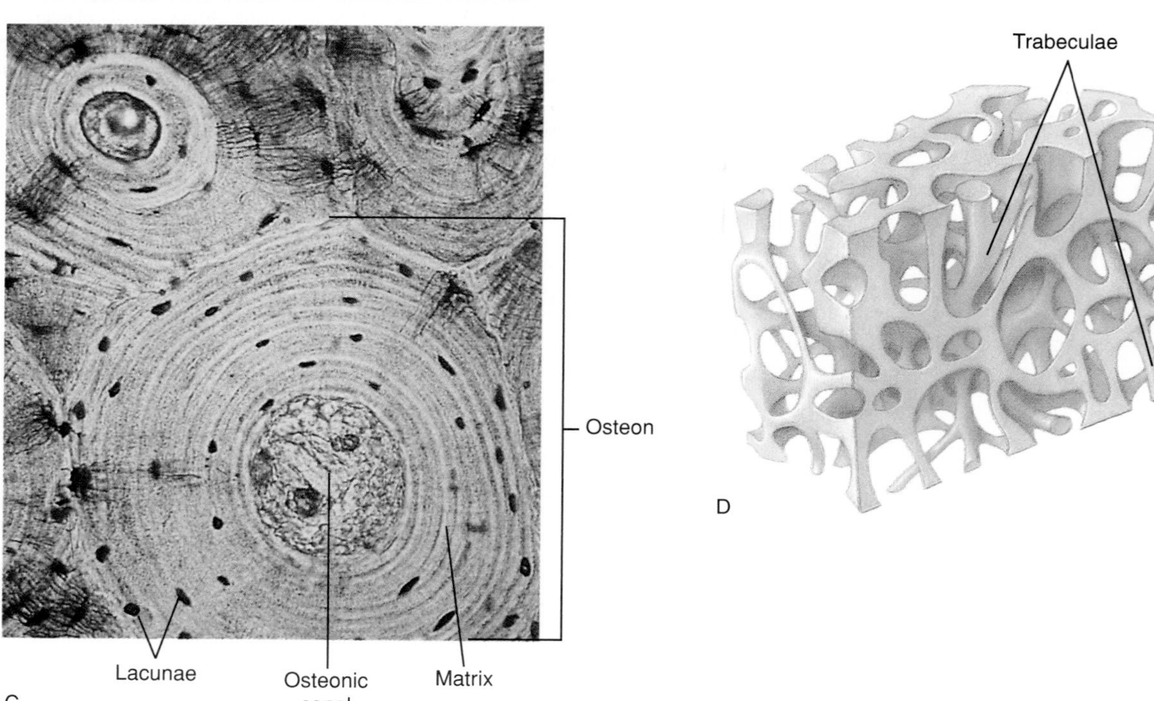

Figure 3-6 The two types of bone tissue: compact and spongy. *A* and *B,* Photograph and drawing of a cross-section of a cranial bone showing the spongy bone tissue in the middle and the compact bone tissue on both sides of the spongy bone. *C,* An enlargement that shows the osteons of compact bone. *D,* An enlargement that shows the trabeculae of spongy bone. (*C* and *D* from Thibodeau GA, Patton KT: *Anatomy and physiology,* ed 5, St Louis, 2003, Mosby.)

- Compact bone is primarily found in the shafts of long bones, where it provides rigidity to the shaft. Compact bone also lines the outer surface of the epiphyses of long bones and the outer surface of all other bones (i.e., short, flat, and irregular bones).

BOX 3-16

The outer surface of a bone is known as its **cortex** or **cortical surface**. When a physician looks at a **radiograph** (i.e., x-ray) of a bone, he or she examines the cortical surface for any break in the margin that would indicate a fracture (i.e., broken bone).

- Compact bone is composed of structural units that are cylindric in shape called **osteons**.
- Each osteon is composed of a central **osteonic canal** in which a blood vessel is located.

BOX 3-17

Osteonic canals are also known as **Haversian canals**. **Volkmann's canals** (also known as *perforating canals*) connect the blood vessel from one osteonic canal to the blood vessel of an adjacent osteonic canal (see Figure 3-8b).

- Bloods vessels provide the nourishment necessary for all living cells, including bone cells (i.e., osteocytes). Therefore osteocytes arrange themselves around the osteonic canal in concentric circles. This arrangement of osteocytes around the osteonic canal is what creates the cylindric shape of an osteon.
- Compact bone is composed of multiple small osteons. This allows for all osteocytes to be close to their blood supply to get their nourishment via diffusion from the blood vessels located within the osteonic canals.

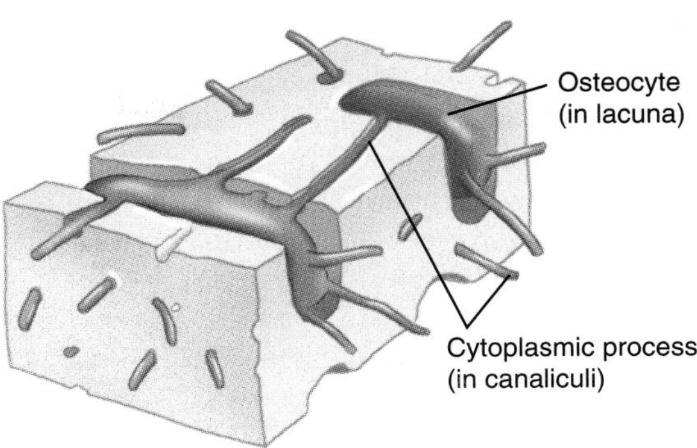

Figure 3-7 Illustration of the concept of osteocytes being located within lacunae and the cytoplasmic processes of the osteocytes communicating with other osteocytes via the canaliculi.

- Each osteocyte is located within a small chamber, surrounded by the matrix of bone. This small chamber is called a **lacuna** (plural: lacunae) (see Figure 3-7).
- Very small canals connect one lacuna to another lacuna. These small canals are called **canaliculi** (singular: canaliculus). Osteocytes send small **cytoplasmic processes** through these canaliculi to communicate with adjacent osteocytes in other lacunae. As a result of these processes, bone cells can communicate very well with each other and bone tissue is very responsive to changes in its environment.

Spongy Bone:

- As stated, spongy bone has many irregular spaces that give it the appearance of a sponge (see Figure 3-6). These spaces allow for a lighter weight while still providing adequate rigidity to the bone.
- Spongy bone is primarily found in the epiphyses of long bones and the center of all other bones (i.e., short, flat, and irregular bones).
  - A small amount of spongy bone is also found within the shafts of long bones (see Figure 3-8b).
- Because spongy bone has many spaces within it that allow for diffusion of nutrients from the blood supply, no need exists for osteonic canals and the ordered arrangement of osteocytes in lacunae around the blood vessel in the osteonic canal. Therefore no need exists for the ordered arrangement of osteons.
- Spongy bone consists of a latticework of bars and plates of bony tissue called **trabeculae** (singular: trabecula). Between these plates are the spaces of spongy bone (see Figure 3-6d).
- When we say that these spaces are irregular, it may give the impression that spongy bone is very haphazard in its arrangement, which is not true. There is a pattern to spongy bone. The trabeculae of spongy bone are arranged in a fashion that allows them to best deal with the compressive forces of weight bearing.

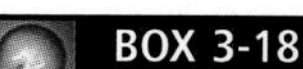

BOX 3-18

The pattern of trabeculae of spongy bone is usually apparent on a radiograph (i.e., x-ray).

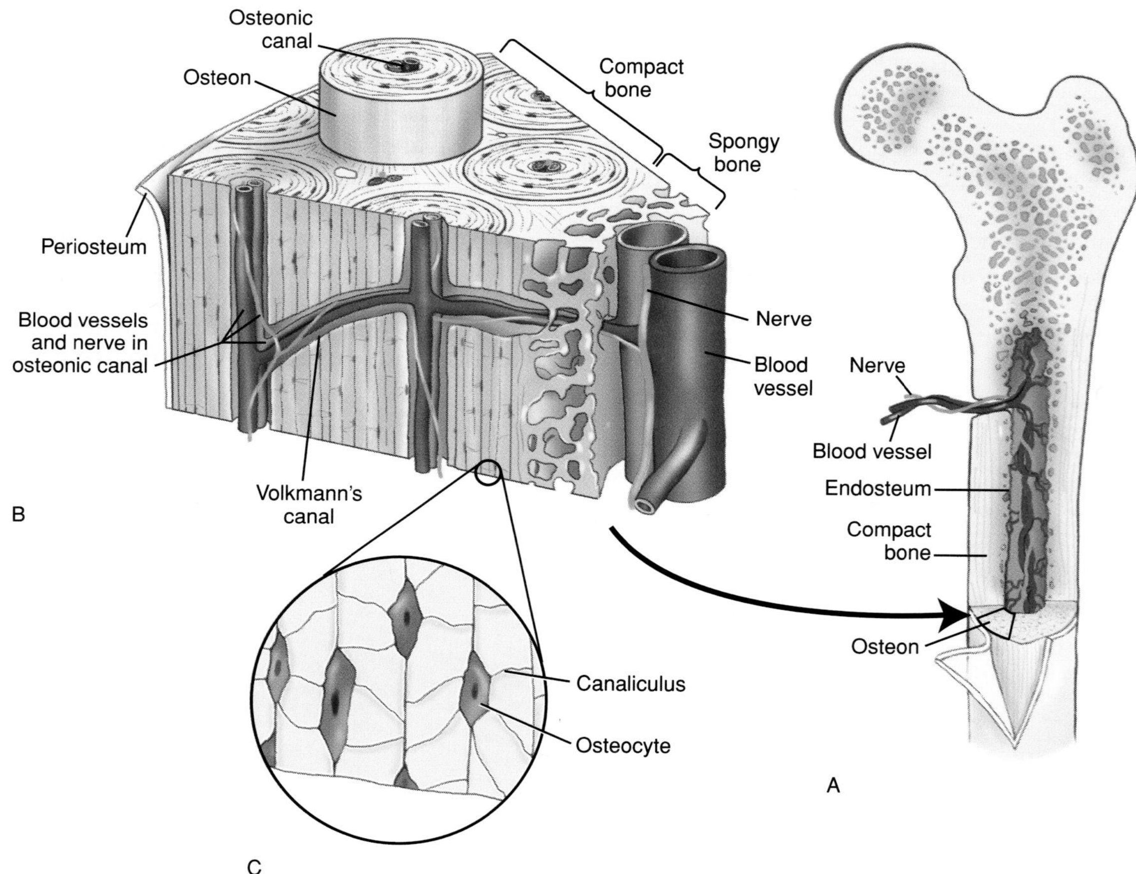

Figure 3-8 *A,* Section of a long bone illustrating the interior of the bone. *B,* Enlargement of a pie-shaped wedge of the shaft of the long bone displaying the osteons of the compact bone, as well as the spongy bone located in the interior of the shaft. *C,* Further enlargement of the compact bony tissue showing the osteocytes (located within the lacunae) that communicate with each other via the canaliculi that connect the lacunae to each other.

☐ 3.6 BONE DEVELOPMENT AND GROWTH

- ❏ When the skeleton begins to form in utero, it is not calcified. Rather, it is composed of cartilage and fibrous structures shaped like the bones of the skeleton. These cartilage and fibrous structures gradually calcify as the child grows (both in utero and after birth) and act as models for development of the mature skeleton.
- ❏ The skeleton forms by two major methods: (1) **endochondral ossification** and (2) **intramembranous ossification**.

Endochondral Ossification:

- ❏ Endochondral ossification, as its name implies, is ossification that occurs within a cartilage model (*chondral* means cartilage).
- ❏ Most bones of the human body develop by endochondral ossification. The steps of endochondral ossification for a long bone are outlined following (Figure 3-9):
  - ❏ The cartilage model of a bone exists.
  - ❏ The cartilage model develops its periosteal lining that surrounds the diaphysis.
  - ❏ The cartilage in the diaphysis gradually breaks down and is replaced with bone tissue by osteoblasts from the periosteum. A region of developing bone tissue is called an **ossification center**. This first region of developing bone in the diaphysis is called the **primary ossification center**.
- ❏ The primary ossification center gradually grows toward the epiphyses, replacing cartilage with bone.
- ❏ **Secondary ossification centers** appear in the epiphyses of the long bone and grow toward the primary ossification center, replacing cartilage with bone.
- ❏ The region between the primary and secondary ossification centers still contain cartilage cells that are producing cartilage tissue, continuing to increase the length of the cartilage model of bone. This region of cartilage growth is called the **epiphysial disc**. Because the epiphysial disc is the region where the model for the future mature bone grows, it is known in lay terms as the **growth plate**.
- ❏ Meanwhile, in the center of the diaphysis, osteoclasts are breaking down the bone tissue, creating the medullary cavity.
- ❏ As the epiphysial disc continues to lengthen the bone by laying down cartilage, the ossification centers keep growing by replacing the cartilage of the epiphysial disc with bone tissue.
- ❏ The pace of the growth of the ossification centers is slightly faster than the growth of new cartilage within the epiphysial disc. When the ossification

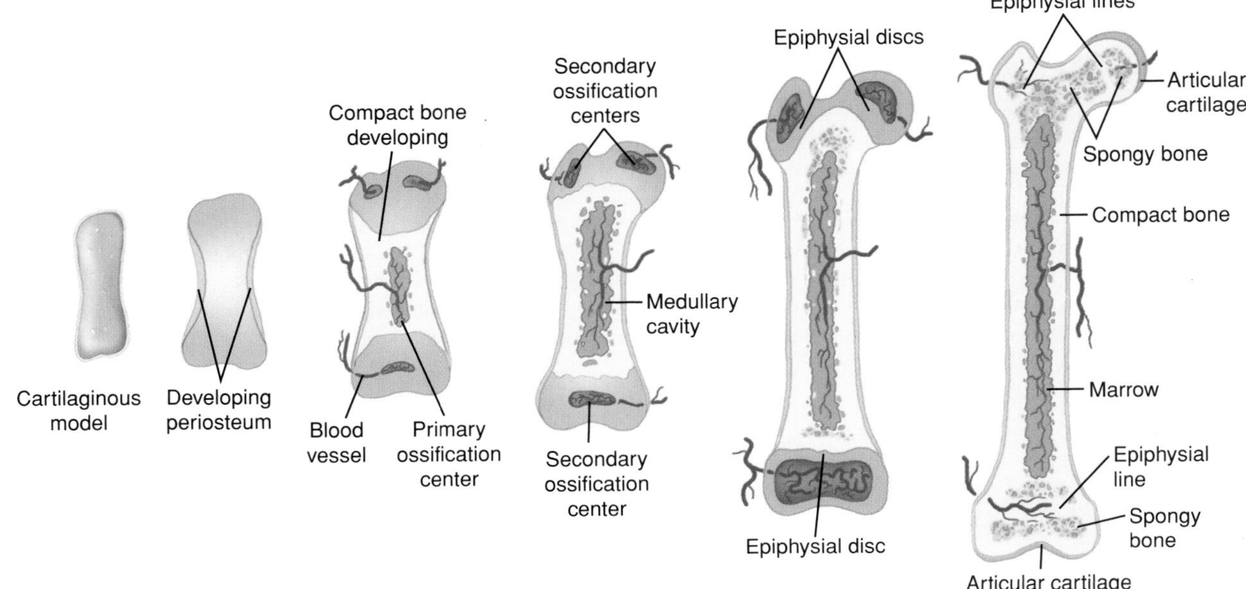

Figure 3-9 The steps of endochondral ossification. Beginning with a cartilaginous model, periosteum forms around the bone; then primary and secondary ossification centers develop in the diaphysis and epiphyses, respectively, and epiphysial discs are located between them. These ossification centers grow toward each other while the epiphysial discs continue to elongate the cartilage model by producing cartilage tissue. When the ossification centers meet, bone growth stops.

centers finally meet, having replaced all the cartilage tissue of the epiphysial disc, bone growth stops (at least in the sense of lengthening) and the bone is mature. This occurs at approximately age 18, when a person is said to stop growing.

BOX 3-19

Although the length of a long bone stops growing at approximately age 18, long bones can continue to thicken into the future by deposition of bone tissue by osteoblasts of the periosteum (and breakdown of bone tissue by osteoclasts of the endosteum).

- A remnant of the epiphysial disc is visible on a radiograph (i.e., x-ray) and is called the **epiphysial line**.

BOX 3-20

By looking at a radiograph (i.e., x-ray), a physician can determine if a person is done growing or if much potential for growth remains, based on how large the epiphysial disc is (i.e., how close the ossification centers are to meeting each other, stopping bone growth).

Intramembranous Ossification:

- Intramembranous ossification, as its name implies, is ossification that occurs within a **membrane** (i.e., a thin sheet or layer of soft tissue); this membrane is composed of fibrous tissue.
- Flat bones of the skull develop by intramembranous ossification. The steps of intramembranous ossification for a flat bone are outlined following:
    - The fibrous membrane model of a bone exists.
    - Regions of osteoblasts develop within the fibrous membrane and begin to lay down bony matrix around themselves, creating spongy bone. These regions of osteoblasts are known as *ossification centers*.
    - A periosteum arises around the membrane and begins to lay down compact bone on both sides of the developing spongy bone within the membrane.
    - The bone is ossified when the entire fibrous membrane has been replaced with bony tissue.
    - Continued growth of flat bones can and does continue into the future by osteoblasts of the periosteum and results in thickening of the flat bones as a person ages. This can usually be seen in the faces of elderly people (Figure 3-10).

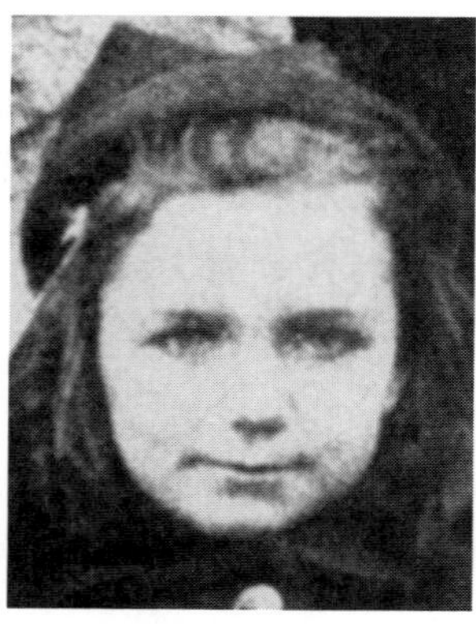
A

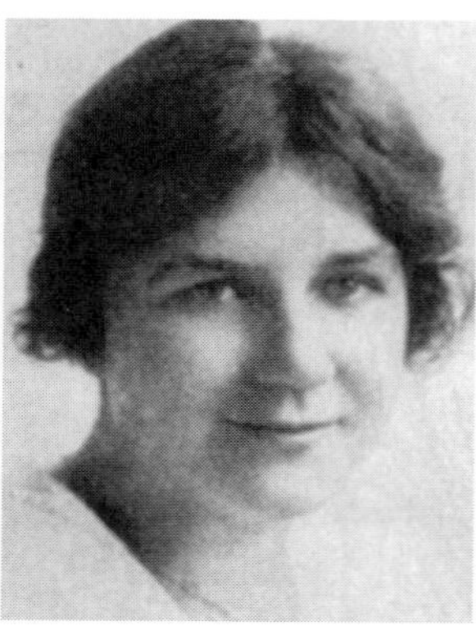
B

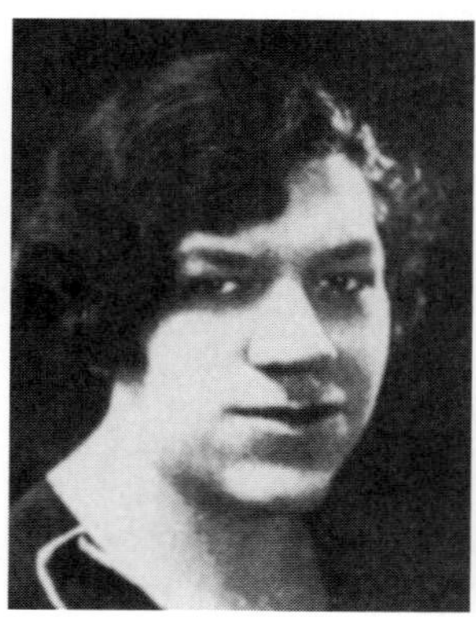
C

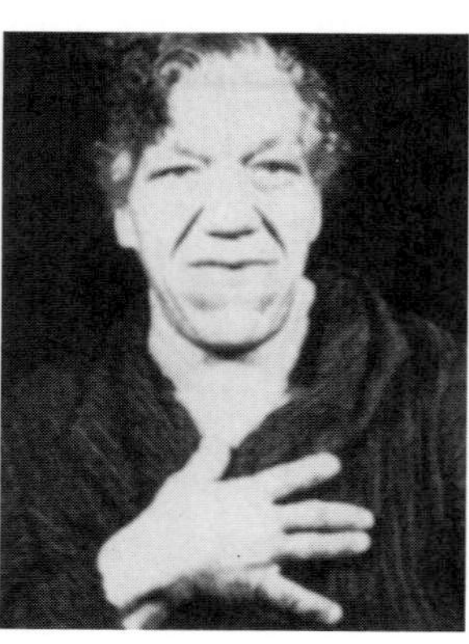
D

Figure 3-10 Four photographs of a woman who suffered from an endocrine disorder called *acromegaly* (an oversecretion of growth hormone in adulthood). In these four photographs from ages 9 years *(A)*, 16 years *(B)*, 33 years *(C)*, and 52 years *(D)*, the changes in facial features because of the continued intramembranous growth of her facial bones are shown. Although this example is extreme as a result of the condition, it illustrates the concept of continued intramembranous growth in adulthood that everyone experiences (to a much smaller degree). (From Hole JW, Jr.: *Hole's human anatomy and physiology*, ed 4. Dubuque, Iowa, 1987, William C. Brown Publishers.)

3.7 FONTANELS

- A **fontanel** is a soft spot on an infant's skull.

> **BOX 3-21**
> The presence of soft spots (i.e., fontanels) means that a therapist doing bodywork must exercise caution when working on the head during infant and child massage.

- These fontanels are soft because they are areas of the primitive fibrous membrane of the skull.
- These regions of fibrous membrane still exist in an infant because the process of intramembranous ossification is not yet complete (see Section 3.6, page 53).

> **BOX 3-22**
> These fontanels prove to be helpful because they allow some movement of the bones of the infant's head (allowing the head to compress to some degree), which allows it to more easily fit through the birth canal during labor. This is helpful to the mother and the child.

- Six major fontanels are found in a child's skull; all of these exist where the parietal bones meet other bones of the skull (Figure 3-11).
  - **Anterior fontanel**: The anterior fontanel is located at the juncture of the two parietal bones and the frontal bone.
    - The anterior fontanel closes at approximately 1 to 2 years of age.
    - The anterior fontanel is also known as the **frontal fontanel**.
  - **Posterior fontanel**: The posterior fontanel is located at the juncture of the two parietal bones with the occipital bone.
    - The posterior fontanel closes at approximately 6 months of age.
    - The posterior fontanel is also known as the **occipital fontanel**.
  - **Anterolateral fontanels** (paired left and right): The anterolateral fontanels are located at the juncture of the parietal, frontal, temporal, and sphenoid bones.
    - The anterolateral fontanels close at approximately 6 months of age.
    - The anterolateral fontanels are also known as the **sphenoid fontanels**.
  - **Posterolateral fontanels** (paired left and right): The posterolateral fontanels are located at the juncture of the parietal, occipital, and temporal bones.
    - The posterolateral fontanels close at approximately 1 year of age.
    - The posterolateral fontanels are also known as the **mastoid fontanels**.

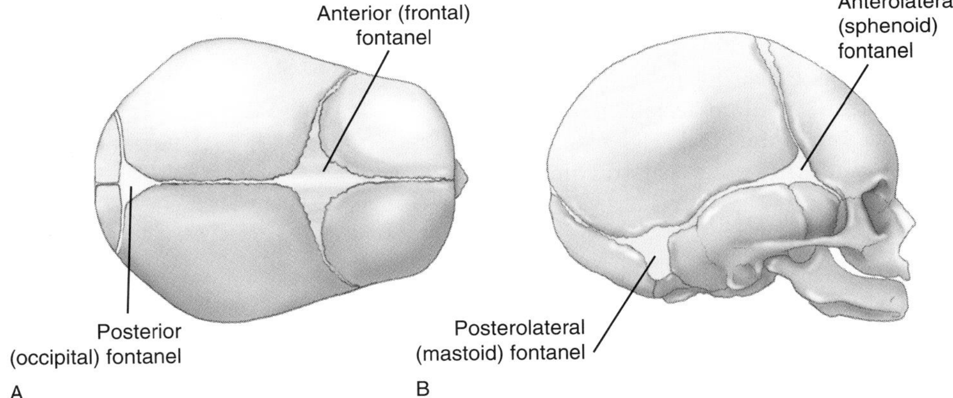

Figure 3-11 *A,* Superior view of an infant's skull; the anterior fontanel is seen between the parietal and frontal bones, and the posterior fontanel is seen between the parietal and occipital bones. *B,* Lateral view of an infant's skull; the anterolateral fontanel is seen between the parietal, frontal, temporal, and sphenoid bones, and the posterolateral fontanel is seen between the parietal, occipital, and temporal bones. (Note: See Section 4.1, Figures 4-3 to 4-7 for views of the skull with labels.)

☐ 3.8 FRACTURE HEALING

- ❑ A fractured bone is a broken bone; a broken bone is a fractured bone; these two terms are synonyms.
- ❑ A *fracture* (i.e., broken bone) is defined as a break in the continuity of a bone.
- ❑ Fractures are usually diagnosed by radiographic examination.
- ❑ When looking at a radiograph (i.e., x-ray) of a bone, the physician pays special attention to the cortical (outer) margin of the bone. If any discontinuity is seen in the cortical margin of a bone, it is diagnosed as fractured.
- ❑ Assuming that the two ends of a fractured bone are well aligned, fracture healing is accomplished by the following steps (Figure 3-12):
    - ❑ When a bone is fractured, blood vessels will also be broken. This causes bleeding in the region and results in a blood clot, which is called a **hematoma**.
    - ❑ Dead fragments of bone are resorbed by the action of osteoclasts.
    - ❑ As the hematoma itself is gradually resorbed, fibrocartilage is deposited in the fracture site. This fibrocartilaginous tissue temporarily holds the two broken ends together and is called a **callus**.
    - ❑ This fibrocartilaginous callus then calcifies, resulting in the formation of a **bony callus**.
    - ❑ Because the bony callus usually results in more bone tissue than was previously present, osteoclasts remodel the bone by resorbing the excessive tissue of the bony callus.
    - ❑ The remodeling process is usually not 100% perfect, and a slight bony callus is usually present for the remainder of the person's lifetime, usually palpable as a bump at the location of the break. However, the fracture is healed and the bone is structurally healthy.

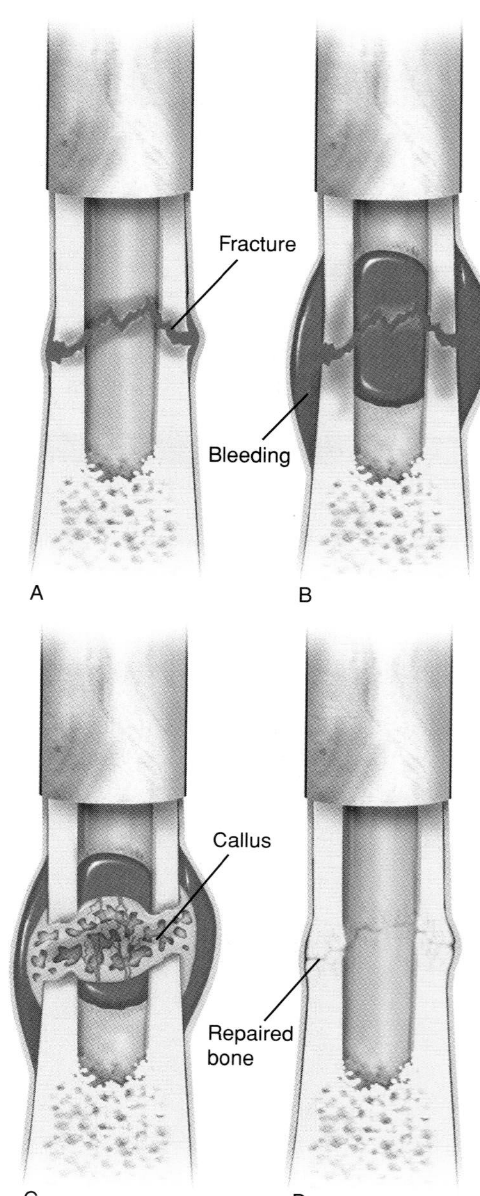

Figure 3-12 The steps that take place during repair of a fractured (i.e., broken) bone. *A,* Fracture of the femur. *B,* Hematoma has formed. *C,* Callus has formed; this callus is initially composed of fibrocartilaginous tissue and then later calcifies to create a bony callus. *D,* Bone repair is complete. A remnant of the bony callus is still evident and would likely be palpable as a bump at the site of the fracture. (From Thibodeau GA, Patton KT: *Anatomy and physiology,* ed 5. St Louis, 2003, Mosby.)

3.9 EFFECTS OF PHYSICAL STRESS ON BONE

- Bone is a dynamic living tissue that responds to the physical demands placed on it. Bone tissue follows **Wolff's law**, which states, "Calcium is laid down in response to stress." Thus according to Wolff's law:
  - If increased physical stress is placed on a bone, then the bone responds by gaining bony matrix and thickening.
  - If decreased physical stress is placed on a bone, then the bone responds by losing bony matrix and thinning.
- The beauty of this principle is that bone can adapt to the demands that are placed on it.
  - If a bone has a great deal of stress placed on it, it will become thicker and stronger so that it will be able to deal with this stress and stay healthy.
    - Imagine the demands placed on the feet of a marathon runner and the need to respond to those demands by thickening the bones of the lower extremities.
  - On the other hand, if a bone has little stress placed on it, the bone does not need to maintain a large amount of matrix and it can afford to lose the unneeded bone mass ("use it or lose it").

BOX 3-23

All living tissue must be maintained with a nutrient supply provided by the cardiovascular system. This places a greater demand and stress on the heart. Further, greater mass of tissue requires greater force by the muscles to be able to move our body through space; this places a greater demand and stress on our muscular system, requiring larger and stronger muscles, which in turn requires more nutrition to be supplied by the cardiovascular system, and so forth. Therefore if any tissue of the body is unneeded, it is in the body's best interest to shed it, hence the wisdom of "use it or lose it."

  - Imagine a sedentary office worker who sits at a desk for the entire workday and never exercises; how necessary it is for the lower extremity bones of this sedentary individual to be as developed and massive as the bones of the marathon runner?

BOX 3-24

When astronauts are seen in their weightless environment in space, they are seen exercising. This is necessary to keep their bones well mineralized, because being in a weightless environment for as little as a few days to a few weeks can cause significant loss of bone mass.

Wolff's Law and the Piezoelectric Effect:

- Wolff's law is explained by the piezoelectric effect.
- When pressure is placed on a tissue, a slight electric charge results in that tissue; this is known as the **piezoelectric effect**. (Note: *Piezo* means *pressure*.)
- The importance of the piezoelectric effect is that while osteoblasts can lay down bone in any tissue that it pleases, osteoclasts are unable to resorb (break down) bone in piezoelectrically charged tissue.
- The result is that a greater bone mass results in the regions of bone that are under greater pressure (i.e., greater patterns of physical stress).
- Therefore Wolff's law, via the piezoelectric effect, explains how and why the trabeculae of spongy bone are laid down along the lines of stress (Figure 3-13). Further, these principles also explain how it is that bones can literally remodel and change their shape in response to the forces placed on them.
- Wolff's law via the piezoelectric effect also explains why it is so important to begin movement as soon as it is safely possible after injury or surgery. Even more universally, Wolff's law explains why movement and exercise is so vital to a healthy skeleton—let alone the rest of our body!

Wolff's Law "Gone Bad":

- Unfortunately, too much of a good thing can occur. When excessive stress is placed on a bone (which often occurs at the joint surfaces of a bone), excessive calcium may be deposited in that bone. As the bone tissue becomes denser and denser, the body starts to place calcium along the outer margins of the bone.
- This can result in what is known as a **bone spur** and the condition that results is called **degenerative joint disease** (**DJD**) or **osteoarthritis** (**OA**) (see Figure 3-14).

BOX 3-25

Degenerative joint disease (DJD) (or osteoarthritis [OA]) is characterized by the breakdown of articular cartilage and the presence of bone spurs on the **subchondral bone** (the bone located immediately under the articular cartilage).

- Although DJD is a condition of the bones and joints, its cause is excessive physical stress on bones and joints.

BOX 3-26 SPOTLIGHT ON DEGENERATIVE JOINT DISEASE

When muscles are chronically tight, they continually pull on their bony attachments. This constant pull creates a stress on the bones and joints, which can contribute to the progression of the arthritic changes of degenerative joint disease (DJD). Further, the pain of tight muscles is very often (but not always) a major part of what is blamed as the pain of DJD. Therefore evaluating the client's lifestyle, the tightness of the musculature, and the stresses placed on the bones by tight muscles is essential for all bodyworkers and trainers.

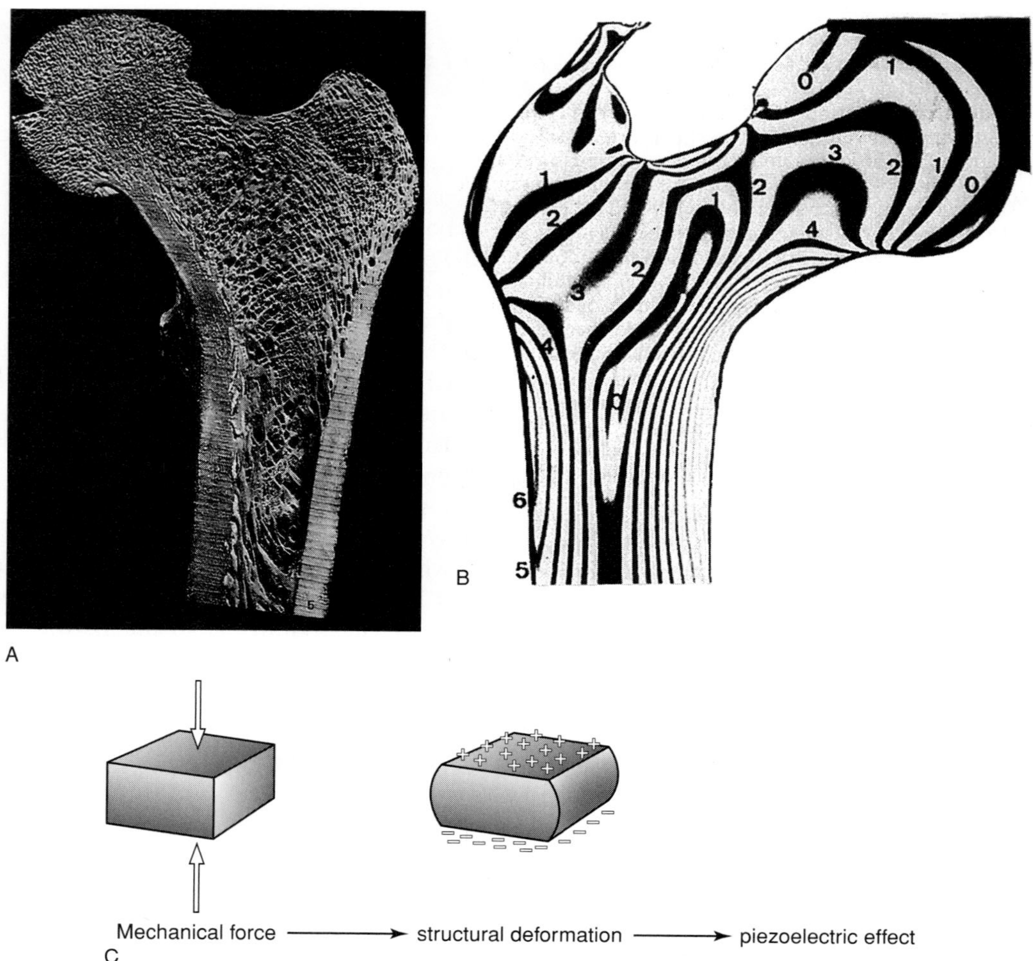

Figure 3-13 *A,* Section of the proximal femur showing the trabecular pattern of the spongy bone. *B,* Lines of stress through the proximal femur appear when the stress of weight bearing is placed on it. The trabeculae of spongy bone will align themselves along these lines of stress as a result of the piezoelectric effect. *C,* Piezoelectric effect (i.e., an electrical charge occurs in a tissue when it is subjected to a mechanical force [a stress] such as weight bearing). (*A* and *B* from Williams PL, ed.: *Gray's anatomy: the anatomical basis of clinical practice,* ed 38. Edinburgh, 1995, Churchill Livingstone. *C* from Oschman JL: *Energy medicine: the scientific basis.* Edinburgh, 2000, Churchill Livingstone.)

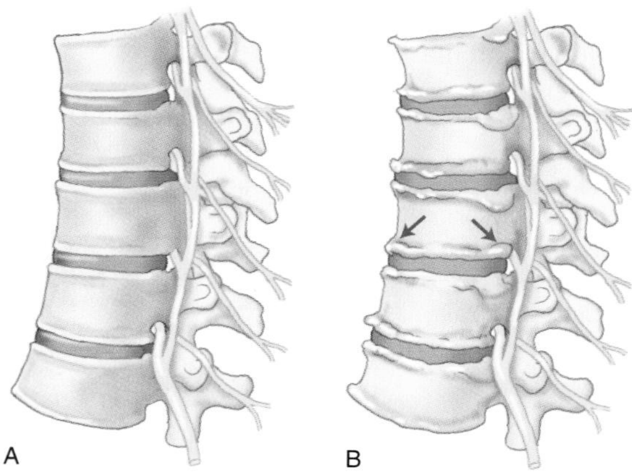

Figure 3-14 *A,* Lateral view of the vertebral column. The contours of the bodies of the vertebrae are smooth, clean, and healthy. *B,* Same view of the vertebral column is shown, this time with the presence of bone spurs (two of the bone spurs are indicated by arrows) at the margins of the vertebrae. The presence of bone spurs is indicative of degenerative joint disease (DJD) (or osteoarthritis [OA]).

☐ 3.10 CARTILAGE TISSUE

- **Cartilage** is a type of tissue that is particularly important to the musculoskeletal system. Some of the roles of cartilage within the musculoskeletal system include the following:
  - Cartilage unites the bones of *cartilaginous joints*.
  - Cartilage caps the joint (articular) surfaces of bones of synovial joints.
  - Intra-articular discs that are located within many synovial joints are composed of cartilage. (For more information on cartilaginous joints, synovial joints, and intra-articular discs, see Sections 6.8, 6.9, and 6.14.)
  - Cartilage provides the framework for developing bones during the process of endochondral ossification (see Section 3.6).
  - Although classified as a *soft tissue*, cartilage is fairly dense and firm; it has attributes of being both partly rigid and partly flexible.
  - Cartilage has a very poor blood supply and therefore has a very poor ability to heal after injury.
  - Most of the blood supply to cartilage comes via diffusion from blood vessels that are located in the **perichondrium**, a fibrous connective tissue that covers cartilage.

BOX 3-27

Articular cartilage has no perichondrium, so its nutrient supply must come from diffusion from the synovial fluid of the joint. For this reason, articular cartilage is particularly bad at healing after an injury or damage.

- Cartilage tissue, like bone tissue, is a type of connective tissue. As such, it is composed of cartilage cells and matrix.
  - The matrix of cartilage is a firm gel with fibers embedded within it.
- Three types of cartilage exist: (1) **hyaline cartilage**, (2) **fibrocartilage**, and (3) **elastic cartilage**.

Cartilage Cells:

- Two types of cartilage cells exist:
  - **Chondroblasts**: Chondroblasts build up cartilage tissue by secreting the matrix tissue of the cartilage.
  - **Chondrocytes**: Once chondroblasts are mature and fully surrounded by the matrix of cartilage, they are called *chondrocytes*.
    - As in bone tissue, the cells of cartilage are said to be located within lacunae.

Matrix:

- By definition, the components of the matrix of a connective tissue can be divided into fibers and ground substance.

Matrix Fibers:

- The fibers of cartilage are collagen and/or elastin fibers.
  - Collagen fibers add to the tensile strength of cartilage.
  - **Elastin fibers** add to the elastic nature of elastic cartilage.

Matrix Ground Substance:

- The ground substance of cartilage in which the fibers are embedded is a firm gel-like organic matrix that is composed of proteoglycan molecules.
- Proteoglycans are protein/polysaccharide substances that are composed primarily of **glucosamine** and **chondroitin sulfate** molecules.
- Proteoglycan molecules have feathery shapes that resemble a bottlebrush in appearance.
- Proteoglycan molecules trap and hold water in the spaces that are located within and between them.

BOX 3-28

Glucosamine and chondroitin sulfate are the building blocks of proteoglycans, which are found in the matrix of most all connective tissues, including cartilage. Taking these substances as nutritional supplements has recently become very popular. Because proteoglycans keep the connective tissue matrix of articular cartilage well hydrated (and therefore thicker and softer), joints are better able to absorb shock without degeneration and damage.

Types of Cartilage:

- Each one of the three types of cartilage has a slightly different structural makeup and therefore is best suited for a specific role in the body (Figure 3-15).

Hyaline Cartilage:

- Hyaline cartilage is the most common type of cartilage and resembles *milky glass* in appearance.
- Hyaline cartilage is often called *articular cartilage* because it is the type of cartilage that usually caps the articular surfaces of the bones of synovial joints.
  - Its role in capping the articular surfaces of bones is to absorb compressive shock that occurs to the joint.

BOX 3-29

In addition to forming the articular cartilage of the joint surfaces of bones, hyaline cartilage is also found in the epiphysial plate of growing bones, forms the soft part of the nose, and is located within the rings of the respiratory passage.

Fibrocartilage:

- ❑ Fibrocartilage, as its name implies, contains a greater density of fibrous collagen fibers and a lesser amount of the chondroitin sulfate ground substance.
- ❑ Therefore fibrocartilage is the toughest form of cartilaginous tissue and is ideally suited for roles that require a great deal of tensile strength (ability to withstand being pulled and stretched).
  - ❑ Fibrocartilage is the type of cartilage that forms the union of most cartilaginous joints.
    - ❑ Examples of cartilaginous joints include the disc joints of the spine and the symphysis pubis joint of the pelvis.
- ❑ Fibrocartilage is also the type of cartilage of which intra-articular discs are made.
  - ❑ Intra-articular discs are found in the sternoclavicular, wrist, and knee joints.

Elastic Cartilage:

- ❑ In addition to collagen fibers, elastic cartilage also contains elastin fibers.
- ❑ Therefore elastic cartilage is best suited for structures that require the firmness of cartilage but also require a great degree of elasticity.
  - ❑ Elastic cartilage gives form to the external ear.
    - ❑ In addition to giving form to the ear, elastic cartilage also gives form to the epiglottis (that covers the trachea when swallowing food) and the eustachian tube (that connects the throat to the middle ear cavity).

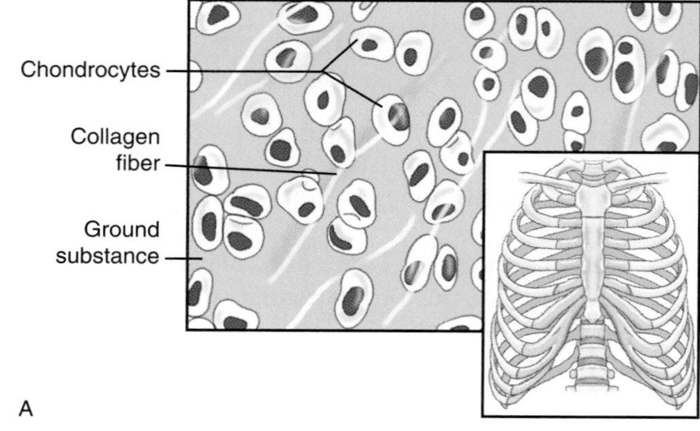

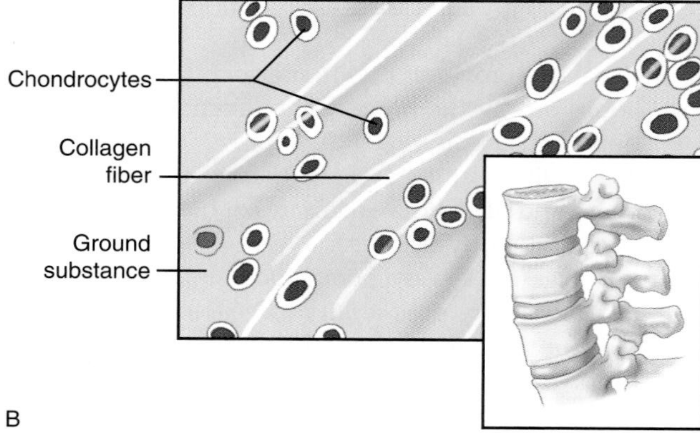

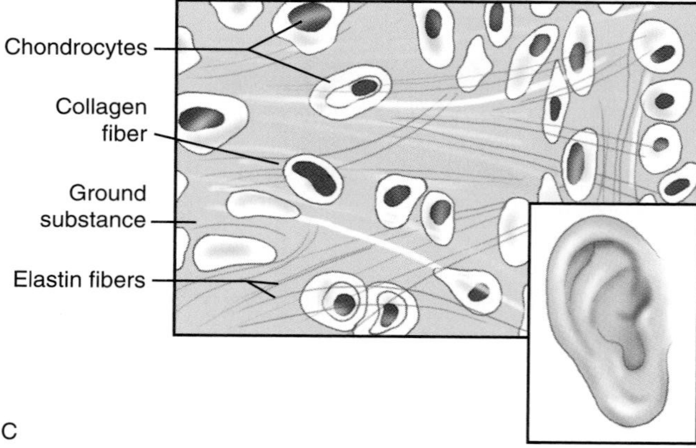

Figure 3-15 *A, Milky-glass* tissue composition of hyaline cartilage, the most common cartilage tissue in the body; inset shows the cartilages of the ribs (examples of hyaline cartilage). *B,* Tissue composition of fibrocartilage, containing a greater density of collagen fibers; inset shows intervertebral discs (examples of fibrocartilage). *C,* Tissue composition of elastic cartilage containing the presence of elastin fibers in addition to collagen fibers; inset shows the ear (cartilage in the ear is an example of elastic cartilage).

3.11 TENDONS AND LIGAMENTS

- A **tendon** connects a muscle to a bone.
- A **ligament** connects a bone to a bone.

BOX 3-30

By definition, a tendon's shape is round and cordlike. If the shape of a tendon is broad and flat, it is termed an **aponeurosis** (plural: aponeuroses). Tendons and aponeuroses are identical in their tissue makeup; they merely differ in shape.

Within the context of the musculoskeletal system, a ligament is defined as connecting a bone to a bone. However, the actual definition of a ligament is broader in that a ligament can attach any two structures (except a muscle and bone) to each other.

- A tendon functions to transmit the pulling force of a muscle to its bony attachment, creating movement.
- A ligament functions to create stability at a joint by holding the bones of the joint together. (For a fuller discussion of the mobility and stability of a joint, see Section 6.3.)
- Both tendons and ligaments are types of dense fibrous connective tissue (Figure 3-16).

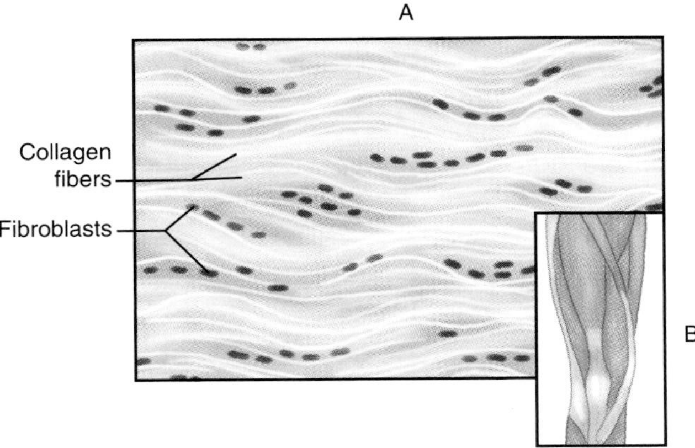

Figure 3-16 Tissue composition of tendons and ligaments (examples of which are shown in the inset). Tendons and ligaments are dense fibrous connective tissue, made up almost entirely of collagen fibers with occasional scattered fibroblast cells.

- Dense fibrous connective tissue is composed of many collagen fibers packed tightly together.
- Very few cells are present; the cells that are present are primarily **fibroblasts**. Fibroblasts create the fibrin threads of collagen.

BOX 3-31 SPOTLIGHT ON BODYWORK AND SCAR TISSUE ADHESIONS

Scar tissue adhesions are made up of fibrin threads of collagen that are created by fibroblasts. Scar tissue adhesions help heal wounded tissues by binding them together. However, they may also be oversecreted by the body, resulting in the loss of normal and healthy mobility of the tissues. Much of the value of bodywork, movement, and exercise is to break up patterns of excessive scar tissue adhesions.

- Some elastin fibers are present in tendons and ligaments.
- Being made up nearly entirely of collagen fibers gives tendons and ligaments extremely strong tensile force (the ability to withstand strong pulling forces without damage or injury).
- This strong tensile force is needed in two situations:
  - It is needed by a tendon when the muscle to which it is attached contracts and pulls on it.
  - It is needed by tendons and ligaments when they are stretched and pulled, because the joint that they cross is moved in the opposite direction as a result of contraction and shortening of the muscles on the opposite side of the joint (resulting in movement of the bones of the joint in the opposite direction).
- Having collagen fibers tightly packed together leaves little space for blood vessels; therefore tendons and ligaments have a poor blood supply and do not heal well after an injury.

BOX 3-32

Except in a few circumstances, it is usually better to break a bone than it is to tear (sprain) a ligament (or rupture a tendon), because bones have a greater blood supply and therefore heal better after an injury. Although bones usually return to 100% function after an injury, ligament tears rarely ever heal fully and some instability of the joint remains into the future. Ironically, after an injury people will often be heard to say something like, "Thank goodness I didn't break the bone. It's just a sprain."

- Because tearing a tendon causes inflammation, it is called **tendinitis**.
- By definition, tearing a ligament is called a **sprain**.

BOX 3-33

Tendinitis can also be spelled *tendonitis.*

Tearing the fibrous capsule of a (synovial) joint is also termed a *sprain,* because the fibrous capsule is ligamentous tissue. In contrast, tearing of a muscle is called a **strain**.

3.12 BURSAE AND TENDON SHEATHS

- Bursae (singular: bursa) and tendon sheaths are located in regions of the body where friction that occurs because of the rubbing of two structures against each other needs to be minimized.
- This is necessary because friction causes the build-up of heat, and excessive heat can cause damage to the tissues.

BOX 3-34

If the ability of a bursa to minimize friction is overcome and the bursa itself becomes inflamed, it is called **bursitis**.

- A **bursa** is a flattened sac of synovial membrane that contains a film of synovial fluid within it. (For more information of synovial membranes and synovial fluid, see Section 6.9.)
- Bursae are often found located between a tendon and an adjacent joint structure, usually a bone.
- Bursae are found in many joints of the body including the shoulder joint and the ankle joint (Figure 3-17a–c).

BOX 3-35

A bursa is usually an independent structure. However, it may be continuous with the synovial membrane of a synovial joint One example is the suprapatellar bursa of the knee joint (see Section 6.9, Figure 6-11c.)

- A **tendon sheath** can be thought of as a sheathlike bursa that envelops a tendon.
  - Just as a sword fits into its sheath, a tendon may be enclosed in a tendon sheath.
- Bursae and tendon sheaths are similar in tissue structure; they differ in shape.
- Because tendon sheaths are constructed of synovial membrane tissue, they are also known as **synovial tendon sheaths**.

BOX 3-36

If the ability of a tendon sheath to minimize friction is overcome and the tendon sheath itself becomes inflamed, it is called **tenosynovitis**. A common form of this condition occurs at the tendon sheath that envelops the abductor pollicis longus and extensor pollicis brevis tendons. With excessive movement of the thumb, these tendons rub against the styloid process at the radius, resulting in a form of tenosynovitis known as *deQuervain's tenosynovitis* (or *deQuervain's disease*).

  - Tendon sheaths are commonly found in the hands and feet, where tendons rub against an adjacent structure such as a bone or a retinaculum (Figure 3-17c–d).
- A **retinaculum** (plural: retinacula) is a thin sheet of fibrous connective tissue that holds down and stabilizes (i.e., retains) a structure. Retinacula are commonly found retaining the tendons of muscles that cross into the hands or the feet. To minimize friction between the tendons and these retinacula, tendon sheaths are located in these regions (see Figure 3-17c). (For more information on retinacula, see Section 8.17.)

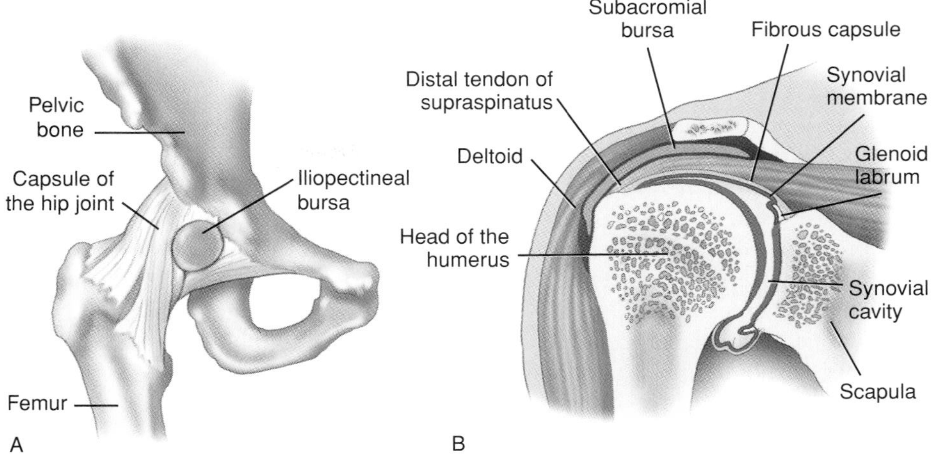

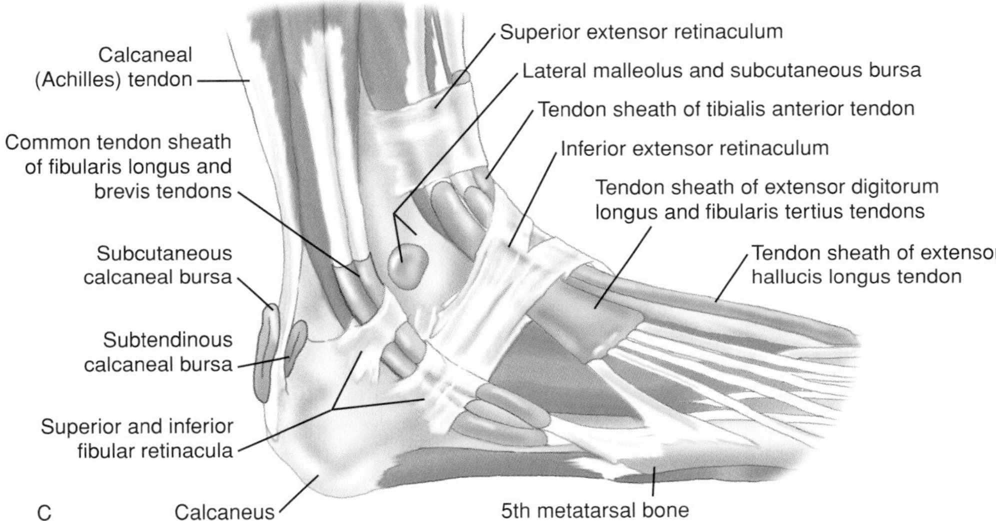

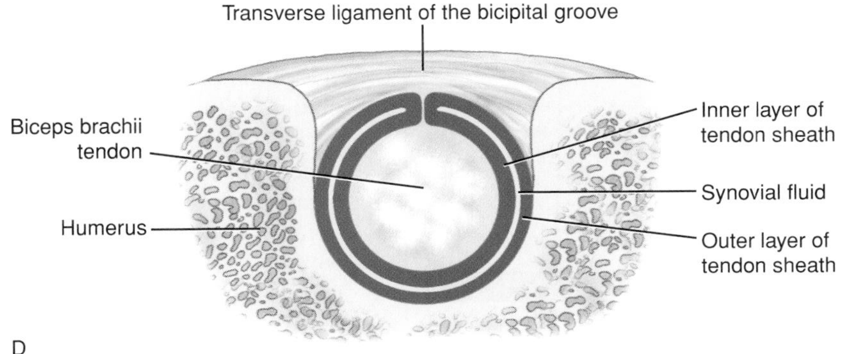

Figure 3-17 *A,* Anterior view with a bursa shown overlying the hip joint. This bursa helps to reduce friction between the capsule of the hip joint and the overlying iliopsoas and pectineus muscles. *B,* Anterior view of a cross-section of a shoulder joint. The subacromial bursa is located between the supraspinatus portion of the rotator cuff tendon inferiorly and the acromion process of the scapula and the deltoid muscle superiorly. The subacromial bursa functions to minimize friction between these structures, thereby maintaining the health of the rotator cuff tendon. *C,* Lateral view of the ankle joint region. A number of bursae and tendon sheaths are seen. Specifically the tendon sheaths function to minimize friction between the tendons that enter the foot and their adjacent structures, including the underlying bones and the overlying retinacula. *D,* Cross-section through the humerus (i.e., bone of the arm) showing a tendon sheath encasing the biceps brachii muscle's tendon as it runs within the bicipital groove of the humerus.

☐ 3.13 PROPERTIES OF SKELETAL TISSUES

To fully understand the nature of skeletal connective tissue and to be able to better deliver therapeutic bodywork and guide clients in exercise, it is helpful to understand the properties that these tissues possess. Following are terms that describe properties of skeletal connective tissues. The degree to which each individual tissue possesses each of the following properties varies.

- ❑ **Stretch**: The ability of a tissue to stretch is simply its ability to become longer without injury or damage. Certainly all *soft* connective tissues of the body need to be able to lengthen and stretch with various body movements. Because tight/taut tissues are generally unable to stretch without damage, a major focus of bodywork and stretching exercises is to gradually stretch and loosen these tight/taut tissues.
- ❑ **Contractility**: The ability to contract is the ability to shorten. This property is unique to muscular tissue; musculoskeletal connective tissues do not possess this ability.

BOX 3-37

The use of the terms *contraction* and *contractility* is problematic when speaking about muscle function, because although the ability to contract is the ability to shorten, not all muscle *contractions* actually result in shortening. (For further study, this topic of muscular contraction is discussed in more detail in Chapter 12.)

- ❑ **Weight bearing**: Weight bearing is the ability of a tissue of the body to bear the compressive force of the weight of the mass of the body that is located above it, without injury or damage. Generally the joints of the lower extremity and the axial body are weight-bearing joints. Because of the great stress of bearing weight, weight-bearing joints generally need to have greater stability so that they are not damaged and injured.
- ❑ **Tensile strength**: The tensile strength of a connective tissue is its ability to withstand a pulling force without injury or damage. Collagen fibers add tensile strength to connective tissues.

BOX 3-38

The ability to stretch and tensile ability are very similar. The difference is that the *stretchability* of a tissue is defined by how long it can become. The *tensile strength* of a tissue is defined by how much pulling force the tissue can withstand without tearing.

- ❑ **Elasticity**: Elasticity of a connective tissue is its ability to return to its normal length after being stretched. For example, after being stretched, a rubber band is elastic because it returns to its original length; similarly, most healthy connective tissues of the body also possess a good degree of elasticity. The presence of elastin fibers adds elasticity to a connective tissue.
  - ❑ **Viscoelasticity**: The term *viscoelasticity* is a synonym for elasticity.
- ❑ **Plasticity**: *Plasticity* is a term that describes the ability of a tissue to have its shape molded or altered, and the tissue then retains that new shape. For example, after stretching bubble gum (that has already been chewed), it is plastic because it does not return to its original shape; rather, it maintains its new shape. Plastic is named for its property of plasticity.
  - ❑ **Viscoplasticity**: The term *viscoplasticity* is a synonym for plasticity.
- ❑ **Elasticity and plasticity compared**: Understanding the concepts of elasticity and plasticity is important when working with soft tissues of the body. Whenever a soft tissue of the body has been altered or deformed in some manner because a force has been applied to it (whether it has been compressed or pulled on) the tissue has a certain elastic ability to return to its original shape; if that elasticity is exceeded, then plasticity describes the fact that the shape of the tissue will stay permanently altered or deformed to some degree. An example is a ligament that is stretched. If it is only slightly stretched, its elastic ability allows it to return to its original length. However, if it is stretched to a greater degree and its elastic ability is exceeded, the tissue will enter its *plastic range* and will become permanently overstretched and lax. This can result in a permanent decrease in stability of the joint where this ligament is located.
- ❑ **Creep**: The term *creep* describes the gradual change in shape of a tissue when it is subjected to a force that is applied to the tissue in a slow and sustained manner. The *creep* of the tissue may be temporary or permanent. If the creep is temporary, then the tissue is sufficiently elastic to return to its original form. If the creep is permanent, then the elasticity of the tissue has been exceeded and the tissue is said to be plastic. The concept of creep may be negative such as when a client changes the tissue shape and structure over time because of poor posture, or it may be positive such as when bodywork and exercise are done to change and correct a client's poor tissue shape and structure.

BOX 3-39 SPOTLIGHT ON BODYWORK AND CREEP

The fact that creep of a tissue tends to occur more readily when a force is applied slowly is one reason why pressure applied during massage and bodywork should not be sudden and forceful; rather the increasing depth of pressure should be done in a slow and incremental manner. This is not to say that deep pressure cannot be delivered, but rather that one should slowly sink into the muscles and fascia when applying deep pressure.

❑ **Thixotropy**: Thixotropy describes the ability of a soft tissue of the body to change from a more rigid **gel state** to a softer more hydrated (i.e., liquid) **sol state.** This concept is particularly important to bodywork and exercise. The matrix component of most connective tissues has a great thixotropic ability to attain more of a sol state (due to the presence of proteoglycans), which is desirable because it allows for greater freedom of blood and nutrient flow and greater freedom of movement. Bodywork and movement applied to body tissues result in a change from gel to sol state.

BOX 3-40

Thixo comes from the Greek word for touch, and *tropy* comes from the Greek word for change. Therefore *thixotropy* literally means *to change by touch*, illustrating the importance of massage and bodywork to this property of tissue!

The term *thixotropy* can be a daunting term for new students. Perhaps a better term is the one coined by Bob King, a distinguished educator in the field of massage and bodywork. He refers to thixotropy as *rejuicification* of the tissue. ☺

❑ **Hysteresis**: Hysteresis describes the process wherein a tissue exhibits fluid loss and minute structural damage as a result of friction and heat buildup when it is worked excessively. Bodywork and exercise that result in hysteresis of a tissue may be any type of stroke, technique, or movement that repetitively and excessively compress or stretch the client's tissue.

REVIEW QUESTIONS

evolve Answers to the following review questions appear on the Evolve website accompanying this book.

1. What are the four major classifications of bones by shape?

2. Give an example of each one of the four major classifications of bones by shape.

3. Name and describe the major structural components of a long bone.

4. What are the five major functions of bones?

5. Which function of bones is most important to the study of musculoskeletal movement and the field of kinesiology?

6. What are the two major components of bone as a connective tissue?

7. What are the functions of osteoblasts and osteoclasts?

8. Compare and contrast compact and spongy bone.

9. Where is compact bone found?

10. Where is spongy bone found?

11. Compare and contrast the two different methods of bone growth (endochondral and intramembranous ossification).

12. What is the importance of fontanels to bodywork?

13. What are the four major fontanels? Where are they located? When does each one close?

14. What are the steps involved in fracture healing?

15. What is Wolff's law, and how does the piezoelectric effect explain it?

16. How do tight muscles relate to Wolff's law, the development of DJD, and the role of a bodyworker or trainer when working on a client who has DJD?

17. What are the three major types of cartilage tissue?

18. What is the role of proteoglycan molecules in cartilage and other connective tissues?

19. What is the definition of a tendon?

20. What is the definition of a ligament?

21. What is the function of fibroblasts?

22. What is the difference between a sprain and a strain?

23. Compare and contrast a tendon with an aponeurosis.

24. Compare and contrast a bursa with a tendon sheath.

25. How does the concept of thixotropy apply to the fields of bodywork, movement, and/or exercise?

26. How do the properties of stretch, tensile strength, elasticity, and plasticity apply to the delivery of bodywork, and/or the performance of exercise?

27. What is the difference between elasticity and plasticity of a tissue?

28. How does the concept of creep apply to the fields of bodywork, movement, and/or exercise?

29. How does the concept of thixotropy apply to the fields of bodywork, movement, and/or exercise?

30. How does the concept of hysteresis apply to the fields of bodywork, movement, and/or exercise?

NOTES

Chapter 4

Bones of the Human Body

CHAPTER OUTLINE

Axial Skeleton
Section 4.1 Bones of the Head
Section 4.2 Bones of the Spine (and Hyoid)
Section 4.3 Bones of the Ribcage and Sternum

Appendicular Skeleton, Lower Extremity
Section 4.4 Entire Lower Extremity
Section 4.5 Bones of the Pelvis and Hip Joint
Section 4.6 Bones of the Thigh and Knee Joint
Section 4.7 Bones of the Leg and Ankle Joint
Section 4.8 Bones of the Foot

Appendicular Skeleton, Upper Extremity
Section 4.9 Entire Upper Extremity
Section 4.10 Bones of the Shoulder Girdle and Shoulder Joint
Section 4.11 Bones of the Arm and Elbow Joint
Section 4.12 Bones of the Forearm, Wrist Joint, and Hand

CHAPTER OBJECTIVES

After completing this chapter, the student should be able to perform the following:

- ❑ List the major divisions of the skeleton.
- ❑ Name and locate the bones of the axial skeleton.
- ❑ Name and locate the bones of the lower extremity skeleton.
- ❑ Name and locate the bones of the upper extremity skeleton.
- ❑ Name and locate the bony landmarks of the axial skeleton.
- ❑ Name and locate the bony landmarks of the lower extremity skeleton.
- ❑ Name and locate the bony landmarks of the upper extremity skeleton.
- ❑ Name and locate the joints of the axial skeleton.
- ❑ Name and locate the joints of the lower extremity skeleton.
- ❑ Name and locate the joints of the upper extremity skeleton.
- ❑ Define the key terms of this chapter.
- ❑ State the meanings of the word origins of this chapter.

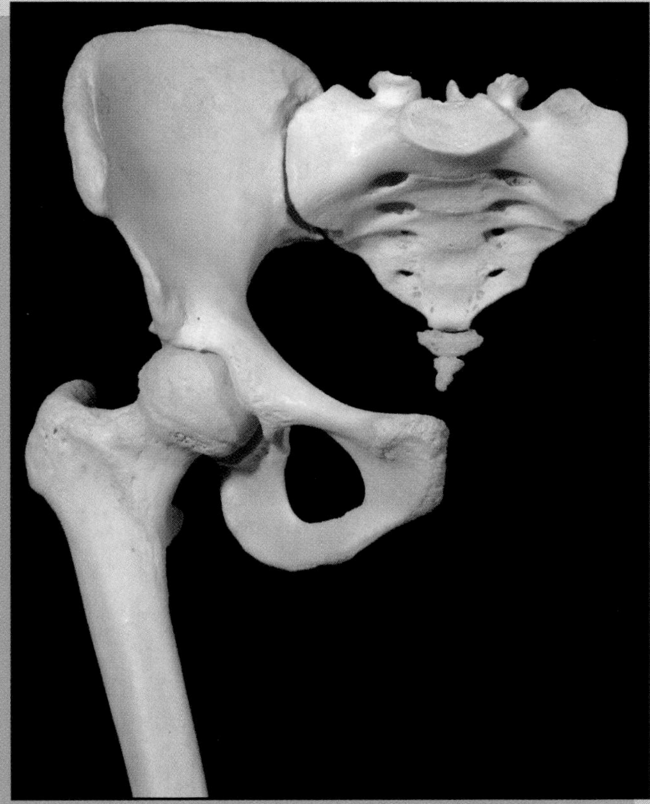

OVERVIEW

The human skeleton is usually said to have 206 bones.

BOX 4-1

The number 206 is variable. Sesamoid bones in addition to the patellae usually exist, and small islets of bone located within the sutures of the skull called **wormian bones** are often present. Further, occasional anomalous bones may exist. Any bone beyond the usual number of 206 may be called a **supernumerary bone**.

This number is based on the axial skeleton having 80 bones and the appendicular skeleton having 126. The axial skeleton makes up the central vertical axis of the body and is composed of the bones of the head, neck, trunk, and the sacrum and coccyx.

BOX 4-2

Another way to look at the axial skeleton is to say that it is composed of the bones of the head, spinal column (the sacrum and coccyx are part of the spinal column), ribcage, and hyoid.

The appendicular skeleton is made up of the appendages that attach onto the axial skeleton (i.e., the upper and lower extremities), including the bones of the shoulder girdle (scapulae and clavicles) and the pelvic girdle (pelvic bones). Figures 4-1 and 4-2 illustrate the axial and appendicular skeletons. Table 4-1 lists the bones of the human body.

Note: Whenever a bone exists on both sides of the body, the right sided bone is shown in this chapter.

TABLE 4-1

Bones of Skeleton (206 Total)

AXIAL SKELETON (80 BONES TOTAL)		APPENDICULAR SKELETON (126 BONES TOTAL)	
Part of Body	**Name of Bone(s)**	**Part of Body**	**Name of Bone(s)**
Skull (28 bones total)		Upper extremities (including shoulder girdle) (64 bones total)	Clavicle (2) Scapula (2) Humerus (2) Radius (2) Ulna (2) Carpals (16) Metacarpals (10) Phalanges (28)
Cranium (8 bones)	Frontal (1) Parietal (2) Temporal (2) Occipital (1) Sphenoid (1) Ethmoid (1)		
Face (14 bones)	Nasal (2) Maxillary (2) Zygomatic (2) Mandible (1) Lacrimal (2) Palatine (2) Inferior nasal conchae (2) Vomer (1)	Lower extremities (including pelvic girdle) (62 bones total)	Pelvic (2) Femur (2) Patella (2) Tibia (2) Fibula (2) Tarsals (14) Metatarsals (10) Phalanges (28)
Ear bones (6 bones)	Malleus (2) Incus (2) Stapes (2)		
Hyoid bone (1)			
Spinal column (26 bones total)	Cervical vertebrae (7) Thoracic vertebrae (12) Lumbar vertebrae (5) Sacrum (1) Coccyx (1)		
Sternum and ribs (25 bones total)	Sternum (1) True ribs (14) False ribs (10)		

From Thibodeau GA, Patton KT: *Anatomy and physiology*, ed 5, St Louis, 2003, Mosby.

KEY TERMS

Accessory (ak-SES-or-ee)
Acetabulum (AS-i-TAB-you-lum)
Acromion (a-KROM-ee-on)
Ala, pl. alae (A-la, A-lee)
Alveolar (al-VEE-o-lar)
Apex, pl. apices (A-peks, A-pi-sees)
Arch (ARCH)
Arcuate (ARE-cue-at)
Articular (are-TIK-you-lar)
Atlanto/atlas (at-LAN-to/AT-las)
Auditory (AW-di-tore-ee)
Auricular (or-IK-you-lar)
Axis (AKS-is)
Base/basilar (BASE/BAZE-i-lar)
Bicipital (bye-SIP-i-tal)
Bifid (BYE-fid)
Calcaneus, pl. calcanei (kal-KAY-nee-us, kal-KAY-nee-eye)
Canine (KAY-nine)
Capitate, capitulum (KAP-i-tate, ka-PICH-you-lum)
Carotid (ka-ROT-id)
Carpal (CAR-pull)
Cervical (SERV-i-kul)
Clavicle (KLAV-i-kul)
Coccyx, pl. coccyges (KOK-siks, KOK-si-jeez)
Concha, pl. conchae (KON-ka, KON-kee)
Condyle (KON-dial)
Conoid (CONE-oid)
Coracoid (CORE-a-koyd)
Cornu, pl. cornua (KORN-oo, KORN-oo-a)
Coronoid (CORE-o-noyd)
Costal (COST-al)
Coxal (COCK-sal)
Cranium (KRAY-nee-um)
Cribriform (KRIB-ri-form)
Crista galli (KRIS-ta GA-li)
Cuboid (KEW-boyd)
Cuneiform (kew-NEE-a-form)
Deltoid (DEL-toyd)
Dens, pl. dentes (DENS, DEN-tees)
Disc (DISK)
Dorsum sellae (DOOR-sum SELL-ee)
Epicondyle (EP-ee-KON-dial)
Ethmoid (ETH-moyd)
Facet (fa-SET)
Femur, pl. femora (FEE-mur, FEM-or-a)
Fibula (FIB-you-la)
Fovea (FOE-vee-ah)
Frontal (FRON-tal)
Glabella (gla-BELL-a)
Glenoid (GLEN-oyd)
Gluteal (GLUE-tee-al)
Hamate (HAM-ate)
Hamulus, pl. hamuli (HAM-you-lus, HAM-you-lie)
Hemifacet (HEM-ee-fa-SET)
Hiatus (hi-ATE-us)
Humerus, pl. humeri (HUME-er-us, HUME-er-eye)
Hyoid (HI-oyd)
Ilium, pl. ilia (IL-lee-um, IL-ee-a)
Incisive (in-SISE-iv)
Infraspinatus (IN-fra-spine-ATE-us)
Inion (IN-yon)
Innominate (i-NOM-i-nate)
Intercostal (IN-ter-KOST-al)
Interosseus (IN-ter-oss-ee-us)
Ischium, pl. ischia (IS-kee-um, IS-kee-a)
Jugular (JUG-you-lar)
Kyphosis (ki-FOS-is)
Lacerum (LA-ser-um)
Lacrimal (LAK-ri-mal)
Lambdoid (LAM-doyd)
Lamina, pl. laminae (LAM-i-na, LAM-i-nee)
Lingula (LING-you-la)
Lordotic (lor-DOT-ik)
Lumbar (LUM-bar)
Lunate (LOON-ate)
Magnum (MAG-num)
Malleolus, pl. malleoli (mal-EE-o-lus, mal-EE-o-lie)
Mamillary (MAM-i-lary)
Mandible (MAN-di-bul)
Manubrium, pl. manubria (ma-NOOB-ree-um, ma-NOOB-ree-a)
Mastoid (MAS-toyd)
Maxilla, pl. maxillae (MAX-i-la, MAX-i-lee)
Meatus (me-ATE-us)
Mental/menti (MEN-tal/MEN-tee)
Metacarpal (MET-a-CAR-pal)
Metatarsal (MET-a-TARS-al)
Mylohyoid (MY-low-HI-oyd)
Nasal (NAY-sul)
Navicular (na-VIK-you-lar)
Nuchal (NEW-kul)
Obturator (OB-tour-ate-or)
Occipital (ok-SIP-i-tal)
Odontoid (o-DONT-oyd)
Olecranon (o-LEK-ran-on)
Optic (OP-tik)
Palatine (PAL-a-tine)
Parietal (pa-RYE-it-al)
Patella, pl. patellae (pa-TELL-a, pa-TELL-ee)
Pedicle (PED-i-kul)
Pelvic bone (PEL-vik)
Petrous (PEE-trus)
Phalanx, pl. phalanges (FAL-anks, fa-LAN-jeez)
Pisiform (PIES-a-form)
Promontory (PROM-on-tor-ee)
Pterygoid (TER-i-goid)

Pubis, pl. pubes (PYU-bis, PYU-bees)
Radius, pl. radii (RAY-dee-us, RAY-dee-eye)
Ramus, pl. rami (RAY-mus, RAY-my)
Sacrum (SA-krum)
Sagittal (SAJ-i-tal)
Scaphoid (SKAF-oyd)
Scapula, pl. scapulae (SKAP-you-la, SKAP-you-lee)
Sciatic (sigh-AT-ik)
Sella turcica (SEL-a TER-si-ka)
Sesamoid (SES-a-moid)
Soleal (SO-lee-al)
Sphenoid (SFEE-noyd)
Spine/spinous (SPINE/SPINE-us)
Squamosal (squaw-MOS-al)
Sternum (STERN-um)
Styloid (STI-loyd)
Subscapular (SUB-SKAP-you-lar)
Subtalar (sub-TAL-ar)
Sulcus, pl. sulci (SUL-kus, SUL-ki)
Superciliary (SOO-per-CIL-ee-ary)
Supernumerary bone (SOO-per-noom-air-ee)
Supraorbital (SOO-pra-OR-bi-tal)
Supraspinatus (SOO-pra-spine-ATE-us)
Sustentaculum (sus-ten-TAK-you-lum)
Suture (SOO-cher)
Symphysis (SIM-fi-sis)
Talus, pl. tali (TA-lus, TA-lie)
Tarsal (TAR-sal)
Temporal (TEM-por-al)
Thoracic (thor-AS-ik)
Tibia, pl. tibiae (TIB-ee-a, TIB-ee-ee
Transverse (TRANS-vers)
Trapezium, trapezoid (tra-PEEZ-ee-um, TRAP-i-zoyd)
Triquetrum (try-KWE-trum)
Trochanter (tro-CAN-ter)
Trochlea (TRO-klee-a)
Tubercle (TWO-ber-kul)
Tuberosity (TWO-ber-OS-i-tee)
Ulna, pl. ulnae (UL-na, UL-nee)
Uncus (UN-kus)
Vomer (VO-mer)
Wormian bones (WWERM-ee-an)
Xiphoid (ZI-foyd)
Zygomatic (ZI-go-MAT-ik)

The following key terms are a number of general terms that are used to describe landmarks on bones. Many bony landmarks are raised aspects of a bone's surface that serve as muscle and/or ligament attachment sites.

Angle—A corner of a bone.
Articular surface—The surface of a bone that articulates with another bone (i.e., the joint surface).
Body—The main portion of a bone; the body of a long bone is the shaft.
Condyle—Rounded bump found at the end of a long bone (part of the epiphysis); usually part of a joint fitting into a fossa of an adjacent bone.
Crest—A moderately raised ridge of bone; often a site of muscle attachment.
Eminence—A raised prominent area of a bone.
Epicondyle—A small bump found on a condyle; often a site of muscle attachment.
Facet—A smooth (usually flat) surface on a bone that forms a joint with another facet or flat surface of an adjacent bone.
Fissure—A cleft or cracklike hole in a bone that allows the passage of nerves and/or vessels.
Foramen—A hole within a bone that allows the passage of nerves and/or vessels (plural: foramina).
Fossa—A depression in a bone that often receives an articulating bone (plural: fossae).
Groove—A narrow elongated depression within a bone, often containing a tendon, nerve, or vessel.
Head—The expanded rounded end (epiphysis) of a long bone; usually separated from the body (i.e., shaft) of the bone by a neck.
Hiatus—An opening in a bone.
Impression—A shallow groove on a bone, often formed by a tendon, nerve, or vessel.
Line—A mildly raised ridge of bone (usually less than a crest); often a site of muscle attachment.
Lip—A raised liplike structure that forms the border of a groove or opening.
Margin—The edge of a bone.
Meatus—A tubelike channel within a bone.
Neck—A narrowed portion of a bone that separates the head from the body (i.e., shaft) of a bone.
Notch—A V-shaped or U-shaped depression in a bone.
Process—A projection of a bone; may be involved with an articulation or may be a site of muscle attachment.
Protuberance—A bump on a bone; often the site of muscle attachment.
Ramus—A portion of bone that branches from the body of the bone (plural: rami).
Sinus—A cavity within a bone.
Spine—A thornlike, sharp, pointed process of a bone; often a site of muscle attachment.
Sulcus—A groove or elongated depression in a bone (plural: sulci).
Trochanter—A large bump on a bone (larger than a tubercle/tuberosity); usually a site of muscle attachment.
Tubercle/tuberosity—A moderately sized bump on a bone; often a site of muscle attachment. A tubercle is usually considered to be smaller than a tuberosity.

WORD ORIGINS

- ❑ Accessory—From Latin *accessorius,* meaning *supplemental*
- ❑ Acetabulum—From Latin *acetum,* meaning *vinegar,* and Latin *abulum,* meaning *small receptacle, cup*
- ❑ Acromion—From Greek *akron,* meaning tip and Greek *omos,* meaning shoulder
- ❑ Ala, pl. alae—From Latin *ala,* meaning *wing*
- ❑ Alveolar—From Latin *alveolus,* meaning *a concavity, a bowl*
- ❑ Apex, pl. apices—From Latin *apex,* meaning *tip*
- ❑ Arch—From Latin *arcus,* meaning *a bow*
- ❑ Arcuate—From Latin *arcuatus,* meaning *bowed, shaped like an arc*
- ❑ Articular—From Latin *articulus,* meaning *joint*
- ❑ Atlanto/atlas—From Greek *Atlas,* the Greek figure, who supports the world (the first cervical vertebra supports the head)
- ❑ Auditory—From Latin *auditorius,* meaning *pertaining to the sense of hearing*
- ❑ Auricular—From Latin *auricula,* meaning *a little ear*
- ❑ Axis—From Latin *axis,* meaning *axis* (an imaginary line about which something revolves)
- ❑ Base/basilar—From Latin *basilaris,* meaning *the base of something*
- ❑ Bicipital—From Latin *bi,* meaning *two,* and Greek *kephale,* meaning *head*
- ❑ Bifid—From Latin *bis,* meaning *twice,* and Latin *findere,* meaning *to cleave*
- ❑ Calcaneus, pl. calcanei—From Latin *calcaneus,* meaning *heel bone*
- ❑ Canine—From Latin *caninus,* meaning *pertaining to a dog* (refers to proximity to canine tooth)
- ❑ Capitate, capitulum—From Latin *caput,* meaning *a small head*
- ❑ Carotid—From Greek *karoun,* meaning *to plunge into sleep or stupor* (because compression of the carotid arteries can result in unconsciousness)
- ❑ Carpal—From Greek *karpos,* meaning *wrist*
- ❑ Cervical—From Latin *cervicalis,* meaning *pertaining to the neck*
- ❑ Clavicle—From Latin *clavicula,* meaning *a small key*
- ❑ Coccyx, pl. coccyges—From Greek *kokkyx,* meaning *cuckoo bird*
- ❑ Concha—From Greek *konch,* meaning *shell*
- ❑ Condyle—From Greek *kondylos,* meaning *knuckle*
- ❑ Conoid—From Greek *konos,* meaning *cone,* and Greek *eidos,* meaning *resemblance*
- ❑ Coracoid—From Greek *korax,* meaning *raven,* and Greek *eidos,* meaning *resemblance*
- ❑ Cornu, pl. cornua—From Latin *cornu,* meaning *horn*
- ❑ Coronoid—From Greek *korone,* meaning *crown,* and Greek *eidos,* meaning *resemblance*
- ❑ Costal—From Latin *costa,* meaning *rib*
- ❑ Coxal—From Latin *coxa,* meaning *hip*
- ❑ Cranium—From Latin *cranium,* meaning *skull*
- ❑ Cribriform—From Latin *cribum,* meaning *sieve,* and Latin *forma,* meaning *shape*
- ❑ Crista galli—From Latin *crista,* meaning *crest* or *plume,* and Latin *gallus,* meaning *rooster*
- ❑ Cuboid—From Greek *kubos,* meaning *cube,* and Greek *eidos,* meaning *resemblance*
- ❑ Cuneiform—From Latin *cuneus,* meaning *wedge,* and Latin *forma,* meaning *shape*
- ❑ Deltoid—From Latin *deltoides,* meaning shaped like a delta (Δ), and Greek *eidos,* meaning *resemblance*
- ❑ Dens, pl. dentes—From Latin *dens,* meaning *tooth*
- ❑ Disc—From Greek *diskos,* meaning *a flat round structure*
- ❑ Dorsum sellae—From Latin *dorsum,* meaning *back,* and Latin *sella,* meaning *saddle* (the dorsum sellae is the posterior wall of the sella turcica)
- ❑ Epicondyle—From Greek *epi,* meaning *upon,* and Greek *kondylos,* meaning *knuckle*
- ❑ Ethmoid—From Greek *ethmos,* meaning *sieve,* and Greek *eidos,* meaning *resemblance*
- ❑ Facet—From French *facette,* meaning *a small face*
- ❑ Femur, pl. femora—From Latin *femur,* meaning *thighbone*
- ❑ Fibula—From Latin *fibula,* meaning *that which clasps or clamps*
- ❑ Fovea—From Latin *fovea,* meaning *a pit*
- ❑ Frontal—From Latin *frontalis,* meaning *anterior*
- ❑ Glabella—From Latin *glaber,* meaning *smooth*
- ❑ Glenoid—From Greek *glene,* meaning *socket,* and Greek *eidos,* meaning *resemblance*
- ❑ Gluteal—From Greek *gloutos,* meaning *buttock*
- ❑ Hamate—From Latin *hamatus,* meaning *hooked*
- ❑ Hamulus, pl. hamuli—From Latin *hamulus,* meaning *a small hook*
- ❑ Hemifacet—From Greek *hemi,* meaning *half,* and French *facette,* meaning *small face*
- ❑ Hiatus—From Latin *hiatus,* meaning *an opening*
- ❑ Humerus, pl. humeri—From Latin *humerus,* meaning *shoulder*
- ❑ Hyoid—From Greek *hyoeides,* meaning *U-shaped*
- ❑ Ilium, pl. ilia—From Latin *ilium,* meaning *groin, flank*
- ❑ Incisive—From Latin *incisus,* meaning *to cut* (refers to proximity to incisor teeth)
- ❑ Infraspinatus—From Latin *infra,* meaning *beneath* (the spine of the scapula)
- ❑ Inion—From Greek *inion,* meaning *back of the neck*
- ❑ Innominate—From Latin *innominatus,* meaning *nameless, unnamed*
- ❑ Intercostal—From Latin *inter,* meaning *between,* and Latin *costa,* meaning *rib*

- ❑ Interosseus—From Latin *inter,* meaning *between,* and Latin *ossis,* meaning *bone*
- ❑ Ischium, pl. ischia—From Greek *ischion,* meaning *hip*
- ❑ Jugular—From Latin *jugularis,* meaning *neck* (refers to jugular vein)
- ❑ Kyphosis—From Greek *kyphos,* meaning *bent, humpback*
- ❑ Lacerum—From Latin *lacerare,* meaning *to tear*
- ❑ Lacrimal—From Latin *lacrimal,* meaning *tear*
- ❑ Lambdoid—From Greek letter *lambda* (λ), and Greek *eidos,* meaning *resemblance*
- ❑ Lamina, pl. laminae—From Latin *lamina,* meaning *a thin flat layer or plate*
- ❑ Lingula—From Latin *lingua,* meaning *tongue*
- ❑ Lordotic—From Greek *lordosis,* meaning *a bending backward*
- ❑ Lumbar—From Latin *lumbus,* meaning *loin, low back*
- ❑ Lunate—From Latin *luna,* meaning *moon*
- ❑ Magnum—From Latin *magnum,* meaning *large*
- ❑ Malleolus, pl. malleoli—From Latin *malleolus,* meaning *little hammer*
- ❑ Mamillary—From Latin *mamma,* meaning *breast*
- ❑ Mandible—From Latin *mandere,* meaning *to chew*
- ❑ Manubrium, pl. manubria—From Latin *manubrium,* meaning *handle*
- ❑ Mastoid—From Greek *mastos,* meaning *breast,* and Greek *eidos,* meaning *resemblance*
- ❑ Maxilla, pl. maxillae—From Latin *maxilla,* meaning *jawbone* (especially the upper one)
- ❑ Meatus—From Latin *meatus,* meaning *a passage*
- ❑ Mental/menti—From Latin *mentum,* meaning *mind*
- ❑ Metacarpal—From Greek *meta,* meaning *after,* and Greek *karpos,* meaning *wrist*
- ❑ Metatarsal—From Greek *meta,* meaning *after,* and from Greek *tarsas,* referring to the *tarsal bones*
- ❑ Mylohyoid—From Greek *myle,* meaning *mill* (refers to molar teeth that grind food), and Greek *hyoeides,* meaning *U-shaped*
- ❑ Nasal—From Latin *nasus,* meaning *nose*
- ❑ Navicular—From Latin *navicula,* meaning *boat*
- ❑ Nuchal—From Latin *nucha,* meaning *back of the neck*
- ❑ Obturator—From Latin *obturare,* meaning *to stop up*
- ❑ Occipital—From Latin *occipitalis,* meaning *back of the head*
- ❑ Odontoid—From Greek *odous,* meaning *tooth,* and Greek *eidos,* meaning *resemblance*
- ❑ Olecranon—From Greek *olecranon,* meaning *elbow*
- ❑ Optic—From Greek *optikos,* meaning *pertaining to the sense of sight* (the optic foramen contains the optic nerve)
- ❑ Palatine—From Latin *palatinus,* meaning *concerning the palate*
- ❑ Parietal—From Latin *parietalis,* meaning *pertaining to the wall of a cavity*
- ❑ Patella, pl. patellae—From Latin *patella,* meaning *a plate*
- ❑ Pedicle—From Latin *pediculus,* meaning *small foot*
- ❑ Pelvic bone—From Latin *pelvis,* meaning *basin*
- ❑ Petrous—From Latin *petra,* meaning *stone*
- ❑ Phalanx, pl. phalanges—From Latin *phalanx,* meaning *a line of soldiers*
- ❑ Pisiform—From Latin *pisum,* meaning *pea,* and Latin *forma,* meaning *shape*
- ❑ Promontory—From Latin *promontorium,* meaning *a projecting process or part*
- ❑ Pterygoid—From Greek *pterygion,* meaning *wing*
- ❑ Pubis, pl. pubes—From Latin *pubes,* meaning *grown up*
- ❑ Radius, pl. radii—From Latin *radius,* meaning *rod, spoke of a wheel*
- ❑ Ramus, pl. rami—From Latin *ramus,* meaning *branch*
- ❑ Sacrum—From Latin *sacrum,* meaning *sacred*
- ❑ Sagittal—From Latin *sagittal,* meaning *arrow* (refers to a posterior/anterior direction)
- ❑ Scaphoid—From Greek *skaphe,* meaning *a skiff* or *boat,* and Greek *eidos,* meaning *resemblance*
- ❑ Scapula, pl. scapulae—From Latin *scapulae,* meaning *shoulder blades*
- ❑ Sciatic—From Latin *sciaticus,* meaning *pertaining to ischium* (i.e., hip)
- ❑ Sella turcica—From Latin *sella,* meaning *saddle,* and Latin *turcica,* meaning *Turkish*
- ❑ Sesamoid—From Greek *sesamon,* meaning *sesame seed,* and Greek *eidos,* meaning *resemblance*
- ❑ Soleal—From Latin *solea,* meaning *sole of the foot*
- ❑ Sphenoid—From Greek *sphen,* meaning *wedge,* and Greek *eidos,* meaning *resemblance*
- ❑ Spine/spinous—From Latin *spina,* meaning *thorn*
- ❑ Squamosal—From Latin *squamosus,* meaning *scaly*
- ❑ Sternum—From Greek *sternon,* meaning *chest, breastbone*
- ❑ Styloid—From Greek *stylos,* meaning *pillar* or *post,* and Greek *eidos,* meaning *resemblance*
- ❑ Subscapular—From Latin *sub,* meaning *under* (referring to the underside [i.e., the anterior side] of the scapula)
- ❑ Subtalar—From Latin *sub,* meaning *under,* and *talar* referring to *the talus*
- ❑ Sulcus, pl. sulci—From Latin *sulcus,* meaning *groove*
- ❑ Superciliary—From Latin *super,* meaning *above,* and Latin *cilium,* meaning *eyebrow*
- ❑ Supraorbital—From Latin *supra,* meaning *above,* and Latin *orbis,* meaning *circle, orb*
- ❑ Supraspinatus—From Latin *supra,* meaning *above* (the spine of the scapula)
- ❑ Sustentaculum—From Latin *sustentaculum,* meaning *support*
- ❑ Suture—From Latin *sutura,* meaning *a seam*
- ❑ Symphysis—From Greek *sym,* meaning *with* or *together,* and Greek *physis,* meaning *nature, body*
- ❑ Talus, pl. tali—From Latin *talus,* meaning *ankle*
- ❑ Tarsal—From Greek *tarsos,* meaning *a broad flat surface*

- ❑ Temporal—From Latin *temporalis,* meaning *pertaining to* or *limited in time* (refers to the temple region of the head)
- ❑ Thoracic—From Greek *thorax,* meaning *chest*
- ❑ Tibia, pl. tibiae—From Latin *tibia,* meaning *the large shinbone*
- ❑ Transverse—From Latin *transversus,* meaning *lying across*
- ❑ Trapezium, trapezoid—From Greek *trapeza,* meaning *a (four sided) table*
- ❑ Triquetrum—From Latin *triquetrus,* meaning *triangular*
- ❑ Trochanter—From Greek *trochanter,* meaning *to run*
- ❑ Trochlea—From Latin *trochlear,* meaning *pulley*
- ❑ Tubercle—From Latin *tuberculum,* or *tuber,* meaning *a small knob, swelling, tumor*
- ❑ Tuberosity—From Latin *tuberositas,* or *tuber,* meaning *a knob, swelling, tumor*
- ❑ Ulna, pl. ulnae—From Latin *ulna,* meaning *elbow*
- ❑ Uncus—From Latin *uncus,* meaning *hook*
- ❑ Vomer—From Latin *vomer,* meaning *ploughshare*
- ❑ Xiphoid—From Greek *xiphos,* meaning *sword,* and Greek *eidos,* meaning *resemblance*
- ❑ Zygomatic—From Greek *zygon,* meaning *to join, a yolk*

Full Skeleton—Anterior View

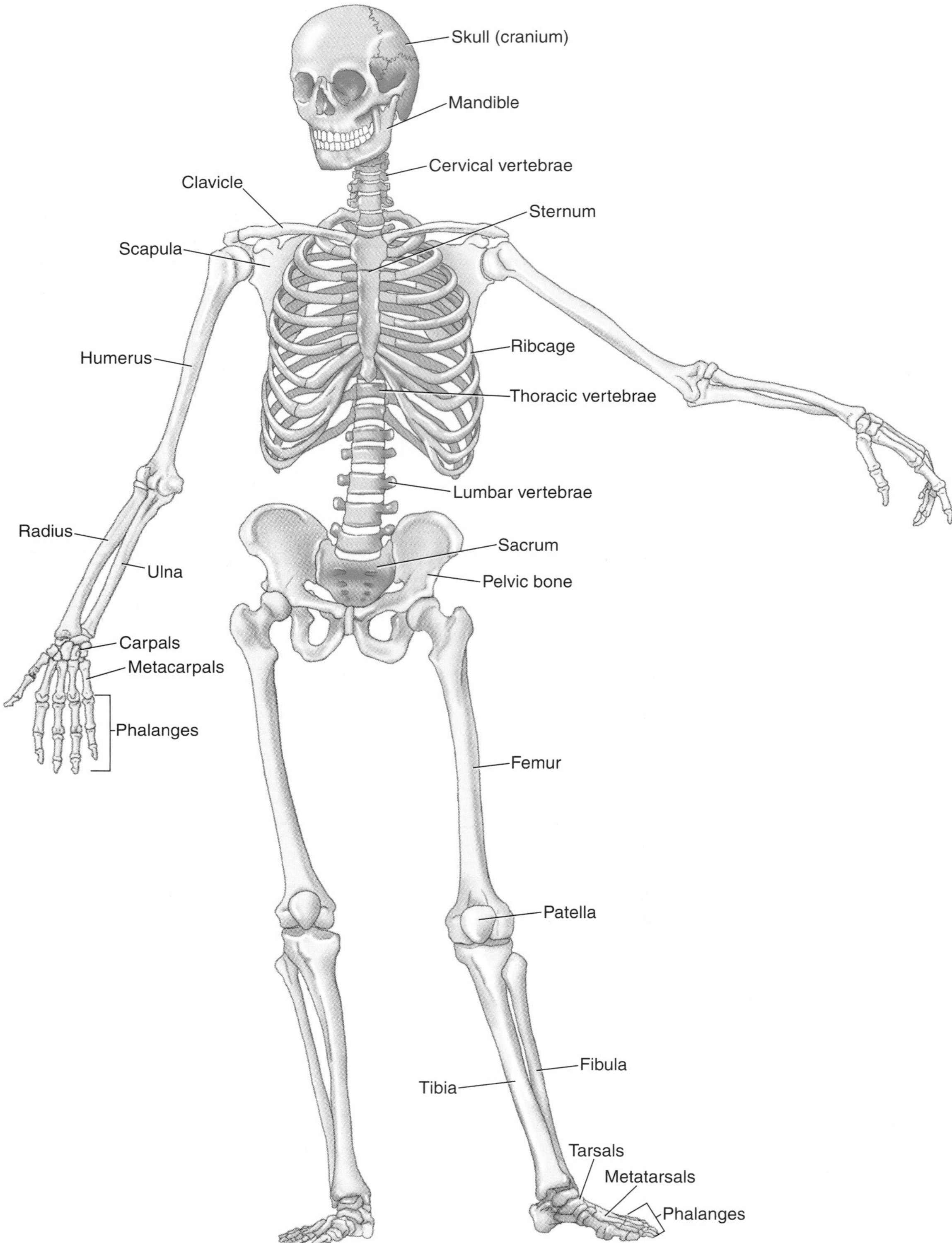

Figure 4-1

Full Skeleton—Posterior View

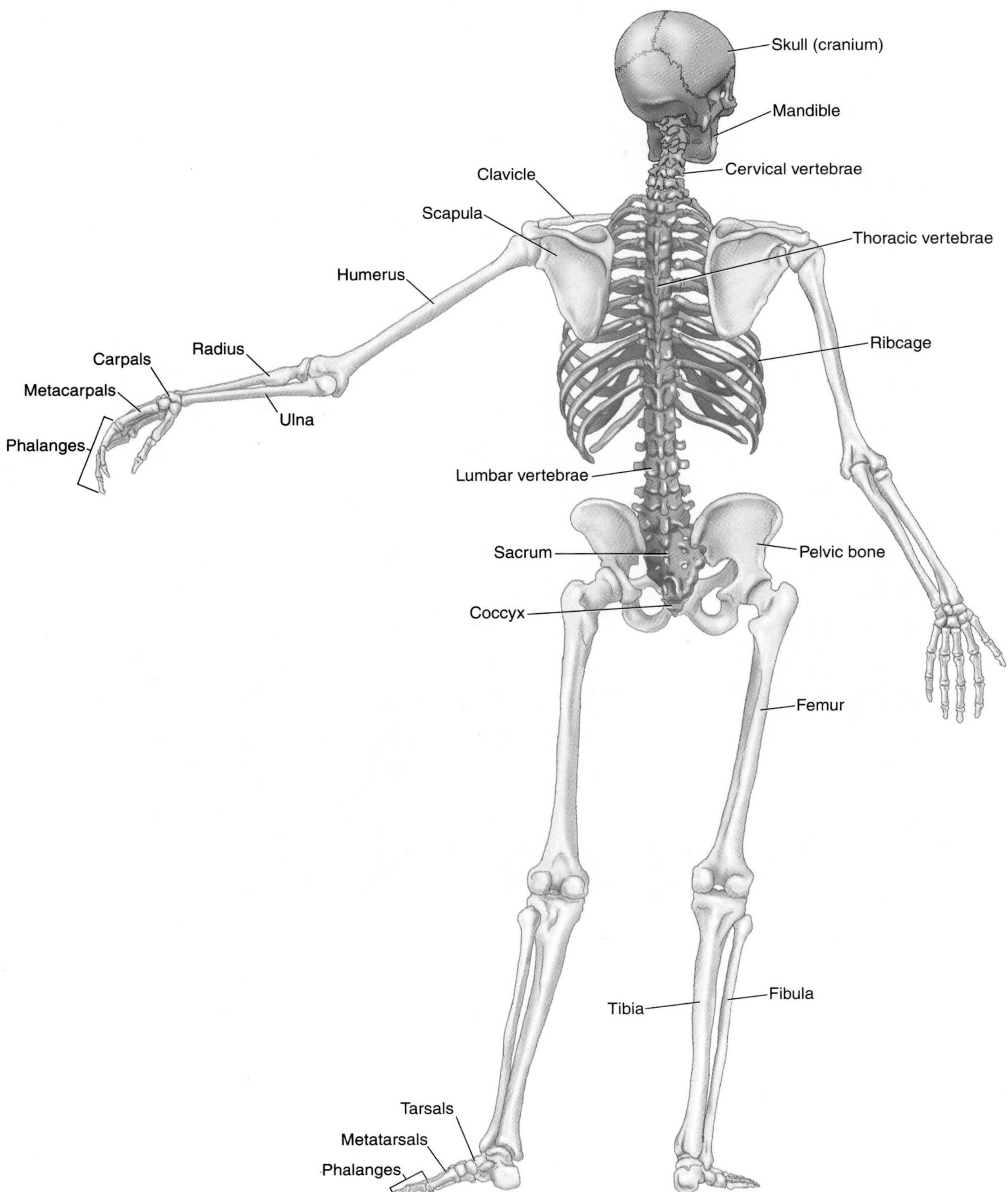

Figure 4-2

☐ 4.1 BONES OF THE HEAD

Skull—Anterior View (colored)

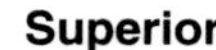

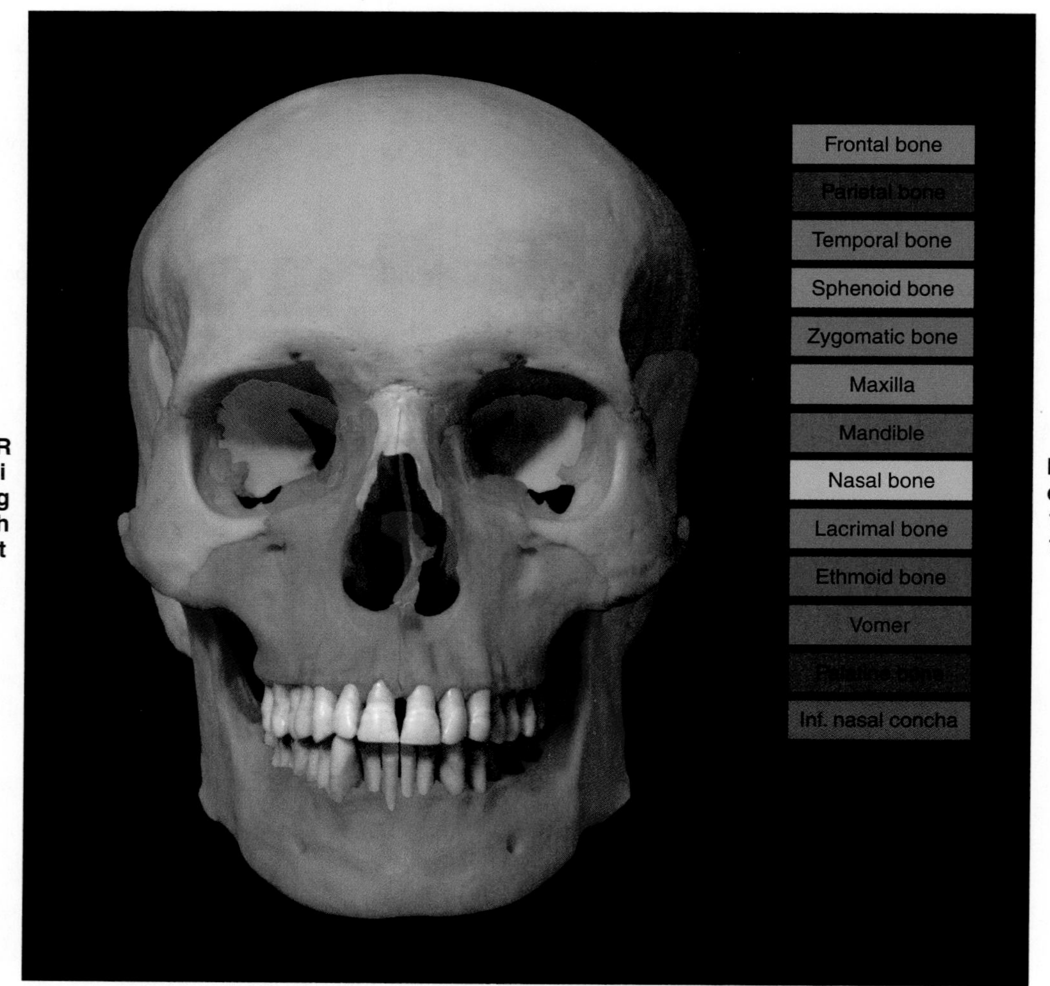

Figure 4-3
Frontal bone
Parietal bone
Occipital bone (not seen)
Temporal bone
Sphenoid bone
Zygomatic bone
Maxilla
Mandible
Nasal bone
Lacrimal bone
Ethmoid bone
Vomer
Palatine bone
Inferior nasal concha

Notes:

1. Embryologically, two maxillary bones (left and right) exist. However, these two bones fuse to form one maxilla (an incomplete fusion results in a cleft palate). For this reason, we may speak of one maxilla (singular) or of two maxillary bones (plural).
2. The frontal, sphenoid, zygomatic, maxillary, lacrimal, and ethmoid bones all have a presence in the orbital cavity.
3. The ethmoid, vomer, and inferior nasal concha are all visible in this anterior view of the nasal cavity.

Skull—Anterior View

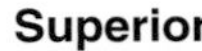

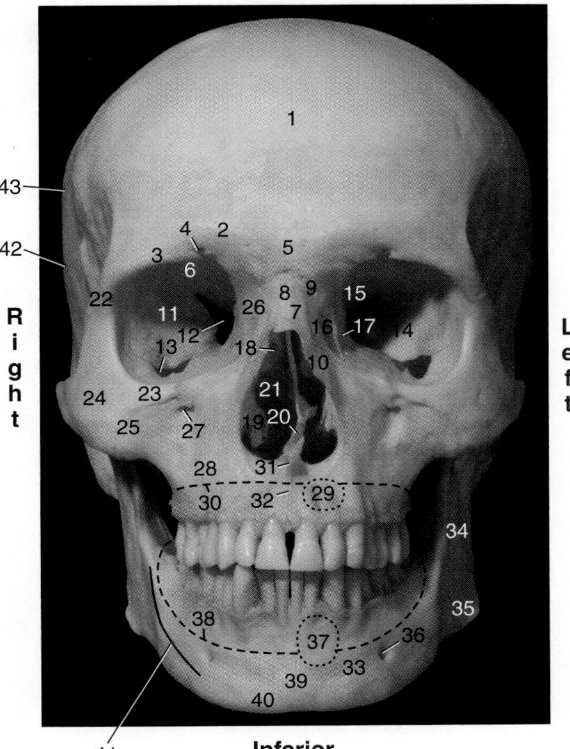

Figure 4-4

1 Frontal bone (#2-6)
2 Superciliary arch
3 Supraorbital margin
4 Supraorbital notch
5 Glabella
6 Orbital surface
7 Nasal bone
8 Internasal suture
9 Frontonasal suture
10 Nasomaxillary suture
11 Orbital cavity
12 Superior orbital fissure
13 Inferior orbital fissure
14 Greater wing of sphenoid
15 Lesser wing of sphenoid
16 Lacrimal bone
17 Ethmoid bone
18 Middle nasal concha (of ethmoid bone)
19 Inferior nasal concha
20 Vomer
21 Palatine bone
22 Frontozygomatic suture
23 Infraorbital margin
24 Zygomatic bone
25 Zygomaticomaxillary suture

Maxilla (#26-31):
26 Frontal process
27 Infraorbital foramen
28 Canine fossa
29 Incisive fossa (indicated by dotted line)
30 Alveolar process (indicated by dashed line)
31 Anterior nasal spine
32 Intermaxillary suture

Mandible (#33-43):
33 Body
34 Ramus
35 Angle
36 Mental foramen
37 Incisive fossa (indicated by dotted line)
38 Alveolar fossa (indicated by dashed line)
39 Symphysis menti
40 Mental tubercle
41 Oblique line (indicated by solid line)
42 Temporal bone
43 Parietal bone

Notes:
1. The term *cranium* is usually considered to be synonymous with the term *skull.* Some sources exclude the mandible and/or other facial bones from the term *cranium.*
2. The glabella is a smooth prominence on the frontal bone, just superior to the nose.
3. The inferior nasal concha is an independent bone. The middle and superior nasal conchae are landmarks of the ethmoid bone.
4. The vomer and ethmoid both contribute to the nasal septum, which divides the nasal cavity into left and right nasal passages.
5. The supraorbital margin is wholly located on the frontal bone; the infraorbital margin is located on the maxilla and the zygomatic bone.

Skull—Right Lateral View (colored)

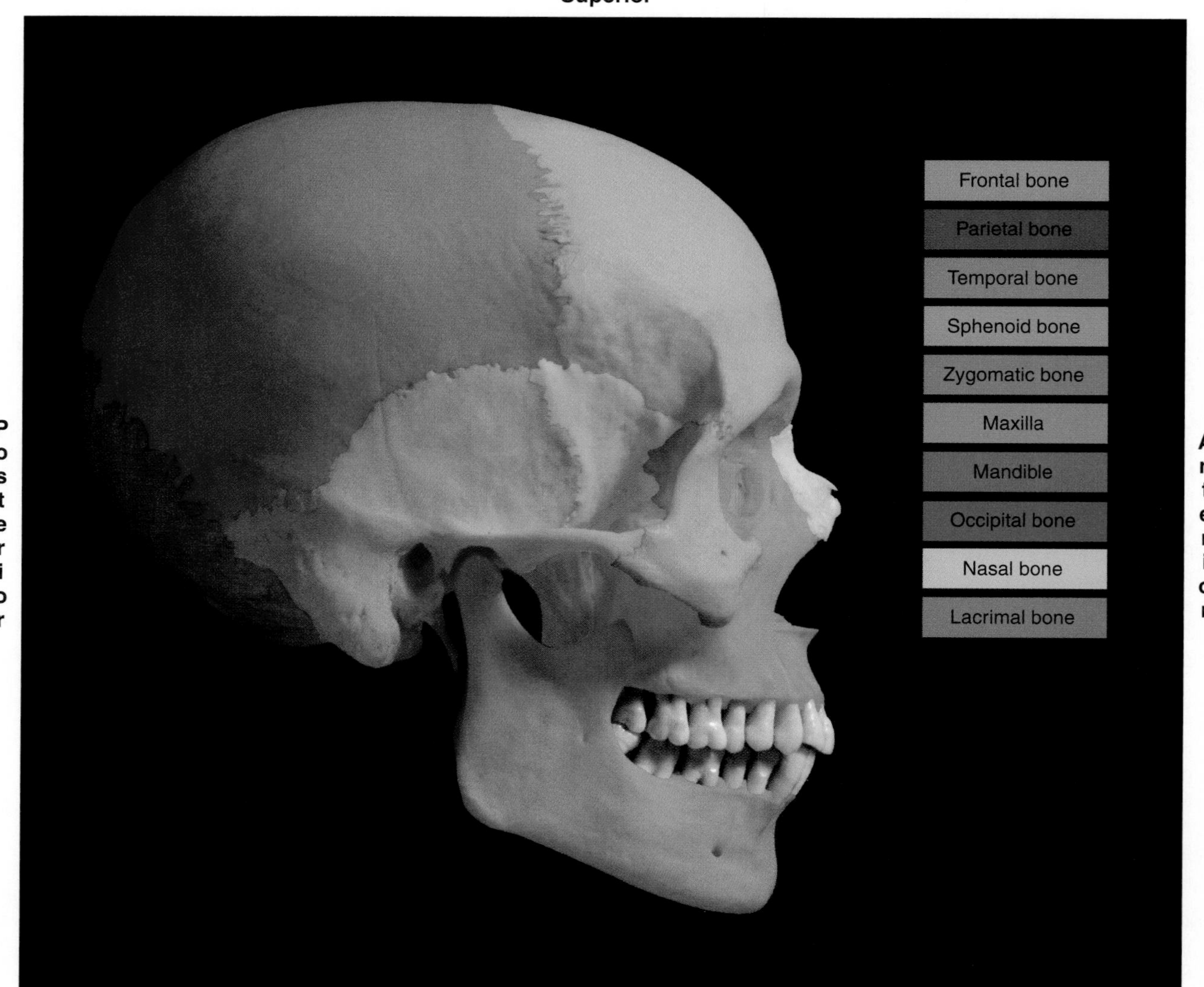

Figure 4-5
Frontal bone
Parietal bone
Temporal bone
Sphenoid bone
Zygomatic bone
Maxilla
Mandible
Occipital bone
Nasal bone
Lacrimal bone

Notes:

1. The occipital bone is often referred to as the *occiput*.
2. In this lateral view, the sphenoid bone is visible posterior to the maxilla (between the condyle and coronoid process of the mandible).

Skull—Right Lateral View

Figure 4-6

1 Frontal bone
2 Glabella
3 Coronal suture
4 Frontozygomatic suture
5 Superior temporal line
6 Parietal bone
7 Lambdoid suture
8 Occipital bone
9 External occipital protuberance (EOP)
10 Temporal bone (#11-14)
11 Mastoid process
12 Styloid process
13 External auditory meatus
14 Zygomatic arch
15 Squamosal suture
16 Zygomaticotemporal suture
17 Temporomandibular joint (TMJ)
18 Greater wing of sphenoid bone
19 Lateral pterygoid plate (of the pterygoid process) of the sphenoid bone
20 Zygomatic bone
21 Nasal bone
22 Maxilla
23 Anterior nasal spine
24 Frontal process of maxilla
25 Lacrimal bone

Mandible (#26-32):
26 Body
27 Angle
28 Ramus
29 Coronoid process
30 Condyle
31 Mental foramen
32 Mental tubercle

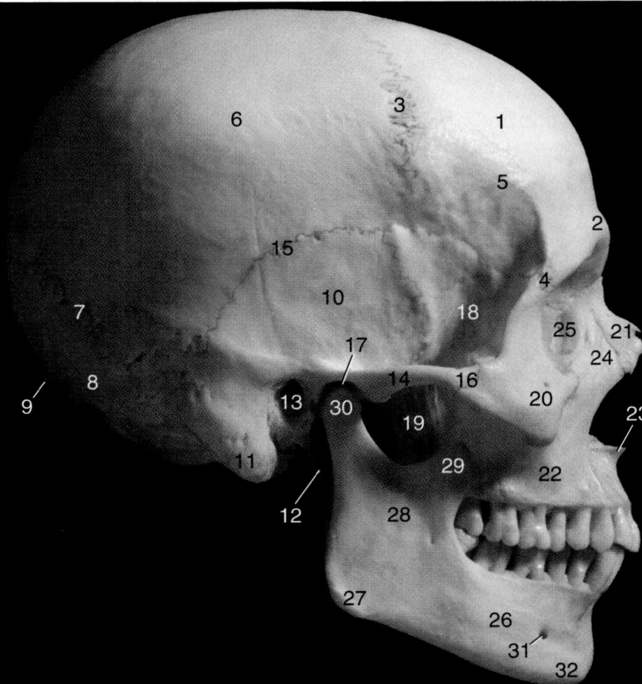

Notes:

1. The temporal fossa (the attachment site of the temporalis muscle) is a broad area of the skull that overlies the temporal, parietal, frontal, and sphenoid bones. The superior margin of the temporal fossa is the superior temporal line, visible on the frontal bone (#5).
2. The external auditory meatus is the opening into the middle ear cavity, which is located within the temporal bone.
3. The zygomatic arch is usually spoken of as being a landmark only of the temporal bone. However, technically the zygomatic arch is a landmark of both the temporal and zygomatic bones formed by the zygomatic process of the temporal bone and the temporal process of the zygomatic bone (see Figure 4-15c).
4. The *squamosal suture* is named for being next to the squamous portion (the superior aspect near the parietal bone) of the temporal bone. The *squamous portion of the temporal bone* is so named because it usually has a scaly appearance (*squamous* means *scaly*).
5. The lateral pterygoid plate (of the pterygoid process) of the sphenoid bone (visible as #19) is the medial attachment site of the lateral and medial pterygoid muscles. The medial pterygoid muscle attaches to its medial surface; the lateral pterygoid muscle attaches to its lateral surface (visible as #19).

Skull—Posterior Views

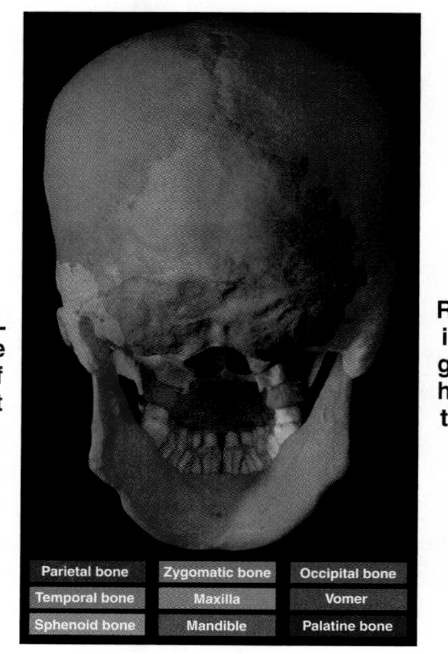

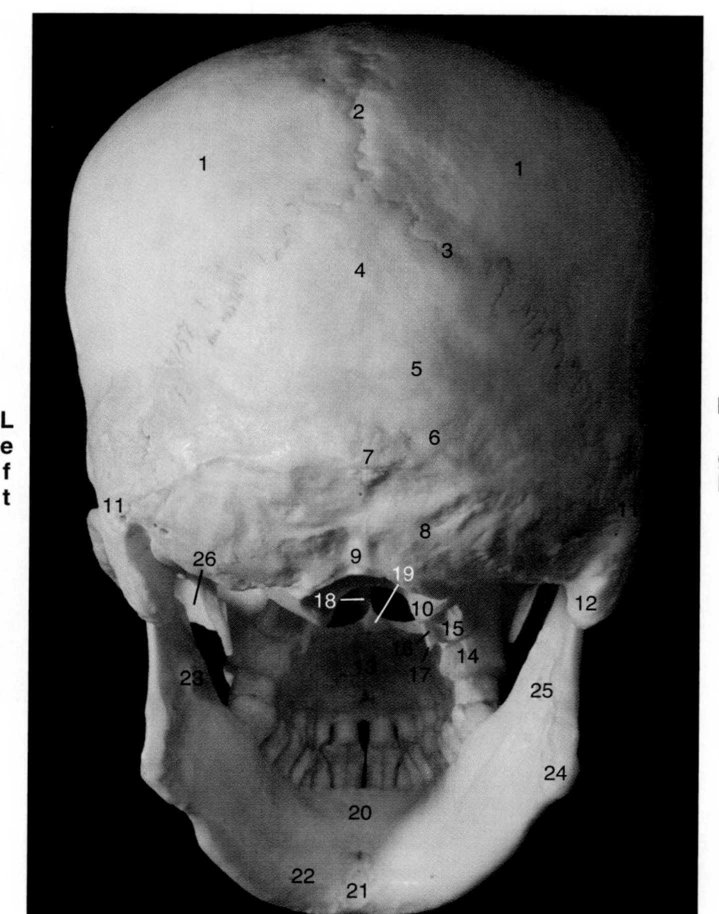

Figure 4-7a and b

1 Parietal bone
2 Sagittal suture
3 Lambdoid suture

Occipital bone (#4-10):
4 Occipital bone
5 Highest nuchal line
6 Superior nuchal line
7 External occipital protuberance (EOP)
8 Inferior nuchal line
9 External occipital crest
10 Condyle
11 Temporal bone
12 Mastoid process of the temporal bone
13 Maxilla
14 Tuberosity of the maxilla

Sphenoid bone (#15-17):
15 Lateral pterygoid plate of the pterygoid process
16 Medial pterygoid plate of the pterygoid process
17 Pterygoid hamulus
18 Vomer
19 Palatine bone

Mandible (#20-25):
20 Mandible
21 Inferior and superior mental spines
22 Mylohyoid line
23 Lingula
24 Angle
25 Ramus
26 Zygomatic bone

Notes:

1. The external occipital protuberance (EOP) is also known as the *inion*.
2. The EOP is located in the middle of the superior nuchal line of the occiput.
3. The lateral and medial pterygoid plates are landmarks of the pterygoid process of the sphenoid bone.
4. The lateral pterygoid muscle attaches to the lateral surface of the lateral pterygoid plate of the sphenoid; the medial pterygoid muscle attaches to the medial surface of the lateral pterygoid plate of the sphenoid.

Skull—Inferior Views

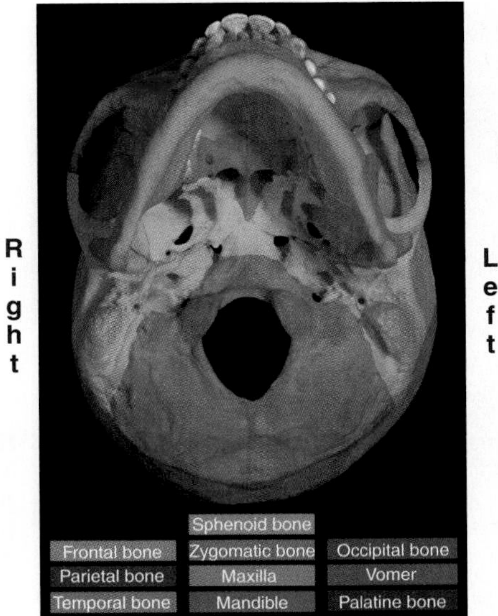

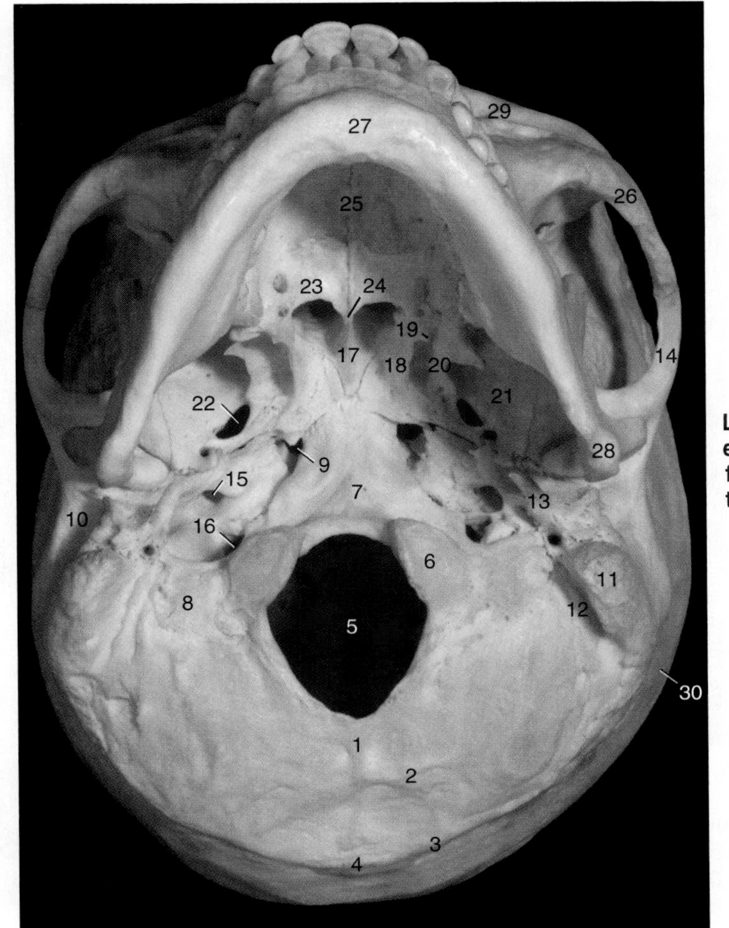

Figure 4-8a and b

Occipital bone (#1-9):

1 External occipital crest
2 Inferior nuchal line
3 Superior nuchal line
4 External occipital protuberance (EOP)
5 Foramen magnum
6 Condyle
7 Basilar part
8 Jugular process
9 Foramen lacerum

Temporal bone (#10-15):

10 Temporal bone
11 Mastoid process
12 Mastoid notch
13 Styloid process
14 Zygomatic arch
15 Carotid canal

16 Jugular foramen (of the occipital bone)
17 Vomer

Sphenoid bone (#18-22):

18 Medial pterygoid plate of pterygoid process
19 Pterygoid hamulus
20 Lateral pterygoid plate of pterygoid process
21 Greater wing of sphenoid
22 Foramen ovale
23 Palatine bone
24 Posterior nasal spine of palatine bones
25 Maxilla
26 Zygomatic bone
27 Mandible
28 Angle of the mandible
29 Frontal bone
30 Parietal bone

Notes:

1. The foramen magnum is the division point between the brain and spinal cord. The brain and spinal cord are actually one structure; superior to the foramen magnum is the brain; inferior to it is the spinal cord.
2. The foramen lacerum is mostly blocked with cartilage, allowing only a small nerve, the nerve of the pterygoid canal, to pass through.
3. The carotid canal provides passageway for the internal carotid artery to enter the cranial cavity.
4. The jugular foramen provides passageway for cranial nerves (CNs) IX, X, and XI to pass from the brain to the neck. Venous blood draining from the brain to the internal jugular vein also passes through the jugular foramen.
5. The foramen ovale provides passageway for the mandibular division of the trigeminal nerve (CN V) to pass from the brain to the neck.

Skull—Internal Views

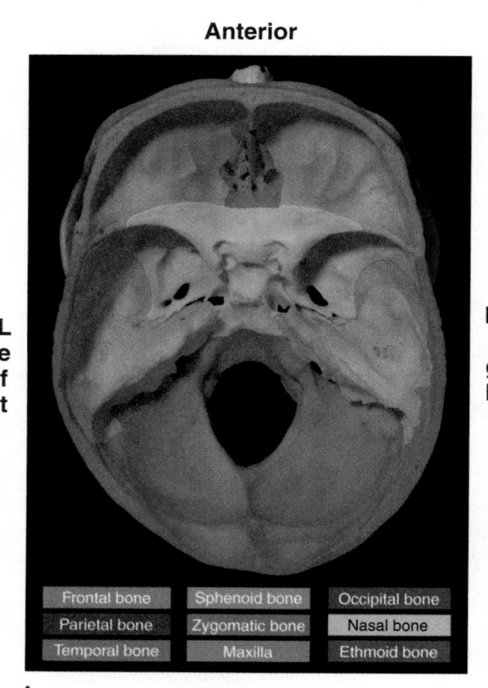

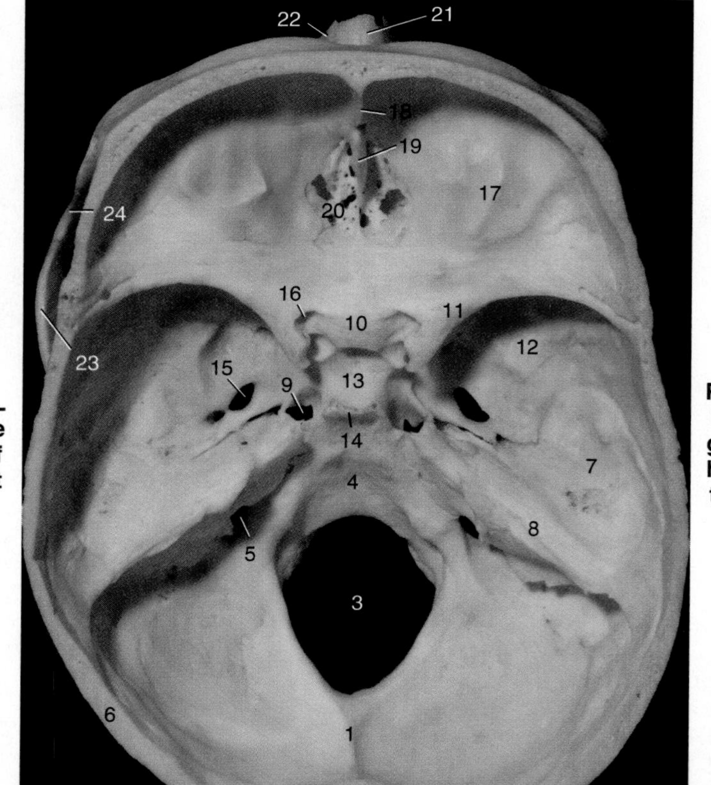

Figure 4-9a and b

Occipital bone (#1-5):

1 Occipital bone
2 Internal occipital protuberance
3 Foramen magnum
4 Basilar part
5 Jugular foramen
6 Parietal bone
7 Squamous part of temporal bone
8 Petrous part of temporal bone
9 Foramen lacerum

Sphenoid bone (#10-16):

10 Sphenoid bone
11 Lesser wing
12 Greater wing
13 Sella turcica
14 Dorsum sellae
15 Foramen ovale
16 Optic foramen
17 Frontal bone (orbital part)
18 Frontal crest
19 Crista galli of ethmoid bone
20 Cribriform plate of ethmoid bone
21 Nasal bone
22 Maxilla
23 Zygomatic arch of temporal bone
24 Temporal arch of zygomatic bone

Notes:

1. The sella turcica of the sphenoid is where the pituitary gland sits (*sella turcica* literally means *Turkish saddle*).
2. The optic foramen allows passage of the optic nerve (cranial nerve [CN] II) from the eye to the brain.
3. From this view, the eyeball is located deep to the orbital part of the frontal bone (#17).
4. The crista galli of the ethmoid is an attachment site of the falx cerebri of the dura mater meninge of the brain.
5. Receptor cells for the sense of smell from the nasal cavity pierce the cribriform plate of the ethmoid bone to connect with the olfactory bulb (CN I) of the brain.
6. The basilar portion of the occiput and the most posterior portion of the sphenoid are often collectively called the *clivus*.

Skull—Sagittal Section and the Orbital Cavity

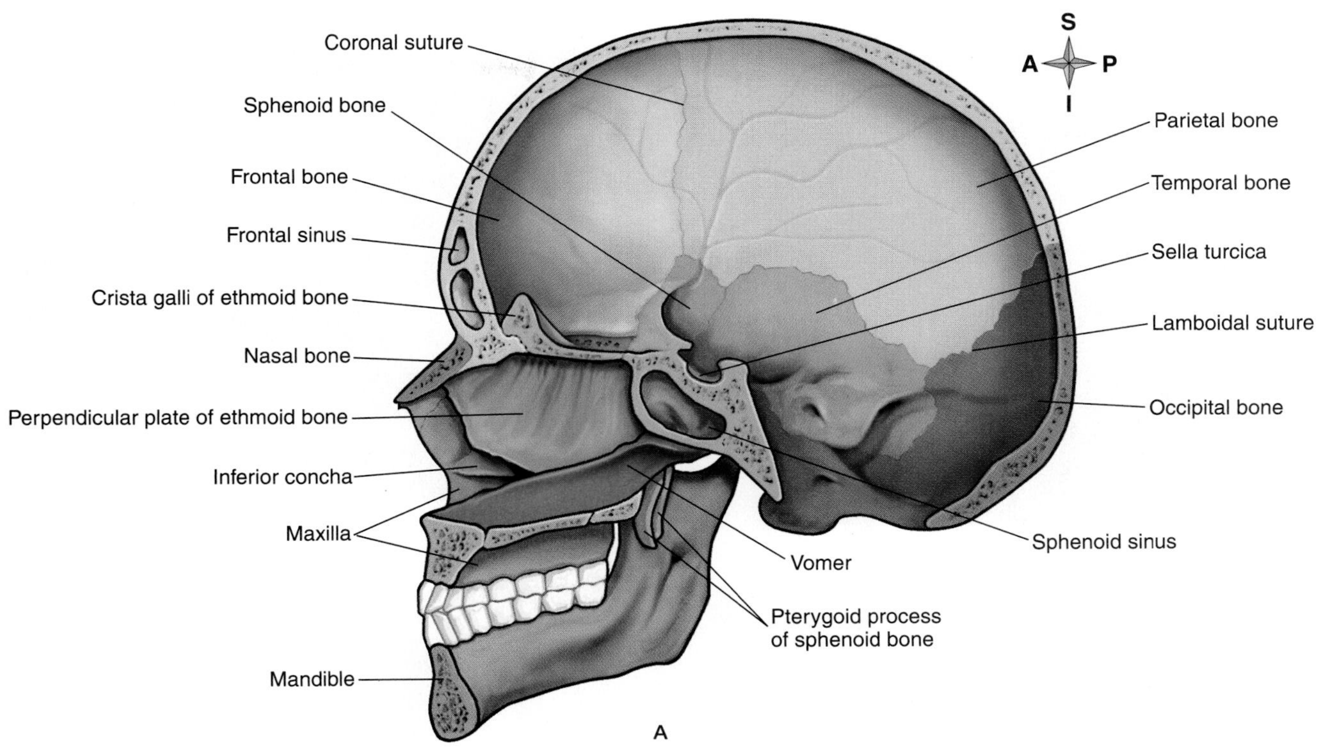

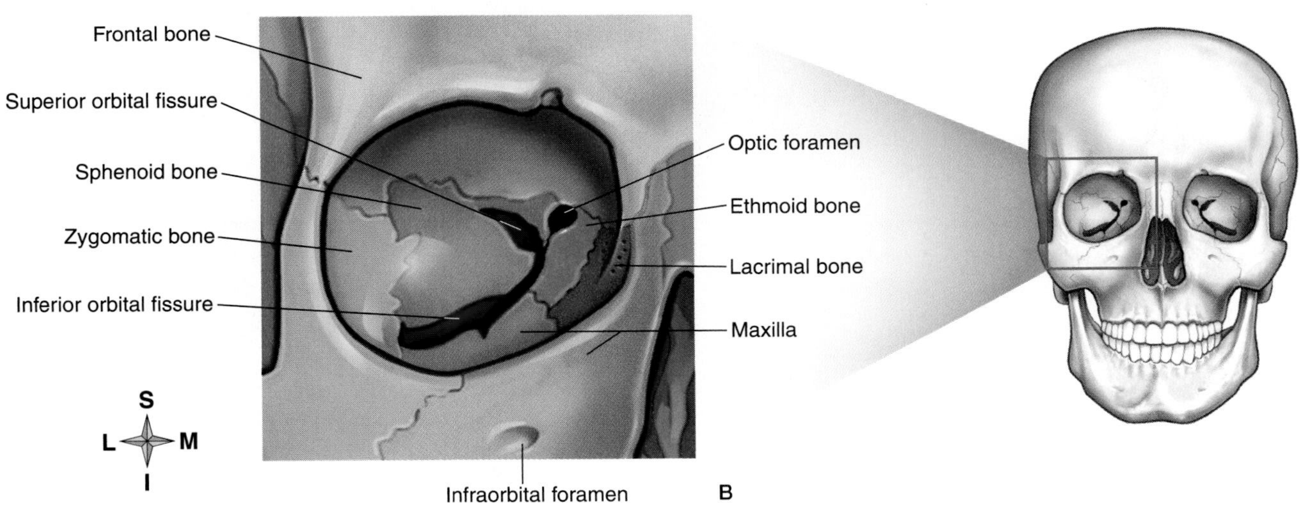

Figure 4-10
A, Right half of the skull viewed from within. *B,* bones that form the right orbit. (Adapted from Thibodeau GA, Patton KT: *Anatomy and physiology*, St Louis, 2003, Mosby.)

Mandible

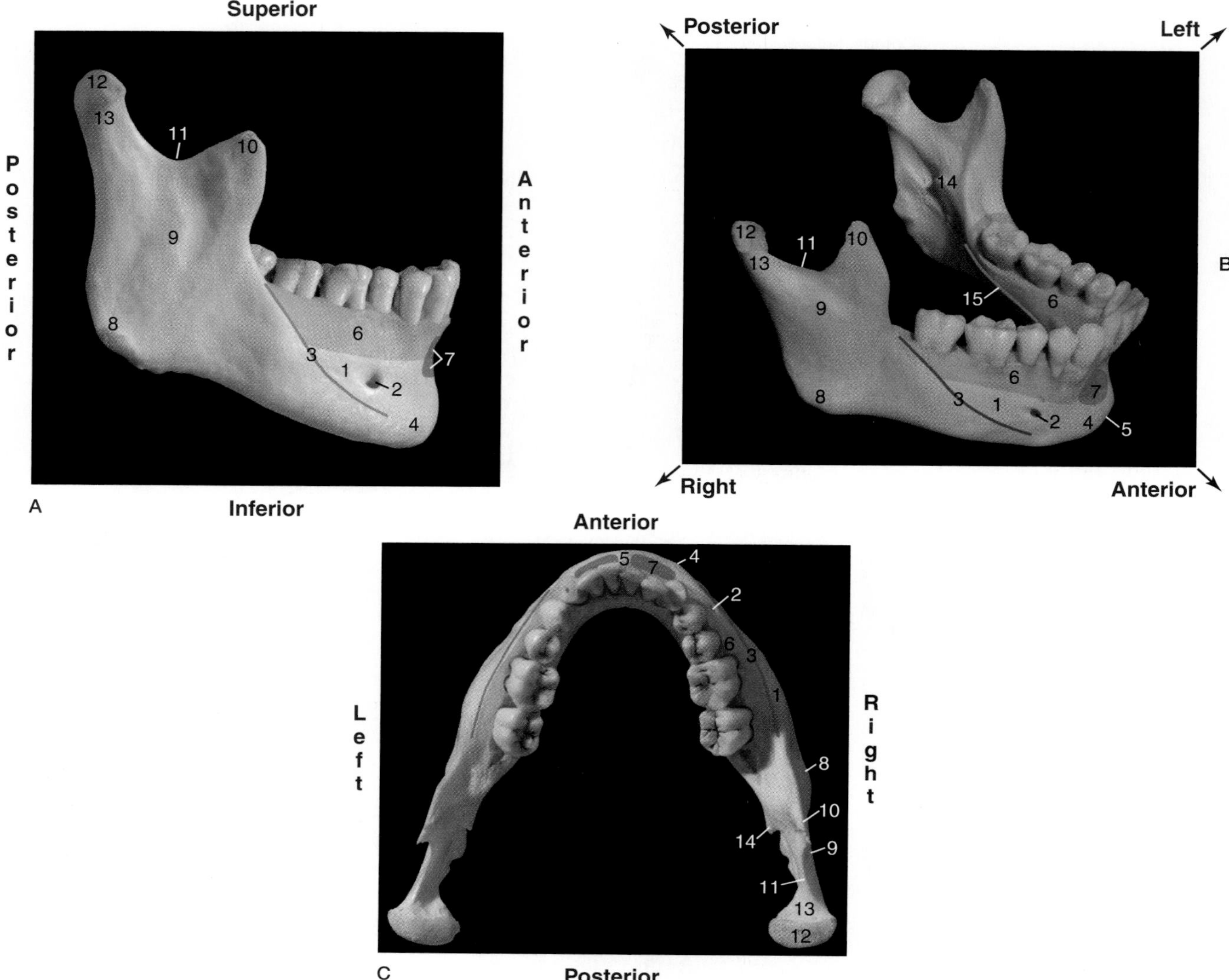

Figure 4-11
A, Right lateral view; *B,* oblique view; *C,* superior view.

1 Body
2 Mental foramen
3 Oblique line
4 Mental protuberance
5 Symphysis menti
6 Alveolar process (indicated in light pink)
7 Incisive fossa (indicated in dark pink)
8 Angle
9 Ramus
10 Coronoid process
11 Mandibular notch
12 Head of condyle
13 Neck of condyle
14 Lingula
15 Mylohyoid line

Notes:

1. The symphysis menti is where the left and right sides of the mandible fuse together.
2. The word *ramus* means *branch.* The ramus of the mandible branches from the body of the mandible.
3. The coronoid process and condyle are landmarks of the ramus of the mandible.
4. The condyle of the mandible articulates with the temporal bone, forming the temporomandibular joint (TMJ).
5. The head of the condyle is easily palpable just anterior to the ear while opening and closing the mouth (elevating and depressing the mandible at the TMJ). Alternately, place your palpating finger inside your ear and press anteriorly while opening and closing the mouth.
6. The mylohyoid line is the attachment site on the internal mandible of the mylohyoid muscle.

Parietal, Temporal, and Frontal Bones

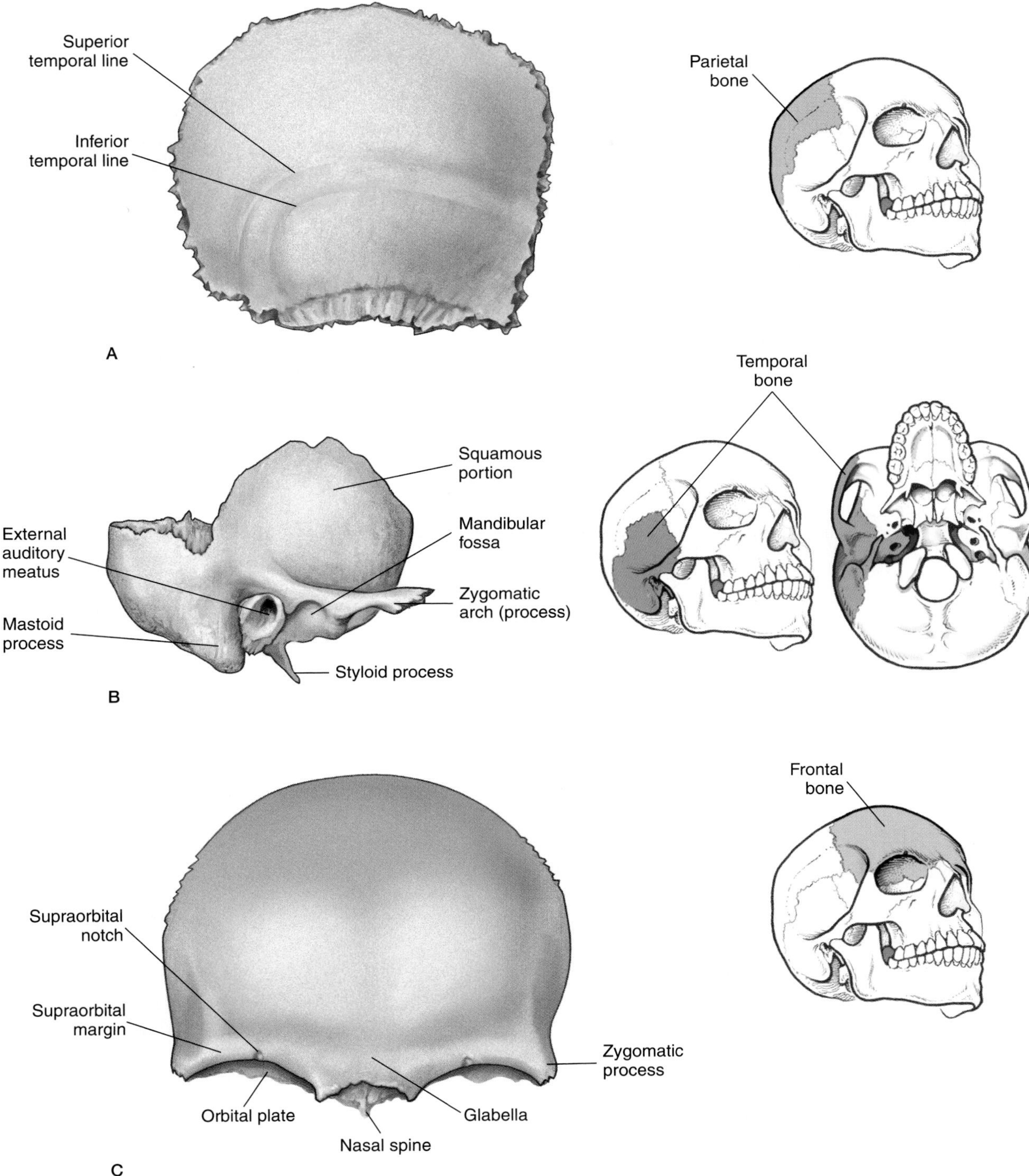

Figure 4-12
A, Lateral view at the right parietal bone. *B,* lateral view of the right temporal bone. *C,* anterior view of the frontal bone. (Modified from Thibodeau GA, Patton KT: *Anatomy and physiology,* St Louis, 2003, Mosby.)

Occipital and Sphenoid Bones

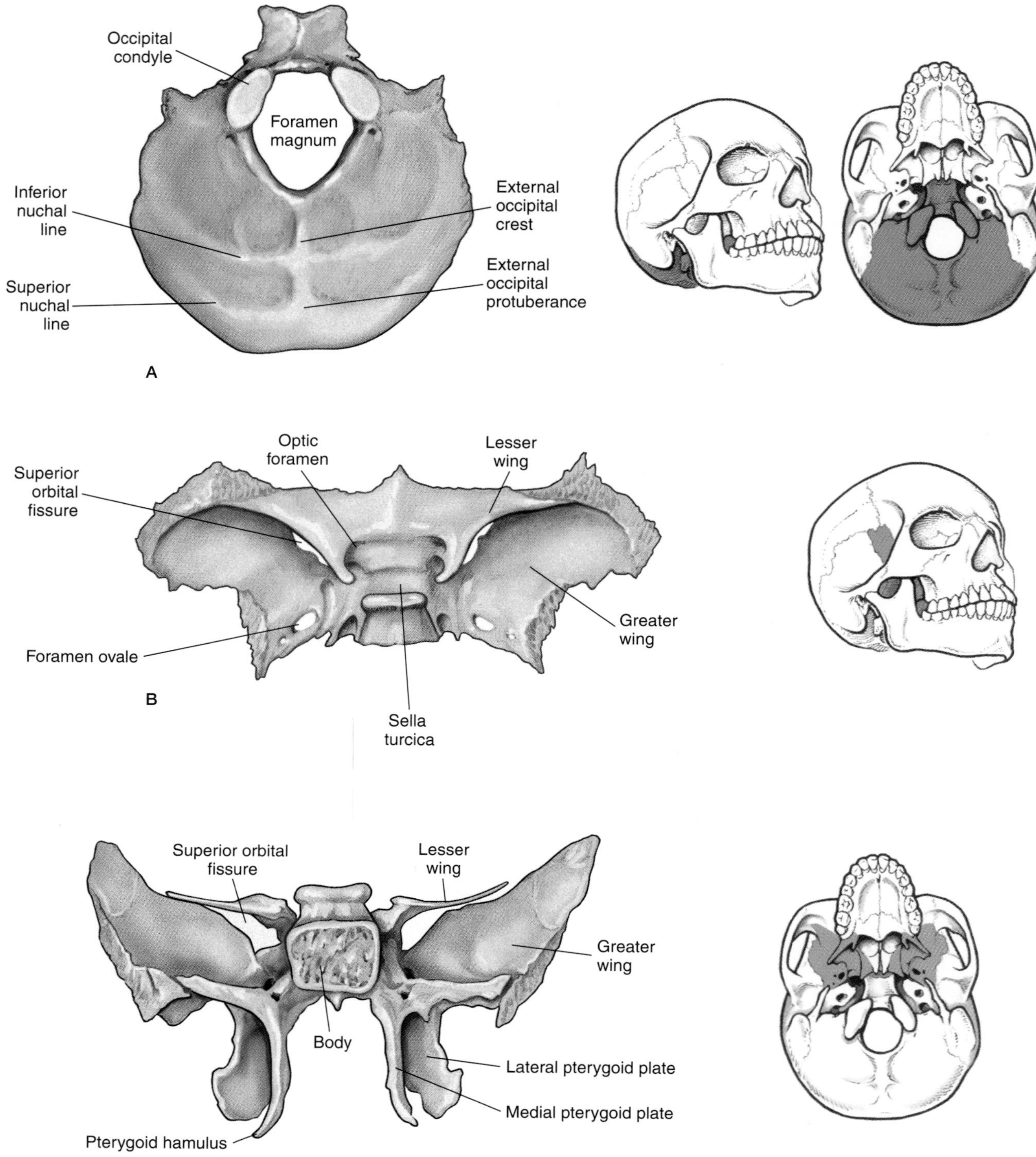

Figure 4-13
A, Inferior view of the occipital bone. *B,* superior view of the sphenoid bone (within the cranial cavity). *C,* posterior view of the sphenoid bone. (Modified from Thibodeau GA, Patton KT: *Anatomy and physiology,* St Louis, 2003, Mosby.)

Ethmoid and Vomer

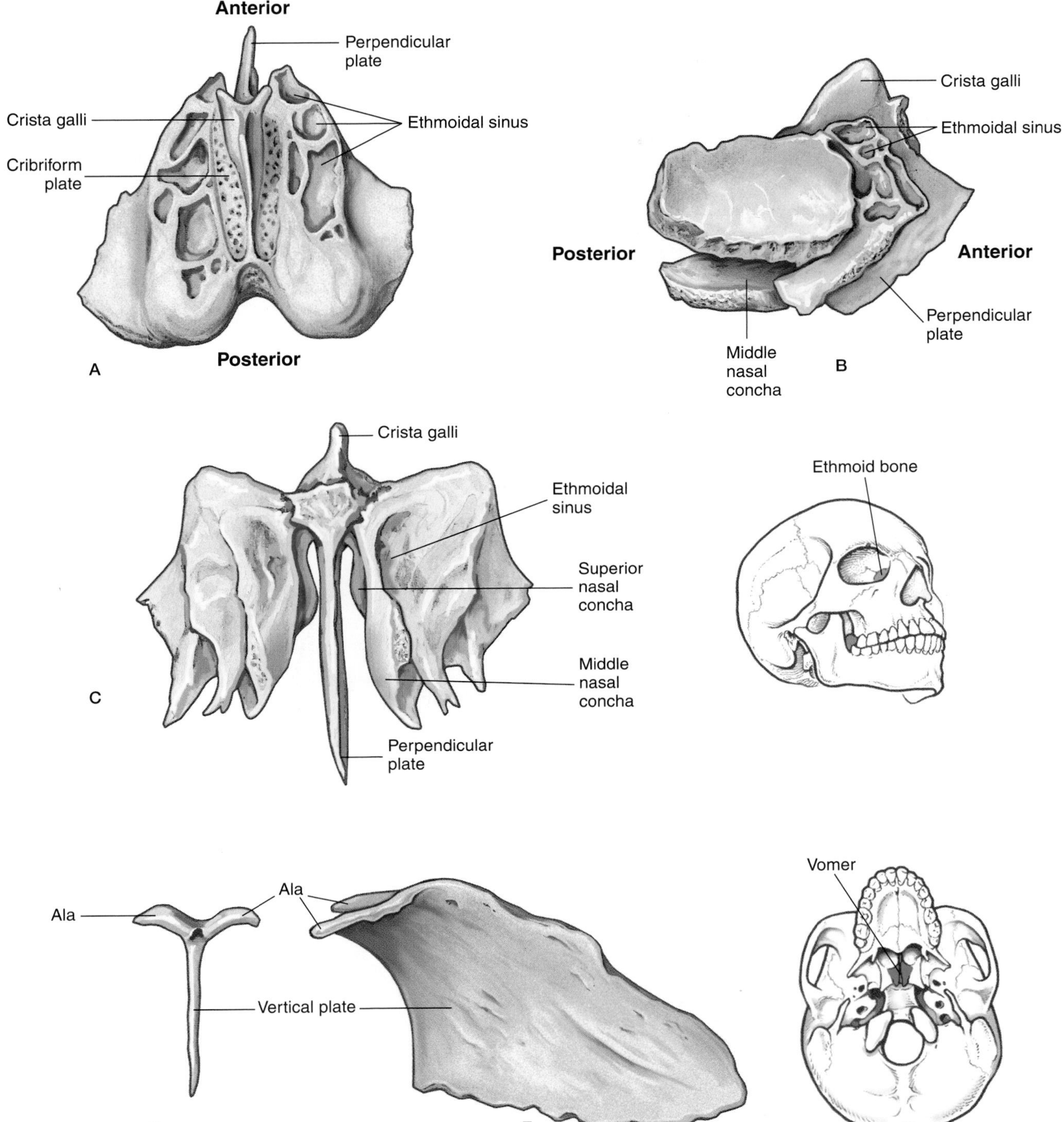

Figure 4-14
A, Superior view of the ethmoid bone. *B,* right lateral view of the ethmoid bone. *C,* anterior view of the ethmoid bone. *D,* anterior view of the vomer. *E,* right lateral view of the vomer. (Modified from Thibodeau GA, Patton KT: *Anatomy and physiology,* St Louis, 2003, Mosby.)

Maxillary and Zygomatic Bones

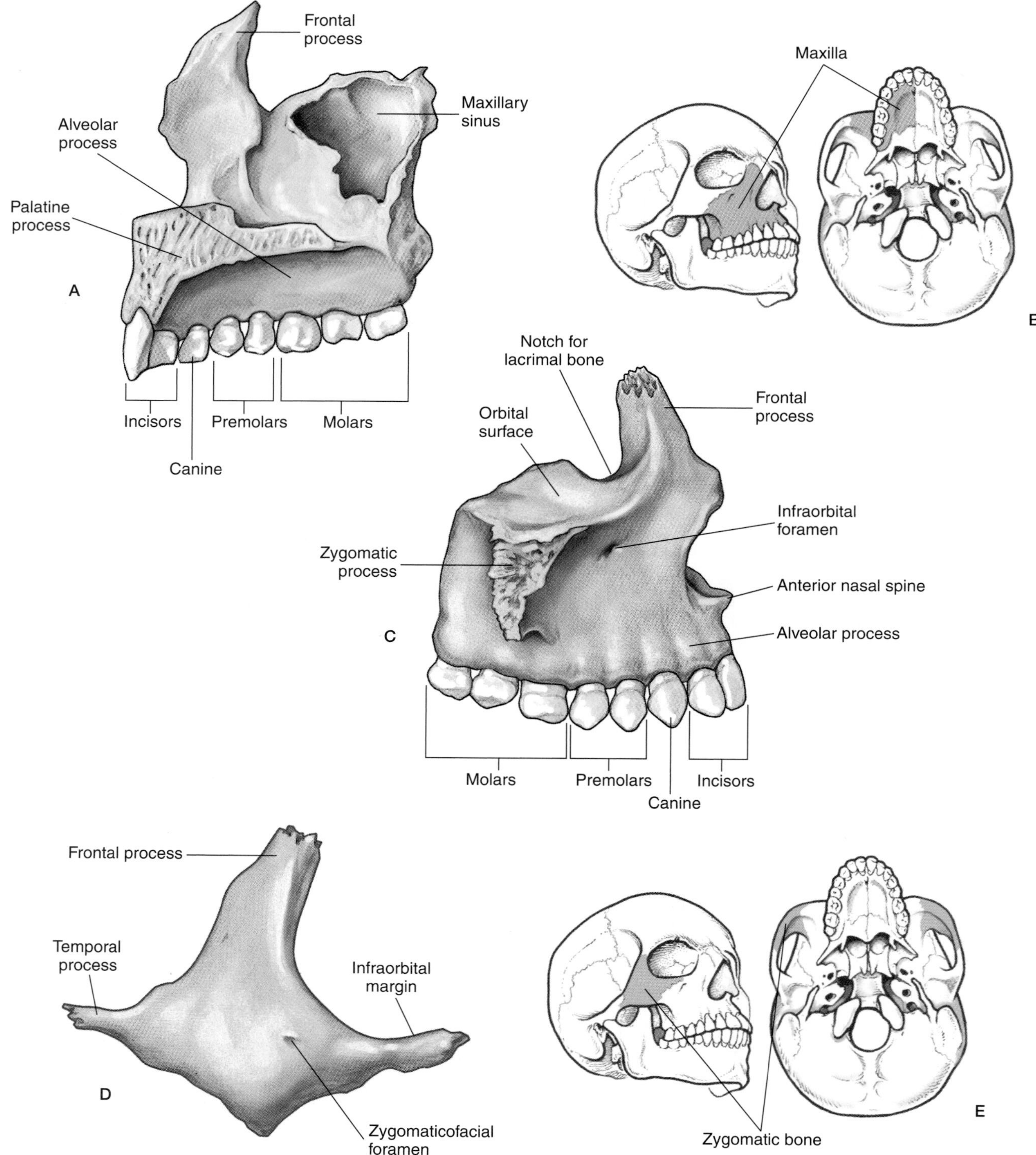

Figure 4-15
A, Medial view of the right maxilla. *B,* lateral view of the right maxilla. *C,* lateral view of the right zygomatic bone. (Modified from Thibodeau GA, Patton KT: *Anatomy and physiology,* St Louis, 2003, Mosby.)

Palatine, Lacrimal, and Nasal Bones

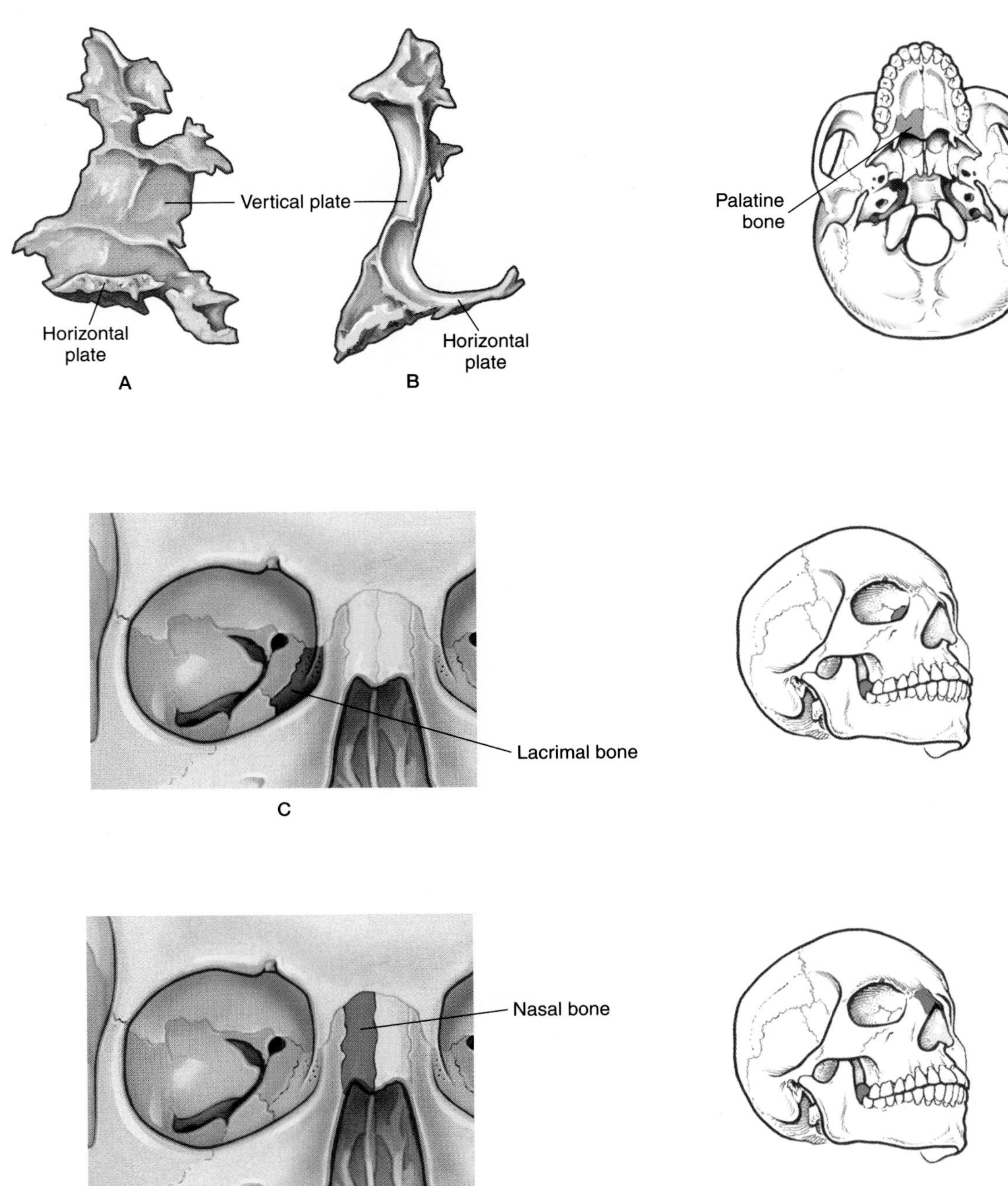

Figure 4-16
A, Medial view of the right palatine bone. *B,* anterior view of the right palatine bone. *C,* anterior view of the right lacrimal bone. *D,* anterior view of the right nasal bone. (From Thibodeau GA, Patton KT: *Anatomy and physiology,* St Louis, 2003, Mosby.)

4.2 BONES OF THE SPINE (AND HYOID)

Spinal Column—Posterior View

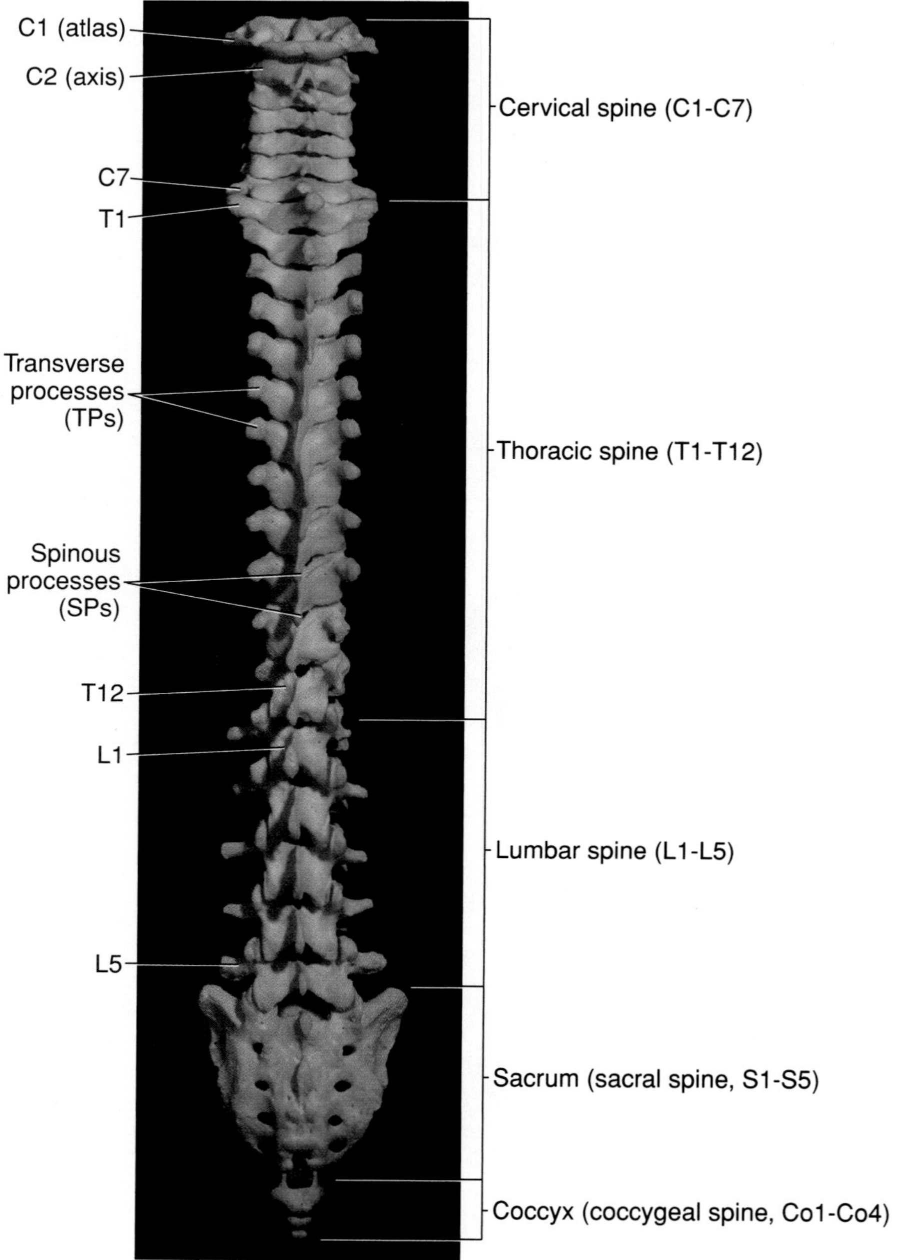

Figure 4-17

Notes:

1. The spine is part of the axial skeleton and is composed of five regions: the cervical, thoracic, lumbar, sacral, and coccygeal spines.
2. The spine has seven cervical vertebrae (named *C1-C7*), 12 thoracic vertebrae (named *T1-T12*), five lumbar vertebrae (named *L1-L5*), one sacrum (composed of five fused sacral vertebrae, named *S1-S5*), and one coccyx (usually composed of four rudimentary vertebrae, named *Co1-Co4*).
3. *Vertebra* is singular; *vertebrae* is plural.
4. The spinal column is composed of 24 vertebrae, a sacrum, and a coccyx.
5. The cervical spine is located within the neck.
6. The thoracic and lumbar spines are located in the trunk.
7. The thoracic spine constitutes the thorax; the lumbar spine constitutes the abdomen.
8. The thoracic spine is defined by having the ribcage attach to it; hence humans have 12 pairs of ribs and 12 thoracic vertebrae.
9. The sacrum and coccyx are located within the pelvis.

Spinal Column—Right Lateral View

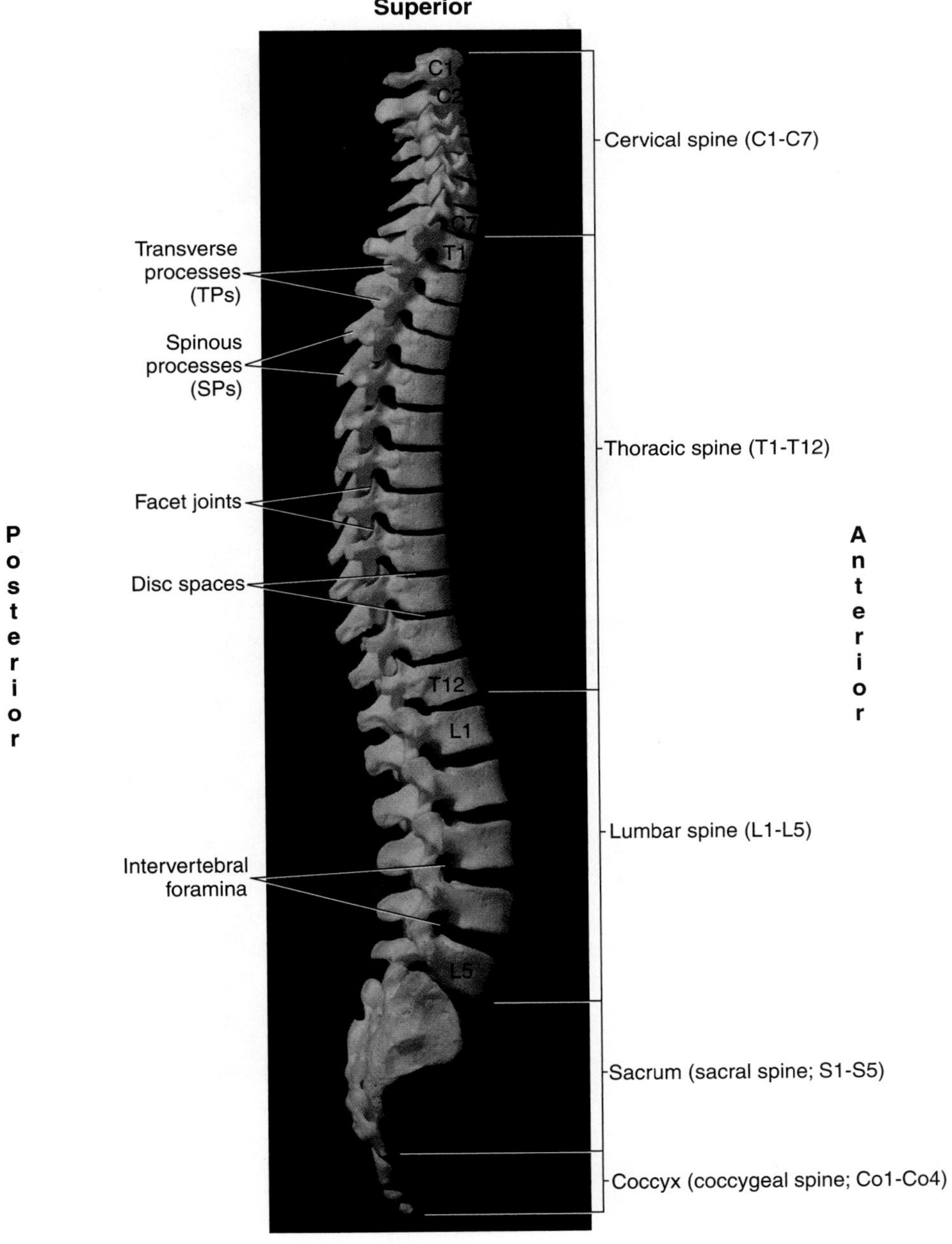

Figure 4-18

Notes:

1. Curves of the spine: The cervical and sacral spines are lordotic (i.e., concave posteriorly); the thoracic and sacral (sacrococcygeal) spines are kyphotic (i.e., concave anteriorly).
2. Generally a disc joint and paired right and left facet joints are found between each two contiguous vertebrae.
3. Intervertebral foramina (singular: foramen) are where spinal nerves enter/exit the spine.
4. Spinous processes (SPs) project posteriorly and are usually easily palpable (Note: The word *spine* means *thorn;* SPs are pointy like thorns).
5. Transverse processes (TPs) project laterally in the transverse plane (hence their name).
6. Because the spine is a weight-bearing structure, the bodies of the vertebrae (the weight-bearing aspect of the spinal column) get progressively larger from superior to inferior.

Cervical Spine and Hyoid

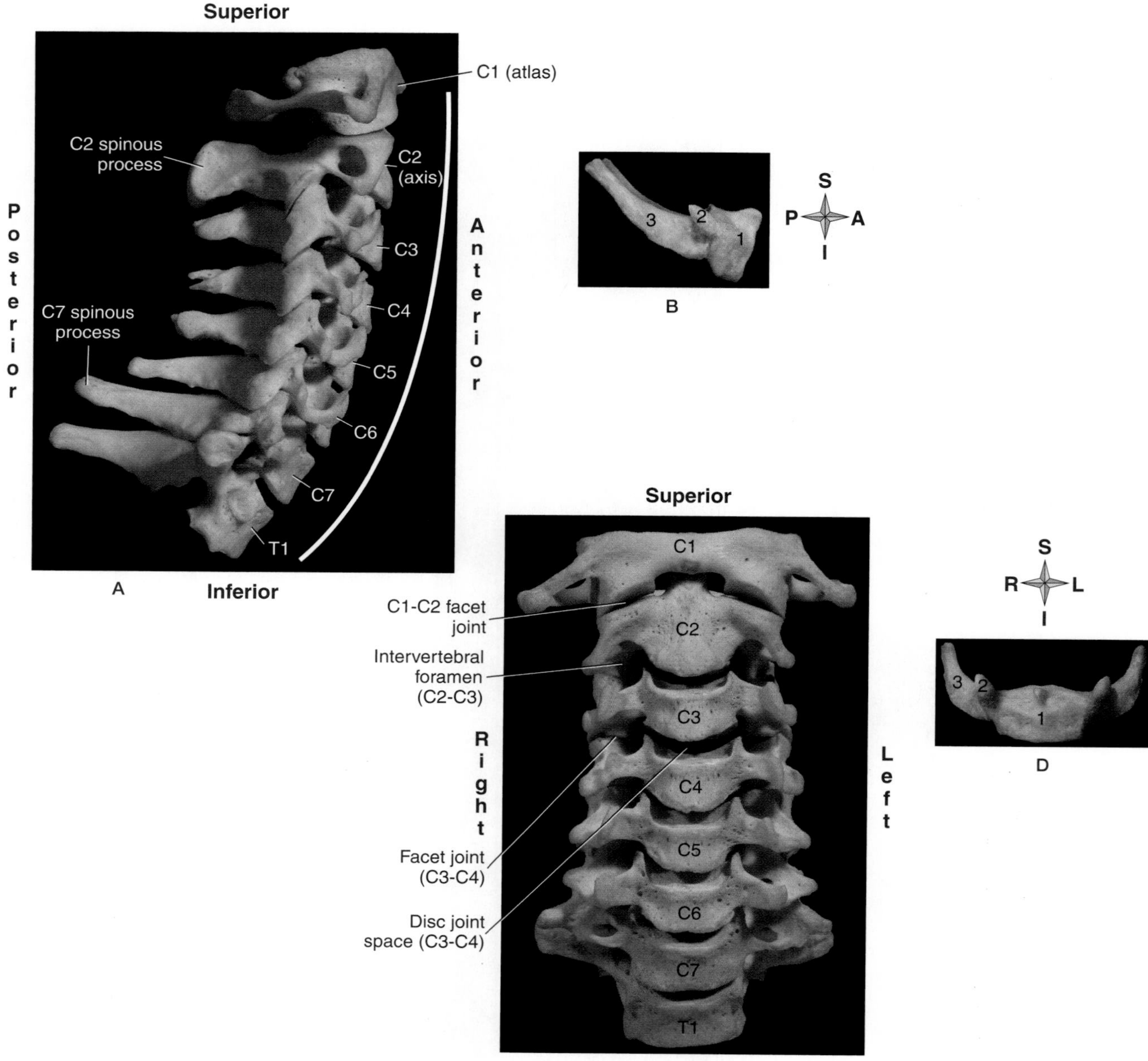

Figure 4-19a, b, c, and d
A, Right lateral view of the cervical spine; *B,* right lateral view of the hyoid bone; *C,* anterior view of the cervical spine, *D,* anterior view of the hyoid bone.

1 Body
2 Lesser cornu
3 Greater cornu

Notes:

1. The hyoid is located at the level of C3 vertebra.
2. The greater cornu and lesser cornu of the hyoid are also known as the *greater* and *lesser horns.*
3. The hyoid bone serves as an attachment site for the hyoid muscle group, as well as many muscles of the tongue.
4. The hyoid is the only bone in the human body that does not articulate with another bone.
5. The lordotic (i.e., concave posteriorly) curve of the cervical spine is indicated by the line drawn in anterior to the cervical spine.
6. The spinous processes (SPs) of C2 and C7 are very palpable and serve as excellent landmarks.

Cervical Spine (continued)

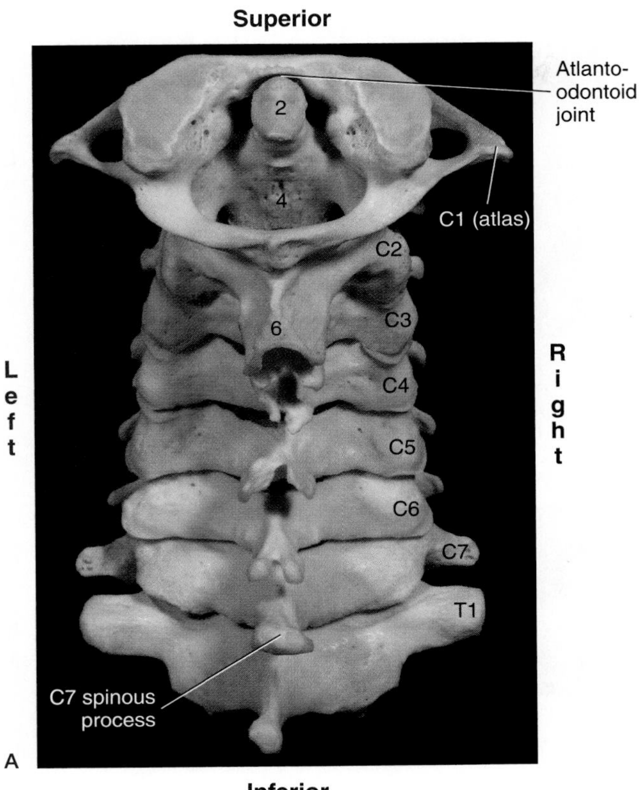

Superior

C2
spinous
process

C2
C3
C4
C5
C6
C7
T1

Intervertebral
foramen
(C3-C4)

C7
spinous
process

B

Inferior
Anterolateral oblique view

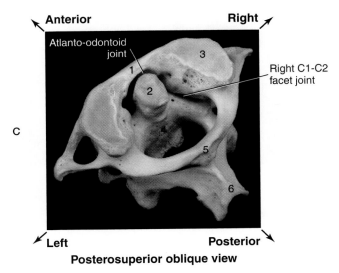

Anterior
Right

Atlanto-odontoid
joint

1
2
3
4
5
6

Right C1-C2
facet joint

C

Left
Posterior

Posterosuperior oblique view

Figure 4-20
A, Posterior view *B,* anterolateral oblique view; *C,* posterosuperior oblique view.

1 Anterior arch of C1 (atlas)
2 Dens of C2 (axis)
3 Superior articular process/facet of C1
4 Body of C2
5 Posterior tubercle of C1
6 Spinous process (SP) of C2

Notes:

1. The oblique view of the cervical spine demonstrates the intervertebral foramina well (the right C3-C4 intervertebral foramen is labeled). The intervertebral foramen is where the spinal nerve enters/exits the spinal cord.
2. The posterosuperior oblique view demonstrates the atlantoaxial joint complex well (Figure 4-20c).

Atlas (C1)

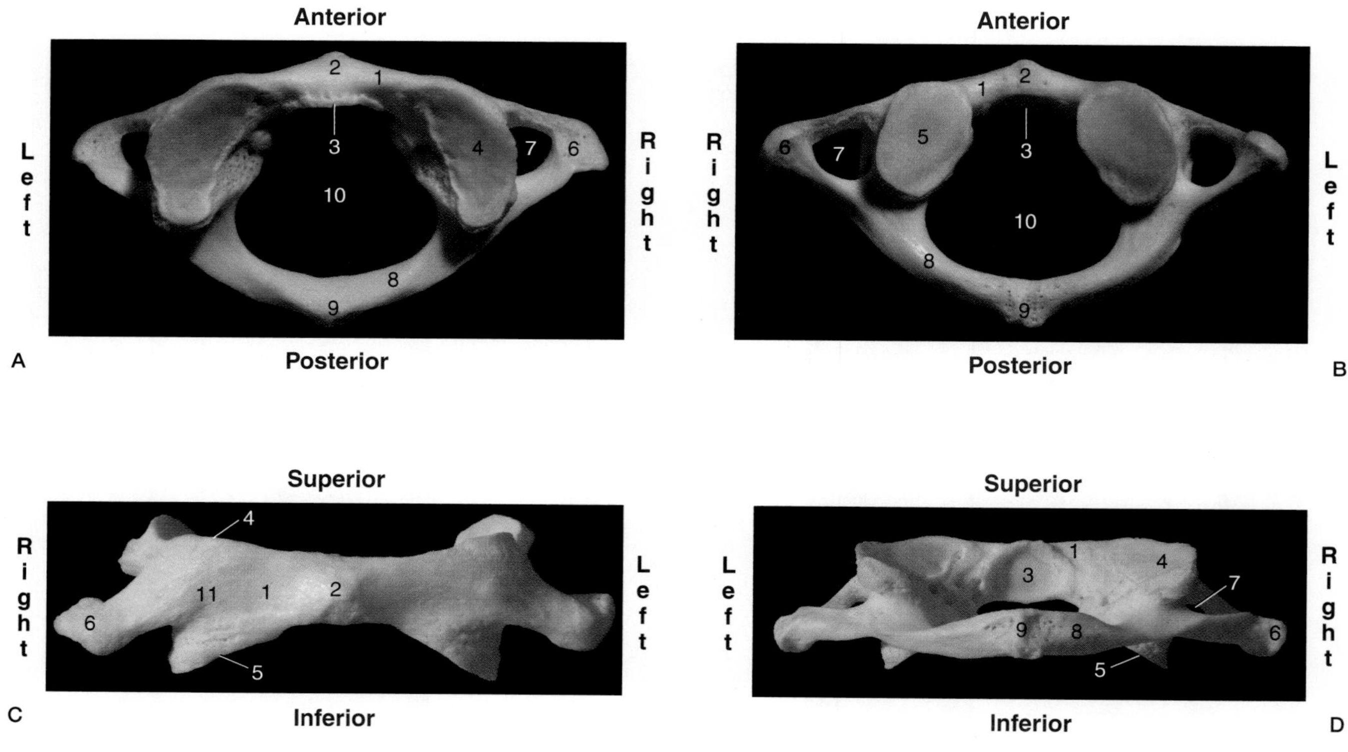

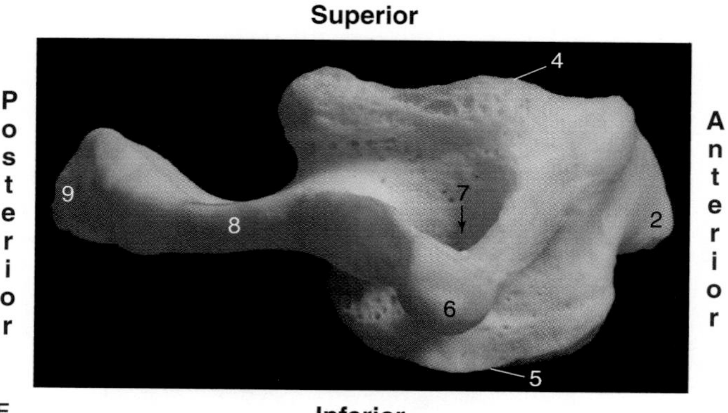

Figure 4-21
A, Superior view; *B,* inferior view; *C,* anterior view; *D,* posterior view; *E,* right lateral view.

1 Anterior arch
2 Anterior tubercle
3 Facet for dens of axis (C2)
4 Superior articular process/facet
5 Inferior articular process/facet
6 Transverse process (TP)
7 Transverse foramen
8 Posterior arch
9 Posterior tubercle
10 Vertebral foramen
11 Lateral mass

Notes:

1. Unlike the other vertebrae, the atlas has no body. What would have been the body of the atlas became the dens of the axis (C2).
2. Also unique to the atlas are the anterior and posterior arches. The centers of these arches have the anterior and posterior tubercles, respectively.
3. The superior articular processes of the atlas articulate with the occipital condyles at the atlanto-occipital joint; the inferior articular processes of the atlas articulate with the superior articular processes of the axis at the atlantoaxial (C1-C2) joint.
4. The superior and inferior articular processes of the atlas create what is termed the *lateral mass* (labeled in the anterior view).

Axis (C2)

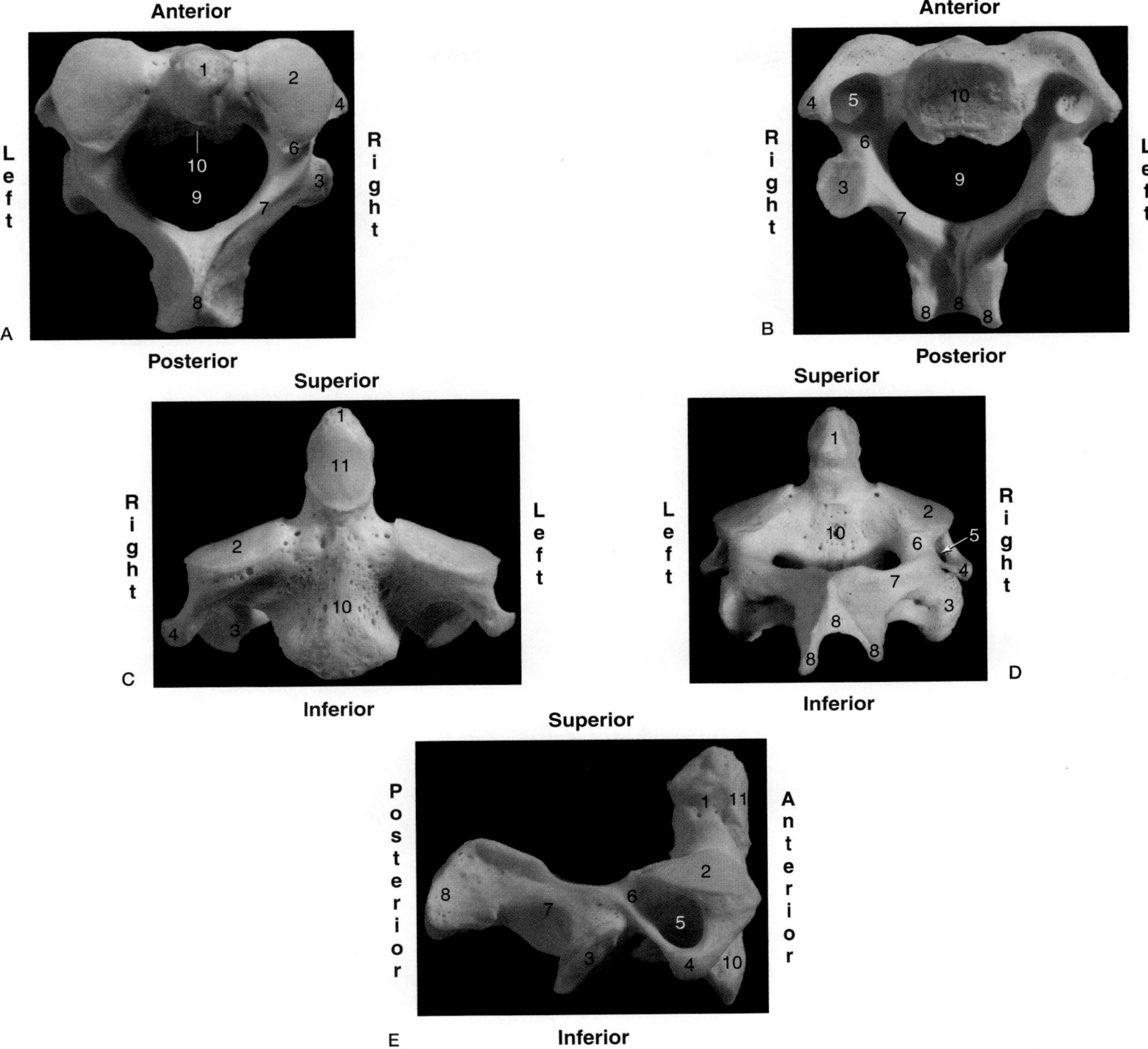

Figure 4-22
A, Superior view; *B,* inferior view; *C,* anterior view; *D,* posterior view; *E,* right lateral view.

1 Dens (odontoid process)
2 Superior articular process/facet
3 Inferior articular process/facet
4 Transverse process (TP)
5 Transverse foramen
6 Pedicle
7 Lamina
8 Spinous process (SP) (bifid)
9 Vertebral foramen
10 Body
11 Facet on dens

Notes:

1. The dens of the axis creates an axis of rotation for the atlas to rotate about, hence the name of *C2* (i.e., the axis).
2. The superior articular processes of the axis articulate with the inferior articular processes of the atlas.
3. The spinous process (SP) of C2 is very large and an excellent landmark when palpating a client's posterior neck. It will be the first large structure felt midline, inferior to the skull.
4. The SP of the axis is bifid. Further, the two bifid points are often asymmetric in size and shape.
5. The facet on the dens articulates with the anterior arch of the atlas, forming the atlanto-odontoid joint.

C5 (Typical Cervical Vertebra)

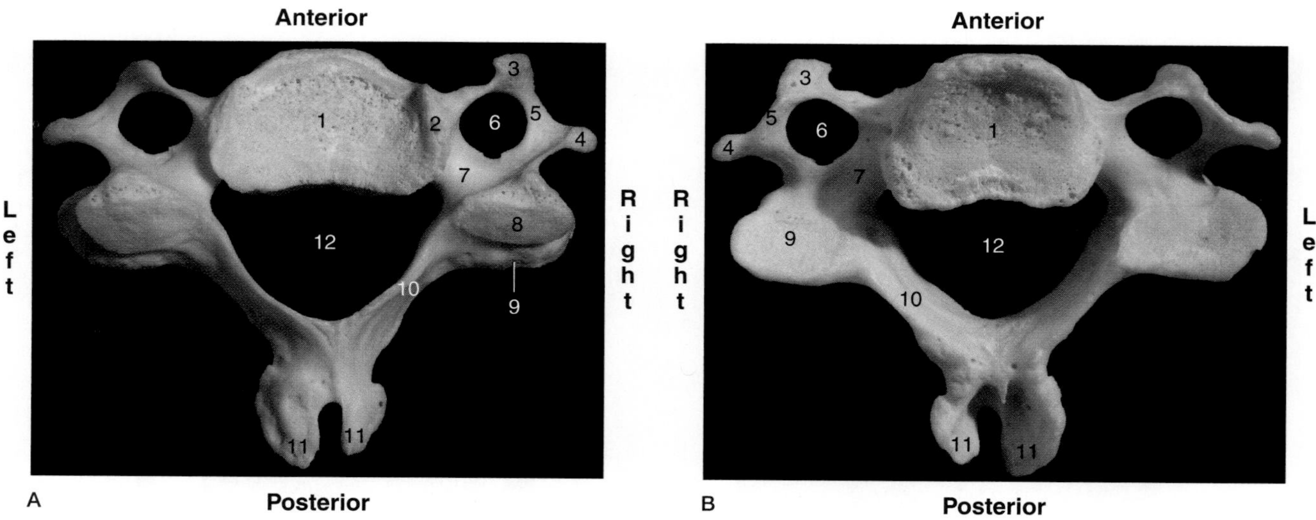

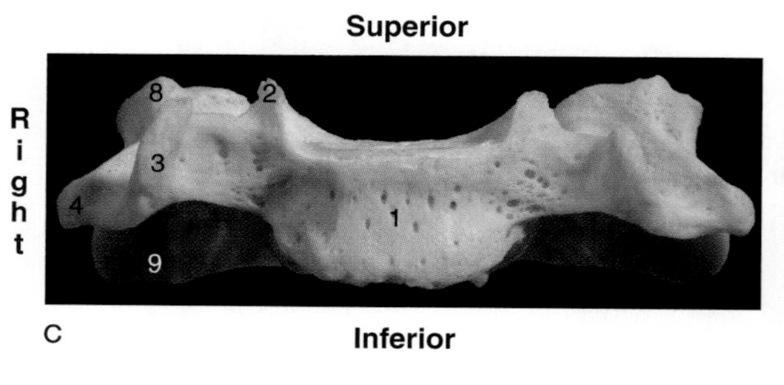

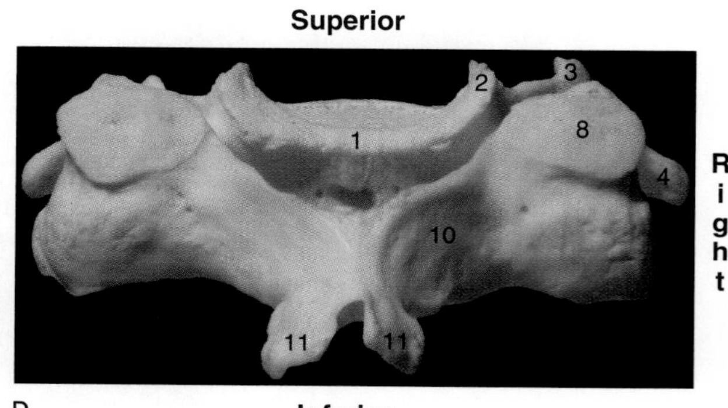

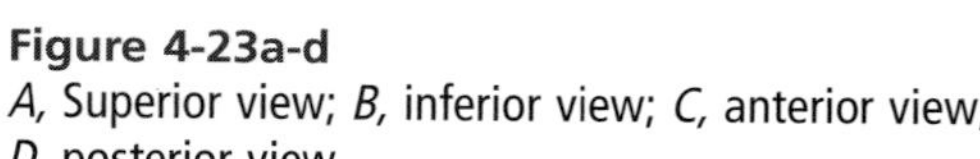

Figure 4-23a-d
A, Superior view; *B,* inferior view; *C,* anterior view; *D,* posterior view.

1 Body
2 Uncus of body
3 Anterior tubercle of transverse process (TP)
4 Posterior tubercle of TP
5 Groove for spinal nerve (on TP)
6 Transverse foramen
7 Pedicle
8 Superior articular process/facet
9 Inferior articular process/facet
10 Lamina
11 Spinous process (SP) (bifid)
12 Vertebral foramen

Notes:

1. The articular process is the entire structural landmark that projects outward from the bone; the articular facet is the smooth articular surface located on the articular process.
2. Plural of foramen is *foramina.*
3. The cervical vertebrae possess a number of structures that the other vertebrae do not: an uncus is located on the left and right sides of the body; they have bifid (i.e., two points on their) spinous processes (SPs); their transverse processes (TPs) have an anterior and posterior tubercle; and they have a foramen located within the TP (hence the name *transverse foramen*).
4. The bifid SP of a cervical vertebra is often asymmetric. This may lead one to conclude on palpatory exam that the vertebra is rotated when it is not.
5. The cervical transverse foramen allows passage up to the skull of the vertebral artery.

C5 (continued) and Cervical Endplates

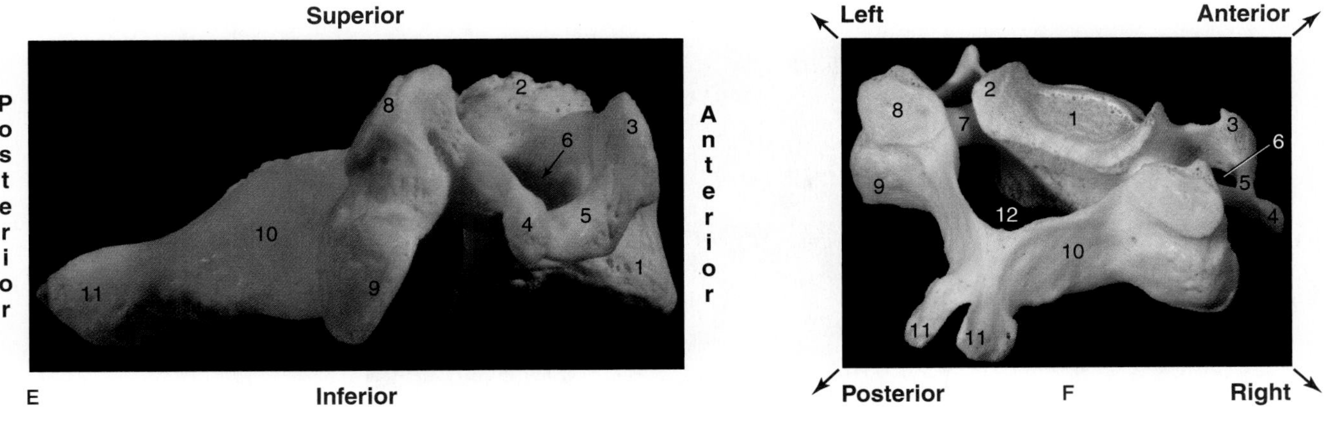

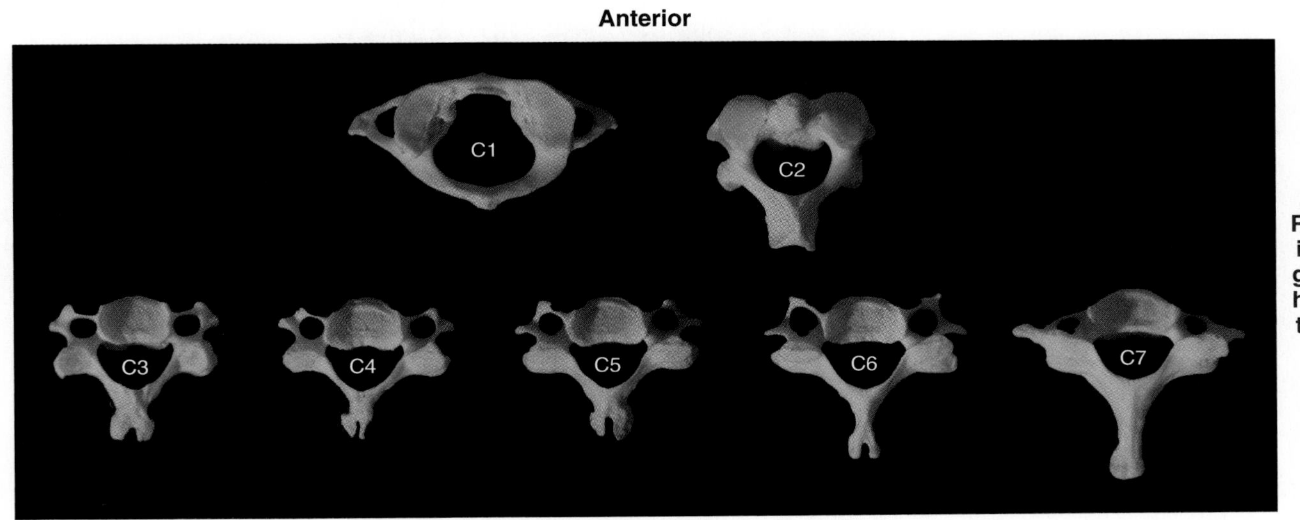

Figure 4-24

Figure 4-23e, f, and Figure 4-24
E, Right lateral view; *F,* oblique posterior view.

1 Body
2 Uncus of body
3 Anterior tubercle of transverse process (TP)
4 Posterior tubercle of TP
5 Groove for spinal nerve (on TP)
6 Transverse foramen
7 Pedicle
8 Superior articular process/facet
9 Inferior articular process/facet
10 Lamina
11 Spinous process (SP) (bifid)
12 Vertebral foramen

Notes:

1. Figure 4-24 shows the superior view of all seven cervical vertebrae (cervical endplate view). The differences from one cervical level to another can be seen.
2. C1 is also known as the *atlas*; C2 is also known as the *axis*.
3. The anterior tubercle of the transverse process (TP) of C6 is larger than the other anterior tubercles and is known as the *carotid tubercle*.
4. The large spinous process (SP) of C7 more closely resembles the SPs of the thoracic vertebrae than it does the other cervical vertebrae. This large SP gives C7 its name, the *vertebra prominens*.

Thoracic Spine—Right Lateral View

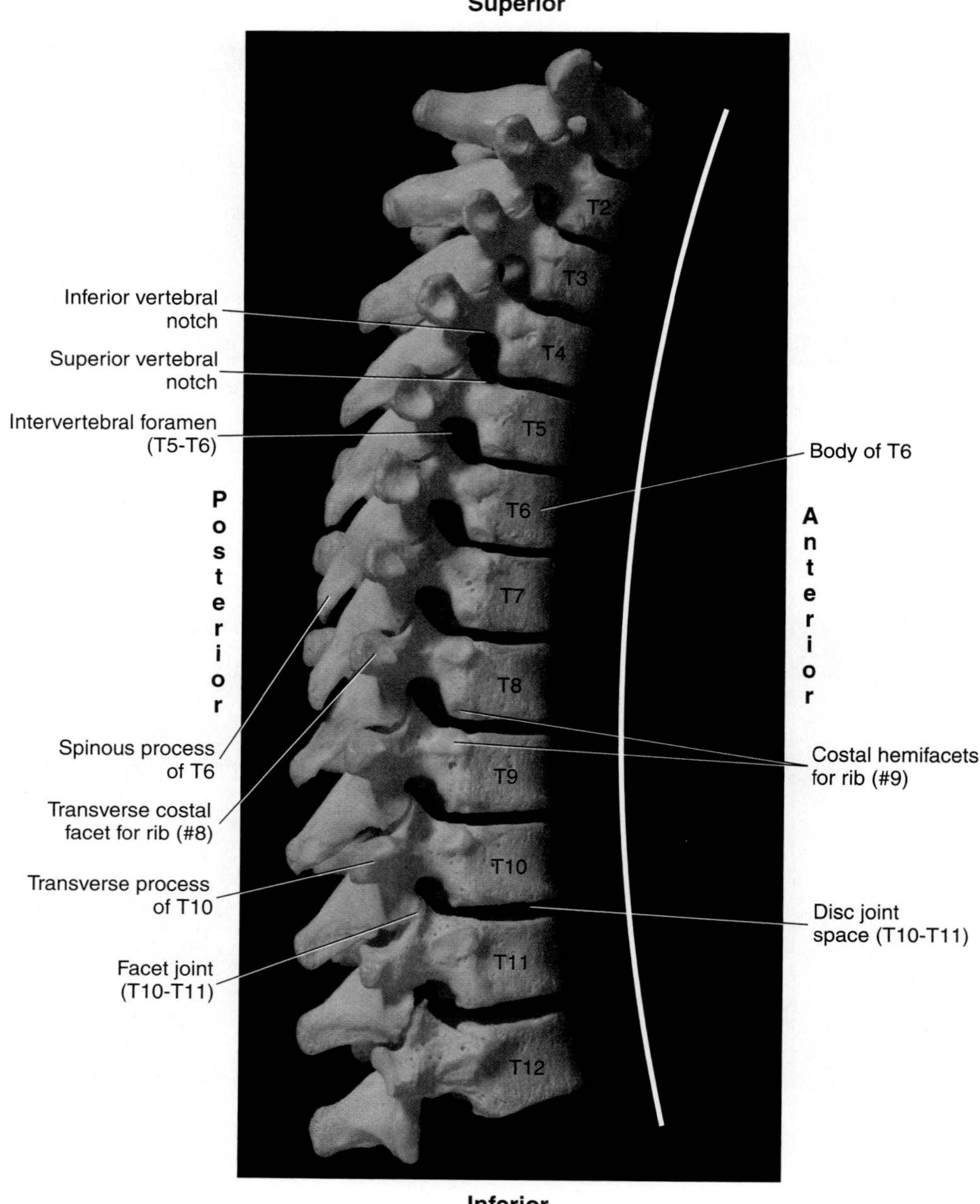

Figure 4-25

Notes:

1. The kyphotic (i.e., concave anteriorly) curve of the thoracic spine is indicated by the line drawn in anterior to the thoracic spine.
2. The lateral view of the thoracic spine demonstrates the intervertebral foramina well (the right T5-T6 intervertebral foramen is labeled). The intervertebral foramen is where the spinal nerve enters/exits the spinal cord.
3. The long downward-slanted orientation of the thoracic spinous processes (SPs), especially of the midthoracic spine, can be seen. The tip of a thoracic SP is at the level of the body of the vertebra below it (e.g., see the body and SP of T6 labeled).
4. The SPs of the thoracic spine are easily palpable (the word *spine* means *thorn* [i.e., a pointy projection]).
5. The vertebral body costal hemifacets for a rib (i.e., for the costovertebral joint) are labeled at the T8-T9 level. They are located on two contiguous vertebral bodies and span across the disc that is located between.
6. The transverse costal facet for a rib (i.e., for the costotransverse joint) is labeled at the T8 level.
7. The gradual increase in size of the thoracic vertebral bodies from T1 to T12 can be seen.

Thoracic Spine—Posterior View

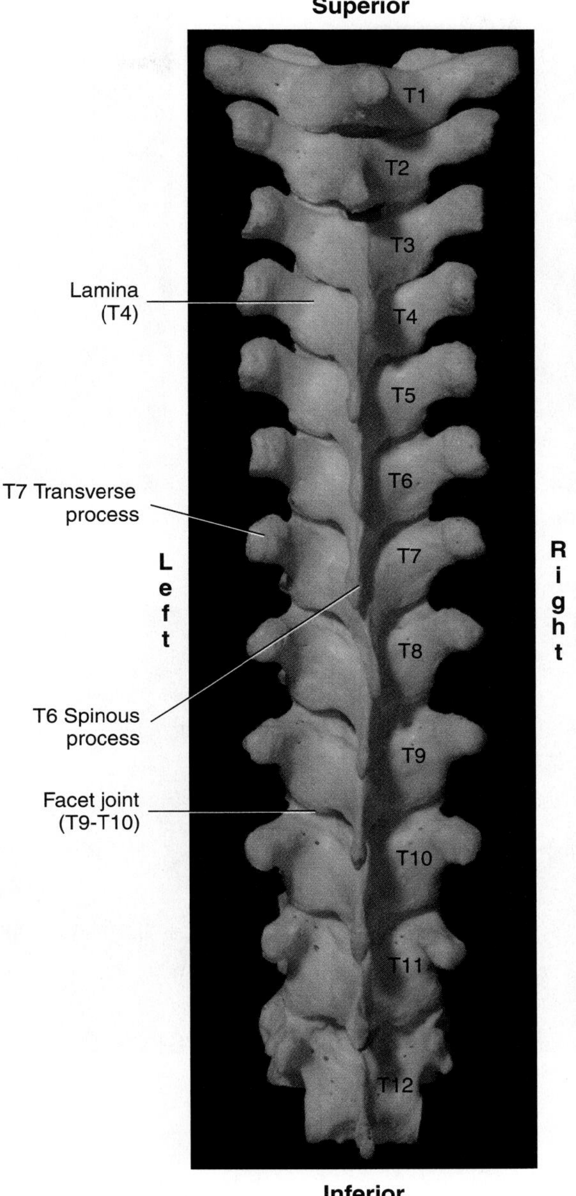

Figure 4-26

Notes:

1. The differences in spinous processes (SPs) from T1 to T12 can be seen.
2. The SP of T6 and the transverse process (TP) of T7 are labeled, illustrating the relative location of a vertebral TP relative to the more palpable SP of the vertebra above. When palpating the thoracic spine (especially the midthoracic spine), the downward slope of the SPs should be kept in mind.
3. The TPs of the spine project laterally into the transverse plane, hence their name.
4. The crooked SP of T7 of this specimen can be seen; bones of the body often have slight asymmetries such as this. A flexible understanding of the shapes of bones is important; otherwise the crooked SP of T7 in this case could be interpreted as a rotated vertebra when in fact it is not.

T5 (Typical Thoracic Vertebra)

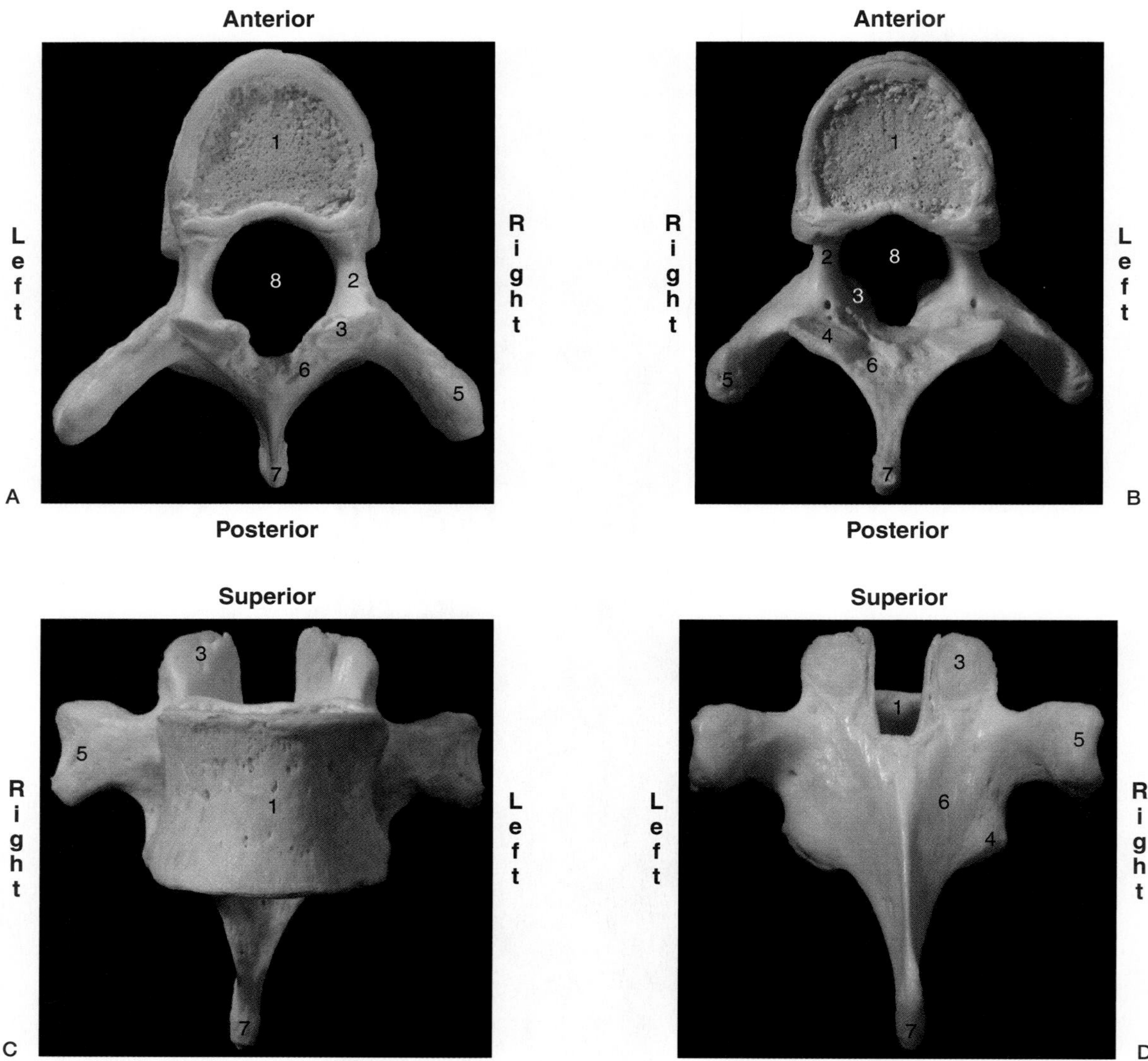

Figure 4-27a-d
A, Superior view; *B,* inferior view; *C,* anterior view; *D,* posterior view.

1 Body
2 Pedicle
3 Superior articular process/facet
4 Inferior articular process/facet
5 Transverse process (TP)
6 Lamina
7 Spinous process (SP)
8 Vertebral foramen

Notes:

1. The pedicle of a vertebra is the structure that connects the body to the rest of the structures of the vertebra. If one looks at the superior or inferior view of a vertebra such that the body is at the bottom of the page, the pedicles may be viewed as the feet (*ped* means *foot*) of a statue that is standing on its base or pedestal (the body of the vertebra being analogous to the base or pedestal of the statue).
2. The articular process is the entire structural landmark that projects outward from the bone; the articular facet is the smooth articular surface located on the articular process.
3. The laminae (singular: lamina) may be viewed as laminating together to form the spinous process (SP) of a vertebra.
4. Plural of foramen is foramina.
5. The vertebral foramina of the spinal column create the spinal canal though which the spinal cord runs.

T5 (continued) and Thoracic Endplates

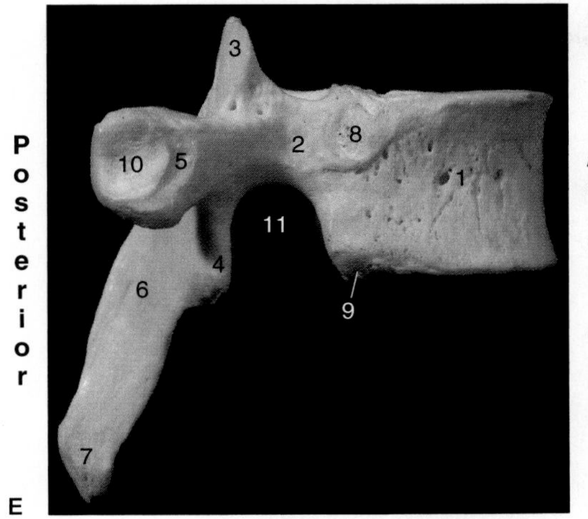

S A
P I

F

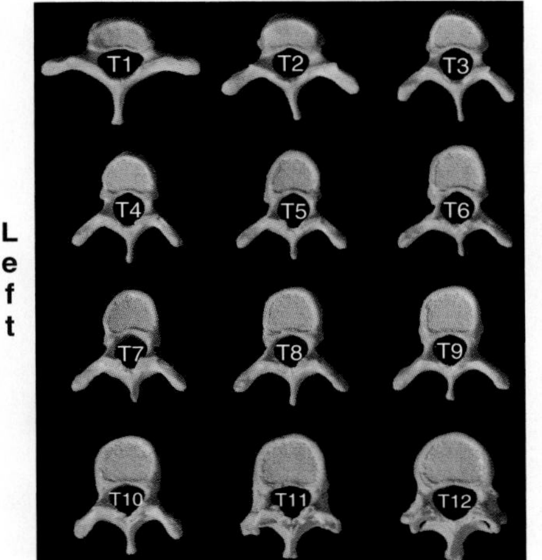

Figure 4-28

Figure 4-27e, f, and Figure 4-28
E, Right lateral view; *F,* posterior oblique view.

1 Body
2 Pedicle
3 Superior articular process/facet
4 Inferior articular process/facet
5 Transverse process (TP)
6 Lamina
7 Spinous process (SP)
8 Superior costal hemifacet
9 Inferior costal hemifacet
10 Transverse costal facet
11 Intervertebral foramen
12 Inferior vertebral notch
13 Superior vertebral notch

Notes:

1. The superior and inferior costal hemifacets on the bodies are the vertebral articular surfaces for the costovertebral joint; the transverse costal facet on the transverse process (TP) is the vertebral articular surface for the costotransverse joint.
2. The lateral view of a thoracic vertebra is ideal for visualizing the intervertebral foramen, which is formed by the inferior vertebral notch of the superior vertebra (see #12) juxtaposed next to the superior vertebral notch of the inferior vertebra (see #13).
3. Figure 4-28 shows a superior view of all twelve thoracic vertebrae (thoracic endplate view). A gradual change in the shape of the thoracic vertebrae is seen from superior to inferior. Specifically, the change in the shape of the spinous processes (SPs) and bodies can be seen.
4. Costal hemifacets on the bodies of thoracic vertebrae usually create the articular surface for the costovertebral joints of ribs #2-10. Usually, T1, T11, and T12 have full facets for ribs #1, 11, and 12, respectively (see Figure 4-25 on page 102).

Lumbar Spine—Right Lateral View

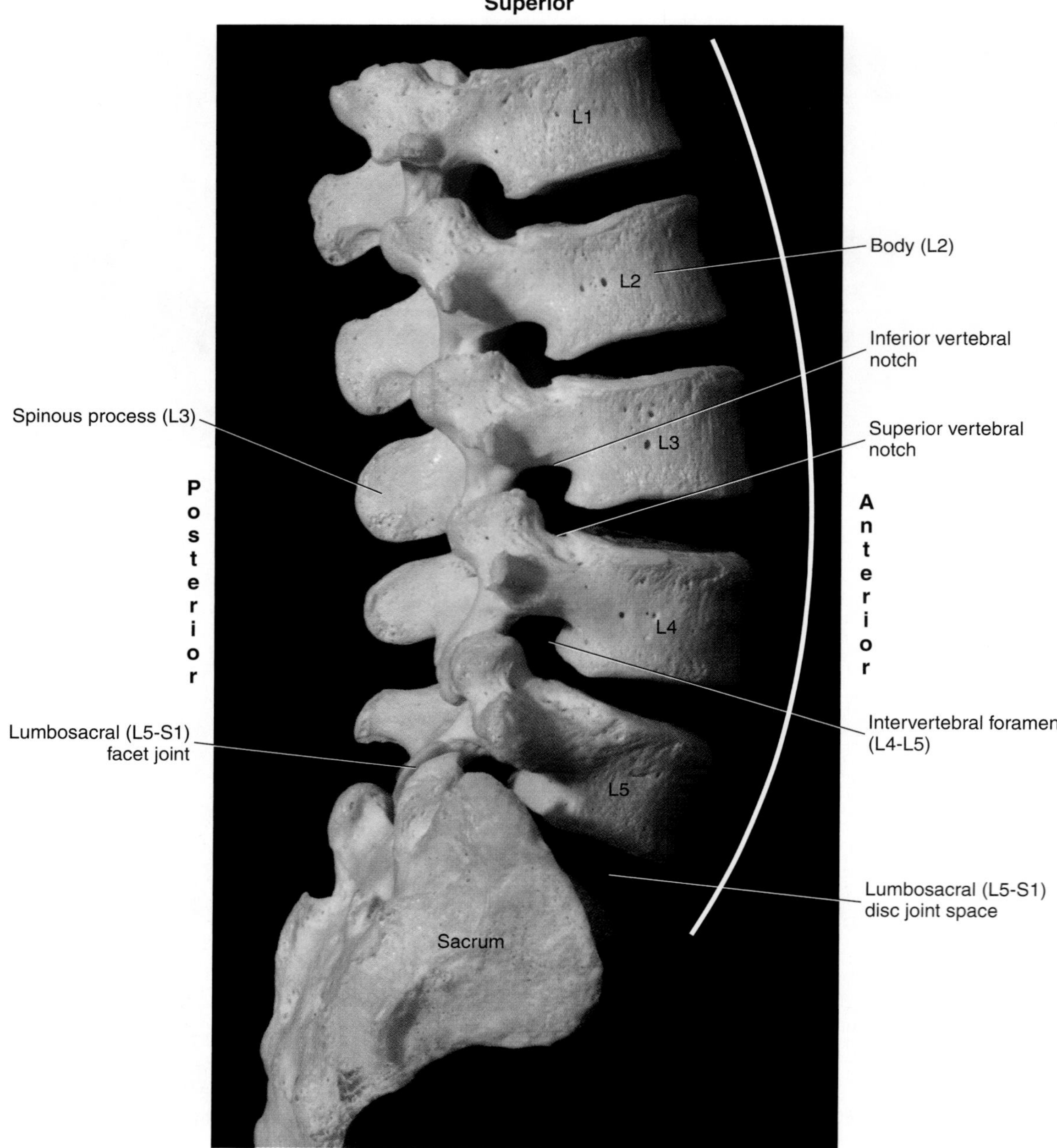

Figure 4-29

Notes:

1. Note the lordotic (concave posteriorly) curve of the lumbar spine (indicated by the line drawn in anterior to the lumbar spine).
2. The lateral view of the lumbar spine demonstrates the intervertebral foramina (the right L4-L5 intervertebral foramen is labeled). The intervertebral foramen is where the spinal nerve enters/exits the spinal cord.
3. Note the large blunt quadrate shaped lumbar spinous processes.
4. The spinous processes of the lumbar spine may be difficult to palpate depending upon the degree of the client's lordotic curve.
5. The disc joint spaces are well visualized in the lateral view.

Lumbar Spine—Posterior View

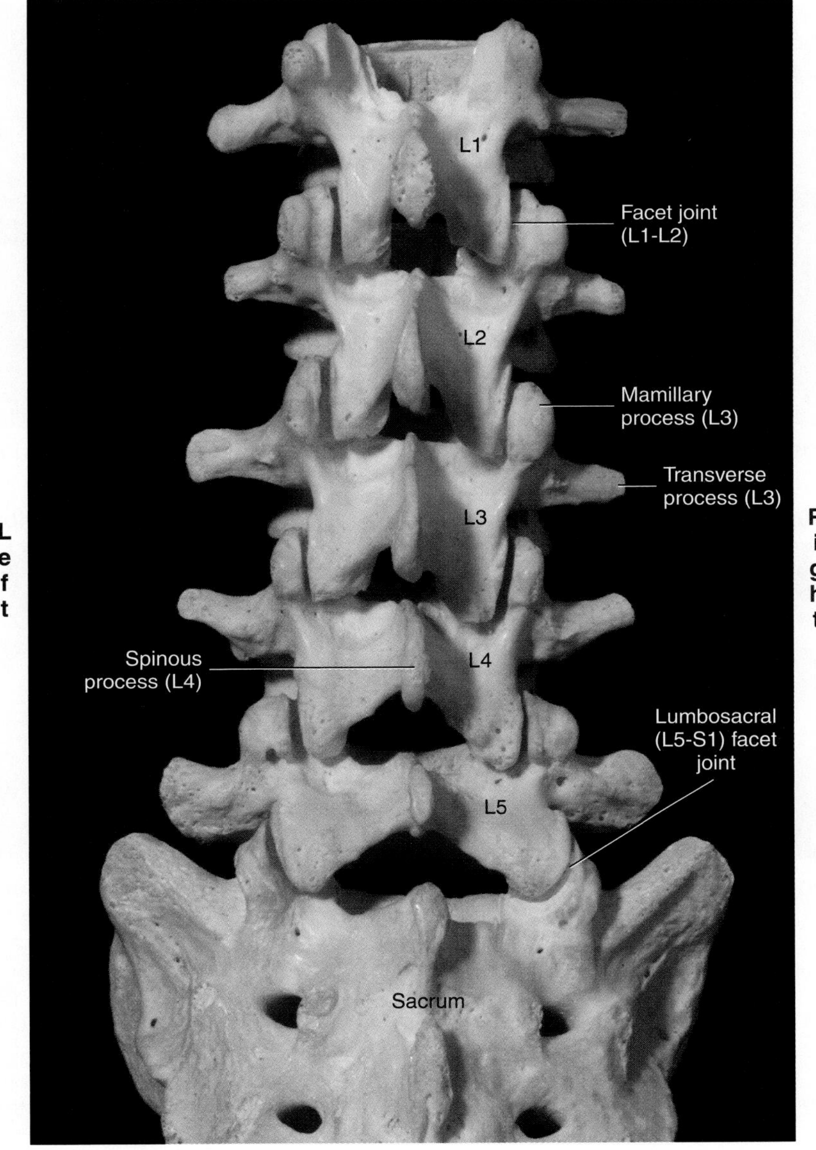

Figure 4-30

Notes:

1. The facet joints of the lumbar spine are well visualized in the posterior view because they are oriented in the sagittal plane.
2. The lumbosacral (L5-S1) facet joints change their orientation; they are oriented more toward the frontal plane than are the other lumbar facet joints.
3. The prominence of the mamillary processes of the lumbar spine can be seen.

L3 (Typical Lumbar Vertebra)

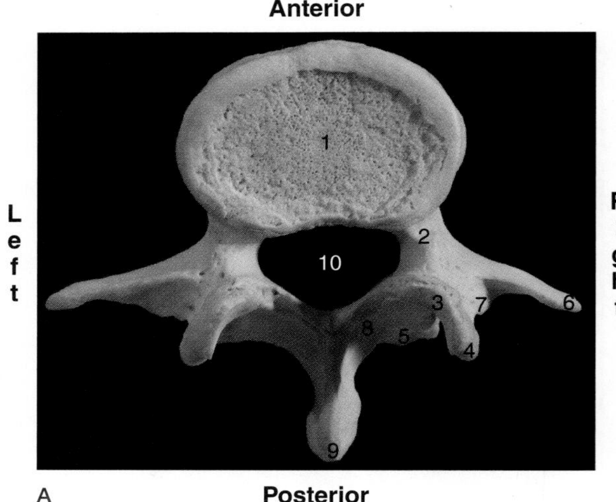

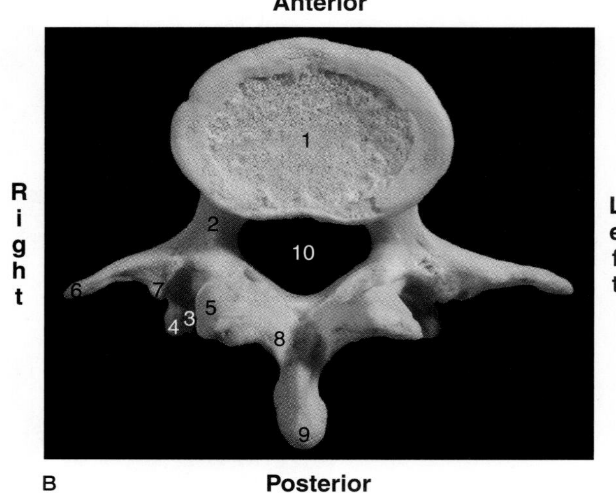

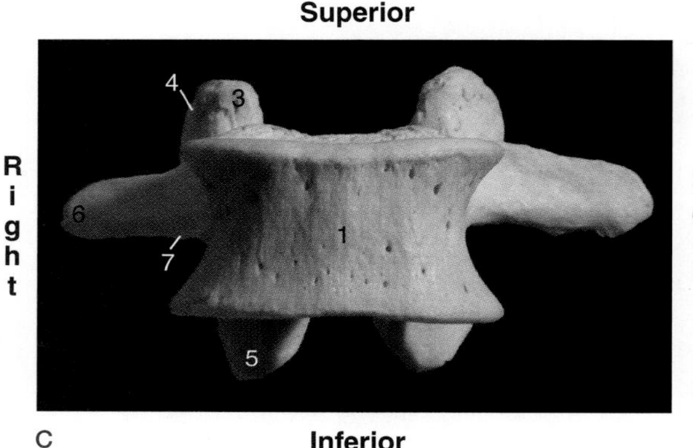

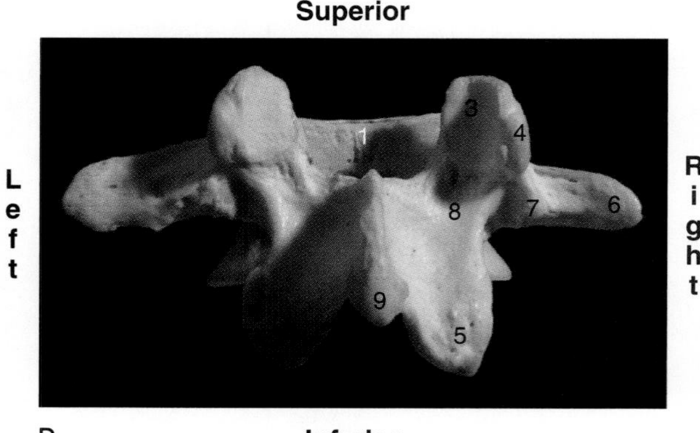

Figure 4-31a-d
A, Superior view; *B,* inferior view; *C,* anterior view; *D,* posterior view.

1 Body
2 Pedicle
3 Superior articular process/facet
4 Mamillary process
5 Inferior articular process/facet
6 Transverse process (TP)
7 Accessory process
8 Lamina
9 Spinous process (SP)
10 Vertebral foramen

Notes:

1. The bodies of lumbar vertebrae are very large because they need to bear all the body weight from above.
2. The articular process is the entire structural landmark that projects outward from the bone; the articular facet is the smooth articular surface located on the articular process.
3. Lumbar vertebrae are unique in that they possess two additional landmarks, mamillary, and accessory processes. The mamillary process is located on the superior articular process; the accessory process is located on the transverse process.
4. Plural of foramen is *foramina.*

L3 (continued) and Lumbar Endplates

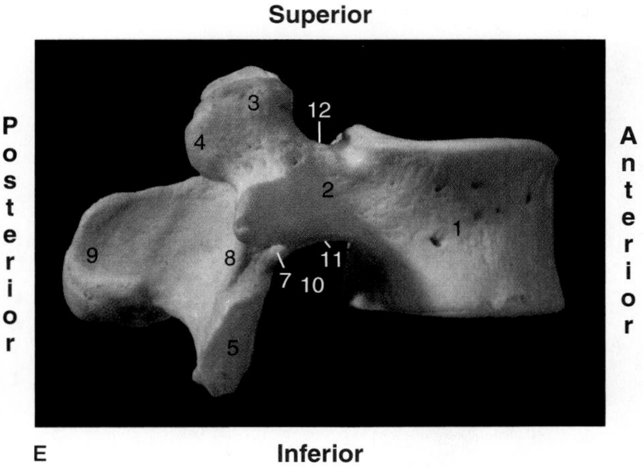

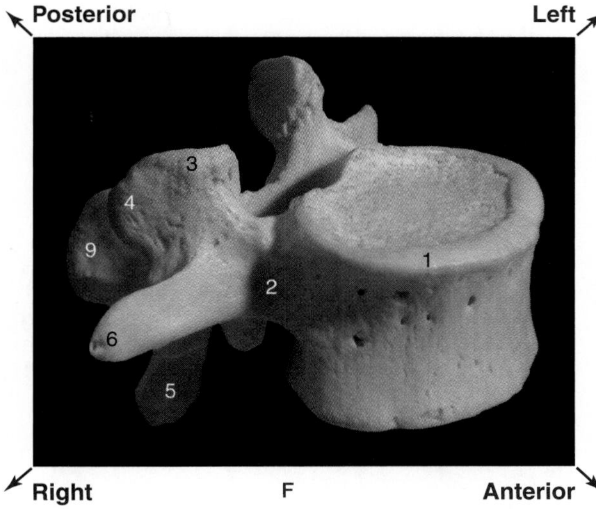

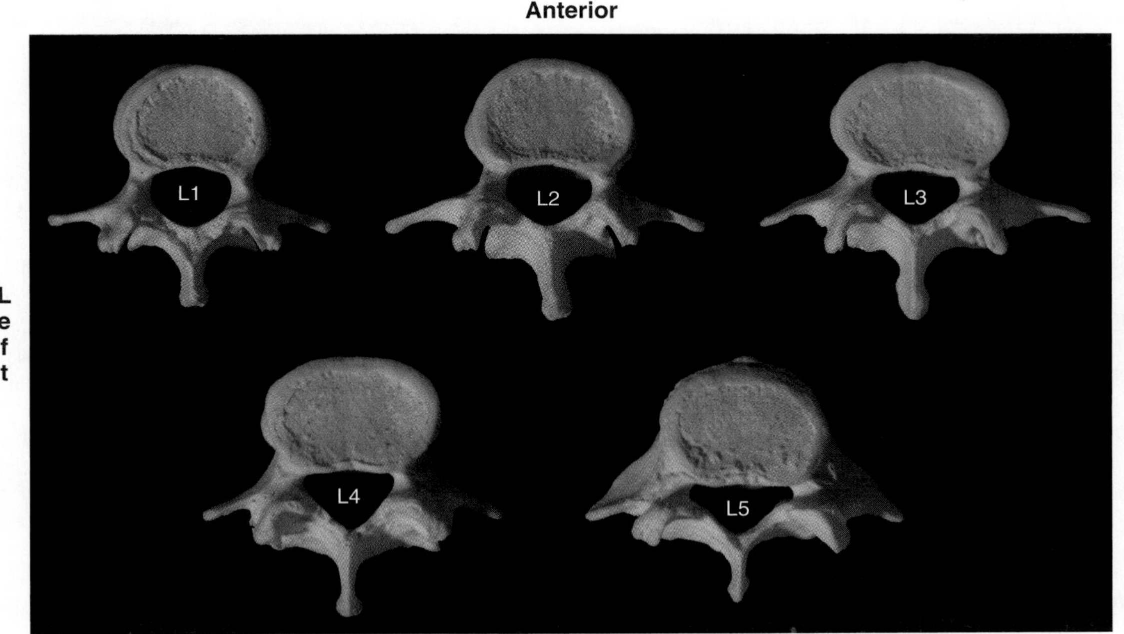

Figure 4-32

Figure 4-31e, f, and Figure 4-32
E, Right lateral view; *F,* anterior oblique view.

1 Body
2 Pedicle
3 Superior articular process/facet
4 Mamillary process
5 Inferior articular process/facet
6 Transverse process (TP)
7 Accessory process
8 Lamina
9 Spinous process (SP)
10 Intervertebral foramen
11 Inferior vertebral notch
12 Superior vertebral notch

Notes:

1. Lumbar vertebrae possess large, blunt, quadrate-shaped spinous processes (SPs), as evident in the lateral view.
2. Figure 4-32 shows a superior view of all five lumbar vertebrae (lumbar endplate view). The transition in shape from superior to inferior can be seen.

Sacrococcygeal Spine

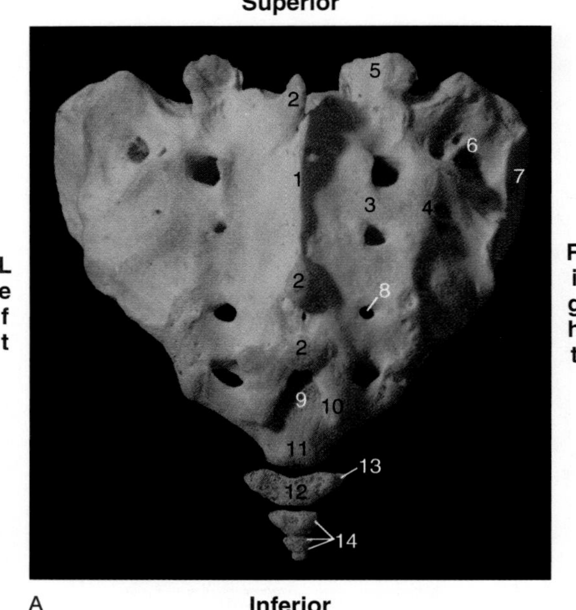

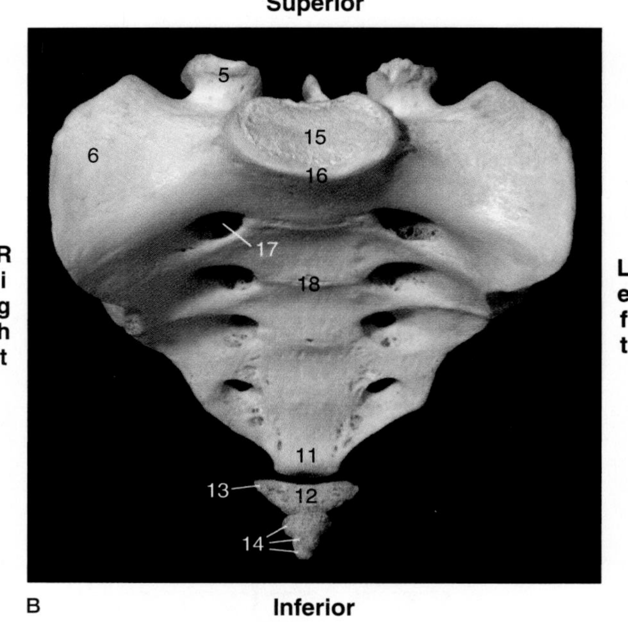

Figure 4-33a and b
A, Posterior view; *B,* anterior view.

1 Median sacral crest
2 Tubercles along the median sacral crest
3 Intermediate sacral crest
4 Lateral sacral crest
5 Superior articular process/facet
6 Ala (wing)
7 Auricular surface (articular surface for ilium)
8 3rd Posterior foramen
9 Sacral hiatus
10 Sacral cornu
11 Apex
12 1st Coccygeal element
13 Coccygeal transverse process (TP)
14 2nd to 4th Coccygeal elements (fused)
15 Sacral base
16 Sacral promontory
17 1st Anterior foramen
18 Fusion of 2nd and 3rd sacral vertebrae

Notes:

1. The sacrum is formed by the fusion of five sacral vertebrae.
2. The sacrum is shaped like an upside-down triangle. The sacral base is located superiorly; the sacral apex is located inferiorly.
3. The medial crest is the fusion of the sacral spinous processes (SPs); the intermediate crest is the fusion of the articular processes; the lateral crest is the fusion of the transverse processes (TPs).
4. The median sacral crest often has projections (remnants of SPs) that are called *sacral tubercles.* This specimen has prominent 1st (asymmetric) and 3rd sacral tubercles.
5. The superior articular processes of the sacrum articulate with the inferior articular processes of L5 (forming the lumbosacral [L5-S1] facet joints).
6. The sacral ala is the winglike superolateral aspect of the sacrum (*ala* means *wing*).
7. Four pairs of posterior and four pairs of anterior sacral foramina exist where sacral spinal nerves enter/exit the spinal canal.
8. The sacral hiatus is the inferior opening of the sacral canal.
9. The coccyx is usually composed of four rudimentary vertebrae; however, the number may vary from two to five. Some sources state that the coccyx is the evolutionary remnant of a tail.

Sacrococcygeal Spine (continued)

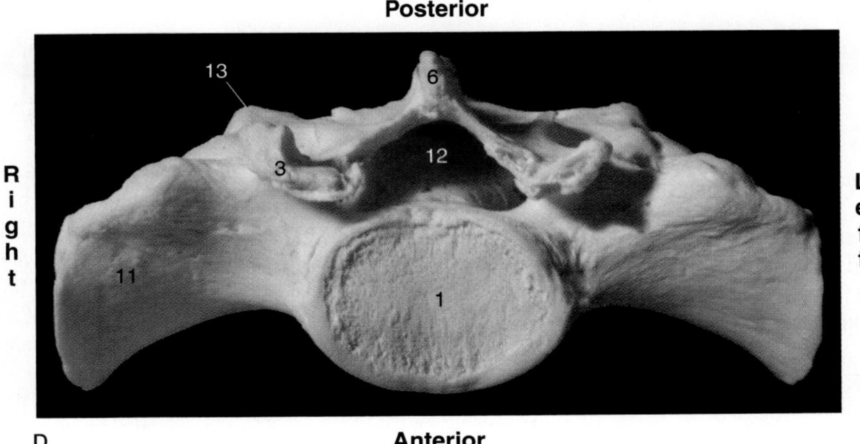

Figure 4-33c-d
C, Right lateral view; *D,* superior view.

1 Base
2 Promontory
3 Superior articular process
4 Auricular surface (articular surface for ilium)
5 1st Posterior foramen
6 (Tubercles of) median sacral crest
7 Cornu
8 Apex
9 1st Coccygeal element
10 2nd to 4th Coccygeal elements
11 Ala (wing)
12 Sacral canal
13 Lateral sacral crest

Notes:

1. The kyphotic (i.e., concave anteriorly) curve of the sacrococcygeal spine is indicated by the line drawn in anterior to the sacrococcygeal spine.
2. The body of L5 sits on the base of the sacrum, forming the lumbosacral (L5-S1) disc joint.
3. The sacral promontory is the portion of the base of the sacrum that projects anteriorly.
4. The cauda equina of nerves from the spinal cord travel through the sacral canal.

☐ 4.3 BONES OF THE RIBCAGE AND STERNUM

Ribcage—Anterior View

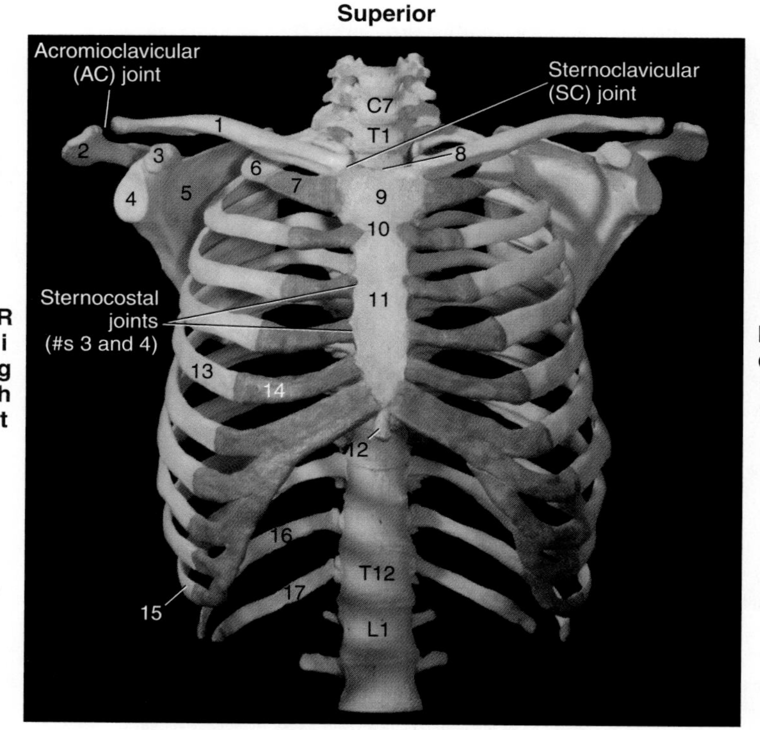

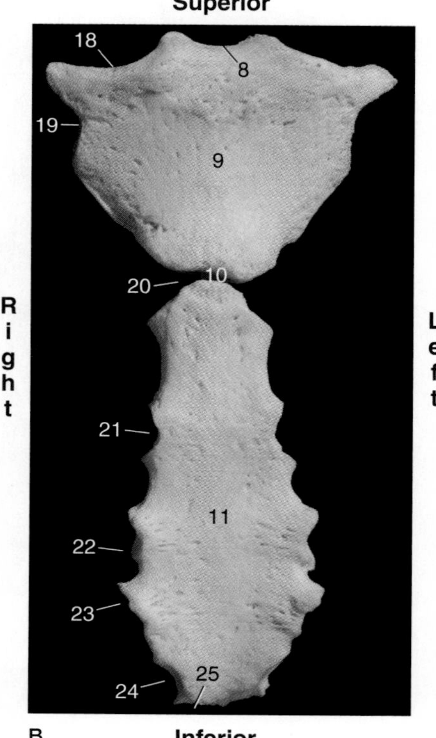

Figure 4-34a and b
1 Clavicle
2 Acromion process
3 Coracoid process
4 Glenoid fossa
5 Subscapular fossa
6 1st Rib
7 Cartilage of 1st rib
8 Sternal notch
9 Manubrium of sternum
10 Sternal angle
11 Body of sternum
12 Xiphoid process of sternum
13 5th Rib
14 Cartilage of 5th Rib
15 10th Rib
16 11th Rib
17 12th Rib
18 Clavicular notch of the manubrium
19 Notch for 1st costal cartilage
20 Notch for 2nd costal cartilage
21 Notch for 3rd costal cartilage
22 Notch for 4th costal cartilage
23 Notch for 5th costal cartilage
24 Notch for 6th costal cartilage
25 Notch for 7th costal cartilage

Notes:

1. The sternal notch is also known as the *jugular notch.*
2. The lateral border of the sternal notch is a good landmark to palpate movement of the sternoclavicular (SC) joint.
3. The sternal angle is also known as the *angle of Louis* and is the joint between the manubrium and body of the sternum. It is located at the junction of the 2nd costal cartilage with the sternum and is often palpable.
4. The xiphoid process remains cartilaginous long into life and is also a landmark used to locate the proper location to administer cardiopulmonary resuscitation (CPR).
5. The ribcage is composed of 12 pairs of ribs. Of these, the first seven pairs (#1-7) are called *true ribs,* because their costal cartilages articulate directly with the sternum. The last five pairs (#8-12) of ribs are called *false ribs,* because they do not articulate directly to the sternum; pairs #8-10 have their cartilage join the costal cartilage of rib #7, and ribs #11 and 12 do not articulate with the sternum at all. Because the last two pairs of false ribs do not attach to the sternum at all, they are called *floating ribs.*
6. The attachment of a rib to the sternum via its costal cartilage is called a *sternocostal joint.*
7. The sternums in *A* and *B* are not the same. The differences in the shape of the manubrium and body of these two specimens can be seen.

Ribcage—Right Lateral View

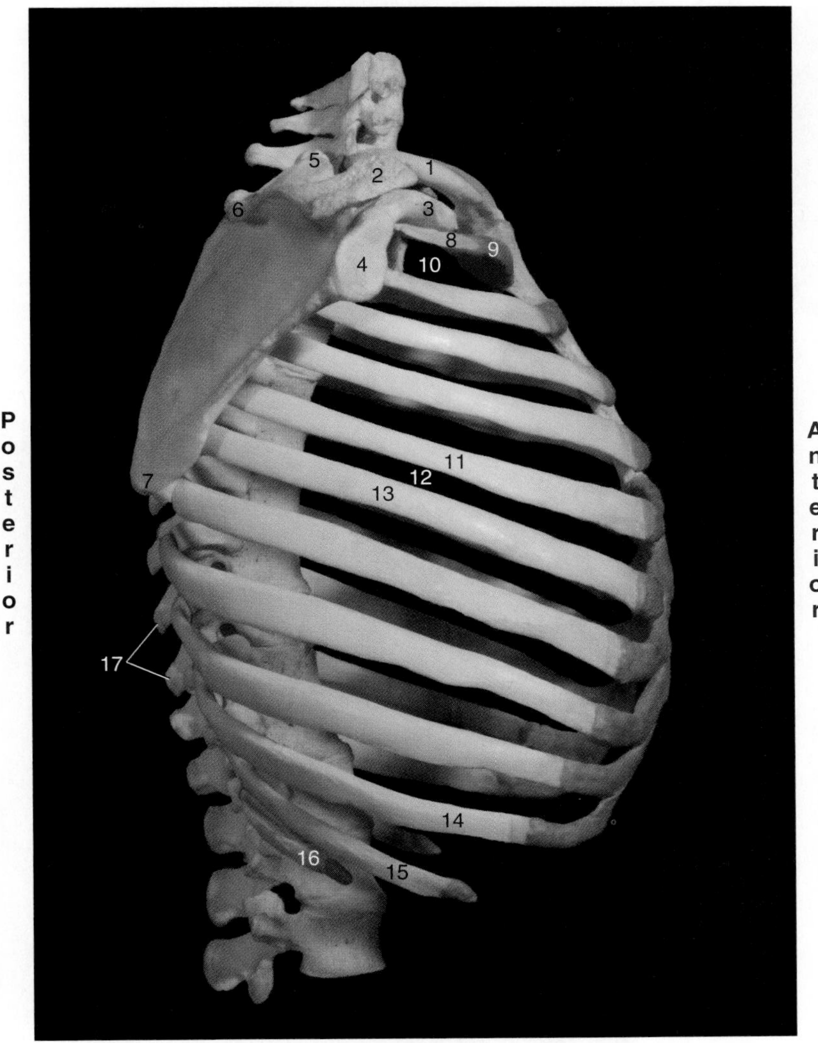

Figure 4-35

1 Clavicle

Scapula (#2-7)

2 Acromion process
3 Coracoid process
4 Glenoid fossa
5 Superior angle
6 Spine of scapula
7 Inferior angle

8 1st Rib
9 Cartilage of 1st rib
10 1st Intercostal space
11 5th Rib
12 5th Intercostal space
13 6th Rib
14 10th Rib
15 11th Rib
16 12th Rib
17 Vertebral transverse processes (TPs)

Notes:

1. The ribs articulate with the spine posteriorly and the sternum anteriorly (except for the floating ribs [#11 and 12], which do not articulate with the sternum.
2. Eleven intercostal spaces are located between the ribs. They are named for the rib that is located superior to the space.
3. The intercostal spaces contain intercostal muscles that often become tight in people with chronic obstructive pulmonary disorders (COPD) such as asthma, emphysema, and chronic bronchitis.
4. The lateral view of the thorax nicely demonstrates the plane of the scapula, which lies neither perfectly in the sagittal nor the frontal plane.

Costospinal Joints

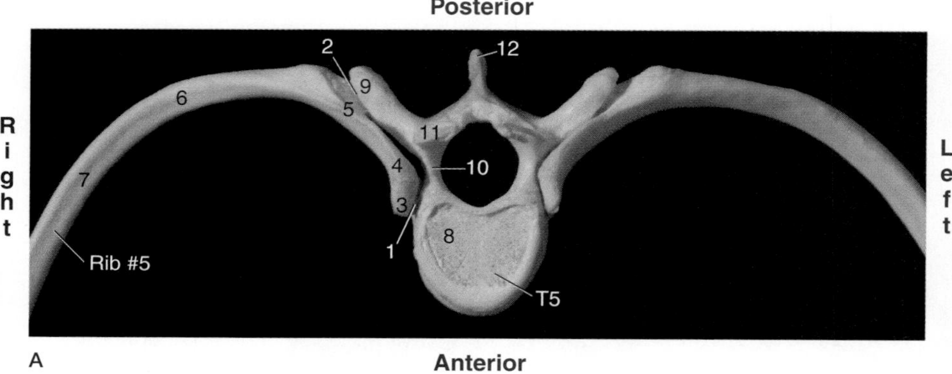

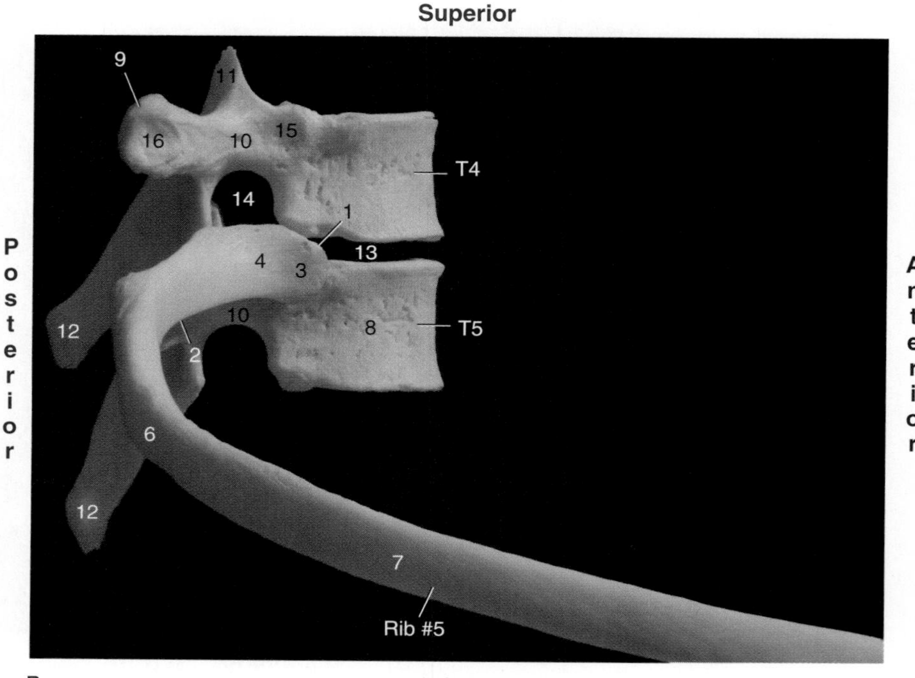

Figure 4-36a and b
A, Superior view; *B,* right lateral view.

1 Costovertebral joint
2 Costotransverse joint
3 Head of rib
4 Neck of rib
5 Tubercle of rib
6 Angle of rib
7 Body of rib
8 Vertebral body
9 Transverse process (TP)
10 Pedicle
11 Superior articular process/facet
12 Spinous process (SP)
13 Disc space (T4-T5)
14 Intervertebral foramen (T4-T5)
15 Costal hemifacet for rib #4
16 Transverse costal facet for rib #4

Notes:

1. A rib articulates with the spinal column in two places, forming two costospinal joints, the costovertebral joint and the costotransverse joint.
2. The costovertebral joint is typically formed by the head of the rib articulating with the (vertebral costal hemifacets of the) bodies of two contiguous vertebrae, as well as the disc that is located between them. Usually ribs #1, 11, and 12 articulate with only one (full vertebral costal facet of a) vertebral body.
3. The costotransverse joint is formed by the tubercle of a rib articulating with the (transverse costal facet of the) transverse process of a vertebra.

Right Ribs

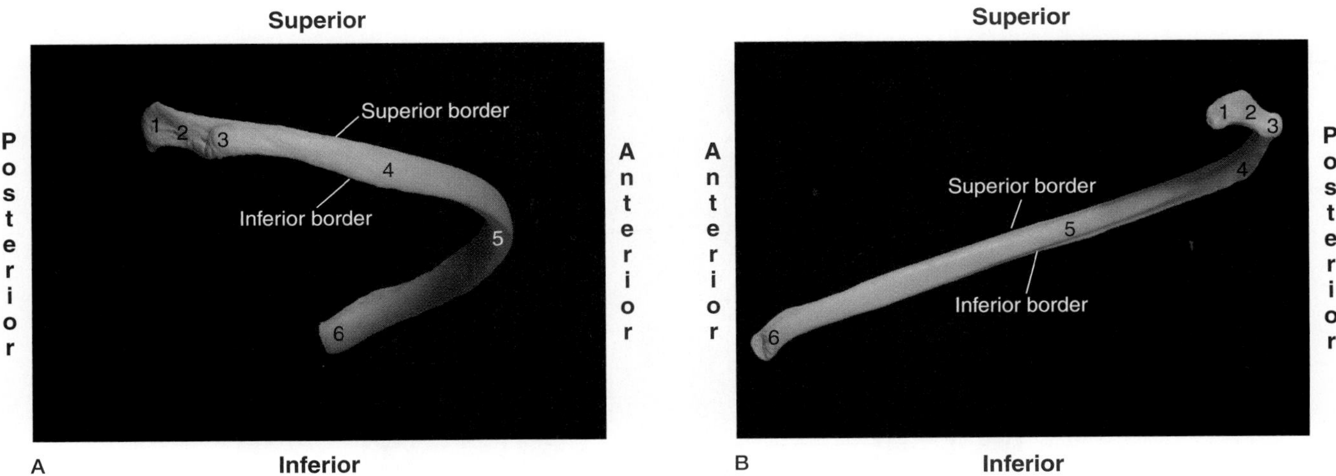

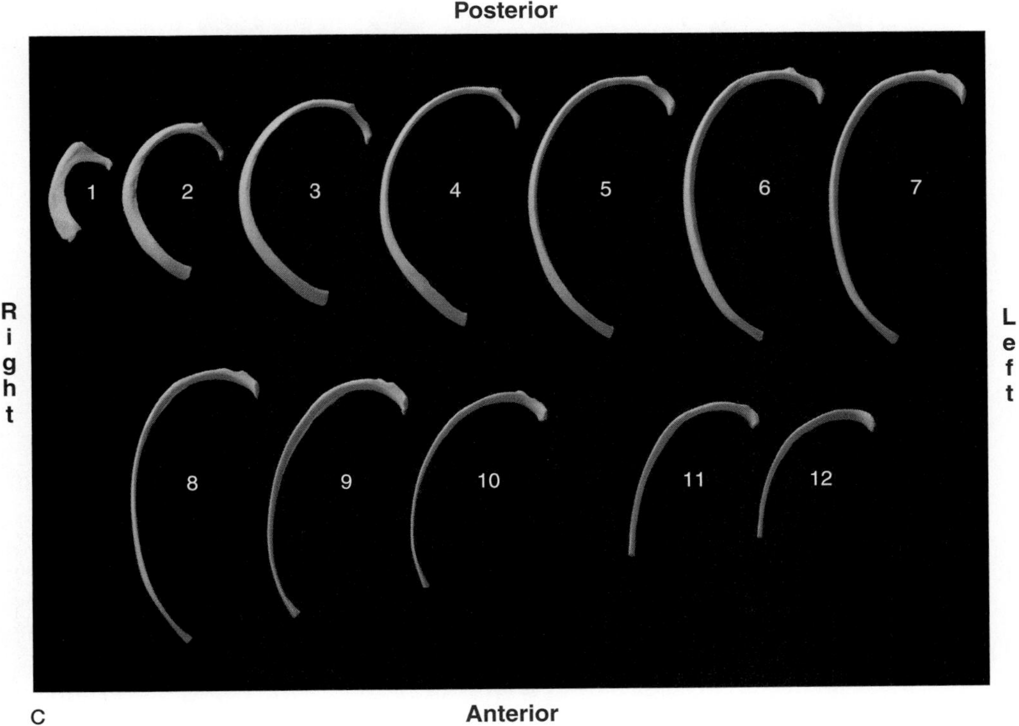

Figure 4-37
A, Posterior view; *B,* medial view; *C,* superior view.

1 Head
2 Neck
3 Tubercle
4 Angle
5 Body
6 Anterior end

Notes:

1. The head of the rib articulates with the vertebral body(ies) to form the costovertebral joint.
2. The tubercle of the rib articulates with the vertebral transverse process (TP) to form the costotransverse joint.
3. The anterior end of the rib meets the sternum via costal cartilage.
4. The first seven pairs of ribs (#1-7) are called *true ribs.*
5. The last five pairs of ribs (#8-12) are called *false ribs.*
6. The last two pairs of false ribs (#11-12) are called *floating ribs.*

☐ 4.4 ENTIRE LOWER EXTREMITY

Right Lower Extremity

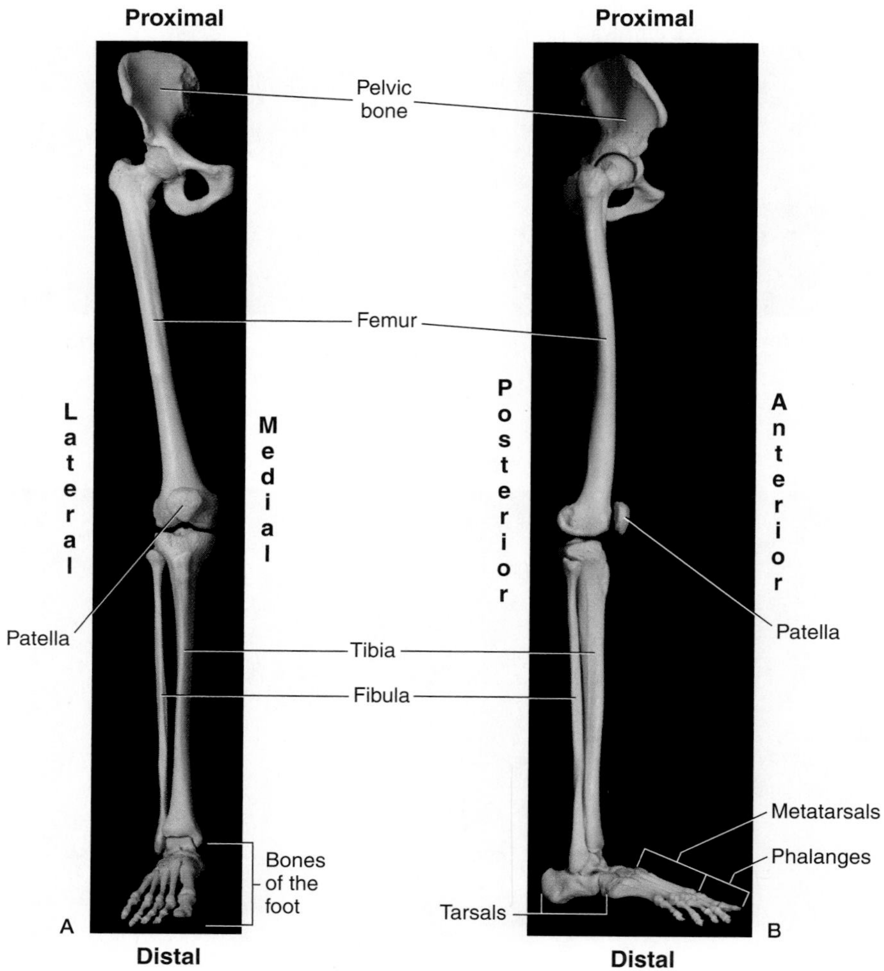

Figure 4-38
A, Anterior view; *B,* right lateral view.

Note:
The femur is in the thigh; the tibia and fibula are in the leg; and the tarsals, metatarsals, and phalanges are in the foot.

☐ 4.5 BONES OF THE PELVIS AND HIP JOINT

Full Pelvis

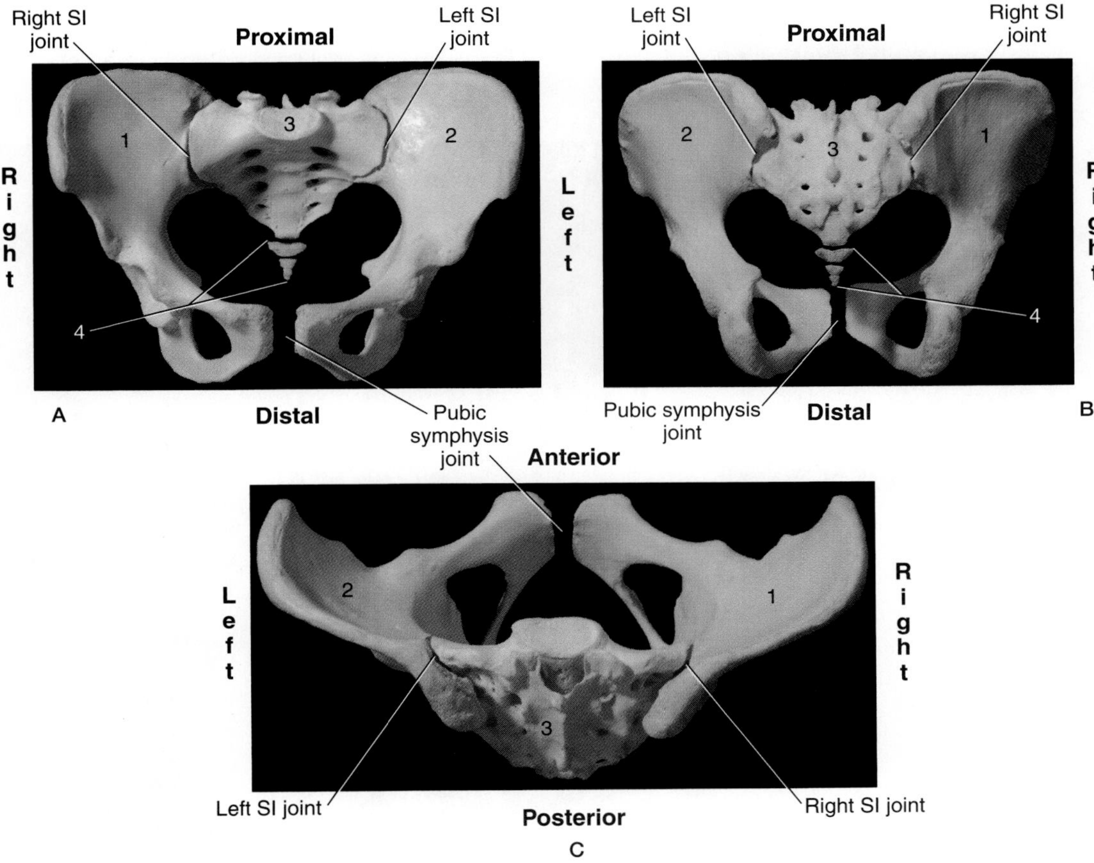

Figure 4-39
A, Anterior view; *B,* posterior view; *C,* superior view.

1 Right pelvic bone
2 Left pelvic bone
3 Sacrum
4 Coccyx

Notes:

1. On the pelvis, either proximal/distal or superior/inferior terminology can be used.
2. There are two sacroiliac (SI) joints, paired left and right. There is one pubic symphysis joint.

Right Pelvic Bone—Anterior Views

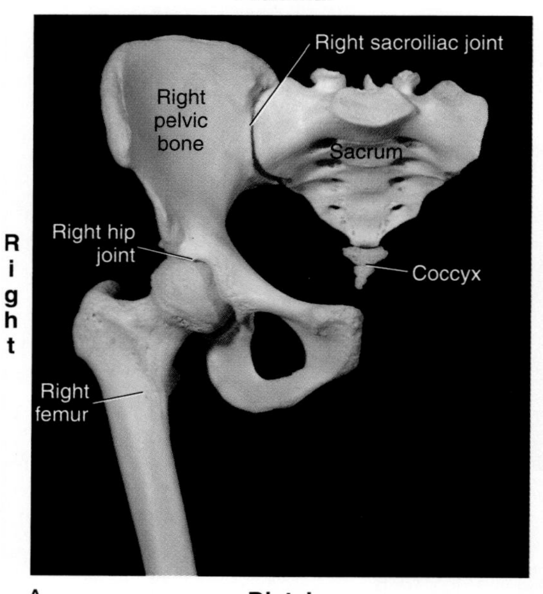

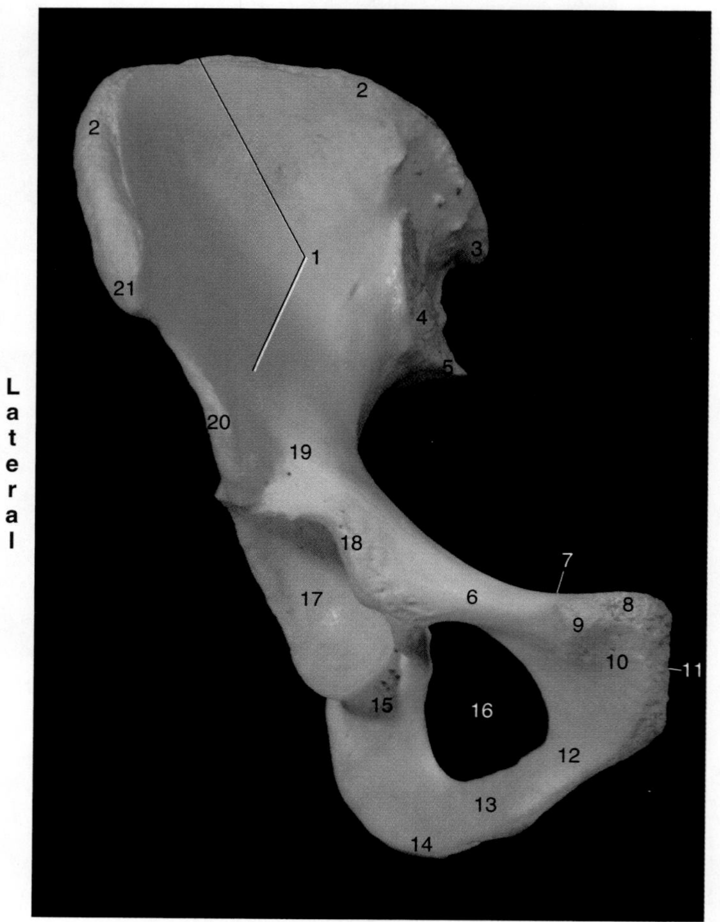

Figure 4-40a and b

1. Wing of the ilium (iliac fossa on internal surface)
2. Iliac crest
3. Posterior superior iliac spine (PSIS)
4. Articular surface for sacroiliac joint
5. Posterior inferior iliac spine (PIIS)
6. Superior ramus of pubis
7. Pectineal line of pubis
8. Pubic crest
9. Pubic tubercle
10. Body of pubis
11. Articular surface for pubic symphysis
12. Inferior ramus of pubis
13. Ramus of ischium
14. Ischial tuberosity
15. Body of ischium
16. Obturator foramen
17. Acetabulum
18. Rim of acetabulum
19. Body of ilium
20. Anterior inferior iliac spine (AIIS)
21. Anterior superior iliac spine (ASIS)

Note:
The articular surface of the ilium for the sacroiliac joint is also known as the *auricular surface,* because is has the shape of an ear (*auricle* means *ear*).

Right Pelvic Bone—Posterior Views

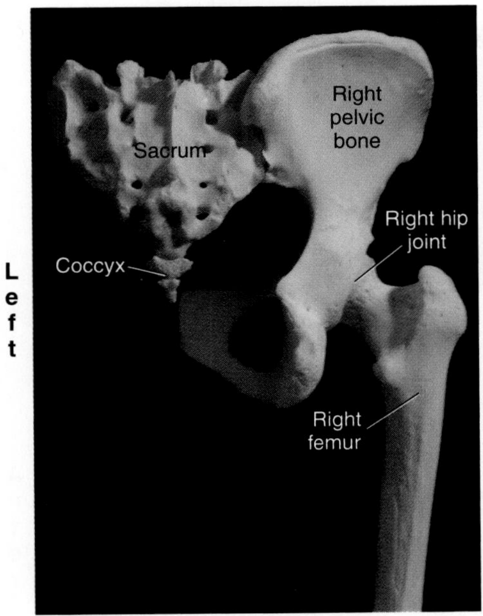

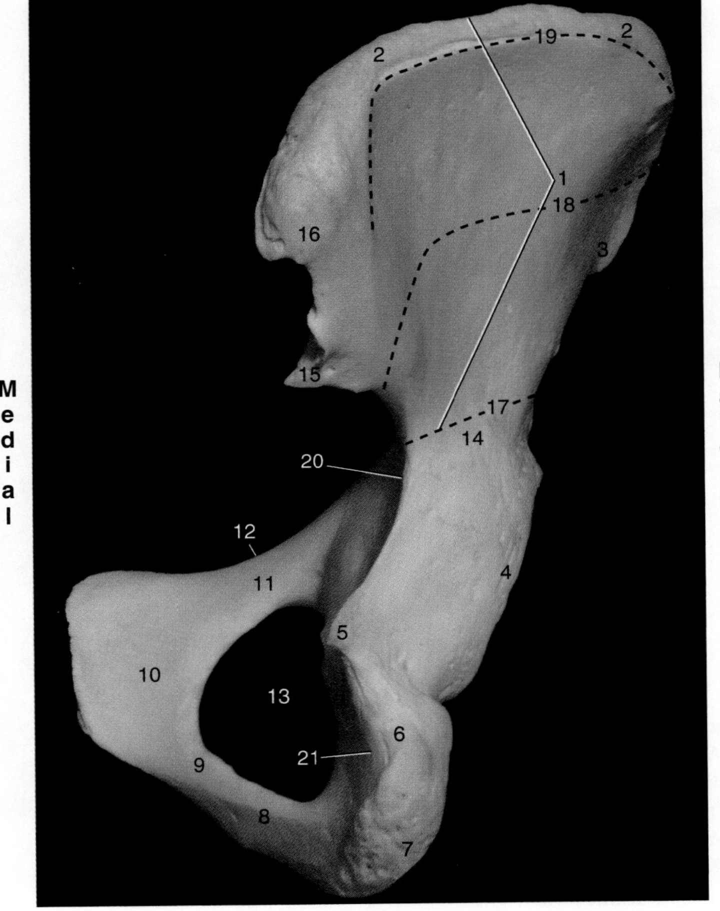

Figure 4-41a and b

1 Wing of the ilium (iliac fossa on internal surface)
2 Iliac crest
3 Anterior superior iliac spine (ASIS)
4 Rim of acetabulum
5 Ischial spine
6 Body of ischium
7 Ischial tuberosity
8 Ramus of ischium
9 Inferior ramus of pubis
10 Body of pubis
11 Superior ramus of pubis
12 Pectineal line of pubis
13 Obturator foramen
14 Body of ilium
15 Posterior inferior iliac spine (PIIS)
16 Posterior superior iliac spine (PSIS)
17 Inferior gluteal line (*dashed line*)
18 Anterior gluteal line (*dashed line*)
19 Posterior gluteal line (*dashed line*)
20 Greater sciatic notch
21 Lesser sciatic notch

Note:
The obturator internus and obturator externus muscles are named for their attachment relative to their obturator foramen.

Right Pelvic Bone—Lateral Views

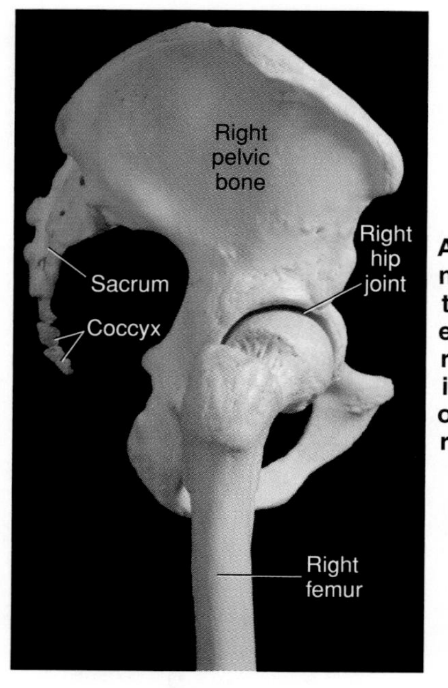

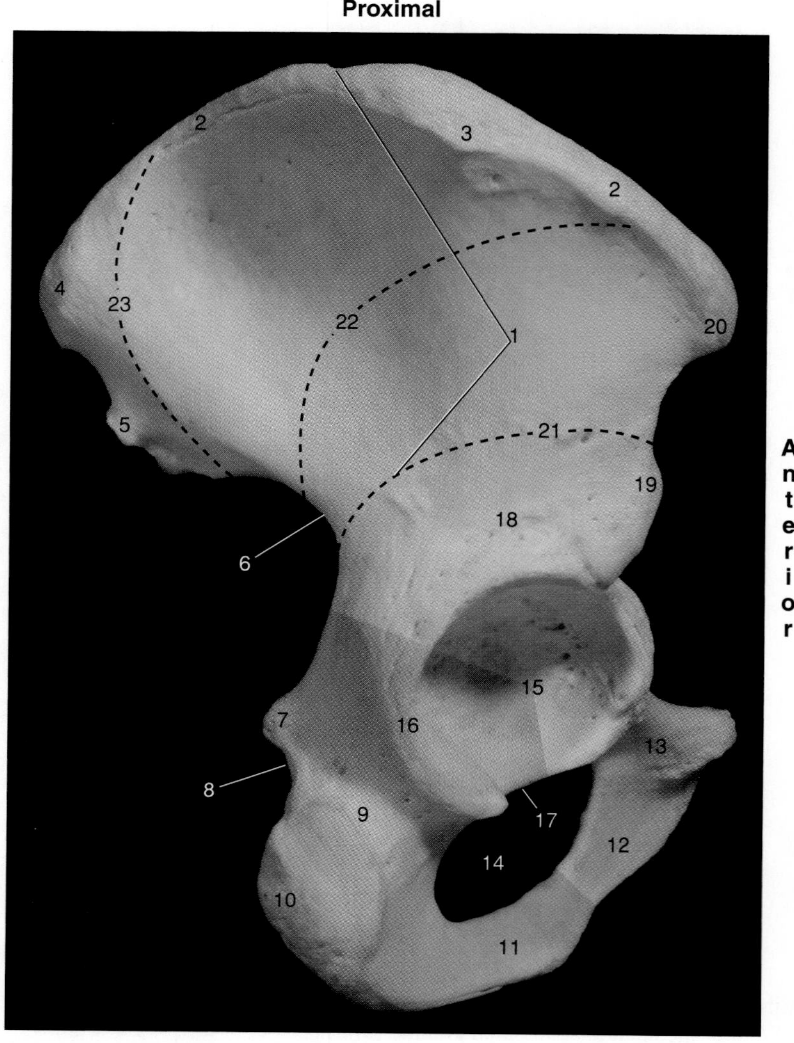

Figure 4-42

1 Wing of the ilium (external/gluteal surface)
2 Iliac crest
3 Tubercle of the iliac crest
4 Posterior superior iliac spine (PSIS)
5 Posterior inferior iliac spine (PIIS)
6 Greater sciatic notch
7 Ischial spine
8 Lesser sciatic notch
9 Body of ischium
10 Ischial tuberosity
11 Ramus of ischium
12 Inferior ramus of pubis
13 Body of pubis
14 Obturator foramen
15 Acetabulum
16 Rim of acetabulum
17 Notch of acetabulum
18 Body of ilium
19 Anterior inferior iliac spine (AIIS)
20 Anterior superior iliac spine (ASIS)
21 Inferior gluteal line (*dashed line*)
22 Anterior gluteal line (*dashed line*)
23 Posterior gluteal line (*dashed line*)

Notes:

1. The pelvic bone is also known as the *coxal, hip,* or *innominate bone.*
2. The pelvic bone is formed by the union of the ilium, ischium, and pubis (see colored shading: the ilium is blue, the ischium is pink, and the pubis is yellow).
3. All three bones of the pelvis (ilium, ischium, and pubis) come together in the acetabulum.
4. The ramus of the ischium (#11) and inferior ramus of the pubis (#12) are often grouped together and called the *ischiopubic ramus.*

Right Pelvic Bone—Medial Views

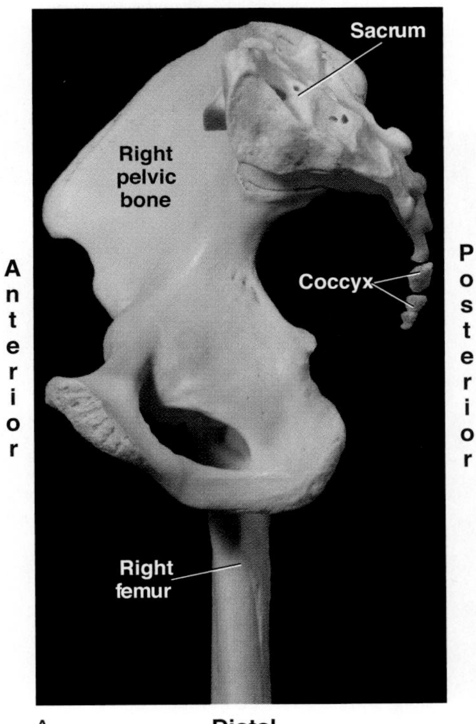

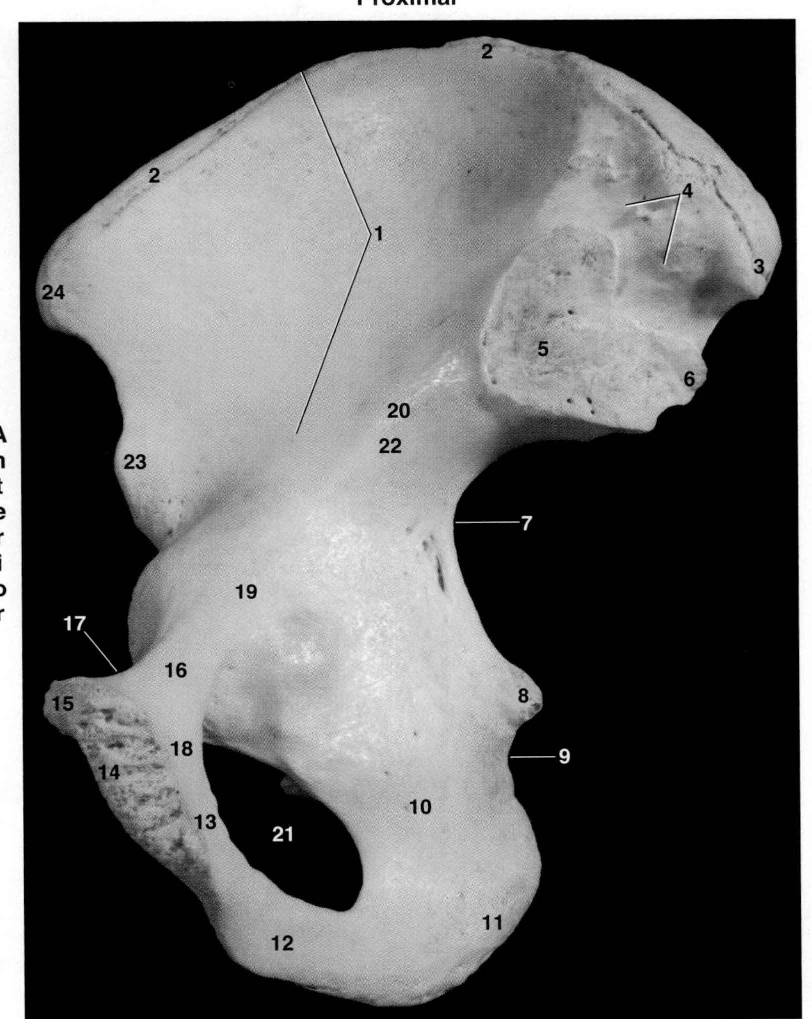

Figure 4-43a and b

1 Wing of the ilium (iliac fossa on internal surface)
2 Iliac crest
3 Posterior superior iliac spine (PSIS)
4 Iliac tuberosity
5 Articular surface of ilium for sacroiliac joint
6 Posterior inferior iliac spine (PIIS)
7 Greater sciatic notch
8 Ischial spine
9 Lesser sciatic notch
10 Body of ischium
11 Ischial tuberosity
12 Ramus of ischium
13 Inferior ramus of pubis
14 Articular surface of pubis for pubis symphysis
15 Pubic tubercle
16 Superior ramus of pubis
17 Pectineal line of pubis
18 Body of pubis
19 Iliopectineal line
20 Arcuate line of the ilium
21 Obturator foramen
22 Body of ilium
23 Anterior inferior iliac spine (AIIS)
24 Anterior superior iliac spine (ASIS)

Note:
The iliopectineal line is located on the ilium and pubis.

□ 4.6 BONES OF THE THIGH AND KNEE JOINT

Right Femur—Anterior and Posterior Views

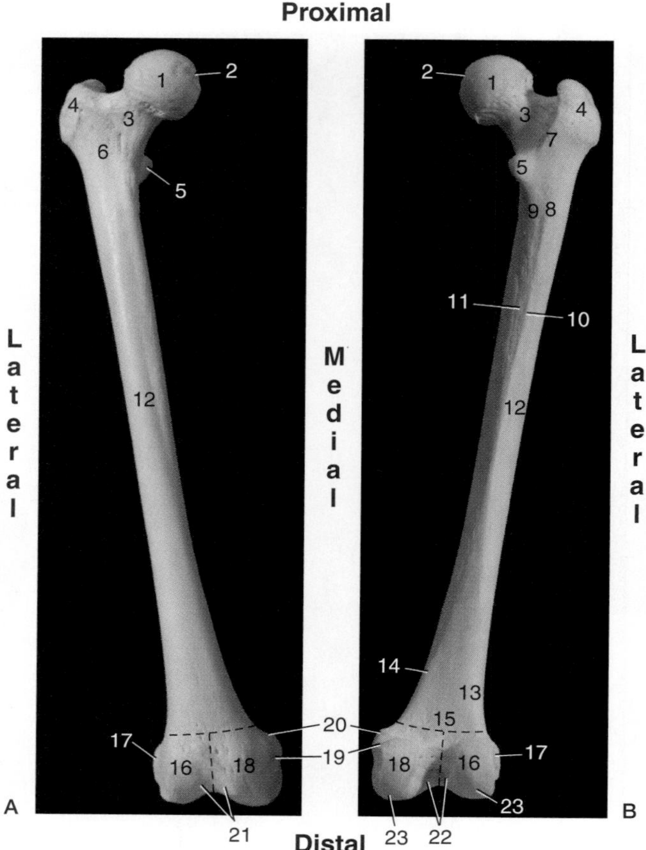

Figure 4-44a and b

1 Head
2 Fovea of the head
3 Neck
4 Greater trochanter
5 Lesser trochanter
6 Intertrochanteric line
7 Intertrochanteric crest
8 Gluteal tuberosity
9 Pectineal line
10 Lateral lip of linea aspera
11 Medial lip of linea aspera
12 Body (shaft)
13 Lateral supracondylar line
14 Medial supracondylar line
15 Popliteal surface
16 Lateral condyle
17 Lateral epicondyle
18 Medial condyle
19 Medial epicondyle
20 Adductor tubercle
21 Articular surface for patellofemoral joint
22 Intercondylar fossa
23 Articular surface for knee (tibiofemoral) joint

Notes:

1. The fovea of the head of the femur is the attachment site for the ligamentum teres of the hip joint.
2. The intertrochanteric line runs between the greater and lesser trochanters anteriorly; the intertrochanteric crest runs between the greater and lesser trochanters posteriorly.
3. The linea aspera is an attachment site for seven muscles. The linea aspera can be looked at as branching proximally to give rise to the gluteal tuberosity and pectineal line, and branching distally to give rise to the lateral and medial supracondylar lines.
4. The gluteal tuberosity is a distal attachment of the gluteus maximus.
5. The pectineal line is the distal attachment of the pectineus.
6. The adductor tubercle is a distal attachment site for the adductor magnus.
7. The borders of the lateral and medial condyles are shown by dashed lines.

Right Femur—Lateral and Medial Views

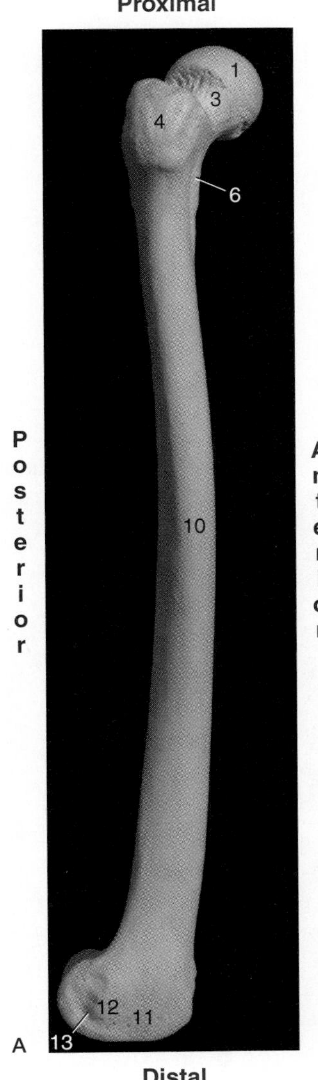

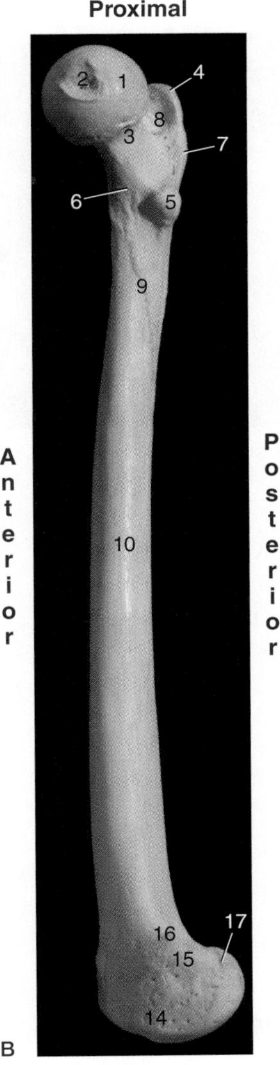

Figure 4-45
A, Lateral view; *B,* medial view.

1 Head
2 Fovea of the head
3 Neck
4 Greater trochanter
5 Lesser trochanter
6 Intertrochanteric line
7 Intertrochanteric crest
8 Trochanteric fossa
9 Pectineal line
10 Body (shaft)
11 Lateral condyle
12 Lateral epicondyle
13 Groove for popliteus tendon
14 Medial condyle
15 Medial epicondyle
16 Adductor tubercle
17 Impression for lateral gastrocnemius

Notes:

1. The shaft of the femur, when viewed from the lateral or medial perspective, is not purely vertical; rather a bow to the shaft exists.
2. The pectineal line of the femur should not be confused with the pectineal line of the pubis (they are the distal and proximal attachments of the pectineus).
3. The femoral condyles articulate with the tibia, forming the knee (i.e., tibiofemoral) joint. The epicondyles are the most prominent points on the condyles.

Right Femur—Proximal and Distal Views

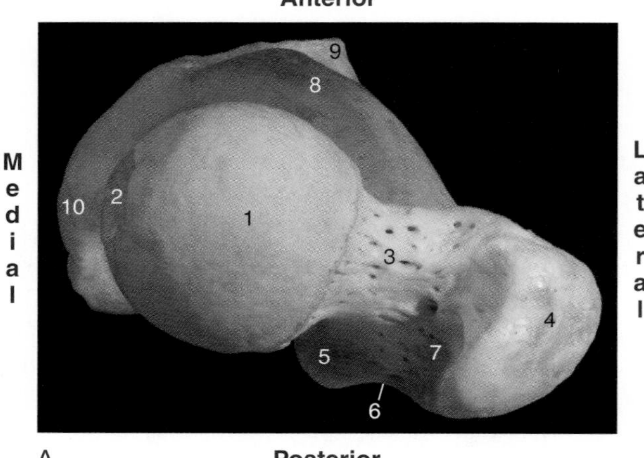

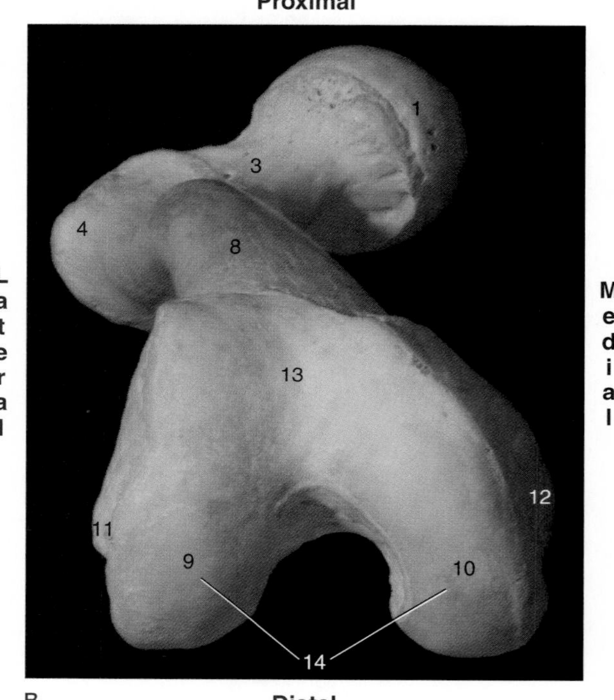

Figure 4-46
A, Proximal (superior) view; *B,* distal (inferior) view.

1 Head
2 Fovea of the head
3 Neck
4 Greater trochanter
5 Lesser trochanter
6 Intertrochanteric crest
7 Trochanteric fossa
8 Body (shaft), anterior surface
9 Lateral condyle
10 Medial condyle
11 Lateral epicondyle
12 Medial epicondyle
13 Articular surface for patellofemoral joint
14 Articular surface for knee (tibiofemoral) joint

Notes:

1. The neck of the femur deviates anteriorly (usually approximately 15 degrees) from the greater trochanter to the head. (see proximal view).
2. The lesser trochanter is medial and it projects somewhat posteriorly as well.
3. From a distal perspective, it is clear that the two condyles of the distal femur are distinct from one another. For this reason, some speak of the knee (i.e., tibiofemoral) joint as having two aspects: a medial tibiofemoral joint and a lateral tibiofemoral joint.

Right Knee Joint and Patella

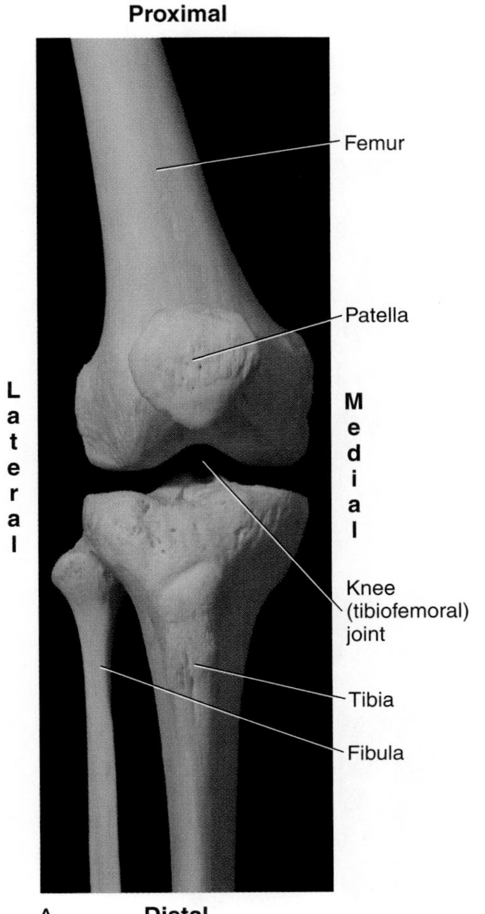

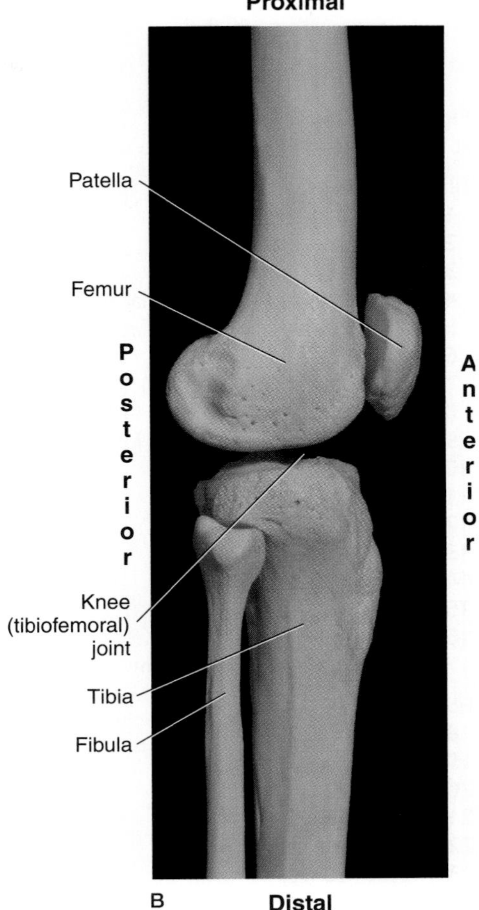

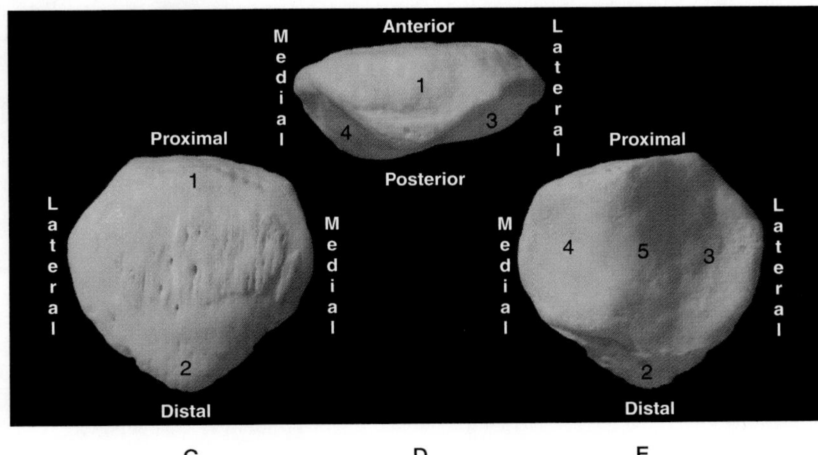

Figure 4-47
A, Anterior view; *B,* lateral view; *C,* anterior view; *D,* proximal (superior) view; *E,* posterior view.

1 Base
2 Apex
3 Facet for lateral condyle of femur
4 Facet for medial condyle of femur
5 Vertical ridge

Notes:
1. The lateral facet of the posterior patella is larger than the medial facet.
2. The articular surfaces of the lateral and medial facets do not extend to the apex of the patella.

☐ 4.7 BONES OF THE LEG AND ANKLE JOINT

Right Tibia/Fibula—Anterior and Proximal Views

Figure 4-48
A, Anterior view; *B,* proximal view.

Tibial Landmarks:

1 Lateral condyle
2 Medial condyle
3 Intercondylar eminence
4 Lateral tubercle of intercondylar eminence
5 Medial tubercle of intercondylar eminence
6 Anterior intercondylar area
7 Posterior intercondylar area
8 Lateral facet (articular surface for knee [i.e., tibiofemoral] joint)
9 Medial facet (articular surface for knee [i.e., tibiofemoral] joint)
10 Tuberosity
11 Impression for iliotibial tract
12 Crest (i.e., anterior border)
13 Interosseus border
14 Medial border
15 Body (shaft)
16 Medial malleolus
17 Articular surface for ankle joint

Fibular Landmarks:

18 Head
19 Neck
20 Interosseus border
21 Body (shaft)
22 Lateral malleolus
23 Articular surface for ankle joint

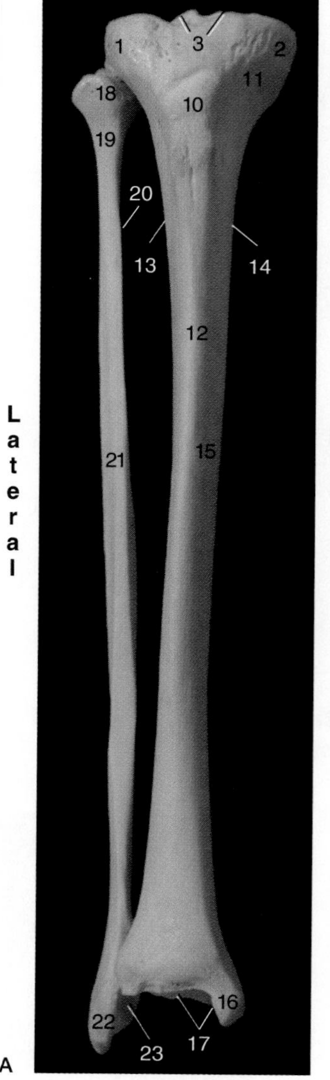

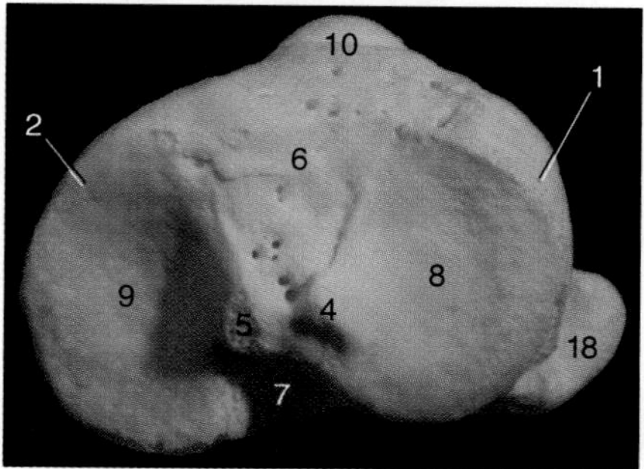

Notes:

1. The entire proximal surface of the tibia is often referred to as the *tibial plateau.*
2. The impression on the tibia for the iliotibial tract is often referred to as *Gerdy's tubercle.*
3. The body (i.e., shaft) of the tibia has three borders: anterior (the crest), medial, and interosseus.
4. The anterior intercondylar area of the tibia is the attachment site of the anterior cruciate ligament; the posterior intercondylar area of the tibia is the attachment site of the posterior cruciate ligament.
5. At the knee joint, the lateral facet of the tibia accepts the lateral condyle of the femur forming the lateral tibiofemoral joint of the knee joint; the medial facet of the tibia accepts the medial condyle of the femur forming the medial tibiofemoral joint of the knee joint.

Right Tibia/Fibula—Posterior and Distal Views

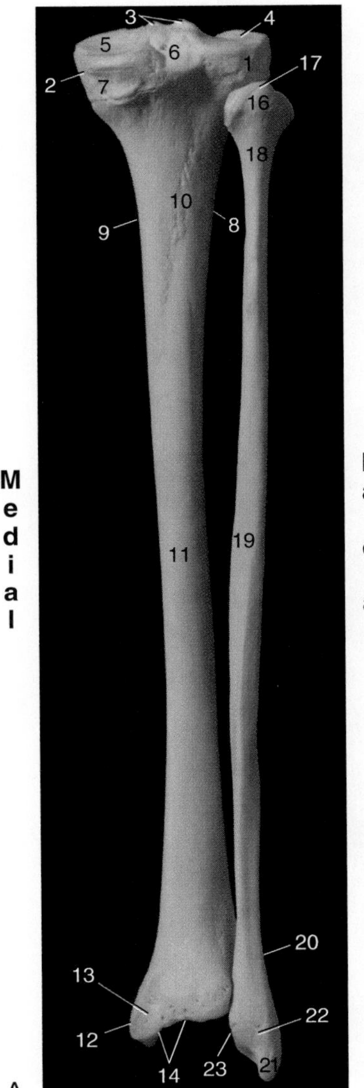

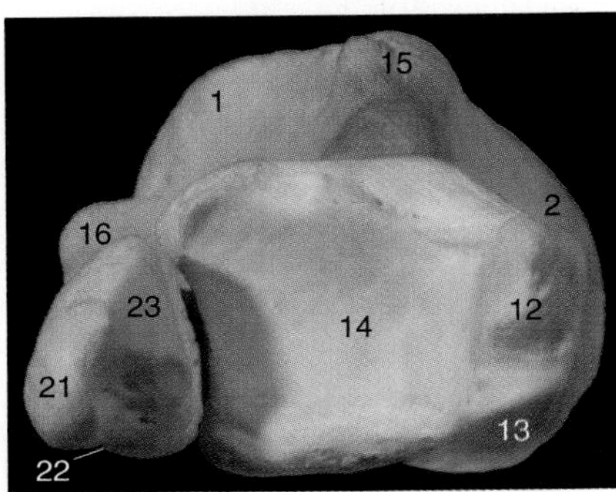

Figure 4-49

Tibial Landmarks:

1 Lateral condyle
2 Medial condyle
3 Intercondylar eminence
4 Lateral facet (articular surface for knee [i.e., tibiofemoral] joint)
5 Medial facet (articular surface for knee [i.e., tibiofemoral] joint)
6 Posterior intercondylar area
7 Groove for semimembranosus muscle
8 Interosseus border
9 Medial border
10 Soleal line
11 Body (shaft)
12 Medial malleolus
13 Groove for tibialis posterior
14 Articular surfaces for ankle joint
15 Tuberosity

Fibular Landmarks:

16 Head
17 Apex of head
18 Neck
19 Body (shaft)
20 Lateral surface
21 Lateral malleolus
22 Groove for fibularis brevis
23 Articular surface for ankle joint

Notes:

1. The apex of the fibular head is also known as the *styloid process of the fibula.*
2. The soleal line of the tibia is part of the proximal attachment of the soleus muscle.
3. The groove for the fibularis brevis is created by the distal tendon of the fibularis brevis muscle as it passes posterior to the lateral malleolus to enter the foot.
4. The lateral malleolus of the fibula extends further distally than the medial malleolus of the tibia. This configuration results in a less eversion range of motion of the foot than inversion.

Right Tibia/Fibula—Lateral Views

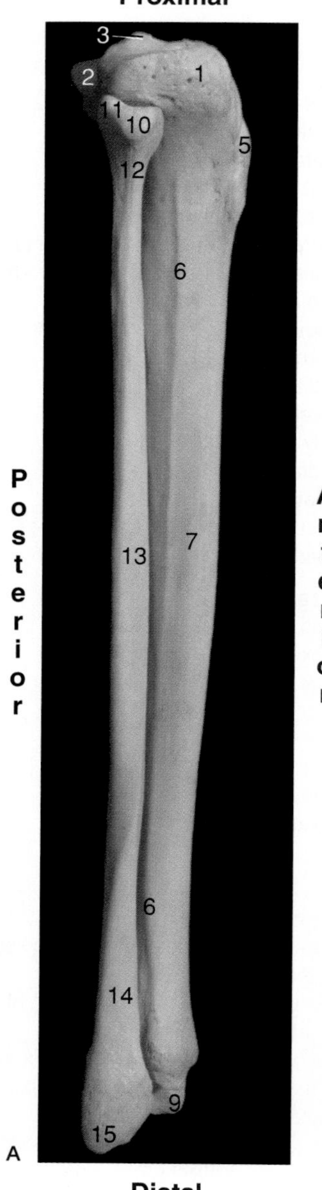

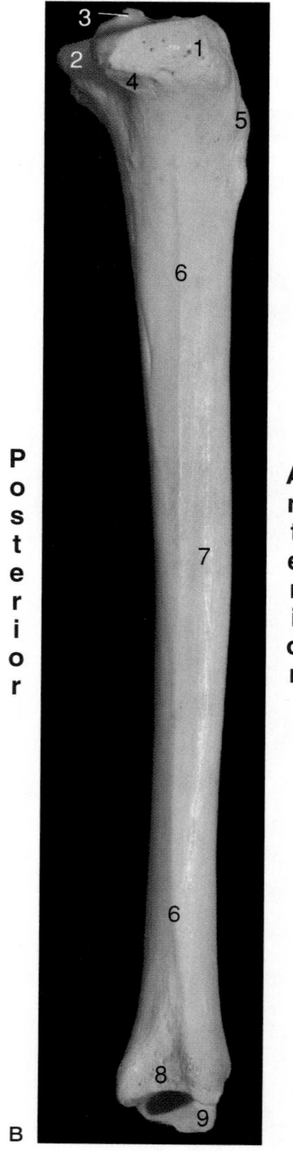

Figure 4-50
A, Right lateral view of the tibia and fibula articulated; *B,* right lateral view of just the tibia.

Tibial Landmarks:

1 Lateral condyle
2 Medial condyle
3 Intercondylar eminence
4 Articular facet for proximal tibiofibular joint
5 Tuberosity
6 Interosseus border
7 Body (shaft)
8 Fibular notch
9 Medial malleolus

Fibular Landmarks:

10 Head
11 Apex of head
12 Neck
13 Body (shaft)
14 Triangular subcutaneous area
15 Lateral malleolus

Notes:

1. The interosseus border on the lateral tibia is the site of attachment for the interosseus membrane of the leg.
2. The triangular subcutaneous area is a triangular area of the distal lateral shaft of the fibula that is palpable through the skin.
3. The articular facet for the proximal tibiofemoral joint on the lateral proximal tibia accepts the head of the fibula.
4. The fibular notch on the lateral distal tibia accepts the distal fibula, forming the distal tibiofibular joint.

Right Tibia/Fibula—Medial Views

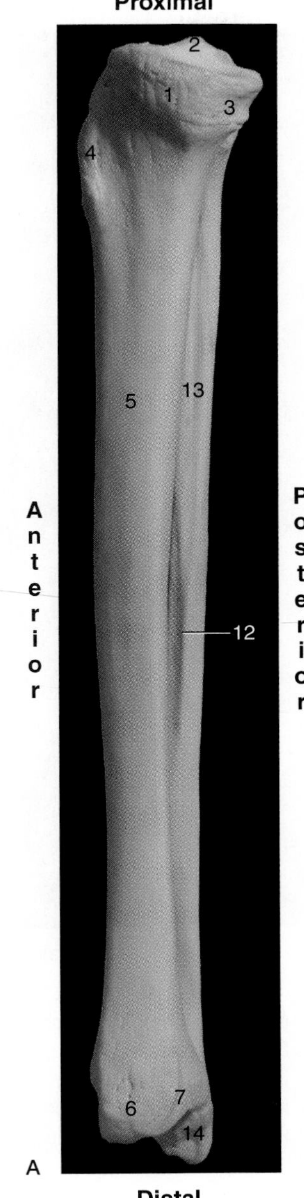

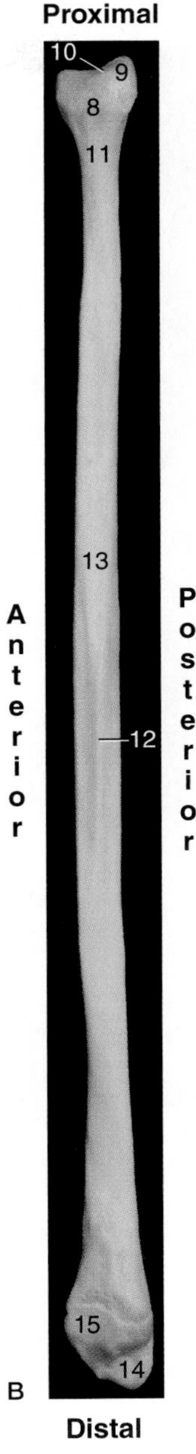

Figure 4-51
A, Medial view of the tibia and fibula articulated; *B,* medial view of just the fibula.

Tibial Landmarks:
- **1** Medial condyle
- **2** Intercondylar eminence
- **3** Groove for semimembranosus muscle
- **4** Tuberosity
- **5** Body (shaft)
- **6** Medial malleolus
- **7** Groove for tibialis posterior muscle

Fibular Landmarks:
- **8** Head
- **9** Apex of head
- **10** Articular surface for proximal tibiofibular joint
- **11** Neck
- **12** Interosseus border
- **13** Body (shaft)
- **14** Lateral malleolus
- **15** Articular surface for ankle joint

Notes:
1. The interosseus border on the medial fibula is the site of attachment for the interosseus membrane of the leg.
2. The medial view of the tibia demonstrates the groove for the semimembranosus muscle proximally and the groove for the tibialis posterior muscle distally.

Right Ankle Joint

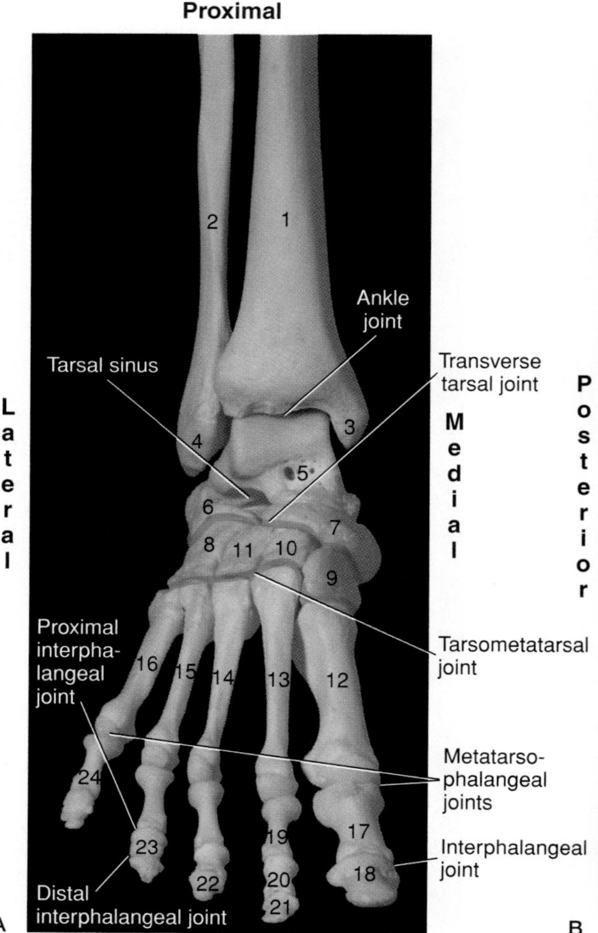

Proximal

2
1
Ankle joint
Transverse tarsal joint
Anterior
5
9
7
10
4
11
12
13
6
8
14
15
16
Tarsal sinus
Tarsometatarsal joint

Distal

Figure 4-52
A, Anterior view; *B,* lateral view.

1 Tibia
2 Fibula
3 Medial malleolus (of tibia)
4 Lateral malleolus (of fibula)
5 Talus
6 Calcaneus
7 Navicular
8 Cuboid
9 1st Cuneiform
10 2nd Cuneiform
11 3rd Cuneiform
12 1st Metatarsal
13 2nd Metatarsal
14 3rd Metatarsal
15 4th Metatarsal
16 5th Metatarsal
17 Proximal phalanx of big toe
18 Distal phalanx of big toe
19 Proximal phalanx of 2nd toe
20 Middle phalanx of 2nd toe
21 Distal phalanx of 2nd toe
22 Distal phalanx of 3rd toe
23 Middle phalanx of 4th toe
24 Proximal phalanx of little toe (i.e., 5th toe)

Notes:

1. The ankle joint is formed by the talus being held between the malleoli of the tibia and fibula. The ankle joint is also known as the *talocrural joint.*
2. The subtalar joint is located between the talus and calcaneus (i.e., under the talus). The subtalar joint is located between tarsal bones; hence it is a tarsal joint.
3. The transverse tarsal joint is composed of the talonavicular joint and the calcaneocuboid joint.
4. The tarsometatarsal joint is located between the cuneiforms and cuboid proximally (posteriorly), and the metatarsals distally (anteriorly).

4.8 BONES OF THE FOOT

Right Subtalar Joint

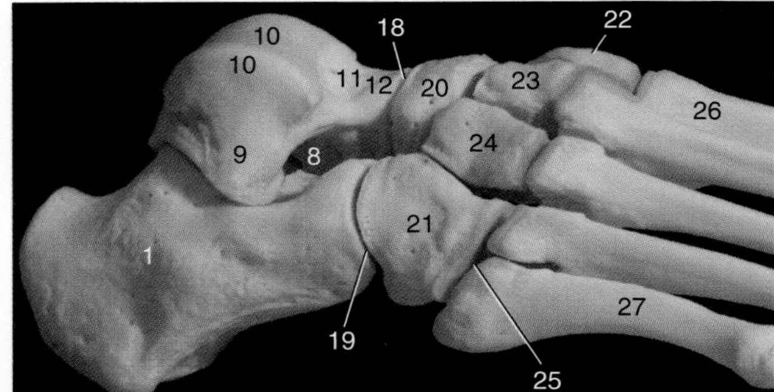

Lateral view

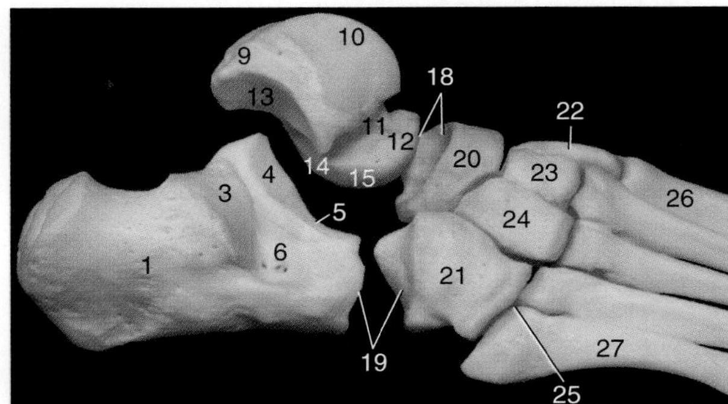

Lateral view, subtalar joint open

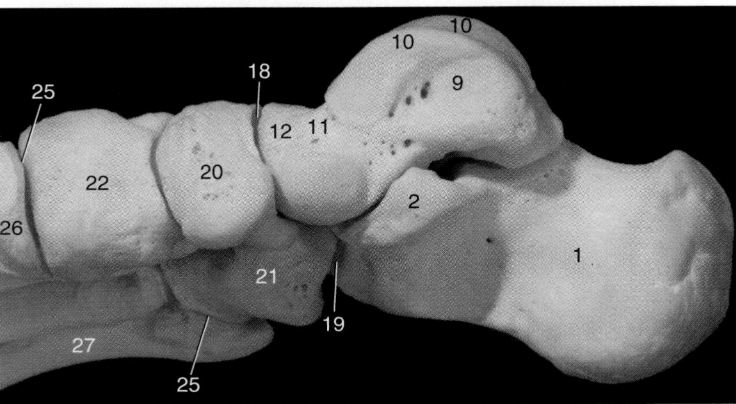

Medial view

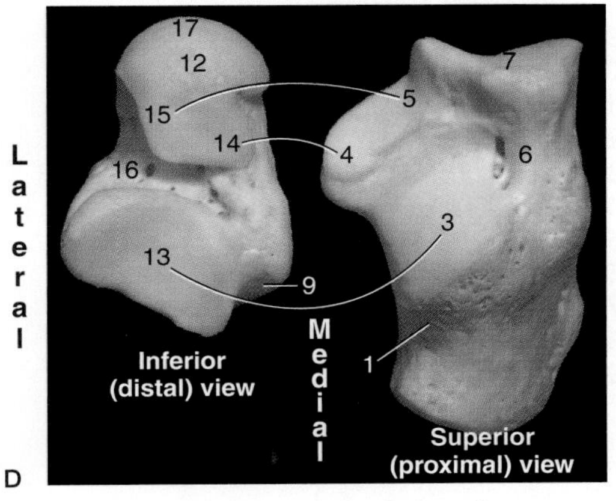

Subtalar joint, articular surfaces

Figure 4-53
A, Right lateral view; *B,* right lateral view, subtalar joint open; *C,* medial view; *D,* subtalar joint, articular surfaces.

1 Calcaneus (#1-7)
2 Sustentaculum tali
3 Calcaneal posterior facet (of subtalar joint)
4 Calcaneal middle facet (of subtalar joint)
5 Calcaneal anterior facet (of subtalar joint)
6 Sulcus (of calcaneus)
7 Articular surface for calcaneocuboid joint (of transverse tarsal joint)
8 Tarsal sinus
9 Talus (#9-17)
10 Articular surface for ankle joint
11 Neck of talus
12 Head of talus
13 Talar posterior facet (of subtalar joint)
14 Talar middle facet (of subtalar joint)
15 Talar anterior facet (of subtalar joint)
16 Sulcus (of talus)
17 Articular surface for talonavicular joint (of transverse tarsal joint)
18 Talonavicular joint (of transverse tarsal joint)
19 Calcaneocuboid joint (of transverse tarsal joint)
20 Navicular
21 Cuboid
22 1st Cuneiform
23 2nd Cuneiform
24 3rd Cuneiform
25 Tarsometatarsal joint
26 1st Metatarsal
27 5th Metatarsal

Notes:

1. The subtalar joint between the talus and calcaneus is composed of three articular surfaces: posterior, middle, and anterior. The posterior articulation is formed by the posterior facets of each bone; the middle articulation is formed by the middle facets of each bone; the anterior articulation is formed by the anterior facets of each bone.
2. The posterior aspect of the subtalar joint is the largest of the three.
3. The tarsal sinus is formed by the sulcus of the calcaneus and the sulcus of the talus.
4. The transverse tarsal joint is formed by the talonavicular and calcaneocuboid joints.

Right Foot—Dorsal View

Figure 4-54

1 Calcaneus
2 Fibular trochlea of calcaneus
3 Articular surface of talus for ankle joint
4 Medial tubercle of talus
5 Lateral tubercle of talus
6 Neck of talus
7 Head of talus
8 Navicular
9 Navicular tuberosity
10 Cuboid
11 Groove for fibularis longus
12 1st Cuneiform
13 2nd Cuneiform
14 3rd Cuneiform
15 Base of 1st metatarsal
16 Body (shaft) of 1st metatarsal
17 Head of 1st metatarsal
18 Tuberosity of base of 5th metatarsal
19 Base of 5th metatarsal
20 Body (shaft) of 5th metatarsal
21 Head of 5th metatarsal
22 Sesamoid bone of big toe
23 Proximal phalanx of big toe
24 Distal phalanx of big toe
25 Base of proximal phalanx of 2nd toe
26 Body (shaft) of proximal phalanx of 2nd toe
27 Head of proximal phalanx of 2nd toe
28 Middle phalanx of 3rd toe
29 Distal phalanx of 4th toe

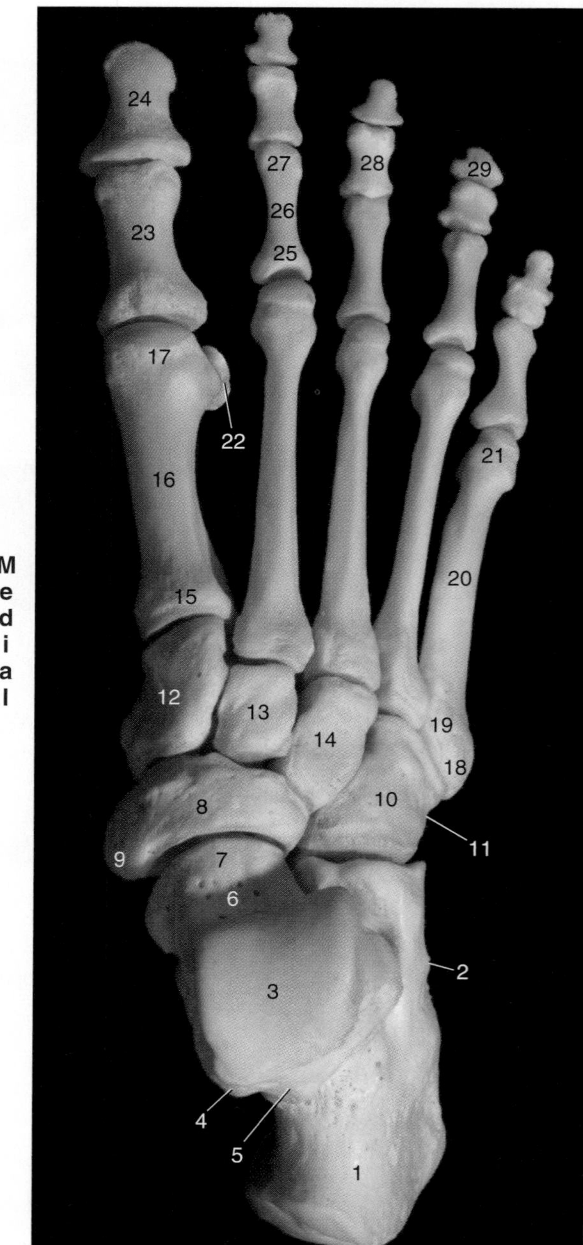

Notes:

1. The word *phalanx* is singular only; plural of phalanx is *phalanges.*
2. The articular surface of the talus for the ankle joint is called the *trochlea* of the talus.
3. The 1st, 2nd, and 3rd cuneiforms are also known as the *medial, intermediate*, and *lateral cuneiforms,* respectively.
4. The 1st cuneiform articulates with the 1st metatarsal; the 2nd cuneiform articulates with the 2nd metatarsal; the 3rd cuneiform articulates with the 3rd metatarsal; and the cuboid articulates with the 4th and 5th metatarsals.
5. All metatarsals and phalanges have a base proximally, a body (i.e., shaft) in the middle, and a head distally.
6. The middle and distal phalanges of the little toe in this specimen have fused together.

Right Foot—Plantar View

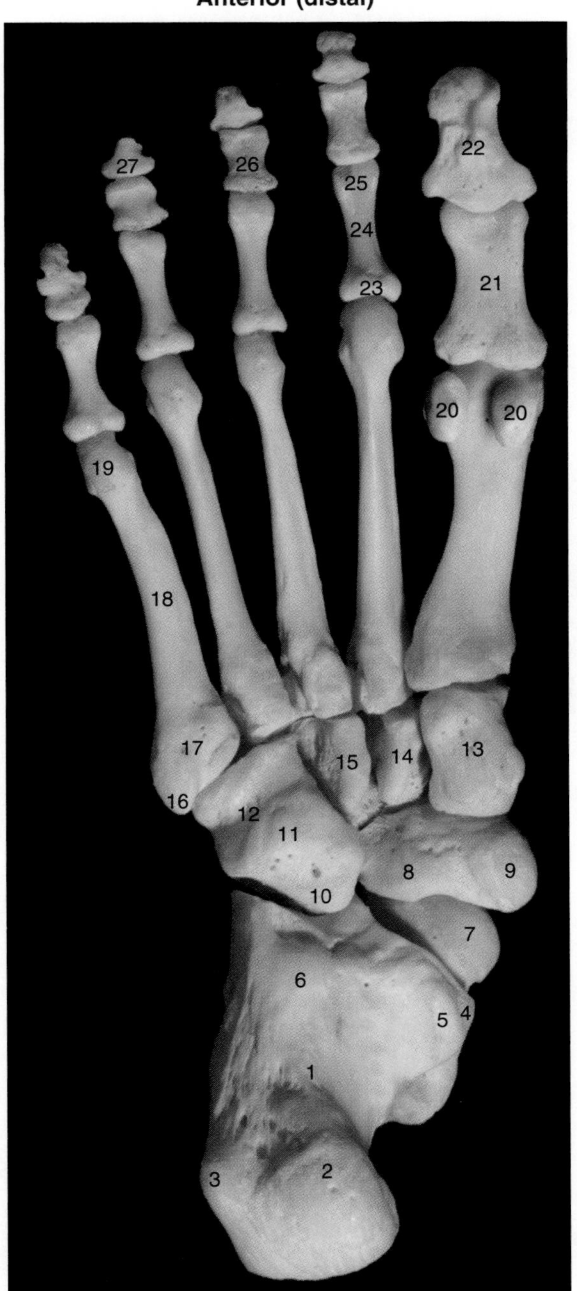

Figure 4-55

1 Calcaneus
2 Medial process of calcaneal tuberosity
3 Lateral process of calcaneal tuberosity
4 Sustentaculum tali of calcaneus
5 Groove for distal tendon of flexor hallucis longus muscle (on sustentaculum tali)
6 Anterior tubercle of calcaneus
7 Head of talus
8 Navicular
9 Navicular tuberosity
10 Cuboid
11 Tuberosity of cuboid
12 Groove for distal tendon of fibularis longus muscle
13 1st Cuneiform
14 2nd Cuneiform
15 3rd Cuneiform
16 Tuberosity of base of 5th metatarsal
17 Base of 5th metatarsal
18 Body (shaft) of 5th metatarsal
19 Head of 5th metatarsal
20 Sesamoid bone of big toe
21 Proximal phalanx of big toe
22 Distal phalanx of big toe
23 Base of proximal phalanx of 2nd toe
24 Body (shaft) of proximal phalanx of 2nd toe
25 Head of proximal phalanx of 2nd toe
26 Middle phalanx of 3rd toe
27 Distal phalanx of 4th toe

Notes:

1. On the calcaneal tuberosity, the medial process is much larger than the lateral process.
2. The base of the 5th metatarsal bone has a large palpable tuberosity.
3. The big toe usually has two sesamoid bones.
4. The groove for the distal tendon of the fibularis longus tendon is clearly visible on the plantar surface of the cuboid demonstrating its passage deep in the plantar foot.
5. The middle and distal phalanges of the little toe have fused together in this specimen.

Right Foot—Medial View

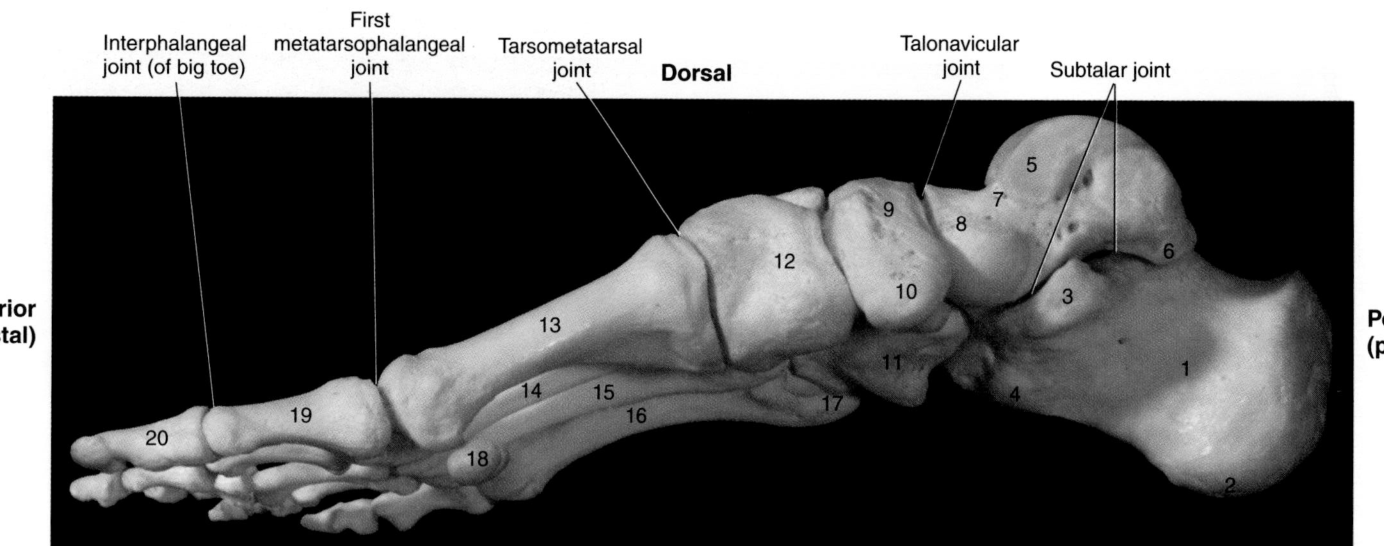

Figure 4-56

1 Calcaneus (medial surface)
2 Medial process of calcaneal tuberosity
3 Sustentaculum tali of calcaneus
4 Anterior tubercle of calcaneus
5 Articular surface of talus for (medial malleolus of) ankle joint
6 Medial tubercle of talus
7 Neck of talus
8 Head of talus
9 Navicular
10 Navicular tuberosity
11 Cuboid
12 1st Cuneiform
13 1st Metatarsal
14 3rd Metatarsal
15 4th Metatarsal
16 5th Metatarsal
17 Tuberosity of base of 5th metatarsal
18 Sesamoid bone of big toe
19 Proximal phalanx of big toe
20 Distal phalanx of big toe

Notes:

1. The sustentaculum tali of the calcaneus forms a ledge on which the talus sits.
2. On the medial side of the foot, the sustentaculum tali of the calcaneus and the navicular tuberosity are easily palpable landmarks.
3. The 2nd metatarsal is not visible in this view.
4. The subtalar joint is located between the talus and the calcaneus.
5. The talonavicular joint (of the transverse tarsal joint) is located between the talus and the navicular.
6. The arch (i.e., medial longitudinal arch) of the foot is apparent in a medial view.

Right Foot—Lateral View

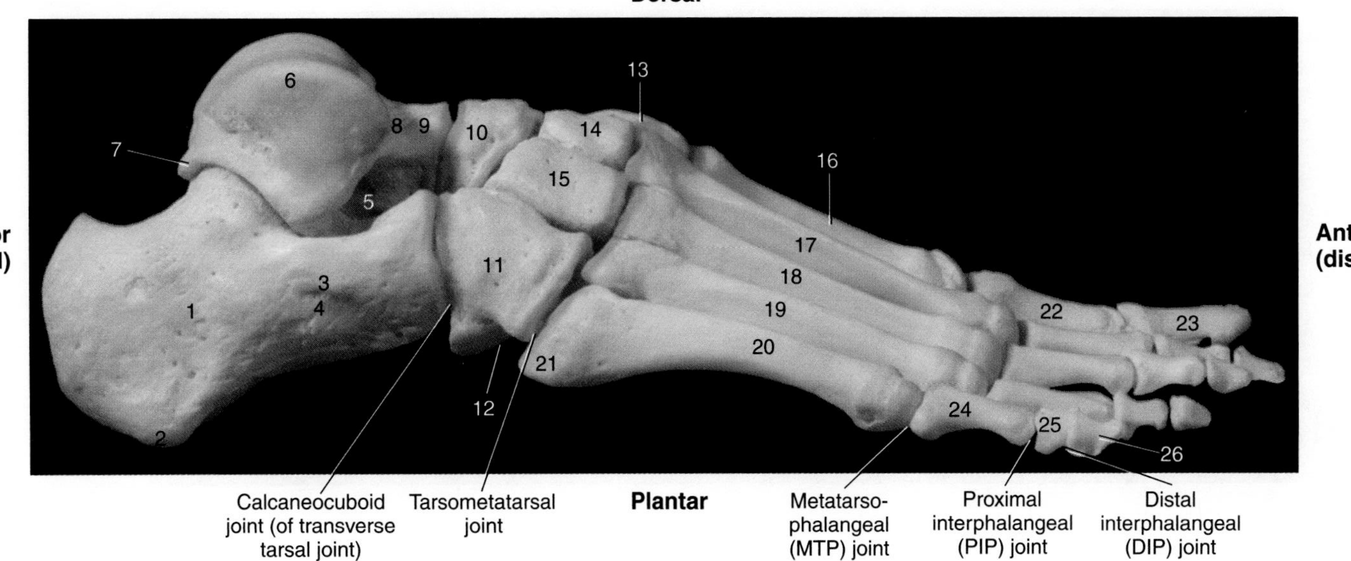

Figure 4-57

1 Calcaneus (lateral surface)
2 Lateral process of calcaneal tuberosity
3 Fibular trochlea
4 Groove for distal tendon of fibularis longus muscle
5 Tarsal sinus
6 Articular surface of talus for (lateral malleolus of) ankle joint
7 Lateral tubercle of talus
8 Neck of talus
9 Head of talus
10 Navicular
11 Cuboid
12 Groove for distal tendon of fibularis longus muscle
13 1st Cuneiform
14 2nd Cuneiform
15 3rd Cuneiform
16 1st Metatarsal
17 2nd Metatarsal
18 3rd Metatarsal
19 4th Metatarsal
20 5th Metatarsal
21 Tuberosity of base of 5th metatarsal
22 Proximal phalanx of big toe
23 Distal phalanx of big toe
24 Proximal phalanx of little toe
25 Middle phalanx of little toe
26 Distal phalanx of little toe

Notes:

1. The tuberosity of the base of the 5th metatarsal is easily palpable on the lateral side of the foot.
2. The subtalar joint is located between the talus and the calcaneus.
3. The tarsal sinus is a space located between the talus and calcaneus.
4. The calcaneocuboid joint of the transverse tarsal joint is located between the calcaneus and the cuboid.
5. The middle and distal phalanges of the little toe are fused together in this specimen.

4.9 ENTIRE UPPER EXTREMITY

Right Upper Extremity

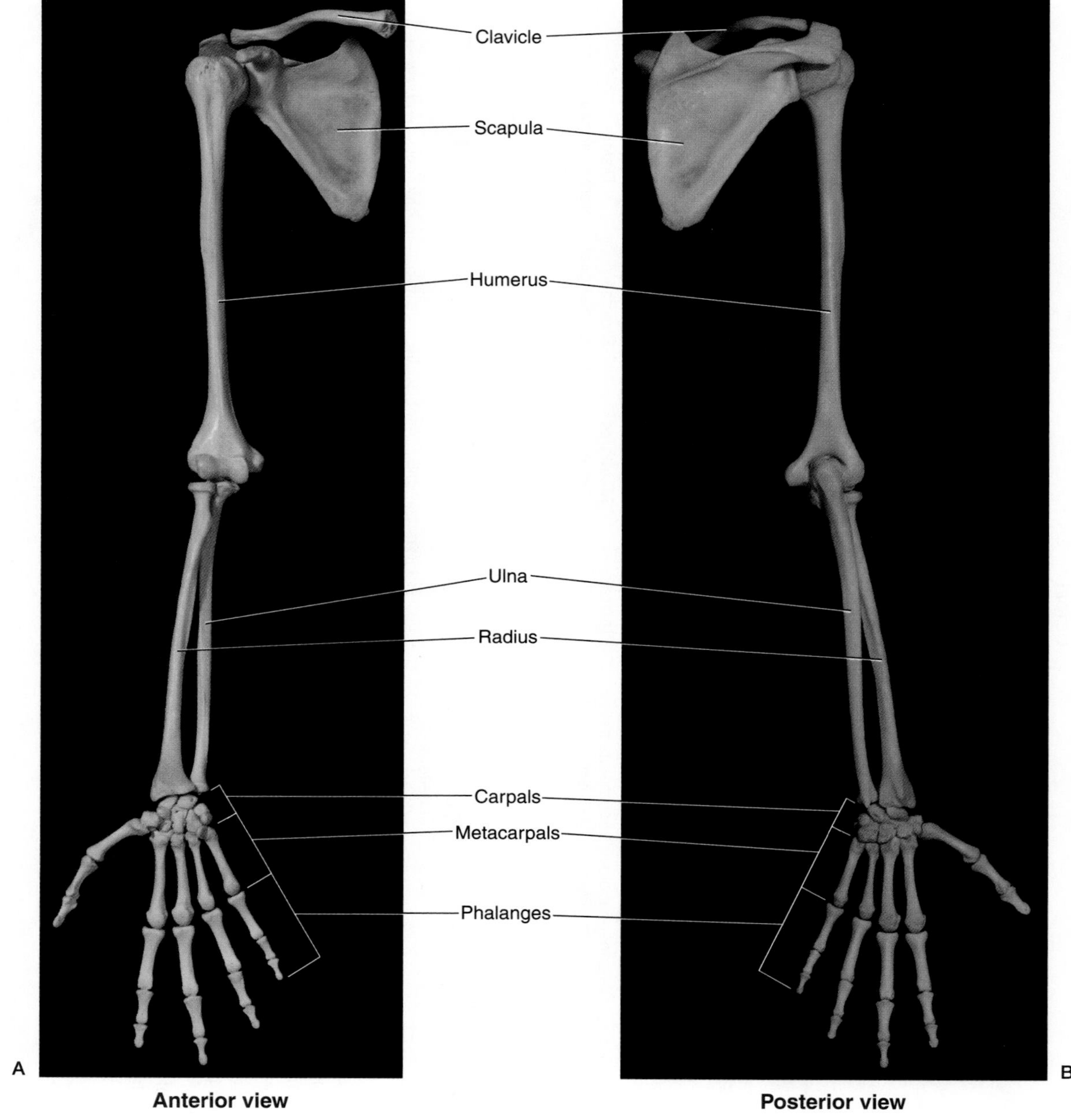

Figure 4-58
A, Anterior view; *B,* posterior view.

Notes:

1. The upper extremity is composed of the bones of the shoulder girdle, arm, forearm, and hand.
2. The shoulder girdle is composed of the scapula and clavicle, and the arm contains the humerus.
3. The forearm contains the radius, which is lateral, and the ulna, which is medial.
4. The hand contains eight carpals, five metacarpals, and 14 phalanges.

☐ 4.10 BONES OF THE SHOULDER GIRDLE AND SHOULDER JOINT

Right Shoulder Joint

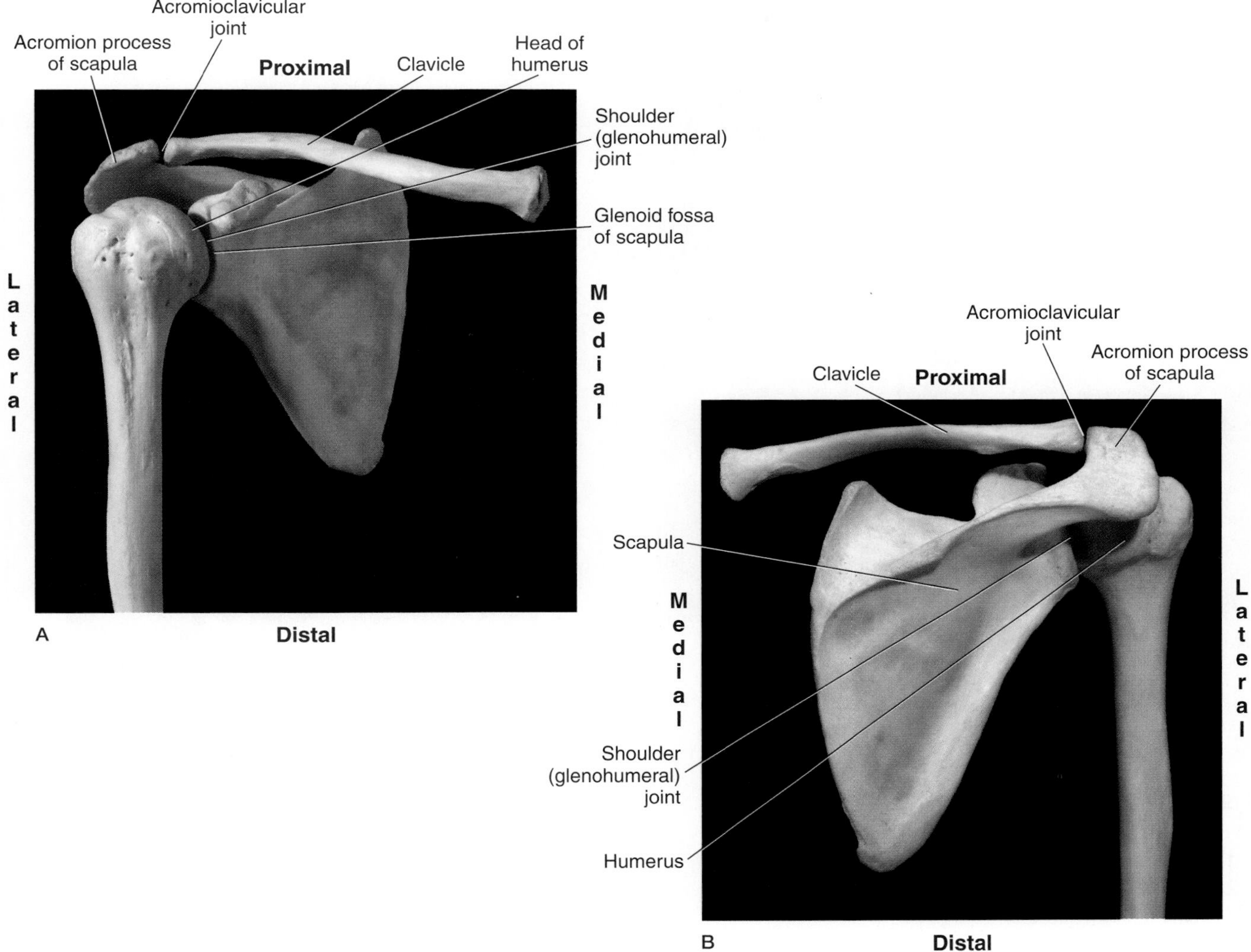

Figure 4-59
A, Anterior view; *B,* posterior view.

Notes:

1. The shoulder joint is formed by the head of the humerus articulating with the glenoid fossa of the humerus. It is also known as the *glenohumeral joint.*
2. Even though the glenohumeral joint is a ball-and-socket joint, the glenoid fossa (i.e., the socket) is shallow.
3. The acromioclavicular (AC) joint is formed by the acromion process of the scapula articulating with the lateral end of the clavicle.

Right Scapula—Posterior and Dorsal Views

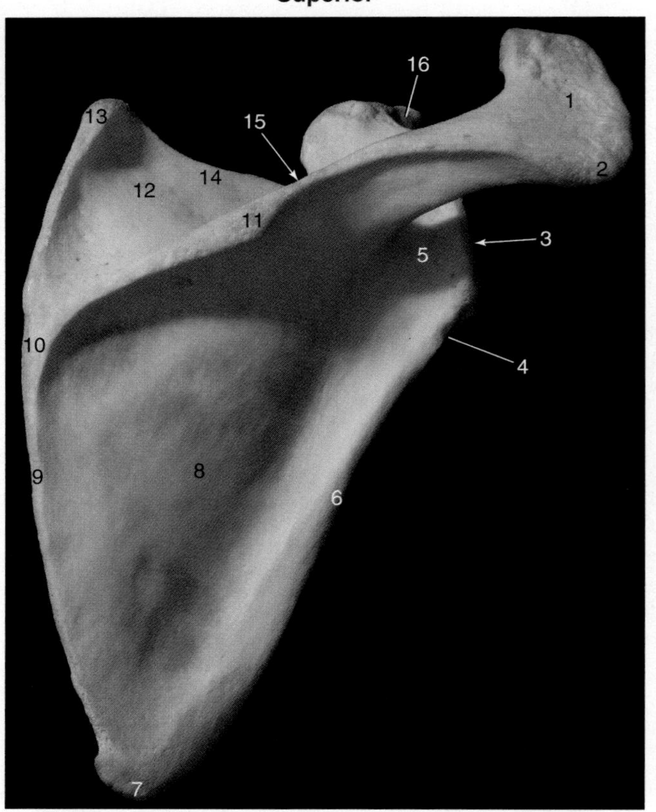

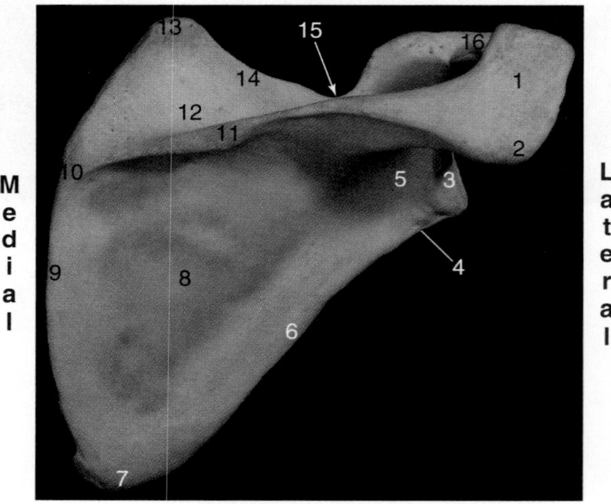

Figure 4-60
A, Posterior view; *B,* dorsal view.

1 Acromion process
2 Acromial angle
3 Glenoid fossa
4 Infraglenoid tubercle
5 Neck
6 Lateral border
7 Inferior angle
8 Infraspinous fossa
9 Medial border
10 Root of the spine
11 Spine
12 Supraspinous fossa
13 Superior angle
14 Superior border
15 Suprascapular notch
16 Coracoid process

Notes:

1. *A* is a pure posterior view of the scapula as it sits on the body; *B* is a view of the dorsal surface of the scapula itself. The difference in these two perspectives can be seen.
2. The medial border is also known as the *vertebral border.*
3. The lateral border is also known as the *axillary border.*
4. The supraspinous and infraspinous fossae are proximal attachment sites of the supraspinatus and infraspinatus muscles.
5. The infraglenoid tubercle and the suprascapular notch are not well developed on this scapula and therefore not well visualized.

Right Scapula—Anterior and Subscapular Views

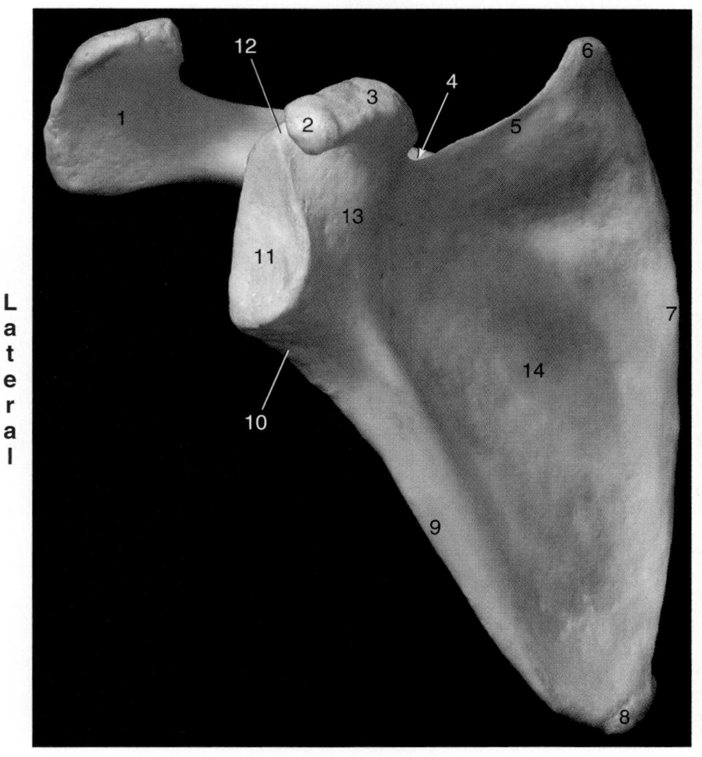

A

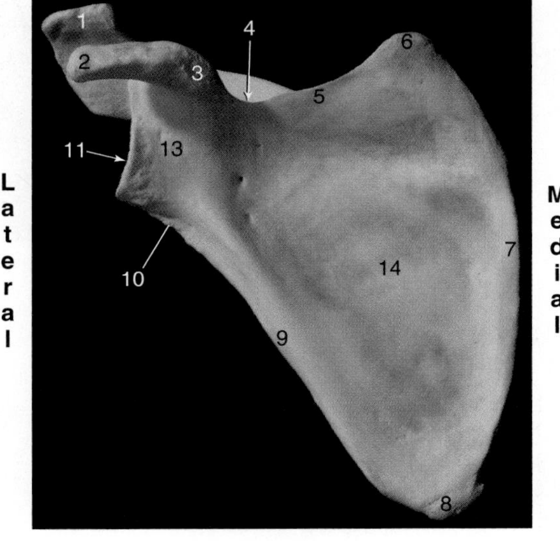

B

Figure 4-61
A, Anterior view; *B,* subscapular view.

1 Acromion process
2 Apex of coracoid process
3 Base of coracoid process
4 Suprascapular notch
5 Superior border
6 Superior angle
7 Medial border
8 Inferior angle
9 Lateral border
10 Infraglenoid tubercle
11 Glenoid fossa
12 Supraglenoid tubercle
13 Neck
14 Subscapular fossa

Notes:
1. *A* is a pure anterior view of the scapula as it sits on the body; *B* is a view of the subscapular (i.e., costal) surface of the scapula itself. The differences in these two perspectives can be seen.
2. The coracoid process projects anteriorly; it also points laterally.
3. The subscapular fossa is the proximal attachment site of the subscapularis muscle.
4. The supraglenoid tubercle is not well developed on this scapula and therefore not well visualized.

Right Scapula—Lateral and Superior Views

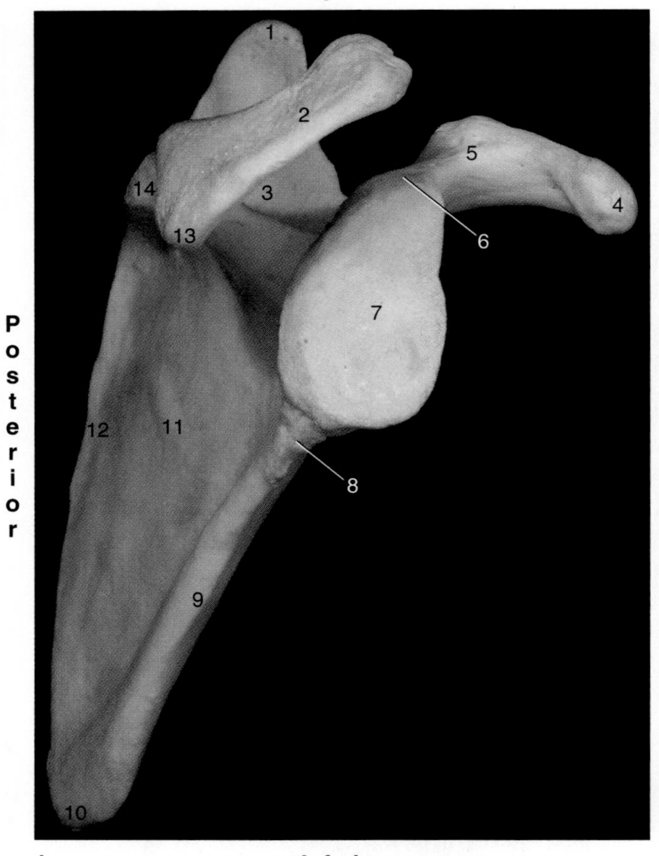

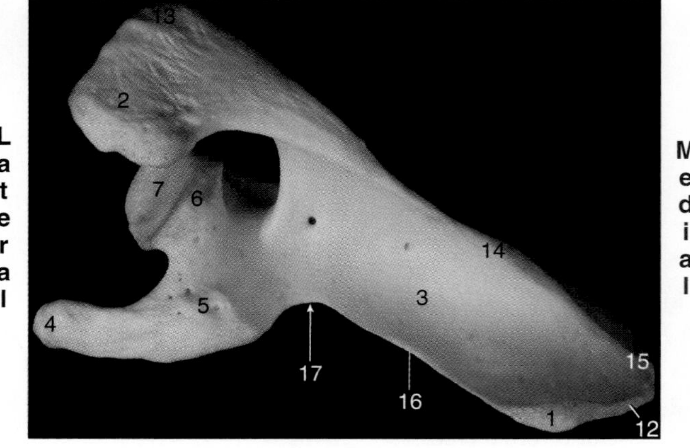

Figure 4-62
A, Lateral view; *B,* superior view.

1 Superior angle
2 Acromion process
3 Supraspinous fossa
4 Apex of coracoid process
5 Base of coracoid process
6 Supraglenoid tubercle
7 Glenoid fossa
8 Infraglenoid tubercle
9 Lateral border
10 Inferior angle
11 Infraspinous fossa
12 Medial border
13 Acromial angle
14 Spine
15 Root of the spine
16 Superior border
17 Suprascapular notch

Notes:

1. The supraglenoid tubercle is the proximal attachment site of the long head of the biceps brachii muscle.
2. The infraglenoid tubercle is the proximal attachment site of the long head of the triceps brachii muscle.

Right Clavicle

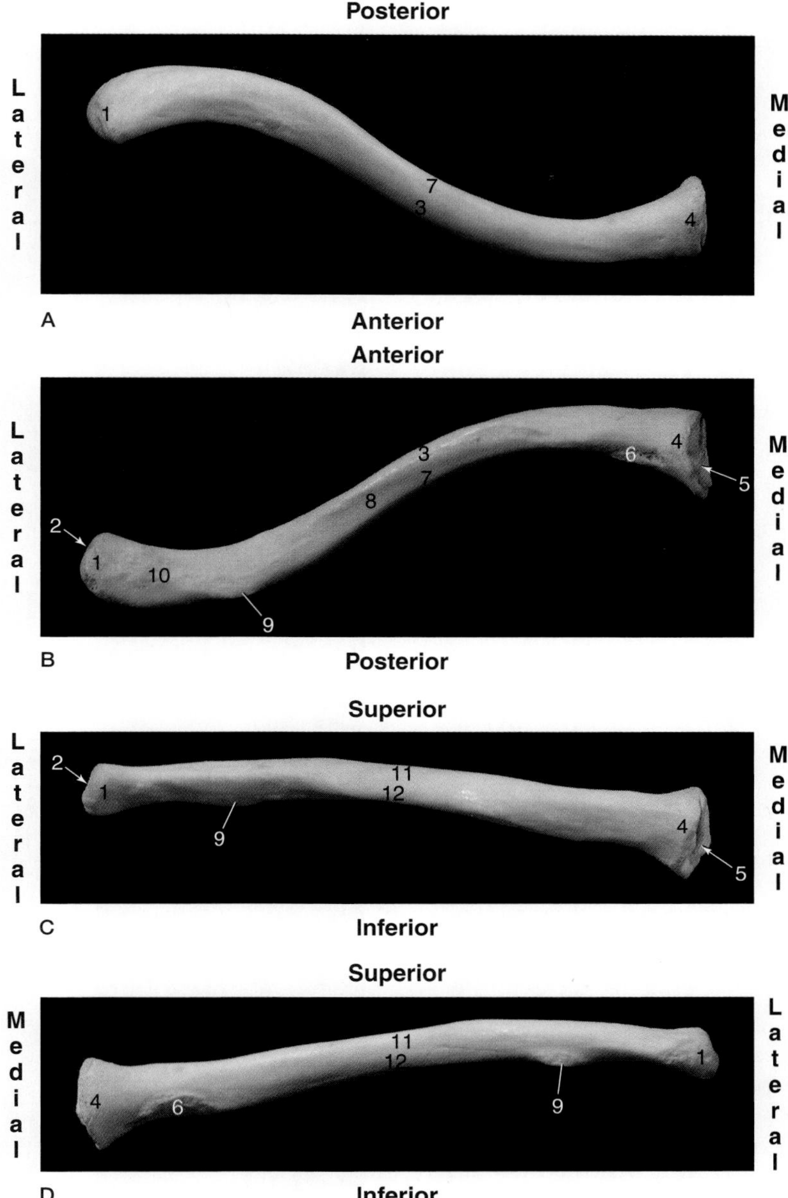

Figure 4-63
A, Superior view; *B,* inferior view; *C,* anterior view; *D,* posterior view.

1 Acromial end
2 Articular surface for acromioclavicular (AC) joint
3 Anterior border
4 Sternal end
5 Articular surface for sternoclavicular joint
6 Costal tubercle
7 Posterior border
8 Subclavian groove
9 Conoid tubercle
10 Trapezoid line
11 Superior border
12 Inferior border

Notes:
1. The acromial end is the lateral (distal) end.
2. The sternal end is the medial (proximal) end.
3. The sternal end of the clavicle is more bulbous, whereas the acromial end is flatter.
4. The medial $^2/_3$ of the clavicle is convex anteriorly; the lateral $^1/_3$ is concave anteriorly.
5. The conoid tubercle is the attachment site of the conoid ligament of the coracoclavicular ligament.
6. The trapezoid line is the attachment site of the trapezoid ligament of the coracoclavicular ligament.
7. The costal tubercle is the attachment site of the costoclavicular ligament.

☐ 4.11 BONES OF THE ARM AND ELBOW JOINT

Right Humerus—Anterior and Posterior Views

Figure 4-64
A, Anterior view; *B,* posterior view.

1 Head
2 Anatomic neck
3 Greater tubercle
4 Lesser tubercle
5 Bicipital groove
6 Surgical neck
7 Deltoid tuberosity
8 Body (shaft)
9 Groove for radial nerve
10 Lateral supracondylar ridge
11 Medial supracondylar ridge
12 Lateral condyle
13 Medial condyle
14 Lateral epicondyle
15 Medial epicondyle
16 Radial fossa
17 Coronoid fossa
18 Olecranon fossa
19 Trochlea
20 Capitulum

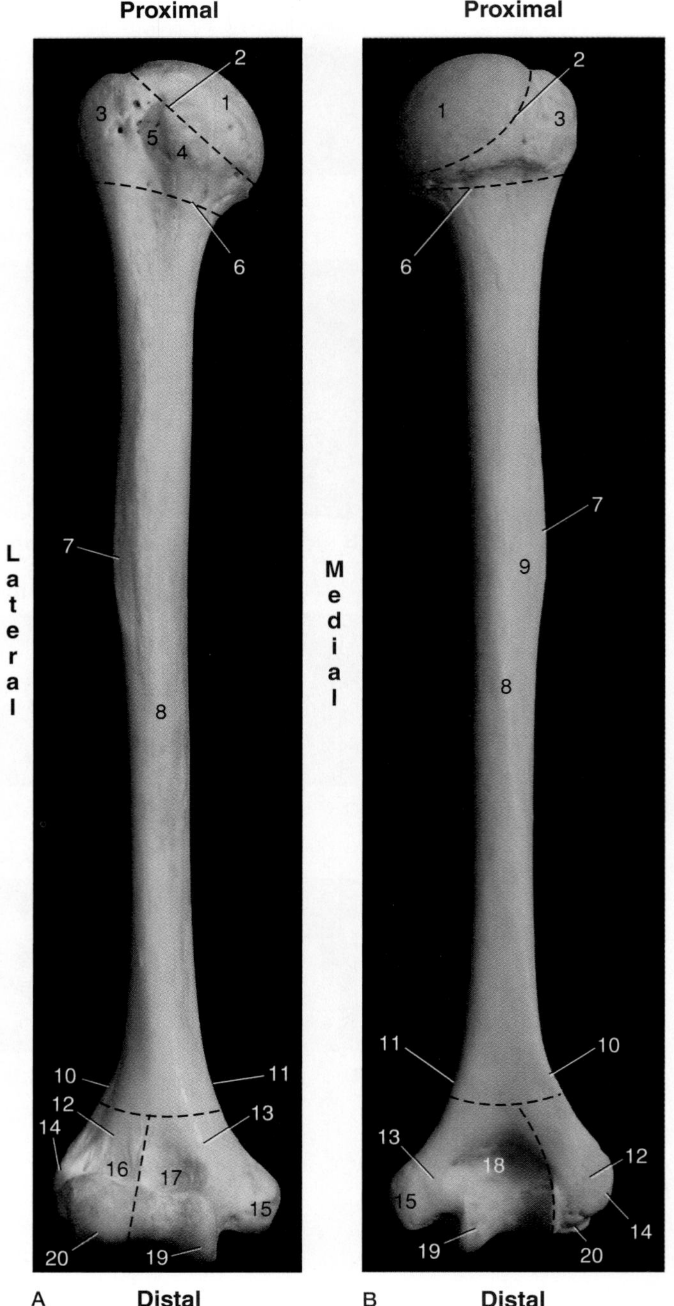

Notes:

1. Proximally, the anatomic and surgical necks are indicated by dashed lines; distally, the borders of the lateral and medial condyles are indicated by dashed lines.
2. The radial and coronoid fossae accept the head of the radius and the coronoid process of the ulna, respectively, when the elbow joint is flexed; the olecranon fossa accepts the olecranon process of the ulna when the elbow joint is extended.
3. The bicipital groove (so named because the biceps brachii long head tendon runs through it) is also known as the *intertubercular groove* (so named because it is located between the greater and lesser tubercles).
4. The groove for the radial nerve is also known as the *spiral groove.*

Right Humerus—Lateral and Medial Views

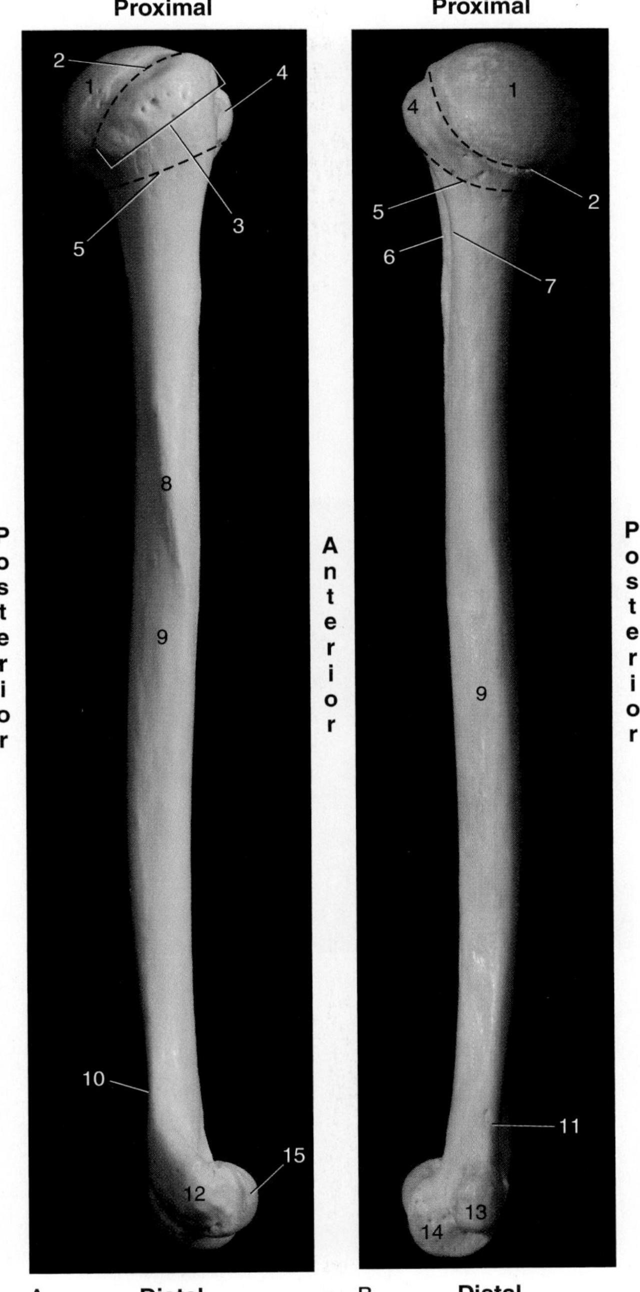

Figure 4-65
A, Lateral view; *B,* medial view.

1 Head
2 Anatomic neck
3 Greater tubercle
4 Lesser tubercle
5 Surgical neck
6 Lateral lip of bicipital groove
7 Medial lip of bicipital groove
8 Deltoid tuberosity
9 Body (shaft)
10 Lateral supracondylar ridge
11 Medial supracondylar ridge
12 Lateral epicondyle
13 Medial epicondyle
14 Trochlea
15 Capitulum

Notes:

1. The anatomic and surgical necks are indicated by dashed lines.
2. The lateral epicondyle and capitulum are landmarks on the lateral condyle; the medial epicondyle and trochlea are landmarks on the medial condyle.
3. The lateral and medial epicondyles are the most prominent points on the lateral and medial condyles, respectively.
4. The medial epicondyle is the attachment site of the common flexor tendon of many of the anterior forearm muscles; the lateral epicondyle is the attachment site of the common extensor tendon of many of the posterior forearm muscles.
5. The deltoid tuberosity is the distal attachment site of the deltoid muscle.

Right Humerus—Proximal and Distal Views

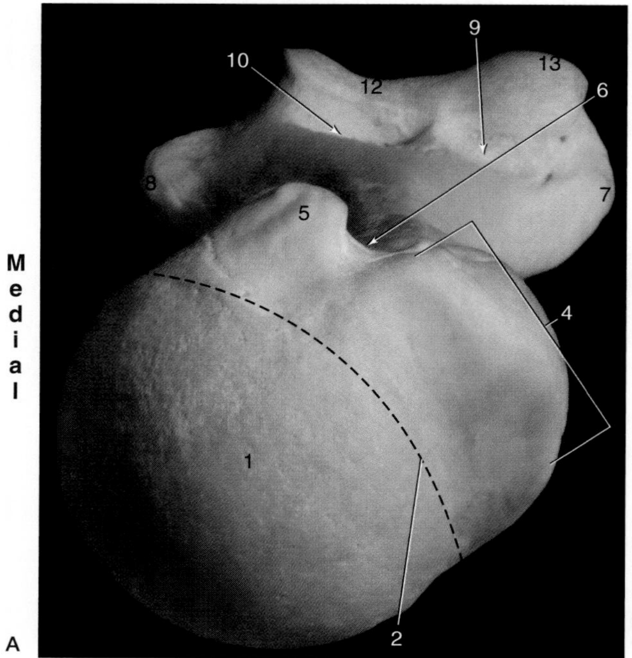

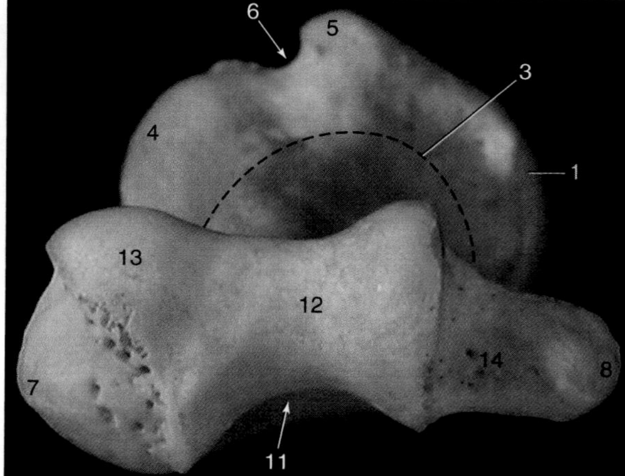

Figure 4-66
A, Proximal (superior) view; *B,* distal (inferior) view.

1 Head
2 Anatomic neck
3 Surgical neck
4 Greater tubercle
5 Lesser tubercle
6 Bicipital groove
7 Lateral epicondyle
8 Medial epicondyle
9 Radial fossa
10 Coronoid fossa
11 Olecranon fossa
12 Trochlea
13 Capitulum
14 Groove for ulnar nerve

Notes:

1. The anatomic and surgical necks are indicated by dashed lines.
2. The ulnar nerve runs in a groove that is located between the medial epicondyle and trochlea of the humerus (it can easily be palpated at this location). The ulnar nerve at this site is often referred to as the *funny bone.*

Right Elbow Joint

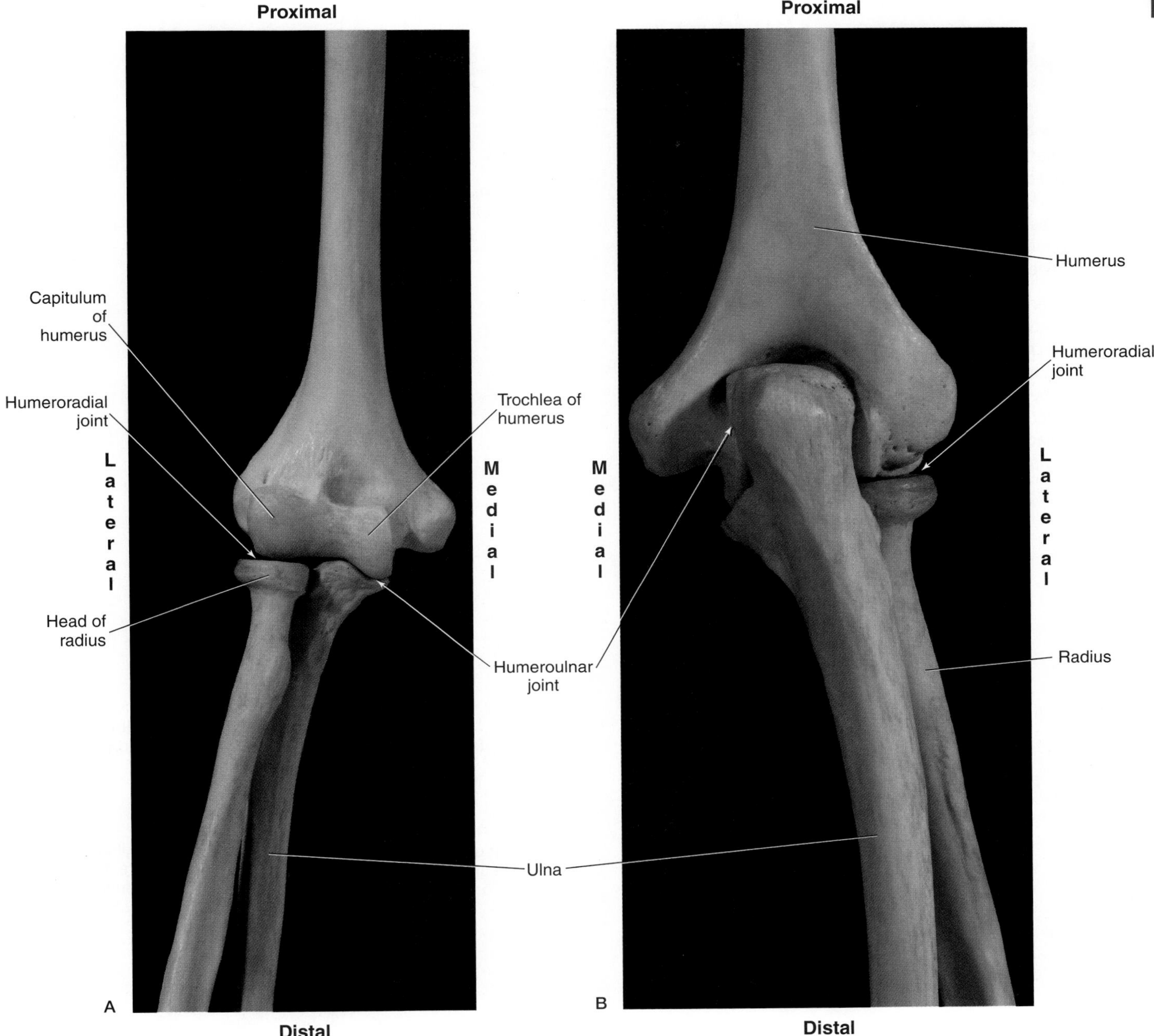

Figure 4-67
A, Anterior view; *B,* posterior view.

Notes:

1. The elbow joint is composed of the humeroulnar and humeroradial joints.
2. The major articulation of the elbow joint is the humeroulnar joint where the trochlea of the humerus articulates with the trochlear notch of the ulna (see Figure 4-68).
3. The humeroradial articulation is not very important functionally to movement at the elbow joint; the humeroradial articulation is formed between the capitulum of the humerus and the head of the radius.
4. The proximal radioulnar joint between the head of the radius and the radial notch of the ulna is anatomically within the same joint capsule as the elbow joint. However, functionally, it is distinct from the elbow joint.

☐ 4.12 BONES OF THE FOREARM, WRIST JOINT, AND HAND

Right Radius/Ulna—Anterior View

Figure 4-68
Landmarks of the Radius
1 Head
2 Neck
3 Tuberosity
4 Interosseus crest
5 Styloid process

Landmarks of the Ulna
6 Olecranon process
7 Trochlear notch
8 Coronoid process
9 Tuberosity
10 Interosseus crest
11 Head
12 Styloid process

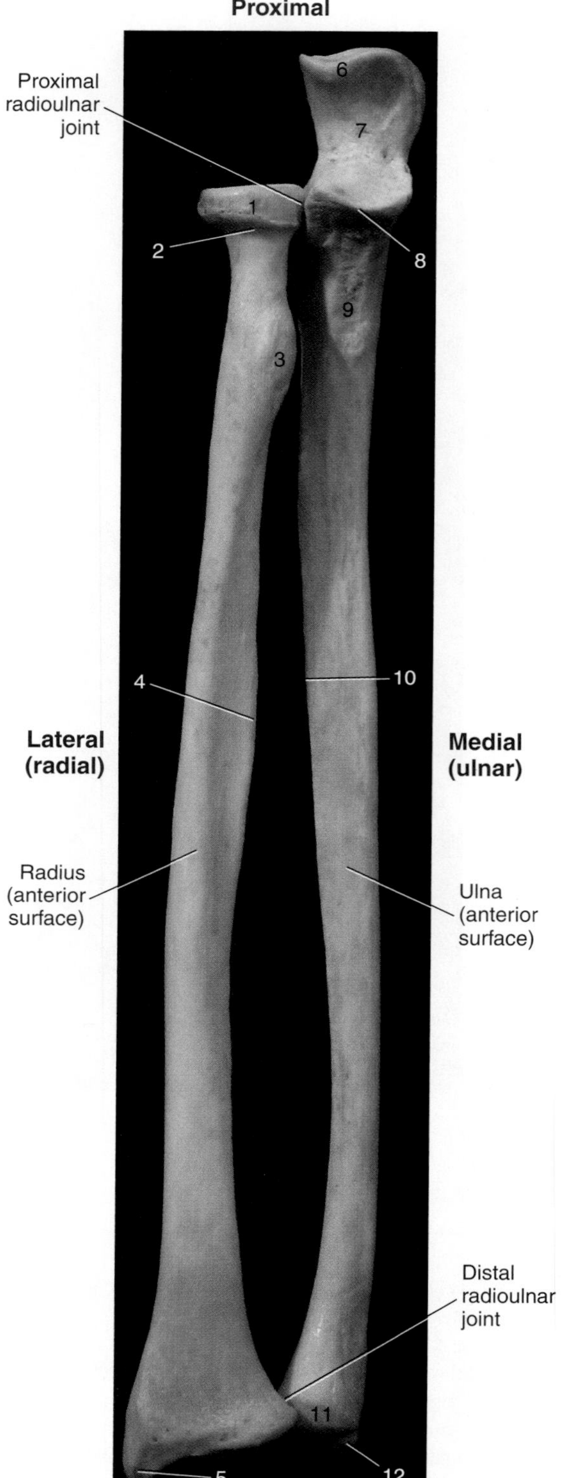

Notes:

1. The radius and ulna articulate with each other both proximally (at the proximal radioulnar joint) and distally (at the distal radioulnar joint).
2. The interosseous crests of the radius and ulna are the attachment sites of the interosseus membrane of the forearm (this interosseus membrane uniting the radius and ulna creates the middle radioulnar joint).
3. The styloid process of the radius projects laterally; the styloid process of the ulna projects posteriorly.

Right Radius/Ulna—Posterior View

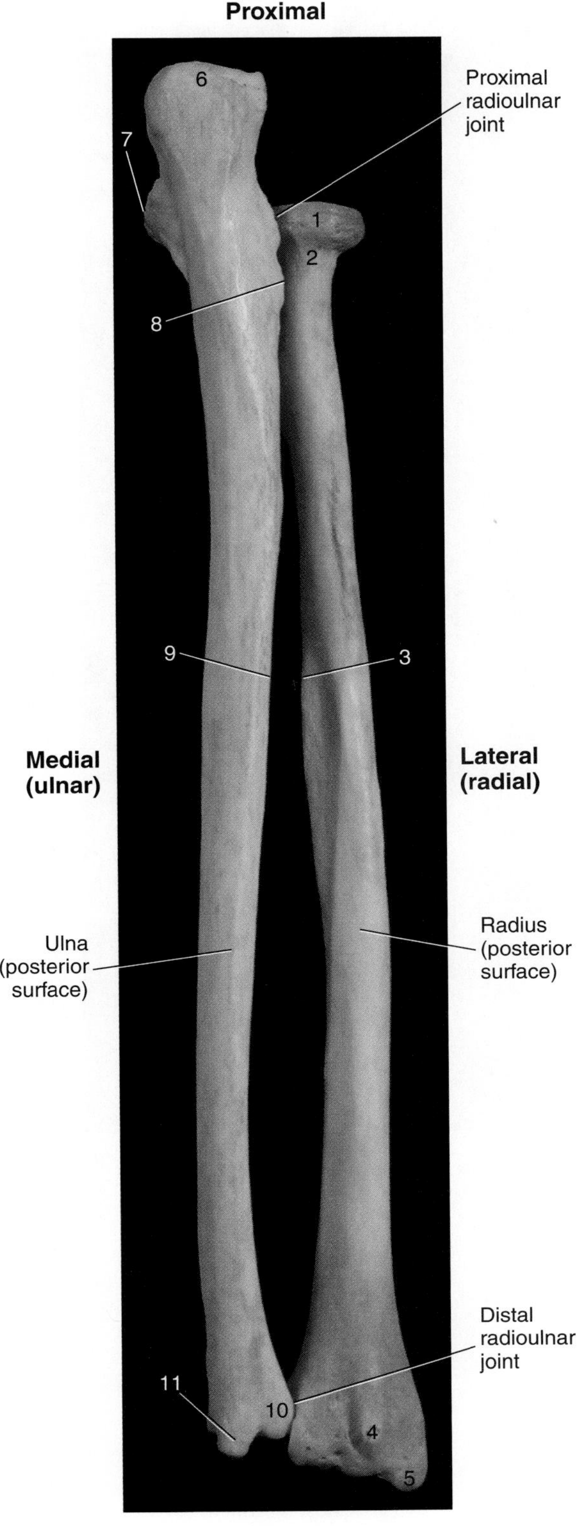

Figure 4-69

Landmarks of the Radius

1 Head
2 Neck
3 Interosseus crest
4 Dorsal tubercle
5 Styloid process

Landmarks of the Ulna

6 Olecranon process
7 Coronoid process
8 Supinator crest
9 Interosseus crest
10 Head
11 Styloid process

Notes:

1. The dorsal tubercle of the radius is also known as *Lister's tubercle.*
2. The distal tendons of the extensors carpi radialis longus and brevis muscles pass between the dorsal tubercle and styloid process of the radius.
3. The distal tendons of the extensor digitorum, extensor indicis, and extensor pollicis longus muscles pass medial to the dorsal tubercle of the radius.
4. The distal tendon of the extensor carpi ulnaris muscle is located within a groove located between the styloid process and head of the ulna.

Right Radius/Ulna—Lateral Views

Figure 4-70
A, Right lateral view of the radius and ulna articulated.
B, Right lateral view of just the ulna.

Landmarks of the Radius:
1 Head
2 Neck
3 Radial tuberosity
4 Grooves for the abductor pollicis longus and extensor pollicis brevis
5 Styloid process
6 Groove for the extensor carpi radialis longus
7 Groove for the extensor carpi radialis brevis
8 Dorsal tubercle

Landmarks of the Ulna:
9 Olecranon process
10 Trochlear notch
11 Coronoid process
12 Radial notch
13 Interosseus crest
14 Tuberosity
15 Supinator crest
16 Head
17 Styloid process

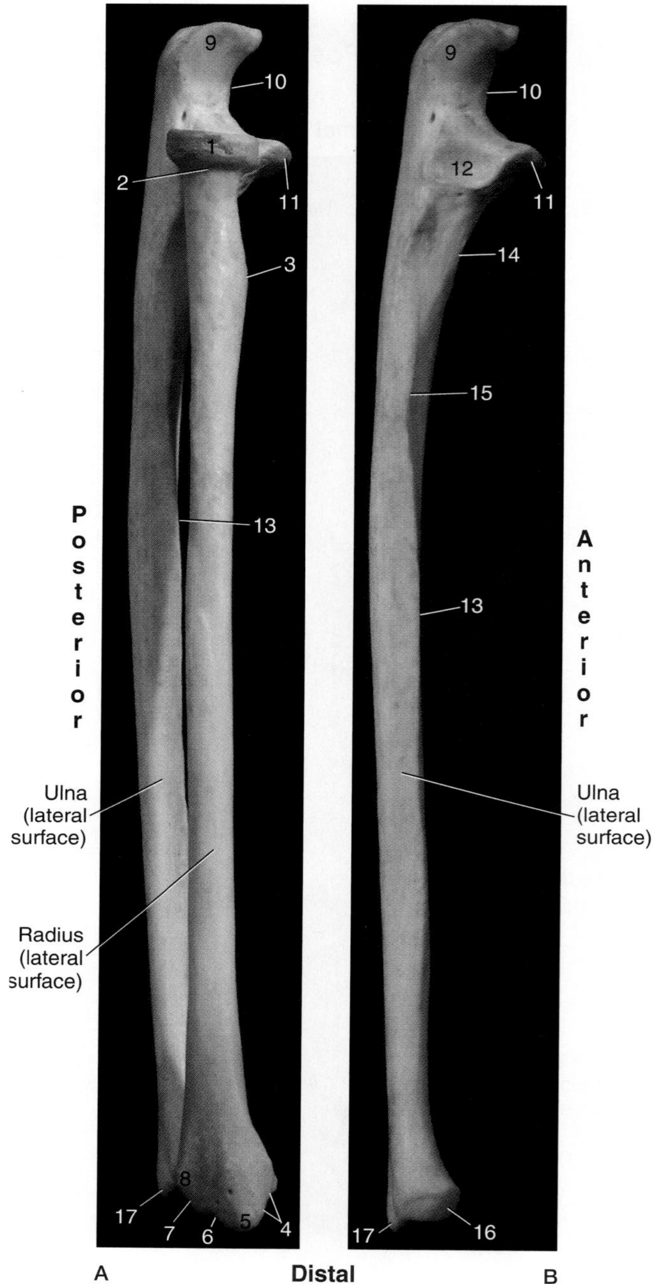

Notes:
1. The head of the radius articulates with the ulna at the radial notch.
2. The lateral view of the ulna *(B)* nicely demonstrates the interosseous crest of the ulna.
3. The grooves for the abductor pollicis longus and extensor pollicis brevis distal tendons are located just anterior to the styloid process of the radius.
4. The tuberosity of the ulna is not well developed on this ulna and therefore is not well visualized.

Right Radius/Ulna—Medial Views

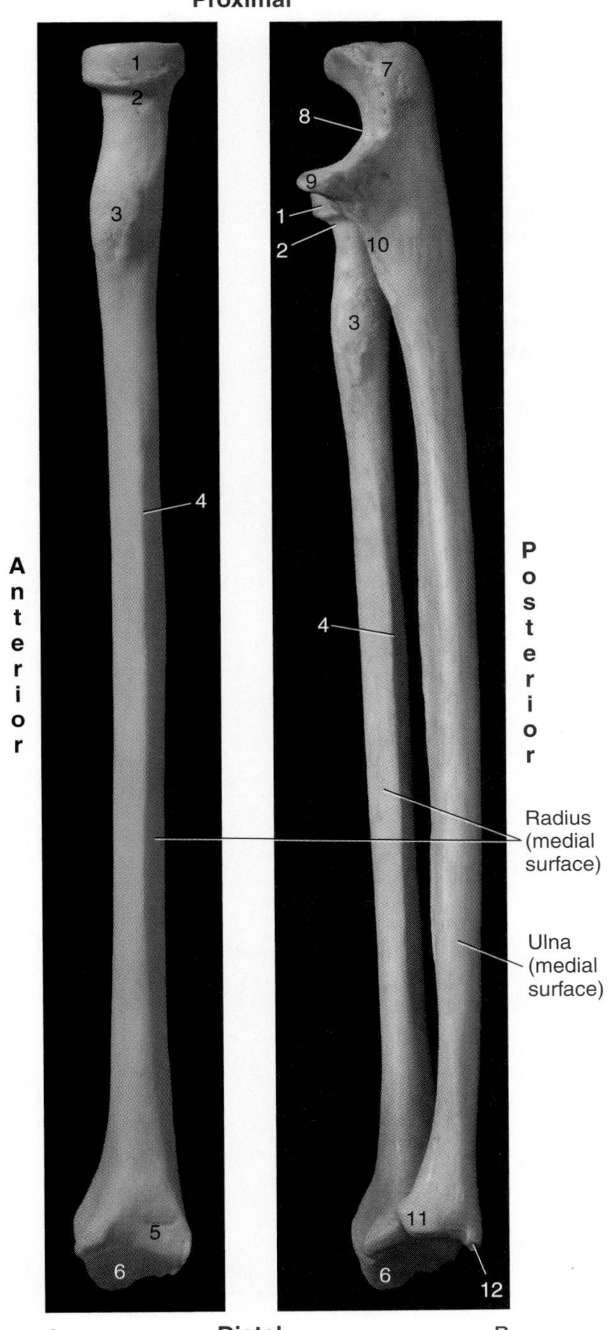

Figure 4-71
A, Medial view of the radius and ulna articulated.
B, Medial view of just the radius.

Landmarks of the Radius:
1 Head
2 Neck
3 Tuberosity
4 Interosseus crest
5 Ulnar notch
6 Styloid process

Landmarks of the Ulna:
7 Olecranon process
8 Trochlear notch
9 Coronoid process
10 Tuberosity
11 Head
12 Styloid process

Notes:
1. The distal end of the ulna articulates with the radius at the ulnar notch of the radius.
2. The medial view of the radius *(B)* nicely demonstrates the interosseous crest of the radius.

Right Radius/Ulna—Pronated

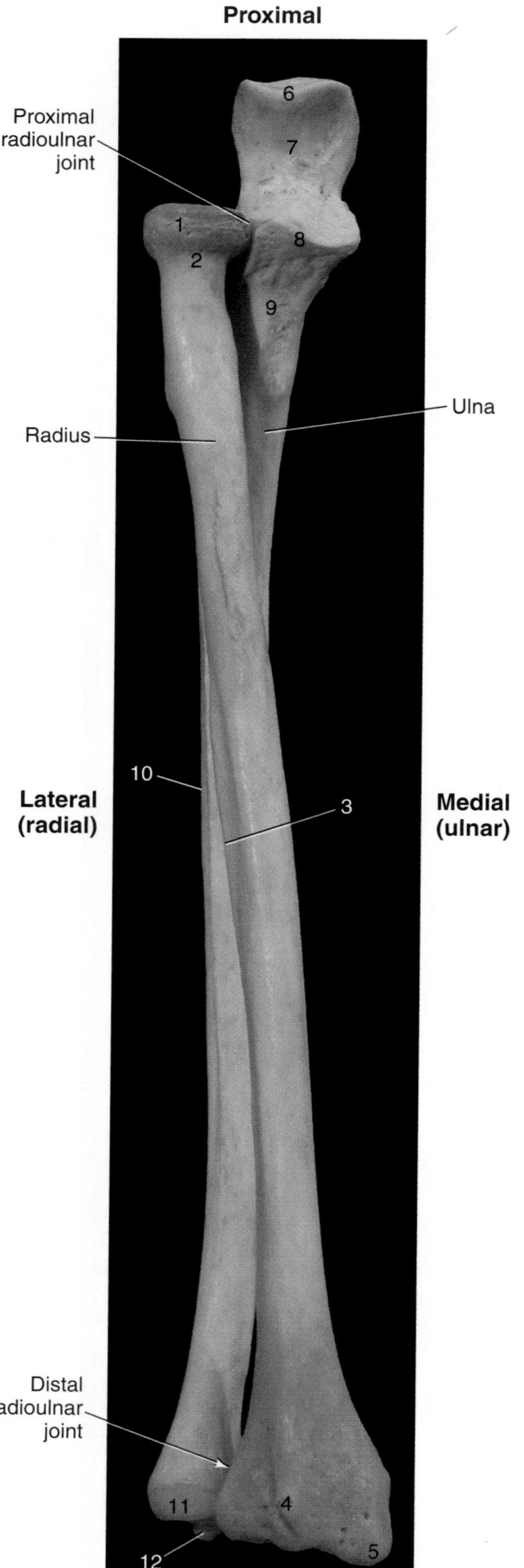

Figure 4-72
Landmarks of the Radius
1 Head
2 Neck
3 Interosseus crest
4 Dorsal tubercle
5 Styloid process

Landmarks of the Ulna
6 Olecranon process
7 Trochlear notch
8 Coronoid process
9 Tuberosity
10 Interosseus crest
11 Head
12 Styloid process

Notes:

1. Pronation of the forearm bones causes the bones to cross each other from the anterior perspective.
2. Pronation and supination of the forearm occur at the radioulnar joints and usually involves a mobile radius moving around a fixed ulna. The head of the radius rotates relative to the ulna and the distal radius swings around the distal ulna (from this anterior perspective, we see the posterior surface of the distal radius).

Right Radius/Ulna—Proximal and Distal Views

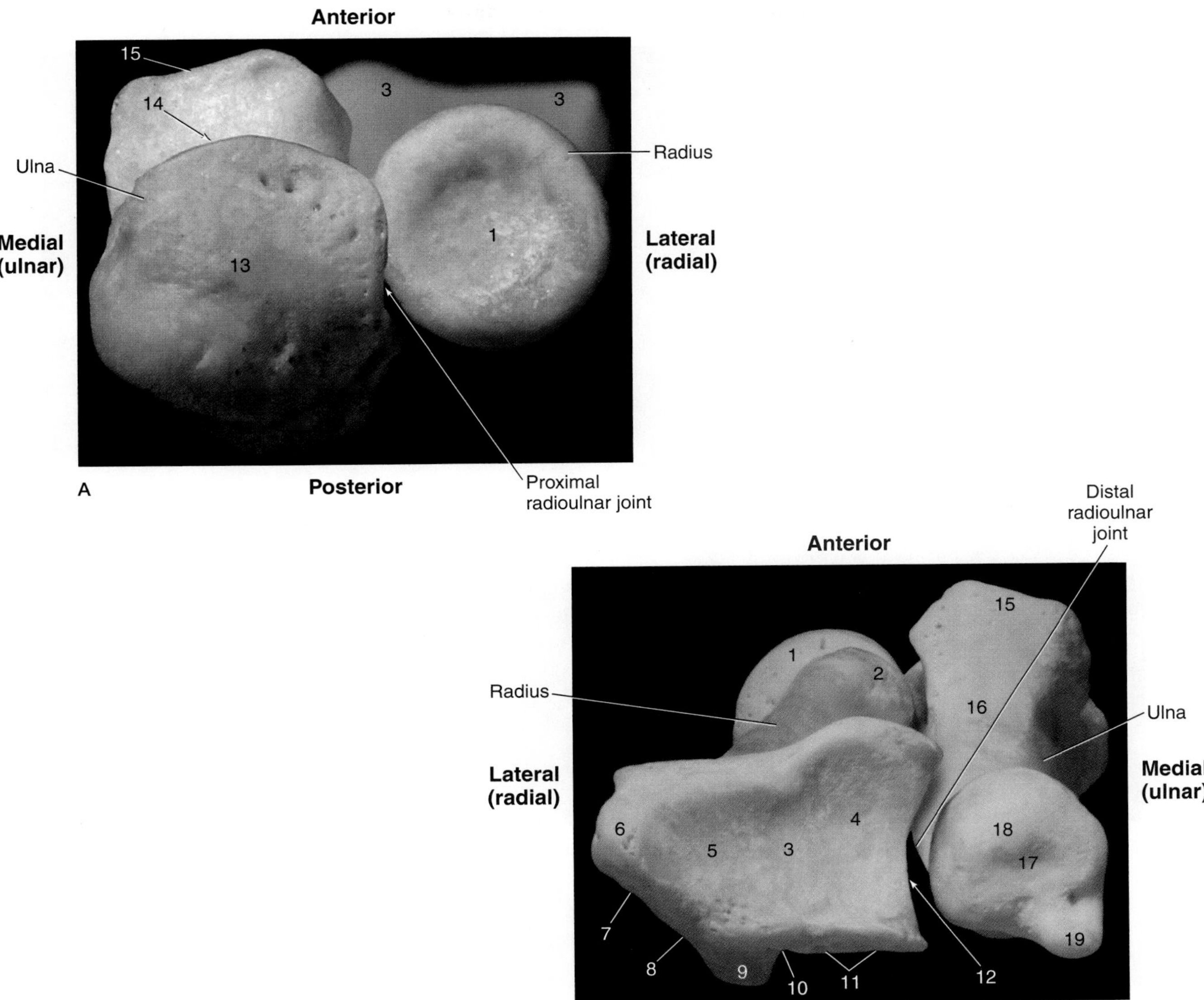

Figure 4-73
A, Proximal (superior) view of the radius and ulna articulated.
B, Distal (inferior) view of the radius and ulna articulated.

Landmarks of the Radius
1 Head
2 Tuberosity
3 Distal end of the radius
4 Articular surface for lunate
5 Articular surface for scaphoid
6 Styloid process
7 Groove for extensor carpi radialis longus tendon
8 Groove for extensor carpi radialis brevis tendon
9 Dorsal tubercle
10 Groove for extensor pollicis longus tendon
11 Groove for extensor digitorum and extensor indicis tendons
12 Ulnar notch

Landmarks of the Ulna
13 Olecranon process
14 Trochlear notch
15 Coronoid process
16 Tuberosity
17 Distal end of the ulna
18 Head
19 Styloid process

Notes:
1. The head of the radius has a concavity at its proximal end to accept the capitulum of the humerus (at the humeroradial joint).
2. The distal end of the ulna articulates with the radius at the ulnar notch of the radius (at the distal radioulnar joint).

Right Carpal Bones (Separated)—Anterior View

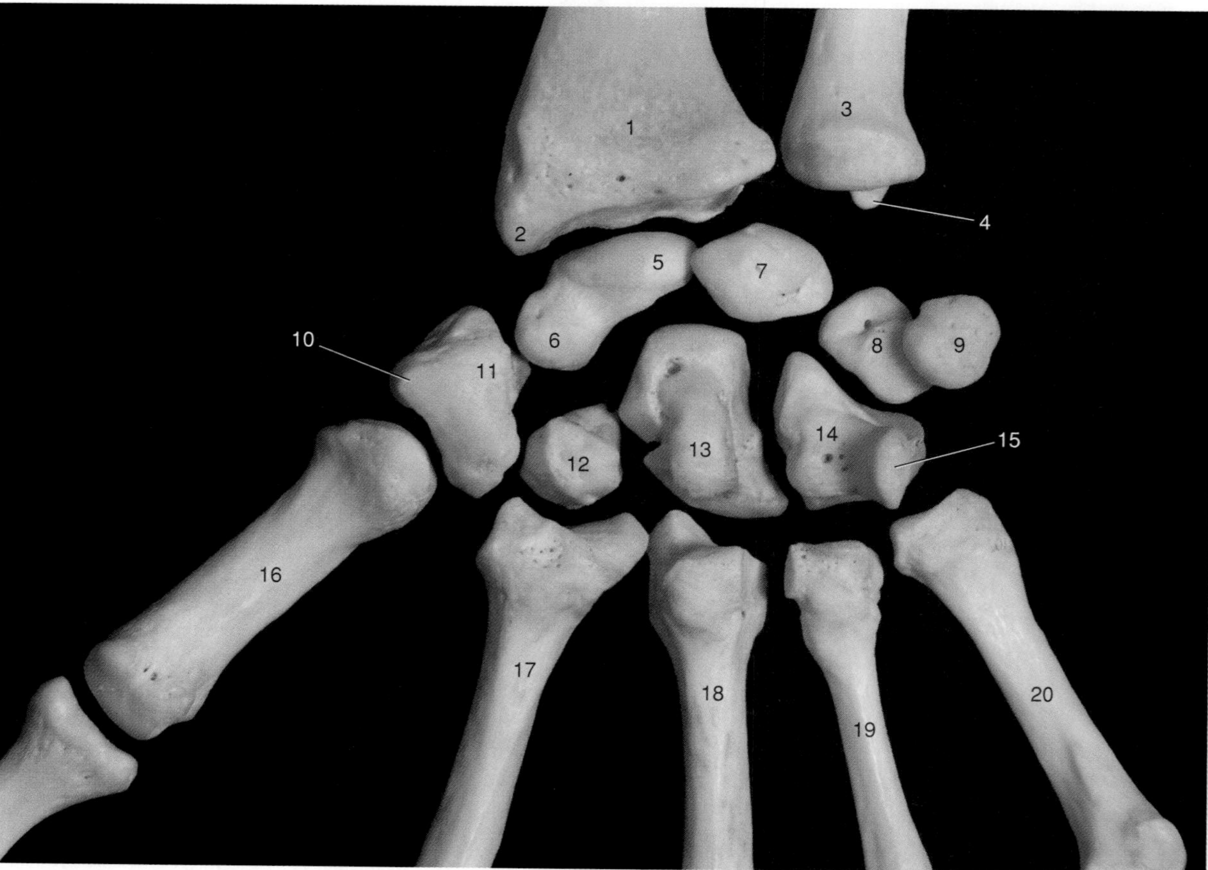

Figure 4-74

1 Radius
2 Styloid process of radius
3 Ulna
4 Styloid process of ulna
5 Scaphoid
6 Tubercle of scaphoid
7 Lunate
8 Triquetrum
9 Pisiform
10 Trapezium
11 Tubercle of trapezium
12 Trapezoid
13 Capitate
14 Hamate
15 Hook of hamate
16 1st Metacarpal (of thumb)
17 2nd Metacarpal (of index finger)
18 3rd Metacarpal (of middle finger)
19 4th Metacarpal (of ring finger)
20 5th Metacarpal (of little finger)

Notes:

1. Eight carpal bones are arranged in two rows: proximal and distal. The proximal row (radial to ulnar) is composed of the scaphoid, lunate, triquetrum, and pisiform; the distal row (radial to ulnar) is composed of the trapezium, trapezoid, capitate, and hamate.
2. A mnemonic can be used to learn the names of the carpal bones. From proximal row to distal row (always radial to ulnar), it is: ***S**ome **L**overs **T**ry **P**ositions **T**hat **T**hey **C**an't **H**andle.*
3. The flexor retinaculum, which forms the ceiling of the carpal tunnel, attaches to the tubercles of the scaphoid and trapezium on the radial side and the hook of the hamate and pisiform on the ulnar side.
4. The pisiform is sesamoid bone (explaining why humans have eight carpal bones and seven tarsal bones).
5. The metacarpal bones are numbered 1 to 5 (numbering begins on the radial [i.e., thumb] side).

Right Carpal Bones (Separated)—Posterior View

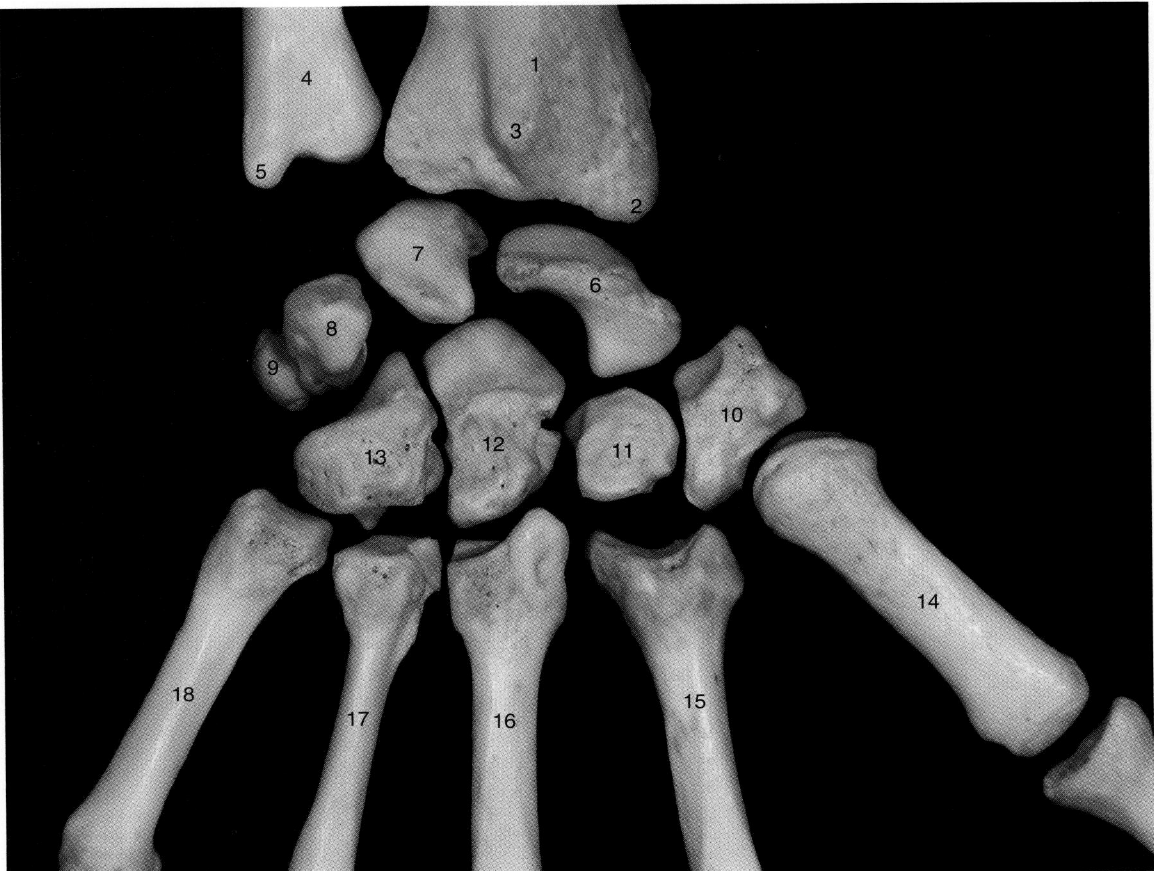

Figure 4-75

1 Radius
2 Styloid process of radius
3 Dorsal tubercle of radius
4 Ulna
5 Styloid process of ulna
6 Scaphoid
7 Lunate
8 Triquetrum
9 Pisiform
10 Trapezium
11 Trapezoid
12 Capitate
13 Hamate
14 1st Metacarpal (of thumb)
15 2nd Metacarpal (of index finger)
16 3rd Metacarpal (of middle finger
17 4th Metacarpal (of ring finger)
18 5th Metacarpal (of little finger)

Notes:

1. The trapezium articulates with the 1st metacarpal (of the thumb); the trapezoid articulates with the 2nd metacarpal (of the index finger); the capitate articulates with the 3rd metacarpal (of the middle finger); and the hamate articulates with the 4th and 5th metacarpals (of the ring and little fingers).
2. The joint between the trapezium and 1st metacarpal (of the thumb) is the 1st carpometacarpal joint, also known as the *saddle joint* of the thumb.
3. At the wrist region, it is the radius that articulates with the carpal bones, not the ulna; the wrist joint is often referred to as the *radiocarpal joint*.
4. The scaphoid is the most commonly fractured carpal bone. The lunate is the most commonly dislocated carpal bone.

Right Wrist/Hand—Anterior View

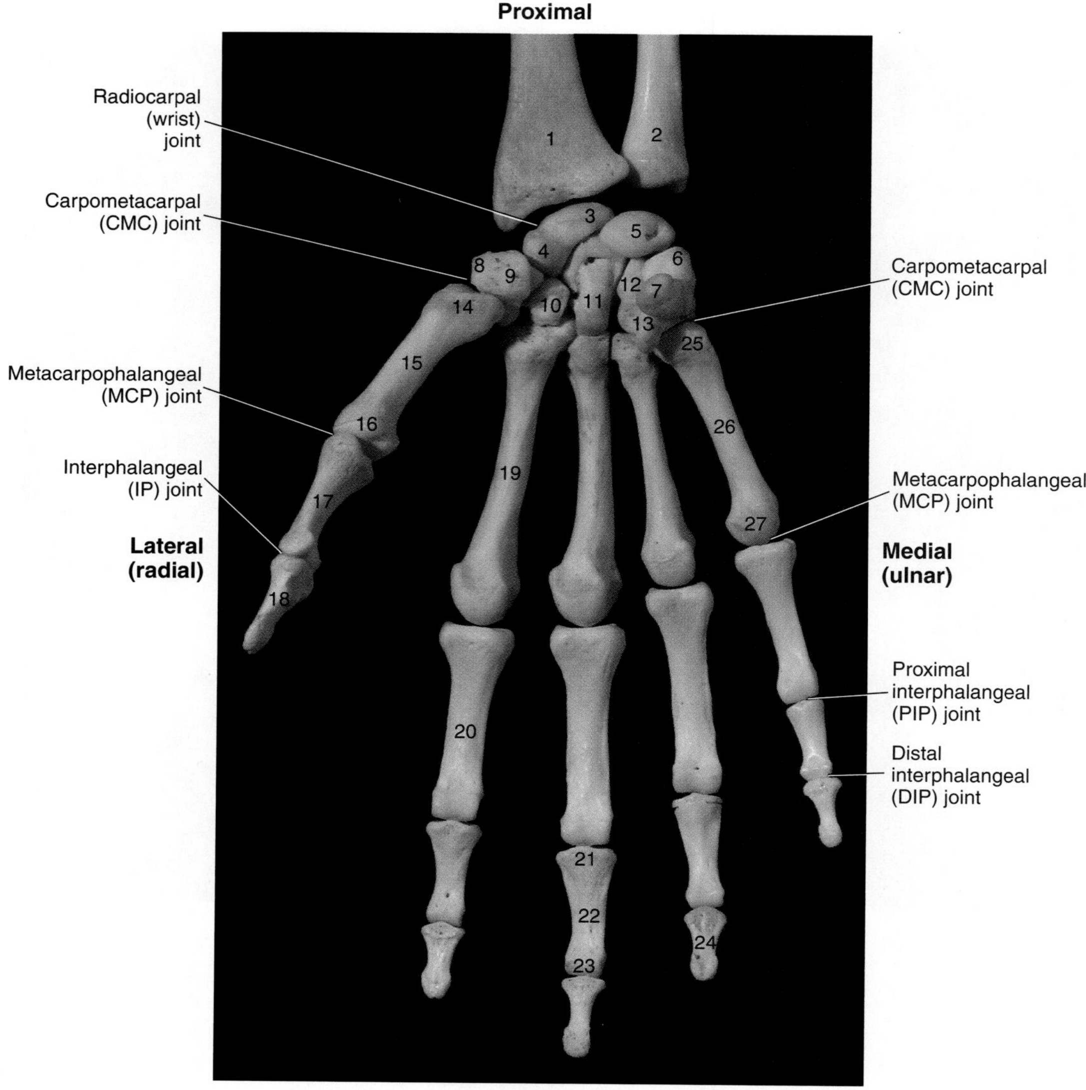

Figure 4-76

1 Radius
2 Ulna
3 Scaphoid
4 Tubercle of scaphoid
5 Lunate
6 Triquetrum
7 Pisiform
8 Trapezium
9 Tubercle of trapezium
10 Trapezoid
11 Capitate
12 Hamate
13 Hook of hamate
14 Base of 1st metacarpal (of thumb)
15 Body (shaft) of 1st metacarpal (of thumb)
16 Head of 1st metacarpal (of thumb)
17 Proximal phalanx of thumb
18 Distal phalanx of thumb
19 2nd Metacarpal (of index finger)
20 Proximal phalanx of index finger
21 Base of middle phalanx of middle finger
22 Body (shaft) of middle phalanx of middle finger
23 Head of middle phalanx of middle finger
24 Distal phalanx of ring finger
25 Base of 5th metacarpal (of little finger)
26 Body (shaft) of 5th metacarpal (of little finger)
27 Head of 5th metacarpal (of little finger)

Notes:

1. The thumb has two phalanges, proximal and distal; the other four fingers each have three phalanges, proximal, middle, and distal.
2. All metacarpals and phalanges have the following landmarks: a base proximally, a body (shaft) in the middle, and a head distally.
3. The length of a metacarpal of a ray is equal to the length of the proximal and middle phalanges of that ray added together; the length of a proximal phalanx of a ray is equal to the length of the middle and distal phalanges of that ray added together.

Right Wrist/Hand—Posterior View

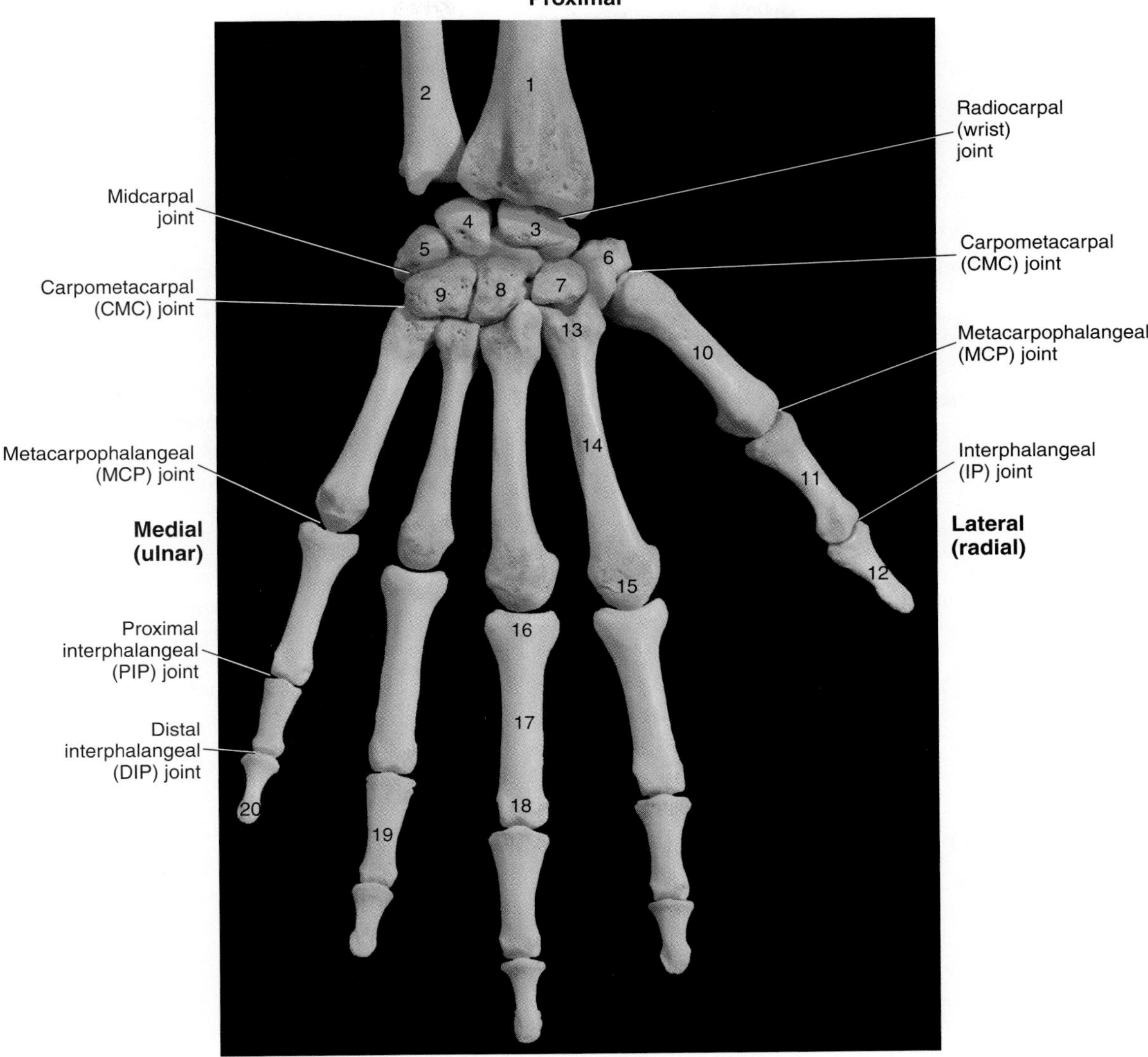

Figure 4-77

1 Radius
2 Ulna
3 Scaphoid
4 Lunate
5 Triquetrum
6 Trapezium
7 Trapezoid
8 Capitate
9 Hamate
10 1st Metacarpal (of thumb)
11 Proximal phalanx of thumb
12 Distal phalanx of thumb
13 Base of metacarpal of index finger
14 Body (shaft) of metacarpal of index finger
15 Head of metacarpal of index finger
16 Base of proximal phalanx of middle finger
17 Body (shaft) of proximal phalanx of middle finger
18 Head of proximal phalanx of middle finger
19 Middle phalanx of little finger
20 Distal phalanx of little finger

Notes:

1. The wrist joint is composed of the radiocarpal and midcarpal joints.
2. The radiocarpal joint is located between the radius and the proximal row of carpal bones. The midcarpal joint is located between the proximal and distal rows of carpal bones. In Figure 4-77, the radiocarpal joint is indicated in green and the midcarpal joint is indicated in yellow.

Right Wrist/Hand—Medial View

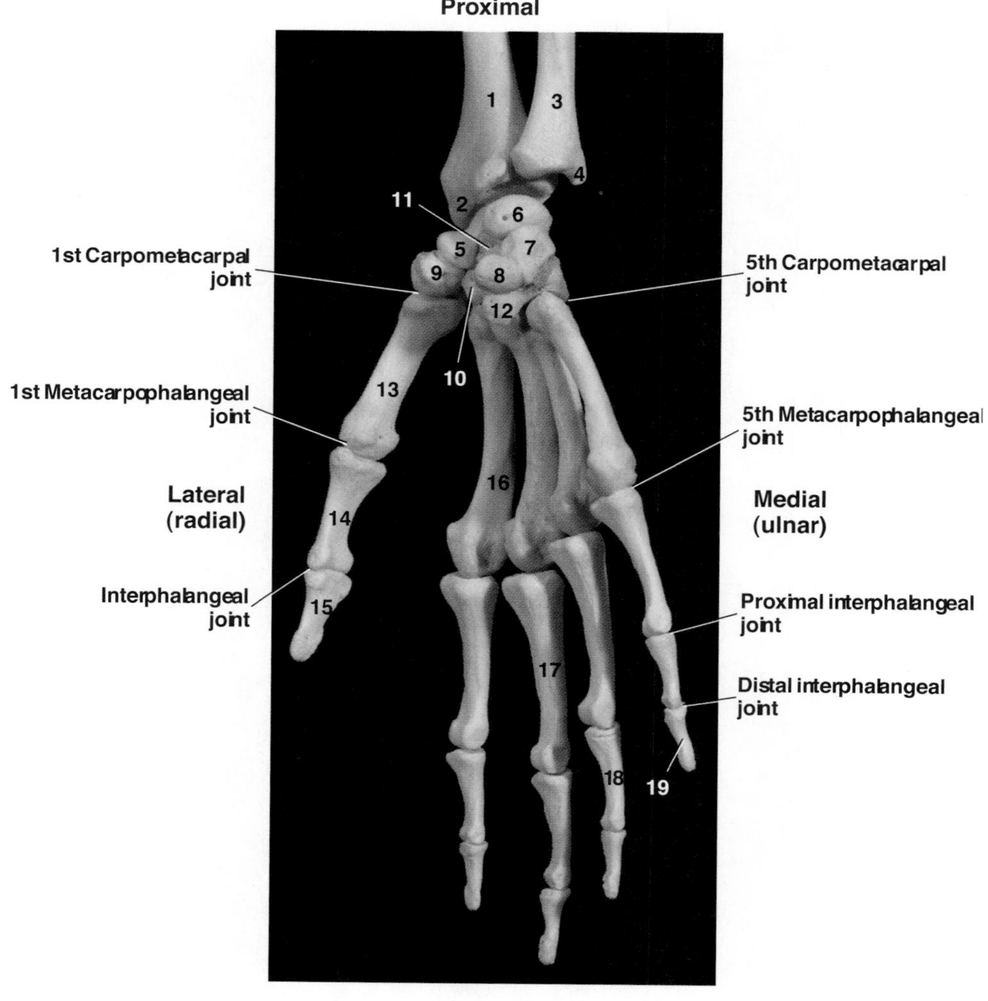

Figure 4-78

1 Radius
2 Styloid process of the radius
3 Ulna
4 Styloid process of the ulna
5 Scaphoid
6 Lunate
7 Triquetrum
8 Pisiform
9 Trapezium
10 Trapezoid
11 Capitate
12 Hamate
13 1st Metacarpal (of thumb)
14 Proximal phalanx of thumb
15 Distal phalanx of thumb
16 Metacarpal of index finger
17 Proximal phalanx of middle finger
18 Middle phalanx of ring finger
19 Distal phalanx of little finger

Notes:

1. The thumb has only two phalanges, hence only one interphalangeal joint.
2. The other fingers have three phalanges, hence two interphalangeal joints, a proximal interphalangeal joint and a distal interphalangeal joint.
3. An interphalangeal joint is often abbreviated as an *IP joint.*
4. The proximal interphalangeal joint is often abbreviated as the *PIP joint.*
5. The distal interphalangeal joint is often abbreviated as the *DIP joint.*
6. The carpometacarpal joint is often abbreviated as the *CMC joint.*
7. The metacarpophalangeal joint is often abbreviated as the *MCP joint.*

Right Wrist/Hand (Flexed) and Carpal Tunnel

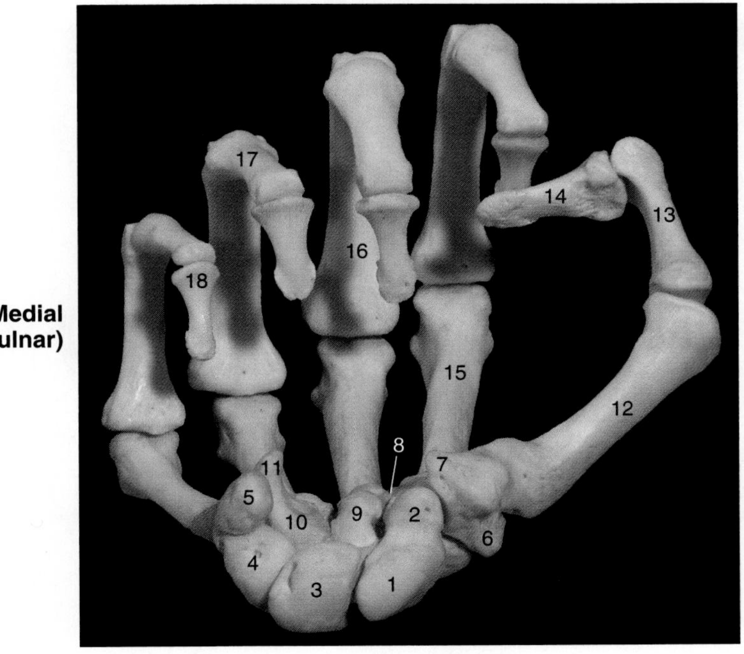

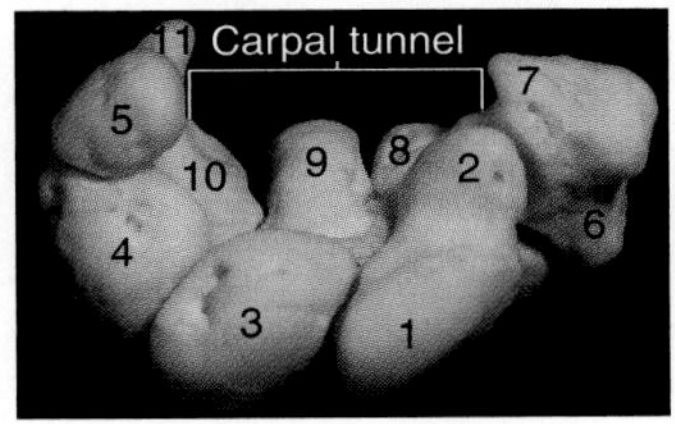

Figure 4-79
A, Proximal view of right wrist and hand with fingers flexed; *B,* proximal view of right carpal tunnel.

1 Scaphoid
2 Tubercle of scaphoid
3 Lunate
4 Triquetrum
5 Pisiform
6 Trapezium
7 Tubercle of trapezium
8 Trapezoid
9 Capitate
10 Hamate
11 Hook of hamate
12 1st Metacarpal (of thumb)
13 Proximal phalanx of thumb
14 Distal phalanx of thumb
15 Metacarpal of index finger
16 Proximal phalanx of middle finger
17 Middle phalanx of ring finger
18 Distal phalanx of little finger

Notes:

1. In figure *A,* the hand is shown with flexion of the fingers at the metacarpophalangeal and interphalangeal joints.
2. Figure *B* is a proximal to distal view demonstrating the tunnel that is formed by the carpal bones known as the carpal tunnel.
3. The flexor retinaculum encloses and forms the ceiling of the carpal tunnel by attaching to the tubercles of the scaphoid and trapezium on the radial side and the pisiform and hook of the hamate on the ulna side.

Chapter 5

Joint Action Terminology

CHAPTER OUTLINE

CHAPTER OBJECTIVES

After completing this chapter, the student should be able to perform the following:

- ❑ With regard to joint motion, explain the function of joints, muscles, and ligaments/joint capsules.
- ❑ Describe the relationship between joint mobility and joint stability.
- ❑ Describe the characteristics of axial motion.
- ❑ Describe the characteristics of nonaxial motion.
- ❑ Describe, compare, and contrast rectilinear and curvilinear motion.
- ❑ Explain the relationship between axial motion and the axis of movement.
- ❑ Describe roll and spin axial motions.
- ❑ Explain the relationship of roll, spin, and glide movements.
- ❑ Be able to state the three components of naming a joint action.
- ❑ Define joint action terms and be able to show examples of each one.
- ❑ Explain the two uses of the term *hyperextension*.
- ❑ Demonstrate and be able to state the component actions of circumduction.
- ❑ Explain how oblique plane movements are broken down into their component cardinal plane actions.
- ❑ Explain the concept of a reverse action and demonstrate examples of reverse actions.
- ❑ Explain how drawing in a vector can help us learn the actions of the muscle.
- ❑ Draw a vector that represents the line of pull of a muscle; and if the muscle's line of pull is oblique, be able to resolve that vector into its component cardinal plane vectors.

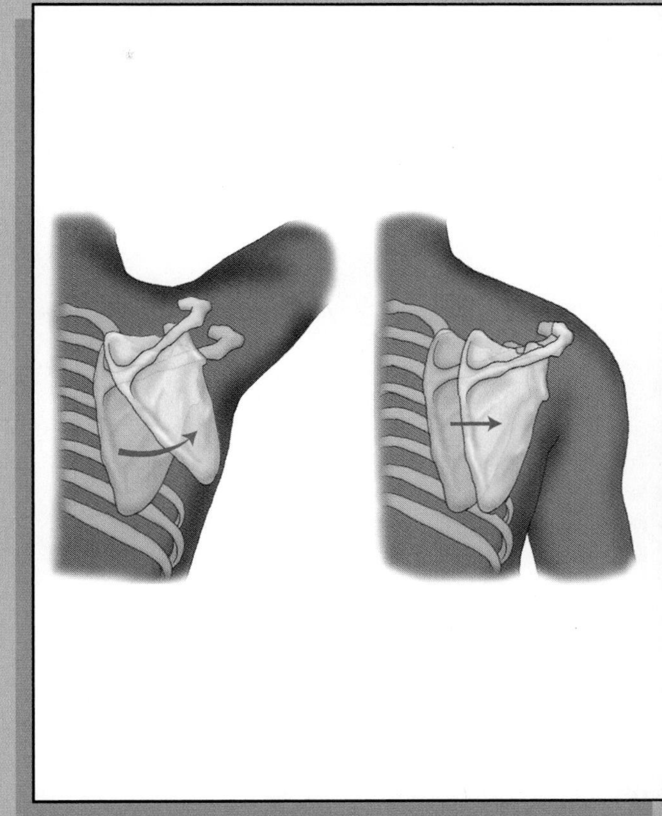

OVERVIEW

Chapter 2 began the discussion of motion in the body. Chapter 5 now continues the exploration of motion in the body. The larger picture of joint function is addressed, axial and nonaxial motions are examined in detail, and the fundamental types of joint movement, (i.e., roll, glide, and spin) are covered. Joint action terminology pairs that describe cardinal plane actions are then presented so that the student is conversant with the language necessary to fully and accurately describe cardinal plane actions of the human body. Finally, oblique plane movement is covered and the concept of breaking an oblique plane movement into its cardinal plane component actions is explained. A strong learning tool to help accomplish this is presented: that is, placing an arrow (vector) along the direction of the fibers of the muscle, from one attachment of the muscle to the other attachment of the muscle. This gives us a visual sense of the overall line of pull of the muscle; resolving this vector into its component vectors then offers us a visual way to figure out the cardinal plane lines of pull and therefore the cardinal plane actions of the muscle.

One other topic, crucial to the understanding of musculoskeletal function, is presented and explored in this chapter; that topic is reverse actions. For too long, students of kinesiology have memorized muscle actions with the flawed belief that one attachment, the origin, always stays fixed, and the other attachment, the insertion, always moves. The concept of reverse actions explains how to look at a muscle's actions in a fundamentally simpler and more accurate way.

From here, Chapter 6 presents a classification of joints of the body, and Chapters 7-9 then regionally examine the joints of the body in much more detail.

KEY TERMS

Abduction (ab-DUK-shun)
Action
Adduction (ad-DUK-shun)
Angular motion
Anterior tilt (an-TEER-ee-or)
Axial motion (AK-see-al)
Circular motion
Circumduction (SIR-kum-DUK-shun)
Contralateral rotation (CON-tra-LAT-er-al)
Curvilinear motion (KERV-i-LIN-ee-ar)
Depression
Dorsiflexion (door-see-FLEK-shun)
Downward rotation
Elevation
Eversion (ee-VER-shun)
Extension (ek-STEN-shun)
Flexion (FLEK-shun)
Gliding motion
Hiking the hip
Horizontal abduction (ab-DUK-shun)
Horizontal adduction (ad-DUK-shun)
Horizontal extension (ek-STEN-shun)
Horizontal flexion (FLEK-shun)
Hyperextension (HI-per-ek-STEN-shun)
Inversion (in-VER-shun)
Ipsilateral rotation (IP-see-LAT-er-al)
Joint action
Lateral deviation
Lateral flexion (FLEK-shun)
Lateral rotation
Lateral tilt
Left lateral deviation
Left lateral flexion (FLEK-shun)
Left rotation
Linear motion
Medial rotation (MEE-dee-al)
Nonaxial motion (NON-AK-see-al)
Oblique plane movements (o-BLEEK)
Opposition (OP-po-ZI-shun)
Plantarflexion (PLAN-tar-FLEK-shun)
Posterior tilt (pos-TEER-ee-or)
Pronation (pro-NAY-shun)
Protraction (pro-TRAK-shun)
Rectilinear motion (REK-ti-LIN-ee-or)
Reposition (REE-po-ZI-shun)
Resolve a vector (VEK-tor)
Retraction (ree-TRAK-shun)
Reverse action
Right lateral deviation
Right lateral flexion (FLEK-shun)
Right rotation
Rocking movement
Rolling movement
Rotary motion
Scaption (SKAP-shun)
Sliding motion
Spinning movement
Supination (SUE-pin-A-shun)
Translation
Upward rotation
Vector (VEK-tor)

WORD ORIGINS

- ❑ Abduct—From Latin *abductus,* meaning *to lead away*
- ❑ Adduct—From Latin *adductus,* meaning *to draw toward*
- ❑ Circum—From Latin *circum,* meaning *circle*
- ❑ Contra—From Latin *contra,* meaning *opposed* or *against*
- ❑ Curv—From Latin *curvus,* meaning *bent, curved*
- ❑ Exten—From Latin *ex,* meaning *out,* and *tendere,* meaning *to stretch*
- ❑ Flex—From Latin *flexus,* meaning *bent*
- ❑ Hyper—From Greek *hyper,* meaning *above, over*
- ❑ Ipsi—From Latin *ipse,* meaning *same* and Latin *latus,* meaning *side*
- ❑ Linea—From Latin *linea,* meaning *a linen thread, a line*
- ❑ Oppos—From Latin *opponere,* meaning *to place against*
- ❑ Pelvis—From Latin *pelvis,* meaning *basin*
- ❑ Rect—From Latin *rectus,* meaning *straight, right*
- ❑ Repos—From Latin *reponere,* meaning *to replace*

5.1 OVERVIEW OF JOINT FUNCTION

- Following is a simplified overview of joint function (For more information on joint function, see Section 6.2.):
  - The primary function of a joint is to allow movement. This is the reason why a joint exists in the first place.
  - The movement that occurs at a joint is created by muscles.

BOX 5-1

The role of a muscle contraction is actually to create a force on the bones of a joint; that force can create movement at a joint. However, the force of the muscle contraction can also stop or modify movement. (For more information on muscle function, see Chapters 11 to 13.)

- Ligaments and joint capsules function to limit excessive movement at a joint.
  - Therefore, the following general rules can be stated:
    - Joints *allow* movement.
    - Muscles *create* movement.
    - Ligaments/joint capsules *limit* movement.
- In addition to allowing movement to occur, joints have three characteristics:
- Weight bearing: Many joints of the body are weight-bearing joints. That is, they bear the weight of the body parts located above them. Most every joint of the lower extremity and all the spinal joints of the axial body are weight-bearing joints. As a rule, weight-bearing joints need to be very stable to support the weight that is borne through them.
- Shock absorption: Joints can function to absorb shock. This is especially important for weight-bearing joints. The primary means by which a joint absorbs shock is due to the cushioning effect of the fluid within the joint cavity.
- Stability: Even though the primary function of a joint is to allow motion to occur, excessive motion would create an unstable joint. Therefore a joint must be sufficiently stable so that it does not lose its integrity and become injured or dislocated.
  - Each joint of the body finds a balance between mobility and stability.
  - Mobility and stability are antagonistic properties: A more mobile joint is less stable; a more stable joint is less mobile.

☐ 5.2 AXIAL AND NONAXIAL MOTION

When a body part moves at a joint, motion of the body part occurs. The body may undergo two basic types of motion: (1) **axial motion** and (2) **nonaxial motion**.

Axial Motion:

- ❏ Axial motion is a motion of a body part that occurs about or around an axis.
- ❏ This type of motion is also known as **circular motion** because the body part moves along a circular path around the axis (in such a manner that a point drawn anywhere on the body part would transcribe a circular path around the axis).
- ❏ With axial motion not every point on the body part moves the same amount. A point closer to the axis moves less (and would transcribe a smaller circle) than a point further from the axis (which would transcribe a larger circle).
- ❏ In other words, with axial motion the body part moves in a circular path around the axis in such as manner that one part of the body part moves more than another part of the body part (Figure 5-1a).

Nonaxial Motion:

- ❏ Nonaxial motion is motion of a body part that does not occur about or around an axis.
- ❏ This type of motion is also known as a **gliding motion** because the body part glides along another body part.
- ❏ With nonaxial motion, every aspect of the body part moves/glides the same amount (i.e., every point on the body part moves in a linear path exactly the same amount in the same direction at the same time as every other point on the body part).
- ❏ In other words, with nonaxial motion the body part does not move around an axis and instead glides as a whole in a linear direction (with every point of the body part moving exactly the same amount as every other point) (Figure 5-1b).
- ❏ In essence, a nonaxial gliding motion is when the entire body part moves as a whole and moves in one direction; an axial circular motion is a circular motion around an axis wherein one aspect of the body part moves more than another aspect of the body part. (For more information on axial motion, see Sections 5.5 through 5.7. For more information on nonaxial motion, see Sections 5.3 and 5.4.)

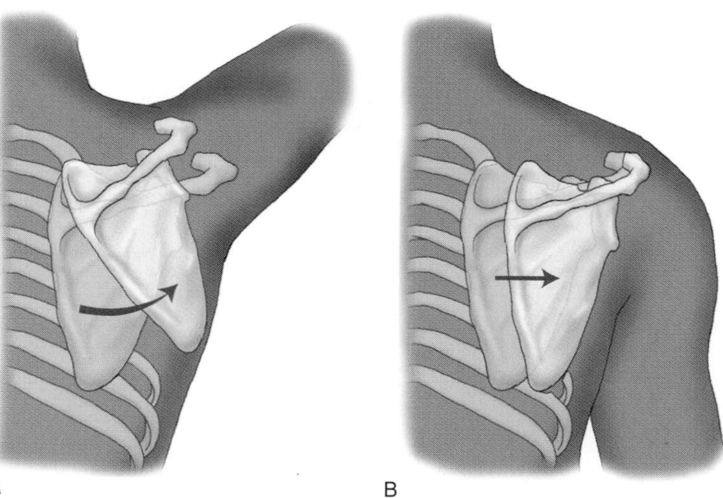

Figure 5-1 *A,* The scapula upwardly rotating, which is an example of axial/circular motion. *B,* The scapula protracting, which is an example of nonaxial/gliding motion.

☐ 5.3 NONAXIAL/GLIDING MOTION

Nonaxial Motion:

- ❑ Nonaxial motion is motion of a body part that does not occur around an axis, hence the name *nonaxial* motion.
- ❑ Nonaxial motion involves a gliding motion (also known as **sliding motion**) because the bone that moves is said to *glide* (or *slide*) along the other bone of the joint.
- ❑ Nonaxial movement of a body part is also known as **translation** of the body part because the entire body part moves the same exact amount; therefore the entire body part can be looked at as changing its location or *translating* its location from one position to another.
- ❑ Nonaxial motion is also known as **linear motion** of a body part because every point on the body part moves in the same linear path, the exact same amount as every other point on the body part (Figure 5-2).
- ❑ In other words, with nonaxial motion the body part does not move around an axis. Instead the entire body part translates its location and glides/slides as a whole in a linear direction along the other bone of the joint.

BOX 5-2

Many synonyms for nonaxial motion exist, such as *glide*, *slide*, *translation*, and *linear motion*. All of these synonyms are used commonly in the field of kinesiology, so it is useful to be familiar with all of them. Further, each one of them is helpful in visually describing a nonaxial motion.

Figure 5-2 shows a nonaxial motion of the scapula (in this case the scapula is protracting). If we pick any point along the scapula and draw a line to demonstrate the path of movement that this point undergoes, we see that this line is identical to the line drawn for the movement of every other point on the scapula. All of these lines would be identical to each other. Therefore one line can be drawn to demonstrate the motion of the entire scapula. This means the entire scapula moves as a whole, the same amount in the same direction at the same time. Because this motion does not occur around an axis, it is called *nonaxial*. Because one line can be drawn to demonstrate this motion, it can also be called *linear motion*.

Figure 5-3 shows other examples of nonaxial linear motion.

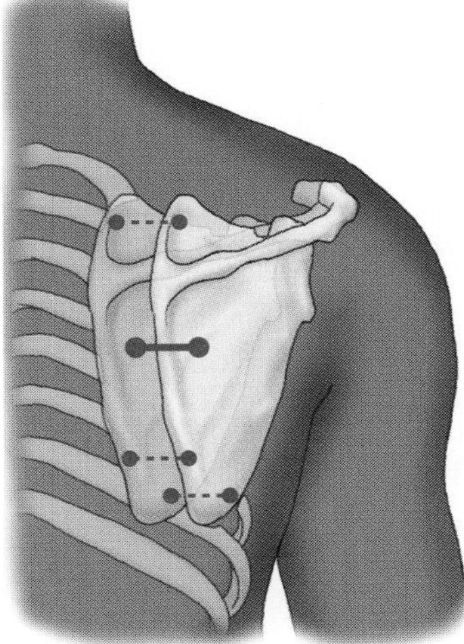

Figure 5-2 The scapula protracting. Three dashed lines have been drawn, representing the motion of three separate points along the scapula; we see that these lines are identical to each other. A bold line has been drawn that demonstrates the motion of the entire scapula. For this reason, nonaxial motion is also termed *linear motion*.

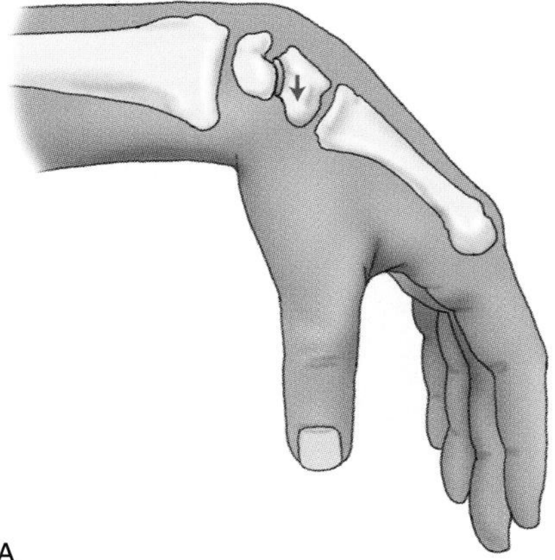

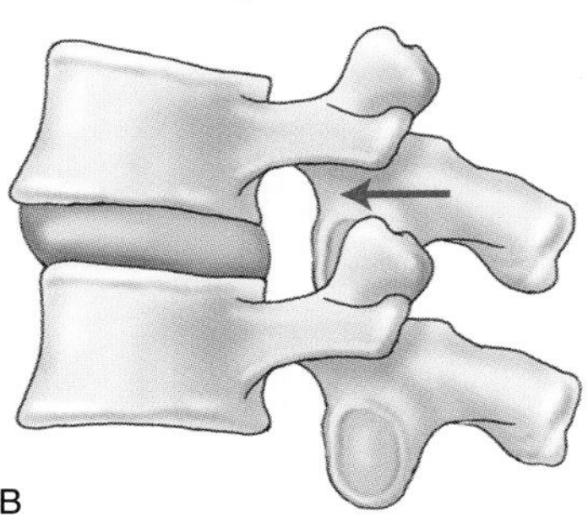

Figure 5-3 *A,* Nonaxial motion of one carpal bone of the wrist along an adjacent carpal bone. *B,* Nonaxial motion of one vertebra along another vertebra at the facet joints of the spine.

☐ 5.4 RECTILINEAR AND CURVILINEAR NONAXIAL MOTION

❑ Two different types of nonaxial linear motion exist: (1) rectilinear and (2) curvilinear.

Figure 5-4 illustrates these two different types of nonaxial linear motion.

❑ In Figure 5-4a, a person is skiing. The person's entire body is moving in a straight line. Because *rect* means straight, motion such as this that occurs in a straight line is termed **rectilinear motion**.

❑ Figure 5-4b illustrates the same skier jumping through the air. Now the person's entire body is moving along a curved line. Because *curv* means *curved*, motion such as this that occurs along a curved line is termed **curvilinear motion**.

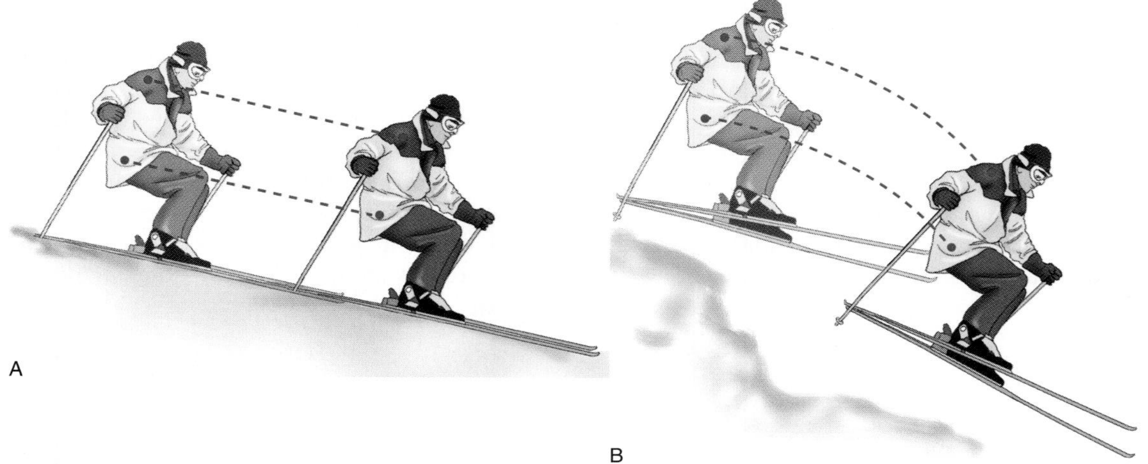

Figure 5-4 Person skiing and demonstrating two different types of nonaxial linear motion of the entire body. *A,* Person gliding along the snow in a straight line. This type of nonaxial linear motion is called *rectilinear motion. B,* Skier's body is now jumping through the air along a curved path. This type of nonaxial linear motion is called *curvilinear motion.*

☐ 5.5 AXIAL/CIRCULAR MOTION

Axial Motion:

- ❏ Axial motion is motion of a body part that occurs around or about an axis, hence the name *axial* motion.
- ❏ Axial motion is also known as *circular motion,* because the body part moves along a circular path around the axis (in such a manner that a point drawn anywhere on the body part would transcribe a circular path around the axis).
- ❏ When moving in a circular path around an axis, not every point on the body part moves an equal amount; points closer to the axis move less than points further from the axis. However, every point on the body part does move along a circular path through the same angle in the same direction (at the same time) as every other point on the body part. Because the direction of motion for every point on the body part is through the same angle, axial motion is also called **angular motion**.
- ❏ One other synonym for axial motion is **rotary motion** (i.e., rotation motion), because the body part moves in a rotary fashion around the axis (Box 5-3).

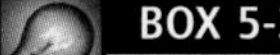

BOX 5-3

As with nonaxial motion, many synonyms for axial motion exist. Because all of them are used, it is necessary to be familiar with all of them. Further, each one of them is useful in its own way toward visually describing axial motion. The one synonym for axial motion that should be avoided or used with caution (at least for the beginning student of kinesiology) is rotary/rotation motion. Use of the word *rotary* or *rotation* in this context can be confusing, because when we start to name the pairs of directional terms used to describe axial motions at joints, the word *rotation* is used again, but is used to describe a certain type of axial movement. For example, *medial rotation* is a term that uses the word *rotation* to describe a certain axial motion; yet *flexion* is a term to describe another axial motion, and *in this context* we do not say that flexion is rotation (even though as an axial movement, it can be described as a *rotary* or *rotation movement*). (For more details, see the section on spin and roll axial movements in this chapter [Section 5.7].)

Figure 5-5 illustrates axial/circular motion of the forearm (in this case the forearm is flexing). We see that every point on the forearm moves along its own circular path; the line of this path for one point along the forearm will not be the same as for any other point along the forearm (i.e., the amount of movement will be different for each point). Therefore this type of motion is not linear. However, the angle that each point on the forearm moves through is the same, hence axial motion is also known as *angular motion.*

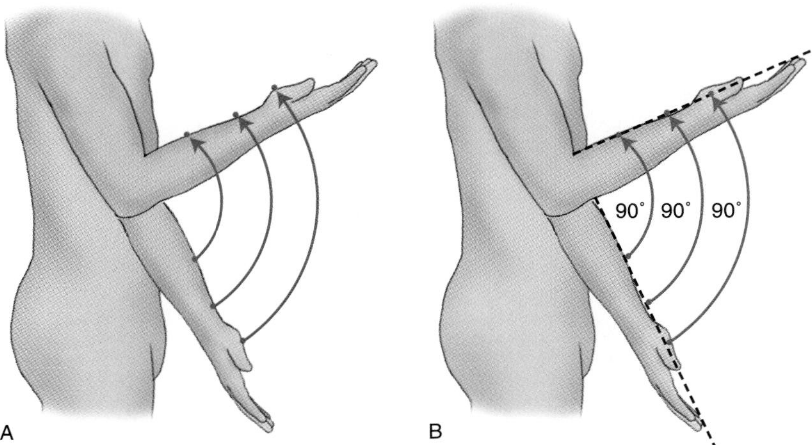

Figure 5-5 *A,* Flexion of the forearm at the elbow joint (a type of axial/circular motion). The paths of movement of three points along the forearm have been drawn. These points do not travel the same amount along the same line of movement; therefore this motion is not linear. *B,* Same axial/circular movement as depicted in *A.* Angles have been drawn in between the forearm and the arm for the three points that were considered in *A.* The angle formed by the motion of each point of the forearm is identical. Because the angle is constant for all points of the forearm, axial motion is also called *angular motion.*

5.6 AXIAL MOTION AND THE AXIS OF MOVEMENT

- With axial motion the body part that is moving moves along a circular path. If we place a point at the center of this circular path, we will have the point around which the body part moves.
- If we now draw a line through this center point that is perpendicular to the plane in which the movement is occurring, we will have the axis of movement for this axial motion.

BOX 5-4

As described in Section 5.5, motion of the body part may be described as rotary, because the body part is rotating around the axis; therefore an axis of movement is often called an *axis of rotation*. For reasons explained in Box 5-3, beginning kinesiology students should avoid use of the term *axis of rotation* and instead use the simpler term, *axis of movement*. (For more on axes, see Sections 2.10 through 2.13.)

- Every axial movement moves around an axis.
- Conversely, an axis is an imaginary line in space around which axial motions occur.

Figure 5-6 illustrates two examples of axial movements and shows the axis for each movement.

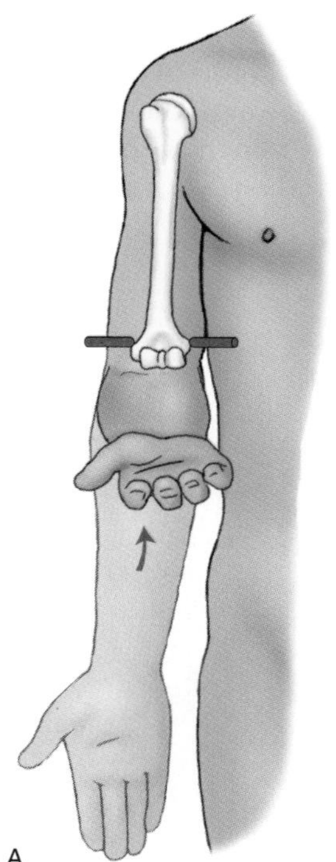

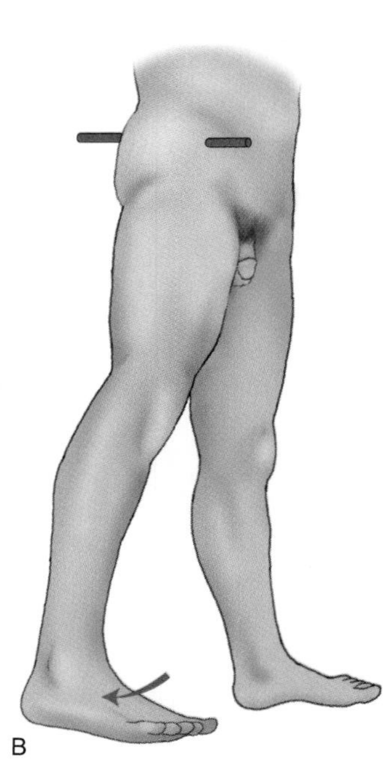

Figure 5-6 *A,* Flexion of the forearm at the elbow joint with the axis of movement drawn in; axis is mediolateral (i.e., medial-lateral) in orientation. *B,* Abduction of the thigh at the hip joint with the axis of movement drawn in; axis is anteroposterior (i.e., anterior-posterior) in orientation. Axes of movement are always perpendicular to the plane in which the motion is occurring.

☐ 5.7 ROLL AND SPIN AXIAL MOVEMENTS

Axial movements can be broadly divided into two categories:

- ❑ One category is where the body part changes its position in space and one end of the bone moves more than the other end of the bone.
  - ❑ This type of axial movement is called a **rolling movement**.
  - ❑ A rolling movement can also be called a **rocking movement** ("rock and roll" ☺).
  - ❑ Figure 5-7a illustrates an example of a rolling movement of the body.
- ❑ The other category is where the body part does not change its position in space; rather it rotates or spins, staying in the same location.
  - ❑ This type of axial movement is called a **spinning movement**.
  - ❑ Spinning movements are generally known as *rotation movements*.
  - ❑ Figure 5-7b illustrates an example of a spin movement of the body.

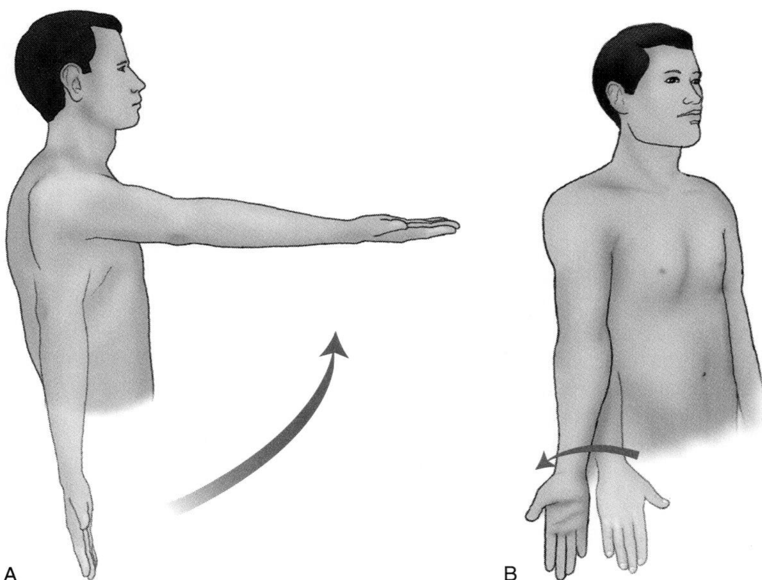

Figure 5-7 *A,* One type of axial motion is called *roll.* This particular motion is flexion of the arm at the shoulder joint. The arm changes position in space, and the distal end of the arm moves more than the proximal end. *B,* Another type of axial motion is called *spin.* This particular motion is lateral rotation of the arm at the shoulder joint. The arm rotates or spins, and it stays in the same location.

BOX 5-5

Flexion of the arm at the shoulder joint is shown here as an example of a roll axial movement. Clearly it is an axial motion because the arm moves around an axis (located at the shoulder joint), and clearly the arm is not spinning, but rather the head of the humerus is rolling within the socket (i.e., glenoid fossa of the scapula) of the shoulder joint to create this motion. However, as will be explained in Section 5.8, flexion also incorporates some nonaxial glide motion so that the head of the humerus does not dislocate by gliding right out of the shoulder joint socket. This concept is true for extension, abduction, adduction, right lateral flexion, and left lateral flexion as well. (See Section 5.8 for a better understanding of the relationship between roll and glide motions.)

☐ 5.8 ROLL, SPIN, AND GLIDE MOVEMENTS COMPARED

- Three fundamental types of movement can occur when one bone moves on another: (1) roll, (2) spin, and (3) glide.
  - Roll and spin are axial movements.
  - Glide is a linear nonaxial movement.

Figure 5-8 depicts all three of these fundamental motions at the joint level. Figure 5-9 draws an analogy for these movements to movements of a car tire.

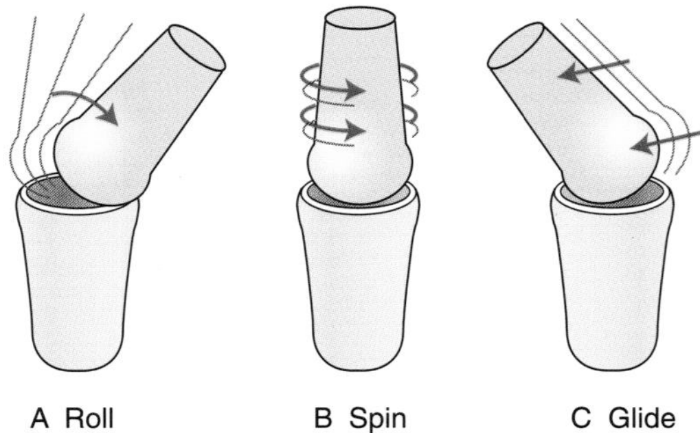

Figure 5-8 *A,* Rolling of one bone on another. *B,* Spinning of one bone on another; spin is an axial movement. *C,* Gliding of one bone on another; glide is a nonaxial movement. This figure shows the fundamental motions of roll, spin, and glide by showing the convex-shaped bone as moving on the concave-shaped bone. However, it is also possible for the concave-shaped bone to move along the convex-shaped bone. (Modeled from Neumann DA: *Kinesiology of the musculoskeletal system: foundations for physical rehabilitation,* St Louis, 2002, Mosby.)

BOX 5-6

Figure 5-8 shows the fundamental motions of roll, spin, and glide by showing the convex-shaped bone as moving on the concave-shaped bone. It is also possible for the concave-shaped bone to move along the convex-shaped bone. When the convex-shaped bone moves relative to the concave-shaped bone, the roll occurs in one direction and the glide occurs in the opposite direction. Conversely, when the concave-shaped bone moves relative to the convex-shaped bone, the roll occurs in one direction and the glide occurs in the same direction.

It is important to realize that these fundamental motions do not always occur independently of each other.

- As a rule, rolling and gliding motions must couple together or the bone that is rolling will dislocate by rolling off the other bone of the joint. For this reason, motions of flexion, extension, abduction, adduction, right lateral flexion, and left lateral flexion are actually made up of a combination of axial roll and nonaxial glide motions (Box 5-5).
- A spinning motion can occur independently. However, it is possible for a motion of the body to incorporate a spinning movement along with a rolling/gliding motion (e.g., when a person simultaneously flexes and laterally rotates the arm at the shoulder joint [both motions depicted in Figure 5-7]).

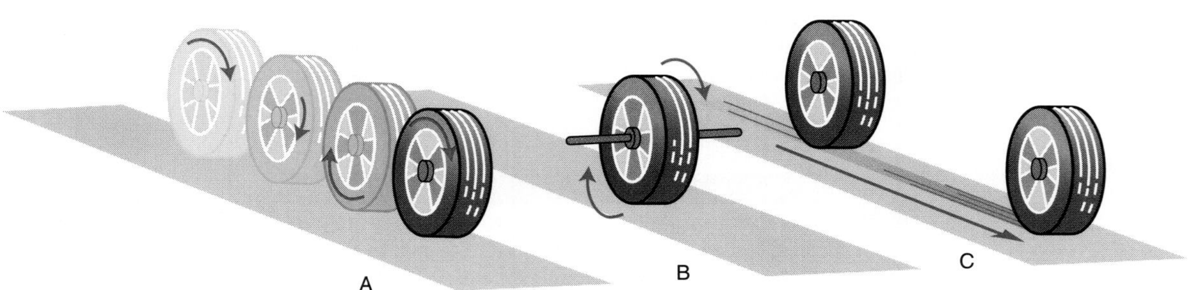

Figure 5-9 To better visualize the fundamental joint motions of roll, spin, and glide, an analogy can be made to a car tire. *A,* Tire that is rolling along the ground. *B,* Tire that is spinning without changing location. *C,* Tire that is gliding (sliding or skidding) along the ground.

5.9 NAMING JOINT ACTIONS—COMPLETELY

- When we want to name a specific movement of the body, we will refer to it as an **action**.
- Because movement of a body part occurs at a joint, the term **joint action** is synonymous with action.
- It is worth noting that most of the commonly thought of actions of the human body are axial (i.e., circular) movements (i.e., the body part that moves at a joint moves in a circular path around the axis of movement).
- Generally the axis of movement is a line that runs through the joint.
- When we describe these movements that occur, we will use terms that indicate the direction that the body part has moved. These terms will come in pairs, and the terms of each pair will be opposite to each other.

BOX 5-7

Joint action terminology pairs of terms are similar to the pairs of terms that are used to describe a location on the body (see Chapter 2 for more details). The difference is that the terms described in Chapter 2 were used to describe a static location on the body, whereas these movement terms are used to describe the direction that a body part is moving during an action that is occurring at a joint.

- Once we know these terms, we will then use three steps to describe an action that occurs:
  1. We will use the directional term describing the direction of the action.
  2. We will then state which body part moved during this action.
  3. We will then state at which joint the action occurred.
- For example, the action that is occurring in Figure 5-10 would be described the following way: Flexion of the right forearm at the elbow joint.
  This tells us three things:
  1. The direction of the action: flexion.
  2. The body part that is moving: the right forearm.
  3. At which joint the action is occurring: the right elbow joint.
- The reader should note that most people and most textbooks do not specify the body part that is moving *and* the joint at which the movement is occurring. For example, the action illustrated in Figure 5-10 is usually referred to as either *flexion of the elbow joint* (and the forearm is left out) or as *flexion of the forearm* (and the elbow joint is left out).

However, naming an action either of these ways can lead to confusion. For example, if we try to describe pronation of the forearm, we can say that the forearm pronated, but we cannot say that the elbow joint pronated because pronation of the forearm does not occur at the elbow joint, it occurs at the radioulnar joints. Therefore in this instance, elbow joint and forearm are not synonymous with each other.

Further, flexion of the elbow joint does not necessarily mean that the forearm moved; the arm can also flex at the elbow joint. In addition, flexion of the forearm does not necessarily mean that the elbow joint flexed; the forearm can also flex at the wrist joint.

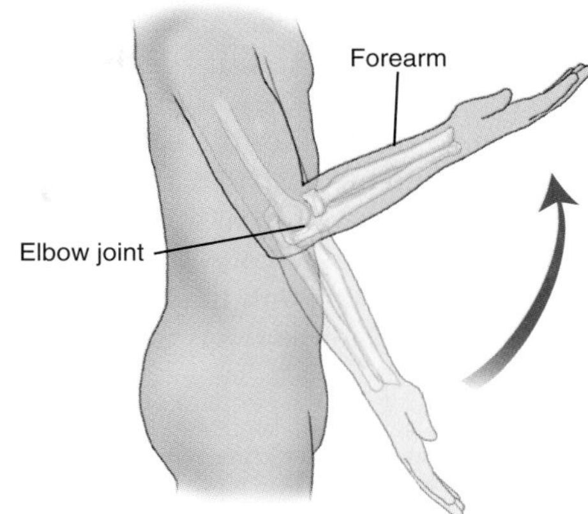

Figure 5-10 Flexion of the right forearm at the elbow joint. Many sources will simply name this action as either *flexion of the right elbow joint* or as *flexion of the right forearm.* However, these phrases are not complete, and unless the context is very clear, confusion may result.

BOX 5-8

Just as forearm and elbow joint are not synonymous with each other because the forearm can also move at the radioulnar joints, confusion can also occur with movements of the foot. The foot can move at the ankle joint, but it can also move at the subtalar joint instead.

The arm flexing at the elbow joint and the forearm flexing at the wrist joint are examples of what is called a *reverse action.* For example, the arm can move at the elbow joint if the forearm is fixed; this motion occurs during a pull-up, as well as whenever we grab a banister or other object and pull ourselves toward it. Movement of the forearm at the wrist joint is not as common, but can occur when the hand is fixed. (For more information on reverse actions, see Section 5.29.)

The advantage to being more complete in naming joint actions is that it requires us to clearly see exactly what is happening with each action of the body that occurs. Therefore to be most clear and eliminate the chance of possible vagueness and confusion, both the body part and the joint at which motion is occurring should be specified.

BOX 5-9

It should be stated that a bone can be named as doing the moving instead of the body part that the bone is within. Most of the time, naming the bone is interchangeable with naming the body part. For example, flexion of the humerus at the shoulder joint is interchangeable with flexion of the arm at the shoulder joint, because it is the humerus that moves when the arm moves. Sometimes naming the bone instead of the body part can actually be advantageous, because it more specifically describes what is actually moving. For example, with pronation/supination of the forearm, it is usually the radius of the forearm that is primarily either pronating or supinating about the ulna. Stating pronation of the radius instead of the pronation of the forearm can actually make the visual picture of what is happening clearer.

☐ 5.10 JOINT ACTION TERMINOLOGY PAIRS

Following are the terms that are used to describe joint actions:

- ❑ These terms come in pairs; each term of a pair is the opposite of the other term of the pair.
- ❑ It is important to remember that these terms do not describe the static location that a body part and/or a joint is in, rather they describe the direction that a body part is moving at a joint. In other words, motion must be occurring for these terms to be used.

BOX 5-10

Joint action terms are sometimes used to describe a static position. For example, it might be said that the client's arm is *in a position of flexion* at the shoulder joint. This is said because relative to anatomic position, the arm is flexed at the shoulder joint. However, this type of use of these motion terms to describe a static position can sometimes lead to confusion. For example, the client with the arm in flexion may have previously been in a position of further flexion, and then the client extended to get to that lesser position of flexion. In other words, knowing a static position does not tell us what joint action was done by the client to get into that position. In addition, because it is more often joint actions that cause injury and not the position that a joint is in, it is best to see and clearly describe what is occurring. Therefore, the best use of these terms is to describe an actual motion that is occurring.

Five major pairs of directional terms are used throughout most of the body:

1. Flexion/extension
2. Abduction/adduction
3. Right lateral flexion/left lateral flexion
4. Lateral rotation/medial rotation
5. Right rotation/left rotation

The following pairs of directional terms are used for certain actions at specific joints of the body.

- ❑ Plantarflexion/dorsiflexion
- ❑ Eversion/inversion
- ❑ Pronation/supination
- ❑ Protraction/retraction
- ❑ Elevation/depression
- ❑ Upward rotation/downward rotation
- ❑ Anterior tilt/downward tilt
- ❑ Opposition/reposition
- ❑ Lateral deviation to the right/lateral deviation to the left
- ❑ Horizontal flexion/horizontal extension

A few additional terms are used when describing joint actions:

- ❑ Hyperextension
- ❑ Circumduction

☐ 5.11 FLEXION/EXTENSION

- **Flexion** is defined as a movement at a joint so that the ventral (soft) surfaces of the two body parts at that joint come closer together.

> **BOX 5-11**
>
> The word *ventral* derives from the word *belly*. The ventral surface of a body part has come to mean the soft "underbelly" aspect of any body part. Generally it is the anterior surface, but in the lower extremity the ventral surface shifts to the posterior surface (and is the plantar surface of the foot). The opposite of ventral is dorsal.

- **Extension** is the opposite of flexion (i.e., the dorsal [harder] surfaces of the body parts come closer together).
  See Figure 5-11 for examples of flexion and extension.
  - Flexion and extension are movements that occur in the sagittal plane.
  - Flexion and extension are axial movements that occur around a mediolateral axis.
  - *Flexion* and *extension* are terms that can be used for the entire body (i.e., the body parts of the axial skeleton and the body parts of the appendicular skeleton).
- Flexion of a body part involves an anterior movement of that body part; extension of a body part involves a posterior movement of that body part.
  - The exception to this rule is at the knee joint and further distally, where flexion is a posterior movement of the body part and extension is an anterior movement.

> **BOX 5-12**
>
> Flexion and extension of the thumb at the saddle joint of the thumb are very unusual in that they occur within the frontal plane. See Section 9.13 for more details regarding movement of the thumb.

- Generally, flexion involves a *bending* at a joint, whereas extension involves a joint straightening out.
  - The word *flexion* comes from the Latin word meaning *to bend*.
  - The word *extension* comes from the Latin word meaning *to straighten out*.
- An easy way to remember flexion is to think of fetal position. When a person goes to sleep in the fetal position, most or all of the joints are in flexion.

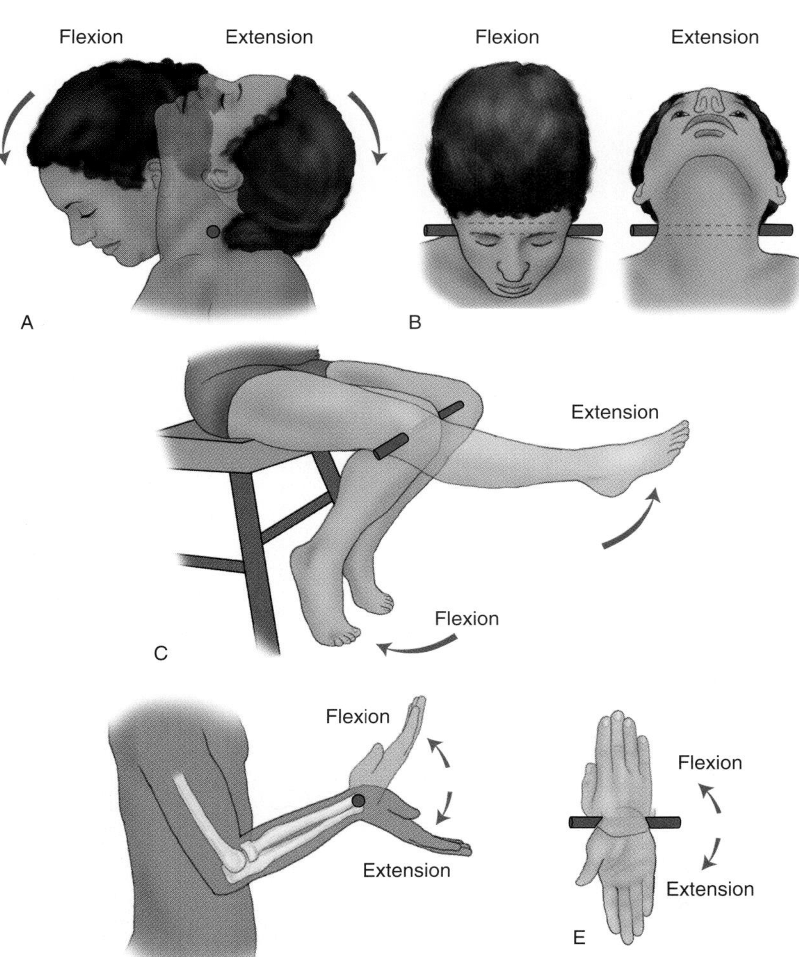

Figure 5-11 Examples of flexion and extension. *A* and *B*, Flexion and extension of the head and neck at the spinal joints. *C*, Flexion and extension of the leg at the knee joint. *D* and *E*, Flexion and extension of the hand at the wrist joint. (Note: In the illustrations, the red tube or red dot represents the axis of movement.)

5.12 ABDUCTION/ADDUCTION

- **Abduction** is defined as a movement at a joint that brings a body part away from the midline of the body. To *abduct* is to take away.

BOX 5-13

The midline of the body is an imaginary line that divides the body into two equal left and right halves.

- **Adduction** is the opposite of abduction; in other words, the body part moves closer toward the midline (it is *added* to the midline).

See Figure 5-12 for examples of abduction and adduction.

- Abduction and adduction are movements that occur in the frontal plane.
- Abduction and adduction are axial movements that occur around an anteroposterior axis.
- *Abduction* and *adduction* are terms that can be used for the body parts of the appendicular skeleton only (i.e., the upper and lower extremities).
- Abduction of a body part involves a lateral movement of that body part; adduction of a body part involves a medial movement of that body part.

BOX 5-14

The fingers and toes do not abduct/adduct relative to the midline of the body. The reference line about which abduction/adduction of the fingers occurs is an imaginary line through the middle finger; the reference line about which abduction/adduction of the toes occurs is an imaginary line through the 2nd toe. Movement of a finger away from the middle finger and movement of a toe away from the 2nd toe is abduction; movement toward these reference lines is adduction. Frontal plane movements of the middle finger itself are termed *radial* and *ulnar* abduction; similar movements of the 2nd toe itself are termed fibular and tibial abduction. Another exception to this rule is abduction/adduction of the thumb. (See Section 9.13 for more details regarding movements of the thumb.)

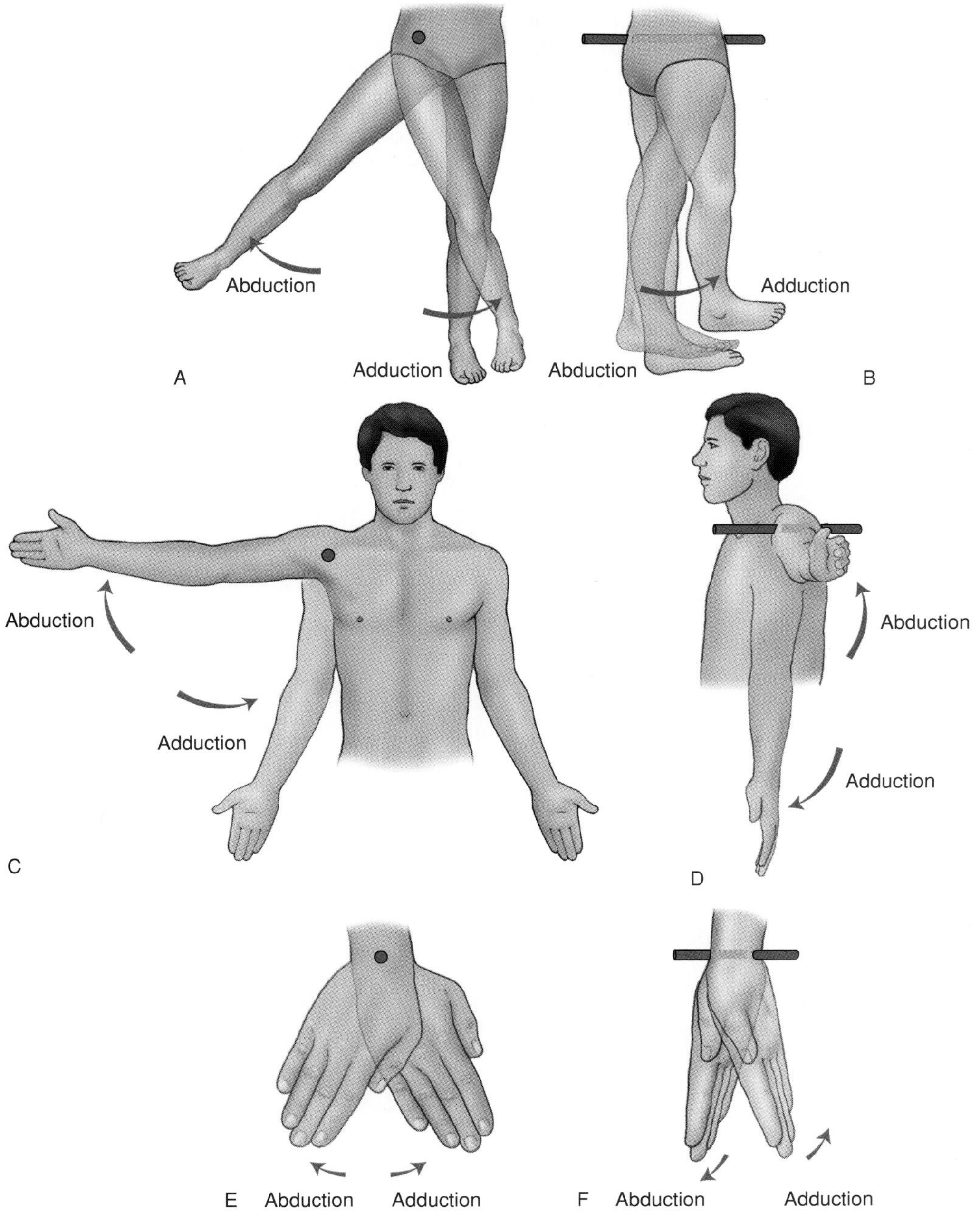

Figure 5-12 Examples of abduction and adduction. *A* and *B,* Abduction and adduction of the thigh at the hip joint. *C* and *D,* Abduction and adduction of the arm at the shoulder joint. *E* and *F,* Abduction and adduction of the hand at the wrist joint. (Note: In the illustrations, the red tube or red dot represents the axis of movement.)

☐ 5.13 RIGHT LATERAL FLEXION/LEFT LATERAL FLEXION

❏ **Right lateral flexion** is defined as a movement at a joint that bends a body part to the right side.

❏ **Left lateral flexion** is the opposite of right lateral flexion; in other words, the body part bends to the left side.

See Figure 5-13 for examples of right lateral flexion and left lateral flexion.

- ❏ Right lateral flexion and left lateral flexion are movements that occur in the frontal plane.
- ❏ Right lateral flexion and left lateral flexion are axial movements that occur around an anteroposterior axis.

❏ *Right lateral flexion* and *left lateral flexion* are terms that can be used for the body parts of the axial skeleton only (i.e., the head, neck, and trunk).

❏ Right lateral flexion of a body part involves a lateral movement of that body part to the right; left lateral flexion of a body part involves a lateral movement of that body part to the left.

❏ **Lateral flexion** is often called *side bending*.

❏ Note: Lateral flexion should not be confused with flexion, although the word *flexion* is contained within the term *lateral flexion*. Flexion is a sagittal plane movement, and lateral flexion is a frontal plane movement.

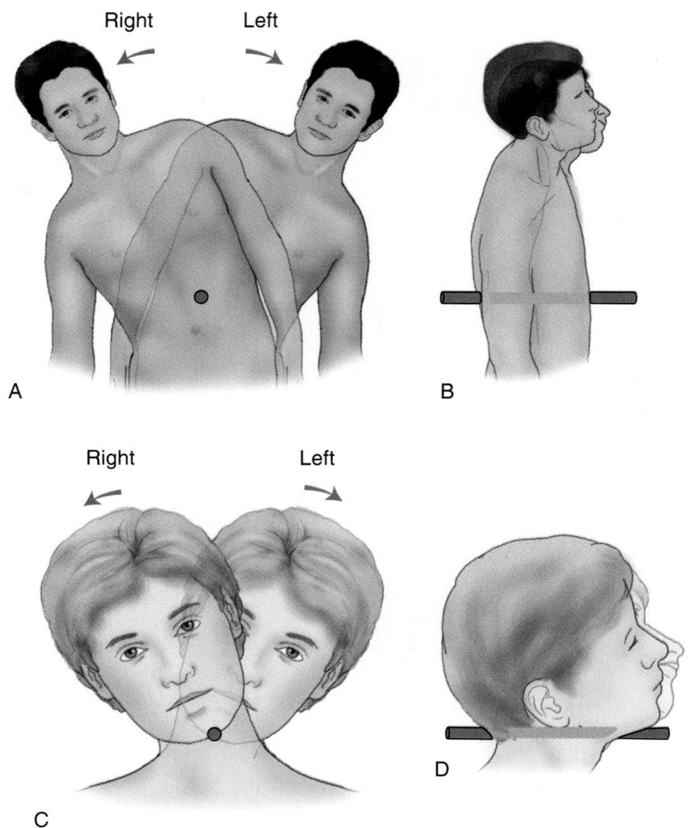

Figure 5-13 Examples of right and left lateral flexion. *A* and *B,* Anterior and lateral views (respectively) of right and left lateral flexion of the trunk at the spinal joints. *C* and *D,* Anterior and lateral views (respectively) of right and left lateral flexion of the neck at the spinal joints. (Note: In the illustrations, the red tube or red dot represents the axis of movement.)

☐ 5.14 LATERAL ROTATION/MEDIAL ROTATION

- **Lateral rotation** is defined as a movement at a joint wherein the anterior surface of the body part rotates away from the midline of the body.
- **Medial rotation** is the opposite of lateral rotation; in other words, the anterior surface of the body part rotates toward the midline of the body.

See Figure 5-14 for examples of lateral rotation and medial rotation.

- Lateral rotation and medial rotation are movements that occur in the transverse plane.
- Lateral rotation and medial rotation are axial movements that occur around a vertical axis.
- *Lateral rotation* and *medial rotation* are terms that can be used for the body parts of the appendicular skeleton only (i.e., the upper and lower extremities only).
- Lateral rotation and medial rotation of a body part involve a rotation (i.e., spin) of the body part around the longitudinal axis that runs through the length of the bone of the body part. When this rotation occurs, the body part does not actually change its physical location in space; rather it stays in the same location and spins or rotates around its own axis.

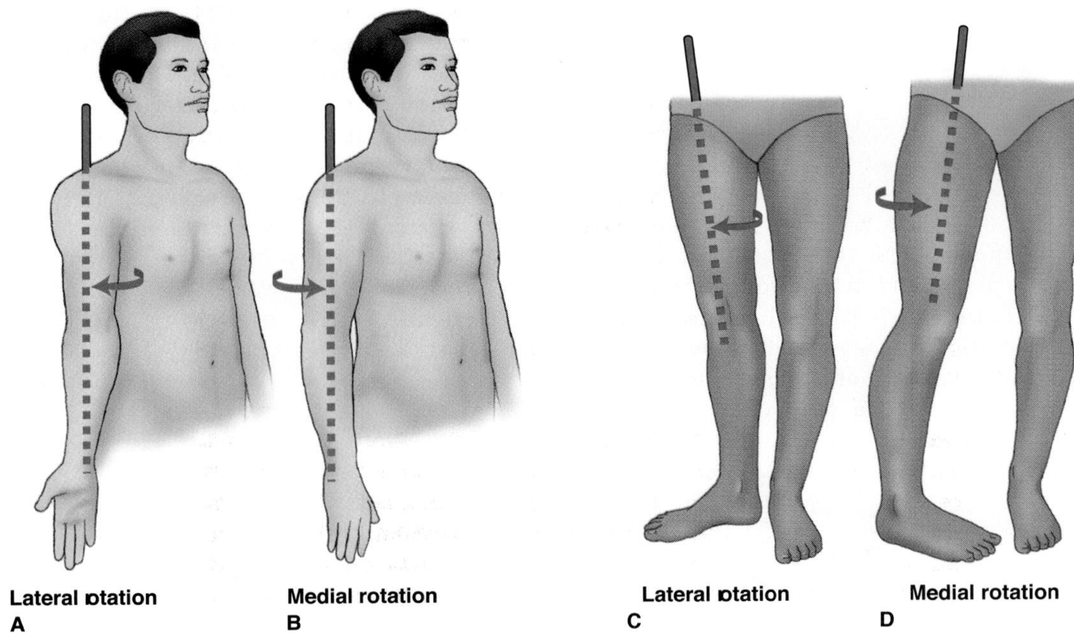

Figure 5-14 Examples of lateral rotation and medial rotation. *A,* Lateral rotation of the arm at the shoulder joint. *B,* Medial rotation of the arm at the shoulder joint. *C,* Lateral rotation of the thigh at the hip joint. *D,* Medial rotation of the thigh at the hip joint. (Note: In all illustrations the red tube and the dashed line represents the axis of movement.)

5.15 RIGHT ROTATION/LEFT ROTATION

- **Right rotation** is defined as a movement at a joint wherein the anterior surface of the body part rotates to the right.
- **Left rotation** is the opposite of right rotation; in other words, the anterior surface of the body part rotates to the left.

See Figure 5-15 for examples of right rotation and left rotation.

- Right rotation and left rotation are movements that occur in the transverse plane.
- Right rotation and left rotation are axial movements that occur around a vertical axis.
- *Right rotation* and *left rotation* are terms that can be used for the body parts of the axial skeleton only (i.e., the head, neck, and trunk).

BOX 5-15

The pelvis can also do right rotation and left rotation. (Note: The pelvis is a transitional body part containing elements of the axial and appendicular skeleton.)

- Right rotation and left rotation of a body part involve a rotation (i.e., spin) of the body part around the longitudinal axis that runs through the length of the bone(s) of the body part. When this rotation occurs, the body part does not actually change its physical location in space; rather it stays in the same location and spins or rotates around its own axis.

Note:

- Two terms are often used when describing the actions of muscles that can rotate an axial body part within the transverse plane. These terms are *ipsilateral rotation* and *contralateral rotation.*
- The terms *ipsilateral rotation* and *contralateral rotation* do not define joint actions; rather, they indicate whether a muscle rotates an axial body part (or the pelvis) toward the same side of the body as where it is located, or toward the opposite side of the body from where it is located.
- A muscle does **ipsilateral rotation** if it rotates an axial body part (or the pelvis) toward the same side of the body as where it is located. For example, the splenius capitis is an ipsilateral rotator because the right splenius capitis rotates the head and neck to the right, and the left splenius capitis rotates the head and neck to the left.
- A muscle does **contralateral rotation** if it rotates an axial body part (or the pelvis) toward the opposite side of the body from where it is located. For example, the sternocleidomastoid is a contralateral rotator because the right sternocleidomastoid rotates the head and neck to the left, and the left sternocleidomastoid rotates the head and neck to the right.

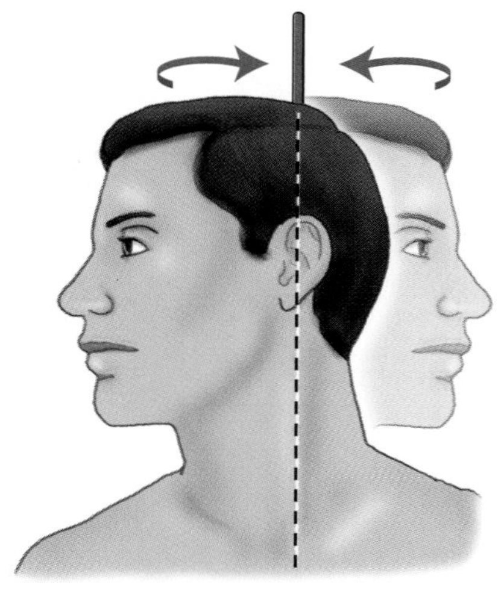

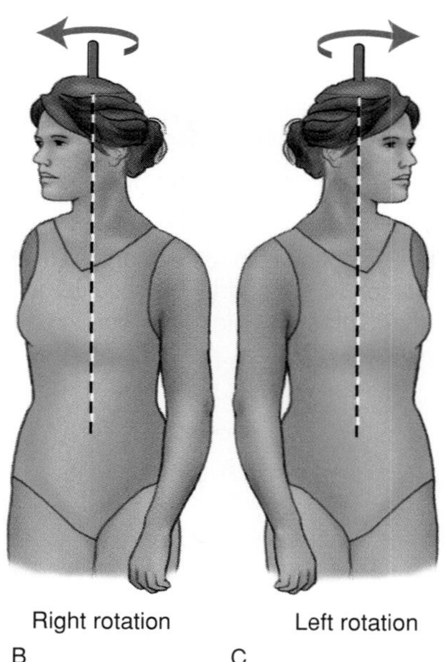

Figure 5-15 Examples of right rotation and left rotation. *A,* Right and left rotation of the head and neck at the spinal joints. *B,* Right rotation of the trunk at the spinal joints. *C,* Left rotation of the trunk at the spinal joints. (Note: In all illustrations the red tube and the dashed line represents the axis of movement.)

☐ 5.16 PLANTARFLEXION/DORSIFLEXION

❑ **Plantarflexion** is defined as the movement at the ankle joint wherein the foot moves inferiorly, toward the plantar surface of the foot.

BOX 5-16

The plantar surface of the foot is the surface that you plant on the ground (i.e., the inferior surface). The dorsal surface is the opposite side of the foot (i.e., the superior surface).

❑ **Dorsiflexion** is the opposite of plantarflexion; in other words, the foot moves superiorly toward its dorsal surface.

See Figure 5-16 for an example of plantarflexion and dorsiflexion.

- ❑ Plantarflexion and dorsiflexion are movements that occur in the sagittal plane.
- ❑ Plantarflexion and dorsiflexion are axial movements that occur around a mediolateral axis.
- ❑ *Plantarflexion* and *dorsiflexion* are terms that are used for the foot moving at the ankle joint.

BOX 5-17

Plantarflexion and *dorsiflexion* are terms that are used in place of flexion and extension. Because the foot is positioned at a 90-degree angle to the rest of the body, movements occur inferiorly and superiorly instead of anteriorly and posteriorly; for this reason, plantarflexion and dorsiflexion are used (instead of flexion and extension) to eliminate the possibility of confusion. When the terms *flexion* and *extension* are used to describe sagittal plane actions of the foot, controversy exists over which term is which. Some sources say that dorsiflexion is flexion, because dorsiflexion is bending of the ankle joint and the word *flexion* means *to bend.* Others sources state that plantarflexion is flexion for two reasons:

1. Flexion is a posterior movement from the knee joint and further distal, and plantarflexion is a posterior movement.
2. Flexion is usually an approximation of two ventral (i.e., soft) surfaces of adjacent body parts, and plantarflexion accomplishes this.

(Note: Dorsiflexion and plantarflexion can also occur to a small degree at the subtalar joint.)

❑ Plantarflexion of a body part involves an inferior movement of that body part; dorsiflexion of a body part involves a superior movement of that body part.

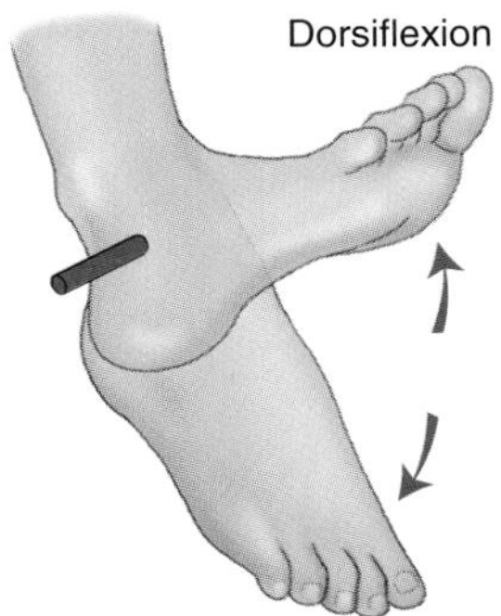

Figure 5-16 Plantarflexion and dorsiflexion of the foot at the ankle joint. (The red tube represents the axis of movement.)

☐ 5.17 EVERSION/INVERSION

- **Eversion** is defined as the movement between tarsal bones wherein the plantar surface of the foot turns away from the midline of the body.
- **Inversion** is the opposite of eversion; in other words, the plantar surface of the foot turns toward the midline of the body.

BOX 5-18

*In*version can be thought of as turning the foot *in*ward, toward the midline of the body. Therefore eversion would be turning the foot outward, away form the midline of the body.

See Figure 5-17 for an example of eversion and inversion.

- Eversion and inversion are movements that occur in the frontal plane.

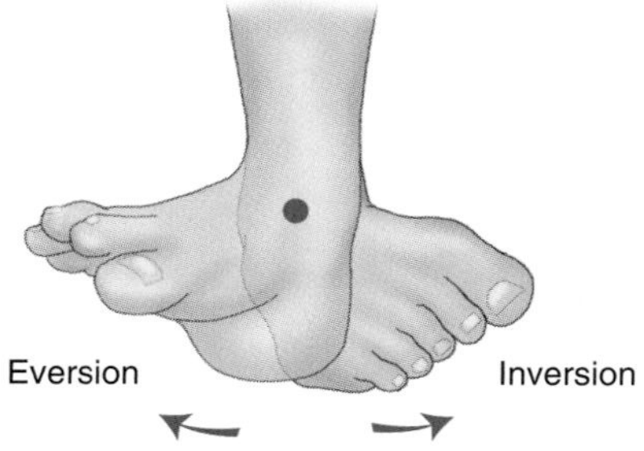

Figure 5-17 Eversion and inversion of the foot at the tarsal joints (i.e., the subtalar joint). (The red dot represents the axis of movement.)

- Eversion and inversion are axial movements that occur around an anteroposterior axis.
- *Eversion* and *inversion* are terms that are used to describe the motion of the foot between tarsal bones. These movements do not occur at the ankle joint.

BOX 5-19

Eversion and inversion occur about the long axis of the foot (i.e., anteroposterior axis). Because rotation actions of a body part occur about the long axis of the body part, this means that eversion and inversion are essentially equivalent to lateral and medial rotation of the foot. Rotations usually occur about a long axis that is vertical, but because the position of the foot is set at a 90-degree angle to the rest of the body, its long axis is anteroposterior (i.e., horizontal).

BOX 5-20

Eversion is an action that is one component of another term, *pronation*, used to describe a broader movement of the foot; inversion is an action that is one component of another term, *supination*, used to describe a broader movement of the foot. (For more details on this, see Section 8.19.)

- The principal tarsal joint is the subtalar joint. For this reason, eversion and inversion are often said to occur at the subtalar joint. For more information on the tarsal joints of the foot, see Sections 8.19 and 8.20.
- Eversion of a body part involves a lateral movement of that body part; inversion of a body part involves a medial movement of that body part.

☐ 5.18 PRONATION/SUPINATION

- **Pronation** is defined as the movement of the forearm wherein the radius crosses over the ulna.

> **BOX 5-21**
>
> Pronation and supination of the forearm are often referred to as *pronation* and *supination of the radius,* because it is the radius that usually does the vast majority of the moving. The ulna does actually move a very small amount. This can be felt if you palpate the distal end of the ulna while doing pronation and supination of the forearm.
>
> Note: If the hand (and therefore the radius) is fixed, it is the ulna that moves relative to the radius during pronation and supination movements of the forearm; this scenario would be an example of reverse actions.

- **Supination** is the opposite of pronation; in other words, the radius uncrosses to return to a position parallel to the ulna.

See Figure 5-18 for examples of pronation and supination.

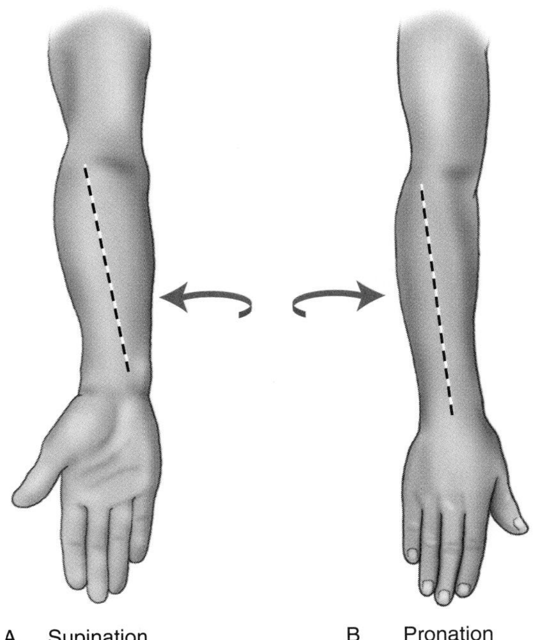

Figure 5-18 Supination and pronation of the right forearm at the radioulnar joints. (The dashed line represents the axis of movement.)

- Pronation and supination are movements that occur in the transverse plane.
- Pronation and supination are axial movements that occur around a vertical axis.
- *Pronation* and *supination* are terms that are used for the radius moving at the radioulnar joints.

> **BOX 5-22**
>
> The axis for pronation and supination is a longitudinal axis that runs approximately from the head of the radius through the styloid process of the ulna (Figure 5-18).
>
> The terms *pronation* and *supination* are also used to describe certain broad movements of the foot. (See Section 8.19 for more details.)

- Pronation of a body part involves two separate motions. The proximal radius medially rotates at the proximal radioulnar joint; and the distal radius moves around the distal end of the ulna.
- In anatomic position, our forearms are fully supinated.
- The practical effect of pronation and supination of the forearm is that it allows us to be able to place the hand in a greater number of positions.

> **BOX 5-23**
>
> Pronation and supination result in an altered position of the distal radius. Because the hand articulates only with the radius, pronation and supination of the forearm result in the hand changing positions. Pronation results in the palm of the hand facing posteriorly; supination results in the palm of the hand facing anteriorly. This altered position of the hand is due to motion at the radioulnar joints; it does not occur at the wrist joint (i.e., radiocarpal joint).

- Note: To avoid confusing pronation/supination of the forearm at the radioulnar joints with medial rotation/lateral rotation of the arm at the shoulder joint, first flex the forearm at the elbow joint to 90 degrees and then perform pronation and supination of the forearm and medial and lateral rotation of the arm at the shoulder joint. The resultant body positions will be markedly different from each other.

5.19 PROTRACTION/RETRACTION

- **Protraction** is defined as a movement at a joint that brings a body part anteriorly.
- **Retraction** is the opposite of protraction; in other words, the body part moves posteriorly (*retraction* literally means to take it back, hence a posterior movement).

See Figure 5-19 for examples of protraction and retraction.

- Protraction and retraction are movements that are considered to occur in the sagittal plane.
- Protraction and retraction can be axial or nonaxial movements depending on the body part. (When the motion is axial, the movement occurs around an axis; when the motion is nonaxial, there is no axis around which the motion occurs.)
- *Protraction* and *retraction* are terms that can be used for the mandible, scapula, and clavicle.

BOX 5-24

The named actions of protraction and retraction can be axial or nonaxial movements, depending on the body part that is moving. Protraction and retraction of the scapula and mandible are nonaxial movements; protraction and retraction of the clavicle are axial movements. (For more information on how these body parts move, see Sections 9.3, 7.2, and 9.4, respectively.)

The tongue and lips may also be said to protract and retract.

Protraction and retraction of the scapula are sometimes referred to as *abduction* and *adduction* of the scapula. The terms *protraction* and *retraction* refer to sagittal plane movements, whereas *abduction* and *adduction* refer to frontal plane movements. The reason for this seeming contradiction in terms is that the scapula lies in a plane that is approximately midway between the sagittal and frontal planes. When the scapula moves in this plane, its movement has a component in both of these planes, hence certain sources choose to describe the motion as *sagittal plane movement* and others choose to describe the motion as *frontal plane movement.* When viewing scapular movement from the anterior or lateral perspectives, the anterior-posterior motion of protraction and retraction is more visible and seems to better describe the scapular movement that is occurring. However, when viewing scapular movement from the posterior perspective, the lateral-medial motion of abduction and adduction away from and toward the midline are more visible and seems to better describe the scapular movement that is occurring. We will use protraction/retraction in this textbook, but we will also reference abduction and adduction. To eliminate this problem, some sources use the term **scaption** to describe the plane of the scapula.

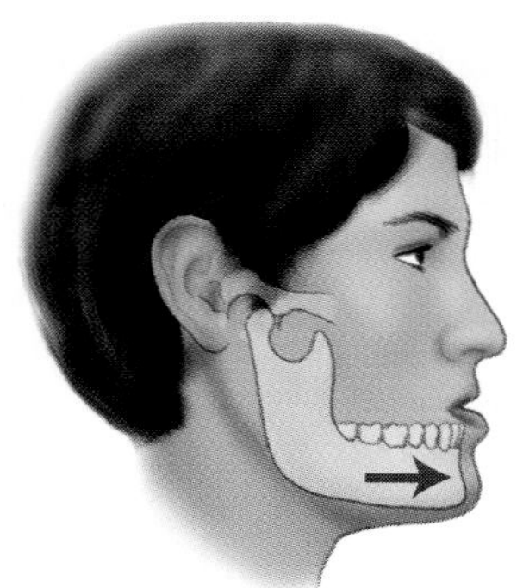

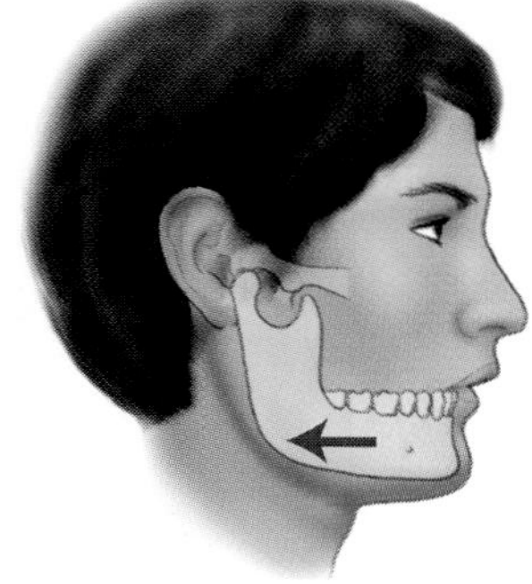

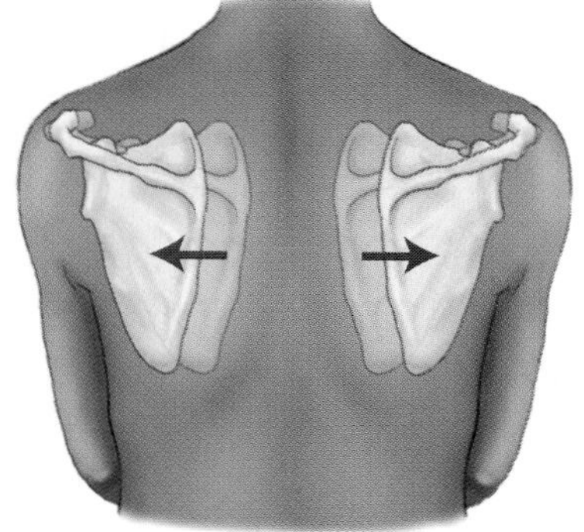

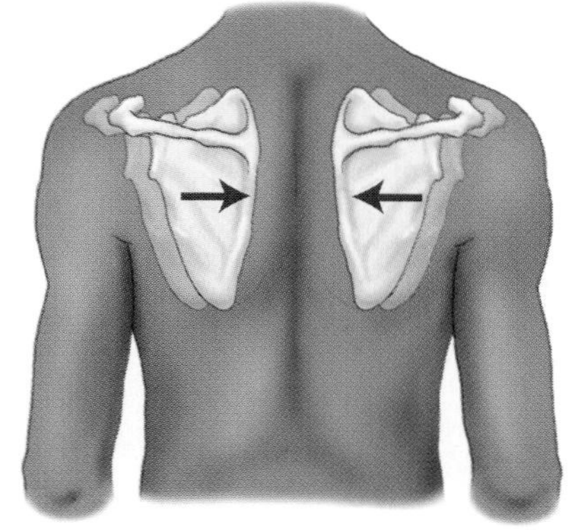

Figure 5-19 Examples of protraction and retraction. *A* and *B,* Protraction and retraction, respectively, of the mandible at the temporomandibular joint (TMJ). *C* and *D,* Protraction and retraction, respectively, of the scapula at the scapulocostal joint (protraction and retraction of the scapula are also known as *abduction and adduction of the scapula*).

5.20 ELEVATION/DEPRESSION

- **Elevation** is defined as a movement at a joint that brings a body part superiorly (*elevate* literally means to bring up).
- **Depression** is the opposite of elevation; in other words, the body part moves inferiorly (*depress* literally means to bring down).

See Figure 5-20 for examples of elevation and depression.

- Elevation and depression are movements that occur in a vertical plane (i.e., sagittal or frontal).
- Elevation and depression can be axial or nonaxial movements depending on the body part. (When the motion is axial, the movement occurs around an axis; when the motion is nonaxial, there is no axis around which the motion occurs.)

BOX 5-25

An example of nonaxial elevation and depression would be the scapula. An example of axial elevation and depression would be the mandible. (For more information on how these body parts move, see Sections 9.3 and 7.2, respectively.)

- *Elevation* and *depression* are terms that can be used for the mandible, scapula, clavicle, and the pelvis.

BOX 5-26

Sometimes the term *elevation* is used more generally to describe movement of a long bone when its distal end elevates. For example, from anatomic position, flexion of the arm is sometimes referred to as *elevation*, because the distal end moves to a position that is higher. Although technically not incorrect, this type of use of the term *elevation* is less precise and therefore less desirable. The term *depression* is sometimes used in a similar manner.

Depression of the pelvis is also known as **lateral tilt** of the pelvis; elevation of the pelvis is also sometimes referred to as **hiking the hip.** (Note: Use of the term *hiking the hip* is not recommended; it can be confusing because *hip* movements are often thought of as thigh movements at the hip joint.) (For more information on the pelvis, see Sections 8.1 through 8.8.)

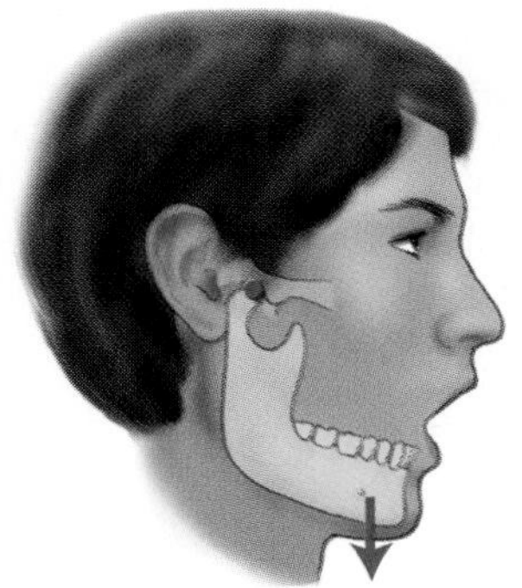

A Depression

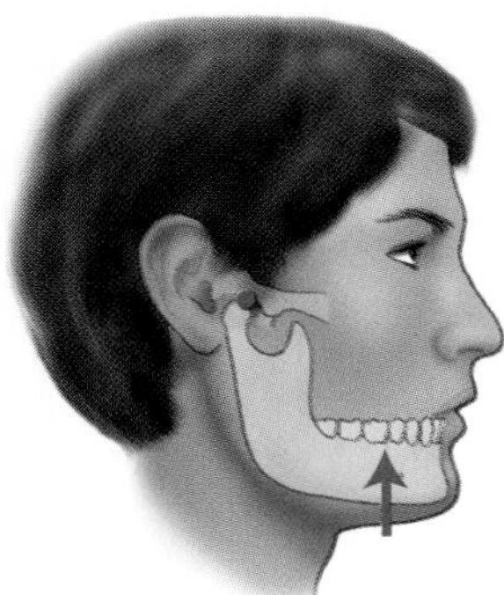

B Elevation

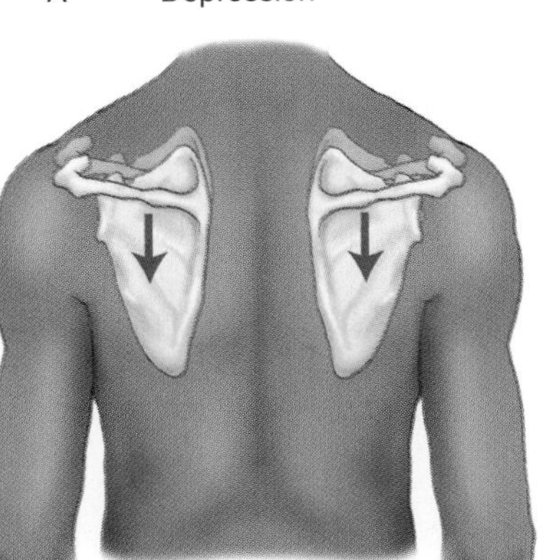

C Depression

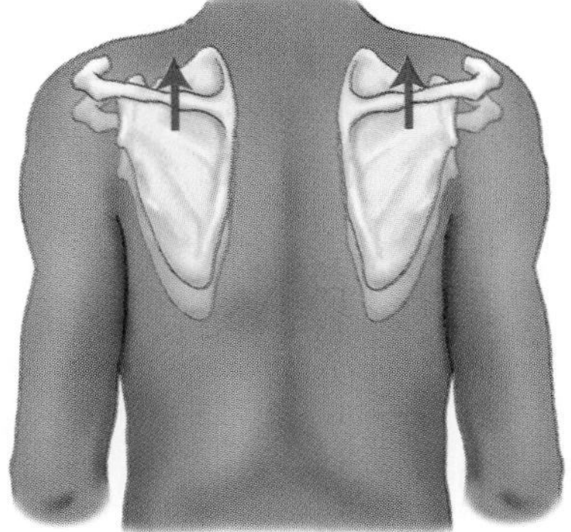

D Elevation

Figure 5-20 Examples of elevation and depression. *A* and *B,* Depression and elevation, respectively, of the mandible at the temporomandibular joint (TMJ) (red dot represents the axis of movement of the mandible). *C* and *D,* Depression and elevation, respectively, of the scapula at the scapulocostal joint.

☐ 5.21 UPWARD ROTATION/DOWNWARD ROTATION

Upward rotation and **downward rotation** are terms that may be used to describe movement of the scapula and the clavicle.

Scapula (Figure 5-21a):

- ❑ Upward rotation is defined as a movement of the scapula wherein the scapula rotates in such a manner that the glenoid fossa orients superiorly.
- ❑ Downward rotation is the opposite of upward rotation; in other words, the scapula rotates to orient the glenoid fossa inferiorly.
  - ❑ Upward rotation and downward rotation of the scapula are axial movements that occur in a vertical plane about an anteroposterior axis.
  - ❑ The importance of upward rotation of the scapula is to orient the glenoid fossa superiorly. This allows the arm to further flex and/or abduct relative to the trunk.

BOX 5-27

The actual plane that the scapula moves within is the plane of the scapula, sometimes called the *scaption plane*, which lies between the sagittal and frontal planes.

According to usual terminology, an action of a body part is the motion of that body part relative to the body part that is directly next to it, with the motion occurring at the joint that is located between them. However, when actions of the *arm* or the *shoulder joint* are spoken of, the entire range of motion of the arm relative to the trunk (not the scapula) is often considered. This lumps the actions of the humerus with the actions of the scapula and clavicle (i.e., the shoulder girdle). Therefore the total motion of the humerus moving at the glenohumeral joint and the shoulder girdle moving at its joints are often considered. Similarly, motion of the *thigh* or the *hip joint* often includes the motion of the pelvic girdle.

Clavicle (Figure 5-21b):

- ❑ Upward rotation may also be used to describe the rotation of the clavicle in which the inferior surface comes to face anteriorly.
- ❑ Being the opposite action, downward rotation returns the inferior surface (now facing anteriorly) back to face inferiorly again.

BOX 5-28

If one were to look at the clavicle from the lateral side, upward rotation would be a counterclockwise motion of the clavicle; downward rotation would be a clockwise motion of the clavicle.

- ❑ Upward rotation and downward rotation of the clavicle are axial movements that occur in a transverse plane around an axis that is approximately mediolateral in orientation.
- ❑ Because of the curve in the distal clavicle, when the clavicle upwardly rotates, the distal end elevates. Therefore one important aspect of upward rotation of the clavicle is to help elevate the shoulder girdle as a whole to facilitate further flexion and/or abduction of the arm relative to the trunk. (For more detailed information on the role of the clavicle [and scapula] in motion of the upper extremity, see Section 9.6.)

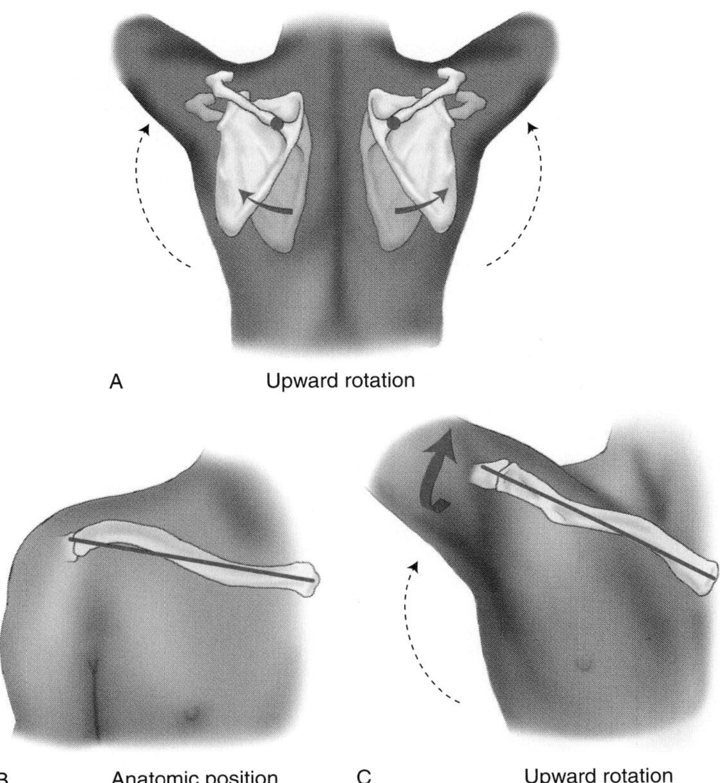

Figure 5-21 Examples of upward rotation and downward rotation. *A,* Upward rotation of the scapulae at the scapulocostal joints from anatomic position (downward rotation of the scapula would be returning to anatomic position). The red dot represents the location of the axis of movement for upward and downward rotation of the scapula. *B,* Clavicle in anatomic position. *C,* Upward rotation of the clavicle at the sternoclavicular joint (downward rotation of the clavicle would be returning to anatomic position). The red line in *B* and *C* represents the axis of movement for upward and downward rotation of the clavicle.

☐ 5.22 ANTERIOR TILT/POSTERIOR TILT

Anterior tilt and **posterior tilt** are terms that may be used to describe movement of the pelvis.

BOX 5-29

Unfortunately many terminology systems exist for naming movements of the pelvis. Because *anterior tilt* and *posterior tilt* are the most common and easiest terms to use when describing sagittal plane movements of the pelvis, this book will use these terms.

- ❑ Anterior tilt is defined as the movement of the pelvis wherein the superior aspect of the pelvis tilts anteriorly (Figure 5-22a).
- ❑ Posterior tilt is defined as the movement of the pelvis wherein the superior aspect of the pelvis tilts posteriorly (Figure 5-22b).
  - ❑ Anterior tilt and posterior tilt are movements that occur in the sagittal plane.

BOX 5-30

The terms *right lateral tilt* and *left lateral tilt* are sometimes used to describe movements of the pelvis in the frontal plane. This book will use the term *depression of the pelvis* (see Sections 8.3 through 8.5) in place of *lateral tilt of the pelvis.*

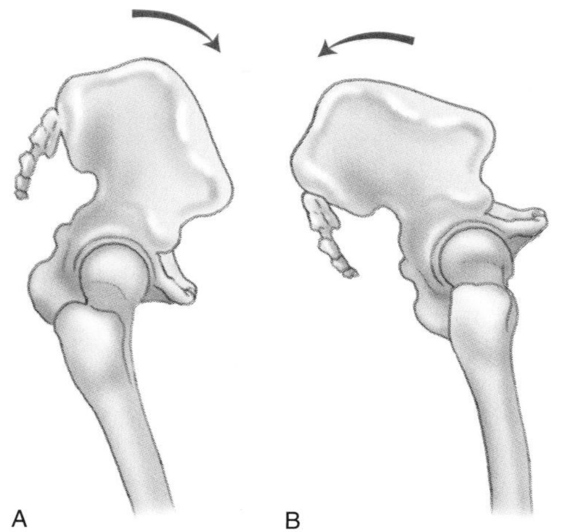

Figure 5-22 *A,* Anterior tilt of the pelvis. *B,* Posterior tilt of the pelvis. Motions are shown as occurring at the hip joint(s).

- ❑ Anterior tilt and posterior tilt are axial movements that occur around a mediolateral axis.
- ❑ *Anterior tilt* and *posterior tilt* are terms that are used for the pelvis moving at the lumbosacral and/or the hip joints.
- ❑ The postural position of anterior/posterior tilt of the pelvis is extremely important because the spine sits on the pelvis; if the amount of anterior/posterior tilt of the pelvis changes, the curves of the spine must change (i.e., increase or decrease) to compensate. (For more information on the effect of the pelvis on the posture of the spine, see Section 8.8.)
- ❑ The word *pelvis* is derived from the Latin word for basin. If one thinks of the pelvis as a basin filled with water, then the word *tilt* refers to where the water would spill out when the pelvis tilts (Figure 5-23).

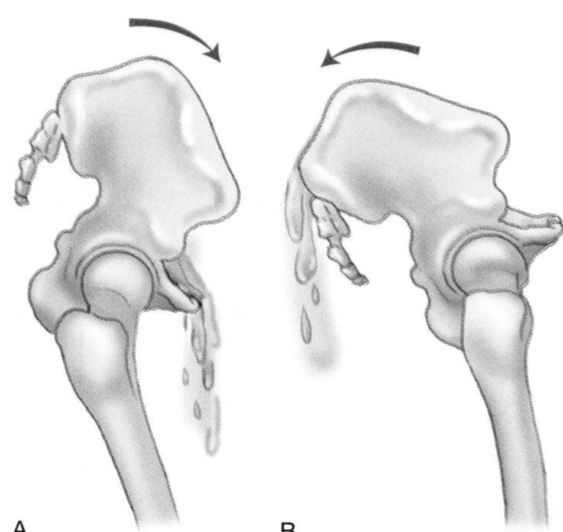

Figure 5-23 *A* and *B,* Water spilling out of the pelvis based on the tilt of the pelvis. To learn the *tilt* actions of the pelvis, it can be helpful to think of the pelvis as a basin that holds water. Whichever way that the pelvis tilts, water will spill out in that direction.

☐ 5.23 OPPOSITION/REPOSITION

- **Opposition** is defined as the movement of the thumb wherein the pad of the thumb meets the pad of another finger (Figure 5-24a).
- **Reposition** is the opposite of opposition; in other words, the thumb returns to its starting position (usually anatomic position) (Figure 5-24b).
  - Opposition is not a specific action; it is a combination of three actions.
    - Opposition is a combination of abduction, flexion, and medial rotation of the metacarpal of the thumb at the saddle joint of the thumb (1st carpometacarpal joint).
  - Reposition is not a specific action; it is a combination of three actions.
    - Reposition is a combination of extension, lateral rotation, and adduction of the metacarpal of the thumb at the saddle joint of the thumb (1st carpometacarpal joint).

BOX 5-31

The cardinal plane component actions of opposition and reposition of the thumb are unusual in that flexion/extension and abduction/adduction do not occur in their usual planes; flexion and extension occur in the frontal plane instead of the sagittal plane, and abduction and adduction occur in the sagittal plane instead of the frontal plane. The reason for this is that the thumb rotated embryologically so that it can be opposed to the other fingers for grasping objects. This can be seen if you look at the orientation of the thumb pad when the thumb is in anatomic or resting position. You will see that the thumb pad primarily faces medially, whereas the pads of the other fingers face anteriorly. Therefore because of this embryologic rotation, flexion/extension and abduction/adduction are named as occurring in planes that are 90 degrees different from the planes that they usually occur within.

Components of Opposition/Reposition (Box 5-31):

- Flexion and extension of the thumb occur in the frontal plane around an anteroposterior axis. With flexion and extension, the thumb moves parallel to the palm of the hand.
- Abduction and adduction of the thumb occur in the sagittal plane around a mediolateral axis. With abduction and adduction, the thumb moves perpendicular to the palm of the hand.
- Medial rotation and lateral rotation of the thumb occur in the transverse plane around a vertical axis.
  - The exact components of opposition (and therefore reposition) can vary depending on the starting position of the thumb and to which finger the thumb is being opposed. (For more information on movement of the thumb, see Section 9.13.)
  - The terms *opposition* and *reposition* are also used to describe movements of the little finger. (For more information on movement of the little finger, see Section 9.12.)

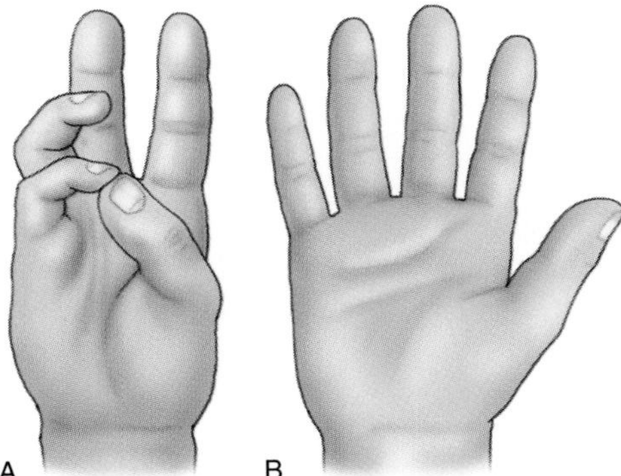

Figure 5-24 *A,* Opposition of the thumb at the saddle joint of the thumb (1st carpometacarpal joint). *B,* Reposition of the thumb at the saddle joint of the thumb (1st carpometacarpal joint).

5.24 RIGHT LATERAL DEVIATION/ LEFT LATERAL DEVIATION

- **Right lateral deviation** is defined as a movement at a joint that brings a body part to the right.
- **Left lateral deviation** is the opposite of right lateral deviation; in other words, the body part moves to the left.
  - Right lateral deviation and left lateral deviation are movements that could be considered to occur in the frontal or the transverse plane.
  - **Lateral deviation** (to the right or left) can be axial or nonaxial movements depending on the body part. (When the motion is axial, the movement occurs around an axis; when the motion is nonaxial, there is no axis around which the motion occurs.)

BOX 5-32

Lateral deviation of the trunk is an axial movement. Lateral deviation of the mandible at the temporomandibular joint (TMJ) is a linear nonaxial movement.

- *Right lateral deviation* and *left lateral deviation* are terms that are used for the mandible and the trunk.

BOX 5-33

Lateral deviation of the trunk occurs as the reverse action of a muscle that crosses the glenohumeral joint from the arm to the trunk (e.g., the pectoralis major or the latissimus dorsi). When the arm stays fixed and the muscle contracts, the trunk moves toward the fixed arm. This movement can occur at the scapulocostal joint if the scapula is fixed to the humerus; in this case the trunk moves relative to the fixed scapula and arm. Alternatively, it can occur at the shoulder joint (i.e., glenohumeral joint); in this case the trunk and scapula move as a unit relative to the fixed humerus. (For more on reverse actions of the trunk at the shoulder joint, see illustrations in Section 7.10.)

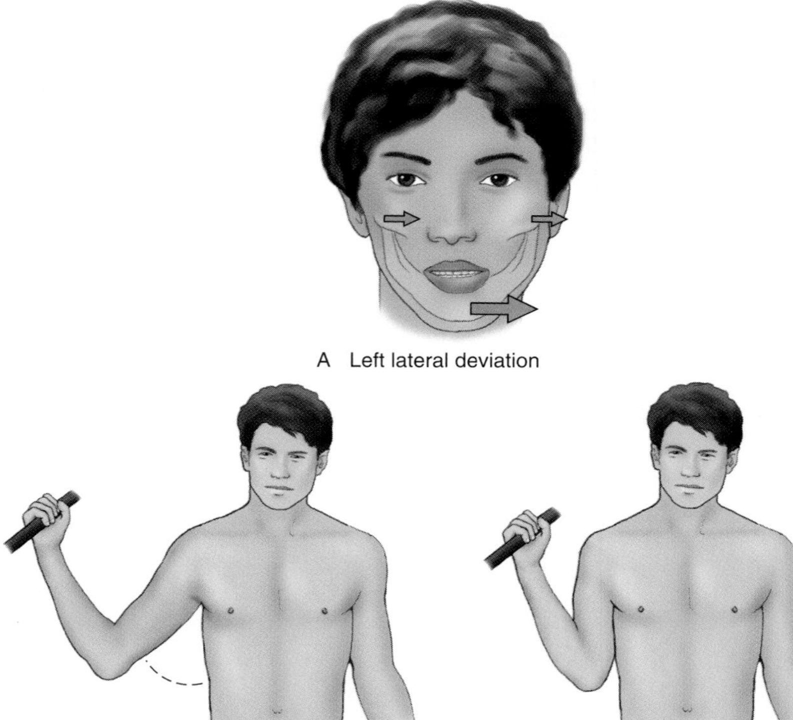

Figure 5-25 Examples of lateral deviation (to the right or left). *A,* Left lateral deviation of the mandible at the temporomandibular joint (TMJ). *B* and *C,* Right lateral deviation of the trunk. In this scenario the hand is holding onto an immovable object and is fixed; when muscles such as the pectoralis major and latissimus dorsi contract, the trunk is laterally deviated to the right, toward the right arm. (Note: The arm has also flexed at the elbow joint.)

☐ 5.25 HORIZONTAL FLEXION/HORIZONTAL EXTENSION

- **Horizontal flexion** is defined as a horizontal movement in an anterior direction of the arm at the shoulder joint or thigh at the hip joint.
- **Horizontal extension** is the opposite of horizontal flexion; in other words, a horizontal movement in a posterior direction of the arm or thigh.

See Figure 5-26 for an example of horizontal flexion and horizontal extension.

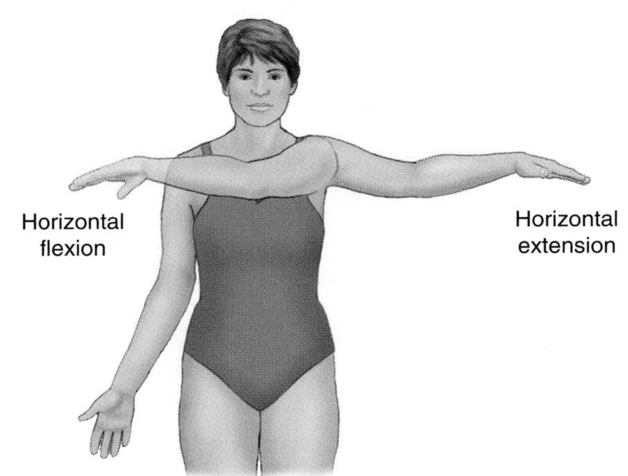

Figure 5-26 Horizontal flexion and horizontal extension of a person's left arm at the shoulder joint.

- Horizontal flexion and horizontal extension are movements that occur once the arm or thigh is first abducted 90 degrees.

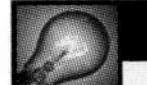

BOX 5-34

Horizontal flexion is also known as **horizontal adduction**; horizontal extension is also known as **horizontal abduction**.

- Horizontal flexion and horizontal extension occur in the transverse plane.
- Horizontal flexion and horizontal extension are axial movements that occur around a vertical axis.
- The terms *horizontal flexion* and *extension* are useful terms created to describe horizontal movements of the arm and/or thigh that commonly occur in many sporting activities (e.g., a baseball swing or tennis forehand or backhand), as well as activities of daily life (e.g., reaching across your body to move an object or perhaps dusting a bookshelf).

☐ 5.26 HYPEREXTENSION

- **Hyperextension** is a term that can be used in two different ways:
  - To denote movement that is beyond what is considered to be a normal or healthy range of motion
  - To describe normal, healthy extension beyond anatomic position
- The prefix *hyper* is used to denote a greater than normal or a greater than healthy amount of something. Therefore hyperextension should theoretically mean an amount of extension of a body part at a joint that is greater than the normal amount or greater than the healthy amount of extension which that joint normally permits. That is the way in which the term *hyperextension* will be used in this book.

BOX 5-35

It should be kept in mind that "normal" and "healthy" are not necessarily the same thing. For example, it is normal for an elderly person in our society to have arteriosclerosis; however, the presence of this condition would not be considered healthy.

- Whether or not hyperextension describes a healthy or unhealthy condition depends on the individual. For example, dancers or contortionists who have extremely flexible muscles and ligaments can hyperextend their joints; this hyperextension would certainly be beyond normal movement, hence the term *hyperextension*, but would not be unhealthy for these individuals. Another person might extend a body part at a joint much less than a dancer or contortionist would and this movement might result in a sprain and/or strain; this hyperextension having caused tissue damage would be considered to be unhealthy.
- Given this reasoning, terms such as *hyperflexion* and *hyperabduction* could also be used in a similar manner to describe any movement that is greater than the normal or healthy amount which that joint will normally permit.
- However, another use of the term *hyperextension* exists. Hyperextension is often used to describe only the particular phase of extension wherein a body part extends beyond anatomic position. In this terminology system, the term *extension* is then reserved for the phase of motion wherein a body part that is first flexed, then extends back toward anatomic position (Figure 5-27). We will not be using this meaning for the term *hyperextension*; however, given how often the term is used in this manner, it is important that any student of kinesiology be familiar with it.

BOX 5-36

Although use of the term *hyperextension* to denote extension beyond anatomic position is fairly common, it is not recommended for two reasons:

1. It is inconsistent with the normal use of the prefix *hyper* (extending beyond anatomic position is not excessive or unhealthy).
2. It is not symmetrical; no other joint action beyond anatomic position is given the prefix *hyper* (e.g., flexion beyond anatomic position is not called *hyperflexion*; abduction beyond anatomic position is not called *hyperabduction*, and so forth).

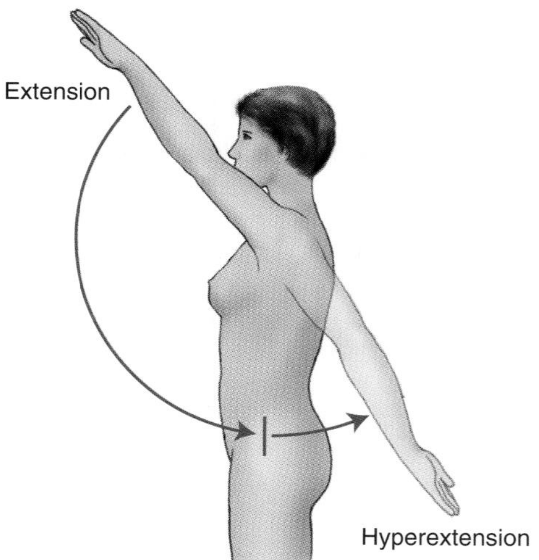

Figure 5-27 Woman extending her arm (that was first flexed) at the shoulder joint toward anatomic position; she then "hyperextends" her arm beyond anatomic position. (Note: This book does not adopt this use of the term *hyperextension*.)

☐ 5.27 CIRCUMDUCTION

- **Circumduction** is a term that is often used when describing joint actions. However, circumduction is not an action; rather it is a combination of actions of a body part that occur sequentially at a joint.
- Circumduction of an appendicular body part involves the frontal and sagittal plane actions of adduction, extension, abduction, and flexion (not necessarily in that order).
- Circumduction of an axial body part involves the frontal and sagittal plane actions of right lateral flexion, extension, left lateral flexion, and flexion (not necessarily in that order).
- A good example of circumduction is shown in Figure 5-28. The arm is seen to first adduct, then extend, then abduct, and then flex (at the shoulder joint). If each of these four motions is performed individually, one after the other, the distal end of the upper extremity will carve out a square, and it will be clear that four separate motions occurred (Figure 5-28a). However, if the same actions are performed, but now the corners of the square are "rounded out," the movement of the upper extremity will now carve out a circle (Figure 5-28b–c).
- Many people erroneously believe that circumduction is or involves some form of rotation. However, no rotation occurs. In Figure 5-28b, the adductors first adduct the arm, then the extensors extend it, then abductors abduct it, and finally the flexors flex it. In this example, it can be seen that circumduction of the arm involves no rotation.

BOX 5-37

The term *circumduction* is used regardless of the sequence of the movements (i.e., using Figure 5-28 as our example); it does not matter if the order is adduction, extension, abduction, and then flexion, or if the order is the opposite (i.e., extension, adduction, flexion, and then abduction). In other words, whether the circles are clockwise or counterclockwise in direction, a circle formed by a sequence of four axial movements is called *circumduction.*

- The arm, thigh, hand, foot, head, neck, trunk, and pelvis can all circumduct.

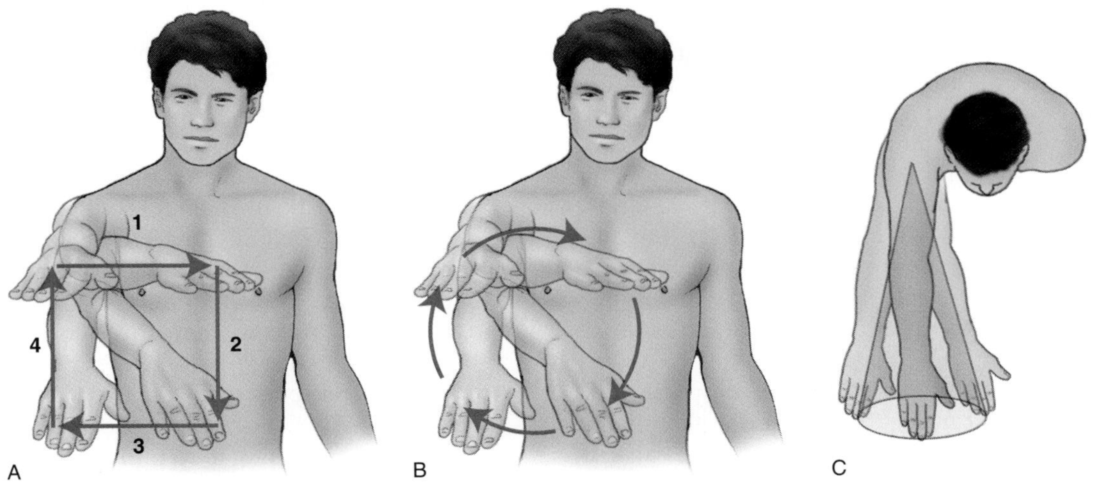

Figure 5-28 Circumduction of the arm at the shoulder joint. *A,* Four separate motions of circumduction carving out a square. *B* and *C,* Circumduction as it typically looks, carving out a circle (*B* is an anterior view; *C* is a superior view).

5.28 NAMING OBLIQUE PLANE MOVEMENTS

- An **oblique plane movement** occurs within an oblique plane.
- An oblique plane is a plane that is not purely sagittal, frontal, or transverse (i.e., an oblique plane is a combination of two or three cardinal planes).
- Naming a joint action that occurs purely in a cardinal plane is simple. We simply name the action that occurred using one of the terms for movement that we have just learned. There is one joint action term that exists for each cardinal plane movement because these joint action terms are defined with respect to cardinal planes.
- However, our body's motions do not always occur within pure cardinal planes; we often move within oblique planes. When describing a movement that occurs within an oblique plane, it is a little more difficult to name this motion.
- When we describe a movement of the human body that occurs in an oblique plane, it is necessary to break the one oblique movement up into the components that can be described by cardinal plane movement terms.
- For example, Figure 5-29 shows a person moving the arm in an oblique plane. This motion is occurring in only one direction; however, that direction is a combination of sagittal plane flexion and frontal plane abduction. We do not have one specific term to describe this one movement; instead we must describe it with two terms by saying that the person has flexed and adducted the arm at the shoulder joint. By our description that includes these two terms, it may seem as if the person made two movements. In reality, the person made only one movement. However, for us to describe that one movement, we have to break that one oblique movement into two separate cardinal plane actions.
- The order in which we say these two components is not important. We can say that the person flexed and adducted the arm at the shoulder joint, or we can say that the person adducted and flexed the arm at the shoulder joint.
- An analogy can be made to geographic directions on a map. If a person is walking northwest, he or she is walking in one direction. In geographic terms, we can state that in one term, *northwest*, which gives the reader the sense that the person is, in fact, walking in one direction (Figure 5-30). However, in kinesiology terminology, we do not combine our joint action terms into one-word combinations like we do in geographic terminology. In the case of Figure 5-29, we cannot say that the person is "flexoabducting" or "abductoflexing." Instead we say that the person flexed and abducted (or abducted and flexed). It is important to realize that the person only moved the arm in one oblique direction, but we describe this one oblique movement by breaking it up into its two pure cardinal plane action components.
- Whenever a person moves a body part in an oblique plane that is a combination of two or three cardinal planes, we must separate that one oblique movement into its two or three pure cardinal plane movements.

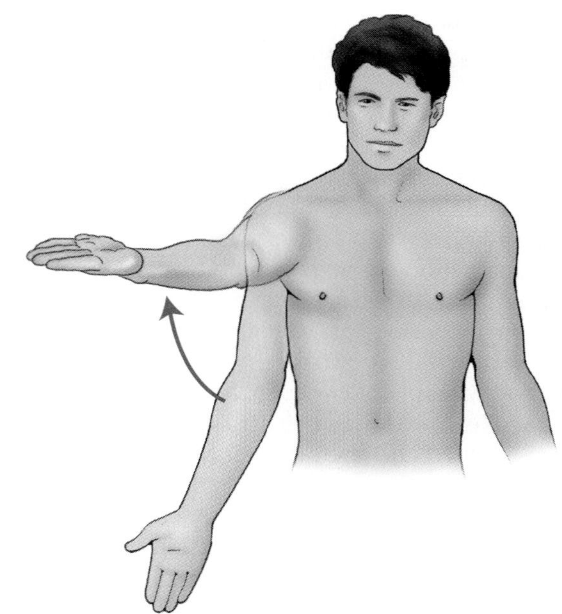

Figure 5-29 Movement that is within an oblique plane that is between the sagittal and frontal planes. This one movement is described as *flexion and abduction of the arm at the shoulder joint* (or *abduction and flexion of the arm at the shoulder joint*; the order does not matter).

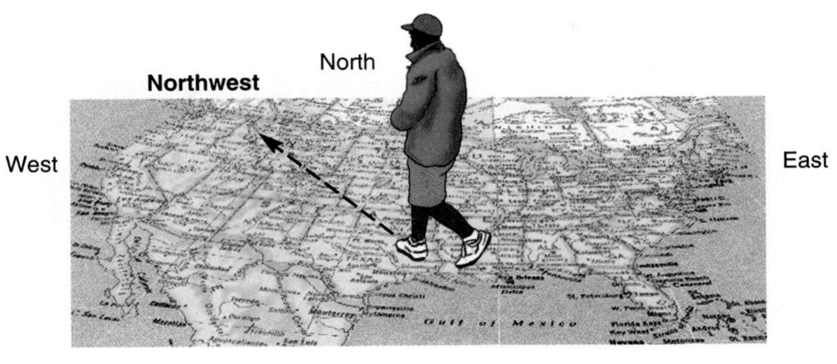

Figure 5-30 Person walking in a northwesterly direction. In geographic terms, this movement is described as *northwest,* instead of saying that the person is walking north and west (or west and north).

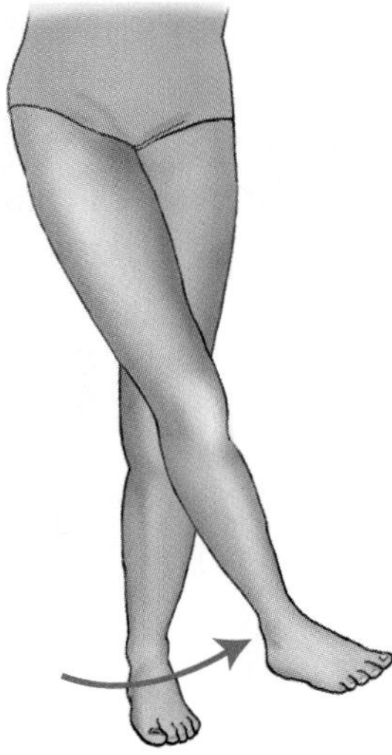

Figure 5-31 Movement occurring within an oblique plane. This oblique plane is a combination of all three cardinal planes; therefore the movement that is occurring has component actions in all three cardinal planes. The person is flexing, adducting, and medially rotating the right thigh at the hip joint (the order that these three actions is listed is not important).

☐ 5.29 REVERSE ACTIONS

❑ A **reverse action** is when a muscle contracts and the attachment that is usually considered to be more fixed; in other words, the origin) moves, and the attachment that is usually considered to be more mobile (i.e., the insertion) stays fixed.

❑ As explained in Chapter 12 (see Section 11.2), whenever a muscle contracts and shortens, it can move either attachment *A* toward attachment *B,* or attachment *B* toward attachment *A*, or it can move both attachments *A* and *B* toward each other. Generally speaking, one of the attachments, call it *attachment A*, will usually do the moving. This is because this attachment, attachment *A,* weighs less than attachment *B* and therefore moves more easily (conversely, attachment *B* is usually heavier and therefore more fixed and will not move as easily). When origin/insertion terminology is used, this attachment that usually moves is called the *insertion* and the other attachment that usually does not move is called the *origin.*

❑ In Figure 5-32a, we see the brachialis, which is a flexor of the elbow joint (the brachialis crosses the elbow joint anteriorly, attaching from the arm to the forearm).

❑ When the brachialis contracts, it will usually move the forearm, not the arm, at the elbow joint, because the forearm is lighter (i.e., less fixed) than the arm. Figure 5-32b illustrates the forearm moving when the brachialis contracts; this action is called *flexion of the forearm at the elbow joint.*

❑ However, in certain circumstances, such as doing a pull-up, the forearm might be more fixed than the arm, and the arm may do the moving instead. Figure 5-32c illustrates the arm moving when the brachialis contracts; this action is called *flexion of the arm at elbow joint.* When the brachialis moves the arm instead of the forearm, it can be called the *reverse action* because it is the opposite action than the action that usually occurs (i.e., the arm is moving instead of the forearm). In origin/insertion terminology the reverse action is said to occur whenever the origin moves instead of the insertion.

> **BOX 5-38**
>
> Interestingly, the action of a muscle that is considered to be its usual action is not always its most common action. Generally it is assumed that the distal attachment of an appendicular body part muscle is the more movable attachment (i.e., the *insertion*). In the upper extremity, this is generally true. However, in the lower extremity we are usually in a weight-bearing position such as standing, walking, or running in which the feet are planted on the ground and therefore more fixed than the more proximal attachment. During the gait cycle, for example, our feet are planted on the ground 60% of the time. Therefore reverse actions in the lower extremity actually occur more often than the usual actions that most students memorize in their beginning kinesiology classes!

❑ It should be emphasized that the reverse action of a muscle is always theoretically possible. Again, a muscle can always move either attachment *A* toward attachment *B* **or** attachment *B* toward attachment *A*.

❑ It is also possible for both attachment *A* and attachment *B* to move. In other words, both the usual and the reverse action can occur at the same time (Figure 5-32d).

> **BOX 5-39**
>
> Understanding the concept of reverse actions of a muscle is not only fundamental to understanding how the musculoskeletal system works but also extremely important when working clinically so that we can best assess muscle contractions and how they relate to the client's health!

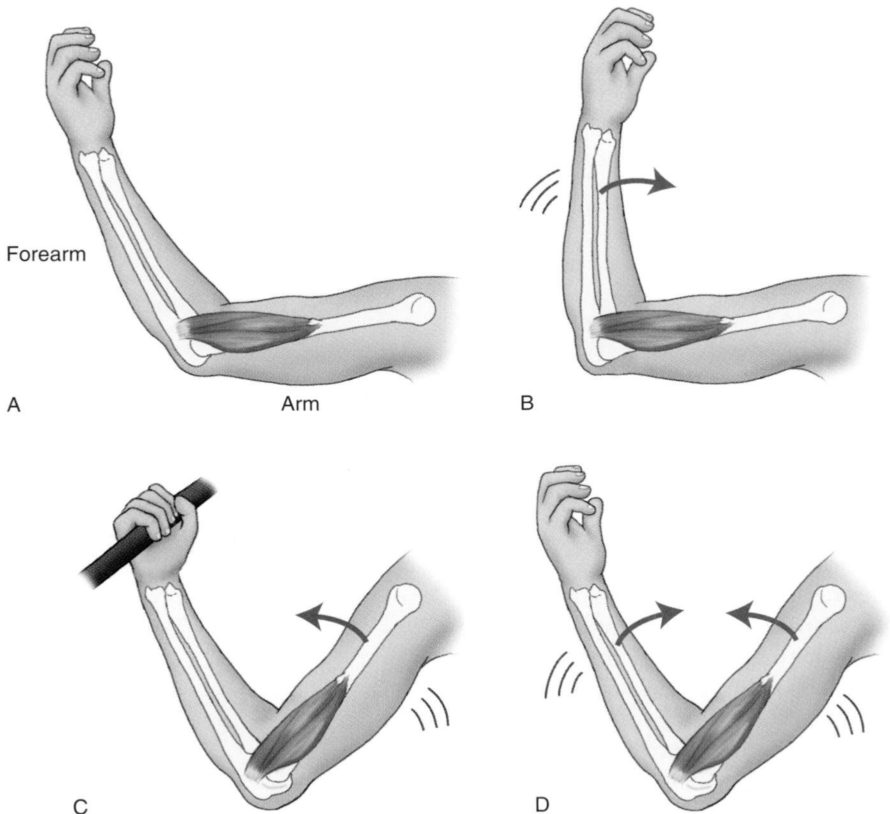

Figure 5-32 *A,* Medial view of the brachialis muscle. *B,* Brachialis muscle contracting and causing flexion of the forearm at the elbow joint. *C,* Brachialis muscle contracting to do a pull-up. In this scenario the hand is fixed to the pull-up bar, so the forearm (being attached to the hand) is now more fixed than the arm; therefore the arm moves instead of the forearm. The resulting action is flexion of the arm at the elbow joint. This action is usually referred to as a *reverse action*, because the attachment that is usually considered to stay fixed did the moving (and the attachment usually considered to move stayed fixed). *D,* Both attachments of the brachialis are moving, so both the forearm and the arm are flexing at the elbow joint; therefore the usual action and the reverse action are occurring at the same time.

☐ 5.30 VECTORS

- A **vector** is nothing more than an arrow drawn to represent the line of pull of a muscle.
- This vector arrow is drawn along the direction of the fibers of the muscle, from one attachment to the other attachment and helps us visually see the action(s) of the muscle.

BOX 5-40

A vector has two components to it. The direction that the arrowhead is pointed tells us the direction of the line of pull of the muscle; the length of the stem of the arrow tells us the magnitude of the muscle's pull (i.e., how far the muscle pulls its attachment). However, in kinesiology textbooks, vectors are often not drawn to scale because it is the direction of the muscle's line of pull represented by the direction of the arrowhead that is usually of primary interest.

Note: The direction that the arrowhead of a vector points can be reversed for reverse actions.

- A very brief understanding of vectors can be helpful toward understanding how to figure out a muscle's actions.
- If that muscle's line of pull is in an oblique plane, vectors can be very helpful toward breaking down and seeing the component cardinal plane actions of that muscle.
- Figure 5-33 illustrates retraction (i.e., adduction) of the scapula at the scapulocostal joint. The direction of the line of pull of the muscle that is creating this action is shown by a vector, which is simply an arrow that is drawn pointing in the direction of the muscle's line of pull. Vectors can be drawn for all muscle lines of pull. Vectors are valuable because they help give us a visual image of the muscle's action.
- In Figure 5-34a, we see that the rhomboids' major and minor muscles also attach to and can move the scapula.
- Figure 5-34b shows a vector that has been drawn in that demonstrates the movement that the rhomboids can have on the scapula.
- In this case, as shown by the vector, the rhomboids' pull on the scapula is diagonal (i.e., oblique). Therefore when the rhomboids contract, they pull the scapula in this diagonal direction.
- Figure 5-34c shows how this diagonal vector can be resolved into its component vectors. We see that to **resolve a vector**, we simply draw in the component vector arrows that begin at the tail of the vector arrow and end at the vector's arrowhead.

BOX 5-41

When an oblique vector is broken down into its cardinal plane component vectors, it is said to be *resolved*. When resolving a vector, note that we must start at the beginning of the tail of the arrow and end at the arrowhead. Being able to resolve a vector that represents the oblique line of pull of a muscle is extremely helpful toward seeing the component cardinal plane actions of the muscle! ☺

- Each of these two component vectors represents the two component cardinal plane actions of this muscle. The horizontal component vector arrow shows that the rhomboids can adduct the scapula; the vertical component vector arrow shows that the rhomboids can elevate the scapula.
- Figure 5-35 illustrates another example of resolving a vector arrow to determine the actions of another muscle (the coracobrachialis muscle).

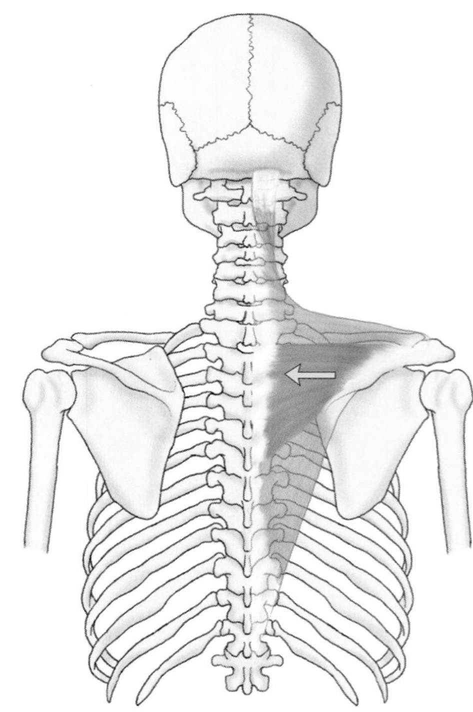

Figure 5-33 Fibers of a muscle (the fibers of the middle trapezius muscle) that can move the scapula (at the scapulocostal joint). Also drawn in is a vector that demonstrates the line of pull of the middle trapezius. The direction that the yellow arrow is pointing represents the muscle's line of pull; in this case it is medial. The fibers of the middle trapezius can pull the scapula medially (i.e., retract the scapula [at the scapulocostal joint]).

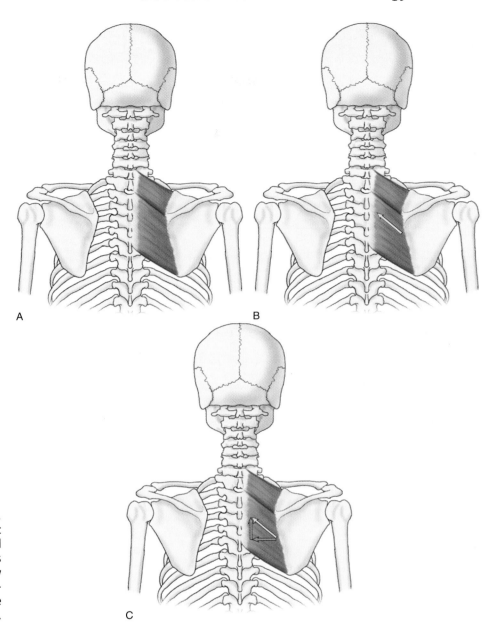

Figure 5-34 *A,* Rhomboid muscles. *B,* Vector arrow drawn in yellow that represents the direction of fibers and resultant line of pull of the rhomboids upon the scapula. *C,* This vector arrow of the rhomboids resolved into component green vectors that represent the cardinal plane actions of the rhomboids.

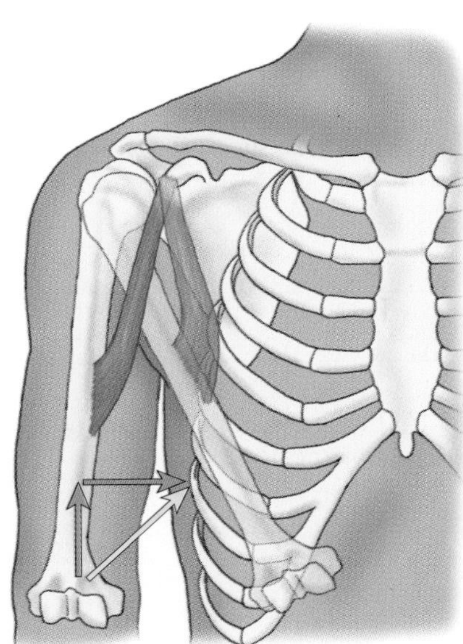

Figure 5-35 Vector analysis of the action(s) of the right coracobrachialis muscle. The yellow arrow represents the overall pull of the coracobrachialis upon the arm at the shoulder joint. Resolving this vector, we draw in a vertical and a horizontal vector (drawn in green) that begin at the tail of the yellow arrow and end at the head of the yellow arrow. The vertical vector represents the muscle's ability to flex the arm; the horizontal vector represents the muscle's ability to adduct the arm. By resolving the vector that represents the line of pull of the coracobrachialis, we see that the coracobrachialis can both flex and adduct the arm at the shoulder joint.

REVIEW QUESTIONS

evolve Answers to the following review questions appear on the Evolve website accompanying this book.

1. What is the primary function of a joint?

2. What is the relationship between the stability and mobility of a joint?

3. What is the main function of a muscle?

4. What is the main function of a ligament?

5. What is the difference between axial and nonaxial motion?

6. Name two synonyms for axial motion.

7. What is the difference between rectilinear and curvilinear motion?

8. What is the difference between curvilinear motion and axial motion?

9. What are the three fundamental ways in which one bone can move along another bone?

10. What three things must be stated to fully name and describe a joint action?

11. What are the five major joint action terminology pairs used to describe motion?

12. What term is used to describe a movement of the scapula at the scapulocostal joint in which the glenoid fossa orients superiorly?

13. What term is used to describe an anterior movement of the mandible at the temporomandibular joint (TMJ)?

14. Within what plane does flexion generally occur?

15. What is the name of the axis for medial and lateral rotation movements?

16. What are the three component cardinal plane actions of opposition of the thumb at the saddle joint of the thumb?

17. What are the two manners in which the term *hyper-extension* can be used?

18. Why is circumduction not an action?

19. How do we describe the actions of a muscle with a line of pull in an oblique plane?

20. What is a reverse action?

21. What is the reverse action of flexion of the right forearm at the elbow joint?

22. What is the reverse action of flexion of the left thigh at the hip joint?

23. What is a vector?

24. How can knowledge of vectors be helpful in the study of kinesiology?

Chapter 6

Classification of Joints

CHAPTER OUTLINE

CHAPTER OBJECTIVES

After completing this chapter, the student should be able to perform the following:

- ❑ Describe the anatomy of a joint and list the three major structural types of joints.
- ❑ Describe the physiology of a joint.
- ❑ With regard to joint physiology (i.e., motion), explain the function of joints, muscles, and ligaments/joint capsules.
- ❑ Explain the distinction between the definitions of a structural joint and a functional joint.
- ❑ Describe the relationship between joint mobility and joint stability; and list the three major determinants of the mobility/stability of a joint.
- ❑ Explain the importance of weight bearing and shock absorption to joints.
- ❑ List and describe the three major structural categories of joints.
- ❑ List and describe the three major functional categories of joints.
- ❑ Explain the relationship between the structural and functional categories of joints.
- ❑ List and describe the three categories of fibrous joints.
- ❑ Give an example of each of the categories of fibrous joints.
- ❑ List and describe the two categories of cartilaginous joints.
- ❑ Give an example of each of the categories of cartilaginous joints.
- ❑ List the structural components of and be able to draw a typical synovial joint.
- ❑ List and describe the four categories of synovial joints.
- ❑ Describe and be able to give examples of the two types of uniaxial synovial joints.
- ❑ Describe and be able to give examples of the two types of biaxial synovial joints.
- ❑ Describe and be able to give examples of triaxial synovial joints.
- ❑ Describe and be able to give examples of nonaxial synovial joints.
- ❑ Explain the purpose of menisci and articular discs and be able to give an example of each one.
- ❑ Define the key terms of this chapter.
- ❑ State the meanings of the word origins of this chapter.

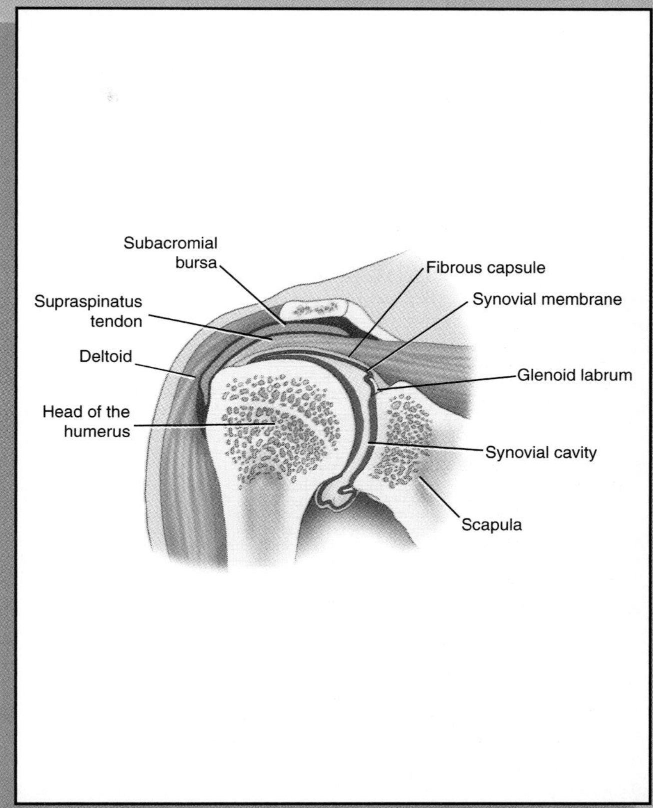

OVERVIEW

The discussion of motion in the body began in Chapter 2 and continued in Chapter 5. Chapter 6 now deepens the exploration of motion by examining the structural and functional characteristics of joints of the body. Specifically, shock absorption, weight bearing, and the concept of mobility versus stability are addressed. This chapter then continues by laying out the classification system for all joints of the body. The three major structural categories of joints (fibrous, cartilaginous, and synovial joints) are each examined. A special emphasis is placed on synovial joints; their four major categories (uniaxial, biaxial, triaxial, and nonaxial synovial joints) are discussed in detail. The chapter concludes with a brief look at the role of articular discs and menisci within joints.

KEY TERMS

Amphiarthrotic joint (amphiarthrosis, pl. amphiarthroses) (AM-fee-are-THROT-ik, AM-fee-are-THROS-is, AM-fee-are-THROS-eez)
Articular cartilage (ar-TIK-you-lar)
Articular disc
Articulation (ar-TIK-you-LAY-shun)
Ball-and-socket joint
Biaxial joint (bye-AK-see-al)
Cartilaginous joint (kar-ti-LAJ-in-us)
Closed-packed position
Compound joint
Condyloid joint (KON-di-loyd)
Congruent (kon-GREW-ent)
Degrees of freedom
Diarthrotic joint (diarthrosis, pl. diarthroses) (DIE-are-THROT-ik, DIE-are-THROS-is, DIE-are-THROS-eez)
Ellipsoid joint (ee-LIPS-oid)
Extra-articular (EKS-tra-ar-TIK-you-lar)
Fibrous joint
Functional joint
Ginglymus joint (GING-la-mus)
Gliding joints
Gomphosis, pl. gomphoses (gom-FOS-is, gom-FOS-ees)
Hinge joint
Intra-articular (IN-tra-ar-TIK-you-lar)
Irregular joints
Joint
Joint capsule (KAP-sool)
Joint cavity
Meniscus, pl. menisci (men-IS-kus, men-IS-KIY)
Mobility
Nonaxial joints (non-AKS-ee-al)
Open-packed position
Ovoid joint (O-void)
Pivot joint
Plane joint
Polyaxial joint (PA-lee-AKS-ee-al)
Saddle joint
Sellar joint (SEL-lar)
Shock absorption
Simple joint
Stability
Structural joint
Suture joint (SOO-chur)
Symphysis joint (SIM-fa-sis)
Synarthrotic joint (synarthrosis, pl. synarthroses) (SIN-are-THROT-ik, SIN-are-THROS-is, SIN-are-THROS-eez)
Synchondrosis joint (SIN-kon-DROS-is)
Syndesmosis, pl. syndesmoses (SIN-des-MO-sis, SIN-des-MO-sees)
Synostosis, pl. synostoses (SIN-ost-O-sis, SIN-ost-O-sees)
Synovial cavity (sin-O-vee-al)
Synovial fluid
Synovial membrane
Synovial joint
Triaxial joint (try-AKS-see-al)
Trochoid joint (TRO-koid)
Uniaxial joint (YOU-nee-AKS-see-al)
Weight-bearing joint

WORD ORIGINS

- ❑ Amphi—From Greek *amphi,* meaning *on both sides, around*
- ❑ Bi—From Latin *bis,* meaning *two, twice*
- ❑ Cavity—From Latin *cavus,* meaning *hollow, concavity*
- ❑ Congruent—From Latin *congruere,* meaning *to come together*
- ❑ Di—From Greek *dis,* meaning *two, twice*
- ❑ Ellips—From Greek *elleipsis,* meaning *oval*
- ❑ Extra—From Latin *extra,* meaning *outside, beyond*
- ❑ Ginglymus—From Greek *ginglymos,* meaning *hinge joint*
- ❑ Intra—From Latin *intra,* meaning *within, inner*
- ❑ Meniscus—From Greek *meniskos,* meaning *crescent moon*
- ❑ Non—From Latin *non,* meaning *not, other than*
- ❑ Ovial—From Latin *ovum,* meaning *egg*
- ❑ Plane—From Latin *planus,* meaning *flat*
- ❑ Poly—From Greek *polys,* meaning *many*
- ❑ Sella—From Latin *sella,* meaning *chair, saddle*
- ❑ Stabile—From Latin *stabilis,* meaning *stationary, resistant to change* (i.e., resistant to movement)
- ❑ Sym—From Greek *syn,* meaning *together, with* (Note: *sym* is the same prefix root as *syn*; *sym* appears before words what begin with *b*, *p*, *ph*, or *m*.)
- ❑ Syn—From Greek *syn,* meaning *together, with*
- ❑ Tri—From Latin *tres,* meaning *three*
- ❑ Uni—From Latin *unus,* meaning *one*

6.1 ANATOMY OF A JOINT

- Structurally, a **joint** is defined as a place of juncture between two or more bones. At this juncture, the bones are joined to each other by soft tissue.
  - In other words, structurally, a **joint** is defined as a place where two or more bones are joined to each other by soft tissue.

BOX 6-1

A typical joint involves two bones; however, more than two bones may be involved in a joint. For example, the elbow joint incorporates three bones: the humerus, radius, and the ulna. Any joint that involves three or more bones of the skeleton is called a **compound joint**. In contrast, the term **simple joint** is sometimes used to describe a joint that has only two bones.

  - The type of soft tissue that connects the two bones of a joint to each other determines the structural classification of the joint. (For more information on the structural classification of joints, see Section 6.6.)

BOX 6-2 SPOTLIGHT ON STRUCTURAL VERSUS FUNCTIONAL JOINTS

Defining a joint as bones connected to each other by soft tissue is a structural definition. As explained in Section 6.2, the function of a joint is to allow movement; so functionally a joint is defined by its ability to allow movement. These structural and functional definitions usually coincide with each other (i.e., a structural joint is a functional joint and a functional joint is a structural joint). However, sometimes they do not perfectly match each other. The scapulocostal joint between the scapula and ribcage is an example of a joint that allows movement between the two bones but is not a structural joint because the bones are not attached to each other by soft tissue (fibrous, cartilaginous, or synovial). For this reason, the scapulocostal joint cannot be defined as a structural joint, but is considered to be a **functional joint**. Another example of the difference between the structural definition of a joint and the functional definition of a joint is the knee joint. Structurally, the distal femur, proximal tibia, proximal fibula, and patella are all connected to each other and enclosed within one joint capsule; therefore all these bones constitute one **structural joint**. However, this one structural joint would be considered to be a number of separate functional joints, because the functional movement of the femur and patella, tibia and femur, and the tibia and fibula are all somewhat independent of each other. Many physiologists/kinesiologists would even divide the tibiofemoral joint (between the tibia and femur) into the medial tibiofemoral joint and the lateral tibiofemoral joint, because the two condyles of the femur move somewhat independently of each other on the tibia!

  - The following are the three major structural classifications of a joint:
    - Fibrous
    - Cartilaginous
    - Synovial
- A joint is also known as an **articulation**.
- Figure 6-1 illustrates the components of a typical joint of the body. (Note: It should be stated that there really is no typical joint of the body. As will be seen later in the chapter, many different types of joints exist, both structurally and functionally.)

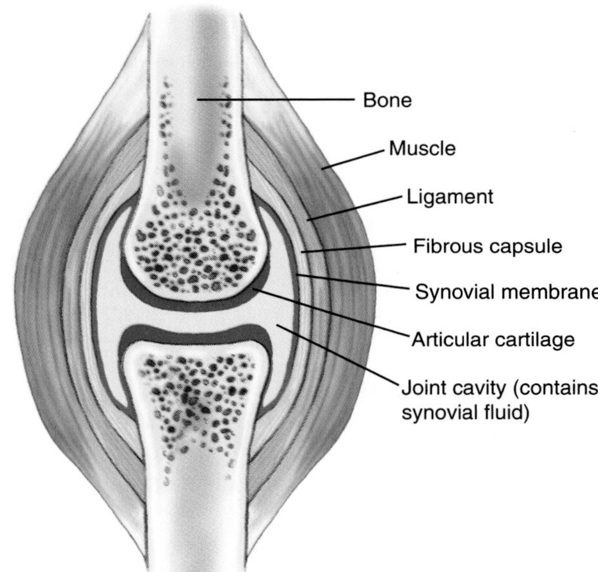

Figure 6-1 Typical joint (in this case a synovial joint is shown). The major features of this joint include a space between the two bones; this space is bounded by a capsule and is filled with fluid. Further, ligaments connect the two bones of the joint to each other, and muscles cross this joint by attaching from one bone of the joint to the other bone of the joint.

☐ 6.2 PHYSIOLOGY OF A JOINT

- The main function of a joint is to allow movement.
- As we have seen, a joint contains a space between the two bones. At this space, the bones can move relative to each other. Figure 6-2 illustrates motion at a joint.

BOX 6-3

There actually are joints in the human body that do not allow movement. However, they exist because they once did allow movement in the past. An example would be the joint between a tooth and the maxilla. When the tooth was "coming in," movement was necessary for the tooth to descend and erupt through the maxilla. However, no movement occurs between the tooth and the maxilla now. Another example that is often given is that of the suture joints of the skull. These joints once required movement to allow the passage of the baby's head through the birth canal of the mother. Once the child has been born and grows to maturity, movement is no longer needed at these suture joints and they often fuse. It must be emphasized that if no movement were needed at a certain point in the body, then there would be no need to have a joint there. Structurally, our body would be far more stable if we had a solid skeleton that was made up of one bone, with no joints located in it at all. However, we do need movement to occur, so at each location where movement is desired, a break or space exists between bones and a joint is formed. It can be useful to think of the Tin Man in the film *The Wizard of Oz*. When he was first found, it was as if he had no joints at all because the spaces of the joints were all rusted together. Then as Dorothy applied oil to each spot, the joints began to function and could once again allow movement. ☺

- When we say that the main function of a joint is to allow movement to occur, the word *allow* must be emphasized. A joint is a passive structure that allows movement to occur; it does not create the movement.
- As will be learned in later chapters, it is the musculature that crosses the joint that contracts to *create* the movement that occurs at a joint.
- In addition, it is the ligaments/joint capsules that connect the bones to each other to keep the bones from moving too far from each other (i.e., dislocating) and therefore *limit* the movement at a joint.

Therefore we can state the following three general rules:

- Joints *allow* movement.
- Muscles *create* movement.
- Ligament/joint capsules *limit* movement.

BOX 6-4

These rules, although generally true, are a bit simplistic. Muscle contractions are the primary means by which joint motion occurs. However, it is more correct is to say that the role of a muscle contraction is actually to create a force on the bones of a joint. That force can create movement at the joint; however, the force of the muscle contraction can also stop or modify movement. A clinical application of this knowledge is that a tight muscle that crosses a joint will limit the motion of the joint by not allowing the bones to move. The motion that will be limited will be the movement in the opposite direction from where this tight muscle is located. For more information on this concept, see Chapter 14.

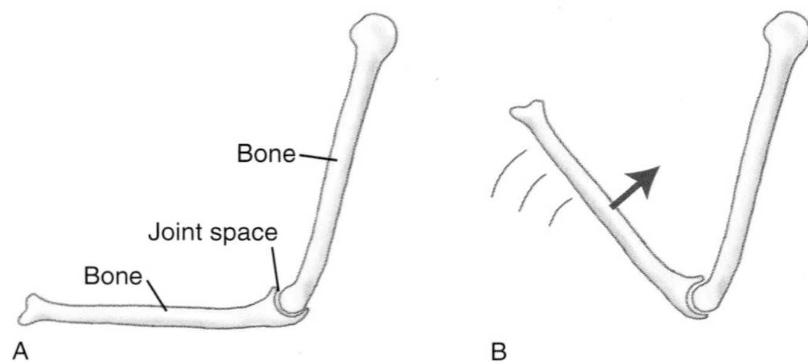

Figure 6-2 Illustration of how motion of one bone relative to the other bone of the joint occurs around the space of the joint.

☐ 6.3 JOINT MOBILITY VERSUS JOINT STABILITY

- By definition, a joint is mobile. However, a joint must also be sufficiently stable so that it maintains its structural integrity (i.e., it does not dislocate).
- Every joint of the body finds a balance between **mobility** and **stability**.
- The more mobile a joint is; the less stable it is.
  - The price to pay for greater mobility is less stability.
  - Less stability means a joint has a greater chance of injury.
- The more stable a joint is; the less mobile it is.
  - The price to pay for greater stability is less mobility.
  - Less mobility means that a joint has a decreased ability to move and locate body parts in certain positions.
- Therefore mobility and stability are antagonistic concepts; more of one means less of the other!

The following are three major factors that determine the balance of mobility and stability of a joint:

- The shape of the bones of the joint
- The ligament/joint capsule complex of the joint (Note: Ligaments and joint capsules are both made up of the same fibrous material and both act to limit motion of a joint, therefore they can be grouped together as the ligament/joint capsule complex.)
- The musculature of the joint

BOX 6-5 SPOTLIGHT ON CLOSED-PACKED AND OPEN-PACKED JOINT POSITIONS

Each joint of the body has a position in which it is most stable; this position is known as its **closed-packed position**. The stable, closed-packed position of a joint is usually the result of a combination of the position of the bones such that they are maximally **congruent** (i.e., their articular surfaces best fit each other) and the ligaments are most taut. These two factors result in a position that restricts motion and therefore increases stability. The **open-packed position** of a joint is the opposite of the closed-packed position; it is the position of the joint wherein the combination of the congruence of the bony fit is poor and the ligaments are lax, resulting in great mobility but poor stability of the joint.

These concepts are well illustrated by comparing the mobility/stability of the shoulder joint to the hip joint. The shoulder joint and hip joint are both the same type of joint—ball-and-socket joint. However, the shoulder joint is much more mobile and much less stable than the hip joint; conversely, the hip joint is much more stabile and much less mobile than the shoulder joint.

Comparing these two joints to each other, we see three things:

1. The bony shape of the socket of the shoulder joint (i.e., the glenoid fossa of the scapula) is much shallower than the socket of the hip joint (i.e., the acetabulum) (Figure 6-3).
2. The ligament/joint capsule complex of the shoulder joint is much looser than the ligament/joint capsule complex of the hip joint.
3. The musculature crossing the shoulder joint is less massive than the musculature crossing the hip joint.

BOX 6-6

Because a muscle crosses a joint (by attaching via its tendons to the bones of the joint), the more massive a muscle is, the more stability it lends to the joint. However, this greater stability also means less mobility. For this reason, people who work out and have very large muscle mass are sometimes referred to as being *muscle-bound*. If the baseline tone of the musculature that crosses a joint is high (i.e., the muscles are tight), stability increases even more and mobility decreases commensurately. (For more information regarding the concept of stabilization of a joint by a muscle, see Section 12.7.)

- The advantage of the greater mobility of the shoulder joint is the greater motion allowing the hand to be placed in a greater variety of positions. However, the disadvantage of the greater mobility of the shoulder joint is a higher frequency of injury.
- The advantage of the greater stability of the hip joint is the low frequency of injury. The disadvantage of the greater stability of the hip joint is the inability to place the foot in as great a variety of positions.

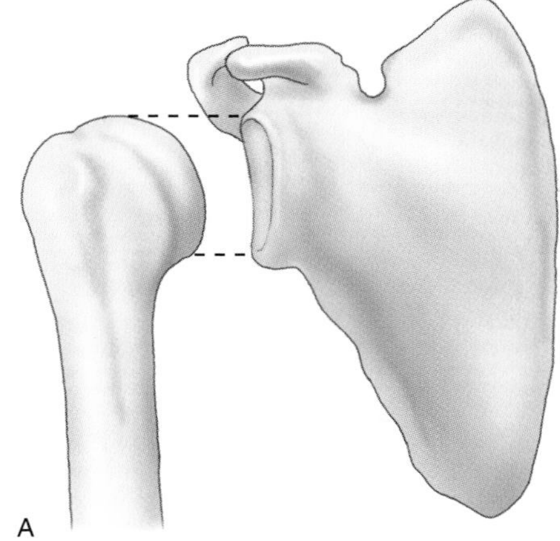

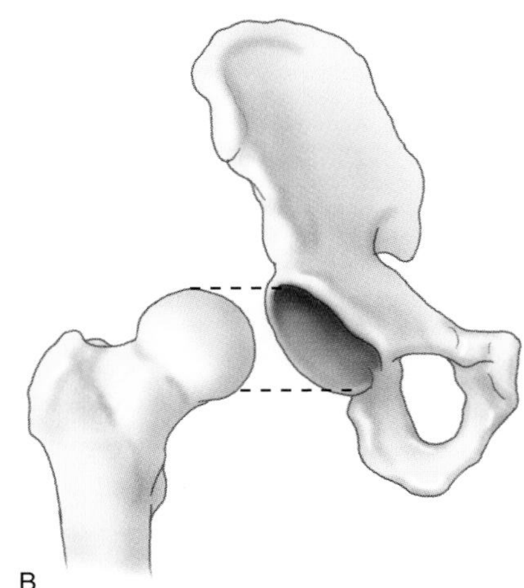

Figure 6-3 *A,* Shallow socket (glenoid fossa of the scapula) of the shoulder joint. *B,* Deep socket (acetabulum of the pelvis bone) of the hip joint. Given the bony shape of these sockets, the shoulder joint allows greater mobility, whereas the hip joint has greater stability. The downside is that the shoulder joint is less stable, and the hip joint is less mobile.

6.4 JOINTS AND SHOCK ABSORPTION

- In addition to allowing motion to occur, a joint may also serve the purpose of **shock absorption** for the body. In addition to the soft tissue located between the bones of a joint, many joints of the body also have fluid located in the capsule of the joint. This fluid can be very helpful toward absorbing shock waves that are transmitted through the joint. (See Section 6.9 for a discussion of synovial joints, which have fluid located within a joint cavity.)
- Although all joints have the ability to absorb shock, lower extremity and spinal joints are especially important for providing shock absorption given the forces that enter our body whenever we walk, run, or jump.
- For example, when we walk, run, or jump and our body weight hits the ground, the force of our body weight hitting the ground causes an equivalent force to be transmitted up through our body. The fluid located in the joints of our lower extremities and the joints of our spine can help to absorb and dampen this shock. Figure 6-4 illustrates this concept.

BOX 6-7

Our joints function to absorb and dampen shock in a similar manner to the shock absorbers of a car. A car's shock absorber is a cylinder filled with fluid. When the car hits a pothole or a bump, the fluid within the shock absorber absorbs and dampens the compression force that occurs (i.e., the shock wave that would otherwise be transmitted to the rest of the car, as well as the people sitting within the car).

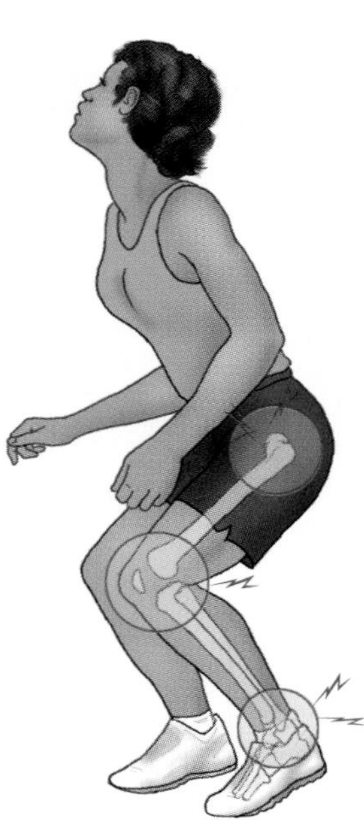

Figure 6-4 Joints of the lower extremity help to absorb shock when a person lands on the ground after having jumped up into the air. All weight-bearing joints, including the joints of the spine, would help with shock absorption in this scenario.

6.5 WEIGHT-BEARING JOINTS

- Many joints of the body are **weight-bearing joints**. A joint is a weight-bearing joint if the weight of the body is borne through that joint.

BOX 6-8

Many textbooks describe weight bearing as another function of some of the joints of our body. Although it is certainly true that many of the joints of our body have the additional function of bearing weight, bearing weight is not a reason for a joint to exist in the first place. Weight bearing places a stress on a joint that requires greater stability. By definition, a joint allows movement, which, by definition, decreases stability. If weight bearing is the goal, and stability is therefore needed, the body would be better off not even having a joint in that location. If, for example, the lower extremity did not have a knee joint, and the entire lower extremity were one bone instead of having a separate femur and tibia, the lower extremity would be much more stable and able to bear the weight of the body through it more efficiently. Having the knee joint allows for movement there and decreases the stability of the lower extremity; therefore it does not help with weight bearing. Of course, once present, the knee joint does now have the added responsibility of bearing weight. Perhaps it is better to say that it is a characteristic, not a function, of some joints that they bear weight.

- All joints of the lower extremities and the joints of the spine are weight-bearing joints. In addition to allowing movement, these joints must also be able to bear the weight of the body parts that are above them.

BOX 6-9

The disc joints of the spine have the major responsibility of weight bearing. The facet joints of the spine are meant primarily to guide movement. (See Section 7.4 for more details.)

- Because of the stress of bearing weight, weight-bearing joints tend to be more stable and less mobile.
- Because a greater proportion of body weight is above joints that are lower in the body, the amount of weight-bearing stress that a joint must bear is greater for the joints that are lower in the body. For example, the upper cervical vertebrae need only bear the weight of the head above them; however, the lower lumbar vertebrae must bear the entire weight of the head, neck, trunk and upper extremities above them. The joints of the ankle and foot have the greatest combined weight of body parts above them and therefore bear the greatest weight.

BOX 6-10

Potentially, the weight-bearing stress on the ankle and foot joints is the greatest. However, because two lower extremities exist, the weight-bearing load on them is divided by two when a person is standing on both feet. Of course, when a person is standing on only one foot, the entire weight of the body is borne through the joints of that side's lower extremity.

- Upper extremity joints (and some other miscellaneous joints) are not usually weight-bearing joints.

Figure 6-5 illustrates the weight-bearing joints of the human body.

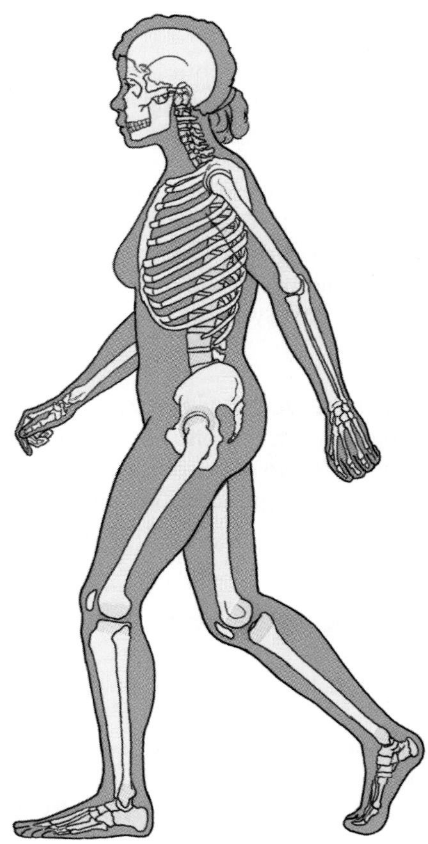

Figure 6-5 Weight-bearing joints of the body. All joints of the lower extremities and the spinal joints of the axial body are weight-bearing joints.

6.6 JOINT CLASSIFICATION

- Joints may be classified based on their structure (i.e., the type of soft tissue that connects the bones to each other).
  - Structurally, joints are usually divided into three categories.
- Joints may also be classified based on their function (i.e., the degree of movement that they allow).
  - Functionally, joints are usually divided into three categories.

Structural Classification of Joints:

- Structurally, joints can be divided into the following three categories: (1) fibrous, (2) cartilaginous, and (3) synovial joints (Table 6-1).
  - A joint in which the bones are held together by a dense fibrous connective tissue is known as a **fibrous joint**.
  - A joint in which the bones are held together by either fibrocartilage or hyaline cartilage is known as a **cartilaginous joint**.
  - A joint in which the bones are connected by a joint capsule, which is composed of two distinct layers (an outer fibrous layer and an inner synovial layer), is known as a **synovial joint**.
- It is worth noting that fibrous and cartilaginous joints have no joint cavity; synovial joints do enclose a joint cavity.

Joints without a Joint Cavity:

- Fibrous: Fibrous joints are joints in which dense fibrous tissue attaches the two bones of the joint to each other.
- Cartilaginous: Cartilaginous joints are joints in which cartilaginous tissue attaches the two bones of the joint to each other.

Joints with a Joint Cavity:

- Synovial: Synovial joints are joints in which a joint capsule attaches the two bones of the joint to each other.
  - This joint capsule has two layers: (1) an outer fibrous layer and (2) an inner synovial membrane layer.
  - This capsule encloses a synovial cavity, which has synovial fluid within it.
  - The articular ends of the bones are lined with hyaline cartilage.

TABLE 6-1

Classification of Joints by Structure

- **Joints without a Joint Cavity**
  - Fibrous
  - Cartilaginous
- **Joints with a Joint Cavity**
  - Synovial

Functional Classification of Joints:

- Functionally, joints can also be divided into three categories: (1) synarthrotic, (2) amphiarthrotic, and (3) diarthrotic (Table 6-2).

BOX 6-11

As in all categories of classification, alternates exist. Another common classification of joints divides them into only two functional categories: (1) synarthroses, lacking a joint cavity, and (2) diarthroses, possessing a joint cavity. Synarthroses are then divided into synostoses (united by bony tissue), synchondroses (united by cartilaginous tissue), and syndesmoses (united by fibrous tissue). Diarthroses are synovial joints (united by a capsule enclosing a joint cavity).

- A joint that allows very little or no movement is known as a **synarthrotic joint** (**synarthrosis**; plural: synarthroses).
- A joint that allows a moderate but limited amount of movement is known as an **amphiarthrotic joint** (**amphiarthrosis**; plural: amphiarthroses).
- A joint that is freely moveable and allows a great deal of movement is known as a **diarthrotic joint** (**diarthrosis**; plural: diarthroses).
- It is worth noting that although general agreement exists among sources as to the classification of joints into three categories based on movement, the exact delineation between these relative amounts of movement may differ at times.
- It is a major principle of anatomy and physiology that structure and function are intimately related to each other.
- It is often said that structure determines function.
- That is, the anatomy of a body part determines what the physiology of the body part will be.

TABLE 6-2

Classification of Joints by Function

❏ Synarthrotic	Synarthrotic joints are joints which allow very little or no movement.
❏ Amphiarthrotic	Amphiarthrotic joints are joints that allow a moderate but limited amount of movement.
❏ Diarthrotic	Diarthrotic joints are joints that are freely moveable and allow a great deal of movement.

- ❏ Relating this to the study of joints, the structure of a joint determines the motion possible at that joint.
- ❏ Therefore although joints may be divided into three categories by structure, and joints may also be divided into three categories by function (i.e., movement), it is important to realize that these three structural and these three functional categories are related to each other.
- ❏ They are only different categories based on whether the perspective is that of an anatomist, who looks at structure, or that of a physiologist or kinesiologist, who looks at function.
- ❏ Therefore the following general correlations can be made:
  - ❏ Fibrous joints are synarthrotic joints.
  - ❏ Cartilaginous joints are amphiarthrotic joints.
  - ❏ Synovial joints are diarthrotic joints.

6.7 FIBROUS JOINTS

- Fibrous joints are joints in which the soft tissue that unites the bones is a dense fibrous connective tissue; hence a fibrous joint has no joint cavity (Table 6-3; Figure 6-6a).
- Fibrous joints typically permit very little or no movement; therefore they are considered to be synarthrotic joints.
- Three types of fibrous joints exist:
  - Syndesmosis joints
  - Suture joints
  - Gomphosis joints

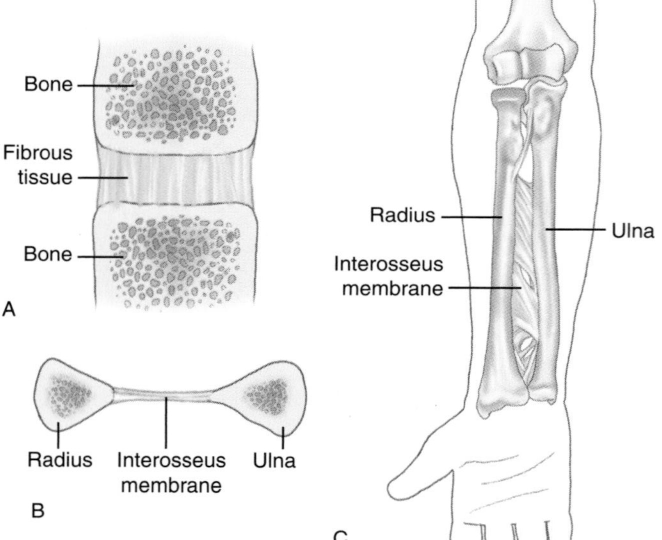

Figure 6-6 *A,* Fibrous tissue that unites the two bones of a fibrous joint. *B,* Cross-sectional view of the interosseus membrane of the forearm. Functionally, the interosseus membrane that unites the radius and ulna is a synarthrotic joint; structurally, it is a fibrous syndesmosis joint. *C,* Anterior view that illustrates the interosseus membrane of the forearm that joins the radius and ulna.

Syndesmosis Joints:

- In a **syndesmosis joint**, a fibrous ligament or fibrous aponeurotic membrane unites the bones of the joint.
- Syndesmoses permit a small amount of movement between the two bones of the joint.
- The interosseus membrane between the radius and ulna is an example of a syndesmosis joint (Figure 6-6b–c).
- The interosseus membrane between the tibia and fibula is another example of a syndesmosis joint.

Suture Joints:

- In a **suture joint**, a thin layer of fibrous tissue unites the two bones of the joint.
- Suture joints are found only in the skull (Figure 6-7).
- A small amount of movement is permitted at these joints early in life.
- The principal purpose of the suture joints is to allow the bones of the skull of a baby to move relative to each other to allow easier passage through the birth canal during delivery of the baby.
- Suture joints are usually considered to allow little or no movement later in life; but controversy exists regarding this.

BOX 6-12

A great deal of controversy exists regarding the ability of suture joints to move. A major premise of craniosacral technique is that suture joints allow an appreciable amount of movement. Part of their technique is to manipulate the bones of the skull at the suture joints for the purpose of aiding the movement of cerebrospinal fluid. Although some degree of motion does remain at the suture joints, study of the skulls of adults shows that these joints do tend to become synostotic as we get older (a **synostosis** is a joint that has fused over with bone).

Gomphosis Joints:

- In a **gomphosis joint**, fibrous tissue unites two bony components with surfaces that are adapted to each other like a peg in a hole (Figure 6-8).
- This type of joint is found only between the teeth and the mandible, or the teeth and the maxilla.
- Gomphoses permit movement of the teeth relative to the mandible or the maxilla early in life; but in an adult, no movement is permitted in a gomphosis joint.

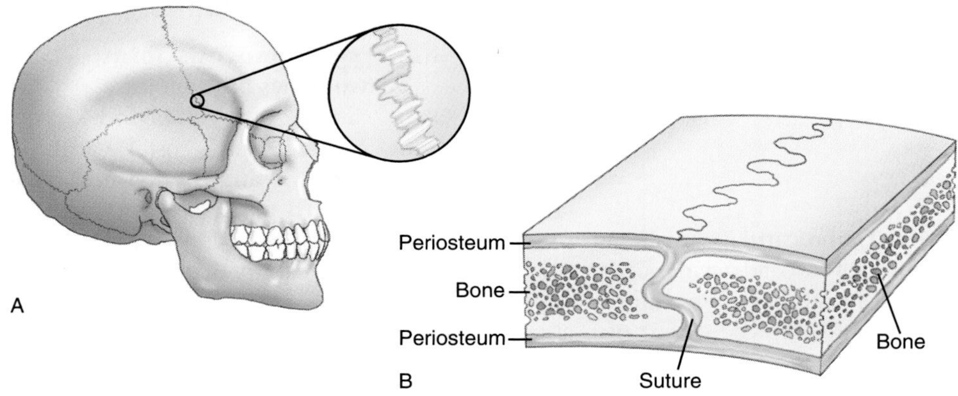

Figure 6-7 *A,* Lateral view that illustrates the coronal suture of the skull that is located between the frontal and parietal bones of the skull. Functionally, this joint is synarthrotic; structurally, this joint is a fibrous suture. *B,* Cross-sectional view of the same suture joint.

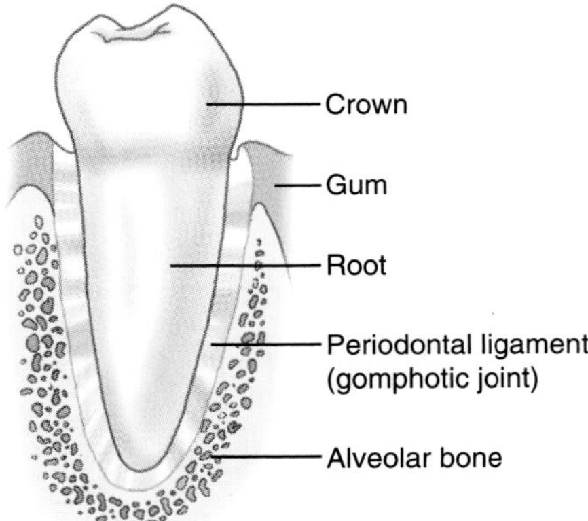

Figure 6-8 View of the joint between a tooth and the adjacent bone. The crown of the tooth is located above the gum line, and the root of the tooth is located below the gum line. The periodontal ligament is the fibrous tissue of the gomphotic joint. Functionally, this joint is synarthrotic; structurally, this joint is a fibrous gomphosis joint.

TABLE 6-3

Types of Synarthrotic Fibrous Joints

Type	Description
❑ Syndesmoses	Bones united by a fibrous ligament or an aponeurosis
❑ Sutures	Bones united by a thin layer of fibrous material
❑ Gomphoses	Peg-in-hole–shaped bones united by fibrous material

6.8 CARTILAGINOUS JOINTS

- Cartilaginous joints are joints in which the soft tissue that unites the bones is cartilaginous connective tissue (either fibrocartilage or hyaline cartilage); hence a cartilaginous joint has no joint cavity.
- Cartilaginous joints typically permit a moderate but limited amount of movement; therefore they are considered to be amphiarthrotic joints.
- Two types of cartilaginous joints exist:
  - Symphysis joints
  - Synchondrosis joints

Symphysis Joints:

- In a **symphysis joint**, fibrocartilage in the form of a disc unites the bodies of two adjacent bones. These fibrocartilaginous discs can be quite thick. Consequently, although not allowing the extent of motion that a diarthrotic synovial joint allows, cartilaginous joints can allow a moderate amount of motion.

BOX 6-13

The term *body* of a bone is usually used to refer to the largest aspect of a bone.

- An example of a cartilaginous symphysis joint is the intervertebral disc joint of the spine (Figure 6-9a).
- Another example is the symphysis pubis joint of the pelvis (Figure 6-9b).

Synchondrosis Joints:

- In a **synchondrosis joint**, hyaline cartilage unites the two bones of the joint.
- An example of a cartilaginous synchondrosis joint is the cartilage (i.e., costal cartilage) that is located between a rib and the sternum (Figure 6-10a).
- The growth plate (i.e., epiphysial disc) of a growing bone may also be considered to be another type of synchondrosis joint that is temporary (Figure 6-10b).

BOX 6-14

Eventually a growth plate (i.e., epiphysial disc) ossifies and only a remnant, the epiphysial line, remains. Many sources do not consider the epiphysial disc of a growing bone to be another type of synchondrosis joint, because the main purpose of the growth plate is growth, not movement. (For more information on growth plates, see Section 3.6.)

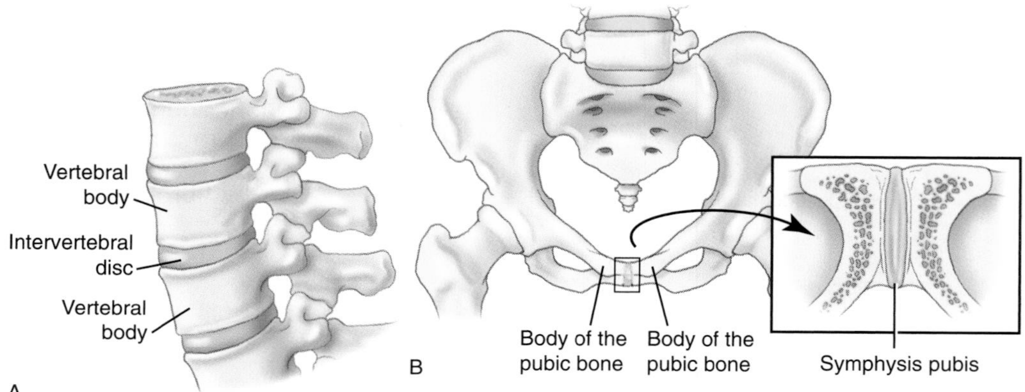

Figure 6-9 *A,* Lateral view that illustrates an intervertebral disc joint located between adjacent vertebral bodies of the spine. Functionally, this joint is amphiarthrotic; structurally, this joint is a cartilaginous symphysis joint. *B,* Anterior view of the pelvis (with a close-up view in the inset box) that illustrates the symphysis pubis joint between the right and left bodies of the pubic bones of the pelvis. Functionally, this joint is amphiarthrotic; structurally, this joint is a cartilaginous symphysis joint.

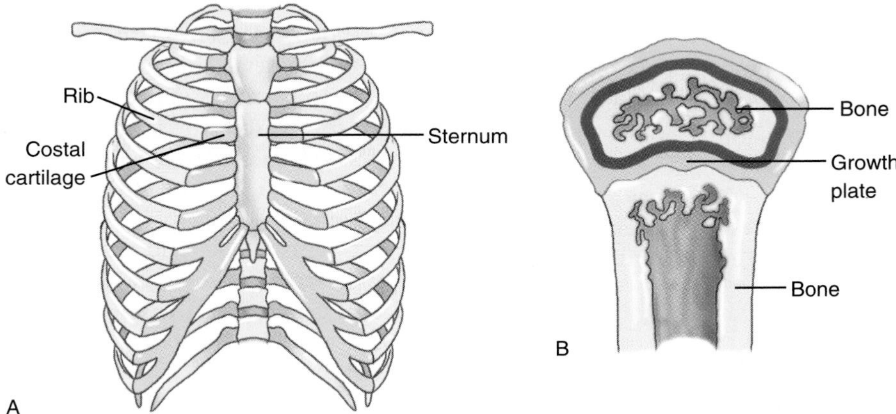

Figure 6-10 *A,* Anterior view of the ribcage. A costal cartilage is an example of a cartilaginous synchondrosis joint that unites a rib with the sternum. Functionally, this joint is amphiarthrotic; structurally, it is a cartilaginous synchondrosis joint. *B,* Growth plate (epiphysial disc) between the adjacent regions of bony tissue of a developing long bone. This is an example of a temporary, cartilaginous synchondrosis joint (eventually, this cartilaginous joint will fuse with bone, leaving only a remnant, the epiphysial line).

6.9 SYNOVIAL JOINTS

- Structurally, synovial joints are the most complicated joints of the body.
- They are also the joints that most people think of when they think of joints. The wrist, elbow, shoulder, ankle, knee, and hip joints are a few examples of synovial joints.

Components of a Synovial Joint:

- The bones of a synovial joint are connected by a **joint capsule**, which encloses a **joint cavity**.
- This joint capsule is composed of two distinct layers: (1) an outer fibrous layer and (2) an inner **synovial membrane** layer (Table 6-4).
- The inner synovial membrane layer secretes **synovial fluid** into the joint cavity, also known as the **synovial cavity**.
- Further, the articular ends of the bones are capped with **articular cartilage** (i.e., hyaline cartilage).
- Synovial joints are the only joints of the body that possess a joint cavity.
- By virtue of the presence of a joint cavity, synovial joints typically allow a great deal of movement; hence they are considered to be diarthrotic joints.

Figure 6-11 illustrates some examples of synovial joints.

TABLE 6-4*

Components of a Synovial Joint

- Outer fibrous layer of the joint capsule
- Inner synovial membrane layer of the joint capsule
- Synovial cavity
- Synovial fluid
- Articular hyaline cartilage lining the articular ends of the bones
- Ligaments
- Muscles

*Note: Table 6-4 lists the structures of a synovial joint. Ligaments and muscles are placed within this table even though they are usually not technically part of the structure of a synovial joint. Their reason for inclusion here is due to their role in the functioning of a synovial joint. Although ligaments and muscles do play a role in the functioning of other joints, given the tremendous motion possible at synovial joints, the role of ligaments and muscles in the functioning of synovial joints is extremely important and vital to the concepts of stability and mobility.

Roles of Ligaments and Muscles to a Synovial Joint:

Ligaments:

- By definition, a ligament is a fibrous structure (made primarily of collagen fibers) that attaches from any one structure of the body to any other structure of the body (except a muscle to a bone).
- In the musculoskeletal field, a ligament is defined more narrowly as attaching from one bone to another bone.
- Therefore ligaments cross a joint, attaching the bones of a joint together.
- Evolutionarily, ligaments of a synovial joint formed as thickenings of the outer fibrous layer of the joint capsule.
  - Some ligaments gradually evolved to be completely independent from the fibrous capsule; other ligaments never fully separated and are simply named as thickenings of the fibrous capsule.
- For this reason, the term *ligamentous/joint capsule complex* is often used to describe the ligaments and the joint capsule of a joint together.
- Synovial joint ligaments are usually located outside of the joint capsule and are therefore **extra-articular**; however, occasionally a ligament is located within the joint cavity and is **intra-articular**.
- Functionally, the purpose of a ligament is to limit motion at a joint.

Muscles:

- By definition, a muscle is a soft tissue structure that is specialized to contract.
- A muscle attaches to the two bones of a joint via its tendons. Therefore a muscle connects the two bones of the joint that it crosses to each other.

BOX 6-15

Some muscles cross more than one joint and do not attach to every bone of each joint that they cross. For example, the biceps brachii crosses the elbow joint that is located between the humerus and radius. Yet even though it does attach distally onto the radius, the biceps brachii does not attach onto the humerus. Instead it continues proximally to cross over the shoulder joint and attaches to the scapula proximally.

- Muscles are nearly always extra-articular.

BOX 6-16

A couple of examples can be found of a tendon of a muscle being located intra-articularly (i.e., within a joint cavity). The long head of the biceps brachii runs through the shoulder (i.e., glenohumeral) joint; the proximal tendon of the popliteus is located within the knee joint.

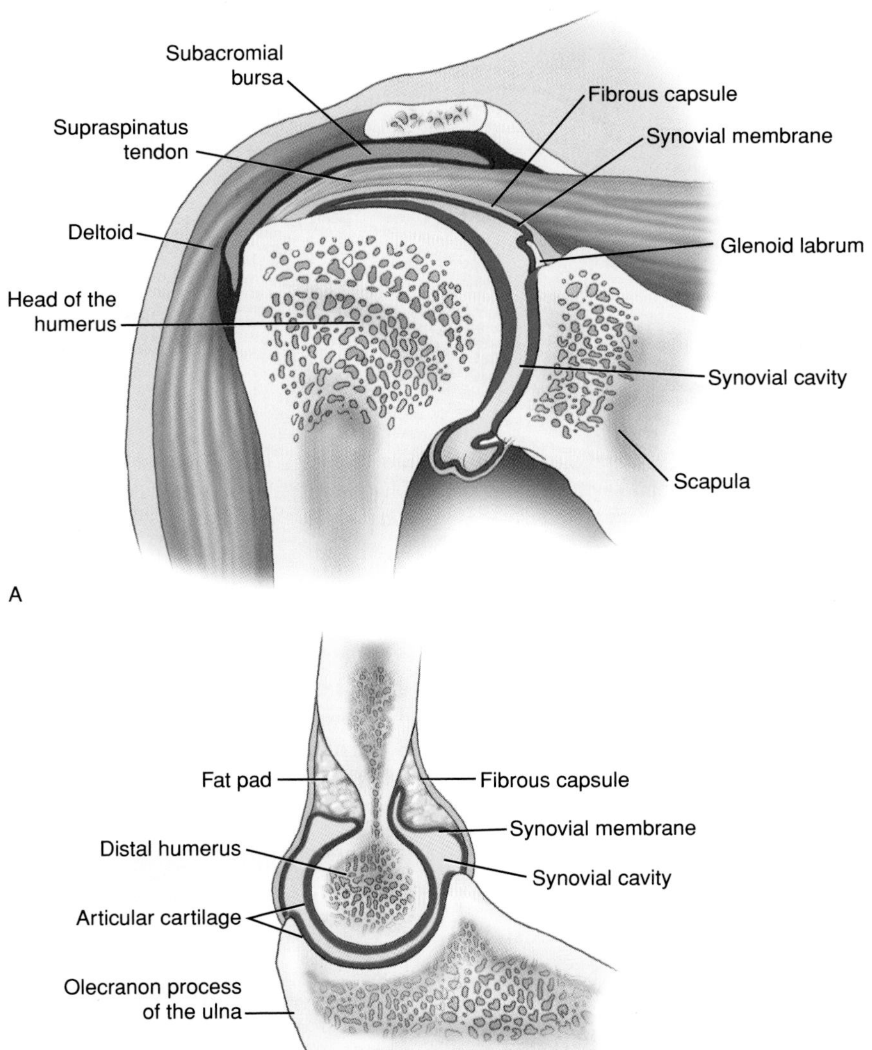

Figure 6-11 Examples of synovial joints. *A,* Anterior view cross-section of the shoulder joint. *B,* Lateral view cross-section of the elbow (humeroulnar) joint.

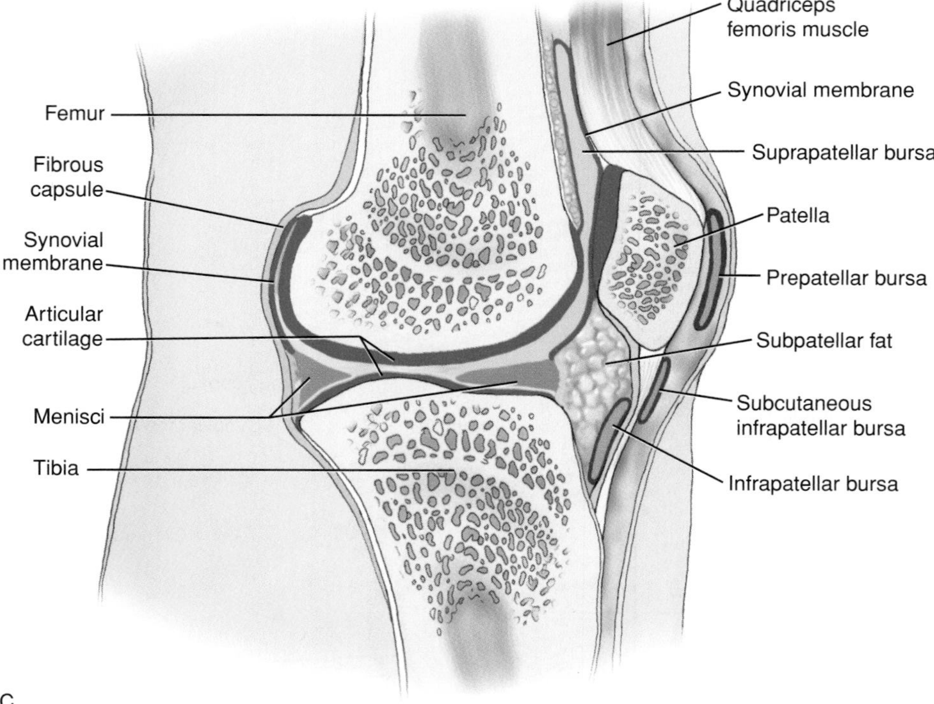

Figure 6-11, cont'd *C,* Lateral view cross-section of the knee joint. Synovial joints possess a capsule that encloses a joint cavity. The capsule has two layers: an outer fibrous layer (shown in beige) and an inner synovial membrane layer (shown in dark blue). The fluid within the joint cavity is shown in light blue.

- The major function of a muscle is to contract and generate a force on one or both bones of a joint. This contraction force can move one or both of the bones and create motion at the joint. (The role that muscles play in the musculoskeletal system is covered in much greater depth in Chapters 11 to 13.)

Classification of Synovial Joints:

- Synovial joints can be divided into four categories based on the number axes of movement that exist at the joint (Table 6-3):

BOX 6-17 SPOTLIGHT ON DEGREES OF FREEDOM

The term **degrees of freedom** is often applied to joints that permit axial motions. When a joint allows motion within one plane around one axis, it is said to possess one degree of freedom. When it allows motion in two planes around two axes, it possesses two degrees of freedom. When it allows motion in three planes around three axes, it possesses three degrees of freedom. If its only type of movement is nonaxial, then it possesses zero degrees of freedom.

1. **Uniaxial joint**: A uniaxial joint allows motion to occur around one axis, within one plane.
2. **Biaxial joint**: A biaxial joint allows motion to occur around two axes, within two planes.
3. **Triaxial joint**: A triaxial joint allows motion to occur around three axes, within three planes.

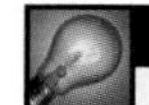

BOX 6-18

A triaxial joint is also known as a **polyaxial** joint.

4. **Nonaxial joint**: A nonaxial joint allows motion to occur within a plane, but this motion is a gliding type of motion and does not occur around an axis.

☐ 6.10 UNIAXIAL SYNOVIAL JOINTS

- ❑ A uniaxial joint allows motion to occur around one axis; this motion occurs within one plane.
- ❑ Two types of uniaxial synovial joints exist:
  - ❑ Hinge joints
  - ❑ Pivot joints

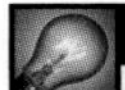

BOX 6-19

A hinge joint is also known as a **ginglymus joint**.
A pivot joint is also known as a **trochoid joint**.

Hinge Joints:

- ❑ A **hinge joint** is a joint in which the surface of one bone is spool-like and the surface of the other bone is concave. The spool-like surface moves within the concave surface of the other bone.
- ❑ A hinge joint is similar in structure and function to the hinge of a door; hence the name, *hinge* joint.
- ❑ An example of a hinge joint is the elbow joint (Figure 6-12a).
- ❑ Another example of a hinge joint is the ankle joint (Figure 6-12b).

Pivot Joints:

- ❑ A **pivot joint** is a joint in which one surface is shaped like a ring, and the other surface is shaped so that it can rotate within the ring.
- ❑ A pivot joint is similar in structure and function to a doorknob.

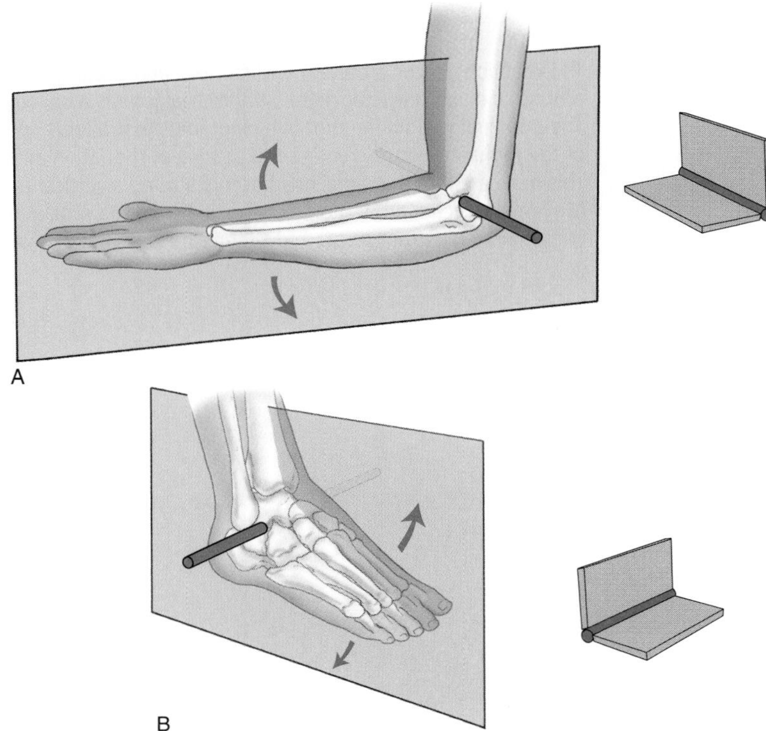

Figure 6-12 *A,* Elbow joint (the humeroulnar joint of the elbow). The elbow joint is a hinge joint that allows only the actions of flexion and extension to occur. These actions occur around a mediolateral axis and occur within the sagittal plane. Movement occurs around only one axis; hence the elbow joint is a uniaxial hinge joint. *B,* Ankle joint. The ankle joint is a hinge joint that allows only the actions of plantarflexion and dorsiflexion to occur. These actions occur around a mediolateral axis and occur within the sagittal plane. Movement occurs around only one axis; hence the ankle joint is a uniaxial hinge joint. A hinge is drawn next to each of these joints demonstrating the similarity in structure of these joints to a hinge. (Note: In all illustrations the red tube represents the axis of movement.)

- An example of a pivot joint is the atlantoaxial joint between the ring-shaped atlas (C1) and the odontoid process (i.e., dens) of the axis (C2) in the cervical spine (Figure 6-13a).

- Another example of a pivot joint is the proximal radioulnar joint of the forearm in which the radial head rotates within the ring-shaped structure created by the radial notch of the ulna and the annular ligament (Figure 6-13b).

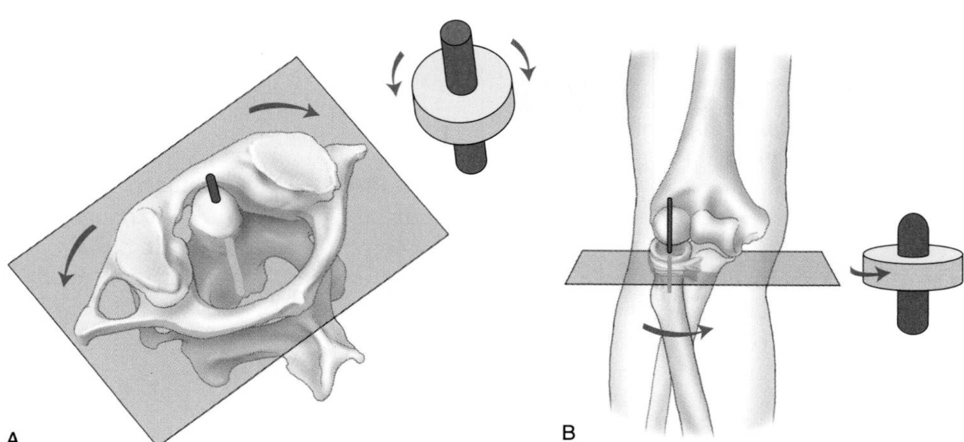

Figure 6-13 *A,* Atlantoaxial joint (formed by the ring-shaped atlas and the odontoid process of the axis). The atlantoaxial joint is a pivot joint that allows only right rotation and left rotation to occur. These actions occur around a vertical axis and occur within the transverse plane. Movement occurs around one axis only; hence the atlantoaxial joint is a uniaxial pivot joint. *B,* Proximal radioulnar joint. The proximal radioulnar joint is a pivot joint that allows only medial and lateral rotation of the head of the radius to occur (creating the actions of pronation and supination of the radius of the forearm). This movement of the radial head occurs around a vertical axis and occurs within the transverse plane. Movement occurs around only one axis; hence the proximal radioulnar joint is a uniaxial pivot joint. (Note: In all illustrations the red tube represents the axis of movement.)

6.11 BIAXIAL SYNOVIAL JOINTS

- A biaxial joint allows motion to occur about two axes; this motion occurs within two planes.
- Two types of biaxial synovial joints exist:
  - Condyloid joints
  - Saddle joints

BOX 6-20

A condyloid joint is also known as an **ovoid joint** or an **ellipsoid joint**.

A saddle joint is also known as a **sellar joint**.

Condyloid Joints:

- In a **condyloid joint**, one bone is concave in shape and the other bone is convex (i.e., oval) in shape. The convex-shaped bone fits into the concave-shaped bone.
- An example of a condyloid joint is the metacarpophalangeal (MCP) joint of the hand (Figure 6-14a–b).
- Another example of a condyloid joint is the radiocarpal joint of the wrist (Figure 6-14c–d).

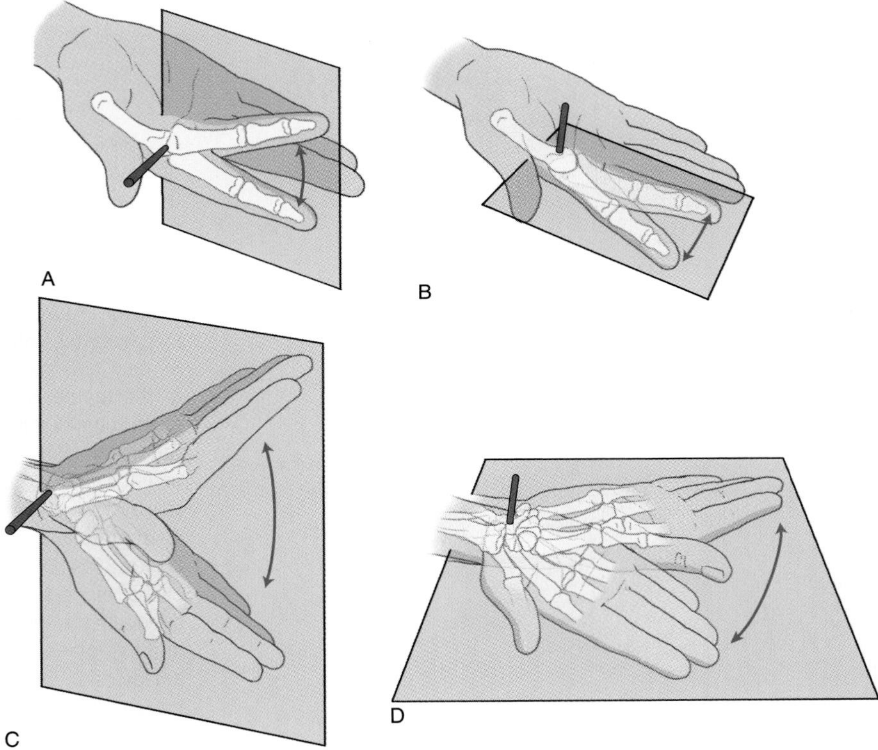

Figure 6-14 Metacarpophalangeal (MCP) joint of the hand. *A,* MCP joint is a condyloid joint that allows the actions of flexion and extension to occur around a mediolateral axis within the sagittal plane. *B,* Actions of abduction and adduction occur around an anteroposterior axis within the frontal plane. Movement occurs around two axes; hence the MCP joint is a biaxial condyloid joint. *C,* Radiocarpal joint of the wrist is a condyloid joint that allows the actions of flexion and extension to occur around a mediolateral axis within the sagittal plane. *D,* Actions of abduction and adduction at the radiocarpal joint of the wrist occur around an anteroposterior axis within the frontal plane. Movement occurs around two axes; hence the radiocarpal joint is a biaxial condyloid joint. (Note: In all illustrations the red tube represents the axis of movement.)

Saddle Joints:

- A **saddle joint** is a modified condyloid joint.
- Instead of having one convex-shaped bone that fits into a concave-shaped bone, both bones of a saddle joint are shaped such that each bone has a convexity and a concavity to its surface; the convexity of one bone fits into the concavity of the other bone and vice versa.
- Saddle joints are similar in structure and function to a person sitting in a Western saddle on a horse.
- The classic example of a saddle joint is the carpometacarpal (CMC) joint of the thumb (Figure 6-15a–b).
- Another example of a saddle joint is the sternoclavicular joint between the manubrium of the sternum and the medial end of the clavicle (Figure 6-15c–d).

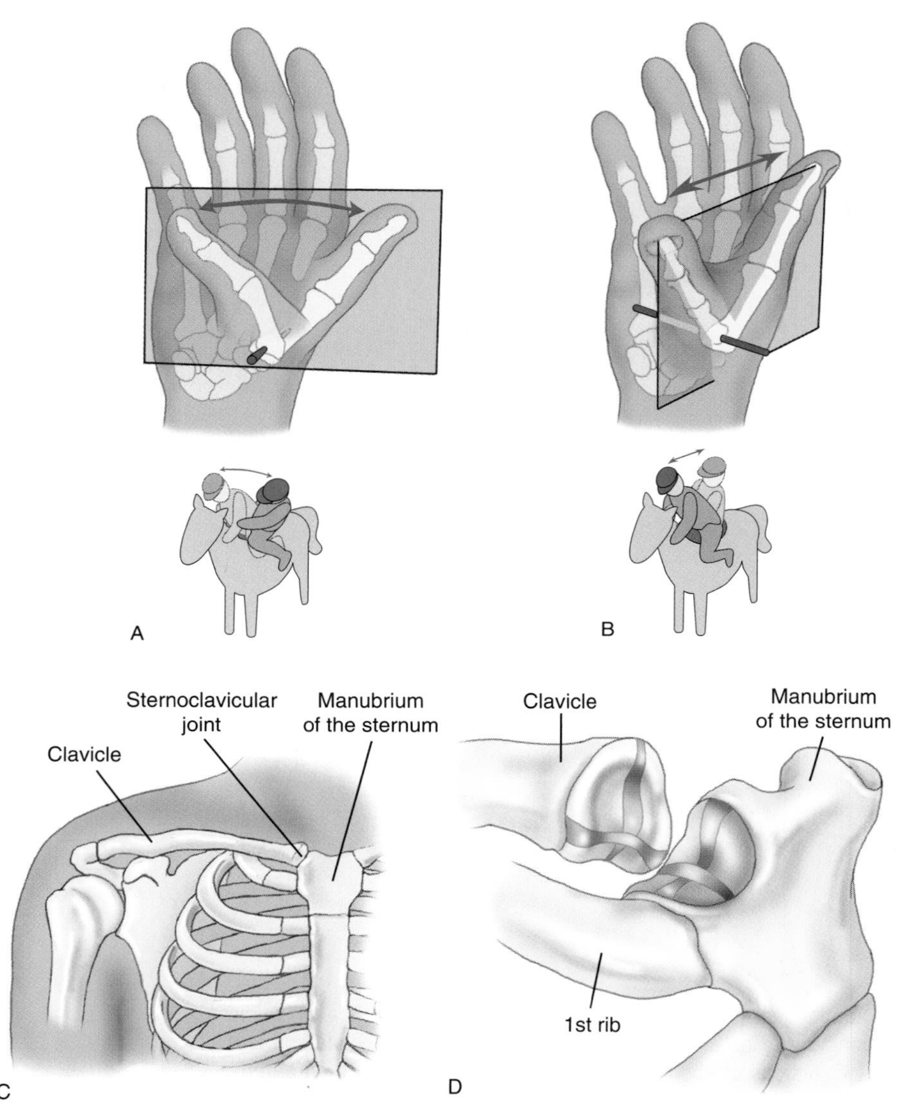

Figure 6-15 Carpometacarpal (CMC) joint of the thumb. *A,* CMC joint is a saddle joint that allows the motions of flexion and extension to occur around an anteroposterior axis within the frontal plane. *B,* CMC joint also allows abduction and adduction to occur around a mediolateral axis within the sagittal plane. Movement occurs around two axes; hence the CMC joint of the thumb is a biaxial saddle joint. An illustration of a person sitting in a Western saddle on a horse has been placed next to each figure, demonstrating the similar structure and movement of the saddle joint of the thumb to a Western saddle. In both illustrations the red tube represents the axis of movement. *C,* Sternoclavicular joint between the manubrium of the sternum and the medial end of the clavicle. *D,* Sternoclavicular joint opened up to visualize the *saddlelike* concave-convex articulating surfaces of both the manubrium and the clavicle. (*A, B, D* modeled from Neumann DA: *Kinesiology of the musculoskeletal system: foundations for physical rehabilitation.* St Louis, 2002, Mosby.)

BOX 6-21

Because of the orientation of the thumb, the terminology for naming actions of the thumb is unusual; flexion and extension occur in the frontal plane, and abduction and adduction occur in the sagittal plane. (For more information on movements of the thumb, see Sections 5.23 and 9.13.)

The saddle joint of the thumb is an interesting joint to classify. It permits a greater degree of movement than a condyloid joint, because it also allows a limited amount of rotation. With this rotation, the saddle joint of the thumb actually moves around three axes in three planes. For this reason, even though it is usually classified as a biaxial joint, it could just as correctly be classified as a triaxial joint. The only difference between the saddle joint of the thumb and a triaxial ball-and-socket joint is that the rotation actions of the saddle joint of the thumb cannot be isolated, as they can be at a ball-and-socket joint. Instead, rotations of the thumb must accompany other actions of the thumb. (For more details, see Section 9.13.)

6.12 TRIAXIAL SYNOVIAL JOINTS

- A triaxial joint allows motion to occur around three axes; this motion occurs within three planes.
- Only one type of triaxial synovial joint exists—the ball-and-socket joint.

Ball-and-Socket Joints:

- In a **ball-and-socket joint**, one bone has a ball-like convex surface that fits into the concave-shaped socket of the other bone.
- An example of a ball-and-socket joint is the hip joint (Figure 6-16).
- Another example of a ball-and-socket joint is the shoulder joint (Figure 6-17).

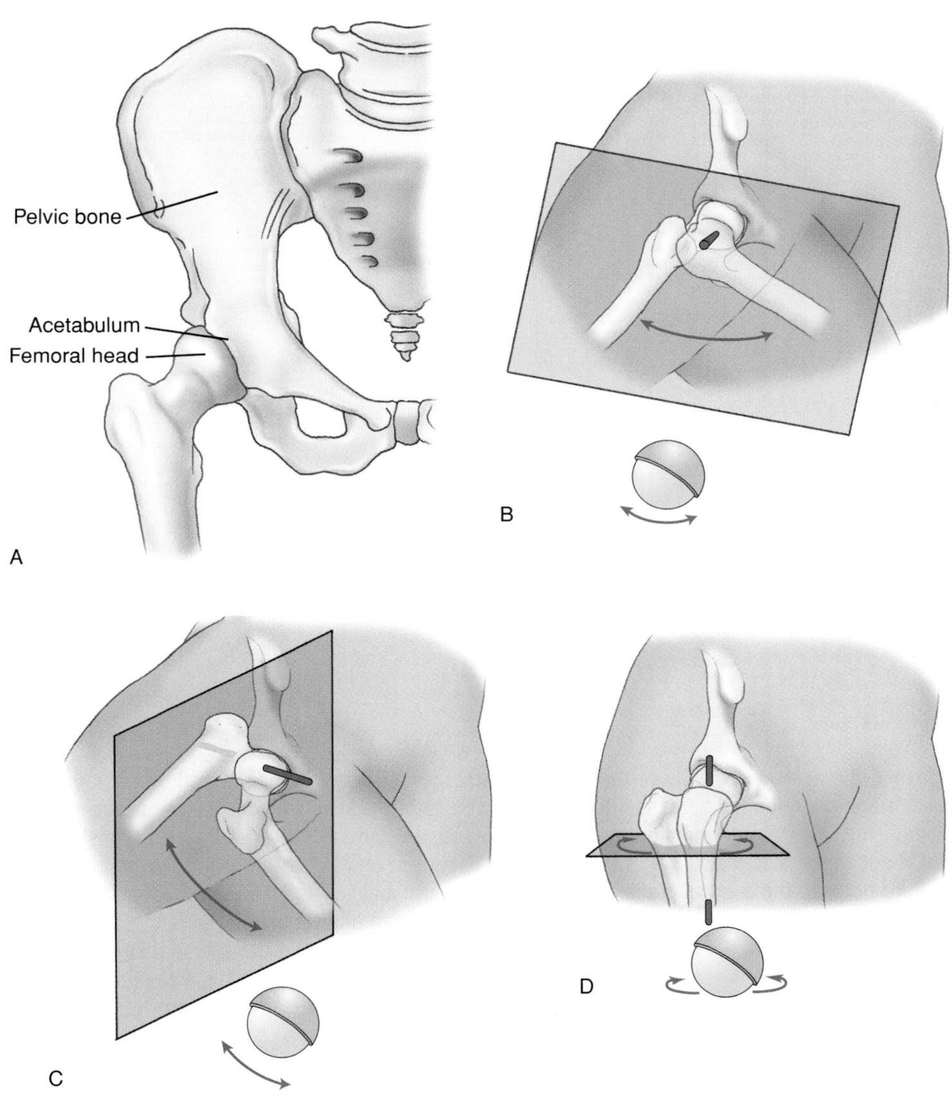

Figure 6-16 *A,* Anterior view of the ball-and-socket joint of the hip. The head of the femur, which is a convex-shaped ball, fits into the acetabulum of the pelvis, which is a concave-shaped socket. *B,* Flexion and extension of the thigh at the hip joint occur in the sagittal plane around a mediolateral axis. *C,* Abduction and adduction of the thigh at the hip joint occur in the frontal plane around an anteroposterior axis. *D,* Lateral rotation and medial rotation of the thigh at the hip joint occur in the transverse plane around a vertical axis. Movement occurs around three axes; hence the hip joint is a triaxial ball-and-socket joint. (Note: In all illustrations the red tube represents the axis of movement.)

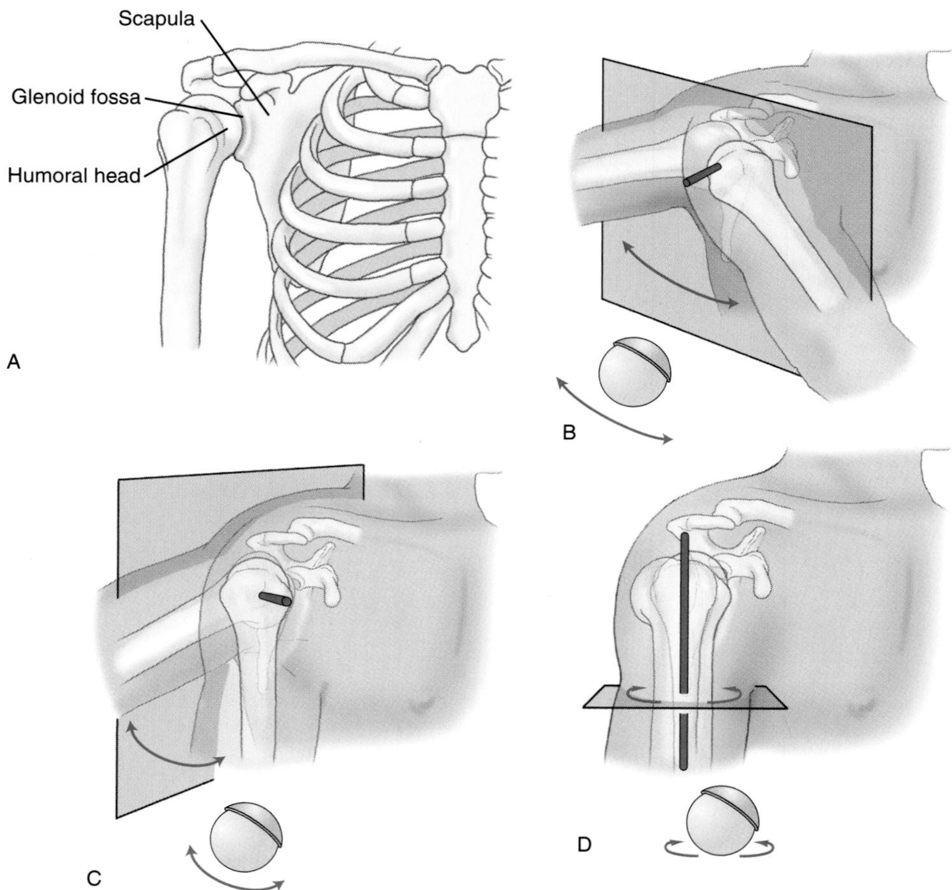

Figure 6-17 *A,* Anterior view of the ball-and-socket joint of the shoulder. Head of the humerus, which is a convex-shaped ball, fits into the glenoid fossa of the scapula, which is a concave-shaped socket. (Note: Comparing this figure with Figure 6-16a, we can see that the socket of the shoulder joint is not as deep as the socket of the hip joint.) *B,* Flexion and extension of the arm at the shoulder joint occur in the sagittal plane around a mediolateral axis. *C,* Abduction and adduction of the arm at the shoulder joint occur in the frontal plane around an anteroposterior axis. *D,* Lateral rotation and medial rotation of the arm at the shoulder joint occur in the transverse plane around a vertical axis. Movement occurs around three axes; hence the shoulder joint is a triaxial ball-and-socket joint. (Note: In all illustrations the red tube represents the axis of movement.)

☐ 6.13 NONAXIAL SYNOVIAL JOINTS

- ❑ A nonaxial joint allows motion to occur within a plane, but this motion does not occur around an axis.
- ❑ The motion that occurs at a nonaxial joint is a gliding movement in which the surface of one bone merely translates (i.e., glides) along the surface of the other bone. (See Sections 5.2 to 5.4 for more information on nonaxial translation motion.)
- ❑ It is important to emphasize that motion at a nonaxial joint may occur within a plane, but it does not occur around an axis; hence the name, *nonaxial* joint.
- ❑ The surfaces of the bones of a nonaxial joint are usually flat or slightly curved.
- ❑ Examples of nonaxial joints are the joints found between adjacent carpal bones (i.e., intercarpal joints) (Figure 6-18).
- ❑ Another example of a nonaxial joint is a facet joint of the spine (Figure 6-19).
- ❑ A nonaxial joint is also known as a **gliding joint**, an **irregular joint**, or a **plane joint**.

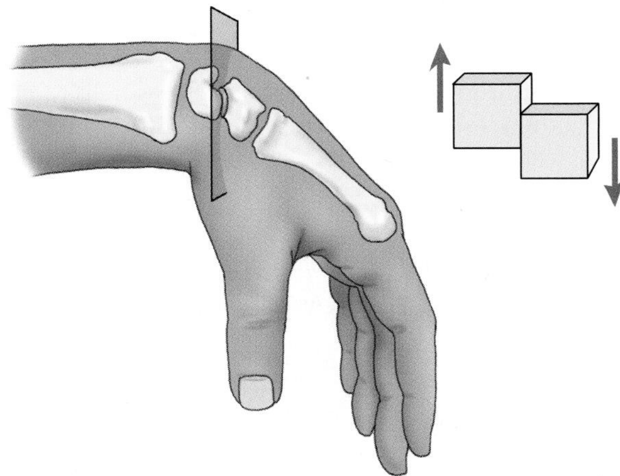

Figure 6-18 Joint between two adjacent carpal bones (an intercarpal joint). The adjacent surfaces of the carpals are approximately flat. When one carpal bone moves relative to another, it glides along the other bone; further, this motion does not occur around an axis. Therefore this type of joint is a nonaxial gliding joint.

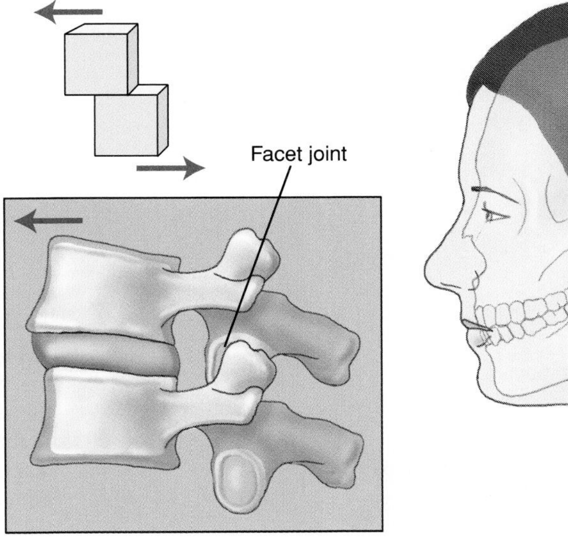

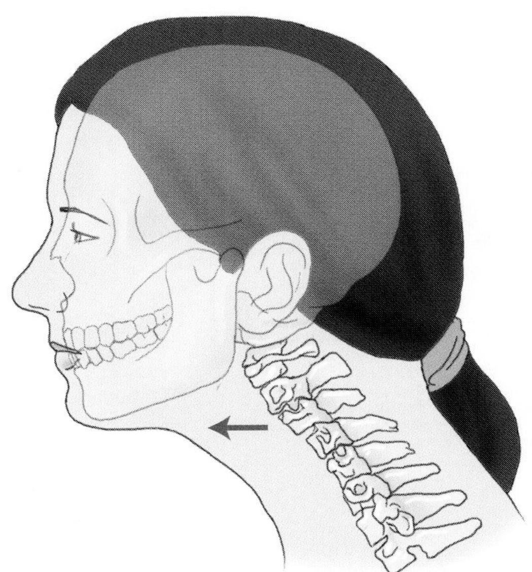

Figure 6-19 Facet joint of the spine. The surfaces of the superior facet (of the inferior vertebra) and the inferior facet (of the superior vertebra) are approximately flat or slightly curved. When one facet moves relative to the other, it glides along the other facet; further, this motion does not occur around an axis. Therefore this type of joint is a nonaxial gliding joint.

6.14 MENISCI AND ARTICULAR DISCS

- Most often, the bones of a joint have opposing surfaces that are **congruent** (i.e., their surfaces match each other). However, sometimes the surfaces of the bones of a joint are not well matched. In these cases the joint will often have an additional intra-articular structure interposed between the two bones.
- These additional intra-articular structures are made of fibrocartilage and function to help maximize the congruence of the joint by helping to improve the fit of the two bones.
- By improving the congruence of a joint, these structures help to do two things:
  - Maintain normal joint movements: Because of the better fit between the two bones of the joint, these structures help to improve the movement of the two bones relative to each other.
  - Cushion the joint: These structures help to cushion the joint by absorbing and transmitting forces (e.g., weight bearing, shock absorption) from the bone of one body part to the bone of the next body part.
- If this fibrocartilaginous structure is ring shaped, it is called an **articular disc**.
- If it is crescent shaped, it is called a **meniscus** (plural: menisci).
- Although these structures are in contact with the articular surfaces of the joints, they are not attached to the joint surfaces but rather to adjacent soft tissue of the capsule or to bone adjacent to the articular surface.
- Articular discs are found in many joints of the body.
  - One example is the temporomandibular joint (TMJ), which has an articular disc located within its joint cavity (Figure 6-20a).
  - Another example is the sternoclavicular joint, which has an articular disc located within its joint cavity (Figure 6-20b).
- Articular menisci are found between the tibia and the femur in the knee joint (Figure 6-21).

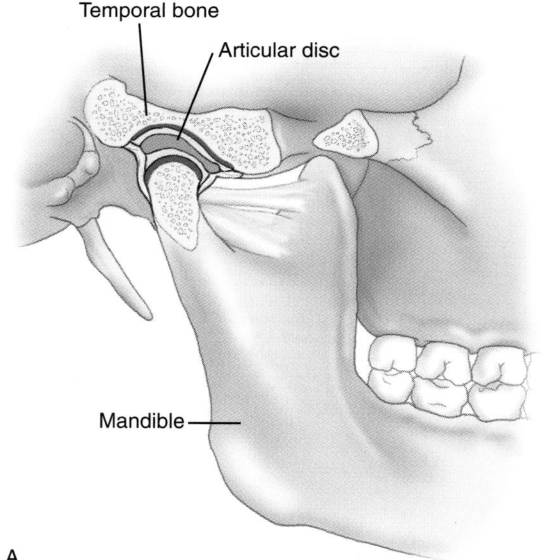

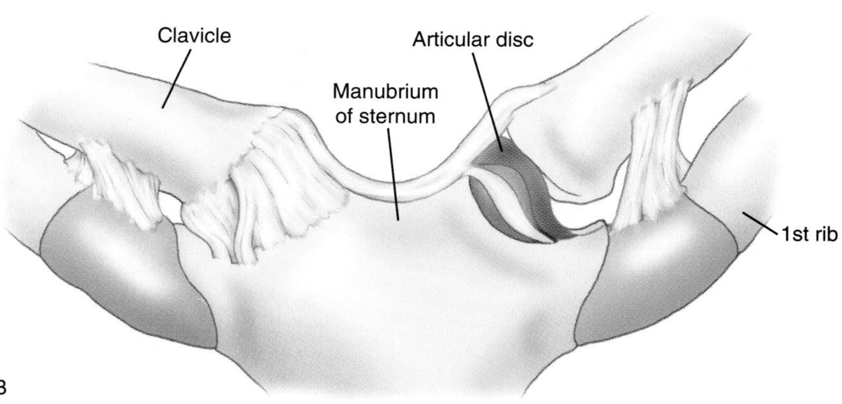

Figure 6-20 *A,* Lateral cross-section view of the temporomandibular joint (TMJ) illustrates the articular disc of the TMJ. *B,* Anterior view of the sternoclavicular joint illustrates the articular disc of the sternoclavicular joint. It can be seen that these articular discs help to improve the fit between the opposing articular surfaces of the joints involved, thereby helping to improve the stability and movement of the joints. By virtue of being a soft tissue, articular discs also aid in absorbing shock and thereby cushioning these joints.

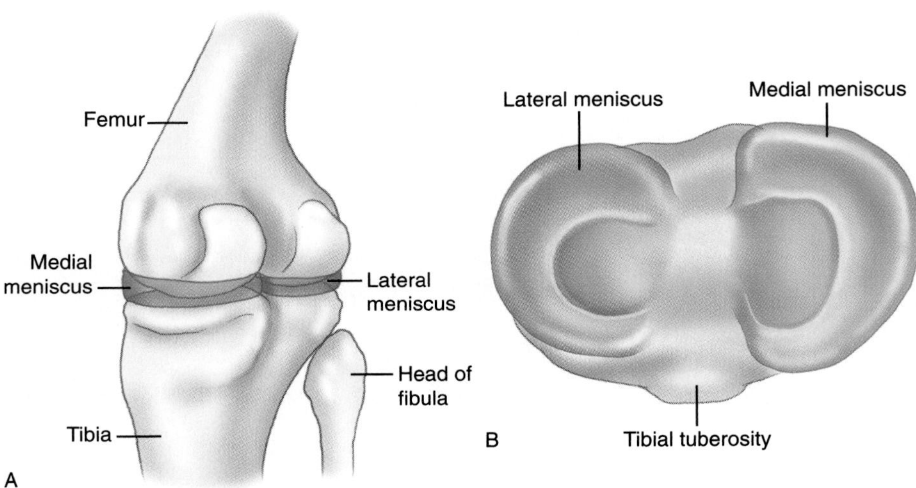

Figure 6-21 *A,* Posteromedial view of the right knee joint; it illustrates the crescent- or *C*-shaped fibrocartilaginous structures called *menisci* that are located between the tibia and femur of the knee joint. A lateral meniscus and a medial meniscus are found in each knee joint. It can be seen that these menisci help to improve the congruence (i.e., fit) between the opposing articular surfaces of the joint, thereby helping to cushion the joint and aid the joint's stability and movement. *B,* Superior view (looking down on) the tibia, illustrating the medial and lateral menisci of the right knee joint.

REVIEW QUESTIONS

evolve Answers to the following review questions appear on the Evolve website accompanying this book.

1. What is the structural definition of a joint?

2. What is the functional definition of a joint?

3. What is the difference between a simple joint and a compound joint?

4. What is the main function of a joint?

5. What is the main function of a muscle?

6. What is the main function of a ligament?

7. What is the relationship between the stability and mobility of a joint?

8. If a joint is more stable, then it is less ____________

9. How do joints absorb shock?

10. Where are most weight-bearing joints of the body located?

11. When classifying joints by structure, what are the three major categories of joints?

12. Which structural category of joints possesses a joint cavity?

13. When classifying joints by function, what are the three major categories of joints?

14. Which functional category of joints allows the most movement?

15. Name the three types of fibrous joints.

16. Name the two types of cartilaginous joints.

17. Give an example in the human body of a fibrous joint, a cartilaginous joint, and a synovial joint.

18. What are the components of a synovial joint?

19. By motion, what are the four major types of synovial joints? Give an example in the human body of each type.

20. Around how many axes does a saddle joint permit motion?

21. In reference to a joint, to what does the term *congruency* refer?

22. Name a joint that has an intra-articular disc.

23. Draw a *typical* synovial joint.

Chapter 7

Joints of the Axial Body

CHAPTER OUTLINE

CHAPTER OBJECTIVES

After completing this chapter, the student should be able to perform the following:

- ❑ Describe the relationship between cranial suture joints and childbirth.
- ❑ List the major muscles of mastication and describe their role in mastication.
- ❑ Explain the possible relationship between TMJ dysfunction and the muscular system.
- ❑ Describe the structure and function of the spine.
- ❑ Define the curves of the spine and describe their development.
- ❑ Describe the structure and function of the median and lateral joints of the spine.
- ❑ State the major difference between the function of the disc joint and the function of the facet joints.
- ❑ Describe the orientation of the planes of the facets in the cervical, thoracic, and lumbar regions of the spine. Further, explain and give examples of how the plane of the facet joints determines the type of motion that occurs at that segmental level.
- ❑ Describe the structure and function of the atlanto-occipital and atlantoaxial joints of the cervical spine.
- ❑ Describe the general structure and function of the cervical spine, thoracic spine, and lumbar spine.
- ❑ List the joints at which rib motion occurs; explain how the movement of a bucket handle is used to describe how rib motion occurs.
- ❑ Describe the roles of the muscles of respiration.
- ❑ Explain the mechanism of thoracic breathing versus abdominal breathing.
- ❑ Describe the structure and function of the thoracolumbar fascia and abdominal aponeurosis.
- ❑ Classify structurally and functionally each joint covered in this chapter.
- ❑ List the major ligaments and bursae of each joint covered in this chapter. Further, explain the major function of each ligament.
- ❑ State the closed-packed position of each joint covered in this chapter.
- ❑ List and describe the actions possible at each joint covered in this chapter.
- ❑ State the range of motion for each axial action of each joint in this chapter.
- ❑ List and describe the reverse actions possible at each joint covered in this chapter.
- ❑ List the major muscles/muscle groups (and their joint actions) for each joint covered in this chapter.
- ❑ Define the key terms of this chapter.
- ❑ State the meanings of the word origins of this chapter.

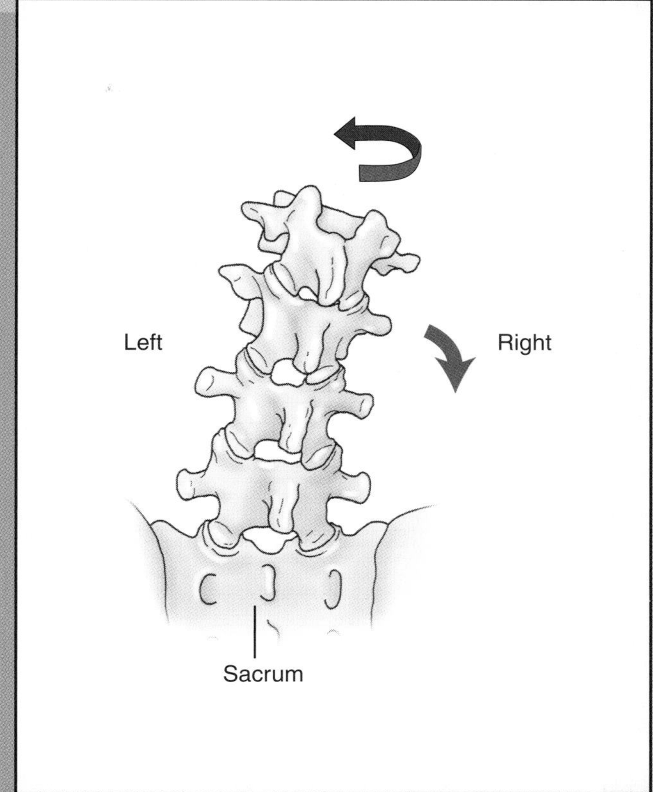

OVERVIEW

Chapters 5 and 6 laid the theoretic basis for the structure and function of joints. Chapters 7 through 9 now examine the structure and function of the joints of the human body regionally. Chapter 7 addresses the joints of the axial body; Chapter 8 addresses the joints of the lower extremity; and Chapter 9 addresses the joints of the upper extremity. Within this chapter, Sections 7.1 and 7.2 cover the suture and temporomandibular joints (TMJs) of the head, respectively. Sections 7.3 through 7.10 then cover the spine. Of these, Section 7.3 begins with a study of the spinal column as an entity, and Section 7.4 covers the general structure and function of spinal joints. Sections 7.5 through 7.10 then sequentially address the various regions of the spine (e.g., cervical, thoracic, lumbar). The last section of this chapter (Section 7.11) addresses the thoracolumbar fascia and abdominal aponeurosis of the trunk.

KEY TERMS

Abdomen (AB-do-men)
Abdominal aponeurosis (ab-DOM-i-nal)
Accessory atlantoaxial ligament (at-LAN-toe-AK-see-al)
Alar ligaments of the dens (A-lar)
Annulus fibrosus (AN-you-lus fi-BROS-us)
Anterior atlanto-occipital membrane (an-TEER-ee-or at-LAN-toe-ok-SIP-i-tal)
Anterior longitudinal ligament
Apical dental ligament (A-pi-kal)
Apical odontoid ligament (o-DONT-oid)
Apophyseal joint (a-POF-i-SEE-al)
Arcuate line (ARE-kew-it)
Atlantoaxial joint (at-LAN-toe-AK-see-al)
Atlanto-occipital joint (at-LAN-toe-ok-SIP-i-tal)
Atlanto-odontoid joint (at-LAN-toe-o-DONT-oid)
Bifid spinous processes (BYE-fid)
Bifid transverse processes
Bucket handle movement
Cervical spine (SERV-i-kul)
Chondrosternal joints (KON-dro-STERN-al)
Costochondral joints (COST-o-KON-dral)
Costocorporeal joint (COST-o-kor-PO-ree-al)
Costospinal joints (COST-o-SPINE-al)
Costotransverse joint (COST-o-TRANS-verse)
Costotransverse ligament
Costovertebral joint (COST-o-VERT-i-bral)
Craniosacral technique (CRANE-ee-o-SAY-kral)
Cruciate ligament of the dens (KRU-shee-it, DENS)
Disc joint
Facet joint (fa-SET)
False ribs
Floating ribs
Forward-head posture
Hyperkyphotic (HI-per-ki-FOT-ik)
Hyperlordotic (HI-per-lor-DOT-ik)
Hypolordotic (HI-po-lor-DOT-ik)
Interchondral ligament (IN-ter-KON-dral)
Interchondral joints
Interspinous ligaments (IN-ter-SPINE-us)
Intertransverse ligaments (IN-ter-TRANS-verse)
Intervertebral disc joint (IN-ter-VERT-i-bral)
Joints of Von Luschka (FON LOOSH-ka)
Kyphosis, pl. kyphoses (ki-FOS-is, ki-FOS-ees)
Kyphotic (ki-FOT-ik)
Lateral collateral ligament (of the temporomandibular joint)
Lateral costotransverse ligament (COST-o-TRANS-verse)
Ligamentum flava, sing. ligamentum flavum (LIG-a-men-tum FLAY-va, FLAY-vum)
Linea alba (LIN-ee-a AL-ba)
Lordosis, pl. lordoses (lor-DOS-is, lor-DOS-ees)
Lordotic (lor-DOT-ik)
Lumbar spine (LUM-bar)
Lumbodorsal fascia (LUM-bo-DOOR-sul)
Lumbosacral joint (LUM-bo-SAY-krul)
Manubriosternal ligament (ma-NOOB-ree-o-STERN-al)
Manubriosternal joint
Medial collateral ligament (of the temporomandibular joint)
Nuchal ligament (NEW-kal)
Nucleus pulposus (NEW-klee-us pul-POS-us)
Posterior atlanto-occipital membrane (pos-TEER-ee-or at-LAN-toe-ok-SIP-i-tal)
Posterior longitudinal ligament
Primary spinal curves
Radiate ligament (of chondrosternal joint) (RAY-dee-at)
Radiate ligament (of costovertebral joint)
Rectus sheath (REK-tus)
Sacral base angle (SAY-krul)
Sacrococcygeal region (SAY-kro-kok-SI-jee-al)
Sacro-occipital technique (SAY-kro-ok-SIP-i-tal)
Scoliosis, pl. scolioses (SKO-lee-os-is, SKO-lee-os-ees)
Secondary spinal curves
Segmental level (seg-MENT-al)
Slipped disc
Sphenomandibular ligament (SFEE-no-man-DIB-you-lar)
Spinal column
Spine
Sternocostal joints (STERN-o-COST-al)
Sternoxiphoid ligament (STERN-o-ZI-foid)
Sternoxiphoid joint
Stylomandibular ligament (STY-lo-man-DIB-you-lar)
Superior costotransverse ligament (sue-PEER-ee-or COST-o-TRANS-verse)
Supraspinous ligament (SUE-pra-SPINE-us)
Swayback (SWAY-back)
Tectorial membrane (tek-TOR-ee-al)
Temporomandibular joint (TEM-po-ro-man-DIB-you-lar)
Temporomandibular joint dysfunction (dis-FUNK-shun)
Temporomandibular ligament (TEM-po-ro-man-DIB-you-lar)
Thoracic spine (thor-AS-ik)
Thoracolumbar fascia (thor-AK-o-LUM-bar FASH-ee-a)
Thoracolumbar spine (thor-AK-o-LUM-bar)
Thorax (THOR-aks)
Transverse ligament of the atlas
True ribs
Uncinate process (UN-sin-ate)
Uncovertebral joint (UN-co-VERT-i-bral)
Vertebral arteries (VERT-i-bral)
Vertebral column
Vertebral endplate (VERT-i-bral)
Vertebral prominens (PROM-i-nens)
Z joints
Zygapophyseal joint (ZI-ga-POF-i-SEE-al)

WORD ORIGINS

- ❑ Alba—From Latin *albus,* meaning *white*
- ❑ Annulus—From Latin *anulus,* meaning *ring*
- ❑ Arcuate—From Latin *arcuatus,* meaning *bowed*
- ❑ Bifid—From Latin *bifidus,* meaning *cleft in two parts*
- ❑ Cervical—From Latin *cervicalis,* meaning *neck*
- ❑ Concavity—From Latin *con,* meaning *with,* and *cavus,* meaning *hollow, concavity*
- ❑ Convexity—From Latin *convexus,* meaning *vaulted, arched*
- ❑ Corporeal—From Latin *corpus,* meaning *body*
- ❑ Costal—From Latin *costa,* meaning *rib*
- ❑ Cruciate—From Latin *crux,* meaning *cross*
- ❑ Flavum—From Latin *flavus,* meaning *yellow*
- ❑ Kyphosis—From Greek *kyphosis,* meaning *bent, hump-back*
- ❑ Linea—From Latin *linea,* meaning *line*
- ❑ Lordosis—From Greek *lordosis,* meaning *a bending backward*
- ❑ Lumbar—From Latin *lumbus,* meaning *loin*
- ❑ Mastication—From Latin *masticare,* meaning *to chew* (Note: This originates from Greek *masten,* meaning *to feed,* which in turn originates from Greek *mastos,* meaning *breast, the first place from which a person receives sustenance.*)
- ❑ Nuchal—From Latin *nucha,* meaning *back of the neck*
- ❑ Nucleus—From Latin *nucleus,* meaning *little kernel, the inside/center of a nut* (Note: Nucleus is diminutive for the Latin word *nux,* meaning *nut.*)
- ❑ Pulposus—From Latin *pulpa,* meaning *flesh*
- ❑ Radiate—From Latin *radius,* meaning *ray, to spread out in all directions*
- ❑ Scoliosis—From Greek *scoliosis,* meaning *curvature, crooked*
- ❑ Thoracic—From Greek *thorax,* meaning *breastplate, chest*
- ❑ Uncinate—From Latin *uncinatus,* meaning *shaped like a hook*
- ❑ Zygapophyseal—From Greek *zygon,* meaning *yoke* or *joining,* and *apophysis,* meaning *offshoot*

☐ 7.1 SUTURE JOINTS OF THE SKULL

❑ The suture joints of the skull are located between most bones of the cranium and also between most bones of the face (Figure 7-1).

Bones:

❑ Suture joints are located between adjacent bones of the cranium and face.

BOX 7-1

All joints between the major bones of the cranium and face (except the temporomandibular joint [TMJ]) are suture joints. Other nonsuture joints of the skull are the joints of the teeth and the joints between middle ear ossicles.

❑ Joint structure classification: Fibrous joint
  ❑ Subtype: Suture joint
❑ Joint function classification: Synarthrotic

Major Motions Allowed:

❑ Nonaxial

Miscellaneous:

❑ Movement at these joints is important during the birth process when the child must be delivered through the birth canal of the mother. Movement of the suture joints allows the child's head to be compressed, allowing for an easier and safer delivery.

❑ Suture joints of the skull allow very little movement in an adult. As a person ages, many suture joints ossify and lose all ability to move.

BOX 7-2

Although suture joints allow little motion, practitioners of **craniosacral technique** and **sacro-occipital technique** assert that this motion is very important. When blockage of this motion occurs, these practitioners manipulate the suture joints of the skull.

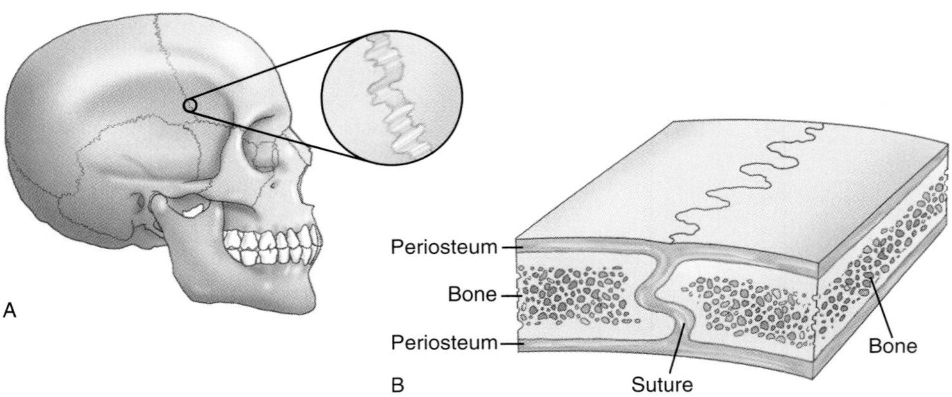

Figure 7-1 Suture joint of the skull. Suture joints are structurally classified as fibrous joints and allow nonaxial motion.

7.2 TEMPOROMANDIBULAR JOINT (TMJ)

Bones:

- The **temporomandibular joint (TMJ)** is located between the temporal bone and the mandible (Figure 7-2).
  - More specifically, it is located between the mandibular fossa of the temporal bone and the condyle of the ramus of the mandible.
- Joint structure classification: Synovial joint
  - Subtype: Modified hinge
- Joint function classification: Diarthrotic
  - Subtype: Uniaxial

Major Motions Allowed:

- The TMJ allows elevation and depression (i.e., axial movements) within the sagittal plane about a mediolateral axis (Figure 7-3).
- The TMJ allows protraction and retraction (i.e., nonaxial anterior and posterior glide movements) (Figure 7-4).
- The TMJ allows left and right lateral deviation (i.e., nonaxial lateral glide movements) (Figure 7-5; Box 7-4).

BOX 7-3

Opening of the mouth involves both depression and protraction (i.e., anterior glide) of the mandible at the TMJ; closing the mouth involves elevation and retraction (i.e., posterior glide).

An easy way to assess the amount of depression that a TMJ should allow (i.e., how wide the mouth can be opened) is to use the proximal interphalangeal (PIP) joints of the fingers. Full depression of the TMJ should allow three PIPs to fit between the teeth.

BOX 7-4

Lateral deviation of the TMJ is actually a combination of spinning and glide. The condyle on the side to which the deviation is occurring spins, and the other condyle glides.

Major Ligaments of the Temporomandibular Joint:

Fibrous Joint Capsule:

- The fibrous capsule (Figure 7-6) thickens medially and laterally, providing stability to the joint there. These thickenings are often referred to as the **medial collateral ligament** and the **lateral collateral ligament** of the TMJ.
- However, the capsule is fairly loose anteriorly and posteriorly, allowing the condyle and disc to freely translate forward and back.

BOX 7-5

LIGAMENTS OF THE TEMPOROMANDIBULAR JOINT (TMJ)

- Fibrous capsule (thickened medially and laterally as the medial and lateral collateral ligaments)
- Temporomandibular ligament (located laterally)
- Stylomandibular ligament (located medially)
- Sphenomandibular ligament (located medially)

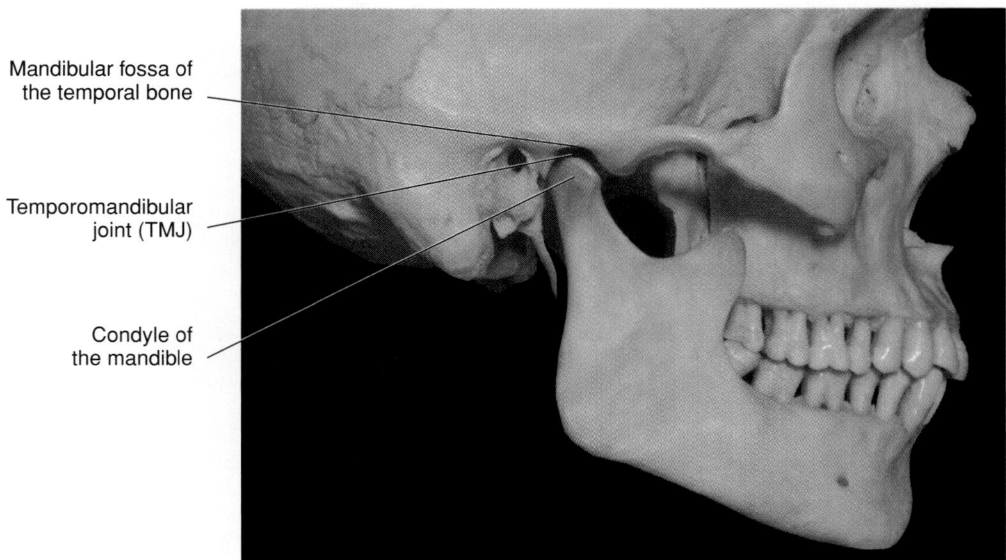

Figure 7-2 Lateral view of the right temporomandibular joint (TMJ). The TMJ is the **j**oint located between the **t**emporal bone and the **m**andibular bone, hence *TMJ.*

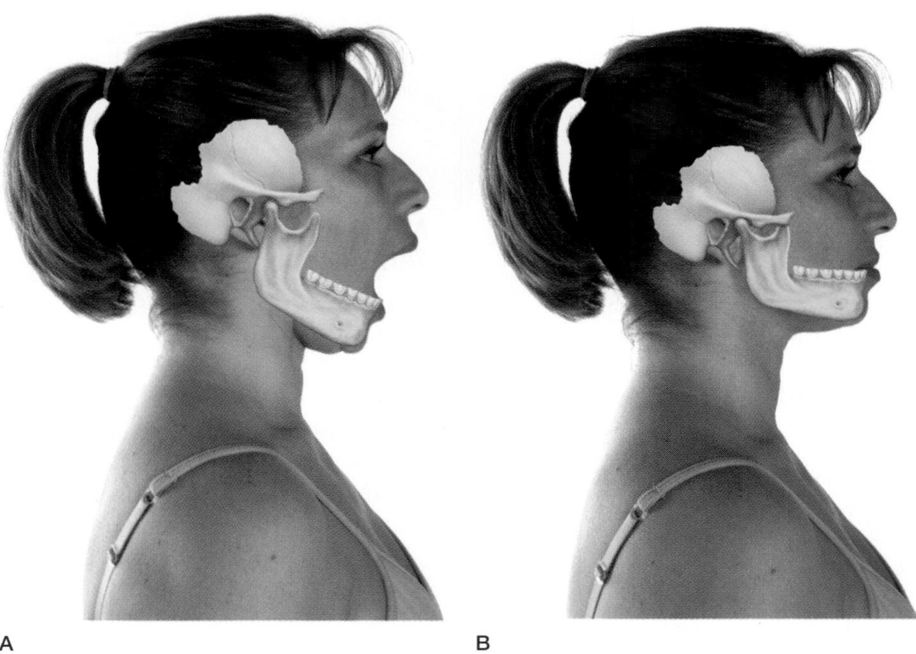

Figure 7-3 *A* and *B,* Lateral views that illustrate depression and elevation, respectively, of the mandible at the temporomandibular joints (TMJs). These are axial motions.

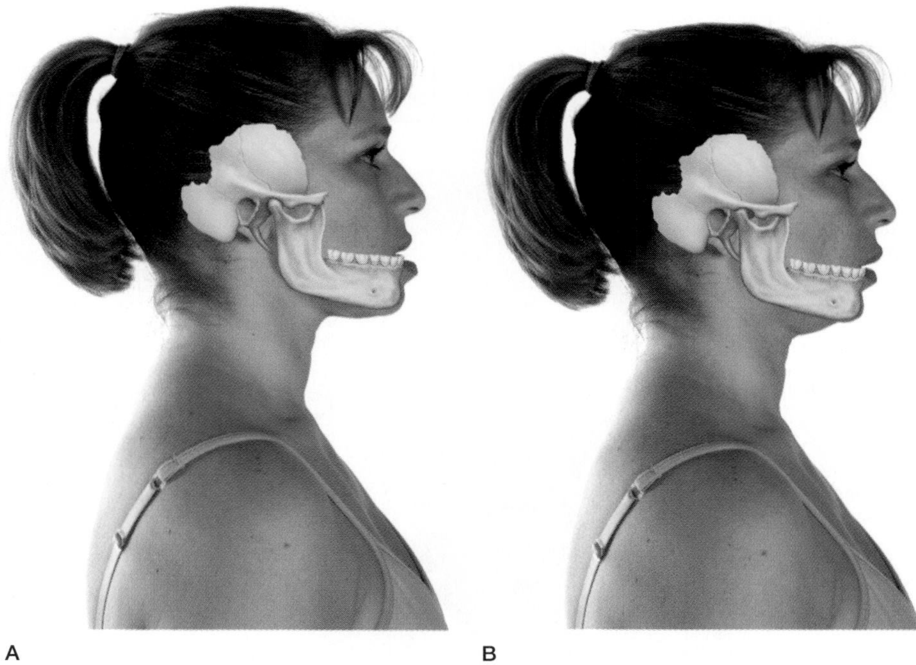

Figure 7-4 *A* and *B,* Lateral views that illustrate protraction and retraction, respectively, of the mandible at the temporomandibular joints (TMJs). These are nonaxial glide motions.

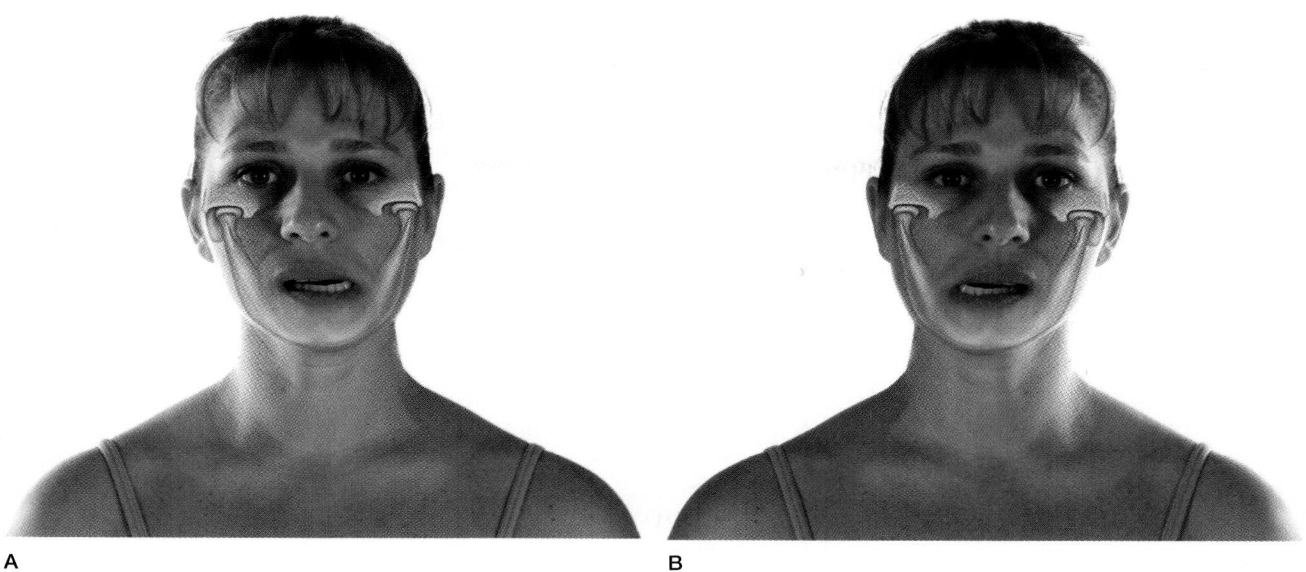

Figure 7-5 *A* and *B,* Anterior views that illustrate right lateral deviation and left lateral deviation, respectively, of the mandible at the temporomandibular joints (TMJs). These are nonaxial glide motions.

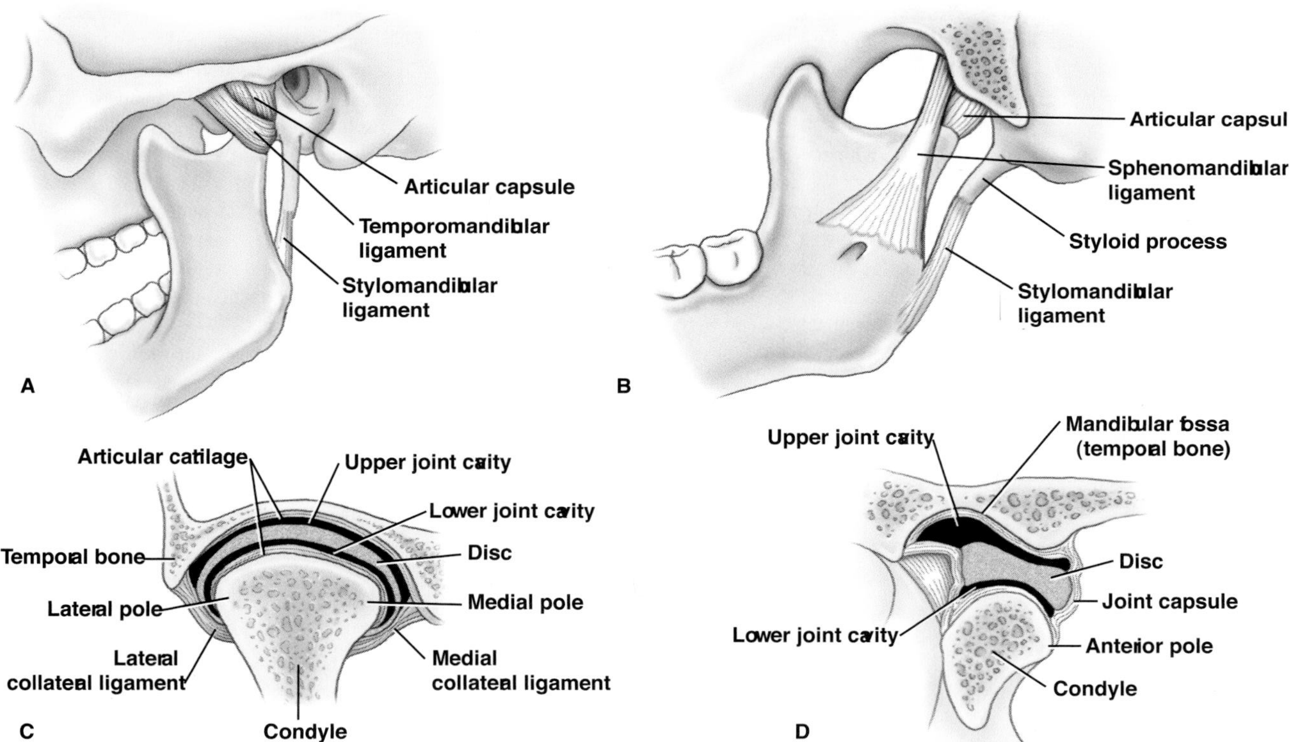

Figure 7-6 *A,* Lateral view of the temporomandibular joint (TMJ). The temporomandibular ligament is located on and stabilizes the lateral side of the TMJ. *B,* Medial view illustrating the stylomandibular and spheno-mandibular ligaments. *C,* Coronal (i.e., frontal) section through the TMJ. The articular disc can be seen to divide the joint into two separate joint cavities: upper and lower. *D,* Sagittal section of the TMJ in the open position. The articular disc can be seen to move anteriorly along with the condyle of the mandible.

- When the mandible depresses at the TMJ, it also protracts (i.e., glides anteriorly). Because the disc attaches into the anterior joint capsule, this motion pulls the disc anteriorly along with the condyle of the mandible.

Temporomandibular Ligament:

- Location: It is located on the lateral side of the joint (Figure 7-6a).
- The temporomandibular ligament is primarily composed of oblique fibers.
- Function: It limits depression of the mandible and stabilizes the lateral side of the joint.
- The temporomandibular ligament is also known as the **lateral ligament** of the TMJ.

BOX 7-6

In addition to stabilizing the lateral side of the capsule of the temporomandibular joint (TMJ), the temporomandibular ligament also stabilizes the intra-articular disc. The superior head of the lateral pterygoid muscle attaches into the disc and exerts a medial pulling force on it. The temporomandibular ligament, being located laterally, opposes this pull, thereby stabilizing the medial-lateral placement of the disc within the joint.

Stylomandibular Ligament:

- Location: It is located on the medial side of the joint (Figure 7-6a–b).
  - More specifically, it is located from the styloid process of the temporal bone to the posterior border of the ramus of the mandible.

Sphenomandibular Ligament:

- Location: It is located on the medial side of the joint (Figure 7-6b).
  - More specifically, it is located from the sphenoid bone to the medial surface of the ramus of the mandible.
- Function: Both the stylomandibular and sphenomandibular ligaments function to limit protraction (i.e., forward translation) of the mandible.

Major Muscles of the Temporomandibular Joint:

- Lateral pterygoid, medial pterygoid, temporalis, and masseter (See figures on page 235 in Box 7-7).

BOX 7-7 SPOTLIGHT ON THE MUSCLES OF MASTICATION

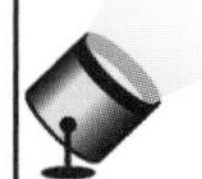

- The term *mastication* means *to chew*, hence muscles of mastication involve moving the mandible at the temporomandibular joint (TMJ), because mandibular movement is necessary for chewing.
- Four major muscles of mastication exist: (1) temporalis, (2) masseter, (3) lateral pterygoid, and (4) medial pterygoid. The temporalis and masseter are located superficially and can be easily accessed when palpating and doing bodywork. The lateral and medial pterygoids are located deeper, and addressing these muscles with bodywork is best done from inside the mouth (see figures in this box on the next page).
- Another group of muscles that is involved with mastication is the hyoid group. The hyoid muscle group is composed of eight muscles: four suprahyoids and four infrahyoids. Three of the four suprahyoids attach from the hyoid bone inferiorly to the mandible superiorly. When these suprahyoids contract, if the hyoid bone is fixed, they move the mandible, hence assisting in mastication. The infrahyoid muscles are also important with respect to mastication. Because the hyoid bone does not form an osseous joint with any other bone of the body (it is the only bone in the human body that does not articulate with another bone), it is quite mobile and needs to be stabilized for the suprahyoids to contract and move the mandible. Therefore when the suprahyoids concentrically contract and shorten to move the mandible at the TMJ, the infrahyoids simultaneously contract isometrically to fix (i.e., stabilize) the hyoid bone. With the hyoid bone fixed, all the force of the pull of the contraction of the suprahyoids will be directed toward moving the mandible.
- In addition to mandibular movement at the TMJ, mastication also involves muscular action by the tongue to move food within the mouth to facilitate chewing. Therefore muscles of the tongue may also be considered to be muscles of mastication.

Continued.

BOX 7-7 SPOTLIGHT ON THE MUSCLES OF MASTICATION—cont'd

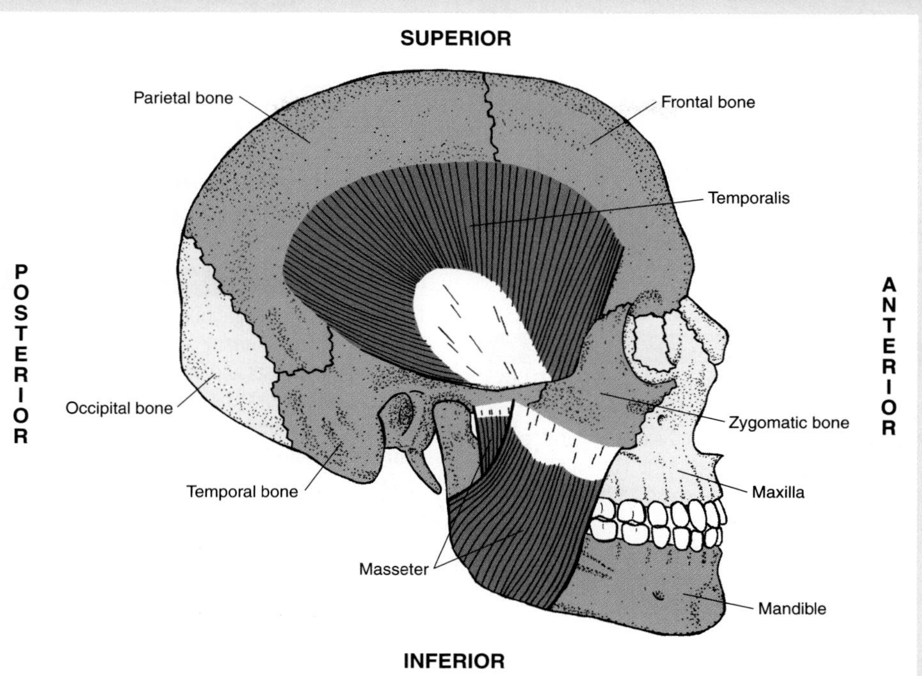

Lateral view of the head. (From Muscolino JE: *The muscular system manual: the skeletal muscles of the human body,* ed 2. St Louis, 2005, Mosby.)

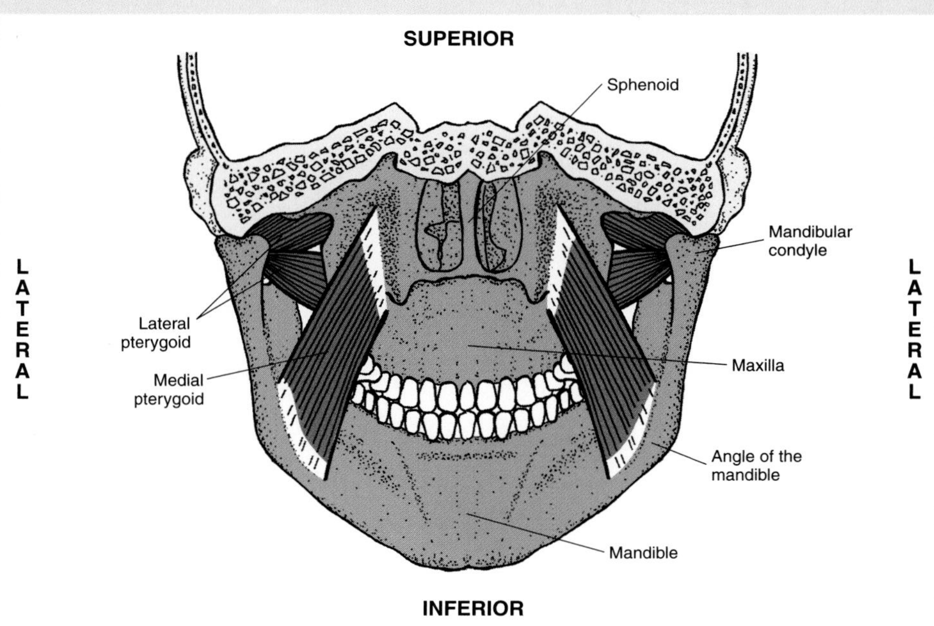

Posterior view of the internal face. (From Muscolino JE: *The muscular system manual: the skeletal muscles of the human body,* ed 2. St Louis, 2005, Mosby.)

Miscellaneous:

- ❑ An intra-articular fibrocartilaginous disc is located within the TMJ (see Figure 7-6c–d).
  - ❑ The purpose of this disc is to increase the congruence (i.e., improve the fit and stability) of the joint surfaces of the temporal bone and mandible.
  - ❑ Being a soft tissue, the disc also serves to cushion the TMJ.
  - ❑ The disc divides the TMJ into two separate joint cavities: (1) an upper cavity and (2) lower cavity.
  - ❑ The intra-articular disc is attached to and moves with the condyle of the mandible.
  - ❑ The intra-articular disc also has attachments into the joint capsule of the TMJ.
- ❑ The lateral pterygoid muscle has tendinous attachments directly into the fibrous joint capsule and the intra-articular disc of the TMJ.
- ❑ **TMJ dysfunction** is a general term that applies to any dysfunction (i.e., abnormal function) of the TMJ.

BOX 7-8

Technically, the lower joint of the temporomandibular joint (TMJ) (between the condyle of the mandible and the intra-articular disc) is a uniaxial joint. The upper joint of the TMJ (between the disc and the temporal bone) is a gliding nonaxial joint. Motions of the TMJ may occur solely at one of these joints, or may occur as a combination of movements at both of these joints.

BOX 7-9

Temporomandibular joint (TMJ) dysfunction has many possible causes. Of these many causes, two may be of special interest to massage therapists and bodyworkers. One is tightness/imbalance of the muscles that cross the TMJ (especially the lateral pterygoid because of its attachment directly into the capsule and disc). The second is **forward-head posture,** a common postural deviation in which the head and often the upper cervical vertebrae are translated anteriorly (i.e., forward). This forward-head posture is believed to create tension on the TMJs as a result of the hyoid muscles being stretched and pulled taut, resulting in a pulling force being placed on the mandible, consequently placing a tensile stress on the TMJs.

☐ 7.3 SPINE

The **spine**, also known as the **spinal column** or **vertebral column**, is literally a column of vertebrae stacked one on top of the other.

Elements of the Spine:

- ❑ The spine has four major regions (Figure 7-7).
- ❑ These four regions contain a total of 26 movable elements.
- ❑ The following are the four regions:
  1. **Cervical spine** (i.e., the neck) containing seven vertebrae (C1-C7)
  2. **Thoracic spine** (i.e., the upper and middle back) containing twelve vertebrae (T1-T12)
  3. **Lumbar spine** (i.e., the low back) containing five vertebrae (L1-L5)
  4. **Sacrococcygeal spine** (within the pelvis) containing one sacrum, which is formed by the fusion of five vertebrae (S1-S5) that have never fully formed, and one coccyx, which is usually four bones (Co1-Co4) that may partially or fully fuse as a person ages

Shape of the Adult Spine Viewed Posteriorly:

- ❑ Viewed posteriorly, the adult spine should ideally be straight (see Figure 7-7a).

BOX 7-10

By definition, any spinal curve that exists from a posterior view is termed a **scoliosis;** a scoliotic curve is a *C*-shaped curvature of the spine that exists within the frontal plane. Ideally, the spine should be straight within the frontal plane; therefore a scoliosis is considered to be a postural pathology of the spine. A scoliosis is named *left* or *right*, based on the side of the curve that is convex. For example, if a curve in the lumbar spine exists that is convex to the left (therefore concave to the right), it is called a *left lumbar scoliosis.* A scoliosis may even have two or three curves (called an *S* or *double-S scoliosis*, respectively); again, each of the curves is named for the side of the convexity.

Shape of the Adult Spine Viewed Laterally:

- ❑ Viewed laterally, the adult spine should have four curves in the sagittal plane (see Figure 7-7b).
- ❑ It has two **primary spinal curves** that are formed first (before birth) and two **secondary spinal curves** that are formed second (after birth).
- ❑ The two primary curves of the spine are the thoracic and sacrococcygeal curves.
  - ❑ These curves are **kyphotic** (i.e., concave anteriorly and convex posteriorly).
- ❑ The two secondary curves of the spine are the cervical and lumbar curves.
  - ❑ These curves are **lordotic** (i.e., concave posteriorly and convex anteriorly).

BOX 7-11

A kyphotic curve is a **kyphosis;** a lordotic curve is a **lordosis.** The terms *kyphosis* and *lordosis* are often misused in that they are used to describe an individual that has an excessive kyphotic or lordotic curve. It is normal and healthy to have a kyphosis in the thoracic and sacral spines and to have a lordosis in the cervical and lumbar spines. An excessive kyphosis should correctly be termed a hyperkyphosis or a **hyperkyphotic curve;** an excessive lordosis should correctly be termed a hyperlordosis or a **hyperlordotic curve.**

Development of the Spinal Curves:

- ❑ When a baby is first born, only one curve to the entire spine exists, which is kyphotic. In effect, the entire spinal column is one large *C*-shaped kyphotic curve (Figure 7-8).
- ❑ Two activities occur during our childhood development that create the cervical and lumbar lordoses:
  1. When a child first starts to lift its head to see the world around it (which is invariably higher), the spinal joints of the neck must extend, creating the cervical lordosis. This cervical lordosis is necessary to bring the position of the head posteriorly so that its weight is balanced over the trunk (see Figure 7-8b).

BOX 7-12

Many people have a **hypolordotic** cervical spine (i.e., decreased cervical lordotic curve), either because it never fully develops or because it is lost after it has developed. This is largely because of the posture of sitting with the head forward when writing (e.g., at a desk). At a very early age we give our children crayons to draw with; then they graduate to pencils in elementary school and pens in high school and beyond. The tremendous number of hours sitting with the neck and head bent (i.e., flexed) over a piece of paper causes a decrease in the extension of the cervical spinal joints, which is a decrease in the cervical lordotic curve. (Note: Many other postures also contribute to a loss of the cervical lordosis.)

  2. Next, when the child wants to sit up (and later stand up), the spinal joints of the low back must extend, creating the lumbar lordosis. This lumbar lordosis is necessary to bring the position of the trunk posteriorly so that its weight is balanced over the pelvis. Otherwise, when the child tries to sit up, he or she would fall forward (see Figure 7-8c).

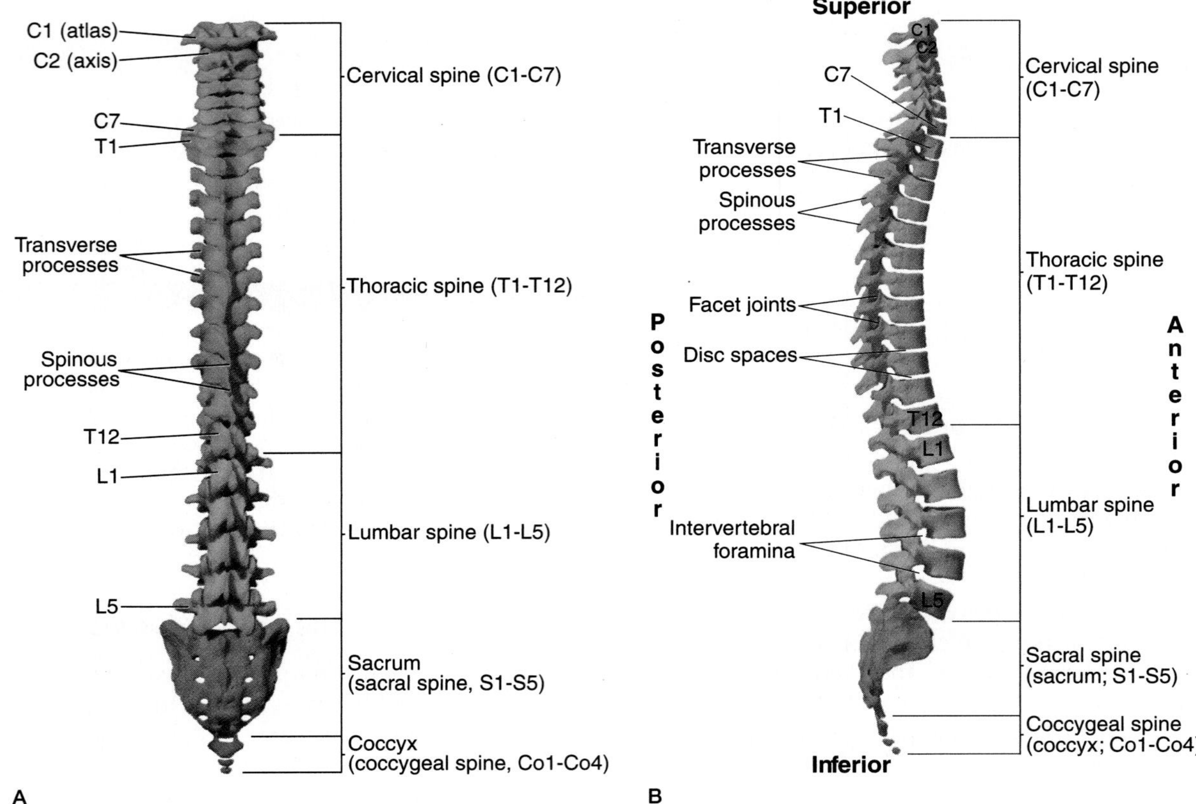

Figure 7-7 *A,* Posterior view of the entire spine. *B,* Right lateral view of the entire spine. The spine is composed of the cervical region containing C1-C7, the thoracic region containing T1-T12, the lumbar region containing L1-L5, and the sacrococcygeal region containing the sacrum and coccyx.

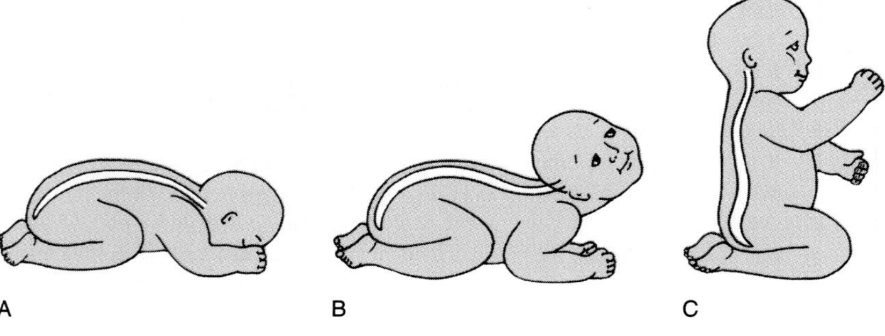

Figure 7-8 The developmental formation of the curves of the spine. *A,* Baby with one *C*-shaped kyphosis for the entire spine. *B,* Baby lifting its head, thereby creating the cervical lordosis of the neck. *C,* Baby sitting up, thereby creating the lumbar lordosis of the low back.

❑ In effect, the cervical and lumbar lordotic secondary curves are formed after birth, whereas the thoracic and sacrococcygeal regions retain their original primary kyphotic curves. The net result is a healthy adult spine that has four curves in the sagittal plane.

BOX 7-13

The four kyphotic and lordotic curves of an adult spine are usually attained at approximately the age of 10 years.

Functions of the Spine:

The spine has four major functions (Figure 7-9):

1. To provide structural support for the body (see Figure 7-9a)
   - ❑ The spine provides a base of support for the head and transmits the entire weight of the head, arms, neck, and trunk to the pelvis.
2. To allow for movement (see Figure 7-9b)

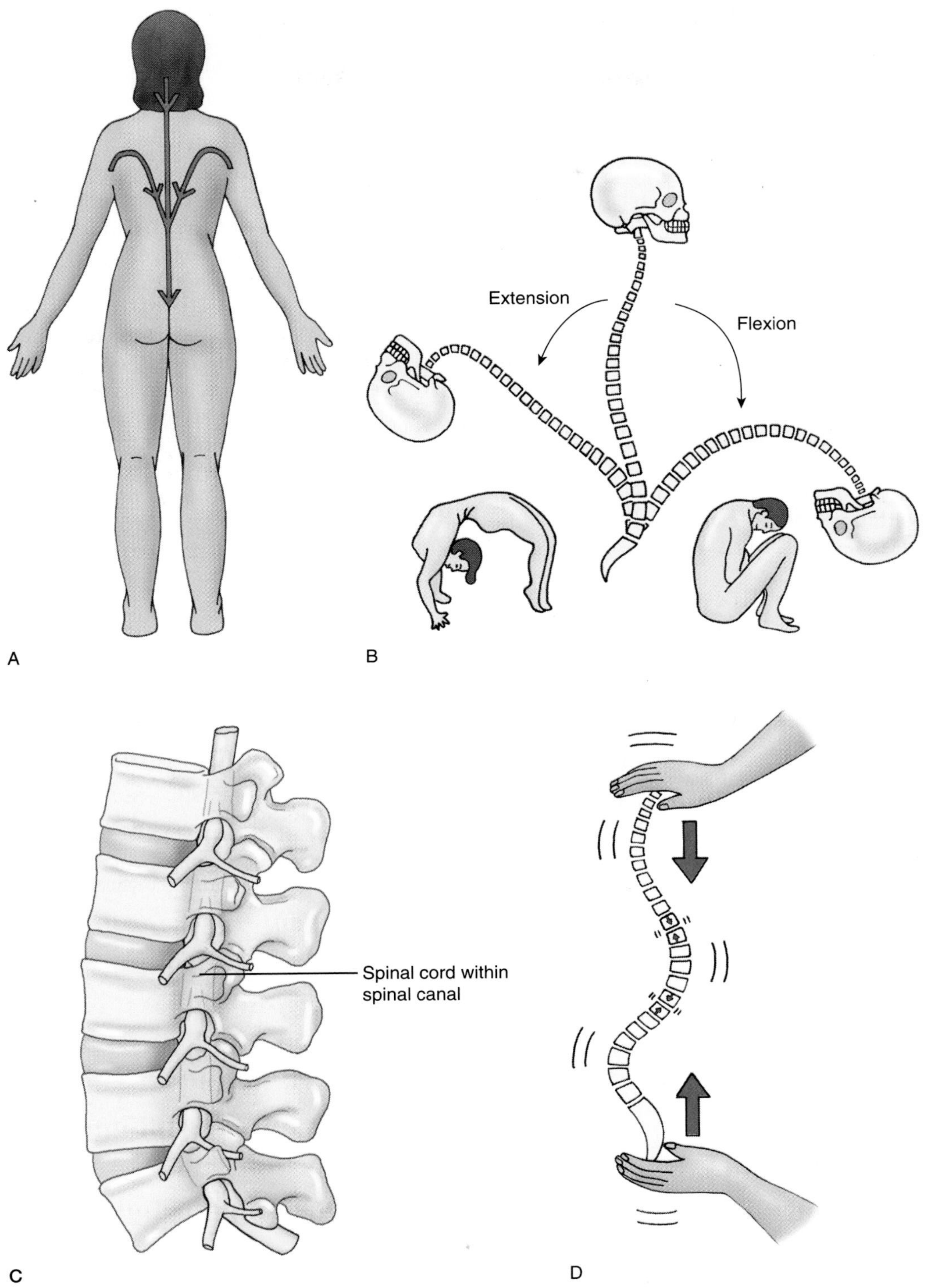

Figure 7-9 The four major functions of the spine. *A,* Posterior view illustrating its weight-bearing function; the lines drawn in indicate the weight of the head, arms, and trunk being borne through the spine and transmitted to the pelvis. *B,* Lateral view demonstrating the tremendous movement possible of the spine (specifically, flexion and extension of the spinal joints are shown). *C,* The spine surrounds and protects the spinal cord located within the spinal canal. *D,* Lateral view that illustrates how the spine can function to absorb shock and compressive forces; both the disc joints themselves and the spinal curves contribute to shock absorption (i.e., absorbing compression force). (*B* modeled after Kapandji IA: *Physiology of the joints: the trunk and the vertebral column,* ed. 2. Edinburgh, 1974, Churchill Livingstone.)

BOX 7-14

As with all joints, the spine must find a balance between structural stability and movement. Generally the more stable a joint is, the less mobile it is; and the more mobile a joint is, the less stable it is. The spine is a remarkable structure in that it can provide so much structural support to the body and yet also afford so much movement!

- ❑ Although each spinal joint generally allows only a small amount of movement, when the movements of all 25 spinal segmental levels are added up, the spine allows a great deal of movement in all three planes (see Table 7-1).
- ❑ The spine allows for movement of the head, neck, trunk, and pelvis. (Illustrations of these motions are shown in Sections 7.5 [head], 7.6 [neck], 7.10 [trunk], and 8.3 through 8.5 [pelvis].)
- ❑ The head can move relative to the neck at the atlanto-occipital joint (AOJ).
- ❑ The neck can move at the cervical spinal joints located within it (and/or relative to the head at the AOJ, or relative to the trunk at the C7-T1 joint).
- ❑ The trunk can move at the thoracic and lumbar spinal joints located within it (or relative to the pelvis at the lumbosacral joint).
- ❑ The pelvis can move relative to the trunk at the lumbosacral joint.

3. To protect the spinal cord (see Figure 7-9c)
   - ❑ Neural tissue is very sensitive to damage. For this reason, the spinal cord is hidden away within the spinal canal and thereby afforded a great degree of protection from damage.
4. To provide shock absorption for the body (see Figure 7-9d)
   - ❑ Being a weight-bearing structure, the spine provides shock absorption to the body whenever a compression force occurs, such as walking, running, and jumping. This is accomplished in two ways:
   - ❑ The nucleus pulposus in the center of the discs absorb this compressive force.
   - ❑ The curves of the spine bend and increase slightly, absorbing some of this compressive force. They then return to their normal posture afterwards.

TABLE 7-1

Average Ranges of Motion of the Entire Spine from Anatomic Position (Including the Atlantooccipital Joint [AOJ] Between the Head and the Neck)*

Flexion	135 Degrees	Extension	120 Degrees
Right lateral flexion	90 Degrees	Left lateral flexion	90 Degrees
Right rotation	120 Degrees	Left rotation	120 Degrees

*No exact agreement exists between sources as to the average or ideal ranges of motion of joints. The ranges given in this text are approximations. Actual ranges of motion vary somewhat from one individual to another. Further, ranges of motion vary enormously with age.

7.4 SPINAL JOINTS

- Spinal joints are joints that involve two contiguous vertebrae (i.e., two adjacent vertebrae) of the spine.
- Naming a spinal joint is usually done by simply naming the levels of the two vertebrae involved. For example, the joint between the fifth cervical vertebra (C5) and the sixth cervical vertebra (C6) is called the *C5-C6 joint.*
- Again, using this example, the C5-C6 joint is one segment of the many spinal joints and is often referred to as a **segmental level** of the spine. The C6-C7 joint would be another; C7-T1 would be the next, and so forth.
- At any one typical segmental level of the spine, one median joint and two lateral joints exist (the median joint is located in the middle, and the lateral joints are located to the sides, hence the names).
- Typically the median joint is an intervertebral disc joint and the lateral joints are the two vertebral facet joints (Figure 7-10).
  - The median spinal joint at the AOJ and atlantoaxial joint (AAJ) are not disc joints (see Section 7.5).
- When movement of one vertebra occurs relative to the contiguous vertebra, this movement is the result of movement at both the intervertebral disc joint and vertebral facet joints.

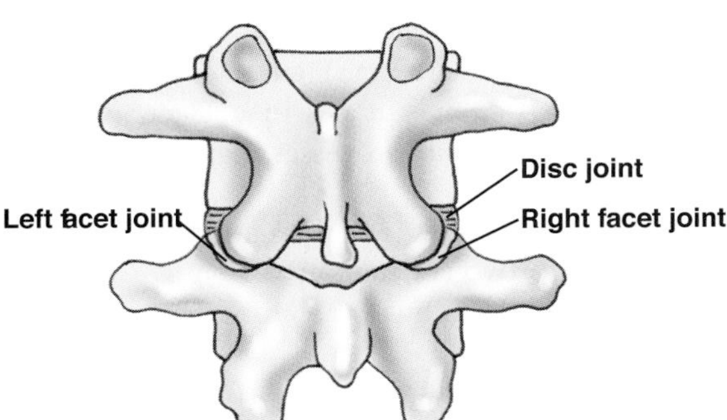

Figure 7-10 The median and lateral spinal joints. The median spinal joint is the disc joint; the lateral spinal joints are the facet joints.

Intervertebral Disc Joint:

- An **intervertebral disc joint** is located between the bodies of two contiguous vertebrae. This joint is often referred to simply as the **disc joint**.
- Joint structure classification: Cartilaginous joint
  - Subtype: Symphysis
- Joint function classification: Amphiarthrotic

Miscellaneous:

- A disc joint is composed of three parts: (1) an outer annulus fibrosus, (2) an inner nucleus pulposus, and (3) the two vertebral endplates (Figure 7-11).
- Discs are actually quite thick, accounting for approximately 25% of the height of the spinal column. The thicker a disc is, the greater its shock absorption ability and the more movement it allows.
- In addition to allowing movement, two major functions of the disc joint are (1) to absorb shock and (2) to bear the weight of the body.
  - The spinal disc joint bears approximately 80% of the weight of the body above it (the other 20% is borne through the facet joints).
- The presence of a disc is also important because it maintains the opening of the intervertebral foramina (through which the spinal nerves travel) by creating a spacer between the two vertebral bodies.

BOX 7-15

If a disc thins excessively, the decreased size of an intervertebral foramen may impinge on the spinal nerve that is located within it. This is commonly known as a *pinched nerve* and may result in referral of pain, numbness, or weakness in the area that this nerve innervates.

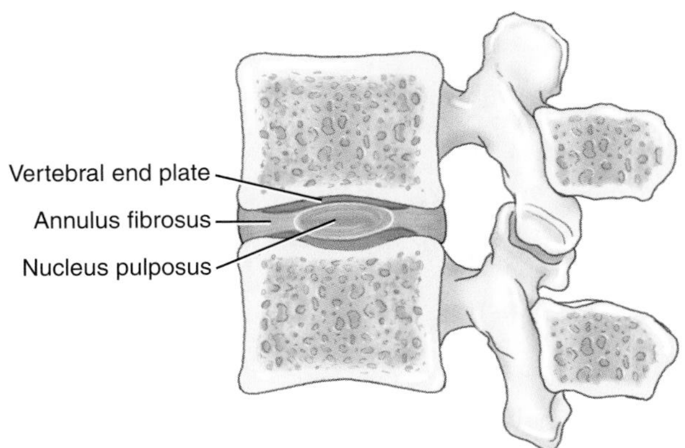

Figure 7-11 The three major components of the intervertebral disc joint: (1) the annulus fibrosus, (2) nucleus pulposus, and (3) the vertebral endplates of the vertebral bodies.

- The outer **annulus fibrosus** is a tough fibrous ring of fibrocartilaginous material that encircles and encloses the inner nucleus pulposus.
  - The annulus fibrosus is composed of up to 10 to 20 concentric rings of fibrous material.
  - These rings are arranged in a basket weave configuration that allows the annulus fibrosus to resist forces from different directions (Figure 7-12).

BOX 7-16

More specifically, the basket weave configuration of the fibers of the annulus fibrosus gives the disc a great ability to resist distraction forces (i.e., a vertical separation of the two vertebrae), shear forces (i.e., a horizontal sliding of one vertebra on the other), and torsion forces (i.e., a twisting of one vertebra on the other).

- The inner **nucleus pulposus** is a pulplike gel material that is located in the center of the disc and is enclosed by the annulus fibrosus.

BOX 7-17

When a disc pathology occurs, it usually involves damage to the annulus fibrosus, allowing the inner nucleus pulposus to bulge or rupture (i.e., herniate) through the annular fibers. The term **slipped disc** is a nonspecific lay term that does not really mean anything. Discs do not "slip," they either bulge or rupture. When this does occur, the most common danger is that the nearby spinal nerve may be compressed in the intervertebral foramen, resulting in a pinched nerve that refers symptoms to whatever location of the body that this nerve innervates.

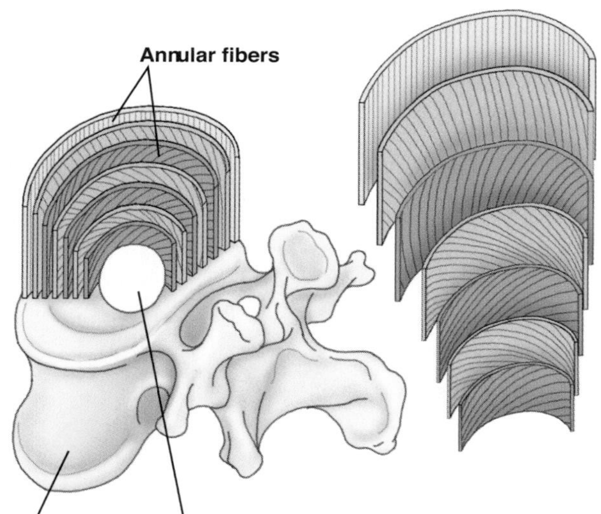

Figure 7-12 The basket weave configuration of the concentric layers of the annulus fibrosus of the intervertebral disc joint. The reader should note how each successive layer has a different orientation to its fibers than the previous layer. Each layer is optimal at resisting the force that runs along its direction. The sum total of having all these varying fiber directions is to resist and stabilize the disc joint along most any line of force to which the joint may be subjected. (Modeled after Kapandji IA: *Physiology of the joints: the trunk and the vertebral column,* ed. 2. Edinburgh, 1974, Churchill Livingstone.)

- The nucleus pulposus has a water content that is 80% or greater.

BOX 7-18

The reason that the nucleus pulposus has such high water content is that it is largely composed of proteoglycans. Therefore given the principle of thixotropy (see Section 3-13), movement of the spine is critically important toward maintaining proper disc hydration and health. (Note: Because disc hydration is responsible for the thickness of the disc, loss of disc hydration would also result in thinning of the disc height and approximation of the vertebral bodies, resulting in an increased likelihood of spinal nerve compression in the intervertebral foramina.)

- The **vertebral endplate** is composed of both hyaline articular cartilage and fibrocartilage, and it lines the surface of the vertebral body. Each disc joint contains two vertebral endplates: one lining the inferior surface of the superior vertebra and the other lining the superior surface of the inferior vertebra.

Vertebral Facet Joints:

- Technically, the correct name for a facet joint is an **apophyseal joint** or a **zygapophyseal joint**. However, these joints of the spine are usually referred to as simply the *facet joints*.

BOX 7-19

Because a facet is a smooth flat surface (think of the facets of a cut stone ring), and the facet joints are formed by the smooth flat surfaces (i.e., the facets) of the articular processes; the name *facet joint* is usually used to refer to these apophyseal (or zygapophyseal) joints of the spine. However, it must be kept in mind that when referring to these joints as facet joints, the context must be clear because other joints in the body involve facets. Facet joints are also often referred to as **Z joints** (*Z* for zygapophyseal).

- A vertebral **facet joint** is located between the articular processes of two contiguous vertebrae.
  - More specifically, a facet joint of the spine is formed by the inferior articular process of the superior vertebra articulating with the superior articular process of the inferior vertebra (Figure 7-13).
- The actual articular surfaces of a facet joint are the facets of the articular processes, hence the name *facet joint*.
- There are two facet joints, paired left and right, between each two contiguous vertebrae.
- Joint structure classification: Synovial joint
  - Subtype: Plane
- Joint function classification: Diarthrotic

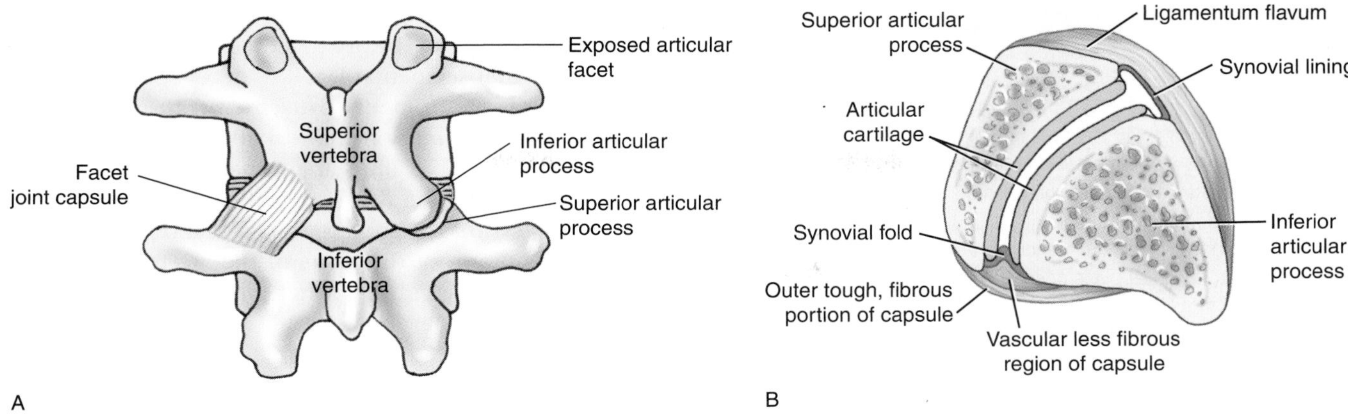

Figure 7-13 The vertebral facet joints. *A,* Posterior view of two contiguous vertebrae. On the left side, the facet joint capsule is seen intact. On the right side, the facet joint capsule has been removed, showing the superior and inferior articular processes; the articular facets of these processes articulate to form a facet joint. The superior articular facet surface of the right articular process of the superior vertebra is also visible and labeled. *B,* Cross-section through a facet joint showing the articular cartilage, fibrous capsule, and synovial lining.

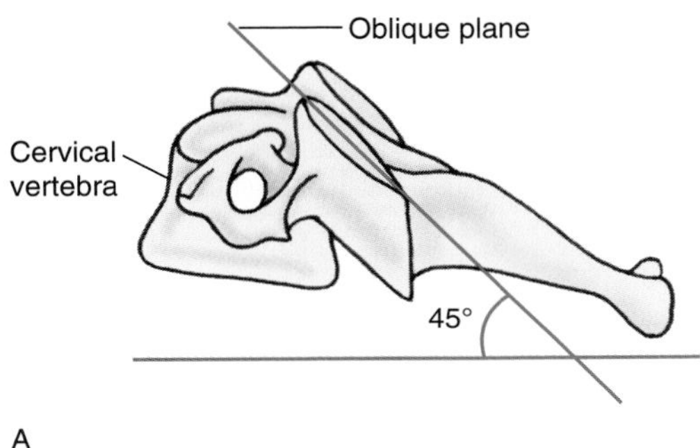

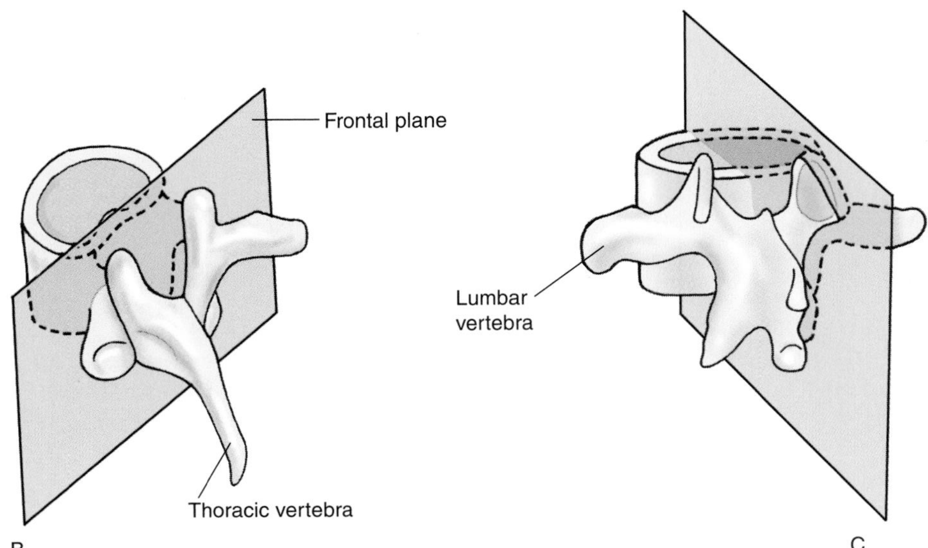

Figure 7-14 General orientation of the planes of the facets for the three regions of the spine. *A,* Lateral view of a cervical vertebra demonstrating the oblique plane of the cervical facet joints, which is approximately 45 degrees between the transverse and frontal planes. *B,* Posterolateral view of a thoracic vertebra demonstrating the frontal plane orientation of the thoracic facet planes. *C,* Posterolateral view of a lumbar vertebra demonstrating the sagittal plane orientation of the lumbar facet planes. The orientation of the facet planes is important because it is the largest determinant of what motion is allowed at the facet joints at that level of the spine.

Miscellaneous:

- ❑ The main purpose of a facet joint is to guide movement.
- ❑ The planes of the facets of the facet joint determine the movement that is best allowed at that level of the spine (Figure 7-14).
- ❑ The cervical facets are generally oriented in an oblique plane that is approximately 45 degrees between the transverse and frontal planes. Therefore these facet joints freely allow transverse and frontal plane motions (i.e., right rotation and left rotation within the transverse plane, and right lateral flexion and left lateral flexion within the frontal plane).

BOX 7-20

The orientation of the cervical facets is often compared with the angle of roof shingles. However, as good as these regional rules for facet orientation are, it should be pointed out that they are generalizations. For example, the facet orientation at the upper cervical spine is nearly perfectly in the transverse plane, not a 45-degree angle like the midcervical region. Further, the orientation of the facet planes is a gradual transition from one region of the spine to the next region. For example, the facet plane orientation of C6-7 of the cervical spine is more similar to the facet plane orientation of T1-2 of the thoracic spine than it is similar to C2-3 of the cervical spine. To determine what motion is best facilitated by the facet planes at any particular segmental level, the facet joint orientation at that level should be observed.

- The thoracic facets are generally oriented within the frontal plane. Therefore these facet joints freely allow right lateral flexion and left lateral flexion within the frontal plane.
- The lumbar facets are generally oriented within the sagittal plane. Therefore these facet joints freely allow flexion and extension within the sagittal plane.

Spinal Joint Segmental Motion—Coupling Disc and Facet Joints:

Comparing and contrasting motion allowed by the disc and facet joints, the following can be stated:

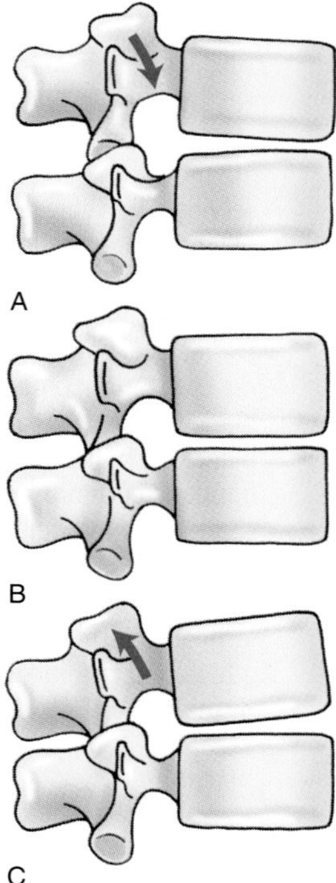

Figure 7-15 Flexion and extension within the sagittal plane of a vertebra on the vertebra that is below it. *A,* Flexion of the vertebra. *B,* Neutral position. *C,* Extension of the vertebra. These motions are a combination of disc and facet joint motion. (Note: All views are lateral.)

- The disc joint and the two facet joints at any particular spinal joint level work together to create the movement at that segmental level.
- Disc joints are primarily concerned with determining the amount of motion that occurs at a particular segmental level; facet joints are primarily concerned with guiding the motion that occurs at that segmental level.
- The thicker that the disc is, the more motion it allows; the orientation of the plane of the facets of that segmental level determines what type of motion is best allowed at that level.

Major Motions Allowed:

- Spinal joints allow flexion and extension (i.e., axial movements) within the sagittal plane around a mediolateral axis (Figures 7-15.

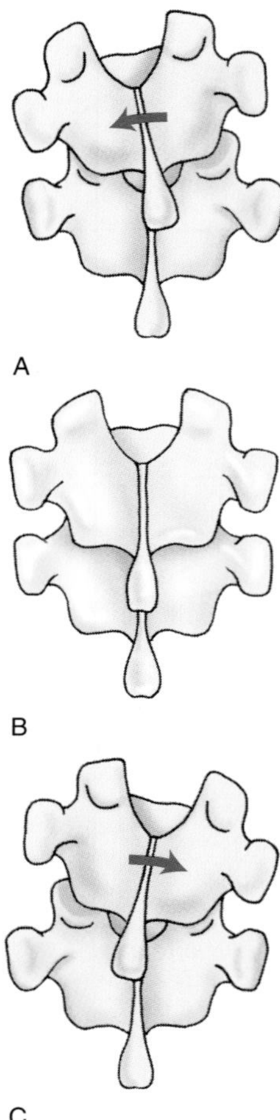

Figure 7-16 Left lateral flexion and right lateral flexion within the frontal plane of a vertebra on the vertebra that is below it. *A,* Left lateral flexion of the vertebra. *B,* Neutral position. *C,* Right lateral flexion of the vertebra. These motions are a combination of disc and facet joint motion. (Note: All views are posterior.)

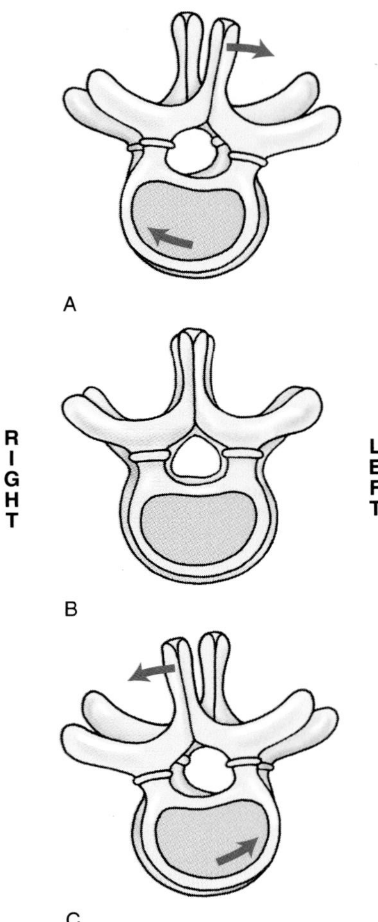

Figure 7-17 Left rotation and right rotation within the transverse plane of a vertebra on the vertebra that is below it. *A,* Left rotation of the vertebra. *B,* Neutral position. *C,* Right rotation of the vertebra. These motions are a combination of disc and facet joint motion. The reader should note that rotation of a vertebra is named for where the anterior aspect of the vertebra (i.e., the body) points. (Note: All views are superior.)

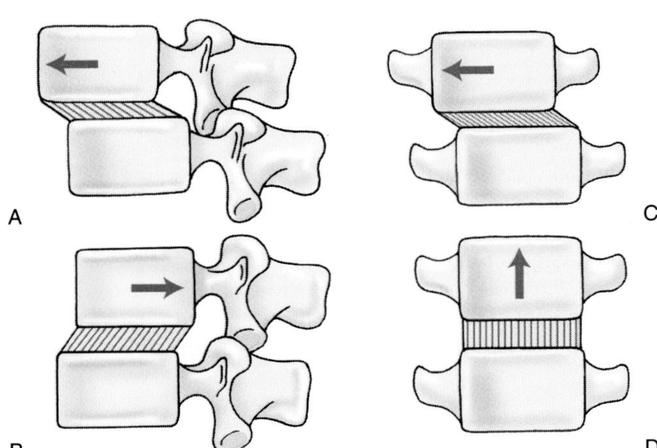

Figure 7-18 Translation motions of a vertebra on the vertebra that is below it. *A,* Anterior translation of the vertebra. *B,* Posterior translation. *C,* Lateral translation to the right of the vertebra (lateral translation to the left would be the opposite motion). *D,* Superior translation of the vertebra (inferior translation would be the opposite motion). All translation motions are a combination of disc and facet joint motion. *A* and *B* are lateral views; *C* and *D* are anterior views.

- ❑ Spinal joints allow right lateral flexion and left lateral flexion (i.e., axial movements) within the frontal plane around an anteroposterior axis (Figure 7-16).
- ❑ Spinal joints allow right rotation and left rotation (i.e., axial movements) within the transverse plane around a vertical axis (Figure 7-17).
- ❑ Spinal joints allow gliding translational movements in three directions (Figure 7-18):
  1. Right-side and left-side translation
  2. Anterior and posterior translation
  3. Superior and inferior translation

BOX 7-21

Perhaps the best visual example of lateral translation of the spinal joints of the neck is the typically thought of "Egyptian" dance movement wherein the head is moved from side to side.

Reverse Actions:

- ❑ Generally when we speak of motion at spinal joints, it is usually the more superior vertebra that is thought of as moving on the more fixed inferior vertebra; this is certainly the usual scenario for a person that is either standing or seated, because the lower part of our body is more fixed in these positions. However, it is possible, especially when lying down, for the more superior vertebrae to stay fixed and to move the more inferior vertebrae relative to the more fixed superior vertebrae of the spine.

Major Ligaments of the Spinal Joints:

The following ligaments provide stability to the spine by limiting excessive spinal motions (Figures 7-19 and 7-20).

BOX 7-22

LIGAMENTS OF THE SPINE

- Fibrous capsules of the facet joints
- Annulus fibrosus of the disc joints
- Anterior longitudinal ligament
- Posterior longitudinal ligament
- Interspinous ligaments
- Supraspinous ligament
- Intertransverse ligaments
- Nuchal ligament

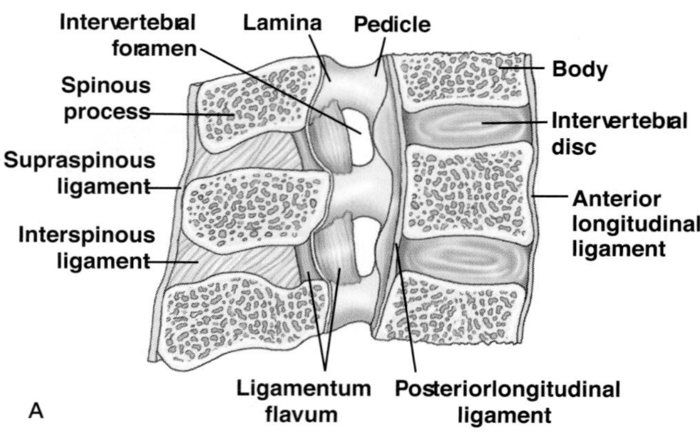

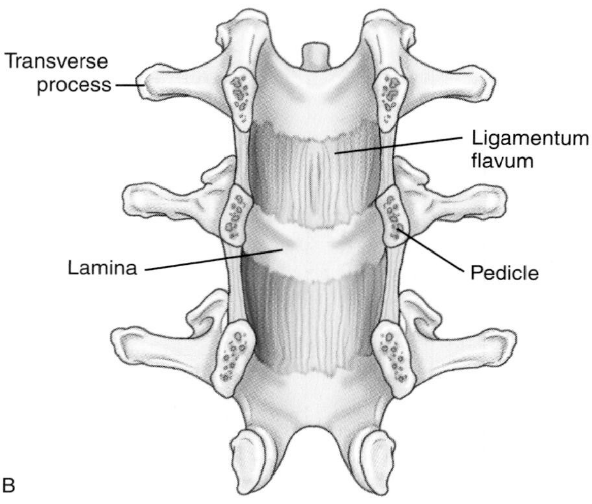

Figure 7-19 Ligaments of the spine. *A,* Lateral view of a sagittal cross-section. The anterior longitudinal ligament runs along the anterior aspect of the vertebral bodies; the posterior longitudinal ligament runs along the posterior aspect of the vertebral bodies. The interspinous ligaments are located between spinous processes; the supraspinous ligament runs along the posterior margin of the spinous processes. The ligamentum flavum runs along the anterior aspect of the laminae (within the spinal canal). *B,* Posterior view of a coronal (frontal) plane cross-section in which all structures anterior to the pedicles have been removed. This view best illustrates the ligamentum flava running along the anterior aspect of the laminae within the spinal canal.

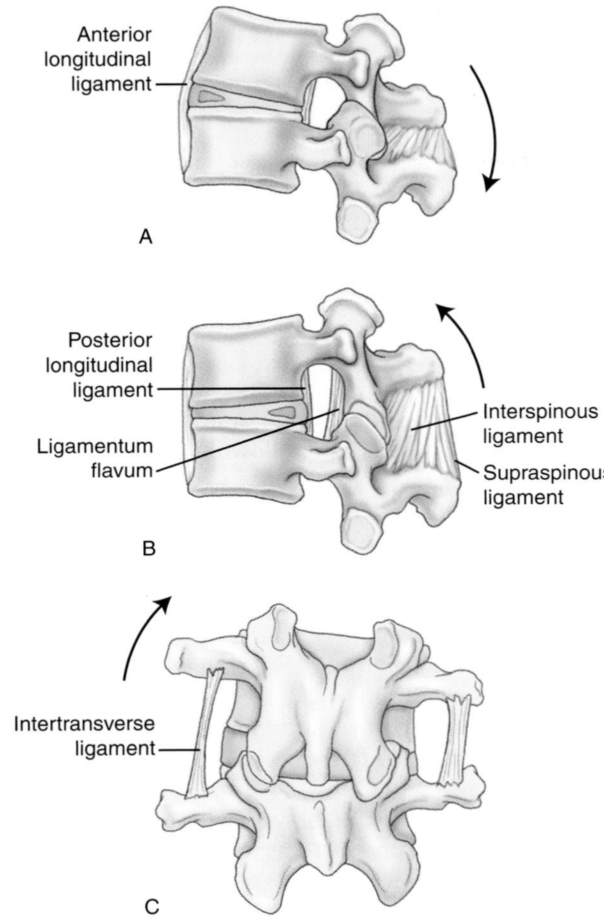

Figure 7-20 Demonstration of how ligaments of the spine limit motion. *A*, The superior vertebra in extension. The anterior longitudinal ligament located anteriorly becomes taut, limiting this motion. *B*, The superior vertebra in flexion. All ligaments on the posterior side (supraspinous, interspinous, ligamentum flavum, and posterior longitudinal ligaments) become taut, limiting this motion. *C*, The superior vertebra in (right) lateral flexion. The intertransverse ligament on the opposite (left) side becomes taut, limiting this motion. (Note: In this position the opposite side [left] facet joint capsule would also become taut, limiting this motion. *A* and *B* are lateral views; *C* is a posterior view.)

❑ Note that in all cases, the ligaments of the spine limit motion that would occur in the opposite direction from where the ligament is located (this rule is true for all ligaments of the body). For example, anterior ligaments limit the posterior motion of vertebral extension; posterior ligaments limit the anterior motion of vertebral flexion. The dividing line for anterior versus posterior is determined by where the center of motion is (i.e., where the axis of motion is located). For sagittal plane motions of the spine, the axis of motion is located between the bodies.

Fibrous Joint Capsules of the Facet Joints:

❑ Location: They are located between articular processes of adjacent vertebrae of the spine (see Figure 7-13a).

❑ Function: They stabilize the facet joints and limit the extremes of all spinal joint motions except extension (and inferior translation [i.e., compression of the two vertebrae wherein they come closer together]).

Annulus Fibrosus of the Disc Joints:

❑ Location: It is located between adjacent vertebral bodies (see Figures 7-11 and 7-19a).

❑ Function: It stabilizes the disc joints and limits the extremes of all spinal motions (except inferior translation).

Anterior Longitudinal Ligament:

❑ Location: The **anterior longitudinal ligament** runs along the anterior margins of the bodies of the vertebrae (see Figure 7-19a).

❑ Function: It limits extension of the spinal joints.

Posterior Longitudinal Ligament:

❑ Location: The **posterior longitudinal ligament** runs along the posterior margins of the bodies of the vertebrae (within the spinal canal) (see Figure 7-19a).

❑ Function: It limits flexion of the spinal joints.

Ligamentum Flava:

❑ Two **ligamentum flava** (singular: ligamentum flavum) are located on the left and right sides of the spinal column.

❑ Location: They run along the anterior margins of the laminae of the vertebrae (within the spinal canal) (see Figure 7-19).

❑ Function: They limit flexion of the spinal joints.

Interspinous Ligaments:

❑ Location: The **interspinous ligaments** are separate short ligaments that run between adjacent spinous processes of the vertebrae (see Figure 7-19a).

❑ Function: They limit flexion of the spinal joints.

Supraspinous Ligament:

❑ Location: The **supraspinous ligament** runs along the posterior margins of the spinous processes of the vertebrae (see Figure 7-19a).

❑ Function: It limits flexion of the spinal joints.

Intertransverse Ligaments:

- ❑ Location: The **intertransverse ligaments** are separate short ligaments that run between adjacent transverse processes of the vertebrae (see Figure 7-20c).
- ❑ Function: They limit contralateral (i.e., opposite sided) lateral flexion of the spinal joints.

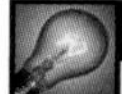

BOX 7-23

Intertransverse spinal ligaments are usually absent in the neck.

Nuchal Ligament:

- ❑ The **nuchal ligament** is a ligament that runs along and between the spinous processes from C7 to the external occipital protuberance of the skull. The nuchal ligament is often described as a combination of the interspinous and supraspinous ligaments of the cervical region.

BOX 7-24

Some of the nuchal ligament's deepest fibers interdigitate into the dura matter. Clinically, this raises the question of whether tension on the nuchal ligament (perhaps from tight muscle insertions) may create an adverse pull on the dura mater.

- ❑ Function: It limits flexion of the spinal joints and provides a site of attachment for muscles of the neck (Figure 7-21).

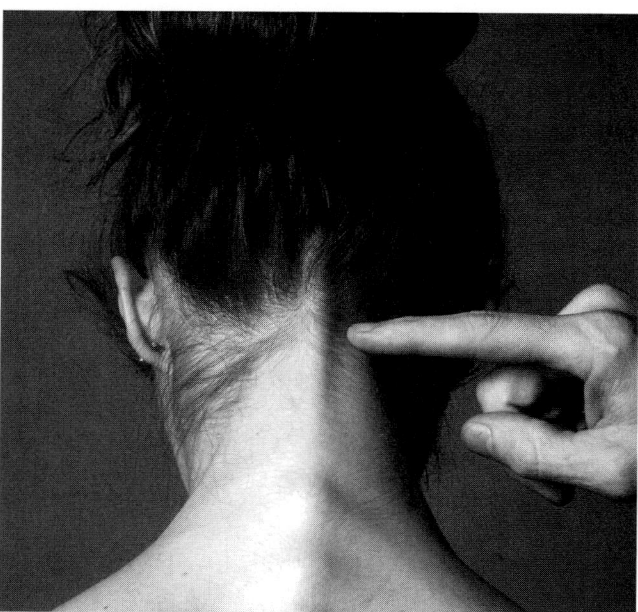

Figure 7-21 Posterior view of a young woman. The nuchal ligament of the cervical region is seen to be taut as she flexes her head and neck at the spinal joints. (From Neumann DA: *Kinesiology of the musculoskeletal system: foundations for physical rehabilitation,* St Louis, 2002, Mosby.

BOX 7-25

Four-legged animals such as dogs have a very taut and stable nuchal ligament. This is necessary to hold their heads and necks from falling into flexion, because their heads and necks are not posturally supported by their trunks.

The trapezius, splenius capitis, rhomboids, serratus posterior superior, and the cervical spinales (of the erector spinae group) all attach into the nuchal ligament of the neck.

A complete list of all muscles is located in the appendix found on page 632.

Major Muscles of the Spinal Joints:

Many muscles cross the spinal joints. Regarding the actions of these muscles, the following general rules can be stated:

- ❑ Muscles that do extension of the spine are located in the posterior trunk and neck and run with a vertical direction to their fibers. The erector spinae group, transversospinalis group, and other muscles in the posterior neck are examples of spinal extensors.
- ❑ Muscles that do flexion of the spine are located in the anterior body and run with a vertical direction to their fibers. The muscles of the anterior abdominal wall and the muscles in the anterior neck are examples of spinal flexors.
- ❑ Muscles that do lateral flexion are located on the side of the body and run with a vertical direction to their fibers. Most all flexors and extensors are also lateral flexors, because they are usually located *anterior and lateral* or *posterior and lateral*. It should be noted that all lateral flexors are ipsilateral lateral flexors (i.e., whichever side of the body that they are located on is the side to which they laterally flex the body part [head, neck, and/or trunk]).
- ❑ Muscles that do rotation are more variable in their location. For example, muscles that do right rotation of the head, neck, or trunk may be located anteriorly or posteriorly; further, they may be located on the right side of the body (in which case they are ipsilateral rotators) or the left side of the body (in which case they are contralateral rotators). Prominent rotators of the trunk include the external and internal abdominal obliques and the transversospinalis group muscles. Prominent rotators of the head and/or neck include the SCM, upper trapezius, splenius capitis and cervicis muscles, as well as the transversospinalis group muscles.

7.5 ATLANTO-OCCIPITAL AND ATLANTOAXIAL JOINTS

Two cervical spinal joints merit special consideration:

- The **atlanto-occipital joint** (AOJ), located between the atlas (C1) and the occiput
- The **atlantoaxial joint** (AAJ or C1-C2 joint), located between the atlas (C1) and the axis (C2)

Atlanto-Occipital Joint:

- The AOJ (Figure 7-22) is formed by the superior articular facets of the atlas (the 1st cervical vertebra [i.e., C1]) meeting the occipital condyles.
  - Therefore the AOJ has two lateral joint surfaces (i.e., two facet joints). Because the atlas has no body, no median disc joint exists as is usual for spinal joints.

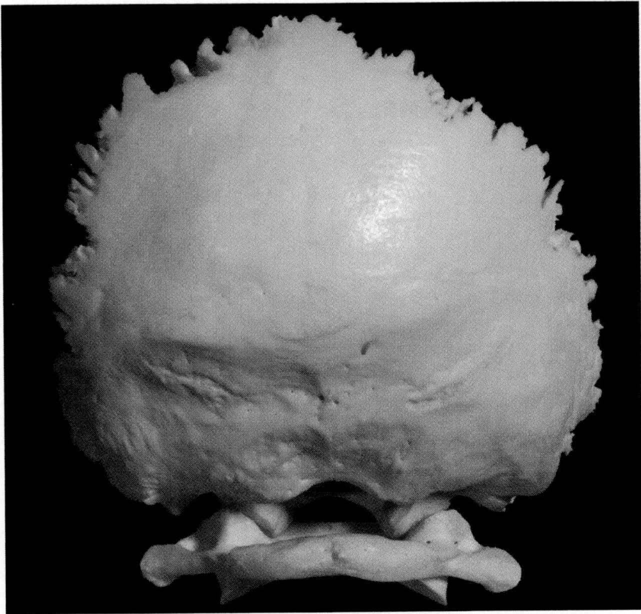

Figure 7-22 Posterior view of the atlanto-occipital joint (AOJ). In this photo, the occipital bone is flexed (i.e., lifted upward) to better view this joint. The AOJ is composed of two lateral joint articulations between the superior articular processes of the atlas and the condyles of the occiput.

- The occipital condyles are convex and the facets of the atlas are concave. This allows the occipital condyles to rock in the concave facets of the atlas.
- Movement of the AOJ allows the cranium to move relative to the atlas (i.e., the head to move on the neck).
- Joint structure classification: Synovial joint
  - Subtype: Condyloid
- Joint function classification: Diarthrotic
  - Subtype: Triaxial

BOX 7-26

The amount of rotation possible at the atlanto-occipital joint (AOJ) is considered to be negligible by many sources. Therefore these sources place the AOJ as being biaxial.

Movement of the Head at the Atlanto-Occipital Joint:

Even though the head usually moves with the neck, the head and neck are separate body parts and can move independently from one another. The presence of the AOJ allows the head to move independently from the neck. When the head moves, it is said to move relative to the neck at the AOJ (Figures 7-23 to 7-25). Following are the movements of the head at the AOJ (the ranges of motion are given in Table 7-2):

- Flexion/extension (i.e., axial movements) in the sagittal plane around a mediolateral axis are the primary motions of the AOJ.

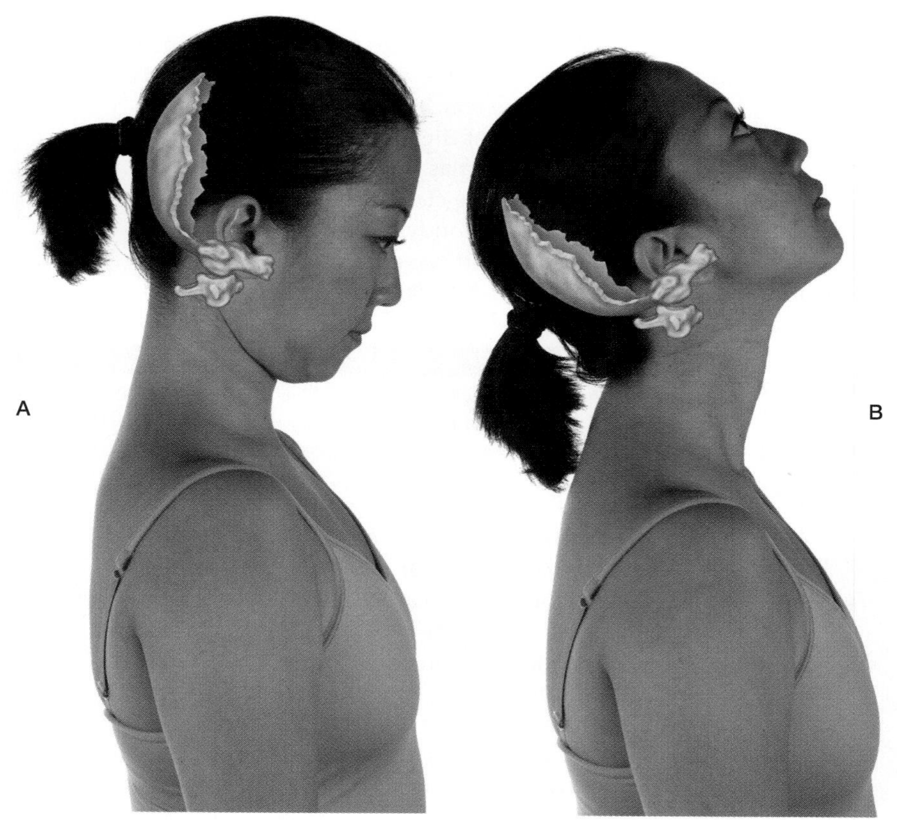

Figure 7-23 Lateral view illustrating sagittal plane motions of the head at the atlanto-occipital joint (AOJ). A illustrates flexion; B illustrates extension. The sagittal plane actions of flexion and extension are the primary motions of the AOJ.

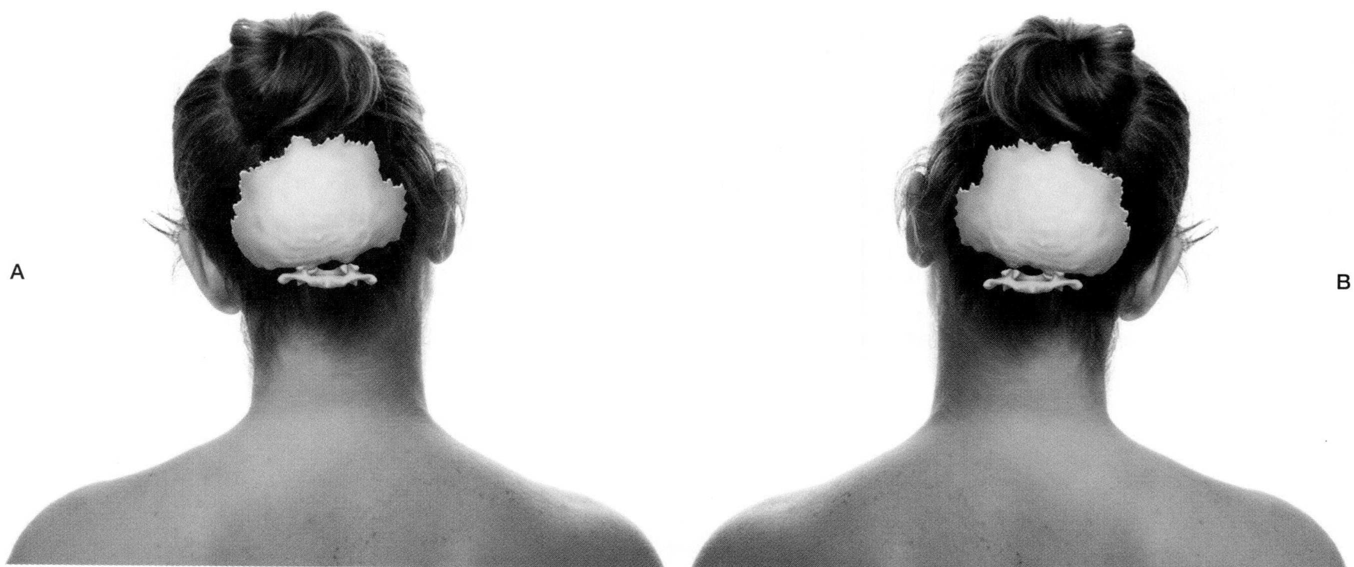

Figure 7-24 Posterior view illustrating lateral flexion motions of the head at the atlanto-occipital joint (AOJ). *A* illustrates left lateral flexion; *B* illustrates right lateral flexion. These actions occur in the frontal plane.

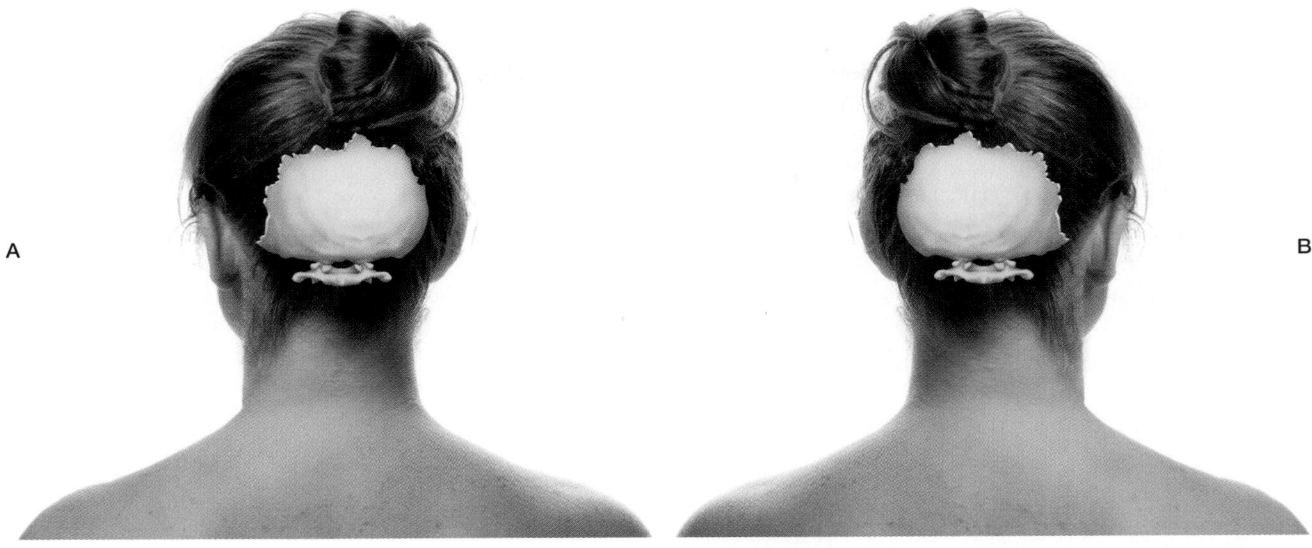

Figure 7-25 Posterior view that illustrates rotation motions of the head at the atlanto-occipital joint (AOJ). *A* illustrates left rotation; *B* illustrates right rotation.These actions occur in the transverse plane.

TABLE 7-2

Average Ranges of Motion of the Head at the Atlantooccipital Joint (AOJ) from Anatomic Position

Flexion	5 Degrees	Extension	10 Degrees
Right lateral flexion	5 Degrees	Left lateral flexion	5 Degrees
Right rotation	5 Degrees	Left rotation	5 Degrees

BOX 7-27
The motion of nodding the head (as in indicating *yes*) is primarily created by flexing and extending the head at the AOJ.

- Right lateral flexion/left lateral flexion (i.e., axial movements) in the frontal plane around an anteroposterior axis are also allowed.
- Right rotation/left rotation (i.e., axial movements) in the transverse plane around a vertical axis are also allowed.

Atlantoaxial (C1-C2) Joint:

- The AAJ allows the atlas (C1) to move on the axis (C2) (Figure 7-26).
- The AAJ is composed of one median joint and two lateral joints.
- The median joint of the AAJ is the **atlanto-odontoid joint**.

BOX 7-28
Intervertebral disc joints are located between bodies of adjacent vertebrae. Because the atlas has no body, there cannot be an intervertebral disc joint between the atlas and axis at the atlantoaxial (C1-C2) joint.

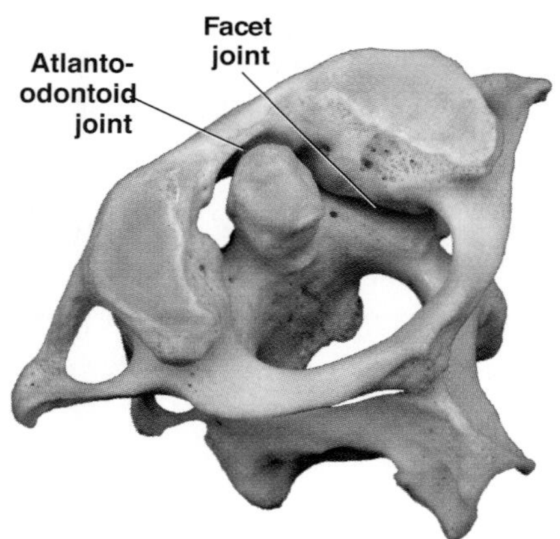

Figure 7-26 Oblique (superior posterolateral) view of the atlantoaxial joint (AAJ) (C1-C2). The AAJ is comprised of three joints: a median atlanto-odontoid joint and two lateral facet joints.

  - The atlanto-odontoid joint is formed by the anterior arch of the atlas meeting the odontoid process (i.e., dens) of the axis.
  - Articular facets are located on the joint surfaces of the atlas and axis (i.e., on the posterior surface of the anterior arch of the atlas and the anterior surface of the dens of the axis).
  - The atlanto-odontoid joint actually has two synovial cavities, one anterior to the dens and the other posterior to the dens.
- The two lateral joints are the facet joints.
  - The facet joints of the AAJ are formed by the inferior articular facets of the atlas (C1) meeting the superior articular facets of the axis (C2).
- Joint structure classification: Synovial joints
  - Subtype: Atlanto-odontoid joint: Pivot joint
  - Lateral facet joints: Plane joints
- Joint function classification: Diarthrotic
  - Subtype: Biaxial

BOX 7-29
The atlanto-odontoid joint itself is often described as a *uniaxial pivot joint*. However, the atlantoaxial joint (AAJ) complex (i.e., the median and two lateral joints) allows motion in two planes around two axes. Therefore all three AAJs, including the atlanto-odontoid joint, technically are biaxial joints.

Movements of the Atlantoaxial Joint:

- Right rotation/left rotation (i.e., axial movements) in the transverse plane around a vertical axis are the primary motions of the AAJ.

BOX 7-30
Approximately half of all the rotation of the cervical spine occurs at the atlantoaxial joint (AAJ). When you turn your head from side to side indicating *no*, the majority of that movement occurs at the AAJ.

- Flexion/extension (i.e., axial movements) in the sagittal plane around a mediolateral axis are also allowed.
- Right lateral flexion/left lateral flexion (i.e., axial movements) are negligible.
- The ranges of motion of the AAJ are given in Table 7-3.

TABLE 7-3

Average Ranges of Motion of the Atlas at the Atlantoaxial Joint (AAJ) (C1-C2 Joint) from Anatomic Position

Flexion	5 Degrees	Extension	10 Degrees
Right lateral flexion	Negligible	Left lateral flexion	Negligible
Right rotation	40 Degrees	Left rotation	40 Degrees

Major Ligaments of the Occipito-Atlantoaxial Region:

The following ligaments all provide stability to the AOJ and AAJ by limiting excessive motion of these joints:

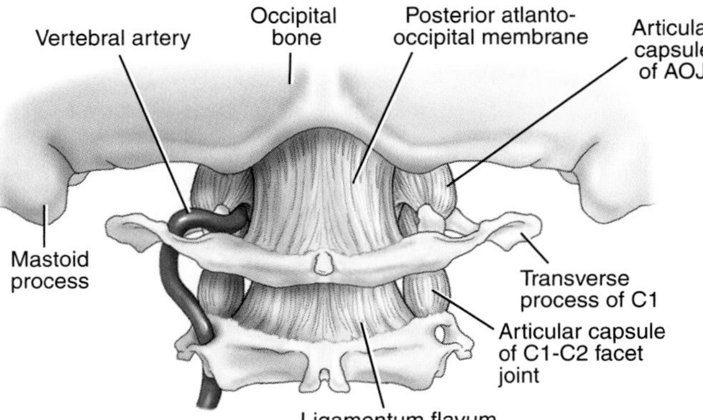

Figure 7-27 Posterior view of the upper cervical region demonstrating the facet joint capsules of the atlanto-occipital joint (AOJ) and atlantoaxial joints (AAJs), as well as the posterior atlanto-occipital membrane between the atlas and occiput. The posterior atlanto-occipital membrane is the continuation of the ligamentum flavum.

BOX 7-31

LIGAMENTS OF THE UPPER CERVICAL (OCCIPITO-ATLANTOAXIAL) REGION

- Nuchal ligament
- Facet joint fibrous capsules of the atlanto-occipital joint (AOJ)
- Facet joint fibrous capsules of the atlantoaxial joint (AAJ)
- Posterior atlanto-occipital membrane
- Tectorial membrane
- Accessory atlantoaxial ligament
- Cruciate ligament of the dens
- Alar ligaments of the dens
- Apical odontoid ligament
- Anterior longitudinal ligament
- Anterior atlanto-occipital membrane

Nuchal Ligament:

- ❑ The nuchal ligament (see Figure 7-21) of the cervical spine continues through this region to attach onto the occiput.
- ❑ Functions: It limits flexion in this region and provides an attachment site for many muscles of the neck.

Posterior Atlanto-Occipital Membrane:

- ❑ Location: The **posterior atlanto-occipital membrane** is located between the posterior arch of the atlas and the occiput.
- ❑ The posterior atlanto-occipital membrane between the atlas and occiput is the continuation of the ligamentum flavum of the spine (Figure 7-27).
- ❑ Function: It stabilizes the AOJ.

Fibrous Capsules of Facet Joints of the Atlanto-Occipital Joints:

- ❑ Location: They are located between the condyles of the occiput and the superior articular processes of the atlas (see Figure 7-27).
- ❑ Function: They stabilize the atlanto-occipital facet joints.

Fibrous Capsules of Facet Joints of the Atlantoaxial Joints:

- ❑ Location: They are located between the inferior articular processes of the atlas and the superior articular processes of the axis (see Figure 7-27).
- ❑ Function: They stabilize the atlantoaxial facet joints.

Tectorial Membrane:

- ❑ Location: The **tectorial membrane** is located within the spinal canal, just posterior to the cruciate ligament of the dens (Figure 7-28a).
- ❑ The tectorial membrane is the continuation of the posterior longitudinal ligament in the region of C2 to the occiput.
- ❑ The **accessory atlantoaxial ligament** (which runs from C2-C1) is considered to be composed of deep fibers of the tectorial membrane (see Figure 7-28a–b).
- ❑ Function: It stabilizes the AAJ and AOJ; more specifically, it limits flexion in this region.

Cruciate Ligament of the Dens:

- ❑ The **cruciate ligament of the dens** attaches the dens of the axis to the atlas and occiput (see Figure 7-28b).

BOX 7-32

The cruciate ligament is given this name because it has the shape of a cross; *cruciate* means cross.

- ❑ It has three parts: (1) a transverse band, (2) a superior vertical band, and (3) an inferior vertical band.
- ❑ The transverse band of the cruciate ligament is often called the **transverse ligament of the atlas**; the superior vertical band of the cruciate ligament is often called the **apical dental ligament** (located directly posterior to the apical odontoid ligament).
- ❑ Location: It is located within the spinal canal, between the tectorial membrane and the alar ligaments

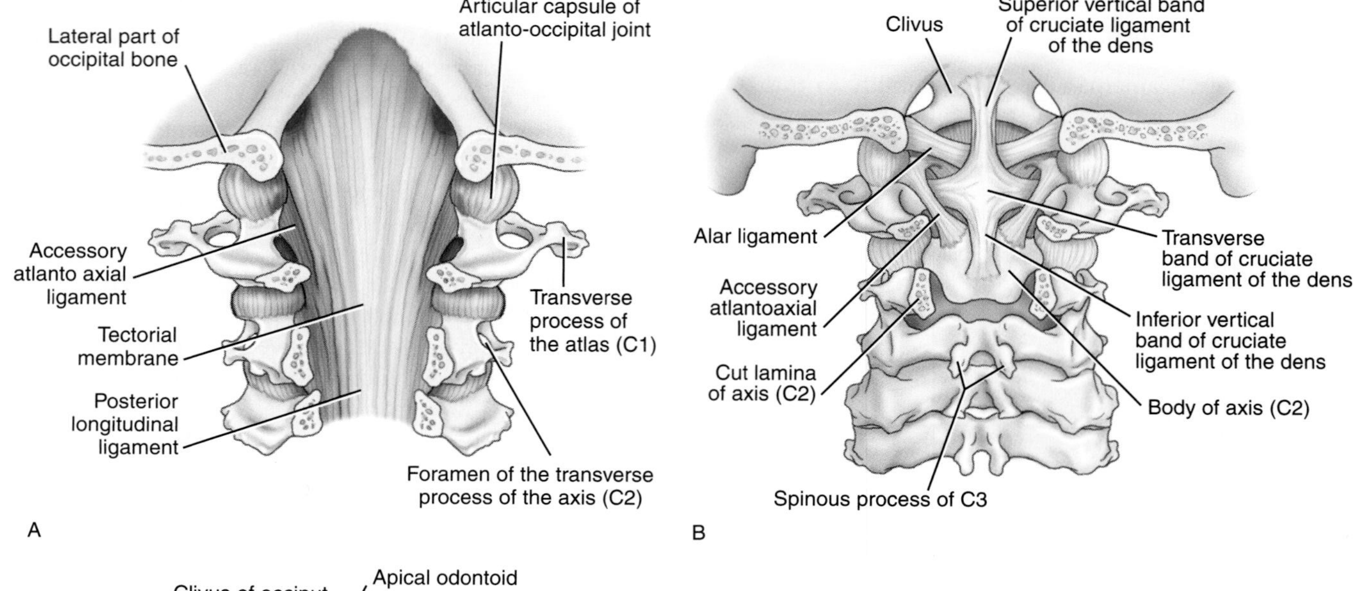

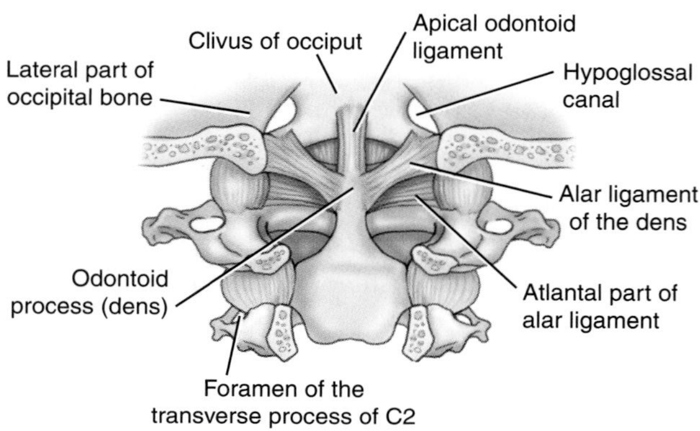

Figure 7-28 Posterior views of the upper cervical region within the spinal canal. *A,* Tectorial membrane that is the continuation of the posterior longitudinal ligament. *B,* Cruciate ligament of the dens located between the axis, atlas, and occiput. The cruciate ligament of the dens has three parts: (1) a superior vertical band, (2) an inferior vertical band, and (3) a transverse band. *C,* Apical odontoid and alar ligaments between the odontoid process of the axis and the atlas and occiput.

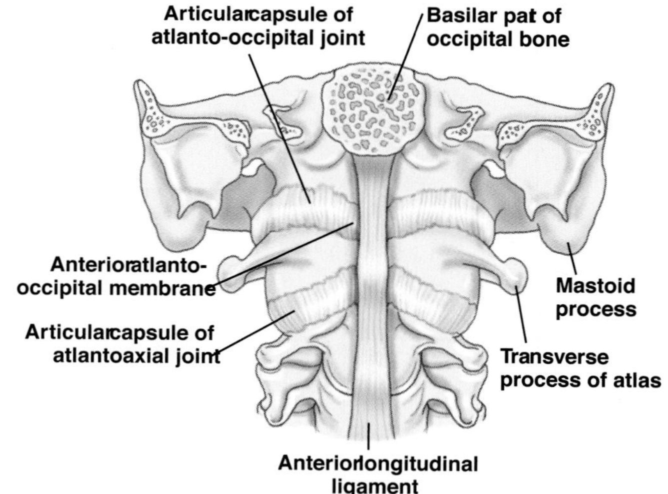

Figure 7-29 Anterior view of the upper cervical region demonstrating the anterior longitudinal ligament and the anterior atlanto-occipital membrane.

(anterior to the tectorial membrane and posterior to the alar ligaments).
- ❑ Functions: It stabilizes the dens and limits anterior translation of the atlas at the AAJ and the head at the AOJ.

Alar Ligaments of the Dens:
- ❑ Two **alar ligaments of the dens** (left and right) exist.
- ❑ Location: They run from the dens to the atlas and occiput (see Figure 7-28b–c).
- ❑ Functions: They stabilize the dens by attaching it to the atlas and occiput, limit right and left rotation of the head at the AOJ and the atlas at the AAJ, and limit superior translation of the head at the AOJ and the atlas at the AAJ.

Apical Odontoid Ligament:
- ❑ Location: The **apical odontoid ligament** runs from the dens to the occiput (see Figure 7-28c).
- ❑ Functions: It stabilizes the dens by attaching it to the occiput and limits superior and anterior translation of the head at the AOJ.

Anterior Longitudinal Ligament:
- ❑ Location: The anterior longitudinal ligament continues through this region, attaching to the body of the axis, the anterior tubercle of the atlas, and ultimately onto the occiput (Figure 7-29).
- ❑ Function: It limits extension in this region.

Anterior Atlanto-Occipital Membrane:
- ❑ Location: The **anterior atlanto-occipital membrane** is located between the anterior arch of the atlas and the occiput (see Figure 7-29).
- ❑ Function: It stabilizes the AOJ.

Major Muscles of the Occipito-Atlantoaxial Region:

Many muscles cross the AOJ and AAJ. (A complete list of muscles of the neck is located in the appendix [see page 632].) Although the functional groups of spinal muscles were addressed in Section 7.4, the following muscles should be specially noted here:
- ❑ Suboccipital group
  - ❑ Rectus capitis posterior major
  - ❑ Rectus capitis posterior minor
  - ❑ Obliquus capitis inferior
  - ❑ Obliquus capitis superior
- ❑ Rectus capitis anterior and rectus capitis lateralis of the prevertebral group

☐ 7.6 CERVICAL SPINE (THE NECK)

- The cervical spine defines the neck as a body part.

Features of the Cervical Spine:

Composition of the Cervical Spine:

- The cervical spine is composed of seven vertebrae (Figure 7-30).
- From superior to inferior, these vertebrae are named C1 through C7.
  - C1: The first cervical vertebra (C1) is also known as the *atlas,* because it holds up the head, much as the Greek mythologic figure Atlas is depicted as holding up the world (Figure 7-31a).

BOX 7-33

Actually, the Greek mythologic figure Atlas was forced by Zeus to hold up the sky, not the Earth. However, in artworks, Atlas is more often depicted as holding up the Earth.

  - C2: The second cervical vertebra (C2) is also known as the *axis,* because the toothlike dens of C2 creates an axis of rotation around which the atlas can rotate (Figure 7-31b). The spinous process of C2 is quite large and is a valuable landmark for palpation.
  - C7: The seventh cervical vertebra (C7) is also known as the **vertebral prominens,** because it is the most prominent cervical vertebra (and often a valuable landmark for palpation).

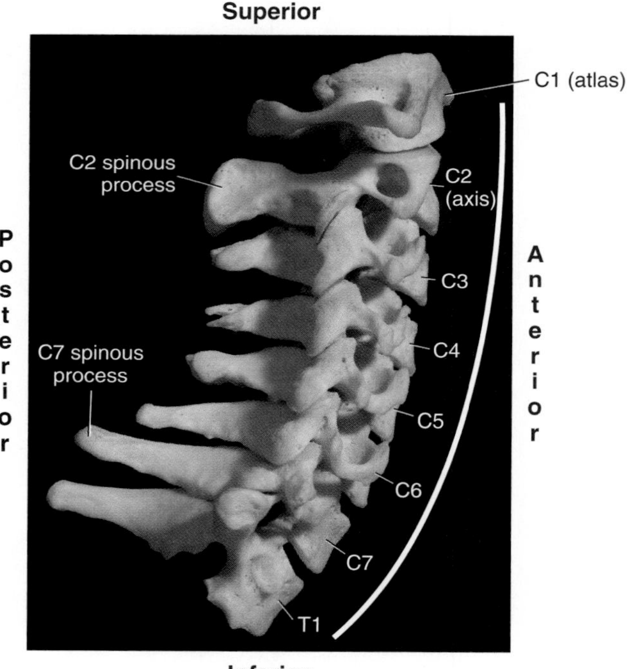

Figure 7-30 Right lateral view of the cervical spine. The reader should note the lordotic curve, which is concave posteriorly (and therefore convex anteriorly).

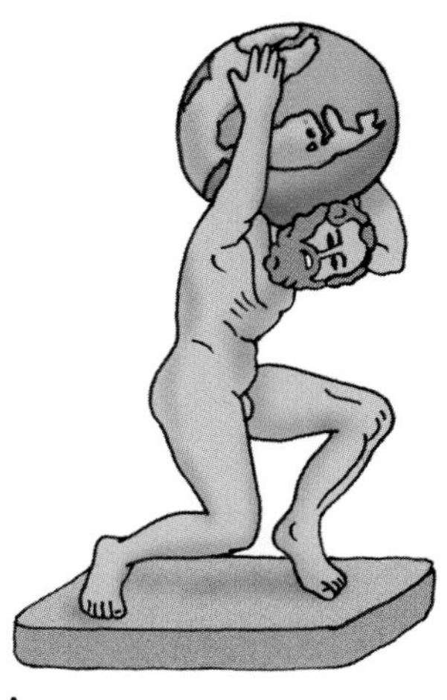

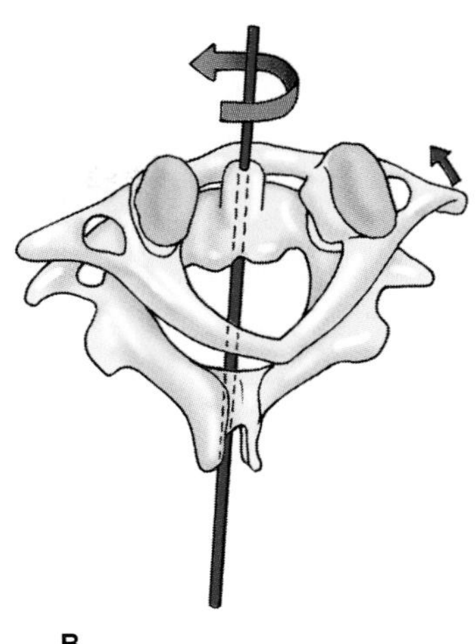

Figure 7-31 *A,* Greek mythologic figure Atlas supporting the world on his shoulder. Similarly, the first cervical vertebra (C1) supports the head. For this reason, C1 is known as the *atlas. B,* Dens of the second cervical vertebra (C2) forming an axis of rotation that the atlas can move around. For this reason, C2 is known as the *axis.*

Special Joints of the Cervical Spine:

- The joint between the atlas and the occiput is known as the *AOJ.*
- The joint between the atlas and the axis is known as the *AAJ* (or the C1-C2 joint). (See Section 7.5 for more information on the AOJ and AAJ.)

Transverse Foramina:

- Cervical vertebrae have transverse foramina in their transverse processes (Figure 7-32a).

BOX 7-34

The cervical transverse foramina allows passage of the two **vertebral arteries** superiorly to the skull (see Figure 7-27). The vertebral arteries enter the cranial cavity to supply the posterior brain with arterial blood. If a client's head and upper neck are extended and rotated, one vertebral artery is naturally pinched off. If the other vertebral artery is blocked because of atherosclerosis or arteriosclerosis, and then the client's head is extended and rotated, the client could lose blood supply to the brain and might experience such symptoms as dizziness, lightheadedness, nausea, or ringing in the ears.

Bifid Spinous Processes:

- The cervical spine has **bifid spinous processes** (i.e., they have two points instead of one) (see Figure 7-32).

BOX 7-35

The presence of bifid spinous processes in the cervical spine may lead an inexperienced massage therapist or bodyworker to believe that a cervical vertebra has a rotational misalignment, when it does not. This is especially true of C2, because its bifid spinous process is so large and often asymmetric in shape.

Bifid Transverse Processes:

- Most transverse processes of the cervical spine are **bifid transverse processes**. The two aspects are called the *anterior and posterior tubercles* (see Figure 7-32).

Uncinate Processes:

- The superior surfaces of the bodies of cervical vertebrae are not flat as in the rest of the spine; rather their lateral sides curve upwards. This feature of the superior cervical body is called an **uncinate process**.
- Where the lateral sides of two contiguous cervical vertebrae meet each other is called an **uncovertebral joint**. (Uncovertebral joints are often called the **joints of Von Luschka**, after the person who first described them.) These uncovertebral joints provide additional stability to the cervical spine because they serve to mildly limit frontal and transverse plane motions of the cervical vertebrae (see Figure 7-32).

Curve of the Cervical Spine:

- The cervical spine has a lordotic curve (i.e., it is concave posteriorly) (see Figure 7-30).

Functions of the Cervical Spine:

- Because only the head is superior to the neck, the cervical region has less of a weight-bearing function than the thoracic and lumbar regions. Having less weight-bearing function means that the cervical spine does not need to be as stable and can allow more movement.
- The cervical spine is the most mobile region of the spine, moving freely in all three planes (Tables 7-4 to 7-6, Box 7-36).
  - One reason that the cervical spine is so very mobile is the thickness of the intervertebral discs. The discs of the cervical spine account for approximately 40% of the height of the neck.

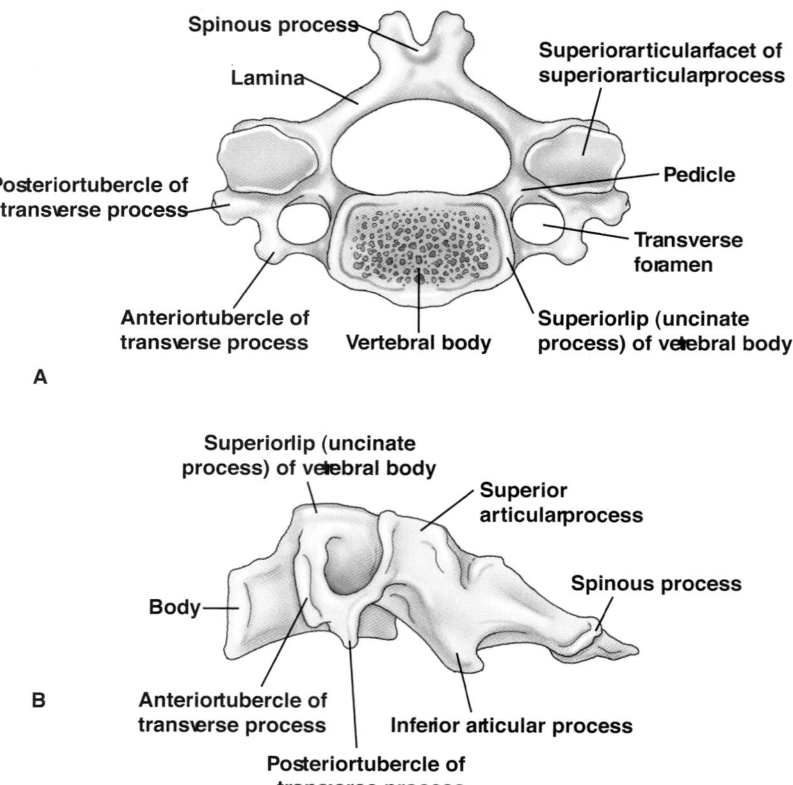

Figure 7-32 *A,* Superior view of a typical cervical vertebra. *B,* Lateral view. The reader should note the bifid spinous and transverse processes.

> **BOX 7-36**
>
> One reason that the cervical spine is so very mobile is the thickness of the intervertebral discs. The discs of the cervical spine account for approximately 40% of the height of the neck.

- The orientation of the cervical facet joints begins in the transverse plane at the top of the cervical spine; this accounts for the tremendous ability of the upper neck to rotate in the transverse plane.
- The cervical facet joints gradually transition from the transverse plane toward the frontal plane so that the facets of the mid- to lower neck are obliquely oriented (similar to shingles on a 45-degree sloped roof) approximately one-half way between the transverse and frontal planes (see Section 7.4, Figure 7-14a).

Major Motions Allowed:

- The cervical spinal joints allow flexion and extension (i.e., axial movements) of the neck in the sagittal plane around a mediolateral axis (Figure 7-33a–b).
- The cervical spinal joints allow right lateral flexion and left lateral flexion (i.e., axial movements) of the neck in the frontal plane around an anteroposterior axis (Figure 7-33c–d).
- The cervical spinal joints allow right rotation and left rotation (i.e., axial movements) of the neck in the transverse plane around a vertical axis (Figure 7-33e–f).
- The cervical spinal joints allow gliding translational movements in all three directions (see Section 7.4, Figure 7-18).

BOX 7-37

Because the facet joints of the cervical spine are oriented between the transverse and frontal planes, when the cervical spine laterally flexes, it ipsilaterally rotates as well. (Note: Remember that vertebral rotation is named for the direction in which the anterior bodies face; the spinous processes would therefore point in the opposite direction.) Therefore these two joint actions of lateral flexion and ipsilateral rotation are coupled together. Consequently, lateral flexion with rotation to the same side is a natural motion for the neck. *A* and *B*, Posterior views. *A* depicts the entire neck and head; *B* is a close-up of two cervical vertebrae.

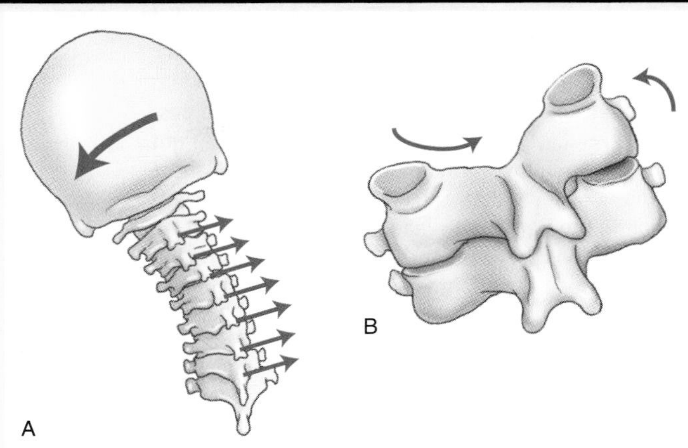

TABLE 7-4

Average Ranges of Motion of the Lower Cervical Spine (C2-C3 Through C7-T1 Joints) from Anatomic Position

Flexion	40 Degrees	Extension	60 Degrees
Right lateral flexion	40 Degrees	Left lateral flexion	40 Degrees
Right rotation	40 Degrees	Left rotation	40 Degrees

TABLE 7-5

Average Ranges of Motion of the Entire Cervical Spine (i.e., the Neck; C1-C2 Through C7-T1 Joints) from Anatomic Position (These Numbers Include the Atlantoaxial Joint [AAJ] [C1-C2] and the Lower Cervical Spine Joints [C2-C3 through C7-T1].)

Flexion	45 Degrees	Extension	70 Degrees
Right lateral flexion	40 Degrees	Left lateral flexion	40 Degrees
Right rotation	80 Degrees	Left rotation	80 Degrees

TABLE 7-6

Average Ranges of Motion of the Entire Cervicocranial Region from Anatomic Position (the Neck and the Head) (These Numbers Include the Entire Cervical Spine [C1-C2 through C7-T1 Joints] and the Head at the Atlanto-occipital Joint [AOJ].)

Flexion	50 Degrees	Extension	80 Degrees
Right lateral flexion	45 Degrees	Left lateral flexion	45 Degrees
Right rotation	85 Degrees	Left rotation	85 Degrees

Figure 7-33 Motions of the neck at the spinal joints. *A* and *B* are lateral views that depict flexion and extension in the sagittal plane, respectively. *C* and *D* are posterior views that depict left lateral flexion and right lateral flexion in the frontal plane, respectively. *E* and *F* are anterior views that depict right rotation and left rotation in the transverse plane, respectively. NOTE: *A-F* depict motions of the entire craniocervical region (i.e., the head at the atlanto-occipital joint and the neck at the spinal joints.)

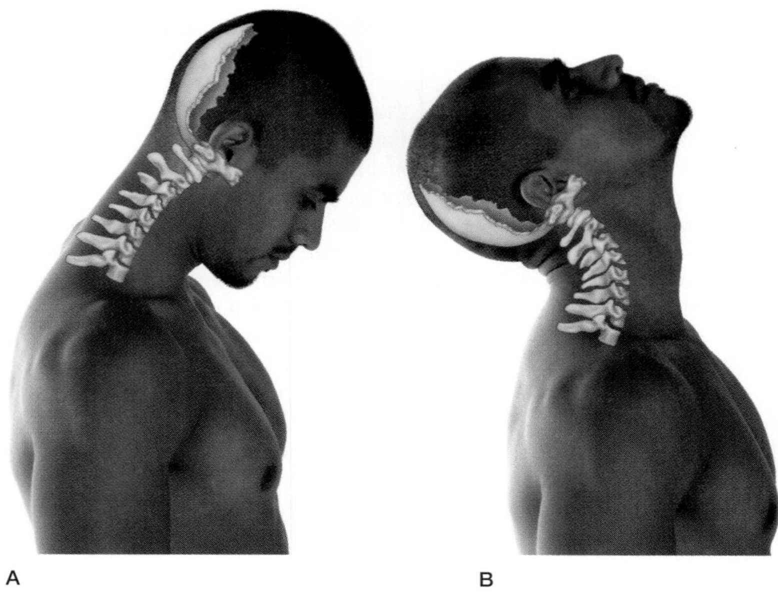

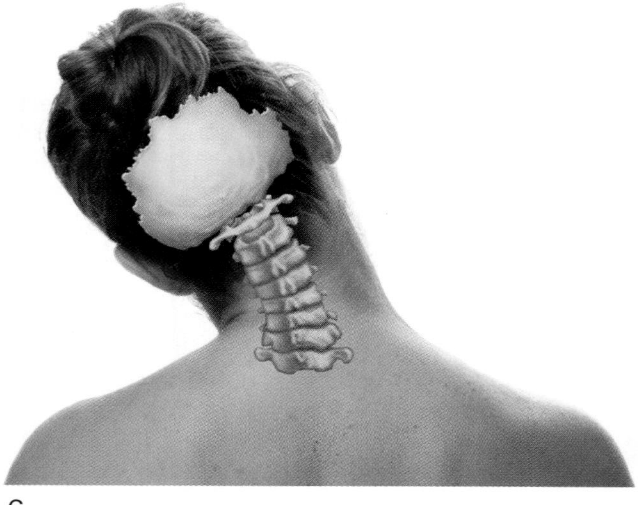

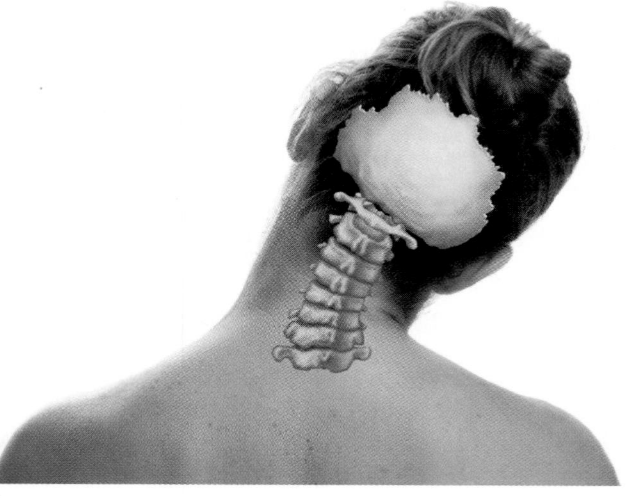

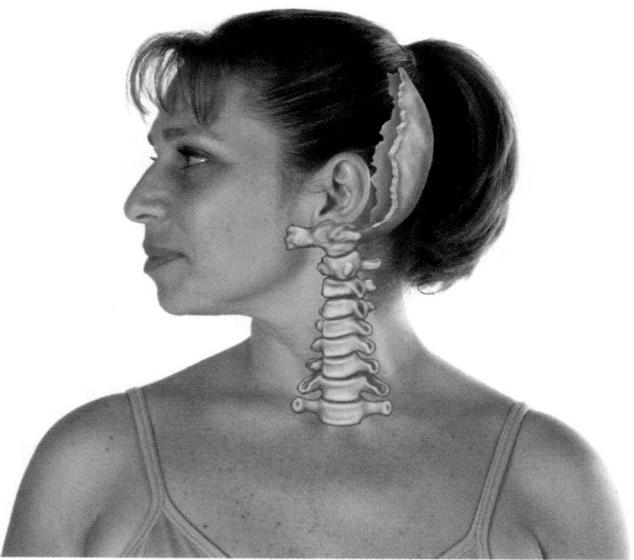

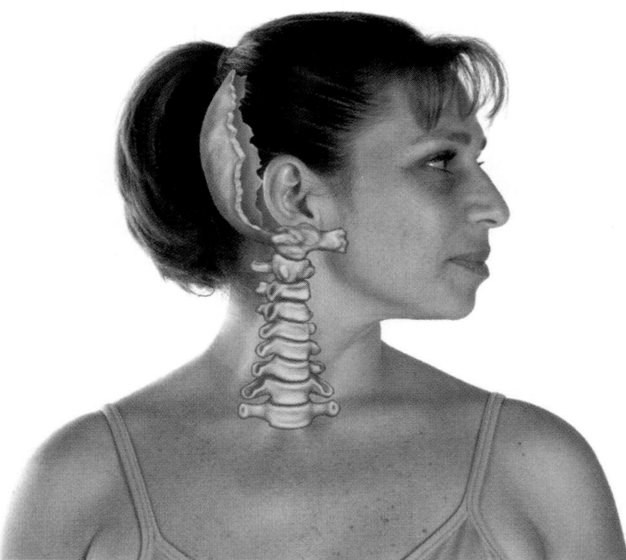

☐ 7.7 THORACIC SPINE (THE THORAX)

❑ The thoracic spine defines the thorax of the body (i.e., the upper part of the trunk).

BOX 7-38

The trunk of the body is made up of the thorax and the abdomen. The **thorax** is the region of the thoracic spine, and the **abdomen** is the region of the lumbar spine.

Features of the Thoracic Spine:

Composition of the Thoracic Spine:

❑ The thoracic spine is composed of twelve vertebrae (Figure 7-34).
  ❑ From superior to inferior, these vertebrae are named T1-T12.

❑ The twelve thoracic vertebrae correspond to the twelve pairs of ribs that articulate with them.

Special Joints (Costospinal Joints):

❑ The ribs articulate with all twelve thoracic vertebrae. Generally each rib has two costospinal articulations with the spine: (1) the costovertebral joint and (2) the costotransverse joint (see Section 7.8, Figure 7-35). (For more detail on the rib joints of the thoracic spine, see Section 7.8.)

BOX 7-39

When describing motion of a rib, instead of stating that the rib moves at the costovertebral and costotransverse joints (and the sternocostal joint), to save time, the term *costospinal joints* will be used to refer to the costovertebral and costotransverse joints collectively.

❑ The **costovertebral joint** is where the rib meets the bodies/discs of the spine.

❑ The **costotransverse joint** is where the rib meets the transverse process of the spine.

❑ Collectively, the costovertebral and costotransverse joints may be called the **costospinal joints**.

❑ Both the costovertebral and costotransverse joints are synovial joints.
  ❑ These joints are nonaxial and allow gliding.
  ❑ These joints both stabilize the ribs by giving them a posterior attachment to the spine, and allow mobility of the ribs relative to the spine.

❑ Note: Ribs #1-10 also articulate with the sternum anteriorly; these joints are called *sternocostal joints*.

Curve of the Thoracic Spine:

❑ The thoracic spine has a kyphotic curve (i.e., it is concave anteriorly) (see Figure 7-34).

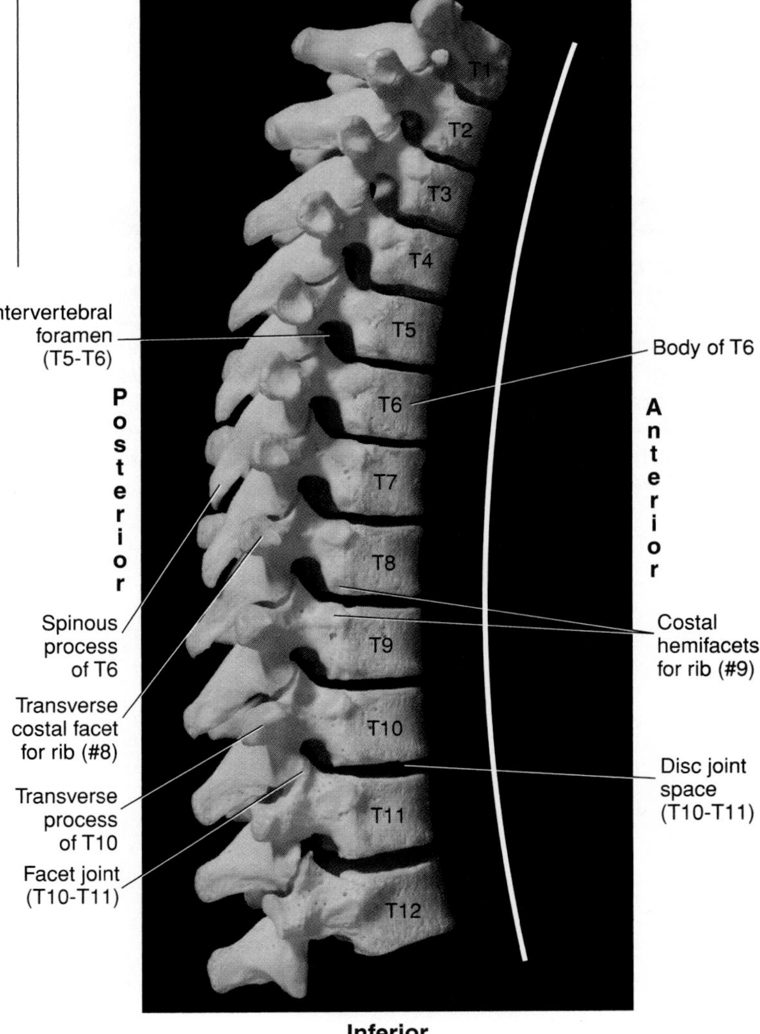

Figure 7-34 Right lateral view of the thoracic spine. The reader should note the kyphotic curve, which is concave anteriorly (and therefore convex posteriorly).

BOX 7-40

As a person ages, it is common for a hyperkyphosis of the thoracic spine to develop. This is largely the result of activities that cause our posture to round forward, flexing the upper trunk (flexion of the upper trunk increases the thoracic kyphosis). It is also due to the effects of gravity pulling the upper trunk down into flexion.

Functions of the Thoracic Spine:

- The thoracic spine is far less mobile than the cervical and lumbar regions (Table 7-7).
- Being less mobile, the thoracic spine is more stable than the cervical and lumbar regions and therefore injured less often.
- The major reason for the lack of movement of the thoracic spine is the presence of the ribcage in this region.
  - The ribcage primarily limits lateral flexion motion in the frontal plane and rotation motion in the transverse plane.
  - Lateral flexion is limited as a result of the ribs of the ribcage crowding into each other on the side to which the trunk is laterally flexed.
  - Rotation is limited as a result of the presence of the rib lateral to the vertebra.
- The spinous processes also limit range of motion of the thoracic spine. Because they are long and oriented inferiorly, they obstruct and limit extension of the thoracic spine.
- The orientation of the thoracic facet joints is essentially in the frontal plane (see Section 7.4, Figure 7-14b), which should allow for ease of lateral flexion motion within the frontal plane; however, because of the presence of the ribcage, lateral flexion is limited.

BOX 7-41

In the lower thoracic region, the facet plane orientation gradually begins to change from the frontal plane to the sagittal plane (which is the orientation that the lumbar facets have). This sagittal orientation facilitates sagittal plane actions (i.e., flexion and extension).

Major Motions Allowed:

See Section 7.10; illustrations in Figure 7-42 demonstrate thoracolumbar motion of the trunk at the spinal joints.

- The thoracic spinal joints allow flexion and extension (i.e., axial movements) of the trunk in the sagittal plane around a mediolateral axis.
- The thoracic spinal joints allow right lateral flexion and left lateral flexion (i.e., axial movements) of the trunk in the frontal plane around an anteroposterior axis.
- The thoracic spinal joints allow right rotation and left rotation (i.e., axial movements) of the trunk in the transverse plane around a vertical axis.
- The thoracic spinal joints allow gliding translational movements in all three directions (see Section 7.4, Figure 7-18).

TABLE 7-7

Average Ranges of Motion of the Thoracic Spine (T1-T2 Through T12-L1 joints) from Anatomic Position*

Flexion	35 Degrees	Extension	25 Degrees
Right lateral flexion	25 Degrees	Left lateral flexion	25 Degrees
Right rotation	30 Degrees	Left rotation	30 Degrees

*As in the cervical spine, when the thoracic spine laterally flexes, it ipsilaterally rotates to some degree as well. Therefore these two actions are coupled together.

7.8 RIB JOINTS OF THE THORACIC SPINE (MORE DETAIL)

- As stated in Section 7.7, the ribs articulate with all twelve thoracic vertebrae posteriorly. The joints between the ribs and the spinal column are known collectively as the *costospinal joints*. Usually, each rib has two articulations with the spine: (1) the costovertebral joint and (2) the costotransverse joint (see Figure 7-35a).
- The costovertebral joint is where the rib meets the vertebral bodies/discs.
- The costotransverse joint is where the rib meets the transverse process of the spinal vertebra.
- Furthermore, most of the ribs articulate with the sternum anteriorly at the sternocostal joints.
- The proper movement of all rib joints is extremely important during respiration. (For more information on respiration, see Box 7-45.)

Costospinal Joints in More Detail:

Costovertebral Joint:

BOX 7-42

The costovertebral joint where a rib articulates with the vertebral body is also known as the **costocorporeal joint.** *Corpus* is Latin for *body.*

- The typical thoracic vertebral body has two costal hemifacets: one superiorly and one inferiorly (see Figure 7-35b).
- The head of the rib therefore forms a joint with the inferior costal hemifacet of the vertebra above and the superior costal hemifacet of the vertebra below, as well as the intervertebral disc that is located between the two vertebral bodies (see Figure 7-35a).

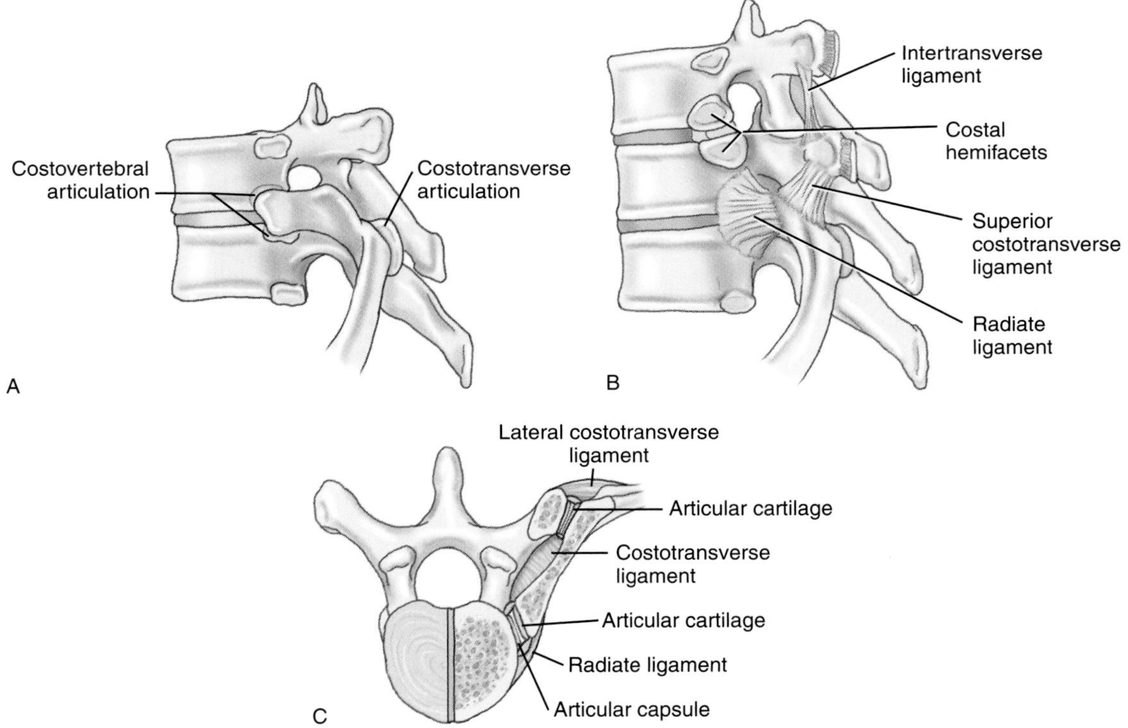

Figure 7-35 Joints between a rib and the spinal column (i.e., costospinal joints). *A,* Lateral view that depicts the costotransverse joint between the rib and transverse process of the vertebra and the costovertebral joint between the rib and bodies/disc of the vertebra. *B,* Lateral view depicting the radiate and superior costotransverse ligaments. *C,* Superior view in which half of the rib-vertebra complex has been horizontally sectioned to expose and illustrate the costospinal joints and the radiate, costotransverse, and lateral costotransverse ligaments.

- The costovertebral joint is stabilized by two ligamentous structures:
  - Its fibrous joint capsule
  - The **radiate ligament** (see Figure 7-35b–c)
- The typical costovertebral joint occurs between ribs #2-10 and the spine.
- The costovertebral joint of rib #1 meets a full costal facet at the superior end of the body of the T1 vertebra (i.e., no hemifacet on the body of C7 exists).
- The costovertebral joints of ribs #11 and #12 meet a full costal facet located at the superior body of T11 and T12, respectively.

Costotransverse Joint:

- The typical thoracic vertebra has a full costal facet on its transverse processes (see Section 4.2, Figure 4-27e).
- The costotransverse joint is where the tubercle of the rib meets the transverse process of the thoracic vertebra.
- The costotransverse joint is stabilized by four ligamentous structures:
  - **A fibrous joint capsule**
  - **A costotransverse ligament:** This long ligament firmly attaches the neck of the rib with the entire length of the transverse process of the same level vertebra (see Figure 7-35c).
  - **A lateral costotransverse ligament:** This ligament attaches the costal tubercle of the rib to the lateral margin of the transverse process of the same level vertebra (see Figure 7-35c).
  - **A superior costotransverse ligament:** This ligament attaches the rib to the transverse process of the vertebra that is located superiorly (see Figure 7-35b).
- The typical costotransverse joints occur between ribs #1-10 and thoracic vertebrae #1-10 of the spine.
- Ribs #11 and #12 do not articulate with transverse processes of the thoracic spine, hence they have no costotransverse joints.

BOX 7-43

LIGAMENTS OF THE COSTOSPINAL JOINTS

Costovertebral Joint:
- Fibrous joint capsule
- Radiate ligament

Costotransverse Joint:
- Fibrous joint capsule
- Costotransverse ligament
- Lateral costotransverse ligament
- Superior costotransverse ligament

Sternocostal Joints:

- Seven pairs of **sternocostal joints** (Figure 7-36) attach ribs to the sternum anteriorly.
- The first seven pairs of ribs attach directly to the sternum via their costal cartilages.
  - These ribs are called **true ribs**.
- The ribs that do not attach directly into the sternum via their own costal cartilages are termed **false ribs**.
  - The 8th through 10th pairs of ribs join the costal cartilage of the 7th rib pair. These ribs are termed *false ribs*.
  - The 11th and 12th rib pairs do not attach to the sternum at all, hence they are free floating anteriorly. These ribs are floating false ribs but are usually referred to simply as **floating ribs**.

Sternocostal Rib Joints:

- Joint structure classification: Cartilaginous joint
  - Subtype: Synchondrosis
- Joint function classification: Amphiarthrotic
  - Subtype: Gliding

Miscellaneous:

- A sternocostal joint can be divided into three separate joints (Figure 7-37):

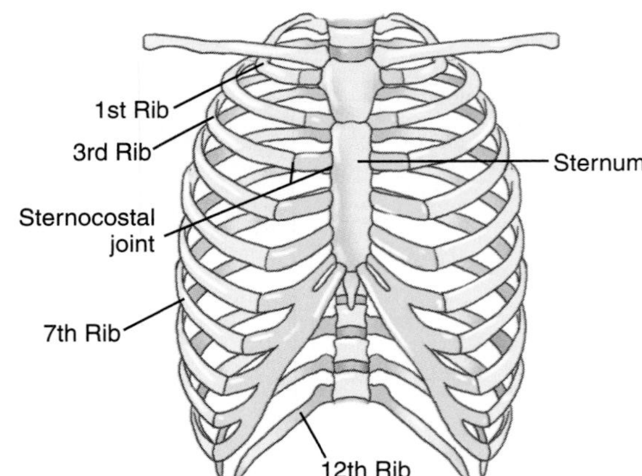

Figure 7-36 Anterior view of the ribcage. The sternocostal joint is located between a rib and the sternum. Seven pairs of sternocostal cartilages exist.

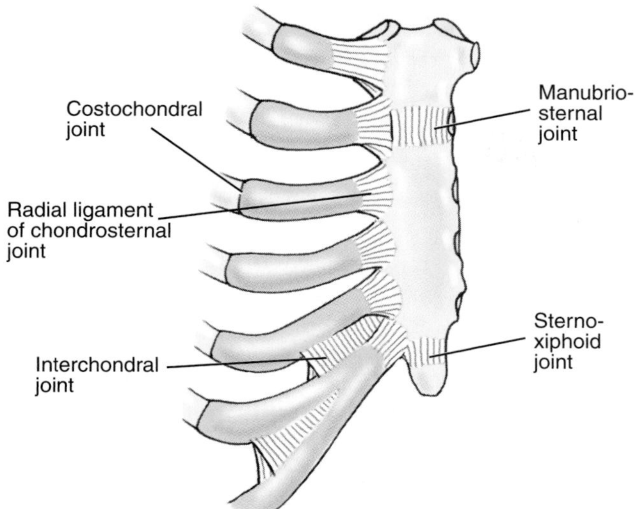

Figure 7-37 Anterior view of the sternum and part of the ribcage on one side of the body. Each sternocostal joint is actually composed of two articulations: (1) the costochondral joint located between a rib and its costal cartilage and (2) the chondrosternal joint located between the costal cartilage and the sternum (in addition, interchondral joints are located between adjacent costal cartilages of ribs #5-10). Further, the manubriosternal and sternoxiphoid joints are located between the three parts of the sternum.

1. **Costochondral joints** are located between the ribs and their cartilages.
   - ❑ A costochondral joint unites a rib directly with its costal cartilage. Neither a joint capsule nor any ligaments are present. The periosteum of the rib gradually transforms into the perichondrium of the costal cartilage. These joints permit very little motion.
   - ❑ Ten pairs of costochondral joints exist (between ribs #1-10 and their costal cartilages).
2. **Chondrosternal joints** are located between the costal cartilages of the ribs and the sternum.
   - ❑ A chondrosternal joint is a gliding synovial joint (except the 1st one, which is a synarthrosis) reinforced by its fibrous joint capsule and a **radiate ligament**.
   - ❑ Seven pairs of chondrosternal joints exist between costal cartilages and the sternum.
3. **Interchondral joints** are located between the costal cartilages of ribs 5-10.
   - ❑ These joints are synovial lined and reinforced by its capsule and an **interchondral ligament**.

Intrasternal Joints

❑ Two intrasternal joints are located between the three parts of the sternum (see Figure 7-37).

1. The **manubriosternal joint** is located between the manubrium and body of the sternum.
2. The **sternoxiphoid joint** is located between the body and xiphoid process of the sternum.
   - ❑ These joints are fibrocartilaginous amphiarthrotic joints that are stabilized by the **manubriosternal ligament** and the **sternoxiphoid ligament**, respectively.

BOX 7-44

LIGAMENTS OF THE STERNOCOSTAL AND STERNAL JOINTS

Chondrosternal Joint:
- Fibrous joint capsule
- Radiate ligament

Interchondral Joint:
- Fibrous joint capsule
- Interchondral ligament

Intrasternal Joints:
- Manubriosternal and sternoxiphoid ligaments

Muscles of the Rib Joints:

❑ Muscles of the rib joints move the ribs at the sternocostal and costospinal joints. Moving the ribs is necessary for the process of respiration (i.e., breathing). Therefore muscles that move ribs are called *muscles of respiration*. To move the ribs, these muscles attach onto the ribs. Any muscle that attaches onto the ribcage may be considered to be a muscle of respiration.

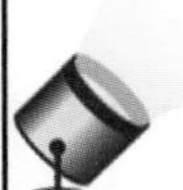

BOX 7-45 SPOTLIGHT ON MUSCLES OF RESPIRATION

Inspiration/Expiration:

Respiration is the process of taking air into and expelling air out of the lungs. Taking air into the lungs is called *inspiration* (i.e., inhalation); expelling air from the lungs is called *expiration* (i.e., exhalation). When air is taken into the lungs, the volume of the thoracic cavity expands; when air is expelled from the lungs, the volume of the thoracic cavity decreases. Therefore any muscle that has the ability to change the volume of the thoracic cavity is a muscle of respiration. Generally the volume of the thoracic cavity can be affected in two ways:

One way is to affect the ribcage by moving the ribs at the sternocostal and costospinal joints. As a general rule, elevating ribs increases thoracic cavity volume (see figure), therefore muscles that elevate ribs are generally categorized as muscles of inspiration. The primary muscle of inspiration is the diaphragm, because it elevates the lower six ribs. Other inspiratory muscles include the external intercostals, scalenes, pectoralis minor, levatores costarum, and the serratus posterior superior. Conversely, muscles that depress the ribs are generally categorized as expiratory muscles and include the internal intercostals, subcostales, and serratus posterior inferior.

The other way in which the volume of the thoracic cavity can be affected is via the abdominal region. In addition to increasing thoracic cavity volume by having the thoracic cavity expand outward when the ribcage itself expands, the thoracic cavity can also expand downward into the abdominal cavity region. Conversely, if the contents of the abdominal cavity push up into the thoracic cavity, the volume of the thoracic cavity would decrease. In this regard, the diaphragm is again the primary muscle of inspiration; when it contracts, in addition to raising the lower ribs, its central dome also drops down against the abdominal contents, thereby increasing the volume of the thoracic cavity. Muscles of expiration that work via the abdominal region are muscles of the abdominal wall, principally amongst these are the rectus abdominis, external abdominal oblique, internal abdominal oblique, and the transversus abdominis.

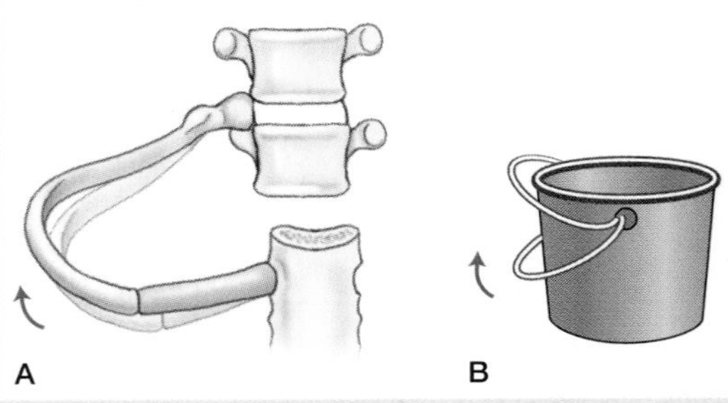

A, Anterior view illustrating the manner in which a rib lifts during inspiration. *B,* The handle of a bucket lifting. Elevation of a rib during inspiration has been described as a **bucket handle movement** because of the similarity of elevation of a rib to the elevation of a bucket handle.

Relaxed versus Forceful Breathing:

Breathing is often divided into two types: (1) relaxed (i.e., quiet) breathing and (2) forceful breathing. During normal healthy relaxed breathing, such as when a person is calmly reading a book, the only muscle that is recruited to contract is the diaphragm. For normal healthy relaxed expiration, no muscles need to contract; instead, the diaphragm simply relaxes and the natural recoil of the tissues that were stretched during inspiration (tissues of the ribcage and abdomen) push back against the lungs, expelling the air. However, when we want to breathe forcefully, such as would occur during exercise, many other muscles of respiration are recruited. These muscles, as already mentioned, act on the thoracic cavity via the ribcage or the abdominal region. Generally speaking, whenever a pathology exists that results in labored breathing (any chronic obstructive pulmonary disorder such as asthma, emphysema, or chronic bronchitis), accessory muscles of respiration are recruited and may become hypertrophic.

Diaphragm Function:

As has been stated, the diaphragm is an inspiratory muscle and increases thoracic cavity volume in two ways: (1) it expands the ribcage by lifting lower ribs, and (2) it drops down, pushing against the abdominal contents in the abdominal cavity. The manner in which the diaphragm is generally considered to function is as follows:

When the diaphragm contracts, the bony peripheral attachments are more fixed and the pull is on the central tendon, which causes the center (i.e., the top of the dome) to drop down (against the abdominal viscera). This raises the volume of the thoracic cavity to allow the lungs to inflate and expand for inspiration. This aspect of the diaphragm's contraction is usually called *abdominal breathing.*

As the diaphragm continues to contract, the pressure caused by the resistance of the abdominal viscera prohibits the central dome from dropping any further and the dome now becomes less able to move (i.e., more fixed). The pull exerted by the contraction of the fibers of the diaphragm now pull peripherally on the ribcage, elevating the lower ribs and causing the anterior ribcage and sternum to push anteriorly. This further increases the volume of the thoracic cavity to allow the lungs to inflate and expand. This aspect of the diaphragm's contraction is usually called *thoracic breathing.*

7.9 LUMBAR SPINE (THE ABDOMEN)

❑ The lumbar spine defines the abdomen of the body (i.e., the lower part of the trunk).

BOX 7-46

Most people think of the abdomen as being located only anteriorly. Actually, the abdomen is the lower (lumbar) region of the trunk that wraps 360 degrees around the body.

Features of the Lumbar Spine:

Composition of the Lumbar Spine:

❑ The lumbar spine is composed of five vertebrae (Figure 7-38).
  ❑ From superior to inferior, these vertebrae are named L1-L5.

Curve of the Lumbar Spine:

❑ The lumbar spine has a lordotic curve (i.e., it is concave posteriorly).

BOX 7-47

When the lumbar spine has a greater than normal lordotic curve, it is called a hyperlordosis. The common lay term for a hyperlordotic lumbar spine is **swayback**. (For more information on swayback, see Section 17.6).

Functions of the Lumbar Spine:

❑ The lumbar spine needs to be stable because it has a greater weight-bearing role than the cervical and thoracic spinal regions.

❑ The lumbar spine is also very mobile. Generally the lumbar spine moves freely in all ranges of motion except rotation (Table 7-8).

❑ The orientation of the lumbar facet joints is essentially in the sagittal plane (see Section 7-4, Figure 7-14c), which allows for ease of flexion and extension motions within the sagittal plane (Box 7-48). This is why it is so easy to bend forward and backward from our low back.

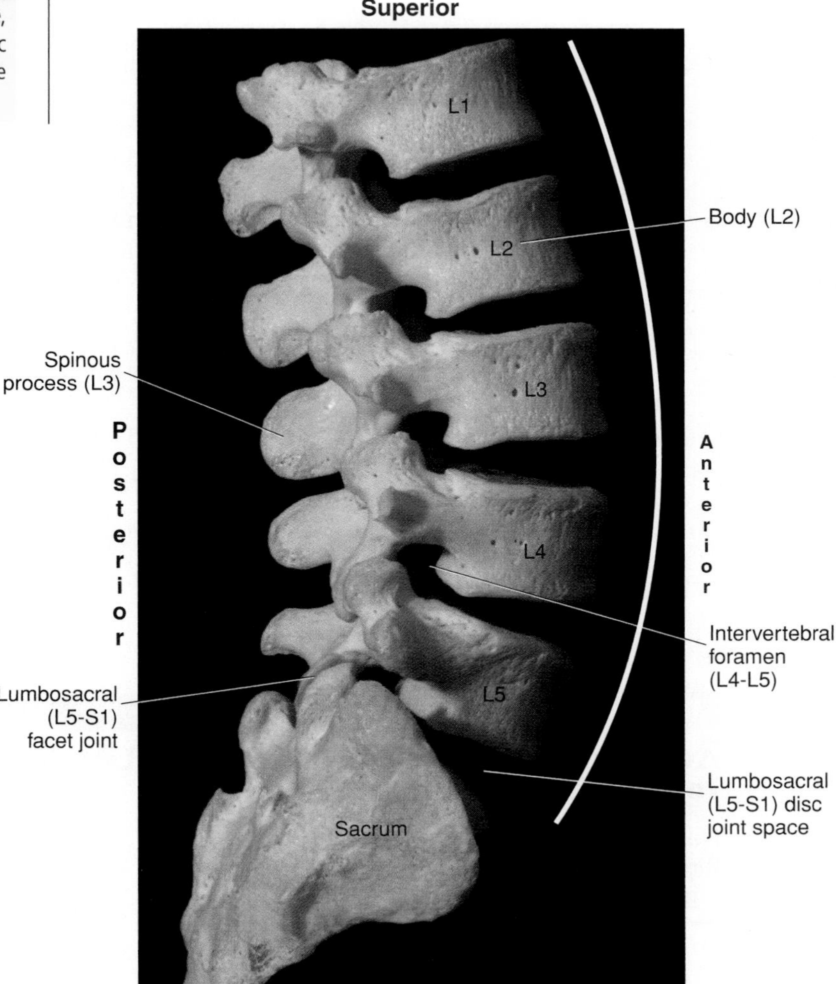

Figure 7-38 Right lateral view of the lumbar spine. The reader should note the lordotic curve, which is concave posteriorly (and therefore convex anteriorly).

BOX 7-48

In the lower lumbar region, the facet plane orientation changes from the sagittal plane back toward the frontal plane. Clinically, this can create problems, because the upper lumbar region facilitates flexion/extension movements in the sagittal plane, but the lumbosacral joint region does not allow these sagittal plane motions as well because their facets are oriented in the frontal plane.

❑ Being both mobile and stable is difficult, because mobility and stability are antagonistic concepts. Usually a joint tends to be either primarily mobile or it tends to be primarily stable. Having to be stable for weight bearing and yet also allow a great amount of mobility is one of the reasons that the low back is so often injured.

Major Motions Allowed:

See Section 7.10; illustrations in Figure 7-41 demonstrate thoracolumbar motion of the trunk.

❑ The lumbar spinal joints allow flexion and extension (i.e., axial movements) of the trunk in the sagittal plane around a mediolateral axis.

❑ The lumbar spinal joints allow right lateral flexion and left lateral flexion (i.e., axial movements) of the trunk in the frontal plane around an anteroposterior axis.

  ❑ Unlike the cervical and thoracic spinal regions, which couple lateral flexion with ipsilateral rotation, the lumbar spine couples lateral flexion with contralateral rotation. An interesting clinical application of this is that when a client has a lumbar scoliosis (a lateral flexion deformity of the spine in the frontal plane), it can be difficult to pick this up on visual examination or palpation because the result of contralateral rotation coupling with lateral flexion is that the spinous processes rotate into the concavity, making it more difficult to see and feel the curvature of the scoliosis (Figure 7-39).

❑ The lumbar spinal joints allow right rotation and left rotation (i.e., axial movements) of the trunk in the transverse plane around a vertical axis.

❑ The lumbar spinal joints allow gliding translational movements in all three directions (see Section 7.4, Figure 7-18).

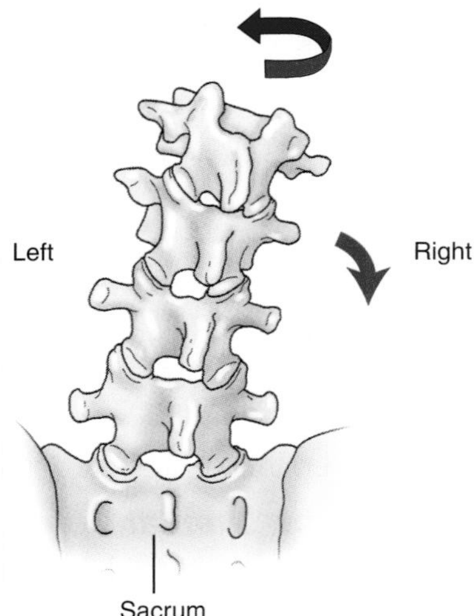

Figure 7-39 Posterior view illustrating the coupling pattern in the lumbar spine of lateral flexion with contralateral rotation. In this figure, the lumbar spine is right laterally flexing and rotating to the left. (Note: Remember that vertebral rotation is named for the direction in which the anterior bodies face; the spinous processes would therefore point in the opposite direction.)

Special Joint:

❑ The joint between the 5th lumbar vertebra and the sacrum is known as the **lumbosacral joint** or L5-S1 joint (see Figure 7-38).

BOX 7-49

The lumbosacral joint is also known as the L5-S1 joint, because it is between the 5th lumbar vertebra and the 1st element of the sacrum. The sacrum is made up of five vertebrae that fused embryologically. Therefore the sacrum can be divided into its five elements, S1-S5 (from superior to inferior).

❑ The lumbosacral joint is not structurally (i.e., anatomically) special. As is typical for intervertebral joints, it is made up of a median disc joint and two lateral facet joints. However, the lumbosacral joint is functionally (i.e., physiologically) special because the lumbosacral joint is not just a joint at which the spine (specifically the 5th lumbar vertebra) can move. It is also the joint at which the pelvis can move relative to the trunk.

TABLE 7-8

Average Ranges of Motion of the Lumbar Spine (L1-L2 Through L5-S1 Joints) from Anatomic Position

Flexion	50 Degrees	Extension	15 Degrees
Right lateral flexion	20 Degrees	Left lateral flexion	20 Degrees
Right rotation	5 Degrees	Left rotation	5 Degrees

BOX 7-50

The pelvis can move relative to the trunk at the lumbosacral joint; the pelvis can also move relative to the thighs at the hip joints. (For motions of the pelvis relative to adjacent body parts, please see Sections 8.3 through 8.5.)

- ❑ Other than the usual ligaments of the spine, stabilization to the lumbosacral joint is provided by the iliolumbar ligaments (see Figure 8-4) and the thoracolumbar fascia (see Section 7-11, Figure 7-42).
- ❑ The lumbosacral joint region is also important because the angle of the sacral base, termed the **sacral base angle** (Figure 7-40), determines the base that the spine sits on; this determines the curvature that the spine has. Therefore the sacral base angle is an important factor toward assessing the posture of the client's spine. (See Section 8.8 for more information on the effect of the sacral base angle on the spine.)

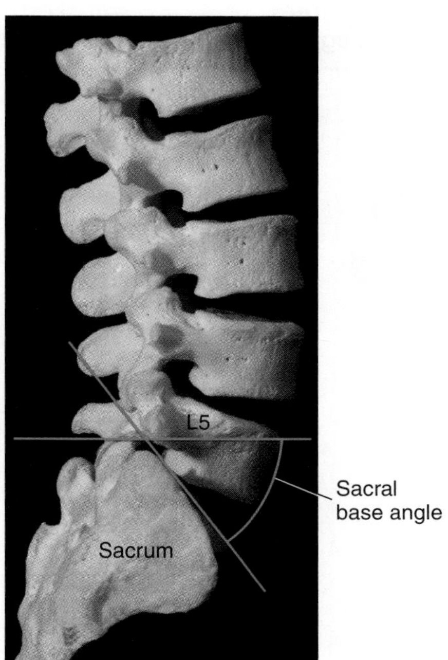

Figure 7-40 Right lateral view of the lumbosacral spine. The sacral base angle is formed by the intersection of a line that runs along the base of the sacrum and a horizontal line. The sacral base angle is important because it determines the degree of curvature that the lumbar spine will have.

☐ 7.10 THORACOLUMBAR SPINE (THE TRUNK)

❑ Given that the thoracic spine and lumbar spine are both located in the trunk, movement of these two regions (i.e., the **thoracolumbar spine**) is often coupled together and often assessed together. Table 7-9 provides the average ranges of motion of the thoracolumbar spine; Figure 7-41 shows the major motions of the thoracolumbar spine (i.e., the trunk).

TABLE 7-9

Average Ranges of Motion of the Thoracolumbar Spine (i.e., the Entire Trunk from Anatomic Position) (These Numbers Include the T1-T2 through L5-S1 Joints.)

Flexion	85 Degrees	Extension	40 Degrees
Right lateral flexion	45 Degrees	Left lateral flexion	45 Degrees
Right rotation	35 Degrees	Left rotation	35 Degrees

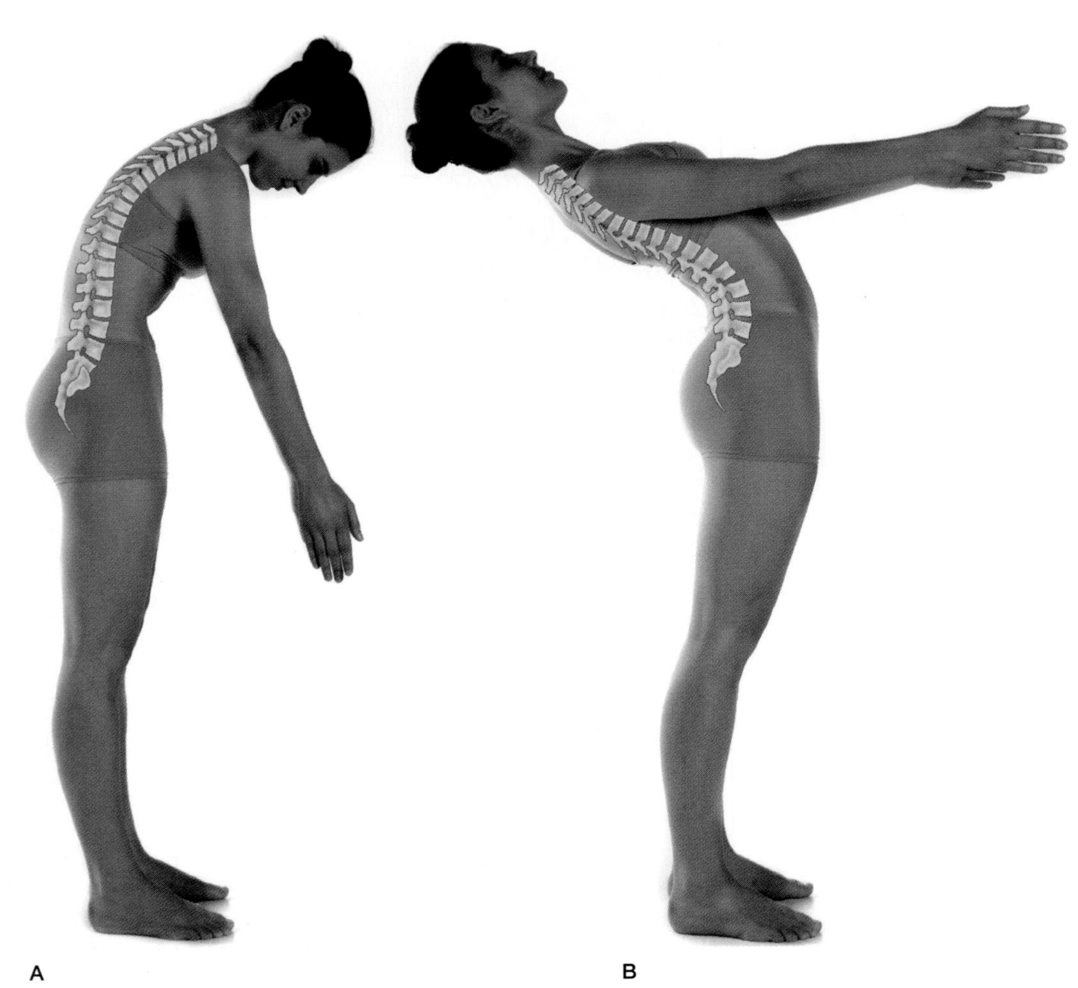

Figure 7-41 Motions of the thoracolumbar spine (trunk) at the spinal joints. *A* and *B* are lateral views that illustrate flexion and extension of the trunk respectively, in the sagittal plane. *C* and *D* are anterior views that illustrate right lateral flexion and left lateral flexion of the trunk respectively, in the frontal plane. *E* and *F* are anterior views that illustrate right rotation and left rotation of the trunk, respectively, in the transverse plane.

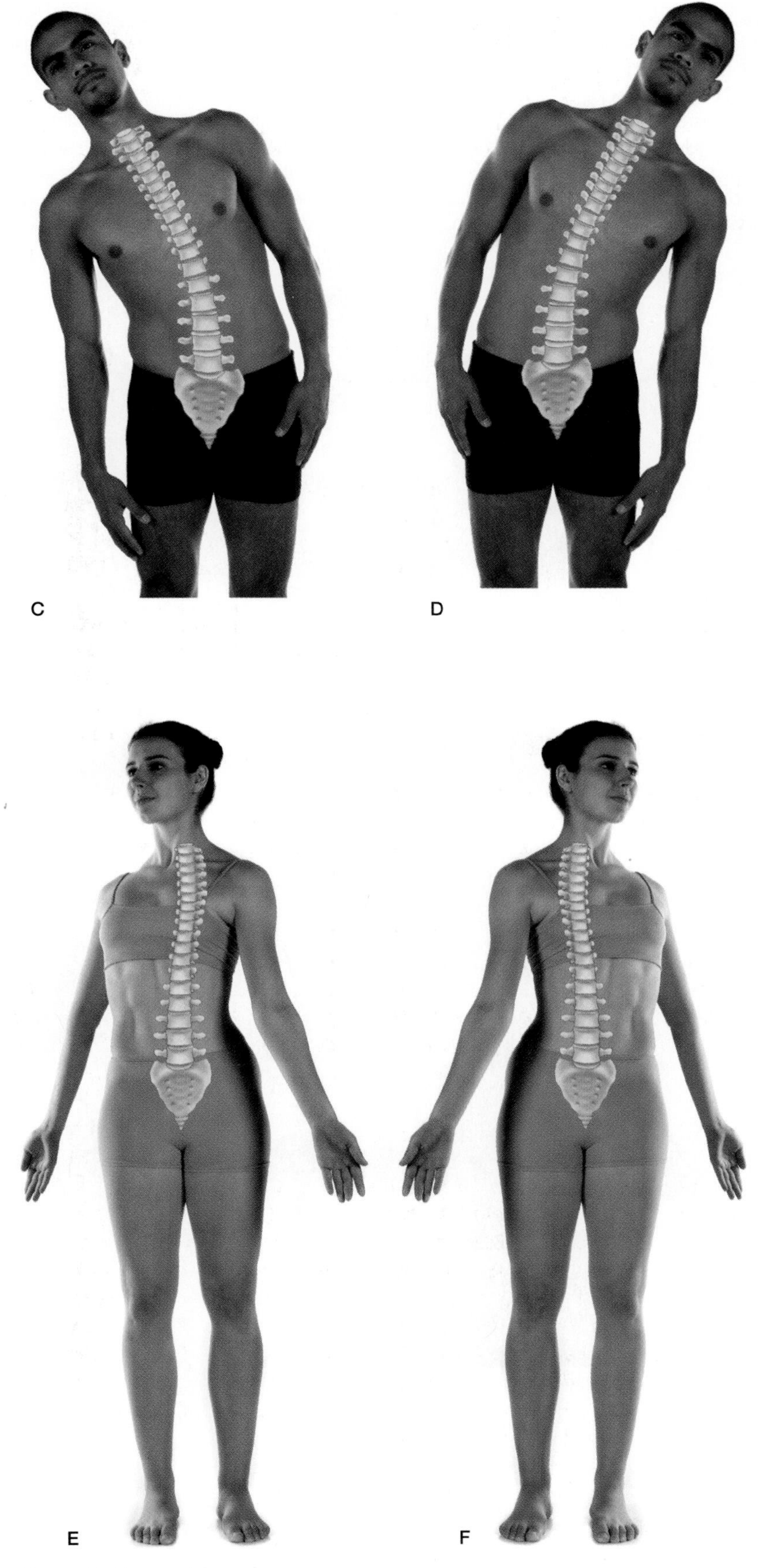

Figure 7-41, cont'd.

BOX 7-51

There are many reverse actions of the trunk that can occur. Reverse actions of the muscles of the thoracolumbar spine (i.e., the trunk) create actions of the pelvis at the lumbosacral joint relative to the trunk (and/or movement of the inferior vertebrae relative to the more superior vertebrae). Reverse actions of the pelvis relative to the trunk are covered in Section 8.6.

Reverse actions in which the trunk moves relative to the arm at the shoulder joint are also possible. In the accompanying illustration, the trunk is seen to move relative to the arm at the shoulder joint. *A* and *B* illustrate neutral position and right lateral deviation of the trunk at the right shoulder joint, respectively; *C* and *D* illustrate neutral position and right rotation of the trunk at the right shoulder joint, respectively; *E* and *F* illustrate neutral position and elevation of the trunk at the right shoulder joint, respectively. In all three cases, note the change in angulation between the arm and trunk at the shoulder joint (for lateral deviation *B* and elevation *F*, the elbow joint has also flexed.)

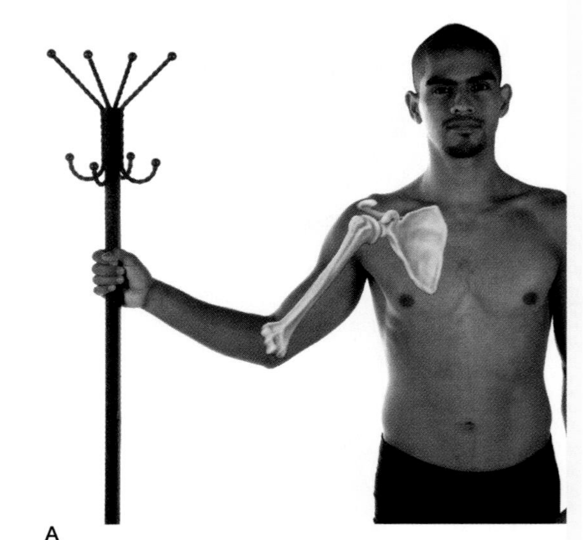

A

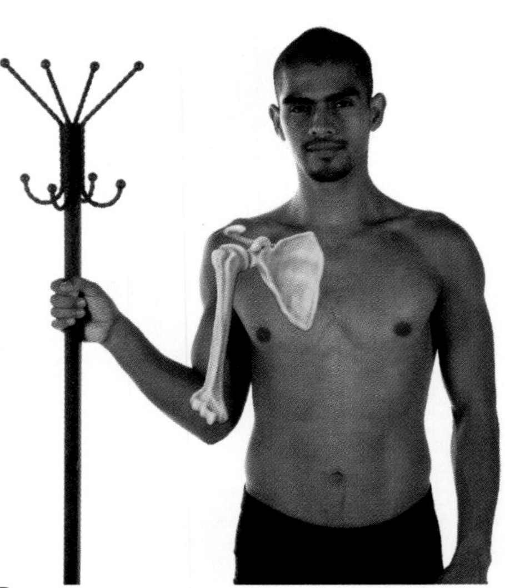

B

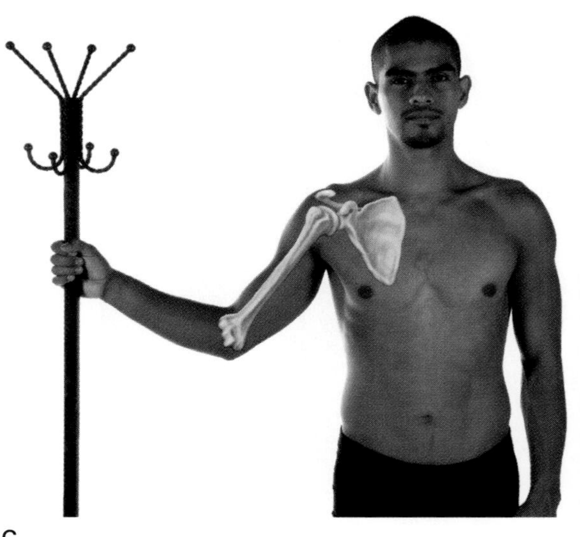

C

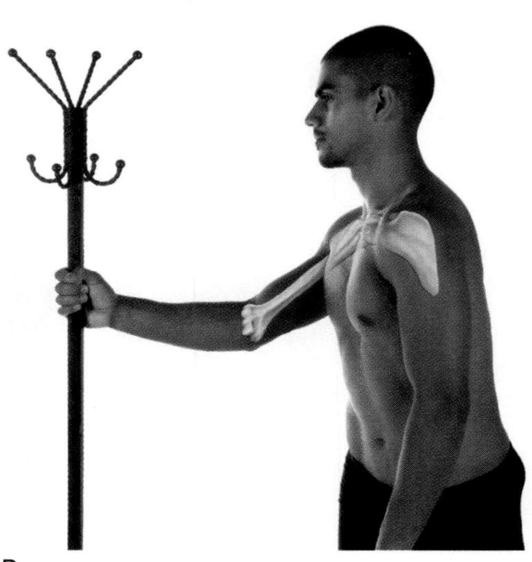

D

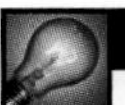

BOX 7-51—cont'd

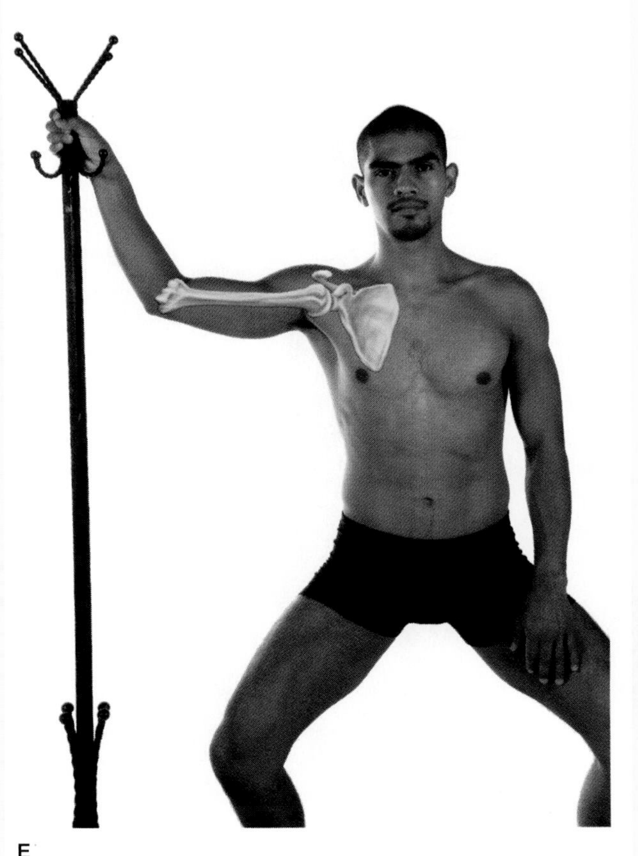

E

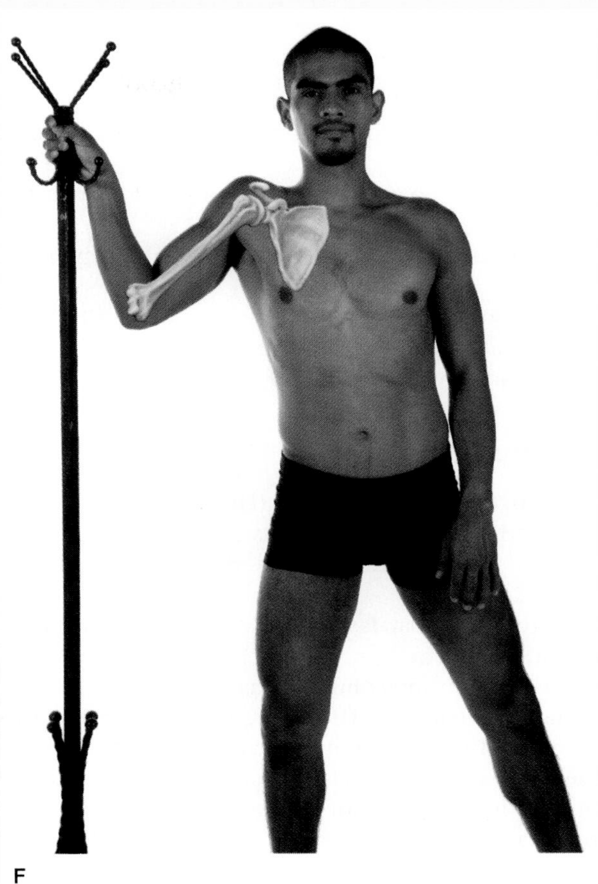

F

7.11 THORACOLUMBAR FASCIA AND ABDOMINAL APONEUROSIS

- The thoracolumbar fascia and abdominal aponeurosis are large sheets of fibrous connective tissue located in the trunk.
- The thoracolumbar fascia is located posteriorly in the trunk.
- The abdominal aponeurosis is located anteriorly in the trunk.
- The functional importance of these structures is twofold:
  - They provide attachment sites for muscles.
  - They add to the stability of the trunk.

Thoracolumbar Fascia:

- The **thoracolumbar fascia** (Figure 7-42a) is located posteriorly in the trunk; as its name implies, it is a layer of fascia located in the thoracic and lumbar regions.
- The thoracolumbar fascia is also known as the **lumbodorsal fascia**.
  - A sheet of thoracolumbar fascia exists on the left and right sides of the body. In other words, two sheets of thoracolumbar fascia exist.
- The thoracolumbar fascia is especially well developed in the lumbar region, where it is divided into three layers: (1) anterior, (2) middle, and (3) deep (Figure 7-42b).
  - The anterior layer is located between the psoas major and quadratus lumborum muscles and attaches to the anterior surface of the transverse processes (TPs).
  - The middle layer is located between the quadratus lumborum and erector spinae group musculature and attaches to the tips of the transverse processes.
  - The posterior layer is located posterior to the erector spinae and latissimus dorsi musculature and attaches to the spinous processes (SPs).

BOX 7-52

The quadratus lumborum and erector spinae group muscles are encased within the thoracolumbar fascia.

The latissimus dorsi attaches into the spine medially via its attachment into the thoracolumbar fascia.

  - All three layers meet posterolaterally where the internal abdominal oblique (IAO) and transversus abdominis (TA) muscles attach into it.
- Inferiorly, the thoracolumbar fascia attaches onto the sacrum and iliac crest.
- Because of its attachments onto the sacrum and ilium, the thoracolumbar fascia helps to stabilize the lumbar spinal joints and the sacroiliac joint.

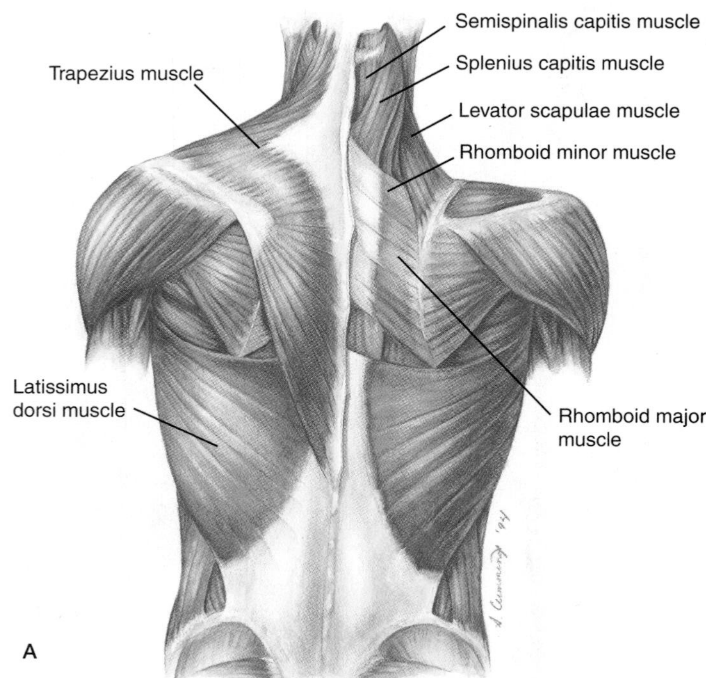

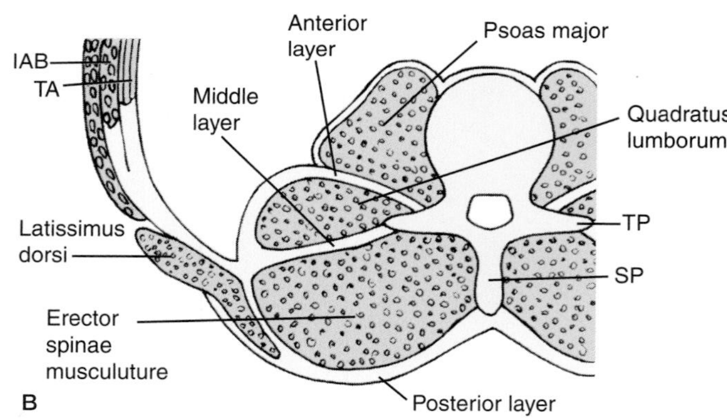

Figure 7-42 *A,* Posterior view of the trunk depicting the thoracolumbar fascia in the thoracolumbar region. *B,* Transverse plane cross-section illustrating the three layers (anterior, middle, and posterior) of the thoracolumbar fascia. (*A* from Cramer GD, Darby SA: *Basic and clinical anatomy of the spine, spinal cord, and ANS,*

Abdominal Aponeurosis:

- The **abdominal aponeurosis** is located anteriorly in the abdominal region (Figure 7-43).
  - An abdominal aponeurosis exists on the left and right sides of the body. In other words, two abdominal aponeuroses (left and right) exist.

❑ The abdominal aponeurosis provides a site of attachment for the external abdominal oblique, internal abdominal oblique, and the transversus abdominis muscles.

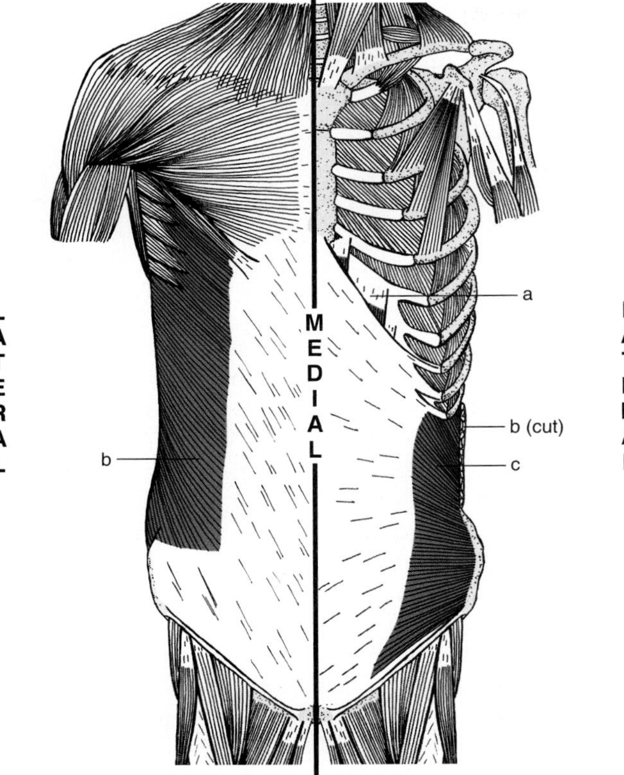

> **BOX 7-53**
>
> The abdominal aponeurosis is often viewed as being an attachment site into which the abdominal wall muscles attach. Viewed another way, it can also be considered to actually be the aponeuroses of these abdominal wall muscles (namely, the external abdominal oblique, internal abdominal oblique, and transversus abdominis muscles bilaterally).

❑ The superior aspect of the abdominal aponeurosis has two layers (anterior and posterior) that encase the rectus abdominis.

❑ The inferior aspect of the abdominal aponeurosis has only one layer that passes superficially (anteriorly) to the rectus abdominis.

> **BOX 7-54**
>
> The border where the abdominal aponeurosis changes its relationship to the rectus abdominis is the arcuate line. The **arcuate line** is a curved line that is located approximately one-half way between the umbilicus and the symphysis pubis.

❑ Because the abdominal aponeurosis covers and/or encases the rectus abdominis, it is also known as the **rectus sheath**.

❑ Where the left and right abdominal aponeuroses meet in the midline is called the **linea alba**, which means *white line*.

❑ The left and right abdominal aponeuroses, by binding the two sides of the anterior abdominal wall together, add to the stability of the trunk.

A

a. Rectus Abdominis
b. External Abdominal Oblique
c. Internal Abdominal Oblique
d. Transversus Abdominis

B

St Louis, 1995, Mosby.)

Figure 7-43 *A,* View of the anterior trunk illustrating the abdominal aponeurosis. The abdominal aponeurosis is a thick layer of fibrous tissue that is an attachment site of the transversus abdominis and external and internal abdominal oblique muscles. *B,* Transverse plane cross-section illustrating the abdominal aponeurosis superiorly and inferiorly in the trunk. The abdominal aponeurosis is also known as the *rectus sheath* because it ensheathes the rectus abdominis muscles. (From Muscolino JE: *The muscular system manual: the skeletal muscles of the human body,* ed 2, St Louis, 2005, Mosby.)

REVIEW QUESTIONS

evolve Answers to the following review questions appear on the Evolve website accompanying this book.

1. What is the relationship between cranial suture joints and childbirth?

2. What are the four major muscles of mastication?

3. What are the four major regions of the spine, and which type of curve is found in each?

4. How many cervical vertebrae are there? How many thoracic vertebrae are there? How many lumbar vertebrae are there?

5. Developmentally, what creates the cervical lordotic curve?

6. Regarding spinal segmental motion, compare and contrast the purpose of the disc joint and the purpose of the facet joints.

7. What is the general orientation of the facet planes of the cervical, thoracic, and lumbar spinal regions?

8. Explain why the anterior longitudinal ligament limits extension of the spinal joints, and the supraspinous ligament limits flexion of the spinal joints.

9. Why is the second cervical vertebra called the *axis*?

10. Name three ligaments of the upper cervical region that stabilize the dens of the axis.

11. Which upper cervical spinous process is the most easily palpable and useful as a palpatory landmark?

12. Why are the coupled actions of extension and rotation of the upper cervical spine potentially contraindicated for clients?

13. The presence of what structure greatly decreases the range of motion of extension of the thoracic spine?

14. What are the two types of costospinal joints?

15. Why is elevation of a rib described as a *bucket handle movement*?

16. Describe the two manners in which the thoracic cavity can expand for inspiration?

17. In which plane is the lumbar spine least mobile?

18. What is the lay term for a hyperlordotic lumbar spine?

19. How is the sacral base angle measured? What is its importance?

20. How many layers does the thoracolumbar fascia have in the lumbar region?

21. Why is the abdominal aponeurosis also known as the *rectus sheath*?

Chapter 8

Joints of the Lower Extremity

CHAPTER OUTLINE

CHAPTER OBJECTIVES

After completing this chapter, the student should be able to perform the following:

- ❑ Describe the structure of the pelvis and explain the difference between intrapelvic motion and motion of the pelvis relative to an adjacent body part.
- ❑ Describe the sacral movements of nutation and counternutation.
- ❑ Describe and compare movements of the pelvis at the lumbosacral and hip joints.
- ❑ Explain the reverse action relationships between pelvic movements and movements of the trunk and thighs.
- ❑ Explain the relationship between pelvic posture (and specifically sacral base angle) and spinal posture.
- ❑ Discuss the meaning of open-chain and closed-chain activities and give examples of each.
- ❑ Explain the concepts of the femoral angle of inclination and femoral torsion angle, and explain the possible consequences of these femoral angulations.
- ❑ Describe and give an example of the concept of femoropelvic rhythm.
- ❑ Explain the concepts of the angulations of the knee joint, namely, genu valgus, genu varum, Q-angle, and genu recurvatum. Further, explain the possible consequences of these knee joint angulations.
- ❑ Describe and give an example of the concept of bowstringing.
- ❑ Describe tibial torsion.
- ❑ List the regions of the foot and the joints of the foot.
- ❑ Compare and contrast the role of stability and flexibility of the foot.
- ❑ Describe the structure and function of the arches of the foot; also, relate the windlass mechanism to the arches of the foot.
- ❑ Define pronation and supination of the foot; list and explain the component cardinal plane actions of pronation and supination.
- ❑ Classify each joint covered in this chapter structurally and functionally.

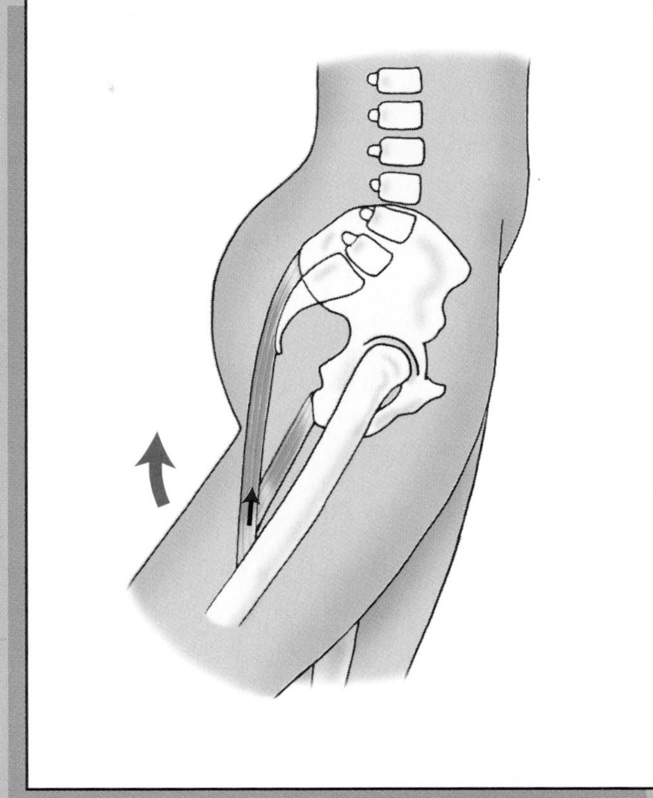

- ❑ List the major ligaments and bursae of each joint covered in this chapter. Further, explain the major function of each ligament.
- ❑ State the closed-packed position of each joint covered in this chapter.
- ❑ List and describe the actions possible at each joint covered in this chapter.
- ❑ List and describe the reverse actions possible at each joint covered in this chapter.
- ❑ List the major muscles/muscle groups (and their joint actions) for each joint covered in this chapter.
- ❑ Define the key terms of this chapter.
- ❑ State the meanings of the word origins of this chapter.

OVERVIEW

While Chapters 5 and 6 laid the theoretical basis for the structure and function of joints, this chapter continues our study of the regional approach of the structure and function of the joints of the body that began in Chapter 7. This chapter addresses the joints of the lower extremity. The lower extremity is primarily concerned with weight bearing and propulsion of the body through space. Toward that end, the joints of the lower extremity must work together to achieve these goals. Sections 8.1 through 8.8 concern themselves with an in-depth examination of the movements of the pelvis. Given the critical importance of the posture of the pelvis to spinal posture, a thorough understanding of the structure and function of the pelvis is crucial. Section 8.9 through 8.11 then cover the hip joint and thigh; and Sections 8.12 through 8.16 cover the knee joint complex and leg. The last 8 sections of this chapter (Sections 8.17 through 8.24) address the structure and function of the ankle joint and foot.

KEY TERMS

Acetabular labrum (AS-i-TAB-you-lar LAY-brum)
Anterior cruciate ligament (an-TEER-ree-or KRU-shee-it)
Anterior talofibular ligament (an-TEER-ree-or TA-low-FIB-you-lar)
Anteversion (AN-tee-ver-shun)
Arch (of the foot)
Arcuate popliteal ligament (ARE-cue-it pop-LIT-ee-al)
Arcuate pubic ligament (PYU-bik)
Bifurcate ligament (by-FUR-kate)
Bony pelvis
Bowleg
Bowstring
Bunion (BUN-yen)
Calcaneocuboid joint (kal-KANE-ee-o-CUE-boyd)
Calcaneocuboid ligament
Calcaneofibular ligament (kal-KANE-ee-o-FIB-you-lar)
Calcaneonavicular ligament (kal-KANE-ee-o-na-VIK-you-lar)
Central stable pillar (of the foot)
Cervical ligament (SERV-i-kul)
Chondromalacia patella (CON-dro-ma-LAY-she-a)
Chopart's joint (SHOW-parz)
Closed-chain activities
Coronary ligaments (CORE-o-nar-ee)
Counternutation (COUN-ter-new-TAY-shun)
Coupled action
Coxa valga (COCKS-a VAL-ga)
Coxa vara (COCKS-a VAR-a)
Coxal bone (COCKS-al)
Coxofemoral joint (COCKS-o-FEM-or-al)
Deep transverse metatarsal ligaments (MET-a-TARS-al)
Deltoid ligament (DEL-toyd)
Distal interphalangeal joints (of the foot) (IN-ter-fa-lan-GEE-al)
Distal intertarsal joints (IN-ter-TAR-sal)
Dorsal calcaneocuboid ligament (DOOR-sul kal-KANE-ee-o-CUE-boyd)
Femoral angle of inclination (FEM-or-al)
Femoral torsion angle (FEM-or-al TOR-shun)
Femoroacetabular joint (FEM-or-o-AS-i-TAB-you-lar)
Femoropelvic rhythm (FEM-or-o-PEL-vik)
Fibular collateral ligament (FIB-you-lar co-LAT-er-al)
Flat foot
Flexor retinaculum (FLEKS-or re-tin-AK-you-lum)
Forefoot (FOUR-foot)
Genu recurvatum (JEN-you REE-ker-VAT-um)
Genu valgum (VAL-gum)
Genu varum (JEN-you VAR-um)
Greater sciatic foramen (sigh-AT-ik)
Greater sciatic notch
Hallux valgus (HAL-uks VAL-gus)
Heel spur
Hindfoot (HIND-foot)
Iliofemoral ligament (IL-ee-o-FEM-or-al)
Iliolumbar ligament (IL-ee-o-LUM-bar)
Inferior extensor retinaculum (ek-STEN-sor re-tin-AK-you-lum)
Inferior fibular retinaculum (FIB-you-lar)
Infrapatellar bursa (IN-fra-pa-TELL-ar BER-sa)
Innominate bone (in-NOM-i-nate)
Intermetatarsal joints (IN-ter-MET-a-TAR-sal)
Intermetatarsal ligaments
Interosseus membrane (of the leg) (IN-ter-OS-ee-us)
Interphalangeal joints (of the foot) (IN-ter-fa-lan-GEE-al)
Ischiofemoral ligament (IS-kee-o-FEM-or-al)
Knock-knees
Lateral collateral ligament (of ankle joint)
Lateral collateral ligament (of interphalangeal joints pedis)
Lateral collateral ligament (of knee joint)
Lateral collateral ligament (of metatarsophalangeal joint)
Lateral longitudinal arch (LON-ji-TOO-di-nal)
Lateral malleolar bursa (ma-LEE-o-lar BER-sa)
Lateral meniscus (men-IS-kus)
Lesser sciatic notch (sigh-at-ik)

Ligamentum teres (LIG-a-MEN-tum TE-reez)
Long plantar ligament (PLAN-tar)
Lower ankle joint
Lumbopelvic rhythm (LUM-bo-PEL-vik)
Lunate cartilage (LOON-ate)
Medial collateral ligament (of ankle joint)
Medial collateral ligament (of interphalangeal joints pedis)
Medial collateral ligament (of knee joint)
Medial collateral ligament (of metatarsophalangeal joint)
Medial longitudinal arch (LON-ji-TOO-di-nal)
Medial malleolar bursa (ma-LEE-o-lar BER-sa)
Medial meniscus (men-IS-kus)
Meniscal horn attachments (men-IS-kal)
Metatarsophalangeal joints (MET-a-TAR-so-fa-lan-GEE-al)
Midfoot
Mortise joint (MOR-tis)
Nutation (new-TAY-shun)
Oblique popliteal ligament (o-BLEEK pop-LIT-ee-al)
Open-chain activities
Patellar ligament (pa-TELL-ar)
Patellofemoral joint (pa-TELL-o-FEM-or-al)
Patellofemoral syndrome
Pelvic girdle (PEL-vik)
Pes cavus (PEZ CAV-us)
Pes planus (PLANE-us)
Pigeon toes
Plantar calcaneocuboid ligament (PLAN-tar kal-KANE-ee-o-CUE-boyd)
Plantar calcaneonavicular ligament (kal-KANE-ee-o-na-VIK-you-lar)
Plantar fascia (PLAN-tar FASH-a)
Plantar fascitis (fash-EYE-tis)
Plantar plate (of interphalangeal joints pedis) (PLAN-tar)
Plantar plate (of metatarsophalangeal joint)
Posterior cruciate ligament (pos-TEER-ree-or KRU-shee-it)
Posterior meniscofemoral ligament (men-IS-ko-FEM-or-al)
Posterior talofibular ligament (pos-TEER-ree-or TA-low-FIB-you-lar)
Prepatellar bursa (PRE-pa-TEL-ar BER-sa)
Proximal interphalangeal joints (of the foot) (IN-ter-fa-lan-GEE-al)
Pubofemoral ligament (PYU-bo-FEM-or-al)
Q-Angle
Ray
Retinacular fibers (re-tin-AK-you-lar)
Retinaculum, pl. retinacula (of the foot/ankle) (re-tin-AK-you-lum, re-tin-AK-you-la)
Retroversion (RET-ro-VER-shun)
Righting reflex
Rigid flat foot
Sacral base angle
Sacroiliac joint (SAY-kro-IL-ee-ak)
Sacroiliac ligaments
Sacrospinous ligament (SAY-kro-SPINE-us)
Sacrotuberous ligament (SAY-kro-TOOB-er-us)
Screw-home mechanism
Short plantar ligament (PLAN-tar)
Sinus tarsus (SIGH-nus TAR-sus)
Spring ligament
Subcutaneous calcaneal bursa (SUB-cue-TANE-ee-us KAL-ka-NEE-al BER-sa)
Subcutaneous infrapatellar bursa (IN-fra-pa-TEL-ar)
Subtendinous calcaneal bursa (sub-TEN-din-us KAL-ka-NEE-al BER-sa)
Subtalar joint (SUB-TAL-ar)
Superior extensor retinaculum (sue-PEE-ree-or eks-TEN-sor re-tin-AK-you-lum)
Superior fibular retinaculum (FIB-you-lar re-tin-AK-you-lum)
Supple flat foot
Suprapatellar bursa (SUE-pra-pa-TEL-ar BER-sa)
Symphysis pubis joint (SIM-fi-sis PYU-bis)
Talocalcaneal joint (TAL-o-kal-KANE-ee-al)
Talocalcaneal ligaments
Talocalcaneonavicular joint complex (TAL-o-kal-KANE-ee-o-na-VIK-you-lar)
Talocalcaneonaviculocuboid joint complex (TAL-o-kal-KANE-ee-o-na-VIK-you-lo-CUE-boyd)
Talocrural joint (TAL-o-KRUR-al)
Talonavicular joint (TAL-o-na-VIK-you-lar)
Tarsal joints (TAR-sal)
Tarsometatarsal joints (TAR-so-MET-a-tars-al)
Tarsometatarsal ligaments
Tibial collateral ligament (TIB-ee-al)
Tibial torsion (TOR-shun)
Tibiofemoral joint (TIB-ee-o-FEM-or-al)
Tibiofibular joints (TIB-ee-o-FIB-you-lar)
Toe-in posture
Toe-out posture
Transverse acetabular ligament (AS-i-TAB-you-lar)
Transverse arch
Transverse ligament (of knee joint)
Transverse tarsal joint (TAR-sal)
Upper ankle joint
Windlass mechanism (WIND-lus)
Y ligament
Zona orbicularis (ZONE-a or-BIK-you-la-ris)

WORD ORIGINS

- ❑ Auricle—From Latin *auris,* meaning *ear*
- ❑ Bifurcate—From Latin *bis,* meaning *two*, and *furca* meaning *fork*
- ❑ Bunion—From Old French *bugne,* meaning *bump on the head*
- ❑ Counter—From Latin *contra,* meaning *against*
- ❑ Coxa—From Latin *coxa,* meaning *hip* or *hip joint*
- ❑ Cruciate—From Latin *crux,* meaning *cross*
- ❑ Deltoid—From the Greek letter *delta,* which is triangular in shape, and *eidos,* meaning *resemblance, appearance*
- ❑ Digit—From Latin *digitus,* meaning *toe* (or *finger*)
- ❑ Hallucis—From Latin *hallucis,* meaning *of the big toe*
- ❑ Hallux—From Latin *hallex,* meaning *big toe*
- ❑ Innominate—From Latin *innominatus,* meaning *unnamed* or *nameless*
- ❑ Labrum—From Latin *labrum,* meaning *lip*
- ❑ Lunate—From Latin *luna,* meaning *moon*
- ❑ Malacia—From Greek *malakia,* meaning *softening* (related Latin *malus,* meaning *bad*)
- ❑ Meniscus—From Greek *meniskos,* meaning *crescent*
- ❑ Nutation—From Latin *annuo,* meaning *to nod*
- ❑ Pedis—From Latin *pes,* meaning *foot*
- ❑ Pelvis—From Latin *pelvis,* meaning *basin*
- ❑ Pes—From Latin *pes,* meaning *foot*
- ❑ Ray—From Latin *radius,* meaning *extending outward (radially) from a structure*
- ❑ Recurvatum—From Latin *recurvus,* meaning *bent back*
- ❑ Retinaculum—From Latin *retineo,* meaning *to hold back, restrain*
- ❑ Sacrum—From Latin *sacrum,* meaning *sacred, holy*
- ❑ Sciatic—From Latin *sciaticus* (which came from Greek *ischiadikos,* which in turn came from *ischion*), meaning *hip*
- ❑ Valga—From Latin *valgus,* meaning *twisted, bent outward, bowlegged*
- ❑ Vara—From Latin *varum,* meaning *crooked, bent inward, knock-kneed*

☐ 8.1 INTRODUCTION TO THE PELVIS AND PELVIC MOVEMENT

- ❑ The pelvis is a body part that is located between the trunk and the thighs (see Section 1.2).
- ❑ The **bony pelvis** is the term that refers to the bones and joints of the pelvis (Figure 8-1).
- ❑ The bones located within the pelvis are the sacrum, coccyx, and the two pelvic bones.
  - ❑ The sacrum is actually five vertebrae that never fully formed, and fused embryologically.
  - ❑ The coccyx is made up of four vertebrae that never fully formed. Usually, these four bones of the coccyx fuse later in life.
  - ❑ Each pelvic bone is composed of an ilium, ischium, and pubis that fused embryologically.

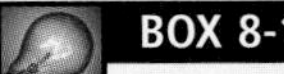

BOX 8-1

The pelvic bone is also known as the **coxal bone**, **innominate bone**, or *hip bone.*

- ❑ The joints that are located within the pelvis are the symphysis pubis and two sacroiliac (SI) joints.
  - ❑ The **symphysis pubis joint** unites the two pubic bones.
  - ❑ Each **sacroiliac (SI) joint** unites the sacrum with the iliac portion of the pelvic bone on that side of the body.
- ❑ The pelvis is a transitional body part that is made up of bones of both the axial skeleton and the appendicular skeleton.
  - ❑ The sacrum and coccyx of the pelvis are axial bones of the spine.
  - ❑ The two pelvic bones (each one composed of an ilium, ischium, and pubis) are appendicular pelvic girdle bones of the lower extremity.
- ❑ The bony pelvis is often referred to as the **pelvic girdle**.

BOX 8-2

A girdle is an article of clothing that encircles the body and provides stabilization. Similarly, the pelvic girdle encircles the body and provides a firm, stable base of attachment for the femurs.

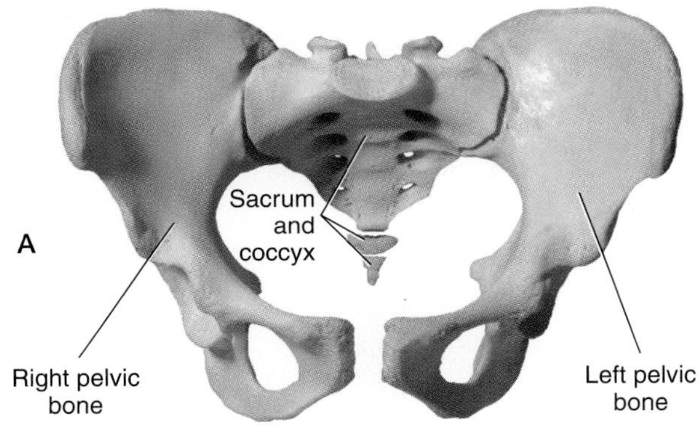

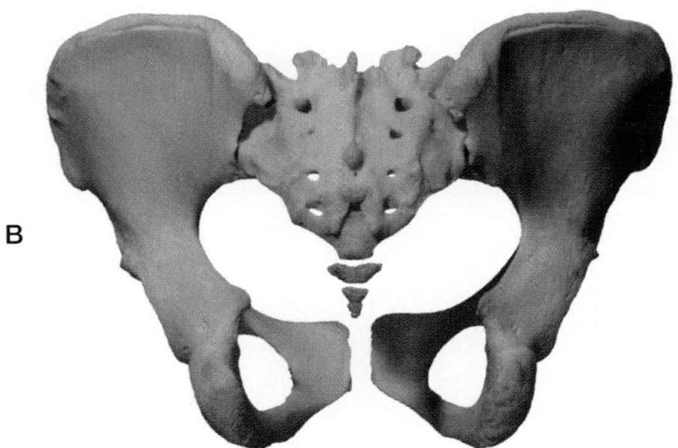

Figure 8-1 *A,* Anterior view of the bony pelvis. *B,* Posterior view. The bony pelvis is composed of the two pelvic bones and the sacrum and coccyx. The pelvic bones are part of the appendicular skeleton; the sacrum and coccyx are part of the axial skeleton. For this reason, the pelvis is considered to be a transitional body part.

Pelvic Motion:

Two types of pelvic motion exist:

- Motion can occur within the pelvis (i.e., intrapelvic motion).
  - This motion can occur at the SI joints and/or at the symphysis pubis joint.
- The entire pelvis can move as one unit relative to an adjacent body part.
  - This motion can occur relative to the trunk at the lumbosacral (L5-S1) joint and/or relative to a thigh at a hip joint or to both thighs at both hip joints.

BOX 8-3

Pelvic motion can be complicated and is often misunderstood. To clearly understand pelvic motion, it is important to be very clear about the basics of defining motion. Motion is defined as movement of one body part relative to another body part at the joint that is located between them. The pelvis is a separate body part from the trunk and can therefore move relative to the trunk at the joint that is located between the pelvis and the trunk (i.e., the lumbosacral [L5-S1] joint). It is also a separate body part from the thighs and can move relative to a thigh at a hip joint (or to both thighs at both hip joints). Given that separate bones within the pelvis are separated by joints, motion within the pelvis is also possible. (For more information on motion within the pelvis, see Section 8-2; for more information on motion between the pelvis and adjacent parts, see Sections 8-3 through 8-5.)

8.2 INTRAPELVIC MOTION (SYMPHYSIS PUBIS AND SACROILIAC JOINTS)

- Because the pelvis has the symphysis pubis and sacroiliac (SI) joints located within it, the bones of the pelvis can move relative to each other at these joints; this is termed *intrapelvic motion*.
- Intrapelvic motion can occur at the symphysis pubis joint and/or the SI joints.

Symphysis Pubis Joint:

- The symphysis pubis joint is located between the two pubic bones of the pelvis.
  - More specifically, it is located between the bodies of the two pubic bones.

BOX 8-4

The name *symphysis pubis* literally means *joining of the bodies of the pubis.*

- Joint structure classification: Cartilaginous joint
  - Subtype: Symphysis joint
- Joint function classification: Amphiarthrotic

Major Motions Allowed:

- Nonaxial gliding

Major Ligaments of the Symphysis Pubis Joint:

Arcuate Pubic Ligament:

- The arcuate pubic ligament spans the pubic symphysis joint inferiorly, stabilizing the joint (Figure 8-2).

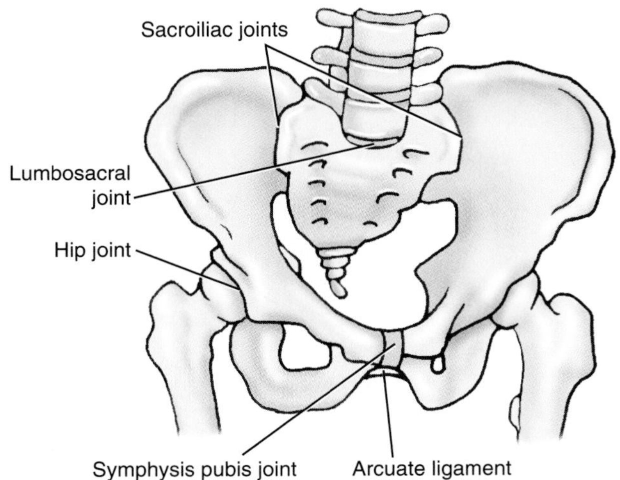

Figure 8-2 Anterolateral view of the pelvis. Both SI joints are seen posteriorly, and the symphysis pubis joint is seen anteriorly. The arcuate ligament of the symphysis pubis joint is also seen.

Miscellaneous:

- The symphysis pubis joint is also stabilized (i.e., reinforced) by the fibrous aponeurotic expansions of a number of muscles of the abdominal wall and the medial thigh.
  - These muscles are the rectus abdominis, external abdominal oblique, internal abdominal oblique, and transversus abdominis of the anterior abdominal wall; as well as the adductor longus, gracilis, and adductor brevis of the medial thigh.
- The end of each pubic bone of the pubic symphysis joint is lined with articular cartilage; these cartilage-covered ends are then joined by a fibrocartilaginous disc.

Sacroiliac Joints:

- Two SI joints exist, paired left and right (see Figure 8-2).
- Each SI joint is located between the sacrum and the iliac portion of the pelvic bone, hence the name SI joint.
  - More specifically, the SI joints unite the *C*-shaped auricular surfaces of the sacrum with the *C*-shaped auricular surfaces of the two pelvic bones.

BOX 8-5

The term *auricular* is Latin for *little ear.* These articular surfaces of the sacrum and ilium are termed *auricular* because they resemble an ear in shape.

- Joint structure classification: Mixed synovial/fibrous joint
  - Subtype: Plane joint
- Joint function classification: Mixed diarthrotic/amphiarthrotic

BOX 8-6

The sacroiliac (SI) joints are unusual in that they begin as diarthrotic, synovial joints; a synovial capsule and cavity are present, the bones are capped with articular cartilage, and the degree of movement allowed is appreciable. However, as a person ages, fibrous tissue is gradually placed within the joint cavity converting this joint to a fibrous, amphiarthrotic joint. The tremendous weight-bearing force from above (see Figure 8-5), wedging the sacrum into the pelvic bones, along with forces transmitted up from the lower extremities, are credited with creating the stresses that cause the changes to this joint.

Major Motions Allowed:

- ❏ Nonaxial gliding
- ❏ Nutation and counternutation (i.e., axial movements) (Figure 8-3)
  - ❏ **Nutation** is defined as the superior sacral base dropping anteriorly and inferiorly, while the inferior tip of the sacrum moves posteriorly and superiorly. Relatively, the pelvic bone tilts posteriorly.
  - ❏ **Counternutation** is defined as the opposite of nutation; the superior sacral base moves posteriorly and superiorly, while the inferior tip of the sacrum moves anteriorly and inferiorly. Relatively, the pelvic bone tilts anteriorly.

BOX 8-7

The amount of motion at the sacroiliac (SI) joints and the biomechanical and clinical importance of SI joint motion are extremely controversial. Many sources, especially in the traditional allopathic world, view SI motion and importance as negligible and unimportant; many sources, especially in the chiropractic and osteopathic world, view the sacrum as the keystone of the pelvis and the motion and importance of the SI joint as perhaps the most important joint of the "low back."

Major Ligaments of the Sacroiliac Joint:

All SI ligaments provide stability to the SI joint (Figure 8-4).

Sacroiliac Ligaments:

- ❏ These ligaments span directly from the sacrum to the ilium
- ❏ Three sets of **sacroiliac (SI) ligaments** exist:
  - ❏ Anterior SI ligaments
  - ❏ Posterior SI ligaments (short and long)
  - ❏ SI interosseus ligaments

Sacrotuberous ligament:

- ❏ The sacrotuberous ligament attaches from the sacrum to the ischial tuberosity.
- ❏ The sacrotuberous ligament does not attach directly from the sacrum to ilium; hence it provides indirect stabilization to the SI joint.

Sacrospinous ligament:

- ❏ The sacrospinous ligament attaches from the sacrum to the ischial spine.
- ❏ The sacrospinous ligament does not attach directly from the sacrum to ilium; hence it provides indirect stabilization to the SI joint.

BOX 8-8

The **greater sciatic notch** and the **lesser sciatic notch** are notches in the posterior contour of the pelvic bone; the dividing point between them is created by the ischial spine. These sciatic notches become sciatic foramina with the presence of the sacrospinous and sacrotuberous ligaments (see Figure 8-4a). (Note: The sciatic nerve exits the pelvis through the **greater sciatic foramen**.)

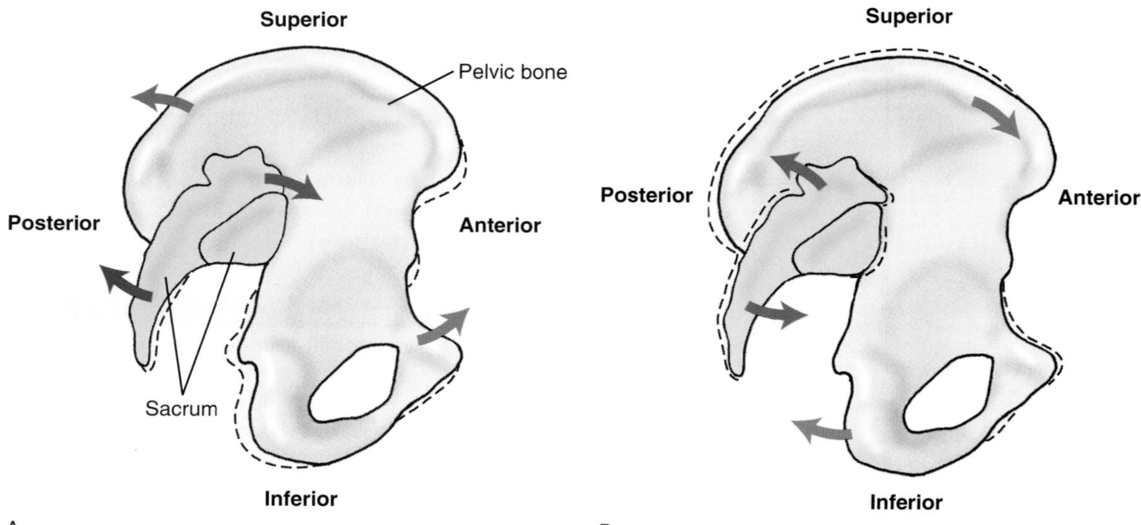

Figure 8-3 The sacrum can move within the pelvis relative to the two pelvic bones. *A,* Intrapelvic motion of nutation wherein the superior end of the sacrum moves anteriorly and inferiorly and the inferior end moves posteriorly and superiorly. Relatively, the pelvic bone tilts posteriorly. *B,* Intrapelvic motion of counternutation wherein the superior end of the sacrum moves posteriorly and superiorly and the inferior end moves anteriorly and inferiorly. Relatively, the pelvic bone tilts anteriorly.

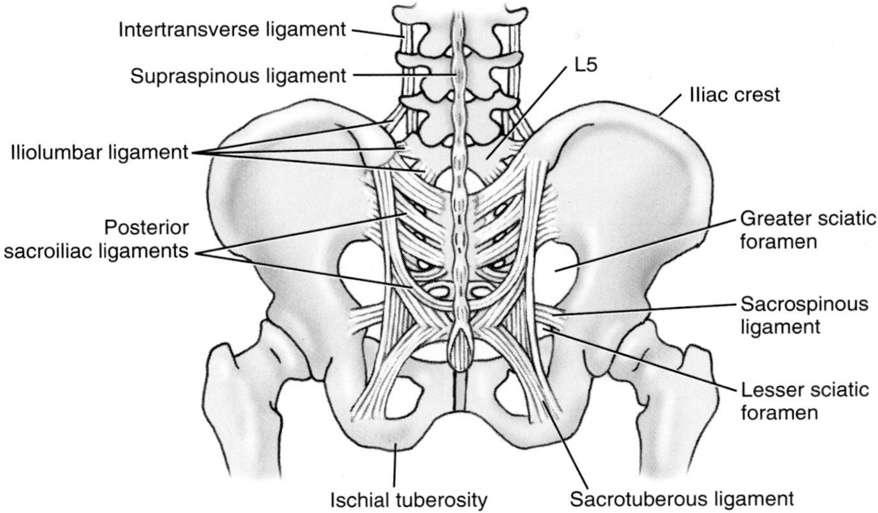

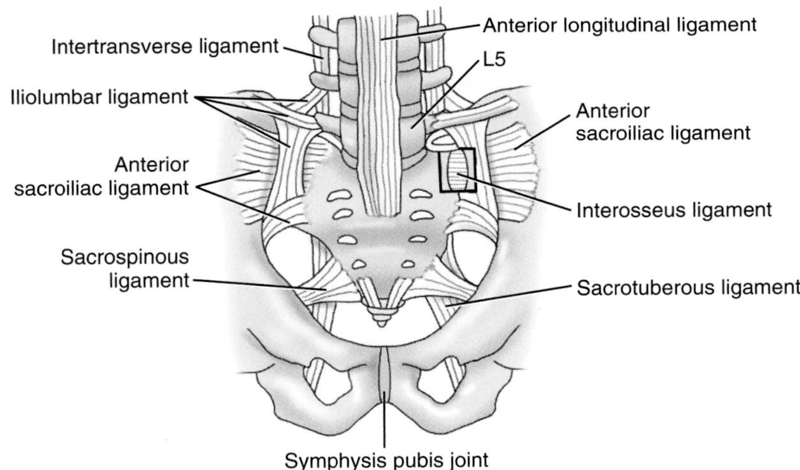

Figure 8-4 *A,* Posterior view of the ligaments of the sacroiliac (SI) joints. The major posterior ligaments of the SI joint are the posterior SI ligaments. Additional stabilization is given to this joint posteriorly by the iliolumbar, sacrotuberous, and sacrospinous ligaments. Note that the sacrospinous ligament separates the greater sciatic foramen from the lesser sciatic foramen. *B,* Anterior view of the ligaments of the SI joints. The major anterior ligaments of the SI joint are the anterior SI ligaments. On the left side (our right side), a small area of the anterior SI ligaments and the bony surfaces of the joint have been partially cut away to reveal the SI interosseus ligaments located within the joint.

Iliolumbar Ligament:

- ❑ The iliolumbar ligament attaches from the lumbar spine to the ilium.
- ❑ The iliolumbar ligament actually has a number of parts that attach the 4th and 5th lumbar vertebrae to the iliac crest.
- ❑ The iliolumbar ligaments indirectly help stabilize the SI joint. They are also important in stabilizing the lumbosacral (L5-S1) joint.

BOX 8-9

LIGAMENTS OF THE SACROILIAC JOINT

- Sacroiliac (SI) ligaments (anterior, posterior, and interosseus)
- Sacrotuberous ligament
- Sacrospinous ligament
- Iliolumbar ligament

Miscellaneous:

- ❑ The SI joint is the joint that is located at the transition of the inferior end of the axial skeleton and the proximal end of the appendicular skeleton of the lower extremity.
- ❑ The SI joints are weight-bearing joints that must transfer the weight of the axial body to the pelvic bones of the lower extremities (Figure 8-5).
- ❑ During pregnancy, the ligaments of the SI joints loosen to allow greater movement so that the baby can be delivered through the birth canal.

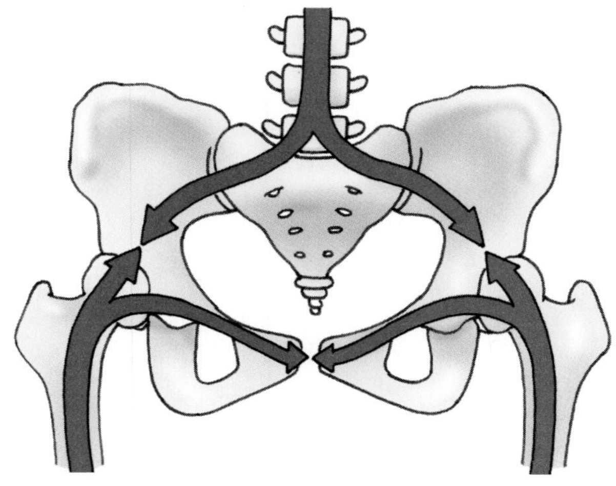

Figure 8-5 Illustration of the forces that are transmitted through the sacroiliac (SI) joint. These forces affect the SI joints from both above and below. Weight-bearing forces from above are represented by the arrow that descends the spine. Forces of impact from below that would occur when walking, running, or jumping are represented by the lines that ascend the femurs. (Modeled from Kapandji IA: *Physiology of the joints: the trunk and the vertebral column,* ed. 2. Edinburgh, 1974, Churchill Livingstone.)

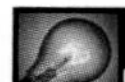

BOX 8-10

The increased looseness of the ligaments of the sacroiliac (SI) joints that occurs during pregnancy often remains throughout the life of the woman. This increased mobility results in a decreased stability of the SI joints and an increased predisposition for low-back problems and pain.

☐ 8.3 MOVEMENT OF THE PELVIS AT THE LUMBOSACRAL JOINT

Motion of the Pelvis at the Lumbosacral Joint:

- ❑ When the pelvis moves as a unit, this motion can occur relative to the lumbar spine of the trunk at the lumbosacral joint.
- ❑ Given that we usually think of the spine as moving at the spinal joints (the lumbosacral joint is a spinal joint), movement of the pelvis at the lumbosacral joint is an example of what is termed a *reverse action*. (See Section 5.29 for information on reverse actions.)
- ❑ If no motion is occurring at the hip joints when the pelvis moves at the lumbosacral joint, then the thighs are fixed to the pelvis and will "go along for the ride," following the movement of the pelvis.

Following are motions of the pelvis at the lumbosacral joint (Figure 8-6; Box 8-11):

- ❑ The pelvis can anteriorly tilt and posteriorly tilt in the sagittal plane around a mediolateral axis.
- ❑ The pelvis can depress or elevate on one side in the frontal plane around an anteroposterior axis.
    - ❑ Note: When the pelvis depresses on one side, the other side of the pelvis elevates (i.e., depression of the right pelvis creates elevation of the left pelvis). Similarly, if the pelvis elevates on one side, then the other side depresses (Box 8-12).
- ❑ The pelvis can rotate to the right or to the left in the transverse plane around a vertical axis.

BOX 8-11

The lumbosacral joint only allows a few degrees of motion. When the pelvis moves at the lumbosacral joint, the rest of the spine will have to begin to move once the motion of the lumbosacral joint has reached its limit. This can be seen in Figures 8-6, *A-F* (the change in the curve of the lumbar spine should be noted).

BOX 8-12

Depression of the pelvis on one side is also called *lateral tilt* (i.e., depression of the right side of the pelvis is called *right lateral tilt of the pelvis*; depression of the left side of the pelvis is called *left lateral tilt of the pelvis*). When describing the side of the pelvis that elevates, it is often called *hiking* the hip or pelvis.

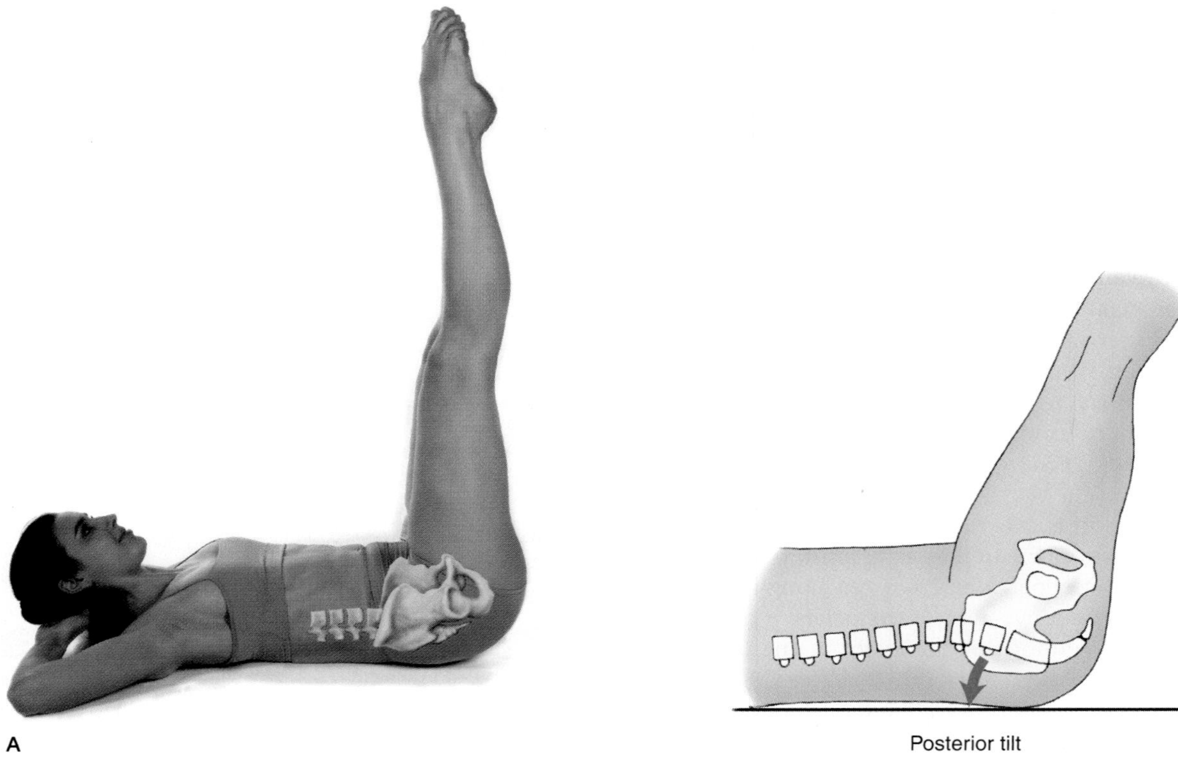

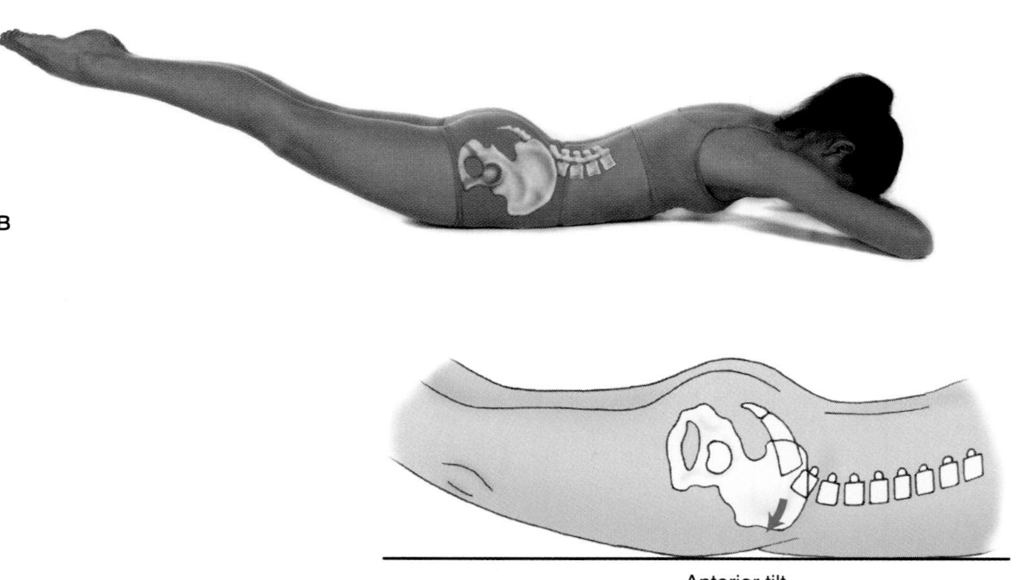

Figure 8-6 Motion of the pelvis at the lumbosacral joint. *A* and *B,* Lateral views illustrating posterior tilt and anterior tilt, respectively, of the pelvis at the lumbosacral joint. (Note: In *A* and *B* no motion is occurring at the hip joints; therefore the thighs are seen to "go along for the ride," resulting in the lower extremities changing their orientation.)

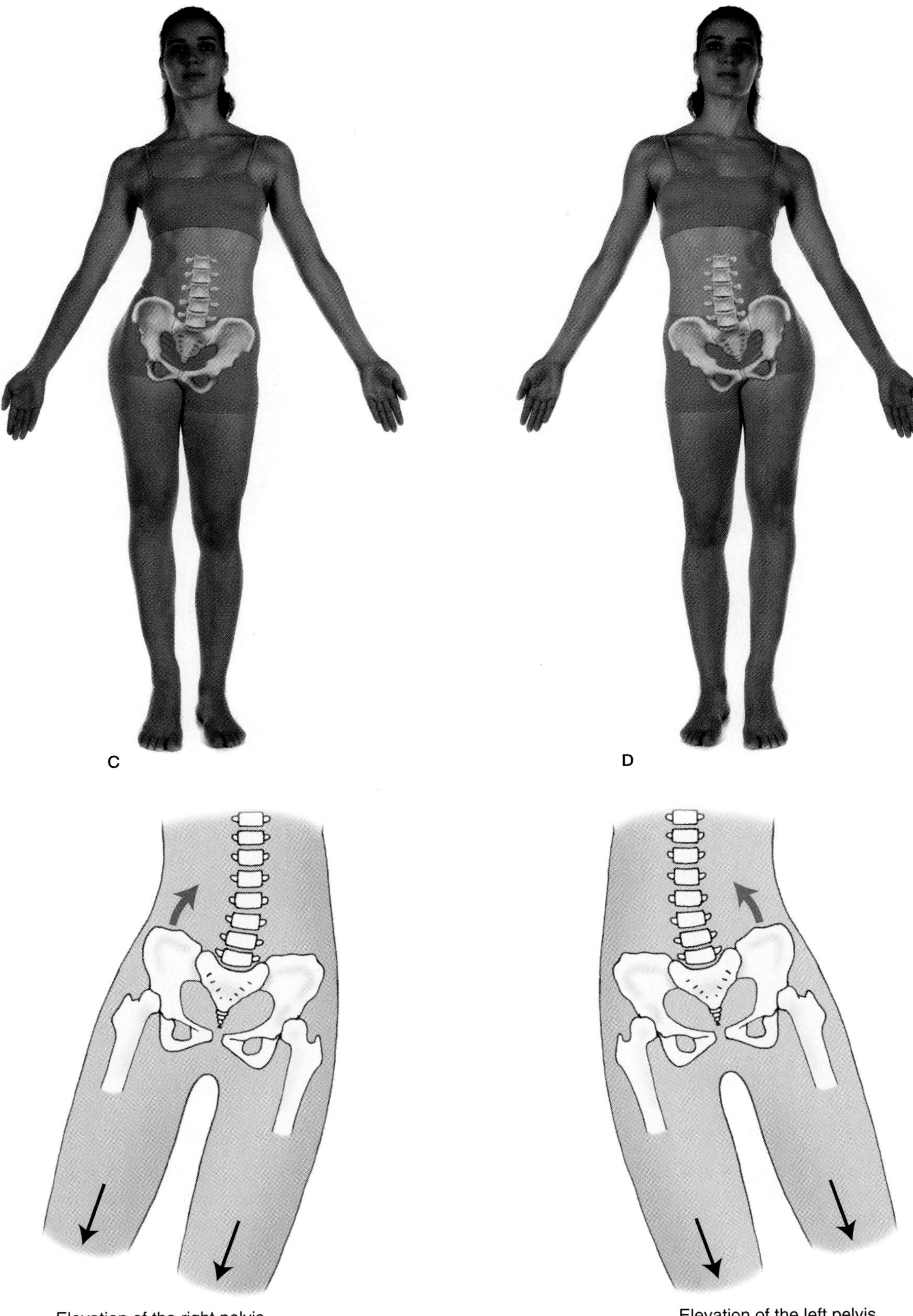

Figure 8-6, cont'd *C* and *D*, Anterior views illustrating elevation of the right pelvis and elevation of the left pelvis, respectively, at the lumbosacral joint. (Note: In the drawn illustration of *C* and *D*, no motion is occurring at the hip joints; therefore, the thighs are seen to "go along for the ride," resulting in the lower extremities changing their orientation.) *Continued*

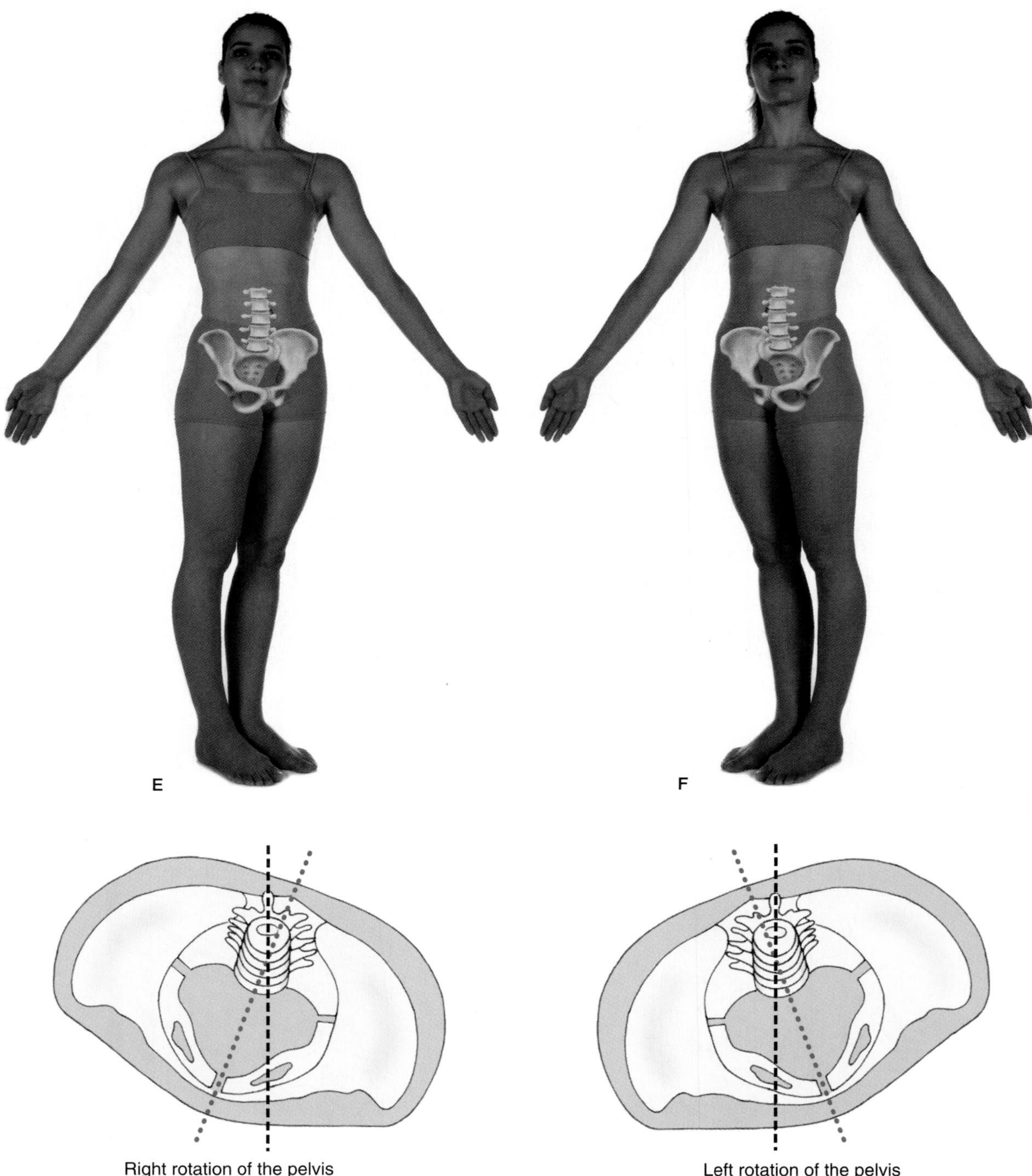

Figure 8-6, cont'd *E* and *F,* Anterior and superior views illustrating rotation of the pelvis to the right and rotation to the left, respectively, at the lumbosacral joint. (Note: In *E* and *F* the dashed black line represents the orientation of the spine and the red dotted line represents the orientation of the pelvis. Given the different directions of these two lines, it is clear that the pelvis has rotated relative to the spine; this motion has occurred at the lumbosacral joint.)

☐ 8.4 MOVEMENT OF THE PELVIS AT THE HIP JOINTS

Motion of the Pelvis as a Unit at the Hip Joints:

- ❑ When the pelvis moves as a unit, this motion can occur relative to the thighs at the hip joints.

BOX 8-13

When the pelvis moves at the hip joints, it is possible for the pelvis to move at both hip joints at the same time; this results in the pelvis changing its position relative to both thighs. It is also possible for the pelvis to move relative to only hip joint. In this case the pelvis moves relative only to that one thigh (at the hip joint located between the pelvis and that thigh); the other thigh stays fixed to the pelvis and "goes along for the ride."

- ❑ Given that we usually think of the thighs as moving at the hip joints, movement of the pelvis at the hip joints is an example of what is termed a *reverse action*. (See Section 5.29 for information on reverse actions.)
- ❑ If no motion is occurring at the lumbosacral joint when the pelvis moves at the hip joints, then the trunk is fixed to the pelvis and will "go along for the ride," following the movement of the pelvis.

BOX 8-14

When a person is standing up and anteriorly tilts the pelvis at the hip joints (and the trunk stays fixed to the pelvis, going along for the ride) to "bend forward," this motion is often incorrectly described as *flexion of the trunk* or *flexion of the spine*. Actually, the trunk never moved in this scenario, because it did not move relative to the pelvis (it merely followed the pelvis). Further, no movement ever occurred at the spinal joints. The entire movement is due to a "flexion" of the hip joint wherein the pelvis anteriorly tilted toward the thighs.

Following are motions of the pelvis at the hip joints (Figure 8-7):

- ❑ The pelvis can anteriorly tilt and posteriorly tilt in the sagittal plane around a mediolateral axis.
- ❑ The pelvis can depress or elevate on one side in the frontal plane around an anteroposterior axis.
- ❑ The pelvis can rotate to the right or to the left in the transverse plane around a vertical axis.

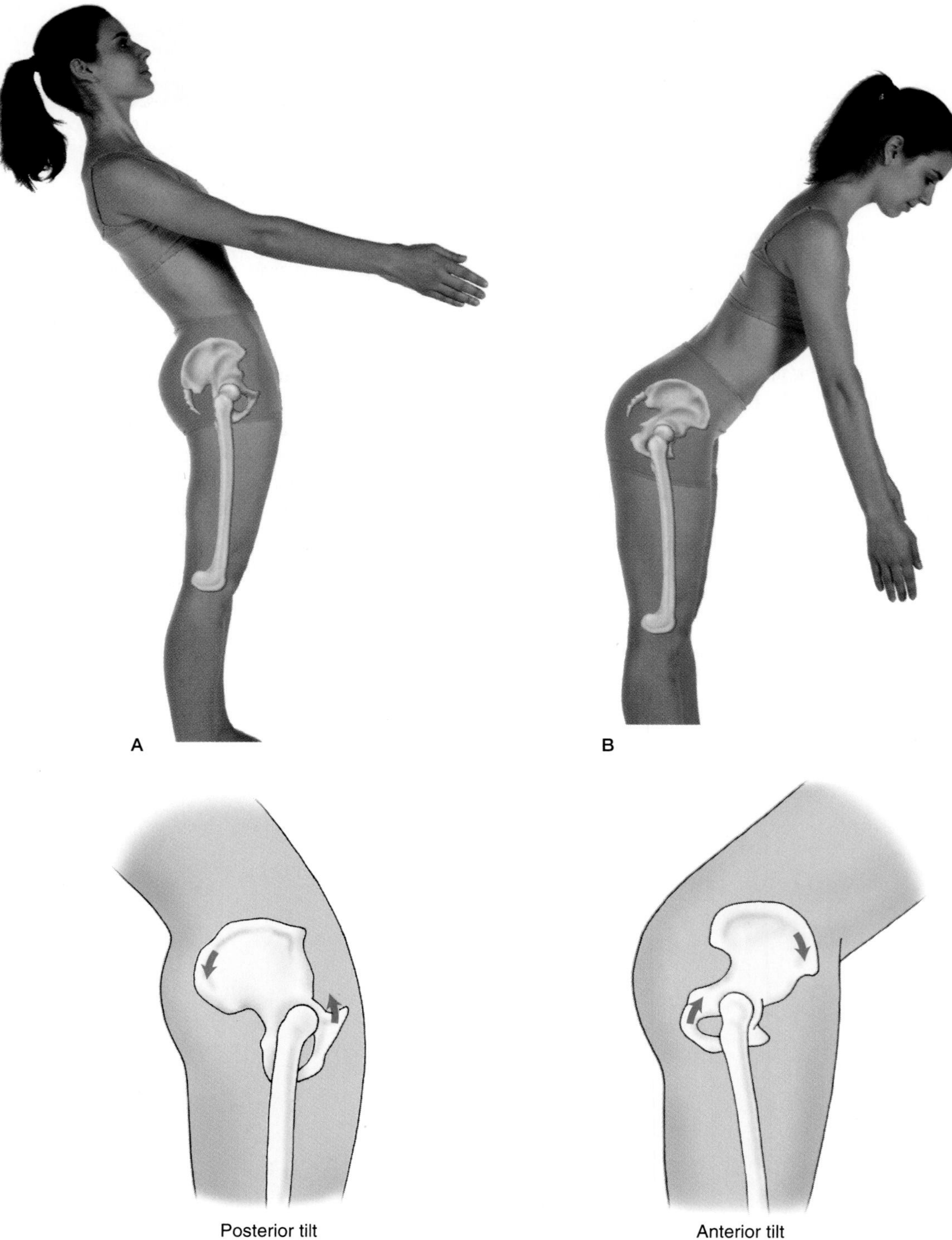

Figure 8-7 Motion of the pelvis at the hip joint. (Note: In *A* to *D* no motion is occurring at the lumbosacral joint; therefore the trunk is seen to "go along for the ride," resulting in the upper body changing its orientation.) *A* and *B,* Lateral views illustrating posterior tilt and anterior tilt, respectively, of the pelvis at the hip joint.

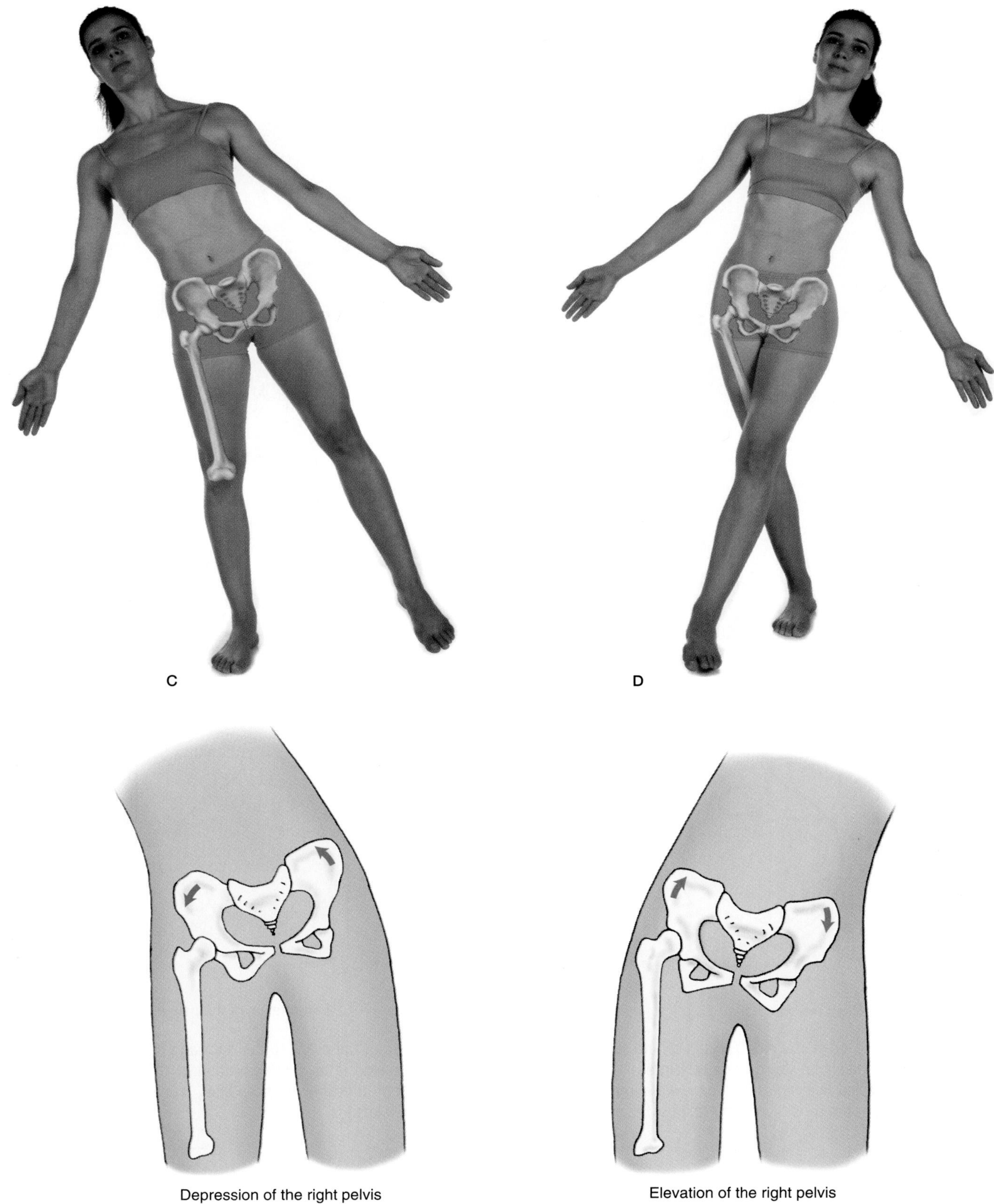

Figure 8-7, cont'd *C* and *D,* Anterior views illustrating depression of the right pelvis and elevation of the right pelvis, respectively, at the right hip joint. (Note: When the pelvis elevates on one side, it depresses on the other, and vice versa.)

Continued

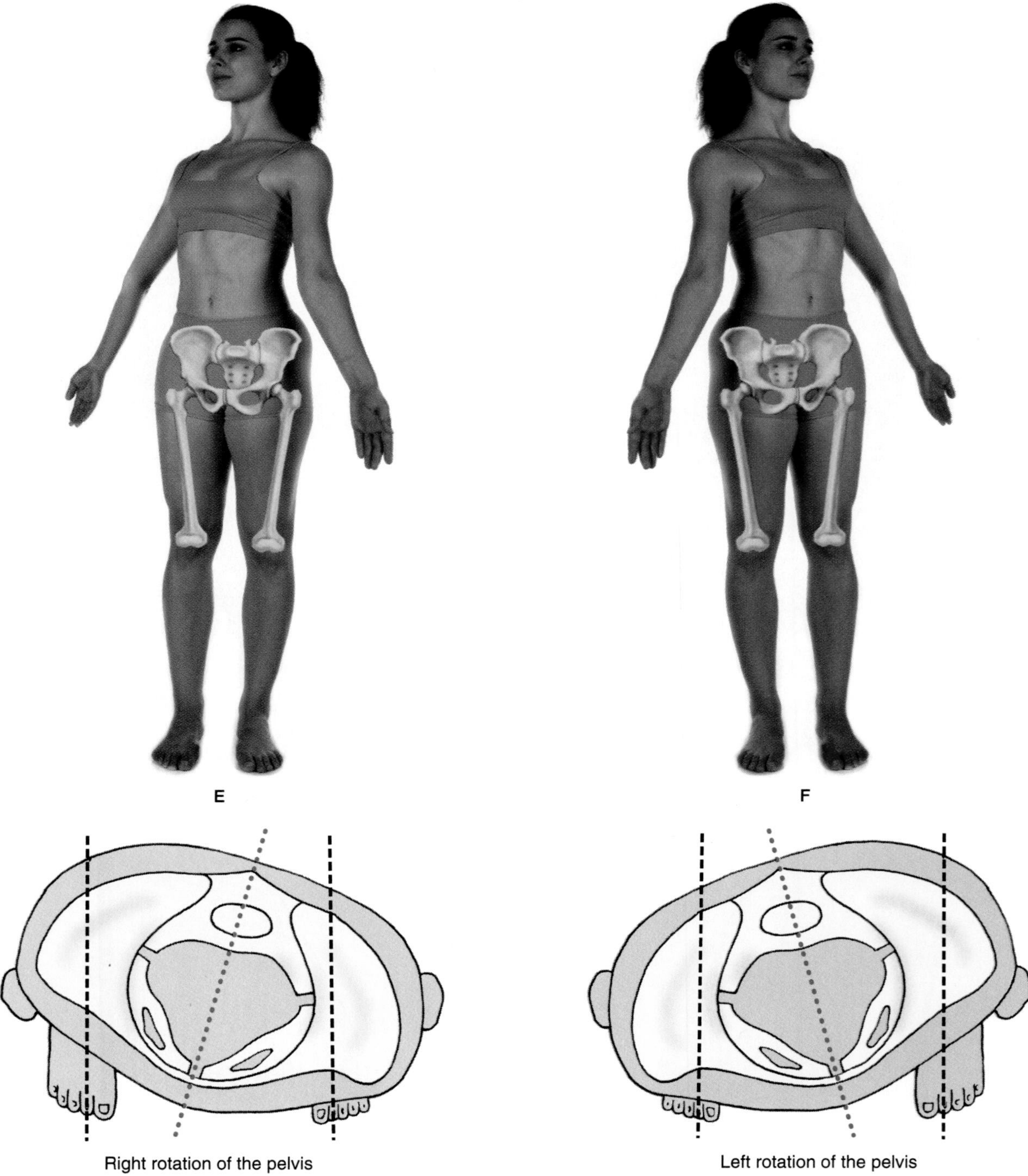

Figure 8-7, cont'd *E* and *F,* Anterior and superior views illustrating rotation of the pelvis to the right and rotation to the left, respectively, at the hip joints. (Note: In *E* and *F* the black dashed line represents the orientation of the thighs and the red dotted line represents the orientation of the pelvis. Given the different directions of these lines, it is clear that the pelvis has rotated relative to the thighs; this motion has occurred at the hip joints.)

8.5 MOVEMENT OF THE PELVIS AT THE LUMBOSACRAL AND HIP JOINTS

Motion of the Pelvis as a Unit at the Lumbosacral and Hip Joints:

- Of course, the pelvis can move as a body part at both the lumbosacral joint and the hips joints at the same time. When this occurs, two things should be noted:
  1. The pelvis moves relative to both the spine and the thigh(s).
  2. The motion has occurred at the both the lumbosacral joint and the hip joint(s) (Figure 8-8). (See Table 8-1 for the average ranges of motion of the pelvis.)

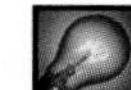

BOX 8-15

As is usual for motion of the pelvis at the lumbosacral joint, when maximum motion possible at this joint is attained by the muscles that move the pelvis at the lumbosacral joint, motion will also occur at the lumbar spinal joints. This can be seen by noting the changes in the lumbar spinal curve.

TABLE 8-1

Average Ranges of Motion of the Pelvis at the Hip and Lumbosacral Joints with the Client Seated and the Thighs Flexed 90 Degrees at the Hip Joint (These Numbers Would be Different if the Client is Standing and Would also Vary Based on Whether the Knee Joint is Flexed or Extended.)

Anterior tilt	30 Degrees	Posterior tilt	15 Degrees
Right depression	30 Degrees	Left depression	30 Degrees
Right rotation	15 Degrees	Left rotation	15 Degrees

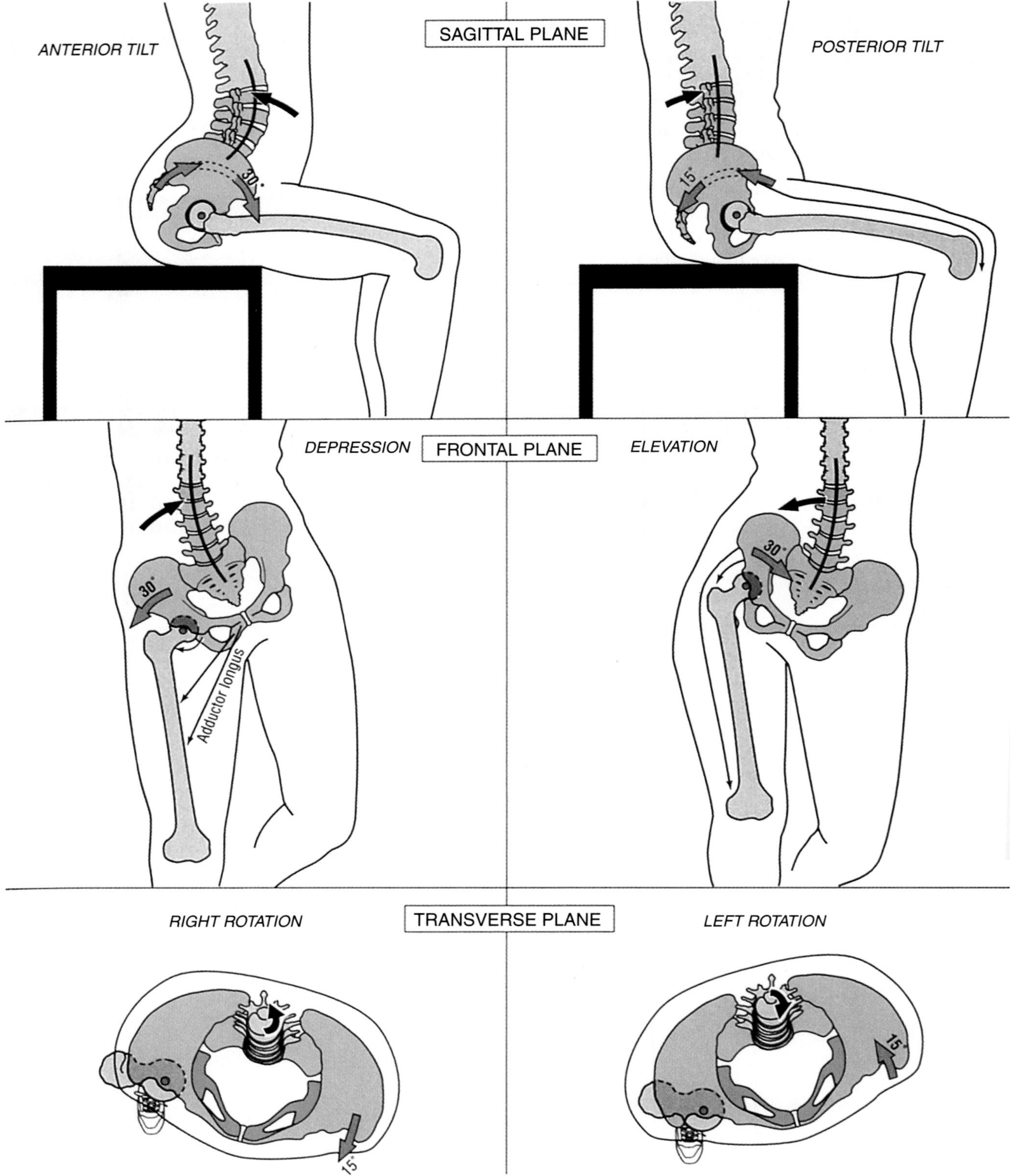

Figure 8-8 Motion of the pelvis at both the lumbosacral joint and the hip joints. (Note: In all illustrations the change in position of the pelvis is relative to both the spine and the femur[s].) *A* and *B,* Illustration of the sagittal plane motions of anterior tilt and posterior tilt, respectively. *C* and *D,* Frontal plane motions of depression and elevation, respectively. *E* and *F,* Transverse plane motions of right rotation and left rotation, respectively. (Modified from Neumann DA: *Kinesiology of the musculoskeletal system: foundations for physical rehabilitation,* St Louis, 2002, Mosby.)

☐ 8.6 RELATIONSHIP OF PELVIC/SPINAL MOVEMENTS AT THE LUMBOSACRAL JOINT

❑ Now that the motion of the pelvis is clearly understood, it is valuable to examine the relationship that pelvic movements have to spinal movements. If we picture the muscles that cross from the trunk to the pelvis (i.e., crossing the lumbosacral joint), then these pelvic movements would be considered the reverse actions of these muscles. Following is the relationship between the pelvis and the spine for the six major movements within the three cardinal planes:

Sagittal Plane Movements:

❑ Posterior tilt of the pelvis at the lumbosacral joint is analogous to flexion of the trunk at the lumbosacral joint. Therefore muscles that do flexion of the trunk also do posterior tilt of the pelvis at the lumbosacral joint (Figure 8-9).

❑ Examples: The muscles of the anterior abdominal wall, such as the rectus abdominis, external abdominal oblique, and the internal abdominal oblique

❑ Anterior tilt of the pelvis at the lumbosacral joint is analogous to extension of the trunk at the lumbosacral joint. Therefore muscles that do extension of the trunk also do anterior tilt of the pelvis at the lumbosacral joint (see Figure 8-9).

❑ Examples: Erector spinae group, transversospinalis group, quadratus lumborum, and latissimus dorsi

Frontal Plane Movements:

❑ Elevation of the right pelvis (which is also depression of the left pelvis) at the lumbosacral joint is analogous to right lateral flexion of the trunk at the lumbosacral joint. Therefore muscles that do right lateral flexion of the trunk also do elevation of the right pelvis (and therefore also depression of the left pelvis) at the lumbosacral joint (Figure 8-10).

❑ Examples: Right erector spinae group, right transversospinalis group, right quadratus lumborum, and right latissimus dorsi

❑ Elevation of the left pelvis (which is also depression of the right pelvis) at the lumbosacral joint is analogous to left lateral flexion of the trunk at the lumbosacral joint. Therefore muscles that do left lateral flexion of the trunk also do elevation of the left pelvis (and therefore also depression of the right pelvis) at the lumbosacral joint (see Figure 8-10).

❑ Examples: Left erector spinae group, left transversospinalis group, left quadratus lumborum, and left latissimus dorsi

Transverse Plane Movements:

❑ Right rotation of the pelvis at the lumbosacral joint is analogous to left rotation of the trunk at the lumbosacral joint. Therefore muscles that do left rotation of the trunk also do right rotation of the pelvis at the lumbosacral joint (Figure 8-11).

❑ Examples: Left-sided ipsilateral rotators of the trunk such as the left erector spinae group and the left internal abdominal oblique; and right-sided contralateral rotators of the trunk such as the right transversospinalis group and the right external abdominal oblique

❑ Left rotation of the pelvis at the lumbosacral joint is analogous to right rotation of the trunk at the lumbosacral joint. Therefore muscles that do right rotation of the trunk also do left rotation of the pelvis at the lumbosacral joint (see Figure 8-11).

❑ Examples: Right-sided ipsilateral rotators of the trunk such as the right erector spinae group and the right internal abdominal oblique; and left-sided contralateral rotators of the trunk such as the left transversospinalis group and the left external abdominal oblique

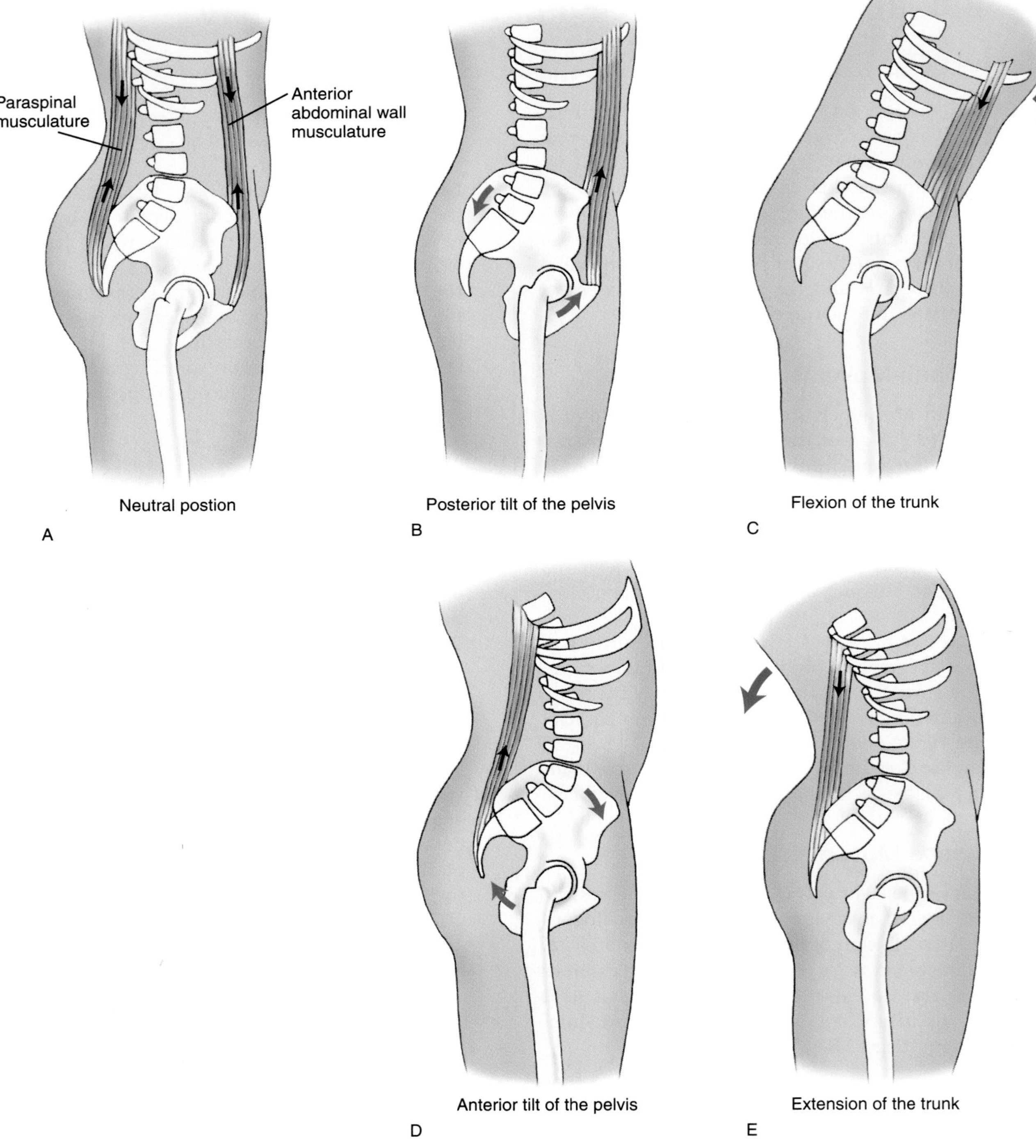

Figure 8-9 Lateral views of two groups of muscles that cross the lumbosacral joint and create sagittal plane actions of the pelvis and trunk; one group is located anteriorly, and the other group is located posteriorly. The anterior group contains the anterior abdominal wall muscles; the posterior group contains the paraspinal musculature (i.e., erector spinae and transversospinalis groups). *A,* Both groups are illustrated; arrows within the muscle groups represent the lines of pull of these muscles. *B* and *C,* Actions of the anterior group on the pelvis and the trunk, respectively; these actions are anterior tilt of the pelvis at the lumbosacral joint and flexion of the trunk at the lumbosacral joint (and the other spinal joints). *D* and *E,* Actions of the posterior group on the pelvis and the trunk; these actions are posterior tilt of the pelvis at the lumbosacral joint and extension of the trunk at the lumbosacral joint (and other spinal joints).

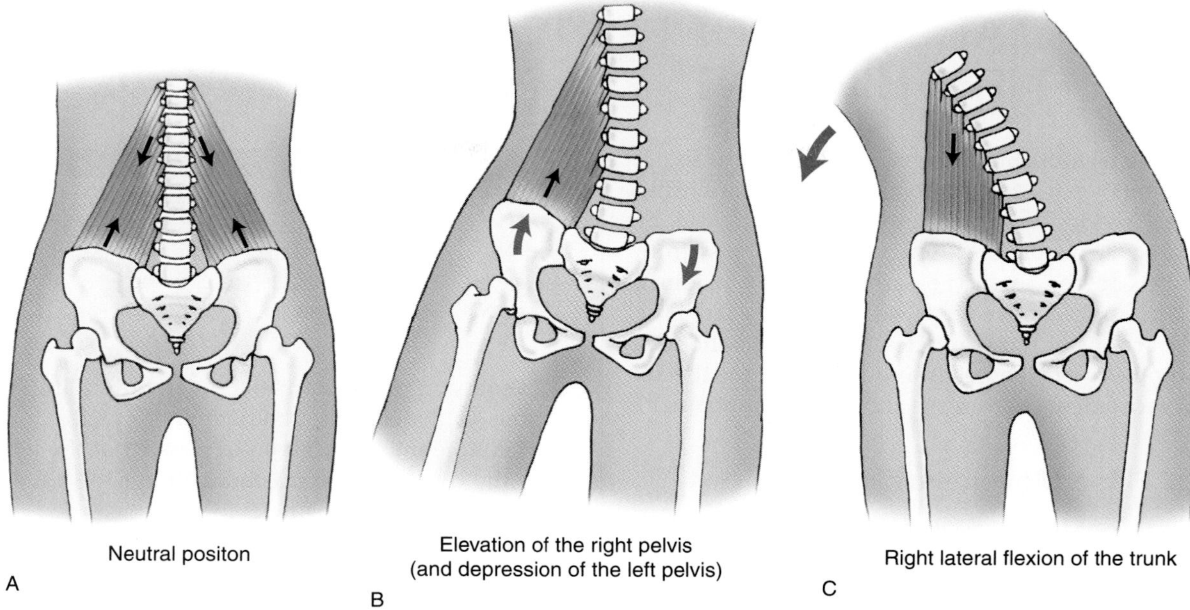

Figure 8-10 Anterior views of musculature that crosses the lumbosacral joint laterally and creates frontal plane actions of the pelvis and trunk at the lumbosacral joint. *A,* Illustration of this musculature bilaterally; the arrows demonstrate the lines of pull of the musculature. *B,* Pelvic action (i.e., elevation of the right pelvis at the lumbosacral joint) created by this musculature on the right side. (Note: When the pelvis elevates on one side, the other side depresses.) *C,* Trunk action (i.e., right lateral flexion of the trunk at the lumbosacral joint and the other spinal joints) created by this musculature on the right side. (Note: The actions for the left-sided musculature are not shown; they would be elevation of the left pelvis and left lateral flexion of the trunk.)

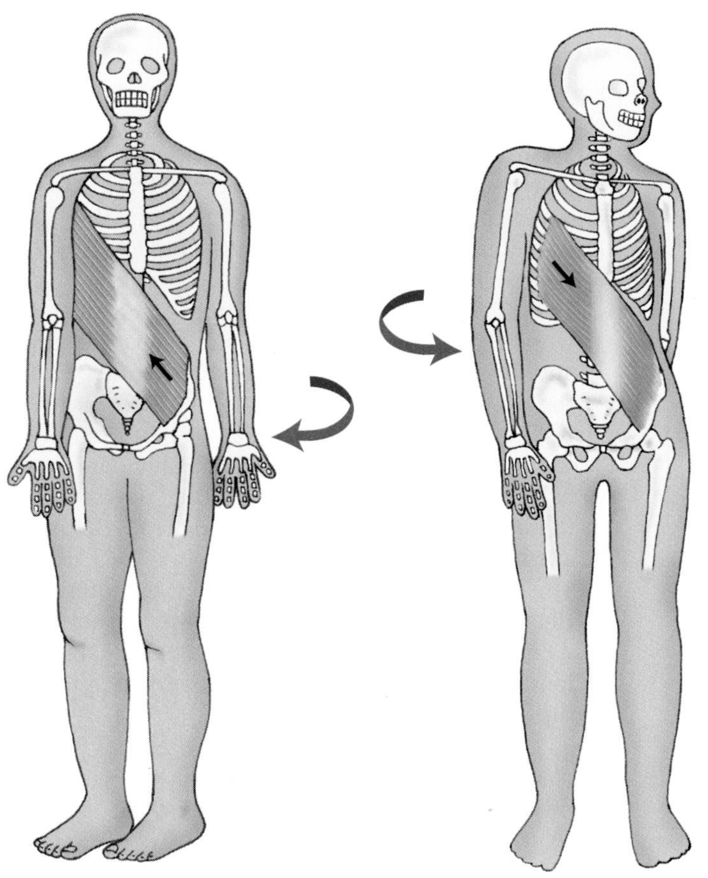

Figure 8-11 Anterior views of musculature that crosses the lumbosacral joint and creates transverse plane actions of the pelvis and trunk at the lumbosacral joint; this musculature is composed of the right-sided external abdominal oblique and the left-sided internal abdominal oblique. *A,* Pelvic action (i.e., right rotation of the pelvis at the lumbosacral joint) created by this musculature. *B,* Trunk action (i.e., left rotation of the trunk at the lumbosacral joint and other spinal joints.) created by this musculature. (Note: The similar musculature of the left-sided external abdominal oblique and right-sided internal abdominal oblique have not been shown. Actions for this musculature would be left rotation of the pelvis and right rotation of the trunk.)

8.7 RELATIONSHIP OF PELVIC/THIGH MOVEMENTS AT THE HIP JOINT

- Just as the relationship of pelvic movements to spinal movements can be compared, the relationship between pelvic and thigh movements can also be compared. If we picture the muscles that cross from the pelvis to the thigh (i.e., crossing the hip joint), then these pelvic movements would be considered the reverse actions of these muscles. Following is the relationship between the pelvis and the thigh for the six major movements within the three cardinal planes:

Sagittal Plane Movements:

- Anterior tilt of the pelvis at the hip joint is analogous to flexion of the thigh at the hip joint. Therefore muscles that do anterior tilt of the pelvis at the hip joint also do flexion of the thigh at the hip joint (Figure 8-12).
  - With flexion of the thigh at the hip joint, the thigh moves up toward the pelvis anteriorly; with anterior tilt of the pelvis at the hip joint, the pelvis moves down toward the thigh anteriorly. The same muscles (i.e., flexors of the hip joint) do both of these actions.
- Posterior tilt of the pelvis at the hip joint is analogous to extension of the thigh at the hip joint. Therefore muscles that do posterior tilt of the pelvis at the hip joint also do extension of the thigh at the hip joint (see Figure 8-12).
  - With extension of the thigh at the hip joint, the thigh moves up toward the pelvis posteriorly; with posterior tilt of the pelvis at the hip joint, the pelvis moves down toward the thigh posteriorly. The same muscles (i.e., extensors of the hip joint) do both of these actions.

Frontal Plane Movements:

- Depression of the right pelvis at the hip joint is analogous to abduction of the right thigh at the hip joint. Therefore muscles that do depression of the right pelvis at the hip joint also do abduction of the right thigh at the hip joint (Figure 8-13.)
  - With abduction of the right thigh at the right hip joint, the right thigh moves up toward the right side of the pelvis laterally; with depression of the right side of the pelvis at the right hip joint, the right side of the pelvis moves down toward the right thigh laterally. The same muscles (i.e., abductors of the right hip joint) do both of these actions.

BOX 8-16

When the right side of the pelvis depresses, the left side must elevate because the pelvis largely moves as a unit. Therefore it can be said that muscles that depress the pelvis on one side of the body also elevate the pelvis on the opposite side of the body (i.e., they are *contralateral elevators* of the pelvis).

- Depression of the left pelvis at the hip joint is analogous to abduction of the left thigh at the hip joint. Therefore muscles that do depression of the left pelvis at the hip joint also do abduction of the left thigh at the hip joint (see Figure 8-13).
  - The reasoning to explain this is identical to depression of the right pelvis (explained previously) except that it is on the left side of the body.

BOX 8-17

Depression of the right side of the pelvis is also known as *right lateral tilt of the pelvis.* The phrase "hiking the (left) hip" is sometimes used to refer to the other side of the pelvis, which has elevated. The same concepts would be true for depression of the left side of the pelvis.

Transverse Plane Movements:

- Right rotation of the pelvis at the hip joints is analogous to medial rotation of the right thigh and lateral rotation of the left thigh at the hip joints. Therefore muscles that do right rotation of the pelvis at the hip joints also do medial rotation of the right thigh and lateral rotation of the left thigh at the hip joints (Figure 8-14).
  - To best visualize this, it is helpful to picture a person who is standing up. If he or she keeps the thighs and lower extremities fixed and rotates the pelvis to the right at both hip joints, then the position that results will be identical to the position obtained if the person were to instead keep the pelvis and upper body fixed and medially rotate the right thigh at the right hip joint and laterally rotate the left thigh at the left hip joint.
  - The result is that muscles that do right rotation of the pelvis at the hip joints are the same muscles that do medial rotation of the right thigh at the right hip joint and lateral rotation of the left thigh at the left hip joint.

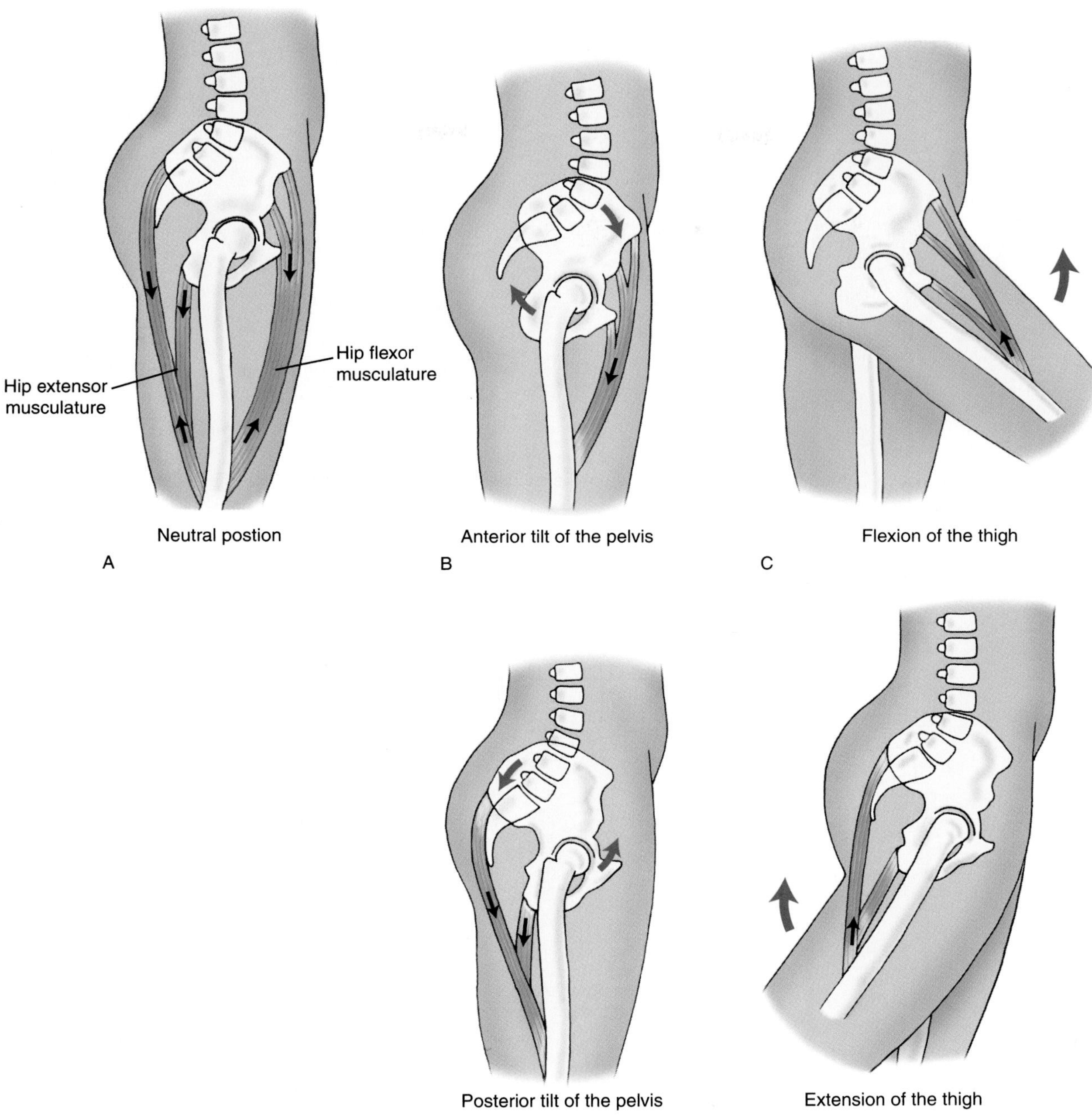

Figure 8-12 Lateral views of two groups of muscles that cross the hip joint and create sagittal plane actions of the pelvis and thigh; one group is located anteriorly and the other group is located posteriorly. The anterior group is composed of what is usually referred to as *hip flexor musculature*; the posterior group is composed of what is usually referred to *hip extensor musculature*. *A,* Both groups are illustrated; arrows within the muscle groups represent the lines of pull of these muscles. *B* and *C,* Actions of the anterior group on the pelvis and the thigh, respectively. These actions are anterior tilt of the pelvis at the hip joint and flexion of the thigh at the hip joint. *D* and *E,* Actions of the posterior group on the pelvis and the thigh; these actions are posterior tilt of the pelvis and extension of the thigh at the hip joint.

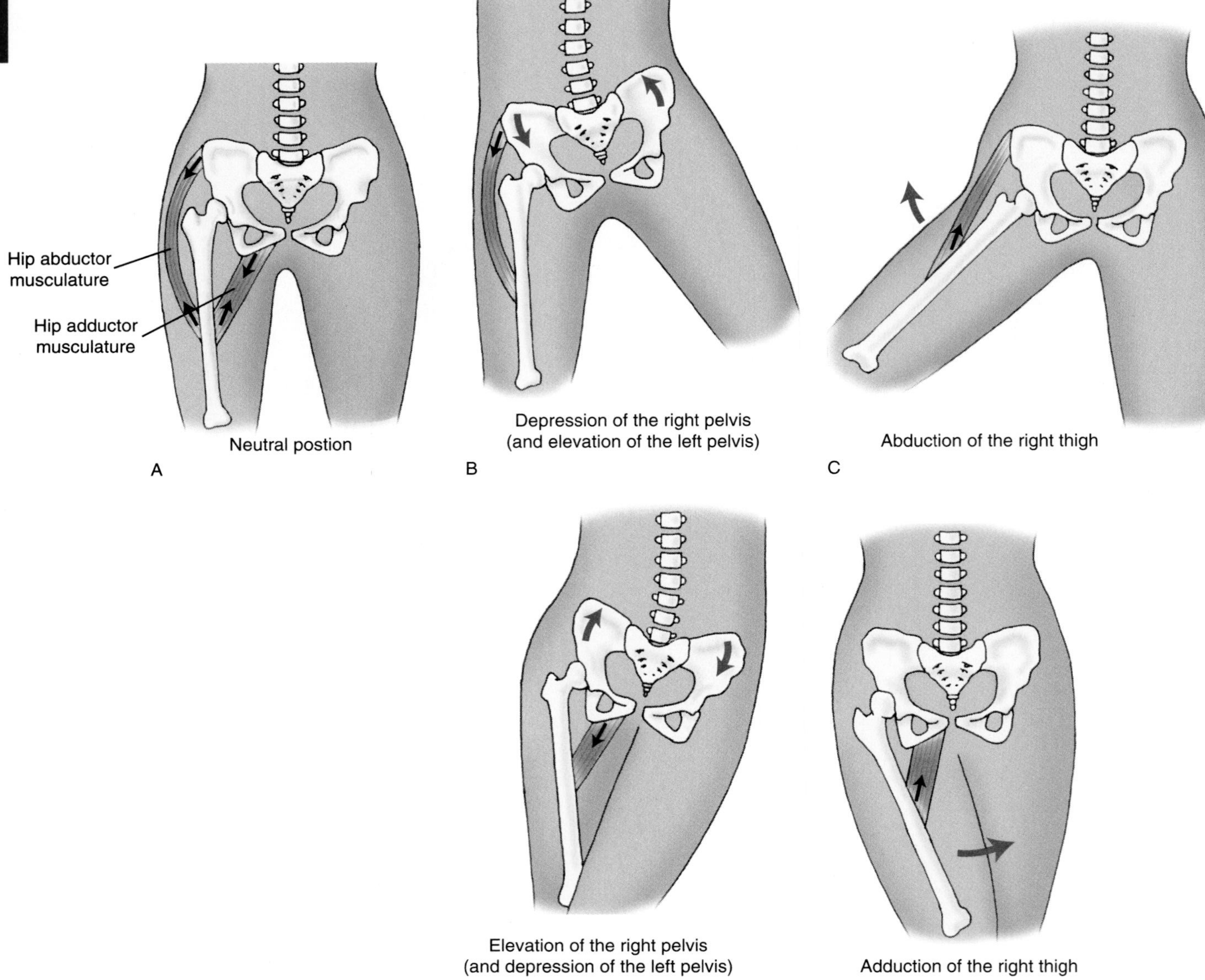

Figure 8-13 Anterior views of musculature that crosses the right hip joint laterally and medially and creates frontal plane actions of the pelvis and thigh at the hip joint. *A,* Both the lateral and medial groups of musculature on the right side of the body; the arrows demonstrate the lines of pull of the musculature. The lateral group is composed of what is usually referred to as *hip abductor musculature*; the medial group is composed of what is usually referred to as *hip adductor musculature. B,* Pelvic action (i.e., depression of the right pelvis) created by the lateral group of musculature. (Note: When the pelvis depresses on the right side, the left side elevates.) *C,* Thigh action (i.e., abduction of the right thigh) created by the lateral group of musculature. *D,* Pelvic action (i.e., elevation of the right pelvis) created by the medial group of musculature. (Note: When the pelvis elevates on the right side, the left side depresses.) *E,* Thigh action (i.e., adduction of the right thigh) created by the medial group of musculature. (Note: The musculature on the left side of the body is not shown.)

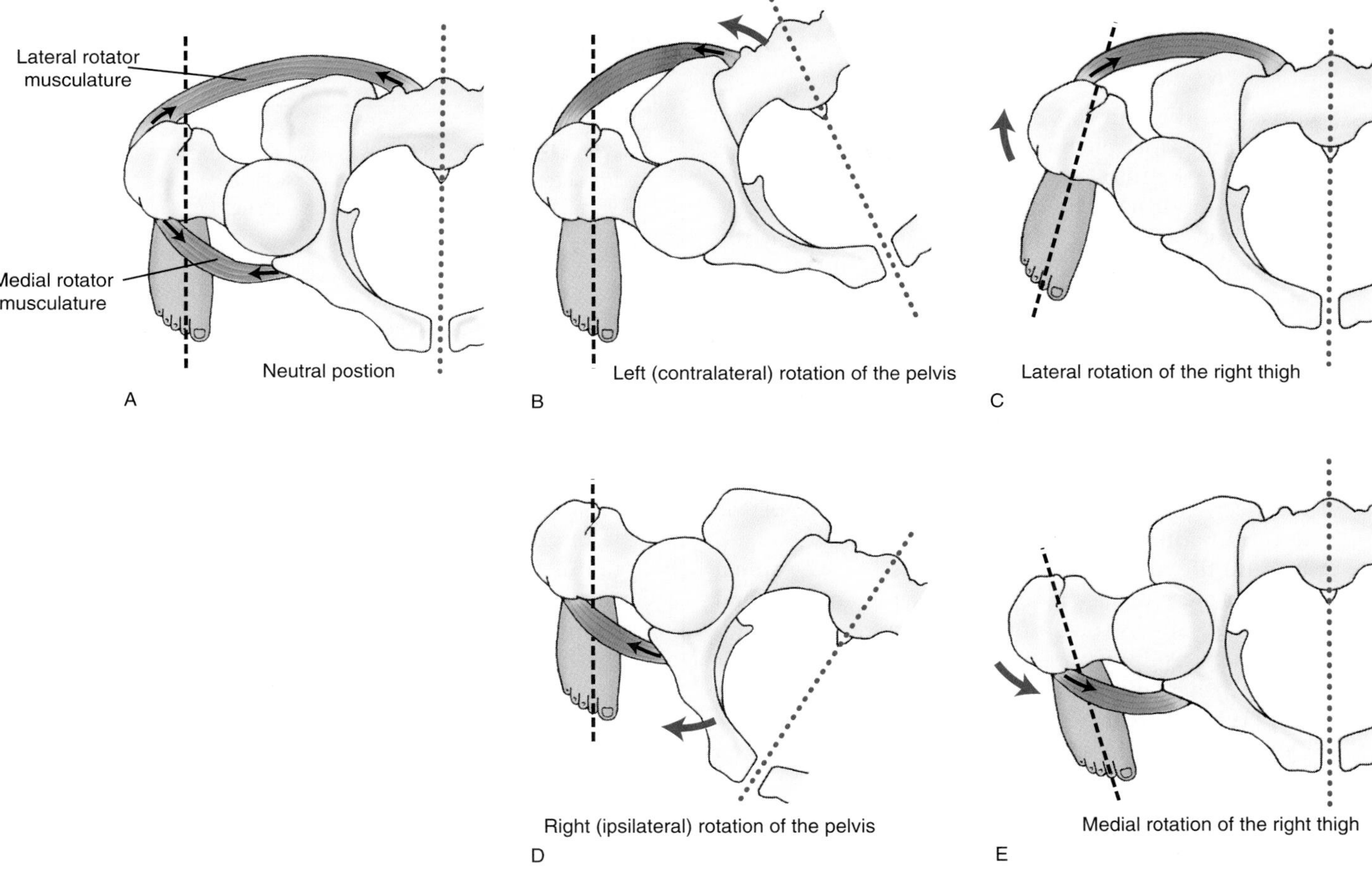

Figure 8-14 Superior views of musculature that crosses the right hip joint and creates transverse plane actions of the pelvis and thigh at the hip joint. *A,* The two groups of musculature: One group is posterior and is often referred to as the *lateral rotators of the hip joint*; the other group is anterior and is often referred to as the *medial rotators of the hip joint. B,* Pelvic action of the posterior musculature, which is left rotation of the pelvis. Given that right-sided musculature created this action, it is contralateral rotation of the pelvis. *C,* Thigh action of the posterior musculature, which is lateral rotation of the thigh created by the posterior musculature. *D,* Pelvic action of the anterior musculature, which is right rotation of the pelvis. Given that right-sided musculature created this action, it is ipsilateral rotation of the pelvis. *E,* Thigh action of the anterior musculature, which is medial rotation of the thigh created by the anterior musculature. In all figures, the black dashed line represents the orientation of the pelvis; the red dotted line represents the orientation of the thigh. (Note: The musculature on the left side of the body is not shown.)

BOX 8-18

Understanding the relationship of pelvic and thigh rotation movements at the hip joint in the transverse plane shows us two things:

1. The lateral rotators of the thigh at the hip joint (e.g., the posterior buttocks muscles like the piriformis or gluteus maximus) do rotation of the pelvis to the opposite side of the body (i.e., they are contralateral rotators of the pelvis at the hip joint). Lateral rotation of the thigh at the hip joint and contralateral rotation of the pelvis at the hip joint are reverse actions of the same muscles.
2. The medial rotators of the thigh at the hip joint (e.g., the anteriorly located TFL and anterior fibers of the gluteus medius) do rotation of the pelvis to the same side of the body (i.e., they are ipsilateral rotators of the pelvis at the hip joint). Medial rotation of the thigh at the hip joint and ipsilateral rotation of the pelvis at the hip joint are reverse actions of the same muscles (see Figure 8-14).

- ❑ Left rotation of the pelvis at the hip joints is analogous to medial rotation of the left thigh and lateral rotation of the right thigh at the hip joints. Therefore muscles that do left rotation of the pelvis at the hip joints also do medial rotation of the left thigh and lateral rotation of the right thigh at the hip joints (see Figure 8-14).
  - ❑ The reasoning to explain this is identical to right rotation of the pelvis at the hip joints (explained previously).
  - ❑ Therefore lateral rotator muscles of the thigh at the hip joint are contralateral rotators of the pelvis at that hip joint (see Figures 8-14b-c); and medial rotator muscles of the thigh at the hip joint are ipsilateral rotators of the pelvis at that hip joint (see Figures 8-14d-e).

☐ 8.8 EFFECT OF PELVIC POSTURE ON SPINAL POSTURE

Sections 8.1 through 8.7 have spent considerable time discussing the kinesiology of the pelvis because the pelvis is probably the most important determinant of the posture and health of the spine.

- When the pelvis tilts, the sacrum tilts because it is a part of the bony pelvis. When the sacrum tilts, the base of the sacrum also tilts; this results in a sacral base that is angled relative to a horizontal line.
- This angulation of the sacral base relative to a horizontal line can be measured by measuring the angle that is created between a line drawn along the top of the sacrum and a horizontal line. This line is called the **sacral base angle**.
- In effect, the sacral base angle is a measure of the degree of anterior tilt of the sacrum.
- Because the sacral base creates a base that the spinal column of vertebrae sits on, any change in the sacral base angle affects the posture of the spine.
- The relationship between the posture and movement of the pelvis and spine is often referred to as **lumbopelvic rhythm**.
- One purpose of the spinal column is to bring the head to a level posture.

BOX 8-19

The head needs to be level so that the inner ear can function as a proprioceptive organ; having the head level also facilitates the sense of vision. The desire of the body to bring the head to a level posture is known as the **righting reflex**.

- If the sacral base were to be perfectly level, the spine could be totally straight and the head would be level. However, if the sacral base tilts, the spine must curve to bring the head to a level posture.
- A sacral base angle of approximately 30 degrees is considered to be normal.
- A sacral base angle that is greater than 30 degrees results in increased spinal curvature; a sacral base angle that is less than 30 degrees results in decreased spinal curvature. (Note: Of course, the spine does not have to compensate for a tilted sacral base [by curving] to bring the head to a level posture. The trunk can "go along for the ride" when the pelvis tilts.) (See Figure 8-7b.)

Figure 8-15 illustrates three different sacral base angles and the concomitant effect that these angles have on spinal posture.

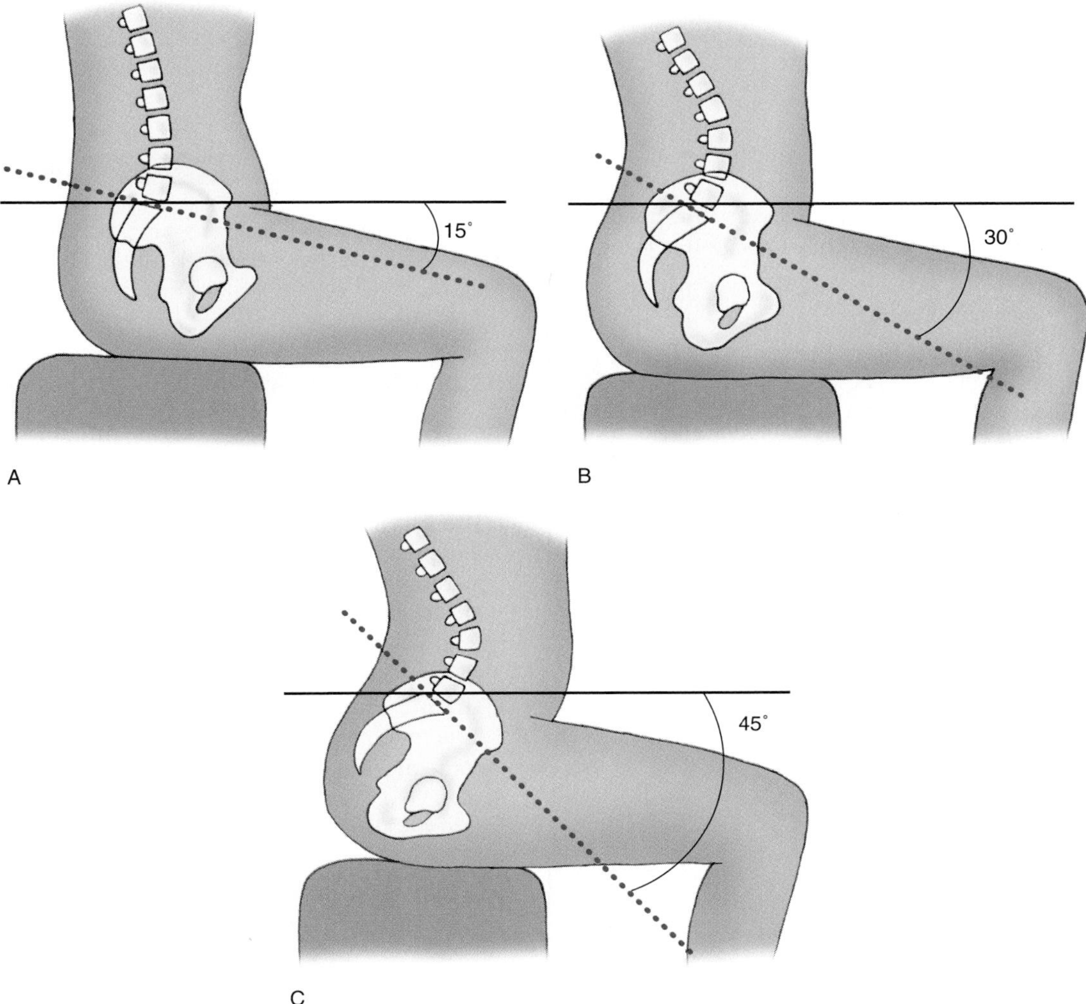

Figure 8-15 Effect on the spinal curve with changes in the sagittal plane tilt angle of the pelvis. When the pelvis tilts in the sagittal plane, it changes the orientation of the base of the sacrum relative to a horizontal line; a measure of this is called the *sacral base angle*. Because the spine sits on the sacrum, any change of the sacral base angle causes a change in the curvature of the spine if the head is to remain level. *A,* Sacral base angle of 15 degrees, which is less than normal. *B,* Normal sacral base angle of 30 degrees. *C,* Increased sacral base angle of 45 degrees. The corresponding changes in the curvature of the lumbar spine with changes in the sacral base angle should be noted.

8.9 HIP JOINT

- The hip joint is also known as the **femoroacetabular joint**.

> **BOX 8-20**
> Another name for the hip joint is the **coxofemoral joint** (i.e., between the coxal bone [the pelvic bone] and the femur).

Bones:

- The hip joint is located between the femur and the pelvic bone (Figure 8-16).
  - More specifically, it is located between the head of the femur and the acetabulum of the pelvic bone.

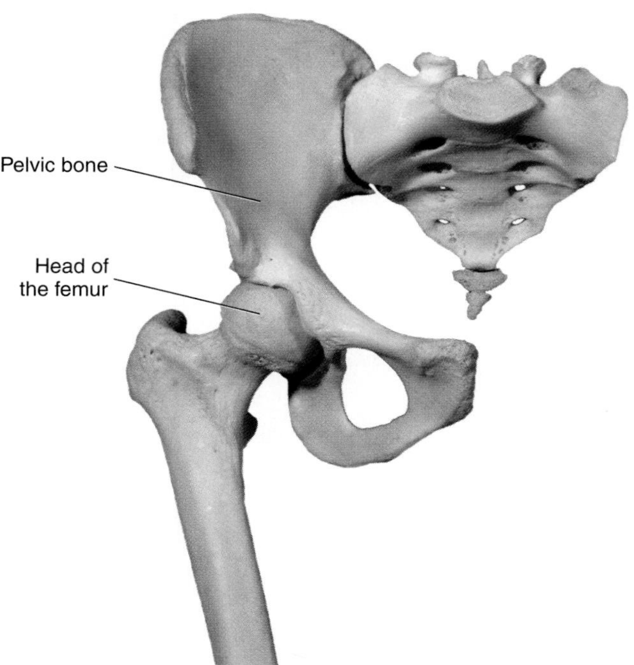

Figure 8-16 Anterior view of the right hip joint. The hip joint is a ball-and-socket joint that is formed by the head of the femur articulating with the acetabulum of the pelvic bone.

> **BOX 8-21**
> All three bones of the pelvic bone (the ilium, ischium, and pubis) contribute to the acetabulum. The word *acetabulum* means *vinegar cup* (vinegar is acetic acid).

- Joint structure classification: Synovial joint
  - Subtype: Ball and socket
- Joint function classification: Diarthrotic
  - Subtype: Triaxial

> **BOX 8-22**
> The socket of the hip joint (formed by the acetabulum of the pelvic bone) is very deep and provides excellent stability but relatively less mobility than a shallower socket like the glenoid fossa of the shoulder joint.

Major Motions Allowed:

The average ranges of motion of the thigh at the hip joint are given in Table 8-2 (Figure 8-17). (For motions of the pelvis at the hip joint, see Section 8-4.)

- The hip joint allows flexion and extension (i.e., axial movements) within the sagittal plane around a mediolateral axis.
- The hip joint allows abduction and adduction (i.e., axial movements) within the frontal plane around an anteroposterior axis.
- The hip joint allows medial rotation and lateral rotation (i.e., axial movements) within the transverse plane around a vertical axis.

Reverse Actions:

- The muscles of the hip joint are generally considered to move the more distal thigh relative to a fixed pelvis. However, closed-chain activities are common in the lower extremity in which the foot is planted on the ground; this fixes the foot/leg/thigh and requires that the pelvis move instead. When this occurs, the pelvis can move at the hip joint instead of the thigh (Box 8-23).

TABLE 8-2

Average Ranges of Motion of the Thigh at the Hip Joint

Flexion	90 Degrees	Extension	20 Degrees
Abduction	40 Degrees	Adduction	20 Degrees
Medial rotation	40 Degrees	Lateral rotation	50 Degrees

Note: Flexion and extension are measured with the knee joint extended; these ranges of motion would change with flexion of the knee joint because of the stretch across the knee joint of multi-joint muscles such as the rectus femoris of the quadriceps femoris group. Medial rotation and lateral rotation are measured with the thigh flexed 90 degrees at the hip joint.

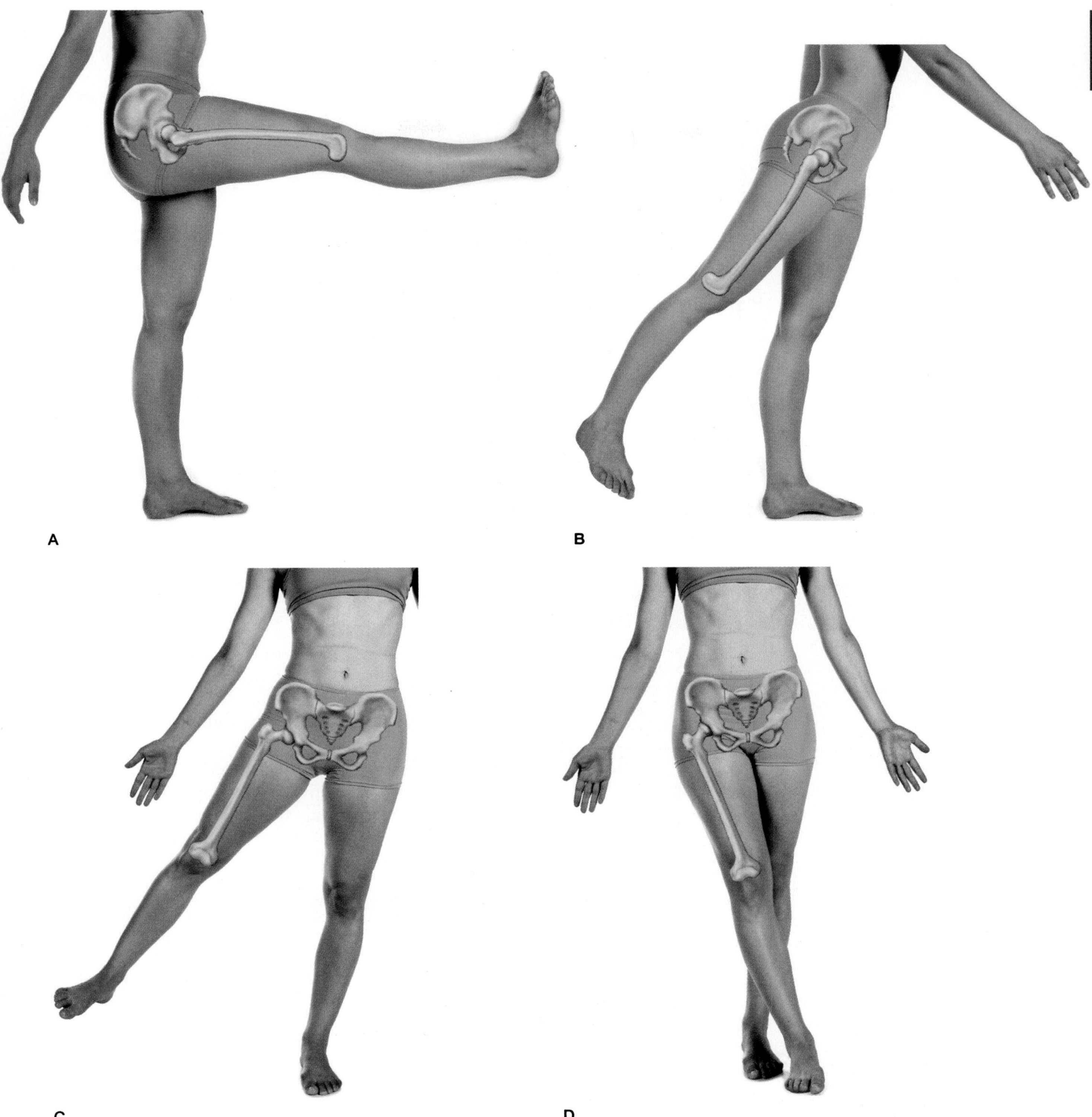

Figure 8-17 Motions of the thigh at the hip joint. *A* and *B,* Flexion and extension, respectively. *C* and *D,* Abduction and adduction, respectively.

Continued

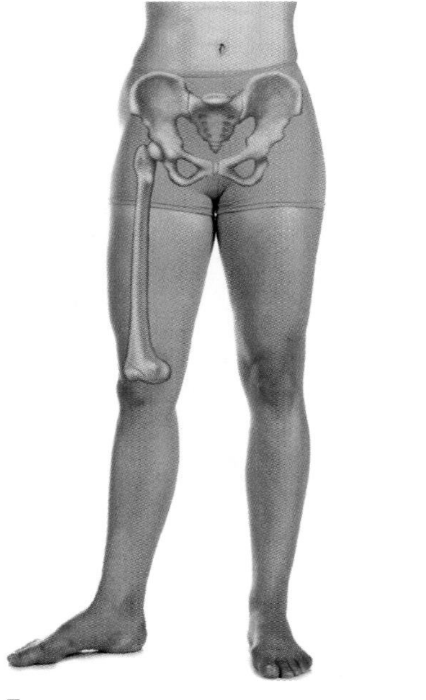

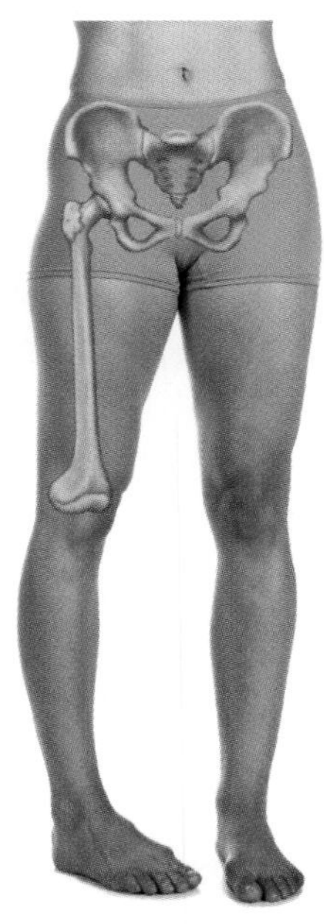

Figure 8-17, cont'd *E* and *F,* Lateral rotation and medial rotation, respectively.

BOX 8-23 SPOTLIGHT ON OPEN AND CLOSED-CHAIN ACTIVITIES

The term **open-chain activity** refers to an activity that is carried out in which the distal bone of a joint is free to move. The term **closed-chain activity** refers to an activity that is carried out in which the distal bone of a joint is fixed in some way, resulting in the proximal bone having to move when movement occurs at that joint. The most common example of a closed-chain activity is when the foot is planted on the ground and is thereby fixed; this results in the leg having to move at the ankle joint, the thigh having to move at the knee joint, and/or the pelvis having to move at the hip joint. Because muscle actions are usually thought of as moving the distal body part relative to the proximal one, these actions that occur with closed-chain activities may be termed *reverse actions.* Closed-chain activities are extremely common in the lower extremity. Although less common, a closed-chain activity may also occur in the upper extremity such as when the hand firmly grasps an immovable object; this results in the forearm moving at the wrist joint, the arm moving at the elbow joint, and/or the shoulder girdle moving at the glenohumeral joint. The terms *open chain* and *closed chain* refer to the idea of a chain of kinematic elements (bones/body parts, usually of the extremities) that are either open ended at their distal end (and therefore free to move distally), or not open ended (i.e., closed) at their distal end so that the distal end cannot move and the proximal end must move instead.

- The reverse actions of the pelvis at the hip joint are anterior tilt and posterior tilt in the sagittal plane, depression and elevation in the frontal plane, and right rotation and left rotation in the transverse plane. These actions were covered in detail in Section 8.4, Figure 8-7.

Major Ligaments of the Hip Joint:

Fibrous Joint Capsule:

- The capsule of the hip joint is strong and dense, providing excellent stability to the joint.
- The capsule contains strong circular deep fibers called the **zona orbicularis** that surround the neck of the femur.
- The fibrous capsule of the hip joint is reinforced by three capsular ligaments, which are named based on their attachments: (1) the iliofemoral, (2) ischiofemoral, and (3) pubofemoral ligaments (Figure 8-18).

BOX 8-24

All three capsular ligaments of the hip joint are twisted as they pass from the pelvic bone to the femur (see Figure 8-18). This twisting reflects the medial rotation twisting that occurs to the shaft of the femur in utero. The result of this femoral twisting is that the ventral (softer) surfaces of the thigh and leg come to face posteriorly instead of anteriorly as in the rest of the body. This also explains why flexion of the leg at the knee joint (and all movements that occur distal to the knee joint) is a posterior movement instead of an anterior movement.

Iliofemoral Ligament:

- The iliofemoral ligament attaches from the ilium to the femur.
  - More specifically, it attaches from the anterior inferior iliac spine (AIIS) to the intertrochanteric line of the femur.

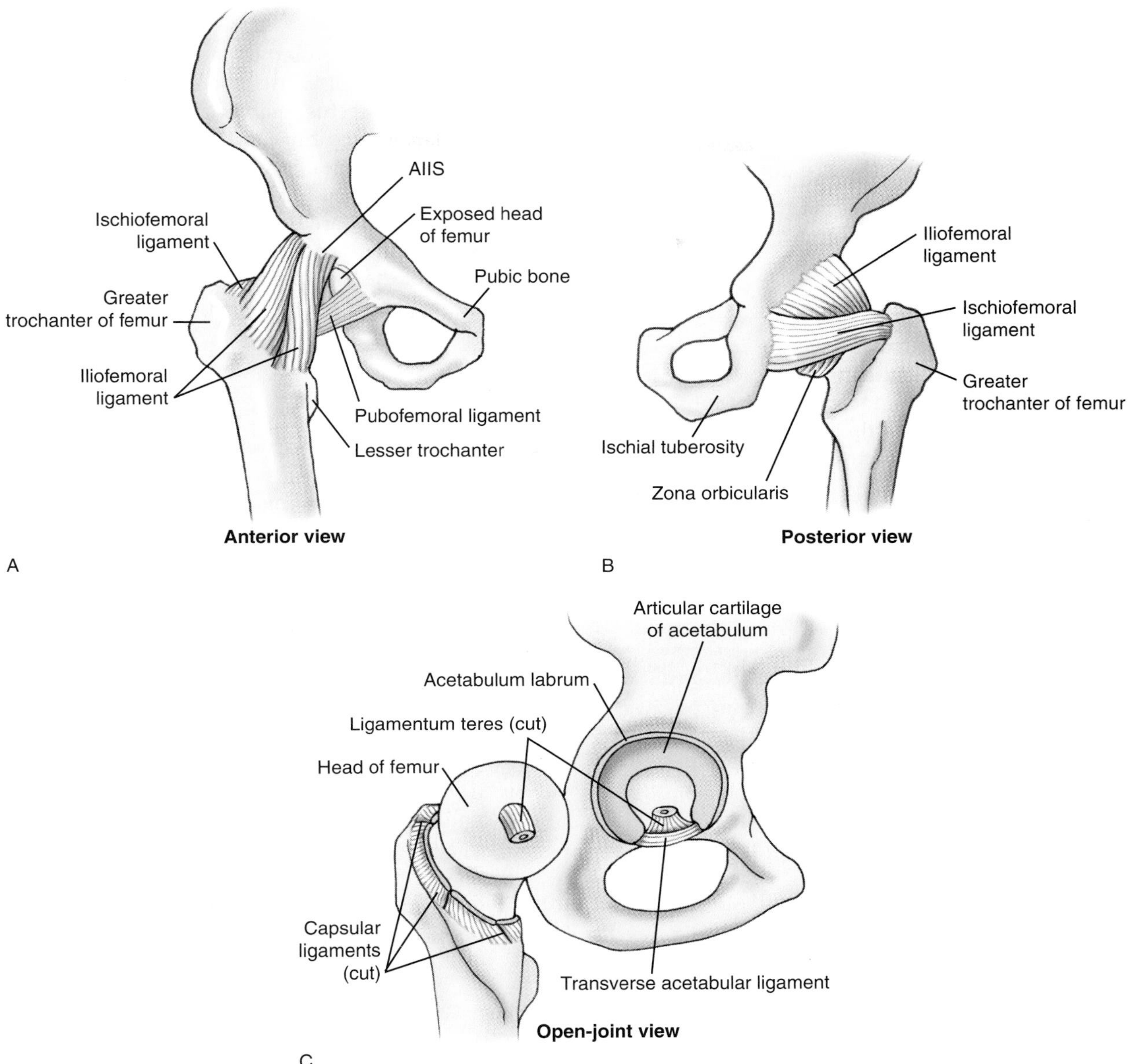

Figure 8-18 Ligaments of the hip joint. The major ligaments are capsular reinforcements called the *iliofemoral, pubofemoral,* and *ischiofemoral ligaments. A,* Anterior view of the hip joint ligaments. *B,* Posterior view. *C,* Joint opened up to illustrate the ligamentum teres and transverse acetabular ligament.

- Location: The iliofemoral ligament is a thickening of the anterosuperior capsule of the hip joint.

Function

- It limits extension of the thigh at the hip joint.
- It limits posterior tilt of the pelvis at the hip joint.
- The iliofemoral ligament is also known as **Y ligament** (because it is shaped like an upside-down letter *Y*).

BOX 8-25

The iliofemoral ligament is one of the thickest and strongest ligaments of the body. It is also a very important ligament, because when someone stands with extension of the hip joint (whether the thigh is extended or the pelvis is posteriorly tilted), his or her body weight leans against the iliofemoral ligament.

Pubofemoral Ligament:

- The pubofemoral ligament attaches from the pubis to the femur.
- Location: The pubofemoral ligament is a thickening of the anteroinferior capsule of the hip joint.

Function

- It limits abduction of the thigh at the hip joint.
- It limits limits extreme extension of the thigh at the hip joint.
- It limits depression (i.e., lateral tilt) of the pelvis at the ipsilateral hip joint.

Ischiofemoral Ligament:

- ❑ The ischiofemoral ligament attaches from the ischium to the femur.
- ❑ Location: The ischiofemoral ligament is a thickening of the posterior capsule of the hip joint.

Function

- ❑ It limits medial rotation of the thigh at the hip joint.
- ❑ It limits extension of the thigh at the hip joint.
- ❑ It limits ipsilateral rotation of the pelvis at the hip joint.

Ligamentum Teres:

- ❑ Location: It is intra-articular, running from the internal surface of the acetabulum to the head of the femur.
- ❑ Function: The ligamentum teres does not substantially increase stability to the hip joint; its purpose is to provide a conduit for blood vessels and nerves to the femoral head.

Closed-Packed Position of the Hip Joint:

- ❑ Full extension

BOX 8-26

LIGAMENTS OF THE HIP JOINT

- Fibrous joint capsule
  - Iliofemoral ligament
  - Ischiofemoral ligament
  - Pubofemoral ligament
  - Zona orbicularis
- Transverse acetabular ligament
- Ligamentum teres

Major Muscles of the Hip Joint:

- ❑ The hip joint is crossed by large muscle groups. Anteriorly, the major muscles are the iliopsoas, tensor fasciae latae, rectus femoris, sartorius, and the more anteriorly located hip joint adductors. Posteriorly are the gluteal muscles, as well as the hamstrings and the adductor magnus. Medially is the hip joint adductor group. Laterally are the gluteal muscles, tensor fasciae lata, and the sartorius. (For a detailed list of the muscles of the hip joint and their actions, see page 632 in the appendix.)

Miscellaneous:

- ❑ The articular cartilage of the acetabulum is crescent-shaped and called the **lunate cartilage** (see Figure 8-18c).
- ❑ A fibrocartilaginous ring of tissue called the **acetabular labrum** surrounds the circumference of the acetabulum.

BOX 8-27

The word *labrum* means *lip*; hence the acetabular labrum runs along the lip of the acetabulum.

- ❑ The acetabular labrum increases the depth of the socket of the hip joint, thereby increasing the stability of the hip joint.
- ❑ The acetabular labrum does not quite form a complete ring; at the inferior margin of the acetabulum, its two ends are connected by the **transverse acetabular ligament** (see Figure 8-18c).

8.10 ANGULATIONS OF THE FEMUR

- The femur is composed of several major components: the head, the neck, and the shaft.
- The relationship of these components is such that they are not arranged in a straight line. The angles that are measured between the head/neck and the shaft of the femur are called *femoral angulations*.
- Two femoral angulations exist:
  - Femoral angle of inclination
  - Femoral torsion angle
- Note: Both the angle of inclination and the torsion angle are properties of the femur and are independent of the actual hip joint. However, abnormal angles of inclination and torsion can alter the functioning of the hip joint by creating compensations of the alignment of the bones at the hip joint and of the musculature of the hip joint.

Femoral Angle of Inclination:

- The **femoral angle of inclination** is the angulation of the head/neck relative to the shaft within the frontal plane (Figure 8-19).
- The angle of inclination is normally approximately 125 degrees.

BOX 8-28

At birth the angle of inclination measures approximately 150 degrees. Because of the stresses of weight bearing, it gradually decreases to the normal adult value of approximately 125 degrees.

- An angle of inclination markedly less than 125 degrees is called a **coxa vara**.
- An angle of inclination markedly greater than 125 degrees is called a **coxa valga**.

BOX 8-29

The term *coxa* refers to the hip; the term *vara* means *turned inward*, and the term *valga* means *turned outward*.

  - Altered angles of inclination result in suboptimal alignment of the femoral head within the acetabulum. This can result in decreased shock absorption ability and increased degenerative changes over time.
  - A coxa valga results in a longer lower extremity; a coxa vara results in a shorter lower extremity.

Femoral Torsion Angle:

- The **femoral torsion angle** is the angulation of the femoral head/neck relative to the shaft within the transverse plane (Figure 8-20).
- The term **anteversion** (or *normal anteversion*) is used to refer to the femoral torsion angle.
- This torsion angle represents the medial rotation of the femoral shaft that occurs embryologically.

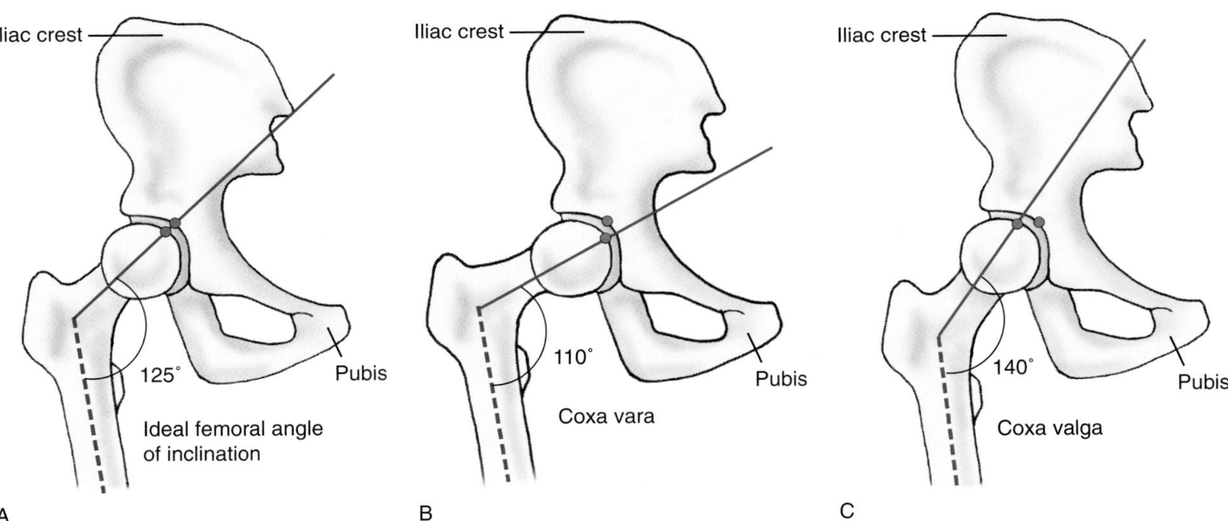

Figure 8-19 Various femoral angles of inclination. (Note: All views are anterior.) *A,* Angle of 125 degrees, which is considered to be normal. *B,* Decreased angle of inclination; this condition is known as *coxa vara*. *C,* Increased angle of inclination; this condition is known as *coxa valga*. The paired blue dots in each figure represent the alignment of the joint surfaces of the femoral head and acetabulum. Ideal alignment occurs at approximately 125 degrees, as seen in *A*.

BOX 8-30

An embryo begins with the limb buds (for the upper and lower extremities) pointed straight laterally. By 2 months of age, the upper and lower limb buds of the embryo adduct (i.e., point more anteriorly). However, the upper limb buds also laterally rotate, bringing the ventral surface of the upper extremities to face anteriorly; whereas the lower limb buds medially rotate, bringing the ventral surface of the lower extremities to face posteriorly. This is the reason why flexion within the lower extremity is a posterior movement from the knee joint and further distally.

- The femoral head and neck actually maintain their position while the shaft twists medially within the transverse plane. The result is a femoral shaft that is twisted medially relative to the head and neck of the femur.

BOX 8-31

As noted in Section 8.9, this torsion of the femoral shaft is apparent by looking at the twisted nature of the fibers of the ligaments of the hip joint (see Figure 8-18a–b).

- The torsion angle is normally approximately 15 degrees.

BOX 8-32

Although the femoral anteversion angle is a measure of the twisting of the femoral shaft that occurs within the transverse plane, its actual angle is a measure of the deviation of the head and neck of the femur from the frontal plane (see Figure 8-20).

- A torsion angle markedly less than 15 degrees is called **retroversion**.
- A torsion angle markedly greater than 15 degrees is called *excessive anteversion*.
  - Femoral retroversion can result in a **toe-out posture**. Toe-out posture is actually lateral rotation of the thigh at the hip joint and is a compensation to try to optimally line up the articular surfaces of the femur and acetabulum.
  - Excessive femoral anteversion can result in a **toe-in posture**, also known as **pigeon toes**. Toe-in posture is actually medial rotation of the thigh at the hip joint and is a compensation to optimally line up the articular surfaces of the joint.
- An altered femoral torsion angle that is uncompensated will result in suboptimal alignment of the femoral head within the acetabulum. This can result in decreased shock absorption ability and increased degenerative changes over time.
  - Toe-in postures are very common in young children, because the femoral torsion angle is higher at birth and gradually decreases through childhood.

BOX 8-33

At birth the femoral torsion angle measures approximately 30 to 40 degrees. Usually by 6 years of age, the torsion angle decreases to the normal adult value of 15 degrees. Because in-toeing is a common compensation for excessive femoral torsion, this postural pattern is common among children. In-toeing is usually outgrown; however, it may be retained throughout adulthood if contractures in the medial rotator muscles and adhesions in certain ligaments develop.

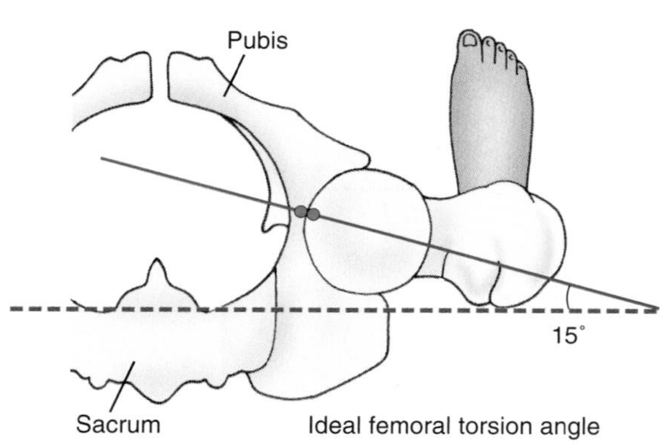

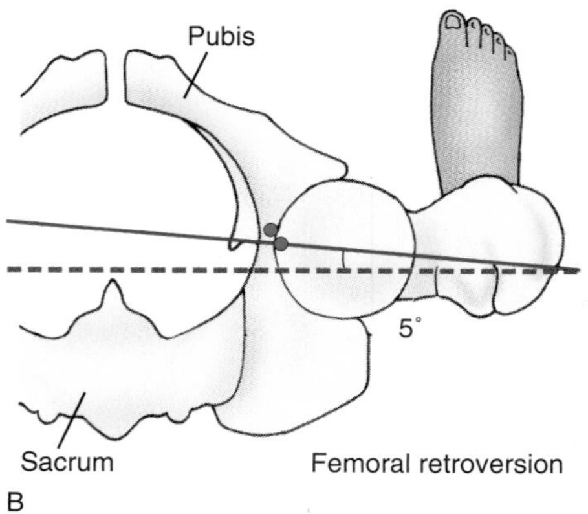

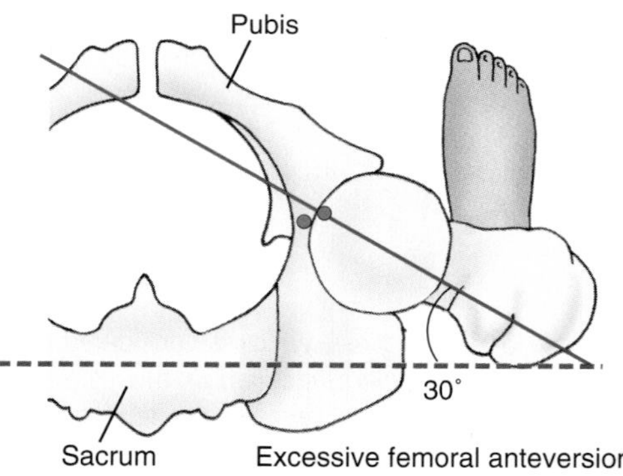

Figure 8-20 Various femoral torsion angles. (Note: All views are superior.) *A,* Angle of 15 degrees, which is considered to be normal. *B,* Decreased torsion angle; this condition is known as *retroversion. C,* Increased torsion angle; this condition is known as *excessive anteversion.* The paired blue dots in each figure represent the alignment of the joint surfaces of the femoral head and acetabulum. Ideal alignment occurs at approximately 15 degrees, as seen in *A.* To achieve optimal alignment in *B,* in which retroversion exists, a toe-out position would occur; to achieve optimal alignment in *C,* in which excessive anteversion exists, a toe-in position would occur.

☐ 8.11 FEMOROPELVIC RHYTHM

- There tends to be a rhythm to how the femur of the thigh and the pelvis move. This coordination of movement between these two body parts is often referred to as **femoropelvic rhythm**.
- Femoropelvic rhythm is an example of the concept of a **coupled action** wherein two different joint actions tend to be *coupled* together (i.e., if one action occurs, the other one tends to also occur).
  - Note: Coupled actions are common between the thigh and pelvis. Coupled actions also occur between the arm and the shoulder girdle (see Section 9.6). The concept of coupled actions is covered in Section 13.12.)
- Generally when the femur is moved, it is often for the purpose of raising the foot up into the air. Given the limitation of the range of motion of the thigh at the hip joint, movement of the pelvis is often created in conjunction with thigh movement to increase the ability of the foot to rise into the air.
  - For example, if a person flexes the right thigh at the hip joint for the purpose of kicking a ball, the actual range of motion of the right thigh at the hip joint is approximately 90 degrees. This is not sufficient for a strong follow-through to the kick. Therefore the pelvis is posteriorly tilted on the left thigh at the left hip joint (the *support limb* side) to increase the range of motion of the kick (Figure 8-21a).
- Note: With femoropelvic rhythm, the nervous system is coordinating two entirely different joint actions to occur together. One joint action is of the thigh at the hip joint; the other joint action is of the pelvis at the other hip joint. These separate actions are coupled together for the larger purpose of raising the foot higher into the air.

The following are common coupled actions that occur between the thigh and the pelvis (see Figure 8-21):

- Thigh flexion at the hip joint is coupled with pelvic posterior tilt at the contralateral (opposite-sided [i.e., the other]) hip joint.
- Thigh extension at the hip joint is coupled with pelvic anterior tilt at the contralateral hip joint.
- Thigh abduction at the hip joint is coupled with pelvic depression at the contralateral hip joint.
- Thigh adduction at the hip joint is coupled with pelvic elevation at the contralateral hip joint.
- Thigh lateral rotation at the hip joint is coupled with pelvic contralateral rotation at the contralateral hip joint.
- Thigh medial rotation at the hip joint is coupled with pelvic ipsilateral rotation at the contralateral hip joint.

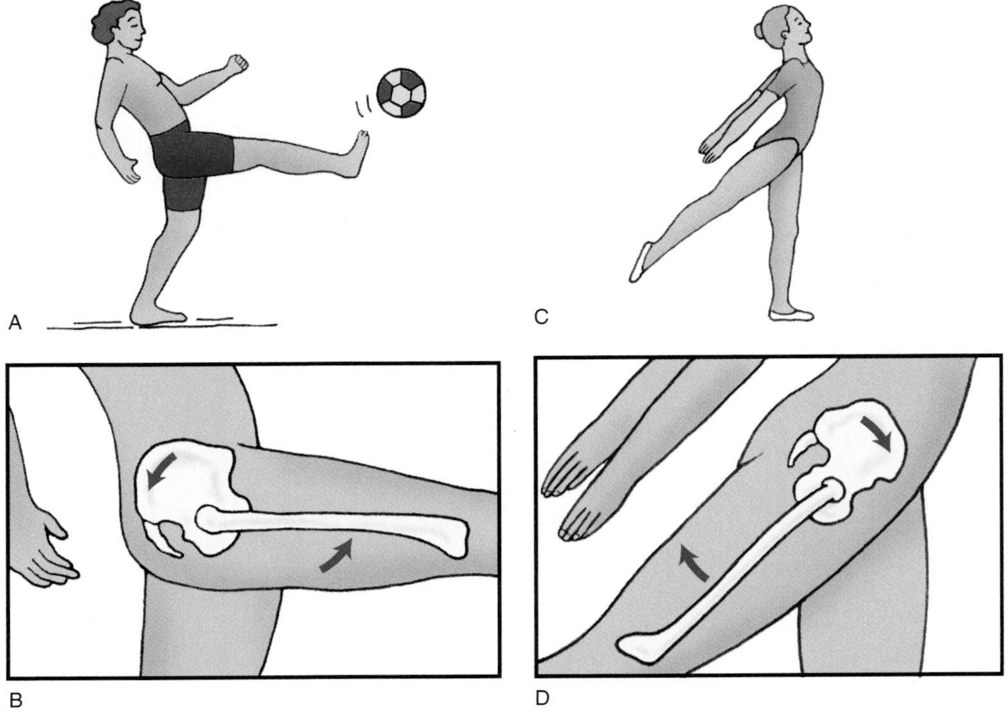

Figure 8-21 Concept of coupled thigh/pelvic actions, known as *femoropelvic rhythm*, in the sagittal plane. *A,* Soccer player who is kicking a soccer ball with his right foot. He accomplishes this by flexing his right thigh at the right hip joint and posteriorly tilting his pelvis at the left (i.e., contralateral) hip joint. These two actions couple together to enable the player to raise his right foot higher in the air. *B,* Ballet dancer who is bringing her right lower extremity up into the air behind her. She accomplishes this by extending her right thigh at her right hip joint and anteriorly tilting her pelvis at her left (i.e., contralateral) hip joint.

☐ 8.12 OVERVIEW OF THE KNEE JOINT COMPLEX

- ❑ The knee joint is actually a joint complex, because more than one articulation exists within the joint capsule of the knee joint (Figure 8-22).
- ❑ The primary articulation at the knee joint is between the tibia and the femur.
  - ❑ This joint is known as the *tibiofemoral joint.*
- ❑ The patella also articulates with the femur within the capsule of the knee joint (see Figure 8-25 in Section 8.14).
  - ❑ This joint is known as the *patellofemoral joint.*
- ❑ The proximal tibiofibular joint between the lateral condyle of the tibia and the head of the fibula is not within the capsule of the knee joint, and the proximal tibiofemoral joint is not very functionally related to the knee joint.
- ❑ Generally when the context is not made otherwise clear, the knee joint is considered to be the tibiofemoral joint.

Bones:

- ❑ The **tibiofemoral joint** is located between the femur and the tibia.
  - ❑ More specifically, it is located between the medial and lateral condyles of the femur and the plateau of the tibia.
  - ❑ Because each condyle of the femur articulates separately with the tibia, some sources consider the tibiofemoral joint to be two joints: (1) the medial tibiofemoral joint and (2) the lateral tibiofemoral joint.
- ❑ The **patellofemoral joint** is located between the patella and the femur.
  - ❑ More specifically, it is located between the posterior surface of the patella and the intercondylar groove of the distal femur.

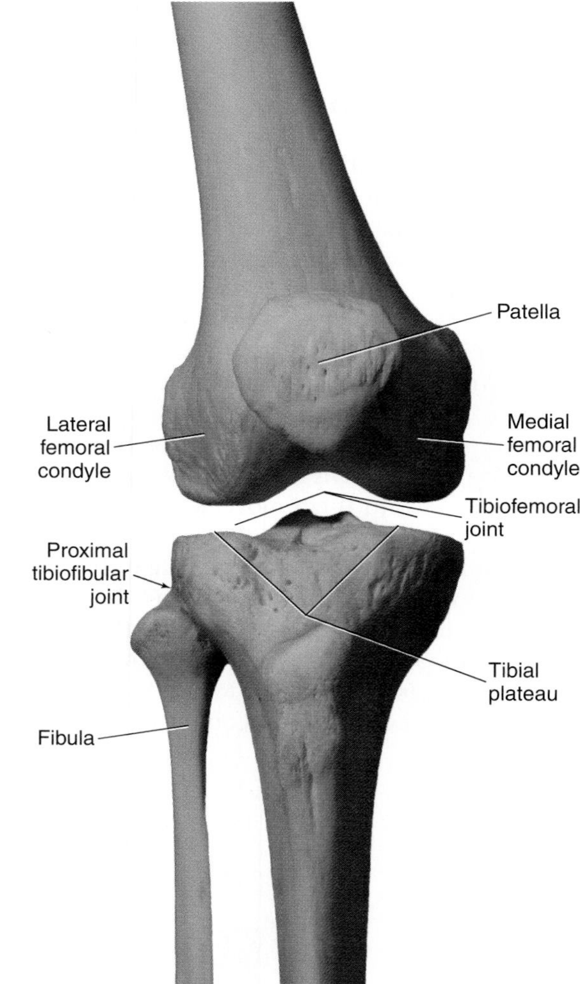

Figure 8-22 Anterior view of the right knee joint. The knee joint is actually a joint complex containing the tibiofemoral joint and the patellofemoral joint.

☐ 8.13 TIBIOFEMORAL (KNEE) JOINT

Bones:

- The tibiofemoral joint is located between the femur and the tibia.
  - More specifically, it is located between the two femoral condyles and the plateau of the tibia.
- The tibiofemoral joint is located within the capsule of the knee joint along with the patellofemoral joint.
- Because each condyle of the femur articulates separately with the tibia, some sources consider the tibiofemoral joint to be two joints, the medial tibiofemoral joint and the lateral tibiofemoral joint.
- Generally when the context is not made otherwise clear, the term *knee joint* refers to the tibiofemoral joint.

Tibiofemoral Joint:

- Joint structure classification: Synovial joint
  - Subtype: Modified hinge joint
- Joint function classification: Diarthrotic
  - Subtype: Biaxial

BOX 8-34

Some sources classify the tibiofemoral joint as a double condyloid joint: the medial condyle of the femur meeting the tibia as one condyloid joint, and the lateral condyle of the femur meeting the tibia as the other condyloid joint.

Major Motions Allowed:

Average ranges of motion of the leg at the knee joint are given in Table 8-3 (Figure 8-23).

- The tibiofemoral joint allows flexion and extension (i.e., axial movements) within the sagittal plane about a mediolateral axis.
- The tibiofemoral joint allows medial rotation and lateral rotation (i.e., axial movements) within the transverse plane around a vertical axis.)
- Medial and lateral rotation of the tibiofemoral joint can only occur if the tibiofemoral joint is in a position of flexion. A fully extended tibiofemoral joint cannot rotate.

BOX 8-35

Rotation of the tibiofemoral (i.e., knee) joint must be carefully described. The leg can rotate when the thigh is fixed, and the thigh can rotate when the leg is fixed. Understanding and naming these reverse actions of rotation of the tibiofemoral joint is important. *Medial rotation* of the leg at the tibiofemoral joint is equivalent to *lateral rotation* of the thigh at the tibiofemoral joint. Similarly, *lateral rotation* of the leg at the tibiofemoral joint is equivalent to *medial rotation* of the thigh at the tibiofemoral joint!

Reverse Actions:

- The muscles of the tibiofemoral joint are generally considered to move the more distal leg on the more proximal thigh. However, closed-chain activities are common in the lower extremity in which the foot is planted on the ground; this fixes the leg and requires that the thigh move instead. When this occurs, the thigh moves at the tibiofemoral joint instead of the leg moving.
- The thigh can flex and extend in the sagittal plane at the tibiofemoral joint.
- The thigh can medially rotate and laterally rotate in the transverse plane at the tibiofemoral joint.

Ligaments of the Tibiofemoral Joint:

- Given the large forces that are transmitted to the tibiofemoral joint, along with the weight-bearing function and the relative lack of bony stability provided by the shape of the bones, the ligaments of the tibiofemoral joint play an important role in providing stability and consequently are often injured (Figure 8-24).

TABLE 8-3

Average Ranges of Motion of the Leg at the Tibiofemoral (i.e., Knee) Joint

Flexion	140 Degrees	(Hyper)extension	5 Degrees
Medial rotation	15 Degrees	Lateral rotation	30 Degrees

Notes: Rotation measurements are done with the tibiofemoral joint in 90 degrees of flexion.
Extension is expressed as (Hyper)extension, because the tibiofemoral joint is fully extended in anatomic position; any further extension is considered to be hyperextension.

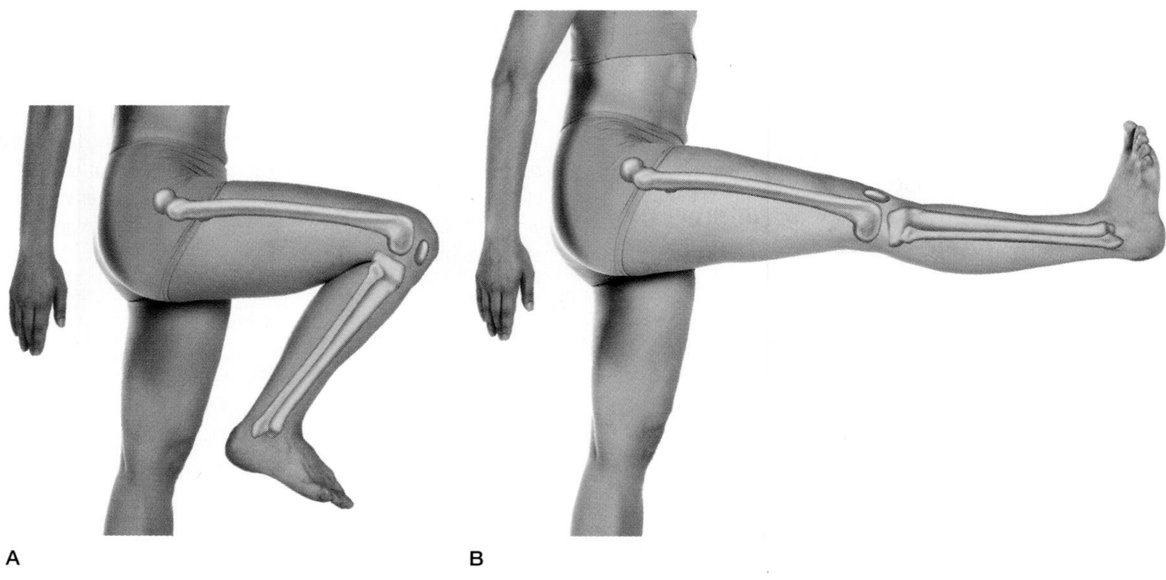

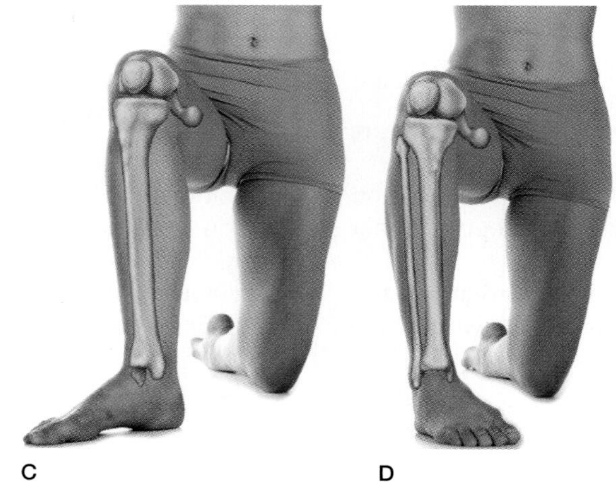

Figure 8-23 Motions possible at the tibiofemoral (i.e., knee) joint. *A* and *B,* Flexion and extension of the leg at the knee joint, respectively. *C* and *D,* Lateral and medial rotation of the leg at the knee joint, respectively. (Note: The knee joint can only rotate if it is first flexed.)

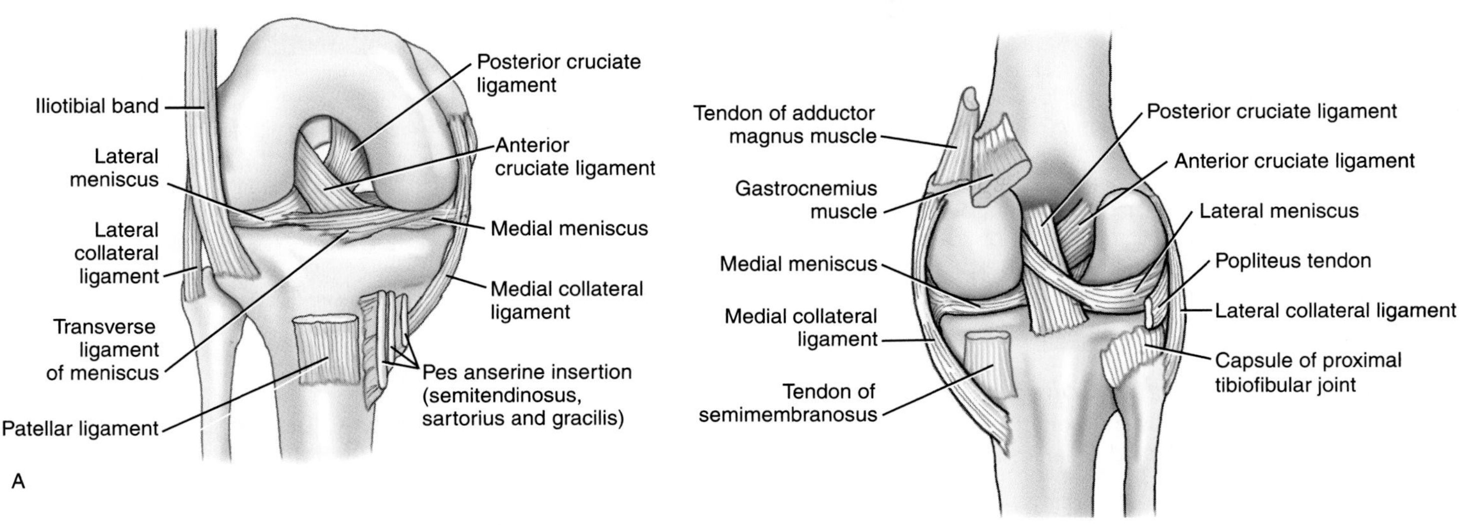

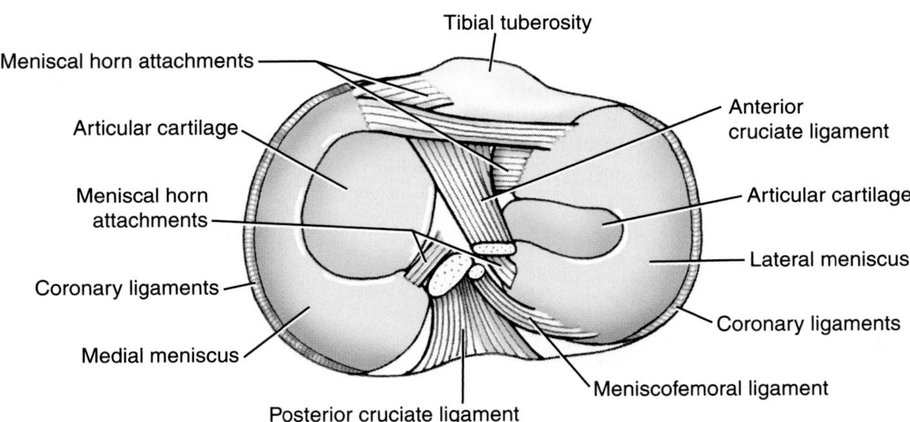

Figure 8-24 Ligaments of the tibiofemoral (i.e., knee) joint. *A,* Anterior view of the ligaments of the tibiofemoral joint. *B,* Posterior view of the ligaments of the tibiofemoral joint. *C,* Superior view of the tibia, demonstrating the menisci and ligaments of the tibiofemoral joint.

Fibrous Joint Capsule:

- The capsule of the tibiofemoral joint extends from the distal femur to the proximal tibia and includes the patella. The proximal tibiofibular joint is not included within the capsule of the knee joint.
- The capsule of the tibiofemoral joint is somewhat lax, but it is reinforced by many ligaments, muscles, and fascia.

BOX 8-36

The anterior capsule of the tibiofemoral joint is reinforced by the distal quadriceps femoris tendon, patella, infrapatellar ligament, and expansions of the quadriceps muscles called medial and lateral **retinacular fibers**. The lateral capsule is reinforced by the lateral collateral ligament, the iliotibial band, and lateral retinacular fibers. The medial capsule is reinforced by the medial collateral ligament, the three pes anserine muscle tendons, and the medial retinacular fibers. The posterior capsule is reinforced by the oblique popliteal ligament, the arcuate popliteal ligament, and fibrous expansions of the popliteus, gastrocnemius, and hamstring muscles.

Medial and Lateral Collateral Ligaments:

- The medial and lateral collateral ligaments are found on both sides (*lateral* means *side*) of the tibiofemoral joint.
- The two collateral ligaments are primarily important for limiting frontal plane movements of the bones of the tibiofemoral joint.

Medial Collateral Ligament:

- The medial collateral ligament attaches from the femur to the tibia.
  - More specifically, it attaches from the medial epicondyle of the femur to the medial proximal tibia.
- The medial collateral ligament is also known as the **tibial collateral ligament**.
- Function: It limits abduction of the leg at the tibiofemoral joint (within the frontal plane).

BOX 8-37

Abduction of the leg at the tibiofemoral joint is defined as a lateral deviation of the leg in the frontal plane; it is not a movement that a healthy tibiofemoral joint allows. A forceful impact from the lateral side, such as "clipping" in football, could abduct the leg and rupture the medial collateral ligament; this is the reason that clipping is illegal. The postural condition wherein the tibiofemoral joint is abducted is called *genu valgum*. (See Section 8.15 for more information.)

Lateral Collateral Ligament:

- The lateral collateral ligament attaches from the femur to the fibula.
  - More specifically, it attaches from the lateral epicondyle of the femur to the head of the fibula.
- The lateral collateral ligament is also known as the **fibular collateral ligament**.
- Function: It limits adduction of the leg at the tibiofemoral joint (within the frontal plane).

BOX 8-38

Adduction of the leg at the tibiofemoral joint is defined as a medial deviation of the leg in the frontal plane; like abduction of the leg, it is not a movement that a healthy tibiofemoral joint allows. A forceful impact from the medial side of the joint would have to occur for the medial collateral ligament to be injured. Because being hit from the medial side is less likely than being hit from the lateral side, the lateral collateral ligament is injured less often than the medial collateral ligament. The postural condition wherein the tibiofemoral joint is adducted is called *genu varum*. (See Section 8-15 for more information.)

Anterior and Posterior Cruciate Ligaments:

- The anterior and posterior cruciate ligaments cross each other (*cruciate* means *cross*). They are named for their tibial attachment.
- The two cruciate ligaments are primarily important for limiting sagittal plane translation movement of the bones of the tibiofemoral joint.

BOX 8-39

The majority of the anterior and posterior cruciate ligaments are located between the fibrous and synovial layers of the tibiofemoral joint capsule. For this reason, they are considered to be intra-articular, yet *extrasynovial*.

BOX 8-40

Anterior and posterior translations of the tibia and femur at the tibiofemoral joint are gliding movements that occur within the sagittal plane. These movements can be assessed by anterior and posterior drawer tests.

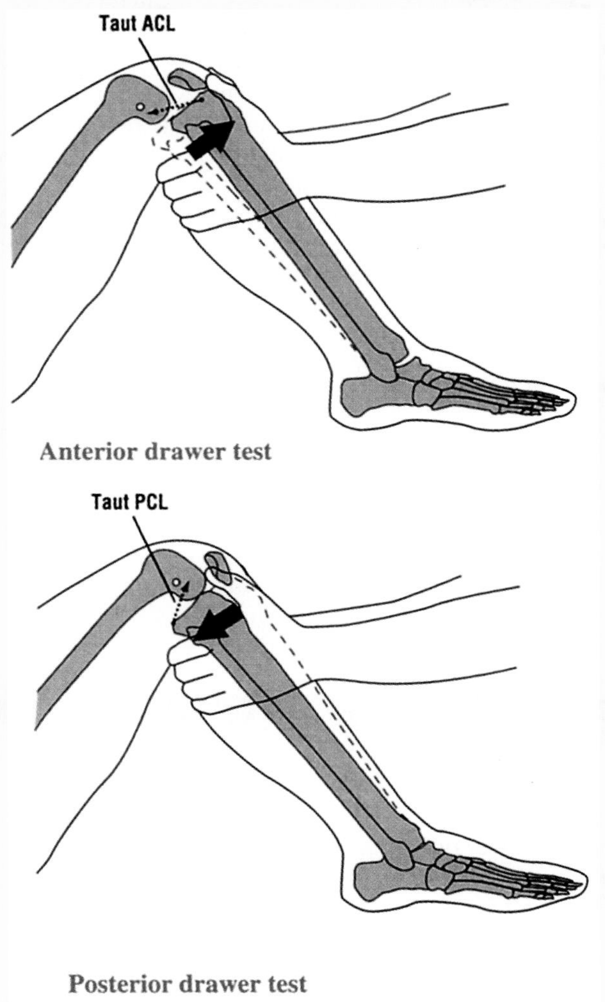

(Figures from Neumann DA: *Kinesiology of the musculoskeletal system: foundations for physical rehabilitation,* St Louis, 2002, Mosby.)

- Together, given the various fibers of the two cruciate ligaments, they are considered able to resist the extremes of every motion at the tibiofemoral joint.

Anterior Cruciate Ligament:

- The **anterior cruciate ligament** attaches from the anterior tibia to the posterior femur (see Figure 8-24).
  - More specifically, it attaches from the anterior tibia to the posterolateral femur, running from the anterior intercondylar region of the tibia to the medial aspect of the lateral condyle of the femur.
- Function: It limits anterior translation of the leg relative to the thigh when the thigh is fixed. It also limits the reverse action of posterior translation of the thigh relative to the leg when the leg is fixed.
- The anterior cruciate ligament becomes taut at the end range of extension of the tibiofemoral joint. Therefore this ligament limits hyperextension of the tibiofemoral joint.
- The anterior cruciate ligament also limits medial rotation of the leg at the tibiofemoral joint (and the reverse action of lateral rotation of the thigh at the tibiofemoral joint).
- Many sources state that the anterior cruciate also limits lateral rotation of the leg at the tibiofemoral joint (and the reverse action of the medial rotation of the thigh at the tibiofemoral joint).

BOX 8-41

The anterior cruciate ligament is the most commonly injured ligament of the tibiofemoral joint. It can be injured in a number of ways. Certainly, any force that anteriorly translates the tibia relative to the femur, or posteriorly translates the femur relative to the tibia, could tear or rupture the anterior cruciate. Hyperextension of the tibiofemoral joint can also tear the anterior cruciate because tibiofemoral joint extension involves an anterior glide of the tibia and/or posterior glide of the femur at the tibiofemoral joint. Strong rotation forces to the tibiofemoral joint (especially medial rotation of the tibia or lateral rotation of the femur) can also tear the anterior cruciate ligament. "Cutting" in sports (a combination of forceful extension and rotation with the foot planted when changing direction while running) is often implicated in anterior cruciate tears because of the forceful rotation necessary.

Posterior Cruciate Ligament:

- The **posterior cruciate ligament** attaches from the posterior tibia to the anterior femur (see Figure 8-24).
  - More specifically, it attaches from the posterior tibia to the anterolateral femur, running from the posterior intercondylar region of the tibia to the lateral aspect of the medial condyle of the femur.
- Function: It limits posterior translation of the leg relative to the thigh when the thigh is fixed. It also limits the reverse action of anterior translation of the thigh relative to the leg when the leg is fixed.
- The posterior cruciate ligament also becomes taut at the extreme end range of flexion of the tibiofemoral joint.

Other Ligaments of the Knee Joint:

Oblique Popliteal Ligament:

- Location: Posterior tibiofemoral joint (see Figure 8-24)
  - More specifically, the **oblique popliteal ligament** attaches proximally from the lateral femoral condyle and distally into fibers of the distal tendon of the semimembranosus muscle.
- Function: It reinforces the posterior capsule of the tibiofemoral joint and resists full extension of the tibiofemoral joint.

Arcuate Popliteal Ligament:

- Location: Posterior tibiofemoral joint (see Figure 8-24)
  - More specifically, the **arcuate popliteal ligament** attaches distally from the fibular head and proximally into the posterior intercondylar region

of the tibia and occasionally into the posterior side of the lateral femoral condyle.

- Function: It reinforces the posterior capsule of the tibiofemoral joint and resists full extension of the tibiofemoral joint.

Patellar Ligament:

- Location: The **patellar ligament** is located between the patella and the tibial tuberosity (see Figure 8-24).
- This ligament is actually part of the distal tendon of the quadriceps femoris group.
- The patellar ligament is also known as the *infrapatellar ligament.*

Ligaments of the Menisci of the Tibiofemoral Joint:

- These ligaments stabilize the medial and lateral menisci by attaching them to adjacent structures.
  - **Meniscal horn attachments**: The four horns of the two menisci are attached to the tibia via ligamentous attachments.
  - **Coronary ligaments**: They attach the periphery of each meniscus to the tibial condyle. These ligaments are also known as the *meniscotibial ligaments.*
  - **Transverse ligament**: It attaches the anterior aspects (i.e., horns) of the two menisci to each other.
  - **Posterior meniscofemoral ligament**: It attaches the lateral meniscus to the femur posteriorly.

BOX 8-42

LIGAMENTS OF THE KNEE JOINT

- Fibrous joint capsule
- Medial (tibial) collateral ligament
- Lateral (fibular) collateral ligament
- Anterior cruciate ligament
- Posterior cruciate ligament
- Oblique popliteal ligament
- Arcuate popliteal ligament
- Patellar ligament
- Meniscal horn attachments
- Coronary ligaments
- Transverse ligament
- Posterior meniscofemoral ligament

Closed-Packed Position of the Tibiofemoral Joint:

- Full extension

Major Muscles of the Tibiofemoral Joint:

- The tibiofemoral joint is crossed by large muscle groups. Anteriorly, the major muscles are the muscles of the quadriceps femoris group; the quadriceps femoris are extensors of the tibiofemoral joint. The gluteus maximus and tensor fasciae latae may also contribute slightly to extension of the tibiofemoral joint via their attachments into the iliotibial band. Posteriorly, the major muscle group is the hamstring group; the two heads of the gastrocnemius are also located posteriorly. These muscles are flexors of the tibiofemoral joint. No muscles move the tibiofemoral joint medially in the frontal plane; however, the three pes anserine muscles (sartorius, gracilis, semitendinosus) help to stabilize the medial side of the tibiofemoral joint. No muscles move the tibiofemoral joint laterally in the frontal plane either; however, the presence of the iliotibial band (which the gluteus maximus and tensor fasciae latae attach into) helps to stabilize the lateral side of the tibiofemoral joint.

Menisci:

- The tibiofemoral joint has two menisci: (1) a **medial meniscus** and (2) a **lateral meniscus** (see Figure 8-24c).
  - The menisci are located within the joint (i.e., intra-articular) on the tibia.
  - They are fibrocartilaginous in structure.
  - The menisci are crescent shaped.
  - The open ends of the menisci are called *horns.*

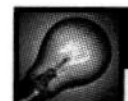

BOX 8-43

The word *meniscus* is Greek for *crescent.*

  - The medial meniscus is shaped like a letter *C*; the shape of the lateral meniscus is closer to the letter *O.*
  - The menisci are thicker peripherally and thinner centrally.
  - The menisci help to increase the congruency of the tibiofemoral joint by transforming the flat tibial plateau into two shallow sockets in which the femoral condyles sit. In this manner, they increase stability of the tibiofemoral joint.
  - The menisci also aid in cushioning and shock absorption of the tibiofemoral joint.
  - Meniscal attachments: The menisci are attached to the tibia at their horns; they are also attached to the tibia along their periphery via coronary ligaments. The transverse ligament attaches the anterior horns of the two menisci to each other. The posterior meniscofemoral ligament attaches the lateral meniscus to the femur.

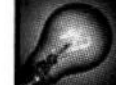

BOX 8-44

The two menisci of the tibiofemoral joint absorb approximately half the weight-bearing force through the tibiofemoral joint.

  - The medial meniscus if more firmly attached to adjacent structures than is the lateral meniscus.
- Note: The menisci do not have a strong arterial blood

supply; therefore they do not heal well after being injured.

BOX 8-45

Because the medial meniscus is more firmly attached to adjacent structures, it has less ability to move freely. This decreased mobility is one reason why the medial meniscus is injured more frequently than the lateral meniscus. The medial meniscus is also attached into the medial collateral ligament (whereas the lateral meniscus is not attached into the lateral collateral ligament); therefore forces that stress the medial collateral ligament may also be transferred to and damage the medial meniscus. The medial collateral ligament and medial meniscus are often injured together.

Miscellaneous:

- ❏ The tibiofemoral joint has many bursae. (See Box 8-46 for a listing of the common bursae of the tibiofemoral joint; see also Section 6.9, Figure 6-11c.)

BOX 8-46

MAJOR BURSAE OF THE TIBIOFEMORAL JOINT

- Suprapatellar bursa (actually part of the joint capsule)
- Prepatellar bursa
- Deep infrapatellar bursa
- Subcutaneous infrapatellar bursa

Bursae are also present between the following:

- Biceps femoris tendon and the fibular collateral ligament (biceps femoris bursa)
- Fibular collateral ligament and the joint capsule (fibular collateral bursa)
- Iliotibial band and the joint capsule (distal iliotibial band bursa)
- Tibial collateral ligament and the pes anserine tendon (anserine bursa)
- Semimembranosus tendon and the joint capsule
- Medial head of gastrocnemius and the joint capsule (medial gastrocnemius bursa)

- ❏ Full extension of the knee joint, unlike the elbow joint, is not stopped by a locking of the bones. Full extension of the knee joint is stopped only by the tension of soft tissues (primarily those located in the posterior knee joint region).
- ❏ The term **screw-home mechanism** describes the fact that during the last 30 degrees of tibiofemoral joint extension (i.e., when the tibiofemoral joint goes into full extension), a concomitant rotation of the tibiofemoral joint must occur. This rotation is either lateral rotation of the leg at the tibiofemoral joint if the thigh is fixed or medial rotation of the thigh at the tibiofemoral joint if the leg is fixed. This associated rotation helps to "lock" the tibiofemoral joint and increase its stability. To initiate flexion of a fully extended tibiofemoral joint, the joint must be "unlocked" with the opposite rotation motion.
  - ❏ By increasing the stability of the tibiofemoral joint, the screw-home mechanism decreases the work of the quadriceps femoris muscle group in maintaining a standing posture at the knee joint.

BOX 8-47

The screw-home mechanism rotation does not have to be created by separate muscular action when the knee joint extends. Rather, it occurs naturally because of the shape of the bones of the tibiofemoral joint, the passive pull of the anterior cruciate ligament, and the relatively greater lateral pull of the quadriceps femoris group. However, unlocking the fully extended tibiofemoral does require active muscular contraction. The popliteus is the muscle that seems to be most important in accomplishing this. If the thigh is fixed (as in *open-chain* movements of the lower extremity), the popliteus medially rotates the leg at the tibiofemoral joint as it begins flexion. If the leg is fixed (as in *closed-chain* movements of the lower extremity), the popliteus laterally rotates the thigh at the tibiofemoral joint as it begins flexion.

☐ 8.14 PATELLOFEMORAL JOINT

Bones:

- ❑ The patellofemoral joint is formed by the articulation between the patella and the femur. (The tibia is not directly involved in the movement of the patella [i.e., with the patellofemoral joint].)
  - ❑ More specifically, the patellofemoral joint is located between the posterior surface of the patella and the intercondylar groove of the femur.
- ❑ The patellofemoral joint is located within the capsule of the knee joint along with the tibiofemoral joint (Figure 8-25).

Major Motions Allowed:

- ❑ Superior and inferior gliding movement (i.e., nonaxial movements) of the patella along the femur are allowed.
- ❑ As the patella moves along the femur, it is usually described as *tracking* along the femur.
- ❑ Two facets exist on the posterior articular surface of the patella. The medial facet moves along the medial condyle of the femur; the lateral facet moves along the lateral condyle of the femur.
- ❑ The major purpose of the patella is to act as an anatomic pulley, changing the line of pull and increasing the leverage and force that the quadriceps femoris muscle group exerts on the tibia (Figure 8-26; Box 8-48).

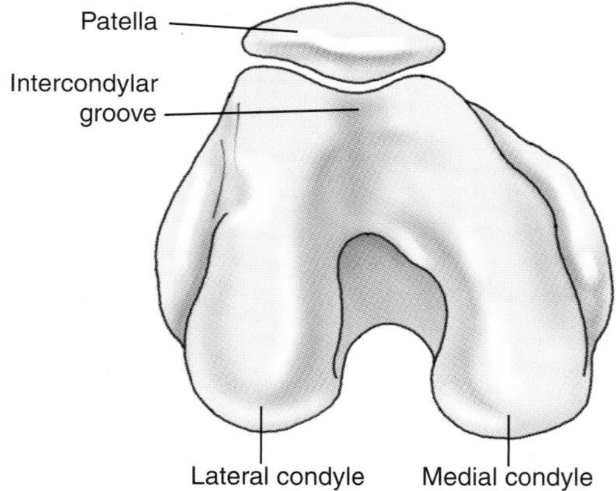

Figure 8-25 Distal view of patellofemoral joint of the right lower extremity. The patella tracks along the intercondylar groove of the femur.

BOX 8-48

Without a patella, the quadriceps femoris group musculature loses approximately 20% of its strength at the knee joint.

- ❑ The patella also functions to reduce friction between the quadriceps femoris tendon and the femoral condyles, and to protect the femoral condyles from trauma.
- ❑ Even though the patellofemoral joint is a separate joint functionally from the tibiofemoral joint, their movements are related. When the tibiofemoral joint extends and flexes, the patella tracks up and down (i.e., moves proximally and distally) along the intercondylar groove of the femur.

BOX 8-49

Ideally, the patella should track perfectly in the middle of the intercondylar groove. However, for a variety of reasons, the patella may not track perfectly. When improper tracking occurs, the patella usually tracks too hard against the lateral condyle of the femur.

- ❑ During forceful extension of the knee joint created by the quadriceps femoris muscle group, not all the force of the quadriceps on the tibia goes toward moving the tibia into extension. Some of the quadriceps femoris contraction force creates a compression of the patella against the femur. For this reason, the articular surface of the patella has the thickest articular cartilage of any joint in the body (Box 8-50).

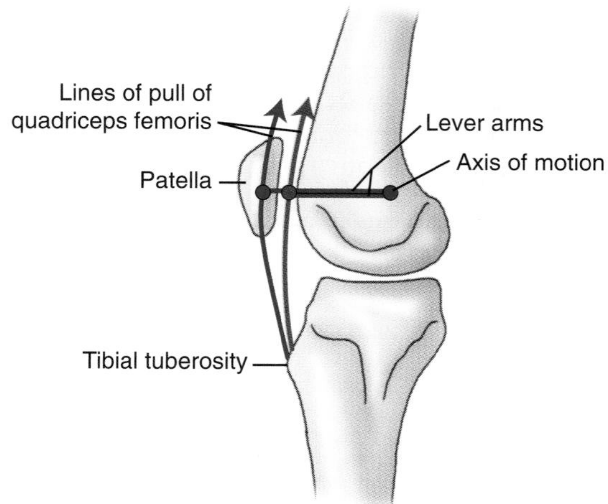

Figure 8-26 Lateral view of the knee joint that illustrates the line of pull and lever arm (i.e., leverage force) of the quadriceps femoris tendon with *(blue lines)* and without *(red lines)* the presence of the patella. The increased leverage of the quadriceps femoris muscle group as a result of the presence of the patella should be noted.

BOX 8-50

The articular surface of the patella has the thickest cartilage of any joint in the body to withstand the compressive force of the patella against the femur, as well as the stress that can occur when the patella does not track perfectly along the intercondylar groove of the femur. Because of the great compressive forces that this joint is subject to, along with the possible improper tracking of the patella, the articular cartilage of the patella often becomes damaged and breaks down. When this occurs, it is called **patellofemoral syndrome** (also known as **chondromalacia patella**). Scraping or sealing the pitted and damaged articular cartilage during arthroscopic surgery is often done to repair this condition.

- ❑ When the knee joint is in full extension, the patella sits proximal to the intercondylar groove and is therefore freely movable. When the knee joint is flexed, the patella is located with the intercondylar groove and its mobility is greatly reduced.

BOX 8-51

Even though the closed-packed position of the knee joint (i.e., tibiofemoral joint) is full extension, the patella itself (i.e., the patellofemoral joint) is most stable when the knee joint is in flexion.

8.15 ANGULATIONS OF THE KNEE JOINT

- The knee joint is composed of several components: the femur, the tibia, and the patella.
- The relationship of these components is such that they are not arranged in a straight line. The angles that are measured between the femur, tibia, and patella are called *knee joint angulations*.
- Three knee joint angulation measurements exist:
  - Genu valgum/varum
  - Q-angle
  - Genu recurvatum

Genu Valgum and Genu Varum:

- The genu valgum/varum angle is the angulation of the shaft of the femur relative to the shaft of the tibia within the frontal plane (Figure 8-27).
- Genu valgum/varum angles are determined by the intersection of two lines: one line runs through the center of the shaft of the femur; the other line runs through the center of the shaft of the tibia.
  - **Genu valgum** is defined as an abduction of the tibia relative to the femur in the frontal plane.

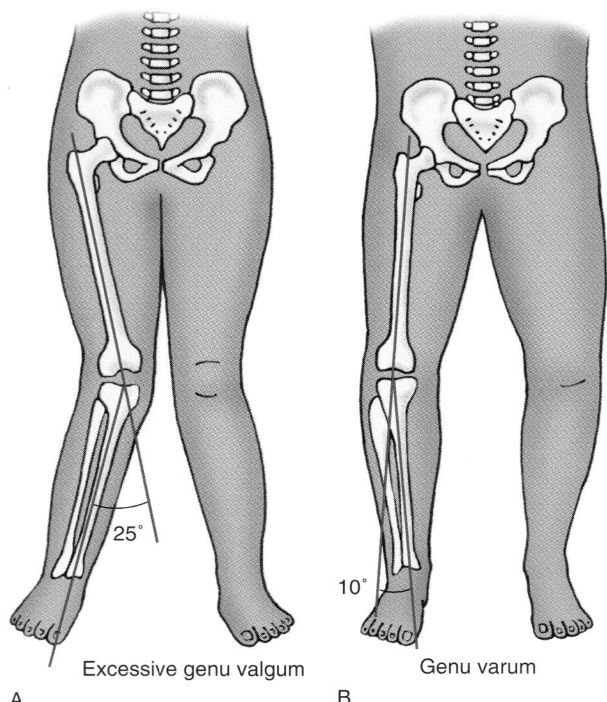

Figure 8-27 Anterior views of genu valgum/varum angulations of the knee joint within the frontal plane. *A,* Genu valgum angle of 25 degrees (i.e., knock-kneed). *B,* Genu varum angle of 10 degrees (i.e., bowlegged). The normal valgum/varum angle is considered to be between 5 and 10 degrees of genu valgum. Genu valgum/varum angles are measured by the intersection of two lines: one passing through the shaft of the femur and the other passing through the shaft of the tibia.

  - **Genu varum** is defined as an adduction of the tibia relative to the femur in the frontal plane.
- It is normal to have a slight genu valgum at the knee joint.
- This normal genu valgum is the result of the femur not being vertical. Because of the angle of inclination of the femur, it slants inward as it descends. When the slanting femur meets the vertical tibia, a genu valgum is formed.
- The normal value for a genu valgum angle is approximately 5 to 10 degrees.

BOX 8-52

The reported number of degrees of genu valgum can vary based on which angle is used to measure the relative positions of the shafts of the femur and tibia. The valgum angle measurement that is used to determine these figures is shown in Figure 8-27.

  - A genu valgum angle greater than 10 degrees is called *excessive genu valgum* or **knock-knees**.

BOX 8-53

Many factors can contribute to an increased genu valgum angle at the knee joint including overpronation of the foot (losing the arch of the foot on weight bearing), a lax medial collateral ligament of the knee, and a hip joint posture of excessive femoral medial rotation and adduction.

  - If a person has a genu varum angle at the knee joint, it is called **bowleg**.
- Excessive genu valgum or varum angles at the knee joint can cause increased stress and damage to the knee joint.

BOX 8-54

An increased genu valgum angle of the knee joint results in excessive compression force at the lateral tibiofemoral joint and excessive tensile (i.e., stretching/pulling) force at the medial tibiofemoral joint. Similarly, an increased genu varum angle of the knee joint results in excessive compression force at the medial tibiofemoral joint and excessive tensile force at the lateral tibiofemoral joint.

Q-Angle:

- Like the angles of genu valgum and genu varum, the Q-angle is also an angulation at the knee joint that exists in the frontal plane.
- The **Q-angle** is determined by the intersection of two lines: one line runs from the tibial tuberosity to the center of the patella; the other line runs from the center of the patella to the anterior superior iliac spine (ASIS) (Figure 8-28).

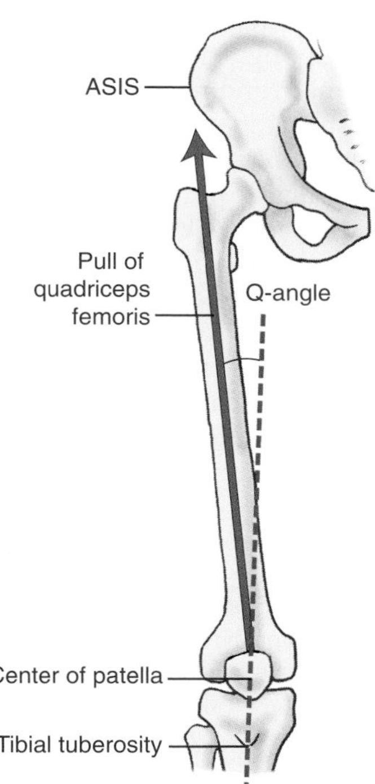

Figure 8-28 Anterior view that illustrates the Q-angle of the knee joint. The Q-angle is formed by the intersection of two lines: one running from the tibial tuberosity to the center of the patella and the other running from the center of the patella to the anterior superior iliac spine (ASIS). The Q-angle represents the pull of the quadriceps femoris muscle group.

- The Q-angle is so named because it represents the angle of pull of the **Q**uadriceps femoris group on the patella.
  - More specifically, the Q-angle measures the lateral angle of pull of the quadriceps femoris group on the patella.
- As the Q-angle increases, so does the lateral pull of the quadriceps femoris group's distal tendon on the patella. The patella is supposed to track smoothly within the center of the intercondylar groove of the femur. However, an increased Q-angle pulls the patella laterally and causes the patella to ride against the lateral side of the intercondylar groove; this may cause damage to the cartilage of the articular posterior surface of the patella (Figure 8-29).

BOX 8-55

Damage to the articular posterior surface of the patella is called either *patellofemoral syndrome* or *chondromalacia patella* (see note in Section 8-14).

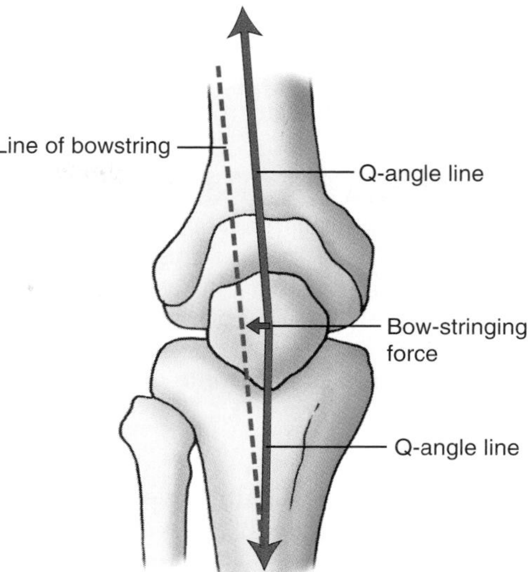

Figure 8-29 Anterior view that demonstrates the effect that the Q-angle has on the patella. The term *bowstringing* is used to describe the lateral pull that occurs on the patella. In this analogy the Q-angle lines represent the bow and the dashed line represents the bowstring. The bowstring force is represented by the distance between the center of the patella and the bowstring. The greater the Q-angle, the greater is the bowstringing force on the patella.

- The normal Q-angle measurement is approximately 10 to 15 degrees.

BOX 8-56

On average, the normal Q-angle for a man is approximately 10 degrees, and the normal Q-angle for a woman is approximately 15 degrees. Women usually have a greater Q-angle because the female pelvis is wider; therefore the line running up to the anterior superior iliac spine (ASIS) would be run more laterally, increasing the Q-angle.

- Because the normal Q-angle is not zero degrees, it reflects the fact that the pull of the quadriceps on the patella is not even; rather it has a bias to the lateral side.

BOX 8-57

The lateral pull on the patella of an increased Q-angle can be explained and measured by something called the **bowstring force**. Just like the string of a bow when under tension is pulled to a position that is a straight line between the two ends of the bow where it is attached, the patella can be looked at as being located within a *string* (in this case the string is the quadriceps femoris muscle group and its distal tendon/patellar ligament) that is pulled straight between its terminal two points of attachment on the tibia and the pelvis (the anterior superior iliac spine [ASIS] is approximately correct and an easy measurement point). Thus the patella can be seen to *bowstring* laterally (see Figure 8-29). (For more on bowstringing, see *Spotlight on Bowstring Force* in Section 8-17.)

- This net lateral pull of the quadriceps femoris group on the patella is due in part to the greater relative strength of the vastus lateralis muscle compared with the vastus medialis muscle.

BOX 8-58

One treatment approach for a client with an increased Q-angle is to recommend that he or she do exercises aimed at specifically strengthening the vastus medialis muscle of the quadriceps femoris group. A strengthened vastus medialis can counter the excessive lateral pull on the patella that occurs with an increased Q-angle. Referral to a physical therapist, chiropractor, or trainer may be necessary to ensure that these exercises are done correctly.

- An increased genu valgum angle (i.e., knock-knees) increases the Q-angle at the knee joint and contributes to the lateral tracking of the patella.

Genu Recurvatum:

- Full extension of the knee joint usually produces an extension beyond neutral (i.e., hyperextension) of approximately 5 to 10 degrees in the sagittal plane.
- **Genu recurvatum** is the term used to describe when the knee joint extends (i.e., hyperextends) in the sagittal plane beyond 10 degrees (Figure 8-30).

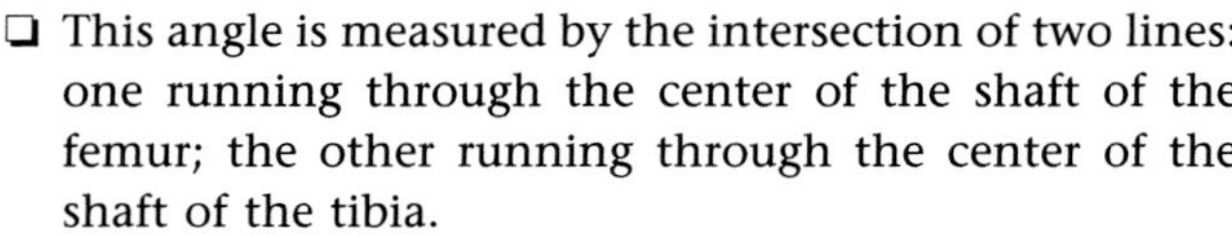

- This angle is measured by the intersection of two lines: one running through the center of the shaft of the femur; the other running through the center of the shaft of the tibia.
- This occurs for two reasons: (1) the shape of the tibial plateau slopes slightly posteriorly, and (2) the fact that the center of a person's body weight falls anterior to the knee joint when a person is standing. Normally this tendency toward extension is resisted by the passive tension of the soft tissue structures of the posterior knee joint. When this passive tension of the soft tissue structures is unable to sufficiently resist these forces of extension and the knee joint extends (i.e., hyperextends) beyond 10 degrees, genu recurvatum results.

BOX 8-59

The advantage to having the center of a person's body weight fall anterior to the knee joint during normal full knee joint extension is that it allows the quadriceps femoris group to relax when standing.

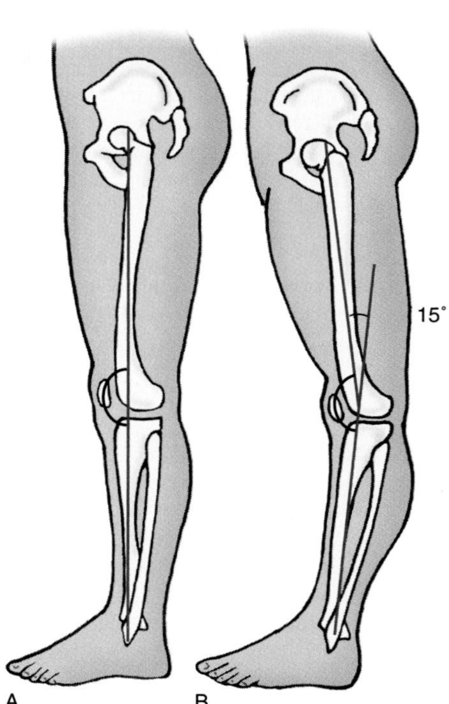

Figure 8-30 Genu recurvatum of the knee joint. *A,* Knee joint that is extended to zero degrees of genu recurvatum (i.e., the femur and tibia are vertically aligned). *B,* Genu recurvatum of 15 degrees. This angle is measured by the intersection of two lines: one running through the center of the shaft of the femur and the other running through the center of the shaft of the tibia.

8.16 TIBIOFIBULAR JOINTS

Bones and Ligaments:

- The **tibiofibular joints** are located between the tibia and the fibula.
- Three tibiofibular joints exist (Figure 8-31):
  - The proximal tibiofibular joint
  - The middle tibiofibular joint
  - The distal tibiofibular joint
- The proximal tibiofibular joint is located between the proximal ends of the tibia and fibula.
  - More specifically, it is located between the lateral condyle of the tibia and the head of the fibula.
  - The proximal tibiofibular joint is a plane synovial joint.
  - Its joint capsule is reinforced by anterior and posterior proximal tibiofibular ligaments.

BOX 8-60

Even though the proximal tibiofibular joint is located close to the knee joint, it is not anatomically part of the knee joint; it has a separate joint capsule. Functionally, it is also not related to the knee joint. Structurally and functionally, all three tibiofibular joints are related to ankle joint movements.

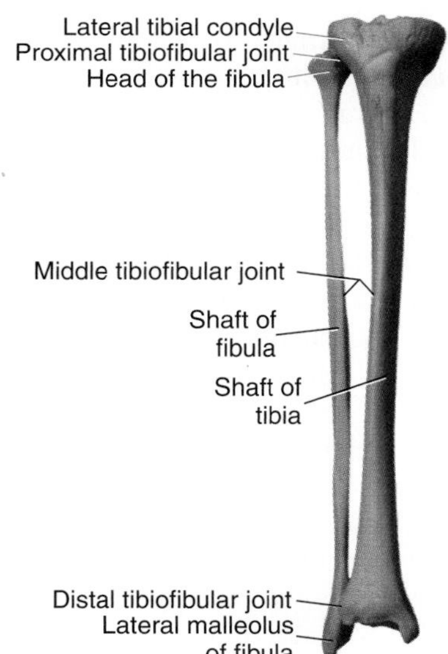

Figure 8-31 Anterior view that illustrates the three tibiofibular joints of the leg. The proximal tibiofibular joint is located between the proximal ends of the tibia and fibula. The middle tibiofibular joint is located between the shafts of the tibia and fibula. The distal tibiofibular joint is located between the distal ends of the tibia and fibula.

- The middle tibiofibular joint is located between the shafts of the tibia and fibula.
  - More specifically, it is created by the **interosseus membrane** uniting the shafts of the tibia and fibula.
  - The middle tibiofibular joint is a syndesmosis fibrous joint.

BOX 8-61

By uniting the shafts of the tibia and fibula together, the interosseus membrane of the leg has two purposes. One is to hold the two bones together so that they can hold the talus between them at the ankle (i.e., talocrural) joint distally. The other is to allow the force of all muscle attachments that pull on the fibula to be transferred to the tibia to move the leg at the knee joint.

- The distal tibiofibular joint is located between the distal ends of the tibia and fibula.
  - More specifically, it is created by the medial side of the lateral malleolus of the fibula articulating with the fibular notch of the distal tibia.
  - The distal tibiofibular joint is a syndesmosis fibrous joint.
  - It is reinforced by the interosseus ligament and the anterior and posterior distal tibiofibular ligaments.

Major Motions Allowed:

- The tibiofibular joints allow superior and inferior glide (i.e., nonaxial movements) of the fibula relative to the tibia.
- The stability of the tibiofibular joints is dependant on the tibia and fibula being securely held to each other.
- The mobility and stability of all three tibiofibular joints are functionally related to movements of the ankle joint. (Note: For more details regarding the relationship between the ankle and tibiofibular joints, see Section 8.18.)
- The stability of the distal tibiofibular joint is particularly important to the functioning of the ankle joint, because the distal ends of the tibia and fibula at the

distal tibiofibular joint must securely hold the talus between them at the ankle joint.

Miscellaneous:

- **Tibial torsion**: The term *tibial torsion* describes the fact that the shaft of the tibia twists so that the distal tibia does not face the same direction that the proximal tibia does.
  - The twisting that the shaft of the tibia undergoes is a lateral torsion.

BOX 8-62

The shafts of both the femur and the tibia undergo twisting or "torsion." However, although the femur twists medially, the tibia twists laterally. (For more on tibial torsion and its effects, see *Spotlight on Tibial Torsion and Talocrural Motion* in Section 8.18.)

- The result of this lateral tibial torsion is that the distal tibia faces somewhat laterally. Therefore motions at the ankle joint (i.e., dorsiflexion and plantarflexion) do not occur exactly within the sagittal plane; rather they occur in an oblique plane.

8.17 OVERVIEW OF THE ANKLE/FOOT REGION

Organization of the Ankle/Foot Region:

Generally the organization of the ankle/foot region is as follows (Figure 8-32):

- The two bones of the leg articulate with the foot at the **talocrural joint** (usually simply referred to as the *ankle joint*).
- The foot is defined as everything distal to the tibia and fibula.
  - The bones of the foot can be divided into tarsals, metatarsals, and phalanges.
  - Just as the carpal bones are the wrist bones, the tarsal bones are known as the *ankle bones*.
- The foot can be divided into three regions: (1) the hindfoot, (2) midfoot, and (3) forefoot.
  - The **hindfoot** consists of the talus and calcaneus, which are tarsal bones.
  - The **midfoot** consists of the navicular, cuboid, and the three cuneiforms, which are tarsal bones.
  - The **forefoot** consists of the metatarsals and phalanges.
- The term **ray** refers (in the foot) to a metatarsal and its associated phalanges; the foot has five rays. (The 1st ray is composed of the 1st metatarsal and the two phalanges of the big toe; the 2nd ray is composed of the 2nd metatarsal and the three phalanges of the 2nd toe, and so forth.)

Functions of the Foot:

- The foot is truly a marvelous structure because it must be both stable and flexible.
- The foot must be sufficiently stable to support the tremendous weight-bearing force from the body above it, absorb the shock from landing on the ground below, and propel the body through space by pushing off the ground. Stability such as this requires the foot to be a rigid structure.
- However, the foot must also be sufficiently flexible and pliable (i.e., mobile) so that it can adapt to the uneven ground surfaces that it encounters.
- Stability and flexibility are two antagonist concepts that the foot must balance to be able to meet these divergent demands.
- Generally weight/shock absorption and propulsion by the foot is a factor of dorsiflexion/plantarflexion of the foot at the ankle (i.e., talocrural joint).
- Generally adapting to uneven ground surfaces is a factor of pronation/supination (primarily composed of eversion/inversion) of the foot at the subtalar joint.
- However, it must be emphasized that the ankle joint region is a complex of joints which must function together to accomplish these tasks. (Note: For more on the functions of the foot during weight bearing and the gait cycle, see Sections 17.12 and 17.13.)
- Movement at the talocrural, subtalar, and transverse tarsal joints must smoothly and seamlessly occur together for proper functioning of the foot!

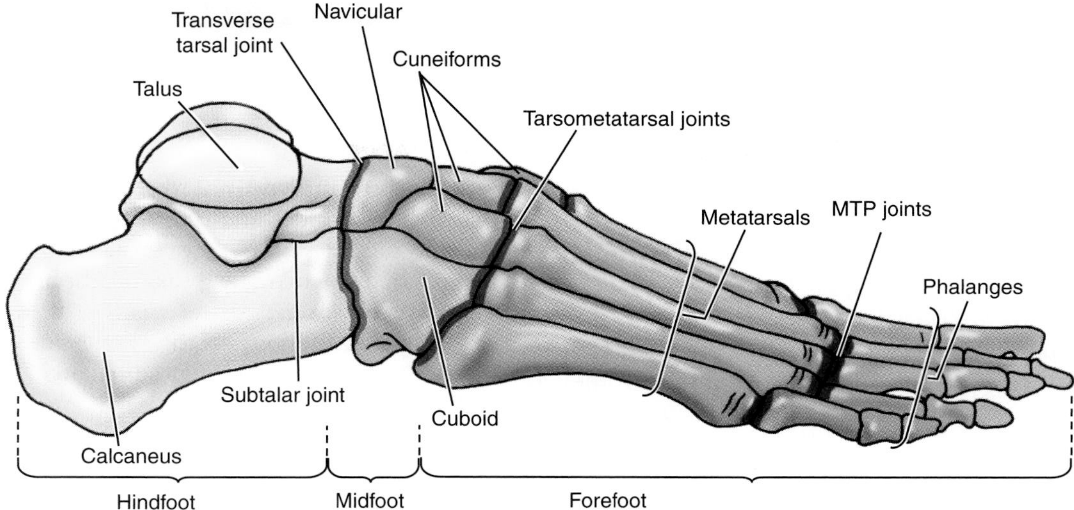

Figure 8-32 The three regions of the foot. The hindfoot is composed of the calcaneus and talus. The midfoot is composed of the navicular, cuboid, and the three cuneiforms. The forefoot is composed of the metatarsals and phalanges. (Note: The major joints of the foot are also labeled.)

Joints of the Ankle/Foot Region:

Ankle Joint:

- The ankle joint is located between the distal tibia/fibula and the talus (see Figure 8-34a in Section 8.18).
  - This joint is usually referred to as the *talocrural joint*.

BOX 8-63

Because the ankle joint involves the distal tibia and fibula meeting the talus, the joints between the tibia and fibula (distal, middle, and proximal tibiofibular joints) are functionally related to the functioning of the ankle joint. (For more on this, see Section 8.18.)

Tarsal Joints:

- **Tarsal joints** are located between tarsal bones of the foot (see Figure 8-32).
- A number of tarsal joints are found in the foot.
- The major tarsal joint is the **subtalar joint**.
  - The subtalar joint is located between the talus and the calcaneus.
- Another important tarsal joint is the **transverse tarsal joint**.
  - The transverse tarsal joint is located between the talus/calcaneus (which are located proximally) and the navicular/cuboid (which are located distally).

- **Distal intertarsal joints** is the term used to describe all other joints formed between the tarsal bones. The individual distal intertarsal joints may also be named for the specific tarsal bones involved (e.g., the cuboidonavicular joint between the cuboid and navicular bone or the intercuneiform joints between the cuneiform bones).

Tarsometatarsal and Intermetatarsal Joints:

- The **tarsometatarsal (TMT) joints** are located between the tarsal bones located proximally and the metatarsal bones located distally (see Figure 8-32).
- **Intermetatarsal joints** are located between the metatarsal bones (see Figure 8-43 in Section 8.22).

Metatarsophalangeal Joints:

- The **metatarsophalangeal (MTP) joints** are located between the metatarsal bones located proximally and the phalanges located distally (see Figure 8-32).

Interphalangeal Joints:

- **Interphalangeal (IP) joints** are located between phalanges (see Figure 8-47 in Section 8.24).
  - **Proximal interphalangeal (PIP) joints** are located between the proximal and middle phalanges of toes #2-5.
  - **Distal interphalangeal (DIP) joints** are located between the middle and distal phalanges of toes #2-5.
  - An IP joint is located between the proximal and middle phalanges of the big toe (toe #1).

Arches of the Foot:

- The foot is often described as having an **arch**. More accurately, it can be described as having three arches (Figure 8-33):

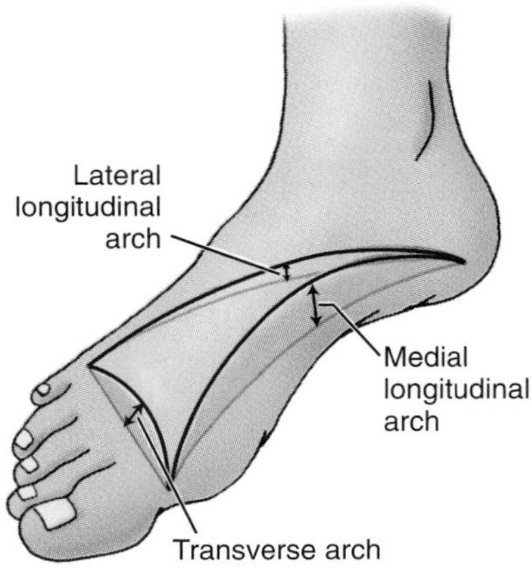

Figure 8-33 The three arches of the foot. Two arches run the length of the foot; they are the medial longitudinal arch, which is the largest arch of the foot, and the lateral longitudinal arch. The 3rd arch runs across the foot; it is the transverse arch.

BOX 8-64

The arch structure of the foot is not present at birth; rather it develops as we age. Most people have their arches developed by approximately 5 years of age.

  - **Medial longitudinal arch**: This arch is the largest arch of the foot and runs the length of the foot on the medial side. This is the arch that is normally referred to when one speaks of "the arch of the foot."
  - **Lateral longitudinal arch**: This arch runs the length of the foot on the lateral side and is not as high as the medial longitudinal arch.
  - **Transverse arch**: This arch runs transversely across the foot.
- Note: Because of the manner in which the bones and joints of the foot tend to function together, motion that affects one arch tends to affect all three arches. (See the discussion of subtalar pronation and supination [Section 8.19] to better understand foot motions that affect the height of the arch[es].) If one arch "drops," then all three arches drop. If one arch "raises," then all three arches raise.

BOX 8-65

The client's arches can be evaluated by simply observing the feet in a weight-bearing position. This can be done from an anterior view in which the height of the arch may be directly observed. This can also be done from a posterior view in which bowing of the calcaneal (i.e., Achilles) tendon is looked at as an indication of the dropping of the arch(es) of the foot. Another very effective way that the arches of the foot can be evaluated is to spread a small amount of oil on the client's feet and then have the client step on colored construction paper. The degree of the arch can be seen by the imprint that the oil leaves on the paper.

- An excessive arch to the foot is called **pes cavus**.
- A decreased arch to the foot is called **pes planus** or described as a **flat foot**.

BOX 8-66

The clinical implications of one foot's arch that drops more than the other foot's arch are many. If one foot's arch is lower than the other foot's arch, then the height of one lower extremity will be less than the other. This will result in a pelvis that is depressed or tilted to one side. This results in a spine that must curve in the frontal plane to bring the head to a level position (which is necessary for vision and proprioceptive balance in the inner ear). This frontal plane curve of the spine is defined as a scoliosis. Therefore evaluation of the arches of a client's feet is extremely important when the client has a scoliosis. A dropped arch will also create structural stresses on the plantar fascia of the foot, as well as the knee joint and hip joint.

Plantar Fascia:

- The foot has a thick layer of dense fibrous tissue on the plantar side known as the **plantar fascia**.

BOX 8-67

Plantar fascitis is a condition wherein the plantar fascia of the foot becomes irritated and inflamed. Because tightening of the intrinsic muscles that attach into the plantar fascia often accompanies this condition, tension is often placed on the calcaneal attachment of the plantar fascia, which can create a **heel spur**. A common cause of plantar fascitis is an overly pronated foot (see Section 8.19). Plantar fascitis usually responds well to soft tissue work.

- The plantar fascia has two layers: (1) superficial and (2) deep.
  - The superficial layer is located in the dermis of the skin of the foot.
  - The deep layer is attached to the calcaneal tuberosity posteriorly and the plantar plates of the MTP joints and adjacent flexor tendons of the toes anteriorly.

BOX 8-68 SPOTLIGHT ON THE WINDLASS MECHANISM

The attachment of the plantar fascia into the flexor tendons of the toes has a functional importance. When we push ourselves off (i.e., *toe-off*) when walking, our metatarsals extend at the metatarsophalangeal (MTP) joints. Because of the attachment of the plantar fascia into the toe flexor tendons, the plantar fascia is pulled taut around the MTP joints. This tension of the plantar fascia then helps to stabilize the arch of the foot and make the foot more rigid, which is necessary when pushing the body forward when walking or running. This mechanism is often called the **windlass mechanism**. A windlass is a pulling mechanism used for lifting the mast of a boat. It consists of a rope that can be tightened by being wound around a cylinder; the tension of the rope then pulls on and lifts the mast. In this case the MTP joint is the cylinder and the rope is the plantar fascia. When the plantar fascia is pulled taut around the MTP, it becomes taut and pulls on the two ends of the arch, increasing the height of the arch.

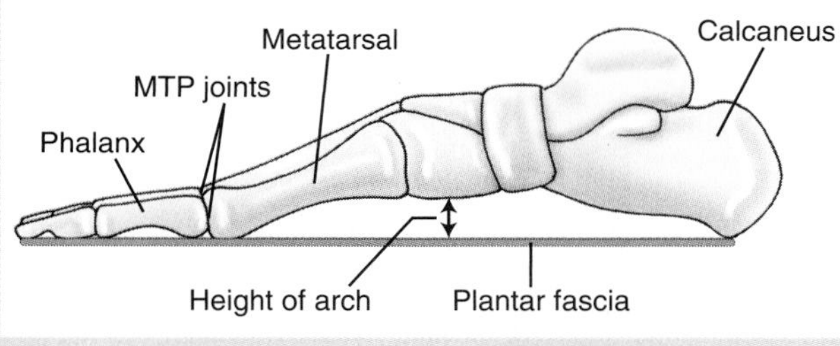

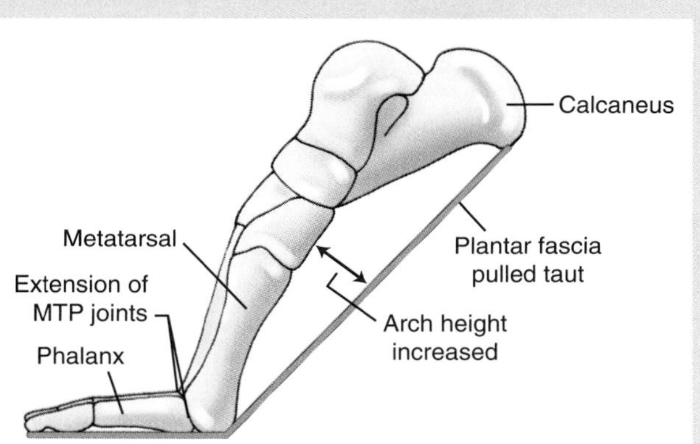

- The main purpose of the plantar fascia is to maintain and stabilize the longitudinal arches of the foot.

BOX 8-69

Many intrinsic muscles of the foot attach into the plantar fascia. By doing so, they help to maintain the tension of the plantar fascia and therefore the arch of the foot. However, walking in shoes (compared with walking barefoot) does not require as much activity from the intrinsic muscles of the foot and may allow them to weaken. Intrinsic musculature weakness could then lead to functional weakness of the plantar fascia and a loss of the normal arch of the foot. An excessive loss of the arch of the foot when weight bearing is defined as an *overly pronating foot* (at the tarsal joints), which can then lead to further problems in the body.

Miscellaneous:

- Many retinacula are located in the ankle region (see Box 8-71). These retinacula run transversely across the ankle and act to hold down and stabilize the tendons that cross from the leg into the foot (see Figure 8-37 in Section 8.18) (Note: In addition to the ankle region, retinacula are also located in the wrist region to hold down the tendons of the muscles of the forearm that enter the hand (see Section 9.10).
- The word *pedis* means *foot.*
- The word *hallucis* or *hallux* means *big toe.*
- The word *digital* refers to toes #2-5 (or fingers #2-5).

BOX 8-70 SPOTLIGHT ON BOWSTRING FORCE

A **retinaculum** (plural: retinacula) acts to hold down (i.e., retain) the tendons of the leg muscles that cross the ankle joint and enter the foot. A number of retinacula are located in the ankle region. Retinacula are needed in the ankle region, because when we contract our leg muscles to move the foot and/or toes, the pull of the muscle belly on its tendon would tend to lift the tendon away from the ankle (i.e., lift it up into the air and away from the body wall) if it were not for a retinaculum holding it down. This phenomenon is called *bowstringing* and weakens the strength of the muscles' ability to move the foot. Therefore the function of the retinacula of the ankle joint region is to hold these tendons down, preventing them from bowstringing away from the body.

Note: The term *bowstring* is used to describe this phenomenon because these tendons act like the string of a bow. A bow is a curved piece of wood with its string attached to both ends of the bow. When the string of a bow is placed under tension, it shortens and lifts away from the bow itself. Therefore the bowstring does not follow the curved contour of the bow; rather it lifts away to form a straight line that connects the two ends of the bow. (Note: The shortest distance between two points is a straight line.) Similarly, the leg and foot are angled relative to each other and can be likened to a curved bow. For example, when the tendons that cross the anterior ankle region are pulled taut (by the contraction of their muscle bellies), they would lift away from the ankle. Therefore we say that this lifting away is caused by the bowstring force, and it can be called *bowstringing.*

☐ 8.18 TALOCRURAL (ANKLE) JOINT

Unless the context is made otherwise clear, when the term *ankle joint* is used, it is assumed that it refers to the talocrural joint.

BOX 8-71

Some sources refer to the talocrural joint as the **upper ankle joint** (the subtalar joint is then referred to as the **lower ankle joint**). The value to this description is that it emphasizes the fact that movements of the foot are primarily dependant on movements at both the talocrural and subtalar joints!

Bones:

- ❑ The talocrural joint is located between the talus and the distal tibia and fibula (Figure 8-34a).
- ❑ More specifically, the talocrural joint is located between the trochlear surface of the dome of the talus and the rectangular cavity formed by the distal end of the tibia and the malleoli of the tibia and fibula.

BOX 8-72

The bony fit of the bones of the ankle joint is so good that many sources consider it to be the most congruent joint of the human body.

- ❑ When describing the shape of the talocrural joint, it is often compared with a **mortise joint** (see Figure 8-34b).

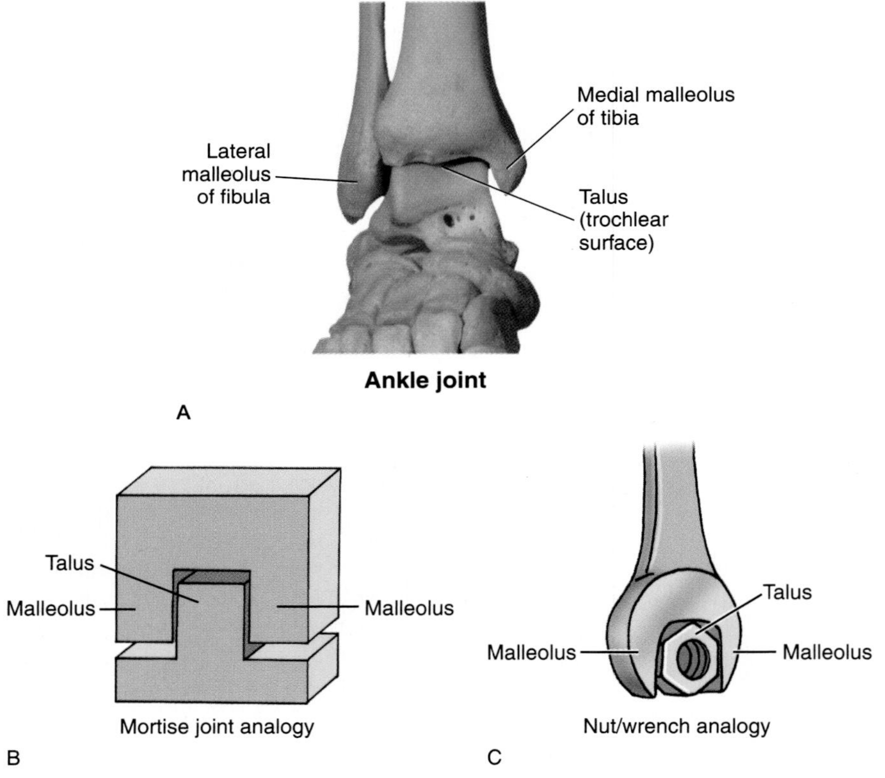

Figure 8-34 Talocrural (i.e., ankle) joint. *A,* Anterior view of the dorsal foot in which we see that the ankle joint is formed by the talus articulating with the distal ends of the tibia and fibula. *B,* Carpenter's mortise joint; the talocrural joint is often compared with a mortise joint. *C,* Nut held in a wrench. The talocrural joint may be compared with a nut held by a wrench. The talus is the nut, and the sides of the wrench are formed by the (malleoli of the) tibia and fibula.

- Perhaps a better analogy to visualize the shape of the talocrural joint is to compare it to a nut being held in a wrench (see Figure 8-34c).

BOX 8-73

A mortise joint was commonly used in the past by carpenters to join two pieces of wood. The mortise was formed by the end of one piece being notched out and the end of the other piece being carved to fit in this notch; a peg was then used to fasten them together. Because of its similarity in shape to a mortise joint, the talocrural (i.e., ankle) joint is often called the *mortise joint* (see Figure 8-34b).

- Joint structure classification: Synovial joint
  - Subtype: Hinge joint
- Joint function classification: Diarthrotic
  - Subtype: Uniaxial

Major Motions Allowed:

Average ranges of motion of the foot at the talocrural joint are given in Table 8-4 (Figure 8-35).

- The talocrural joint allows dorsiflexion and plantarflexion (i.e., axial movements) within the sagittal plane around a mediolateral axis (Boxes 8-74 and 8-75).

BOX 8-74 SPOTLIGHT ON TIBIAL TORSION AND TALOCRURAL MOTION

Actually, dorsiflexion and plantarflexion of the foot at the ankle joint do not occur perfectly within the sagittal plane. Because of the twisting of the tibia known as *tibial torsion*, talocrural motion occurs slightly in an oblique plane (tibial torsion is measured by the difference between the axis of the knee joint and the axis of the ankle joint). For this reason, talocrural joint motion is often listed as triplanar. However, use of the term *triplanar* can be misleading. Triplanar refers to the fact that its motion is across all three cardinal planes. However, the talocrural joint is uniaxial (with one degree of freedom); its motion is in *one* oblique plane around *one* oblique axis.

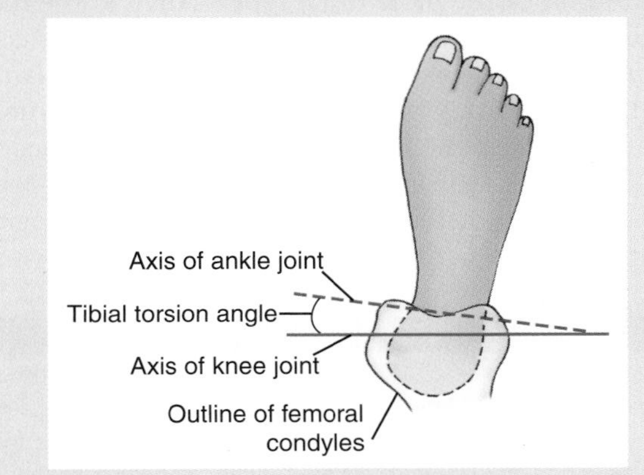

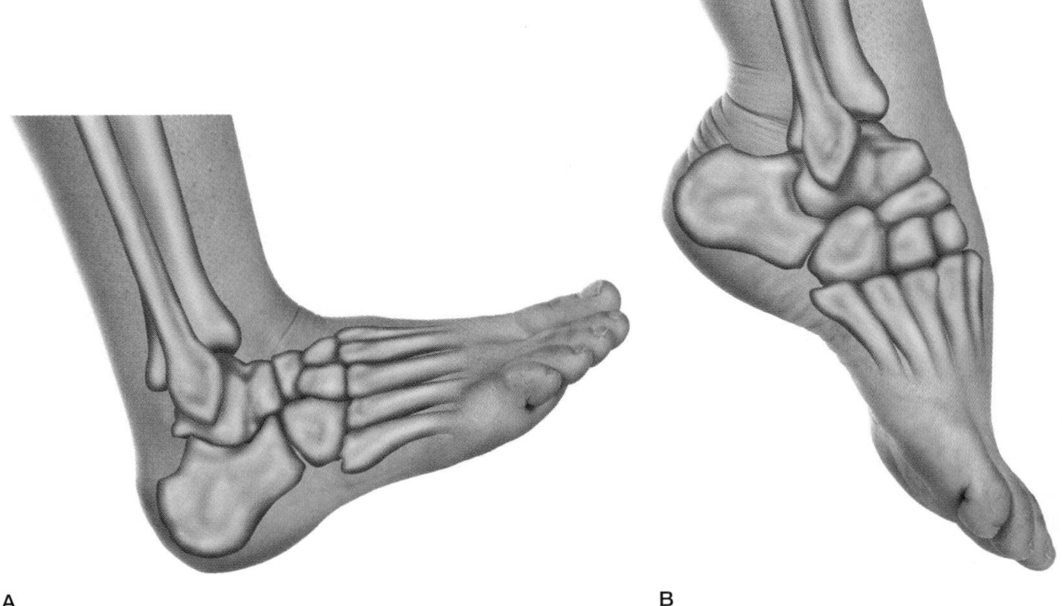

Figure 8-35 *A* and *B*, Dorsiflexion and plantarflexion of the foot at the talocrural (i.e., ankle) joint, respectively.

TABLE 8-4

Average Ranges of Motion of the Foot at the Talocrural Joint

Dorsiflexion	140 Degrees	Plantarflexion	5 Degrees

Note: The amount of dorsiflexion varies based on the position of the knee joint. Because the gastrocnemius (a plantarflexor of the ankle joint) crosses the knee joint posteriorly, if the knee joint is flexed, the gastrocnemius would be slackened and more dorsiflexion would be allowed at the talocrural joint.

BOX 8-75

Functioning of the ankle and tibiofibular joints is related. The dome of the talus is not uniform in size; its anterior aspect is wider than the posterior aspect. When the foot dorsiflexes, the wider anterior aspect of the dome of the talus moves between the distal tibia and fibula; this creates a force that tends to push the tibia and fibula apart. The motion and stability of the tibiofibular joints are necessary to absorb and counter this force.

Reverse Actions:

- The muscles of the talocrural joint are generally considered to move the more distal foot relative to the more proximal leg. However, closed-chain activities are common in the lower extremity in which the foot is planted on the ground; this fixes the foot and requires that the leg move relative to the foot instead. When this occurs, the leg can move at the talocrural joint instead of the foot.
- The leg can dorsiflex and plantarflex in the sagittal plane at the talocrural joint.

BOX 8-76

In a closed-chain activity when the leg moves at the talocrural joint instead of the foot, dorsiflexion of the leg at the talocrural joint is defined as the leg moving anteriorly toward the dorsum of the foot; plantarflexion of the leg at the talocrural joint is defined as the leg moving posteriorly away from the dorsum of the foot.

Major Ligaments of the Talocrural Joint:

Fibrous Joint Capsule:

- The capsule of the talocrural joint is thin and does not offer a great deal of stability to the talocrural joint.

Medial and Lateral Collateral Ligaments:

- The medial and lateral collateral ligaments are found on both sides (*lateral* means *side*) of the talocrural joint (Figure 8-36).
- The collateral ligaments are primarily important for limiting frontal plane movements of the bones of the talocrural joint.

Medial Collateral Ligament:

- The **medial collateral ligament** is also known as the **deltoid ligament** (see Figure 8-36a).

BOX 8-77

The deltoid ligament is so named because it has a delta (i.e., triangular) shape; it fans out in a triangular shape from the tibia to three tarsal bones.

- It attaches from the tibia to the calcaneus, talus, and the navicular bone.
  - More specifically, it attaches from the medial malleolus of the tibia proximally, and then it fans out to attach to the medial side of the talus, the sustentaculum tali of the calcaneus, and the navicular tuberosity.
- Function: It limits eversion of the foot at the talocrural joint (within the frontal plane).
  - The deltoid ligament is a taut, strong ligament that does a very effective job of limiting eversion sprains of the ankle joint.

BOX 8-78

In addition to the presence of the deltoid ligament, the fact that the lateral malleolus of the fibula extends down further distally than does the medial malleolus of the tibia also significantly helps to limit excessive eversion at the ankle joint. For this reason, eversion sprains of the ankle (i.e., talocrural) joint are very uncommon.

Lateral Collateral Ligament:

- The lateral collateral ligament is actually a ligament complex composed of three ligaments: (1) the anterior talofibular ligament, (2) the posterior talofibular ligament, and (3) the calcaneofibular ligament (see Figure 8-36b).
- All three lateral collateral ligaments attach proximally to the fibula.
  - More specifically, all three attach proximally to the lateral malleolus of the fibula.
- Distally, the anterior talofibular ligament attaches to the anterior talus; the posterior talofibular ligament attaches to the posterior talus; and the calcaneofibular ligament attaches to the lateral surface of the calcaneus.
- Function: The lateral collateral ligament limits inversion of the foot at the talocrural joint (within the frontal plane).

BOX 8-79

Given that the medial malleolus does not extend very far distally, the lateral collateral ligaments are the only line of defense against inversion sprains of the ankle joint; therefore inversion sprains are much more common than eversion sprains. Of the three lateral collateral ligaments, the anterior talofibular ligament is the most commonly sprained ligament. In fact, the anterior talofibular ligament is the most commonly sprained ligament of the human body. The reason that this particular lateral collateral ligament is more often sprained is that inversion sprains usually occur as a person is moving forward, which couples a plantarflexion motion to the foot along with the inversion. This places a particular stress on the more anteriorly placed anterior talofibular ligament.

BOX 8-80

LIGAMENTS OF THE TALOCRURAL JOINT

- Fibrous joint capsule
- Medial collateral ligament (deltoid ligament)
- Lateral collateral ligament complex
  - Anterior talofibular ligament
  - Posterior talofibular ligament
  - Calcaneofibular ligament

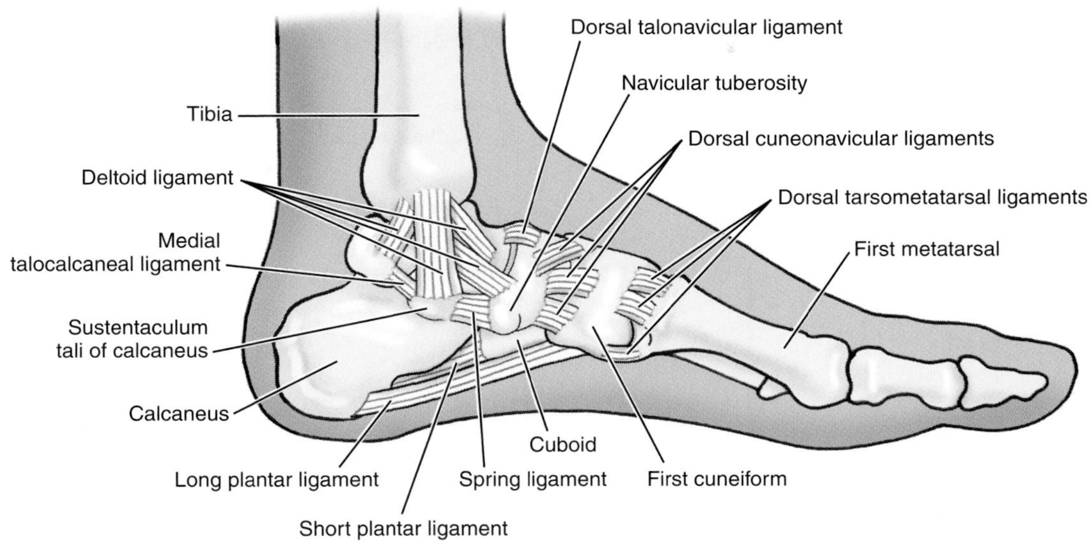

A

Anterior tibiofibular ligament
Tibia
Lateral collateral ligament
Posterior talofibular ligament
Calcaneofibular ligament
Anterior talofibular ligament
Fibula
Dorsal talonavicular ligament
Posterior tibiofibular ligament
Dorsal cuneonavicular ligament
Dorsal tarsometatarsal ligaments
Interosseus talocalcaneal ligament
Dorsal intermetatarsal ligaments
Calcaneus
Dorsal calcaneocuboid ligament
Short plantar ligament
Dorsal cuneocuboid ligament
Long plantar ligament
Bifurcate ligament

B

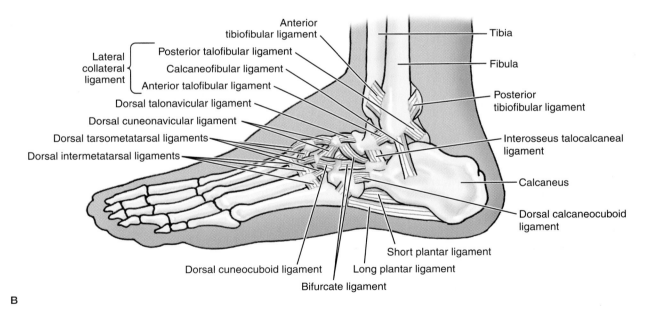

Figure 8-36 Ligaments of the left talocrural (i.e., ankle) and tarsal joints. *A,* Medial view—The major ligament of the medial talocrural joint is the mediolateral collateral ligament (also known as the *deltoid ligament*). *B,* Lateral view—The major ligament of the lateral talocrural joint is the lateral collateral ligament. The lateral collateral ligament is actually a ligament complex composed of three separate ligaments.

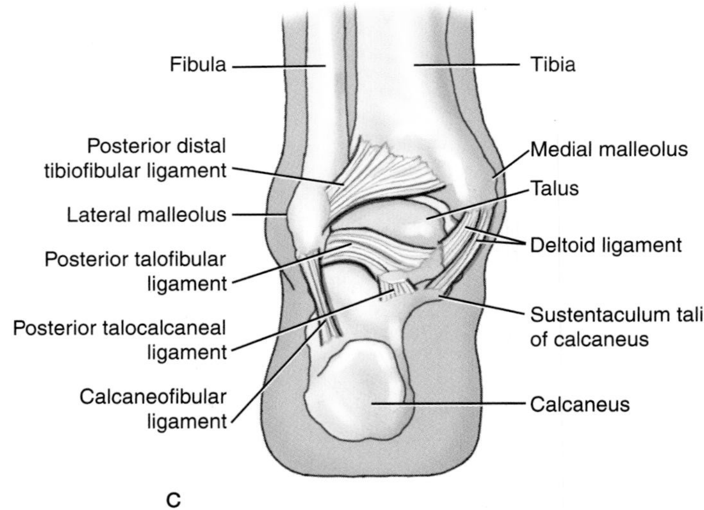

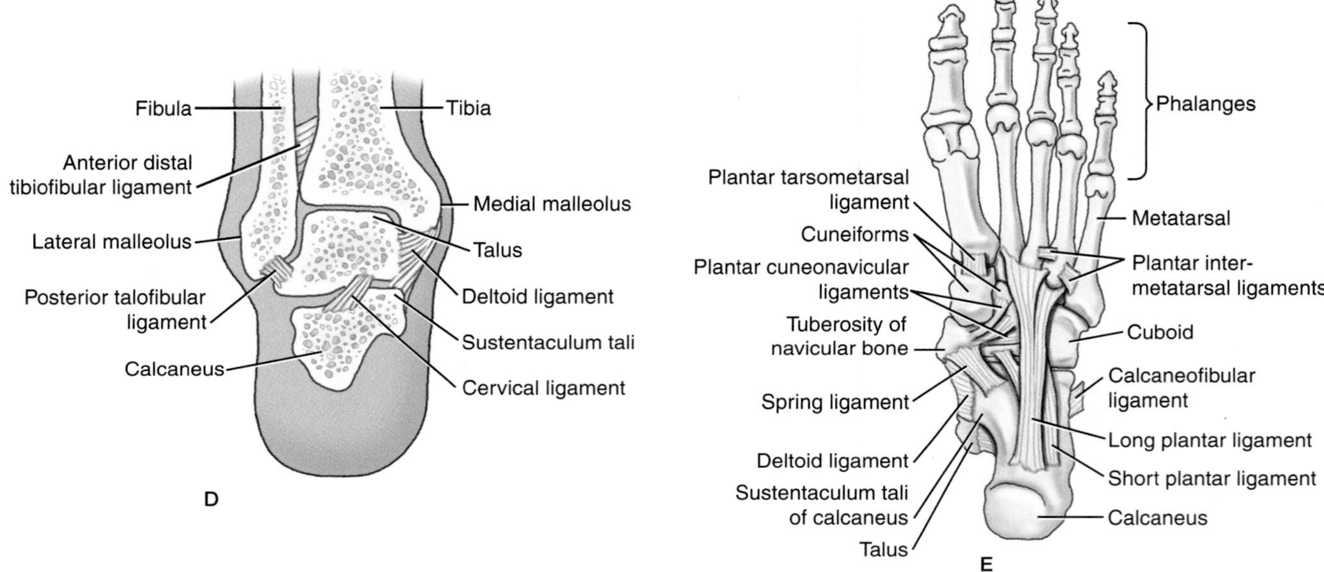

Figure 8-36, cont'd *C* and *D*, Posterior views. (Note: *D* is a frontal plane section through the bones.) *E*, Plantar view of the underside of the foot.

Closed-Packed Position of the Talocrural Joint:

❑ Dorsiflexion

Major Muscles of the Talocrural Joint:

❑ The talocrural joint is crossed anteriorly by all muscles that pass anterior to the malleoli; these are the muscles of the anterior compartment of the leg (tibialis anterior, extensor digitorum longus, extensor hallucis longus, and fibularis tertius). It is crossed posteriorly by all muscles that pass posterior to the malleoli; these are the muscles located in the lateral and posterior compartments of the leg (gastrocnemius, soleus, "Tom, Dick, and Harry" muscles, [i.e., tibialis posterior, flexor digitorum longus, and flexor hallucis longus], and the fibularis longus and brevis). The talocrural joint is crossed laterally by the fibularis muscles (fibularis longus, brevis, and tertius) and medially by the "Tom, Dick, and Harry" muscles.

Miscellaneous:

Bursae of the Talocrural Joint:

❑ The talocrural joint has many bursae (Figure 8-37). (See Table 8-5 for a listing of the common bursae of the talocrural joint.)

TABLE 8-5

Major Bursae and Retinacula of the Talocrural Joint (see Figure 8-37):

Bursae:
- Medial malleolar bursa (subcutaneous)
- Lateral malleolar bursa (subcutaneous)
- Subcutaneous calcaneal (Achilles) bursa
- Subtendinous calcaneal (Achilles) bursa

Retinacula:
- Superior extensor retinaculum
- Inferior extensor retinaculum
- Flexor retinaculum
- Superior fibular retinaculum
- Inferior fibular retinaculum

Retinacula of the Talocrural Joint:

❑ Retinacula are located both anteriorly and posteriorly at the ankle joint (see Figure 8-37). These retinacula function to hold down the tendons that cross the ankle joint and prevent bowstringing of these tendons. (Note: For more information on bowstringing, see *Spotlight on Bowstring Force* in Section 8.17.) (See Table 8-5 for a listing of the retinacula of the talocrural joint.)

Tendon Sheaths:

❑ Tendon sheaths are found around most tendons that cross the ankle joint to minimize friction between these tendons and the underlying bony structures (see Figure 8-37).

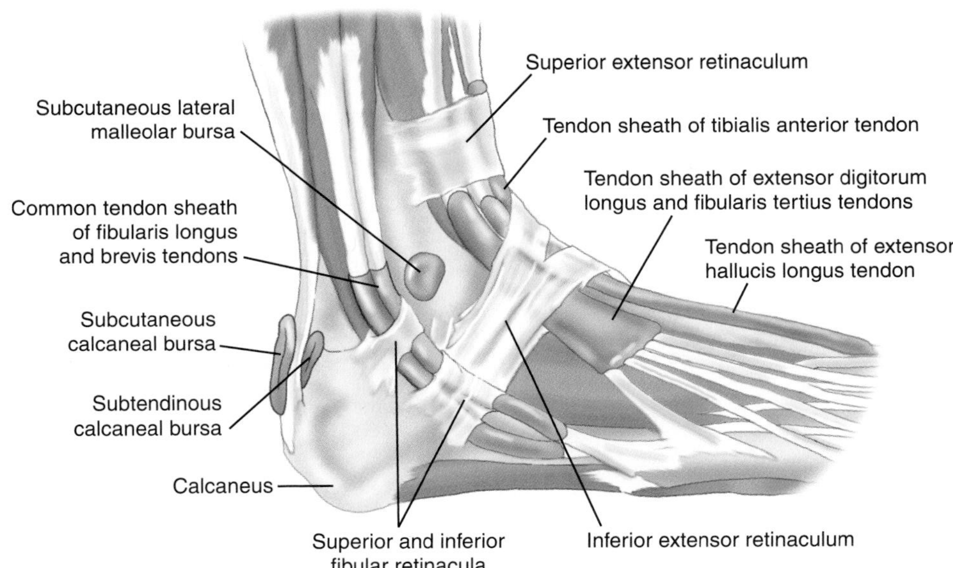

Figure 8-37 Lateral view that illustrates most of the bursae, tendon sheaths, and retinacula of the talocrural (i.e., ankle) joint.

8.19 SUBTALAR TARSAL JOINT

Bones:

- Tarsal joints are located between tarsal bones of the foot.
- The major tarsal joint of the foot is the subtalar joint.
  - The subtalar joint is located, as its name implies, under the talus. Therefore, it is located between the talus and the calcaneus (Figure 8-38).

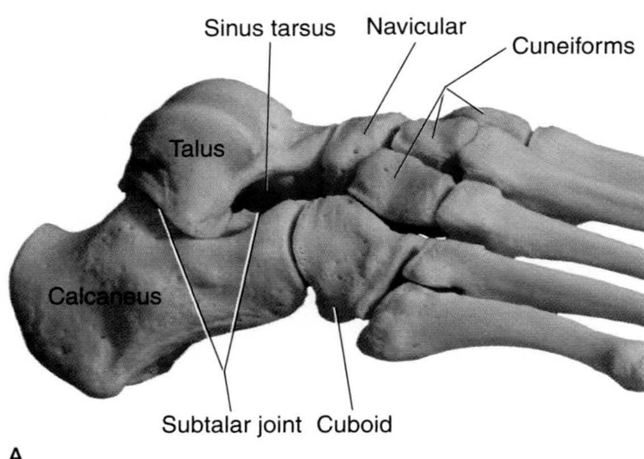

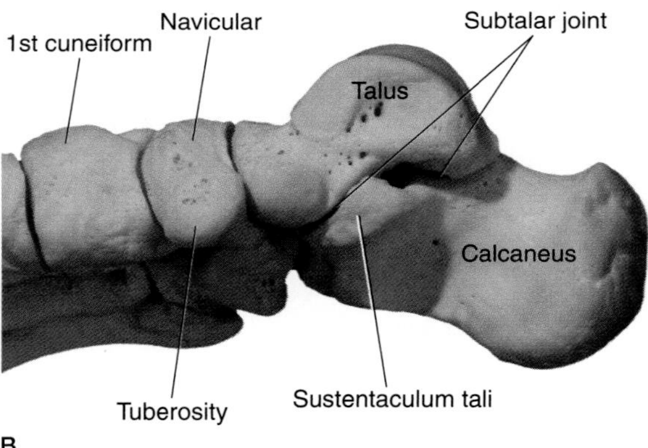

Figure 8-38 Subtalar joint located between the talus and the calcaneus. (Note: *Subtalar* means *under the talus.*) *A,* Lateral view. *B,* Medial view. The sinus tarsus is a large cavity located between the talus and calcaneus and is visible on the lateral side.

BOX 8-81

On the medial side of the foot, the talus is supported by the sustentaculum tali of the calcaneus. The sustentaculum tali is one of two easily palpable landmarks of the medial foot; the other is the tuberosity of the navicular (see Figure 8-38b).

- Therefore the subtalar joint is also known as the **talocalcaneal joint**.
- The subtalar joint is sometimes referred to as the lower ankle joint (the talocrural joint being the upper ankle joint).

Subtalar Joint Articulations:

- The subtalar joint is actually composed of three separate talocalcaneal articulations (between the talus and calcaneus) (Figure 8-39).
  - These articulations are facet articulations that are either slightly concave/convex or flat is shape.
  - The largest articulation is between the posterior facets of the talus and calcaneus.

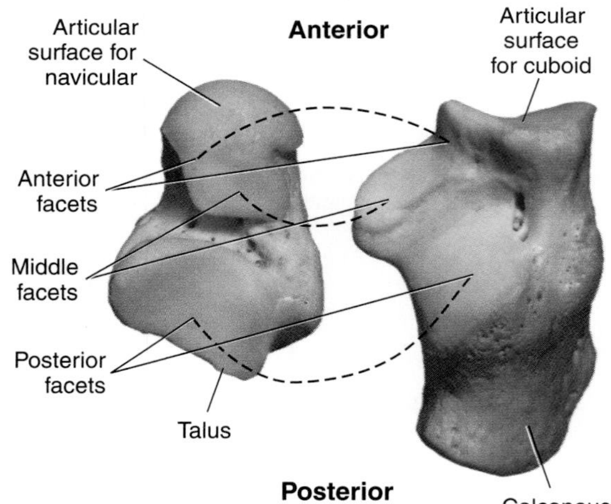

Figure 8-39 An "open-book" photo illustrating the facets of the subtalar joint (showing the superior surface of the calcaneus and the inferior surface of the talus). The subtalar joint is actually composed of three separate articulations. (Note: Each bone has three facets on its subtalar articular surface.) The two posterior facets are the largest of the six. Dashed lines illustrate how the facets line up with each other.

- The other two articulations are between the anterior facets and middle facets of the talus and calcaneus.
- Between the talus and calcaneus, a large cavity exists called the **sinus tarsus**, which is visible from the lateral side.
  - Joint structure classification: Synovial joint(s)
  - Joint function classification: Diarthrotic
    - Subtype: Uniaxial

BOX 8-82

The posterior articulation of the subtalar joint has its own distinct joint capsule, whereas the anterior and middle articulations of the subtalar joint share a joint capsule with the talonavicular joint.

BOX 8-83

The subtalar joint is often referred to as being *triplanar* because it allows movement across all three cardinal planes. However, its motion is in one oblique plane around one axis; hence it is uniaxial. Therefore the subtalar joint is triplanar and uniaxial.

Major Motions Allowed:

Average ranges of motion of the foot at the subtalar joint are given in Table 8-6 (Figure 8-40).

- The subtalar joint allows pronation and supination (i.e., axial movements) in an oblique plane around an oblique axis.

BOX 8-84

The axis for subtalar motion is oblique and is located 42 degrees (i.e., anterosuperior) off the transverse plane and 16 degrees (i.e., anteromedial) off the sagittal plane.

- The oblique plane movements of pronation and supination can be broken up into their component cardinal plane actions.

BOX 8-85

Description of subtalar joint motion varies greatly from one source to another. Some sources state that eversion is pronation and inversion is supination. Technically, this is not true. Eversion and inversion are the principle cardinal plane components of the larger oblique plane pronation and supination actions (see Figure 8-40). It should be emphasized that the component cardinal plane actions of the pronation and supination cannot be isolated at the subtalar joint. All three components of pronation must occur at the subtalar joint when the foot pronates, and all three components of supination must occur at the subtalar joint when the foot supinates.

- Pronation of the foot at the subtalar joint is composed of eversion, dorsiflexion, and abduction of the foot.
- Supination of the foot at the subtalar joint is composed of inversion, plantarflexion, and adduction of the foot.
  - Eversion/inversion of the foot at the subtalar joint occur within the frontal plane around an anteroposterior axis.
  - Dorsiflexion/plantarflexion of the foot at the subtalar joint occur within the sagittal plane around a mediolateral axis.
  - Abduction/adduction of the foot at the subtalar joint occur with the transverse plane around a vertical axis.

Reverse Actions:

- The previously discussed actions describe the components of pronation and supination when the more proximal talus/leg is fixed and the more distal calcaneus/foot is free to move (because the foot is not weight bearing [i.e., it is an open-chain activity]). However, when the foot is planted on the ground, the bones of the foot become somewhat fixed and the manner in which the components of pronation and

TABLE 8-6

Average Ranges of Motion of the (Non–weight-Bearing) Foot at the Subtalar Joint

Pronation:		Supination:	
Eversion	10 Degrees	Inversion	20 Degrees
Dorsiflexion	2.5 Degrees	Plantarflexion	5 Degrees
Abduction	10 Degrees	Adduction	20 Degrees

Note: Determining the relative amounts of eversion/inversion and so forth requires an agreed on neutral position of the subtalar joint. Subtalar neutral position is controversial and not agreed on by all sources. The numbers reflect the guideline that subtalar neutral is a position that allows twice as much inversion as eversion.

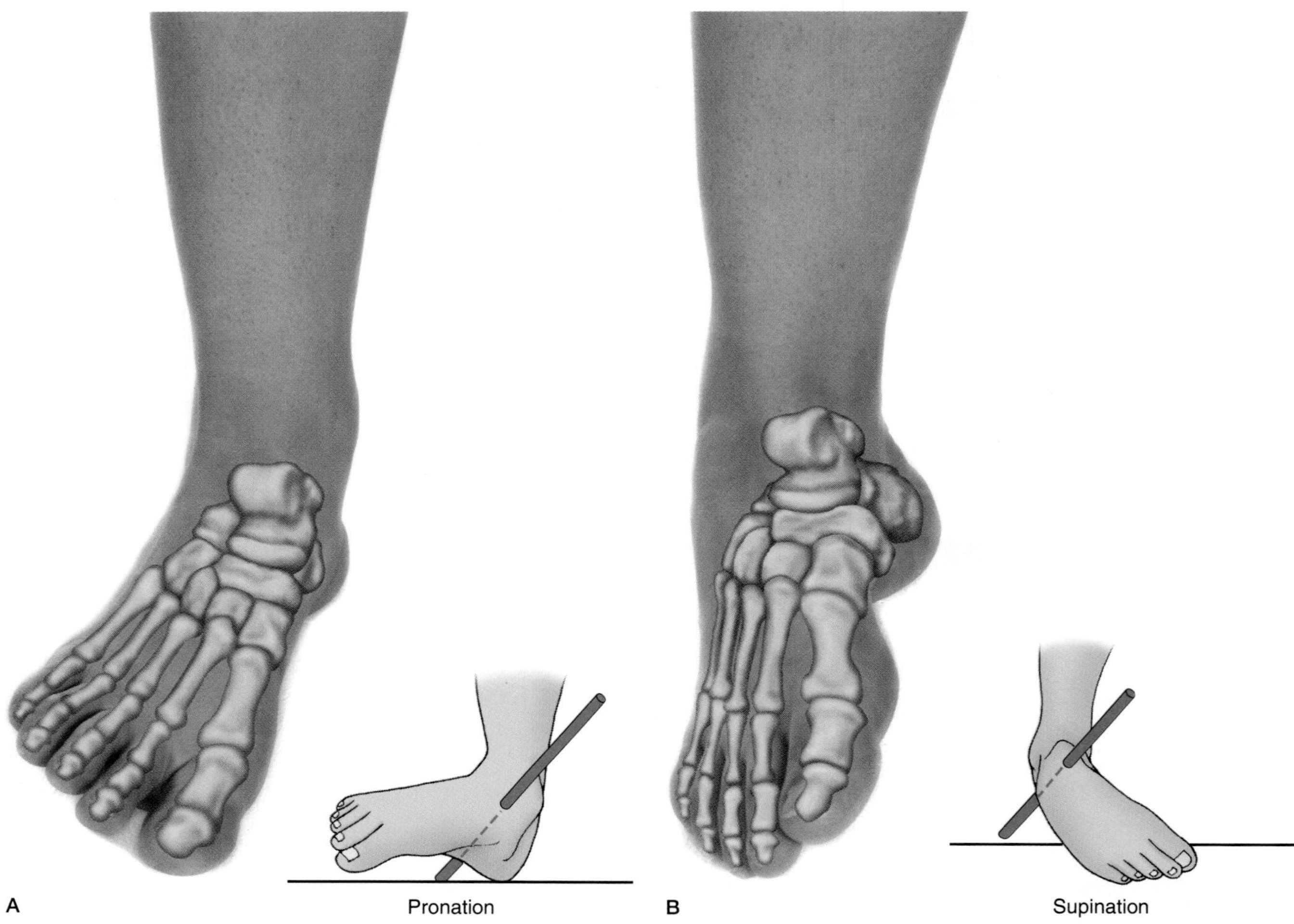

Figure 8-40 Motion of the foot at the subtalar joint. *A,* Pronation of the foot. Pronation is an oblique plane movement composed of three cardinal plane components: (1) eversion, (2) dorsiflexion, and (3) abduction of the foot. *B,* Supination of the foot. Supination is an oblique plane movement composed of three cardinal plane components: (1) inversion, (2) plantarflexion, and (3) adduction of the foot.

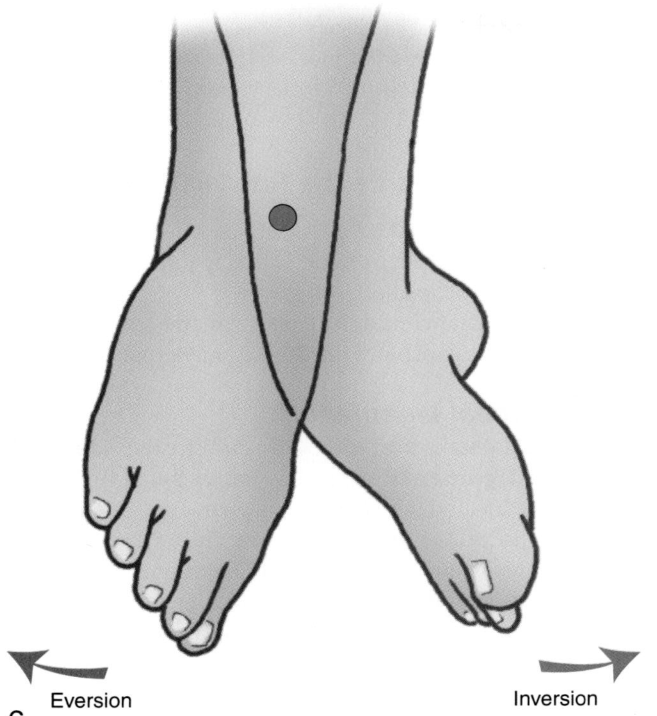

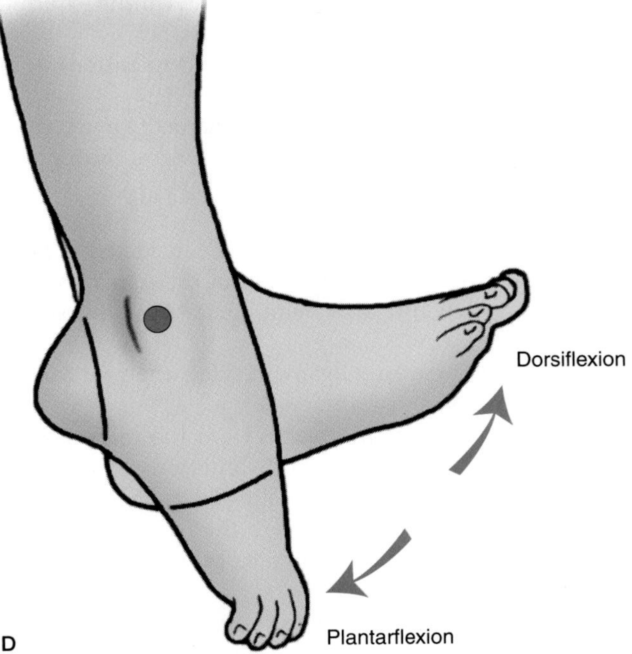

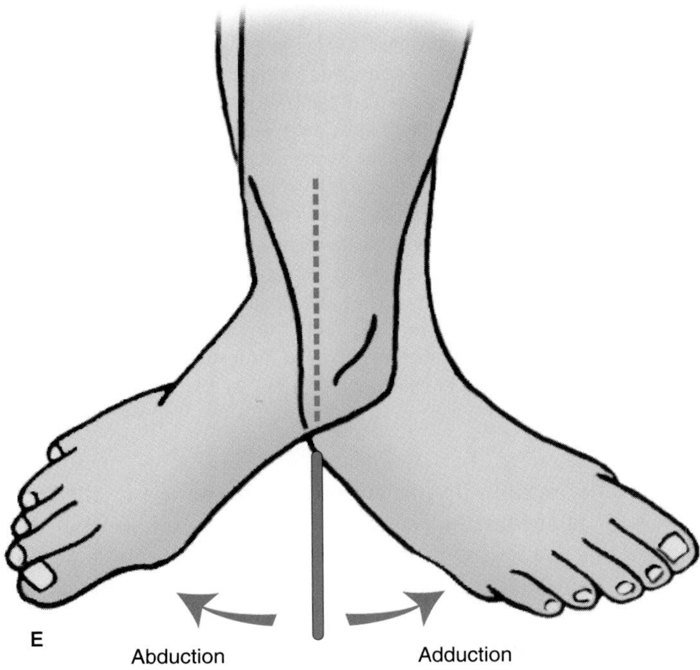

Figure 8-40, cont'd *C,* Frontal plane components of eversion/inversion. *D,* Sagittal plane components of dorsiflexion/plantarflexion. *E,* Transverse plane components of abduction/adduction. In *A, B,* and *E,* the red tube represents the axis for that motion. (Note: In *C* and *D,* the axis is represented by the red dot.)

supination of the foot at the subtalar joint are carried out changes to some degree:

- When we stand and the foot is weight bearing, as a result of being locked between the body weight from above and the fixed bones of the foot on the ground below, the motion of the calcaneus is limited but not completely fixed. In weight bearing, the calcaneus is free to evert/invert (in the frontal plane) only. Because the calcaneus cannot carry out the other two components of pronation/supination (in the sagittal and transverse planes), the more proximal talus must move relative to the calcaneus at the subtalar joint for these other two aspects of pronation and supination. When the talus carries out the aspect of dorsiflexion or plantarflexion that occur in the sagittal plane, this motion can be absorbed at the talocrural joint, because the talocrural joint allows movement in the sagittal plane; therefore this motion is not transmitted up to the leg. However, because the talocrural joint does not allow any transverse plane rotation, when the talus now moves relative to the calcaneus at the subtalar joint in the transverse plane, the bones of the leg must move along with the talus; this results in a rotation of the leg.

BOX 8-86

In a weight-bearing foot, when the subtalar joint pronates and supinates, some of the force of these motions is transferred up to the leg, requiring the leg to rotate within the transverse plane. When the weight-bearing foot pronates, the leg medially rotates; when the weight-bearing foot supinates, the leg laterally rotates. These rotation movements of the leg will then create a rotation force/stress at the knee joint and may affect the health of the knee joint. Because more people overly pronate (which manifests as a flat foot on weight bearing) than overly supinate, the knee joint is often subjected to medial rotation stress from below. Given that the knee joint does not allow rotation when it is extended, much of this (medial) rotation force will then be transmitted up to and affect the functioning and health of the hip joint. Therefore correction of an overly pronating foot may be extremely important toward correcting knee and hip joint problems. One solution to correct an overly pronating foot is to recommend orthotics to the client; another solution might be to recommend that the muscles of supination (i.e., inversion) of the foot at the subtalar joint be strengthened.

- Summing up pronation and supination of the subtalar joint in a weight-bearing foot, we see that the calcaneus everts/inverts relative to the talus at the subtalar joint in the frontal plane, the talus dorsiflexes/plantarflexes relative to the tibia/fibula at the talocrural joint in the sagittal plane, and the talus and leg (fixed together) medially rotate/laterally rotate relative to the thigh at the knee joint or the talus/leg and thigh (fixed together) medially rotate/laterally rotate relative to the pelvis at the hip joint in the transverse plane.

BOX 8-87

Pronation of the weight-bearing foot results in a visible drop of the arches of the foot. People who overly pronate during weight bearing are often said to be flat footed. These people actually do have an arch when not weight bearing, but this arch is lost on weight bearing. For this reason, their condition is more accurately described as being a **supple flat foot**. A **rigid flat foot** is a foot that is flat all the time and is not a result of excessive pronation on weight bearing.

Major Ligaments of the Subtalar Joint:

Fibrous Joint Capsule:

- The posterior aspect of the subtalar joint has its own distinct joint capsule.
- The anterior and middle aspects of the subtalar joint share a joint capsule with the talonavicular joint.

Talocalcaneal Ligaments:

- Medial, lateral, posterior, and interosseus **talocalcaneal ligaments** exist (see Figures 8-36a-b).
- They are located between the talus and calcaneus; their specific locations are indicated by their names.
- The interosseus talocalcaneal ligament is located within the sinus tarsus of the subtalar joint; its function is to limit eversion (i.e., pronation) of the subtalar joint.

Cervical Ligament:

- Location: The **cervical ligament** is located within the sinus tarsus of the subtalar joint, running from the talus to the calcaneus (see Figure 8-36d).
- Function: It limits inversion (i.e., supination) of the subtalar joint.
- Note: The cervical ligament is named for its attachment onto the neck of the talus (*cervical* means *neck*).

Spring Ligament:

- The **spring ligament** is usually considered to be primarily important as a ligament of the transverse tarsal joint; however, it also helps to stabilize the subtalar joint (see Figure 8-36a–e).
- Location: The spring ligament spans the subtalar joint inferiorly (on the plantar side).
- The spring ligament attaches from the calcaneus posteriorly to the navicular bone anteriorly.
  - More specifically, it attaches from the sustentaculum tali of the calcaneus to the navicular bone.
- Function: It limits eversion (i.e., pronation) of the subtalar joint.
- Because of its attachment sites, the spring ligament is also known as the *plantar calcaneonavicular ligament*.

Medial Collateral Ligament of the Talocrural Joint:

- ❑ It is also known as the *deltoid ligament* (see Figure 8-36a). (Note: For more information on the medial collateral ligament of the talocrural joint, see Section 8.18.)
- ❑ It limits eversion (i.e., supination) of the subtalar joint.

Lateral Collateral Ligament Complex of the Talocrural Joint:

- ❑ It is composed of the anterior talofibular, posterior talofibular, and calcaneofibular ligaments (see Figure 8-36b). (Note: For more information on the lateral collateral ligament of the talocrural joint, see Section 8.18.)
- ❑ It limits inversion (i.e., pronation) of the subtalar joint.

BOX 8-88

LIGAMENTS OF THE SUBTALAR JOINT

- Fibrous joint capsule(s)
- Talocalcaneal ligaments (medial, lateral, posterior, interosseus)
- Cervical ligament
- Spring ligament

Note: The medial collateral ligament and the lateral collateral ligament complex of the talocrural joint also help stabilize the subtalar joint.

Closed-Packed Position of the Subtalar Joint:

- ❑ Supination

Miscellaneous:

- ❑ It must be emphasized that in the weight-bearing foot, motion of the subtalar joint cannot occur in isolation. Its motion is intimately tied to the transverse tarsal joint and the talocrural joint, as well as every other joint of the foot and the knee and hip joints.

☐ 8.20 TRANSVERSE TARSAL JOINT

Bones:

- The transverse tarsal joint, as its name implies, runs transversely across the tarsal bones.
- The transverse tarsal joint is actually a compound joint, meaning that it is composed of two joints that are collectively called the *transverse tarsal joint*.
  - The two joints of the transverse tarsal joint are (1) the **talonavicular joint**, which is located between the talus and navicular bone, and (2) the **calcaneocuboid joint**, which is located between the calcaneus and cuboid.

> **BOX 8-89**
> Of the two joints of the transverse tarsal joint, the talonavicular joint is much more mobile than the calcaneocuboid joint.

  - Both of these joints are synovial joints.
  - The talonavicular joint shares its joint capsule with one of the joint capsules of the subtalar joint.
  - The calcaneocuboid joint has its own distinct joint capsule.
  - The transverse tarsal joint is also known as the *midtarsal* or **Chopart's joint**.

Major Motions Allowed:

- Once the subtalar tarsal joint is understood, it is possible to simplify the discussion of the transverse tarsal joint.
- The motions possible at the transverse tarsal joint are pronation and supination (which can be divided into their component cardinal plane actions as explained in Section 8.19).
- Any motion at the subtalar joint requires motion to occur at the transverse tarsal joint as well.
- In fact, the named motions that occur at the subtalar joint are the same named motions that occur at the transverse tarsal joint.
- The interrelationship between the subtalar and transverse tarsal joints can be understood by looking at the bones involved in each of these joints. The talus of the subtalar joint is also part of the talonavicular joint of the transverse tarsal joint; the calcaneus of the subtalar joint is also part of the calcaneocuboid joint of the transverse tarsal joint. Therefore movement of either the talus or the calcaneus requires movement at the transverse tarsal joint when these more distal navicular and cuboid bones are fixed in a weight-bearing foot.
- In addition, recall that the subtalar joint has two joint capsules; of these, the anterior one is shared with the talonavicular joint of the transverse tarsal joint.

> **BOX 8-90**
> Because the talus shares a joint capsule with both the calcaneus and the navicular bone, and because motions of the subtalar and transverse tarsal joints are so intimately linked, some sources like to describe foot motion as occurring at the **talocalcaneonavicular (TCN) joint complex**. Indeed, given the interrelationship of the cuboid of the transverse tarsal joint as well, one could describe foot motion as occurring at the **talocalcaneonaviculocuboid (TCNC) joint complex**!

Ligaments of the Transverse Tarsal Joint:

- A number of ligaments help to stabilize the transverse tarsal joint. By virtue of stabilizing the transverse tarsal joint, these ligaments also help to indirectly limit motion and thereby stabilize the subtalar joint. Ligaments of the transverse tarsal joint include the following:

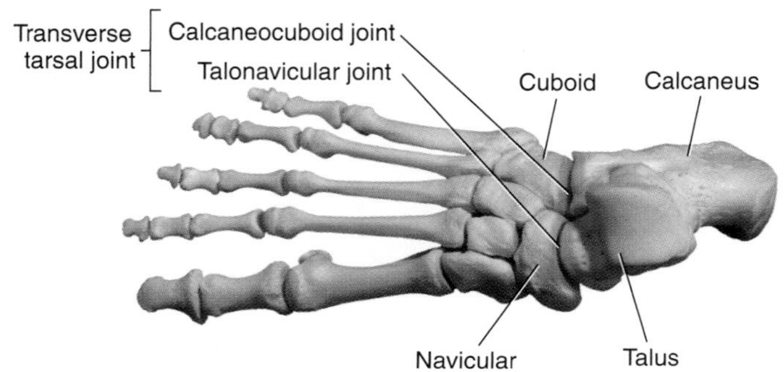

Figure 8-41 Dorsal view of the foot illustrating the transverse tarsal joint. The transverse tarsal joint is actually a joint complex composed of the talonavicular joint and the calcaneocuboid joint.

- **The spring ligament**: The spring ligament (covered in Section 8.19) literally forms the floor of the talonavicular joint (of the transverse tarsal joint) (see Figure 8-36a-b).
  - The spring ligament is also known as the **plantar calcaneonavicular ligament**.
- **The long plantar ligament**: This ligament runs the length of the foot on the plantar side (see Figure 8-36,a-b and e).
- **The short plantar ligament**: This ligament runs deep to the long plantar ligament on the plantar side of the foot between the calcaneus and the cuboid (see Figure 8-36a-b and e).
  - The short plantar ligament is also known as the **plantar calcaneocuboid ligament**.
- **The dorsal calcaneocuboid ligament**: This ligament is located between the calcaneus and cuboid on the dorsal side (see Figure 8-36b).
- **The bifurcate ligament**: This *Y*-shaped ligament is located on the dorsal side of the foot (see Figure 8-36b).
  - Its medial band attaches from the calcaneus to the navicular bone. Its lateral band attaches from the calcaneus to the cuboid.
  - The medial band is also known as the lateral **calcaneonavicular ligament**.
  - The lateral band is also known as the **calcaneocuboid ligament**.

BOX 8-91

LIGAMENTS OF THE TRANSVERSE TARSAL JOINT

- Fibrous joint capsule(s)
- Spring ligament
- Long plantar ligament
- Short plantar ligament
- Dorsal calcaneocuboid ligament
- Bifurcate ligament
  - Calcaneonavicular ligament
  - Calcaneocuboid ligament

Closed-Packed Position of the Transverse Tarsal Joint:

- Supination

8.21 TARSOMETATARSAL JOINTS

Bones:

- The tarsometatarsal (TMT) joints are located between the distal row of tarsal bones and the metatarsal bones.
- Five TMT joints exist (Figure 8-42):
  1. The 1st TMT joint is located between the 1st cuneiform and the base of the 1st metatarsal.
  2. The 2nd TMT joint is located between the 2nd cuneiform and the base of the 2nd metatarsal.
  3. The 3rd TMT joint is located between the 3rd cuneiform and the base of the 3rd metatarsal.
  4. The 4th TMT joint is located between the cuboid and the base of the 4th metatarsal.
  5. The 5th TMT joint is located between the cuboid and the base of the 5th metatarsal.
- Each metatarsal and its associated phalanges make up a ray of the foot.
- The TMT joints are plane synovial joints.
- Only the 1st TMT joint has a well-developed joint capsule.
- The 2nd and 3rd TMT joints share a joint capsule.
- The 4th and 5th TMT joints share a joint capsule.
  - The base of the 2nd metatarsal is set back further posteriorly than the other metatarsal bones, causing it to be wedged between the 1st and 3rd cuneiforms.
  - This position of the 2nd metatarsal decreases mobility of the 2nd TMT joint. Therefore the 2nd TMT joint is the most stable of the five TMT joints.
  - As a result, the 2nd ray of the foot is the **central stable pillar** of the foot.

BOX 8-92

Because the 2nd ray of the foot is the most stable of the five rays, an imaginary line through it is the reference line for abduction and adduction of the toes. In the hand, the 3rd ray is the most stable and is the reference line for abduction and adduction of the fingers.

- The more peripheral rays are the most mobile.
  - The 1st ray is the most mobile, followed by the 5th, 4th, 3rd, and 2nd rays (in that order).

Major Motions Allowed:

- The TMT joints allow dorsiflexion/plantarflexion and inversion/eversion.
  - Dorsiflexion occurs when the distal end of the metatarsal moves dorsally; plantarflexion is the opposite motion.
  - Inversion occurs when the plantar side of the ray turns inward (i.e., medially) toward the midline of the body; eversion is the opposite action.
- These motions of the metatarsal bones at the TMT joints are important toward allowing the foot to conform to the uneven surfaces of the ground on which we stand and walk.

BOX 8-93

When the metatarsals dorsiflex, the 1st ray inverts and the 3rd to 5th rays evert, and the foot flattens to meet the ground. When the metatarsals plantarflex, the 1st ray everts and the 3rd to 5th rays invert, and the arch contour of the foot raises, allowing the foot to mold around a raised surface.

- In addition to the fibrous joint capsules, the TMT joints are stabilized by **TMT ligaments** (see Figure 8-36a-b and e).
  - Dorsal, plantar, and interosseus TMT ligaments exist.

BOX 8-94

LIGAMENTS OF THE TARSOMETATARSAL LIGAMENTS

- Fibrous joint capsule
- Tarsometatarsal (TMT) ligaments (dorsal, plantar, and interosseus)

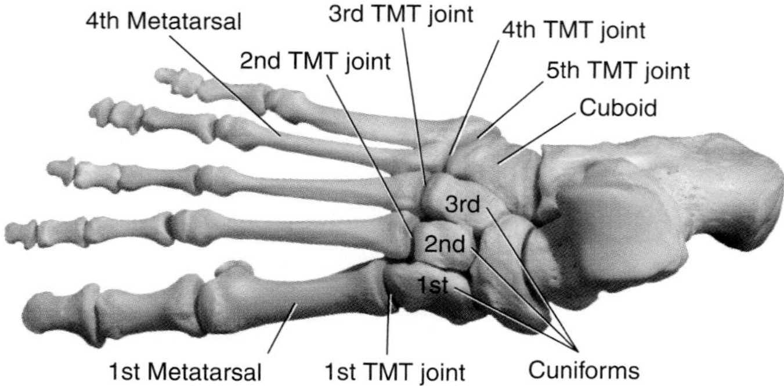

Figure 8-42 Dorsal view that illustrates the tarsometatarsal (TMT) joints of the foot. As the name indicates, TMT joints are located between the tarsal bones and the metatarsal bones. Five TMT joints are located between the three cuneiforms and cuboid proximally and the five metatarsal bones distally. The TMT joints are numbered from the medial to the lateral side of the foot as MTP joints #1-5.

8.22 INTERMETATARSAL (IMT) JOINTS

Bones and Ligaments:

- Intermetatarsal (IMT) joints are located between the metatarsal bones of the foot (Figure 8-43).
  - Proximal intermetatarsal joints and distal intermetatarsal joints exist.
  - All five metatarsal bones articulate with each other, both proximally at their bases and distally at their heads.

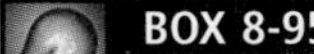

BOX 8-95

The proximal intermetatarsal joint between the big toe and the 2nd toe is not usually well formed. Although ligaments are present, the joint cavity is not usually fully formed.

- The proximal intermetatarsal joints are stabilized by their fibrous joint capsules and **intermetatarsal ligaments** (see Figures 8-36b, and 8-43b).
  - Dorsal, plantar, and interosseus intermetatarsal ligaments connect the base of each metatarsal to the base of the adjacent metatarsal(s).

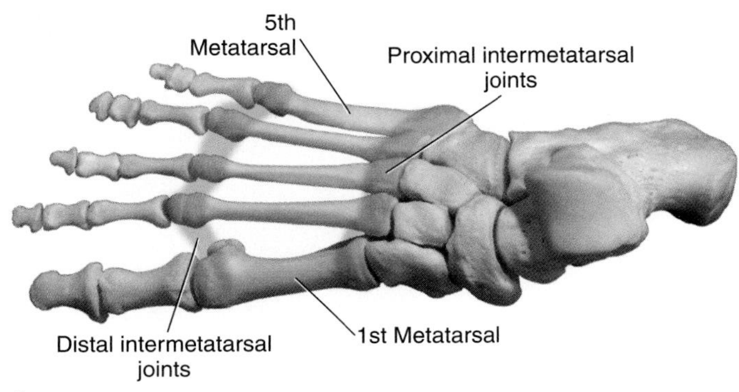

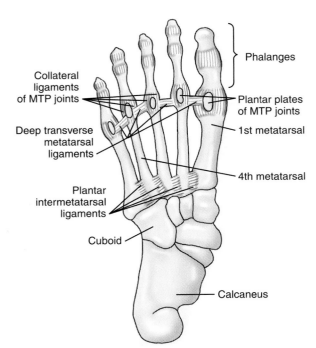

Figure 8-43 Intermetatarsal joints of the foot (i.e., proximal and distal intermetatarsal joints). As the name indicates, intermetatarsal joints are located between metatarsal bones. *A,* Dorsal view. *B,* Plantar view illustrates the ligaments of the plantar surface of the forefoot. The plantar intermetatarsal ligaments of the proximal intermetatarsal joints and the deep transverse metatarsal ligaments of the distal intermetatarsal joints are illustrated and labeled. (Note: The plantar plates and collateral ligaments of the metatarsophalangeal [MTP] joints are also illustrated and labeled.)

- The distal intermetatarsal joints are stabilized by their joint capsules and **deep transverse metatarsal ligaments** (see Figure 8-43b).

BOX 8-96

The deep transverse metatarsal ligaments that connect the distal ends of the metatarsals to each other hold the big toe in the same plane as the other toes; therefore the big toe cannot be opposed. In the hand, the deep transverse metacarpal ligaments connect only the index through little fingers, leaving the thumb free to be opposable. Therefore the foot is designed primarily for weight bearing and propulsion, whereas the hand is designed primarily for manipulation (i.e., fine motion). In theory, the only difference between the potential coordination of the hand and the foot is the ability to oppose digits.

BOX 8-97

LIGAMENTS OF THE INTERMETATARSAL JOINTS

- Fibrous joint capsules
- Intermetatarsal ligaments (dorsal, plantar, and interosseus)
- Deep transverse metatarsal ligaments

Major Motions Allowed:

- These intermetatarsal joints are plane synovial articulations that allow nonaxial gliding motion of one metatarsal relative to the adjacent metatarsal(s).
- Because motion at a TMT joint requires the metatarsal bone to move relative to the adjacent metatarsal bone(s), intermetatarsal joints are functionally related to TMT joints.

☐ 8.23 METATARSOPHALANGEAL JOINTS

Bones:

- ❑ The MTP joints are located between the metatarsals and the phalanges of the toes.
- ❑ More specifically, they are located between the heads of the metatarsals and the bases of the proximal phalanges of the toes.
- ❑ Five MTP joints exist (Figure 8-44):
    1. The 1st MTP joint is located between the 1st metatarsal and the proximal phalanx of the big (1st) toe.
    2. The 2nd MTP joint is located between the 2nd metatarsal and the proximal phalanx of the 2nd toe.
    3. The 3rd MTP joint is located between the 3rd metatarsal and the proximal phalanx of the 3rd toe.
    4. The 4th MTP joint is located between the 4th metatarsal and the proximal phalanx of the 4th toe.
    5. The 5th MTP joint is located between the 5th metatarsal and the proximal phalanx of the little (5th) toe.
- ❑ Joint structure classification: Synovial joint
    - ❑ Subtype: Condyloid
- ❑ Joint function classification: Diarthrotic
    - ❑ Subtype: Biaxial

Major Motions Allowed:

The average ranges of sagittal plane motion of the toes at the MTP joints are given in Table 8-7 (Figure 8-45).

BOX 8-98

The sagittal plane motions of flexion and extension of the toes at the metatarsophalangeal (MTP) joints is much more important than the actions of abduction and adduction of the toes at the MTP joints. Most people have very poor motor control of abduction and adduction of their toes.

- ❑ The MTP joint allows flexion and extension (i.e., axial movements) within the sagittal plane around a mediolateral axis.
- ❑ The MTP joint allows abduction and adduction (i.e., axial movements).

BOX 8-99

Normally, abduction and adduction movements occur within the frontal plane around an anteroposterior axis. However, because the foot is oriented perpendicular to the leg, abduction and adduction of the toes occur within the transverse plane around a vertical axis.

- ❑ The reference for abduction/adduction of the toes at the MTP joints is an imaginary line drawn through the 2nd toe when it is in anatomic position. Movement toward this imaginary line is adduction; movement away from this imaginary line is abduction.
    - ❑ Because frontal plane movement of the 2nd toe in either direction is away from this imaginary line, both directions of movement are termed *abduction*. Lateral movement of the 2nd toe is termed *fibular abduction*; medial movement of the 2nd toe is termed *tibial abduction*.

Reverse Actions:

- ❑ The muscles of the MTP joints are generally considered to move the more distal (proximal phalanx of the) toe relative to a fixed metatarsal bone. However, closed-chain activities are common in the lower extremity in which the foot is planted on the ground; this fixes the toes and requires that the metatarsals (and the entire foot) move relative to the toes instead. This reverse action of the MTP joints occurs every time that we "toe off" when we walk or run; our toes stay fixed on the ground and our foot hinges at the MTP joints instead, allowing the heel to rise off the ground.

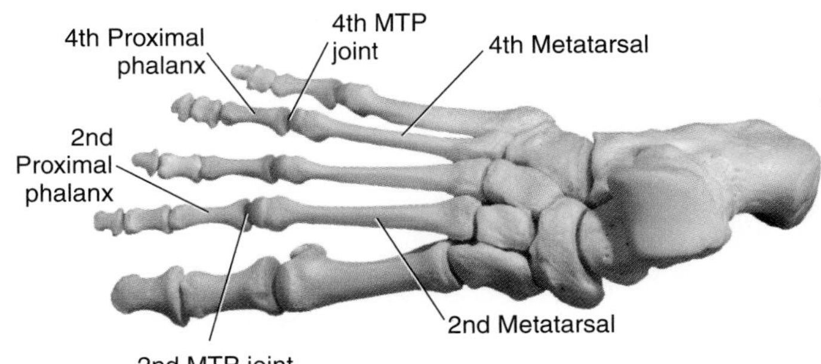

Figure 8-44 Dorsal view illustrating the metatarsophalangeal (MTP) joints of the foot. Five MTP joints are located between the metatarsals and the proximal phalanges of each ray of the foot. They are numbered from the medial (i.e., big toe) side to the lateral (i.e., little toe) side as MTP joints #1-5.

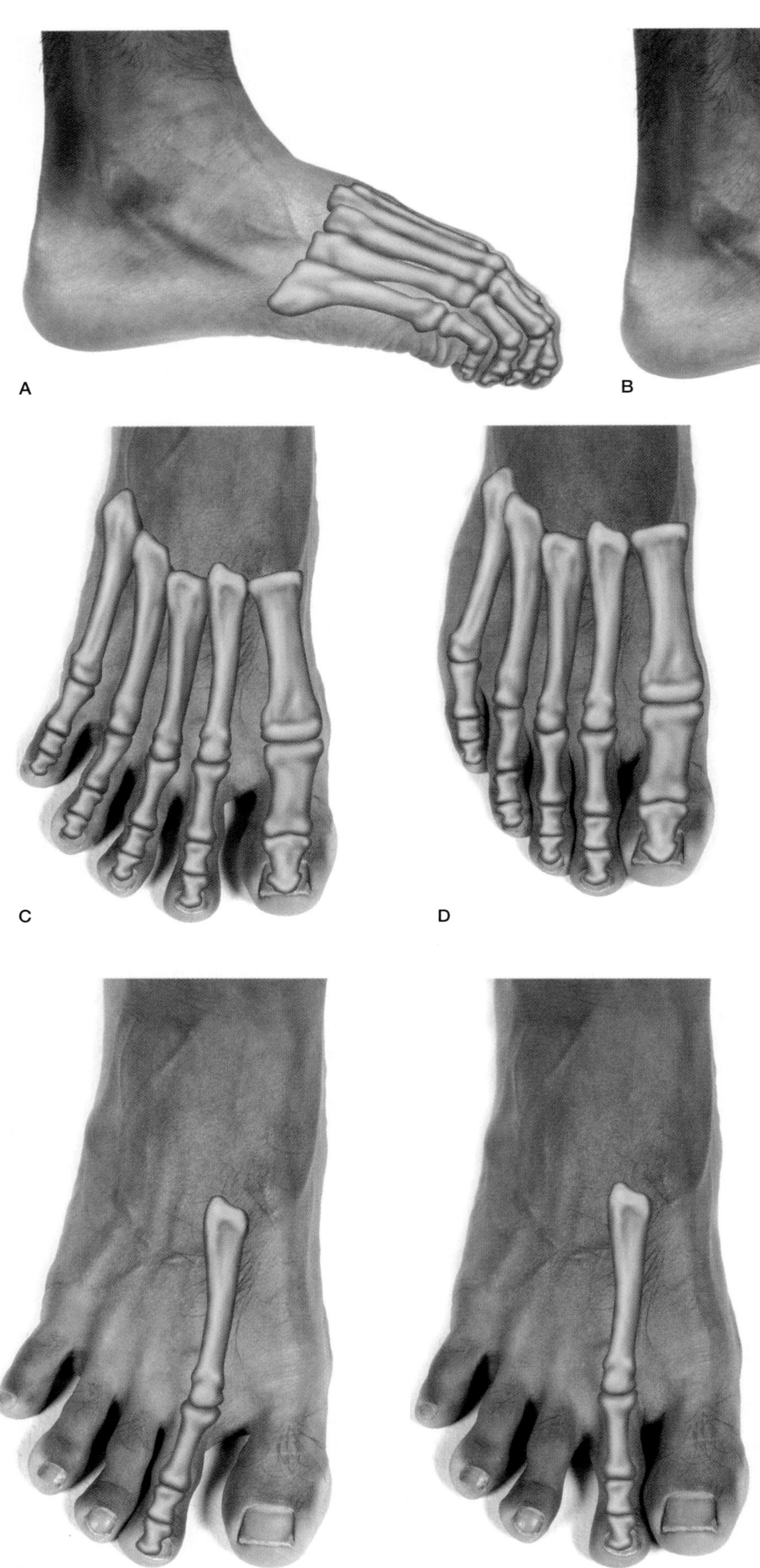

Figure 8-45 Motion of the toes at the metatarsophalangeal (MTP) joints. *A* and *B,* flexion and extension of the toes respectively (at both the MTP and interphalangeal [IP] joints). *C* and *D,* abduction and adduction of the toes at the MTP joints. The reference line for abduction and adduction of the toes is an imaginary line through the center of the 2nd toe when it is in anatomic position. Toes #1, 3, 4, and 5 abduct away from the 2nd toe and adduct toward it. The 2nd toe abducts in either direction it moves. *E,* Fibular abduction of the 2nd toe at the MTP. *F,* Tibial abduction of the 2nd toe at the MTP.

TABLE 8-7

Average Ranges of Sagittal Plane Motion of the Toes at the Metatarsophalangeal (MTP) Joints

Toes #2-5:			
Extension	60 Degrees	Flexion	40 Degrees
Big Toe (Toe #1):			
Extension	80 Degrees	Flexion	40 Degrees

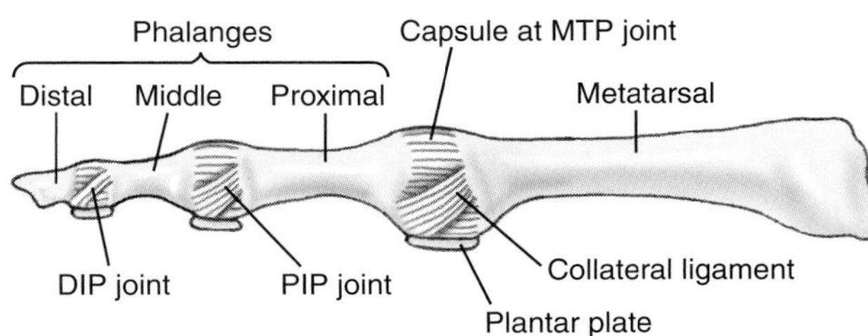

Figure 8-46 Fibrous capsule, collateral ligament, and plantar plate of the metatarsophalangeal (MTP) joint. (Note: These structures are also illustrated for the proximal interphalangeal [PIP] and distal interphalangeal [DIP] joints.)

Ligaments of the Metatarsophalangeal Joints:

Fibrous Joint Capsule:

❑ The capsule of the MTP joint is stabilized by collateral ligaments and the plantar plate (Figure 8-46).

Collateral Ligaments:

❑ The **medial collateral ligament** and the **lateral collateral ligament** are thickenings of the joint capsule and are located on their respective side of the MTP joint.

Plantar Plate:

❑ The **plantar plate** is a thick, dense, fibrous tissue structure located on the plantar side of the MTP joint.

❑ The plantar plate's main function is to protect the head of the metatarsal during walking.

  ❑ This is necessary because when the foot pushes off the ground, the metatarsal moves relative to the toe, exposing the articular surface of the head of the metatarsal to the ground. The plantar plate is placed between the head of the metatarsal and the ground.

BOX 8-100

LIGAMENTS OF THE METATARSOPHALANGEAL JOINT

- Fibrous joint capsule
- Medial collateral ligament
- Lateral collateral ligament
- Plantar plate

Closed-Packed Position of the Metatarsophalangeal Joint:

❑ Extension

Major Muscles of the Metatarsophalangeal Joint:

❑ The MTP joint is crossed by both extrinsic muscles (that originate on the leg) and intrinsic muscles (wholly located within the foot).

❑ Major flexors include the flexors digitorum and hallucis longus, the flexors digitorum and hallucis brevis, quadratus plantae, and flexor digiti minimi pedis, as well as the lumbricals pedis, plantar interossei, and the dorsal interossei pedis.

❑ Major extensors include the extensors digitorum and hallucis longus and the extensors digitorum and hallucis brevis.

❑ Major adductors are the plantar interossei and the adductor hallucis.

❑ Major abductors are the dorsal interossei pedis, as well as the abductor hallucis and abductor digiti minimi pedis.

Miscellaneous:

❑ The MTP joints are analogous to the metacarpophalangeal (MCP) joints of the hands. However, most

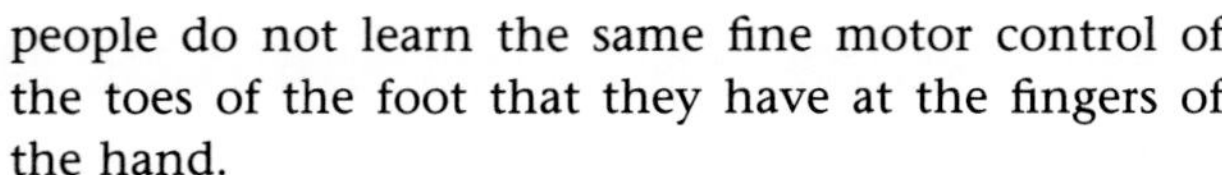

people do not learn the same fine motor control of the toes of the foot that they have at the fingers of the hand.

- **Hallux valgus** is a deformity of the big toe in which the big toe (i.e., the hallux) deviates laterally (in the valgus direction) at the MTP joint.
  - Hallux valgus also often involves a medial deviation of the 1st metatarsal.
  - The deformity of hallux valgus exposes the head of the 1st metatarsal to greater stress resulting in inflammation of the bursa located there. In time this leads to fibrosis and excessive bone growth on the medial (and perhaps dorsal) side of the 1st metatarsal's head; this is called a **bunion**.

BOX 8-101

Hallux valgus, which is a lateral deviation of the big toe of the foot, may be genetically predisposed to occur in certain individuals. However, overly pronated feet and incorrect footwear (high heels and/or shoes with a triangular front [i.e., toe box] that pushes the big toe laterally) seem certain to cause and/or accelerate this condition!

☐ 8.24 INTERPHALANGEAL JOINTS OF THE FOOT

- Interphalangeal (IP) joints pedis (i.e., of the foot) are located between phalanges of the toes (Figure 8-47).
  - More specifically, each IP joint is located between the head of the more proximal phalanx and the base of the more distal phalanx.

BOX 8-102

Interphalangeal (IP) joints are found in both the foot and the hand. To distinguish these joints from each other, the words pedis (denoting *foot*) and *manus* (denoting *hand*) are used.

- The big toe has one IP joint. It is located between the proximal and distal phalanges of the big toe.
- Because toes #2-5 each have three phalanges, two IP joints are found in each of these toes.
  - The IP joint located between the proximal and middle phalanges is called the *PIP joint* (pedis).
  - The IP joint located between the middle and distal phalanges is called the *DIP joint* (pedis).
  - In total, nine IP joints are found in the foot (one IP, four PIPs, and four DIPs).

BOX 8-103

When motion occurs at an interphalangeal (IP) joint of the foot, we can say that a toe has moved at the proximal or distal interphalangeal (DIP) joint. To be more specific, we could say that the distal phalanx moved at the DIP joint and/or that the middle phalanx moved at the proximal interphalangeal (PIP) joint.

- Joint structure classification: Synovial joint
  - Subtype: Hinge
- Joint function classification: Diarthrotic
  - Subtype: Uniaxial

Major Motions Allowed:

The average ranges of motion of the toes at the IP joints are given in Box 8-104 (see Figure 8-45 in Section 8.23).

BOX 8-104

AVERAGE RANGES OF MOTION OF THE INTERPHALANGEAL (IP) JOINTS

Proximal Interphalangeal (PIP) Joints
- From a neutral position, flexion of the proximal interphalangeal (PIP) joints (and the IP joint of the big toe) is limited to approximately 90 degrees and tends to be less in the more lateral toes.
- From a neutral position, the PIP joints (and the IP joint of the big toe) do not allow any further extension.

Distal Interphalangeal (DIP) Joints
- From a neutral position, flexion of the distal interphalangeal (DIP) joints is limited to approximately 45 degrees and tends to be less in the more lateral toes.
- From a neutral position, the DIP joints do allow a small amount of further extension (i.e., hyperextension).

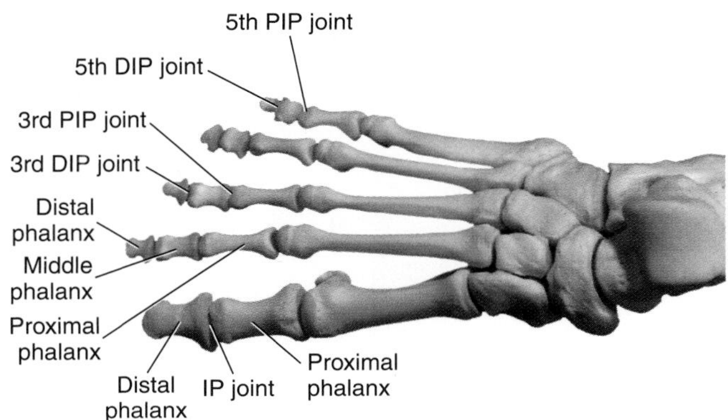

Figure 8-47 Dorsal view that illustrates the interphalangeal (IP) joints of the foot. Except for the big toe, which has only one IP joint, each toe has two IP joints: (1) the proximal interphalangeal (PIP) joint and (2) the distal interphalangeal (DIP) joint. Further the IP joints are numbered 1 to 5 from the medial (i.e., big toe) side to the lateral (i.e., little toe) side. (Note: In this photo, the 5th DIP joint [of the little toe] has fused.)

- ❑ The IP joints allow flexion and extension (i.e., axial movements) within the sagittal plane around a mediolateral axis.

Reverse Actions:

- ❑ The muscles of the IP joints are generally considered to move the more distal phalanx of a toe relative to the more proximal one. However, it is possible to move the more proximal one relative to the more distal one.

Ligaments of the Interphalangeal Joints of the Foot:

As in the MTP joints, each IP joint has a capsule that is thickened and stabilized by medial and lateral collateral ligaments; plantar plates are also present. These structures are usually not as well developed as they are in the MTP joints (see Figure 8-46).

- ❑ **Fibrous capsule**
- ❑ **Medial collateral ligament**
- ❑ **Lateral collateral ligament**
- ❑ **Plantar plate**.

BOX 8-105

LIGAMENTS OF THE INTERPHALANGEAL JOINTS

- Fibrous capsules
- Medial collateral ligaments
- Lateral collateral ligaments
- Plantar plates

Closed-Packed Position of the Interphalangeal Joints of the Foot:

- ❑ Extension

Major Muscles of the Interphalangeal Joints:

- ❑ The IP joints are crossed by both extrinsic and intrinsic muscles of the foot.
- ❑ Major flexors include the flexors digitorum and hallucis longus and the flexor digitorum brevis, as well as the quadratus plantae.
- ❑ Major extensors include the extensors digitorum and hallucis longus, the extensor digitorum brevis, and the lumbricals pedis, plantar interossei, and the dorsal interossei pedis. (Some of the aforementioned muscles do not cross the DIP joint.)

Miscellaneous:

- ❑ Other than the fact that toes are quite a bit shorter than fingers, the IP joints of the foot are analogous to the IP joints of the hand. However, most people do not learn the same fine motor control of the toes of the foot that they have at the fingers of the hand.

REVIEW QUESTIONS

evolve The answers to the following review questions are available on the Evolve site that accompanies this book.

1. When intrapelvic motion occurs, at what joint(s) does it occur?

2. When motion of the pelvis occurs relative to an adjacent body part, this motion occurs at what joint(s)?

3. What name is given to the motion of the sacrum wherein the sacral base drops anteriorly and inferiorly?

4. What are the names given to the transverse plane motions of the pelvis at the lumbosacral joint?

5. What are the names given to the sagittal plane motions of the pelvis at the hip joint?

6. A muscle that can do lateral flexion of the trunk at the lumbosacral joint can do what action of the pelvis at the lumbosacral joint?

7. A muscle that can do lateral rotation of the thigh at the hip joint can do what action of the pelvis at the hip joint?

8. What effect does an excessively anteriorly tilted pelvis usually have on the lumbar spine?

9. What are the three major ligaments that stabilize the hip joint?

10. Why are closed-chain activities more common in the lower extremities? What effect does this have on the actions of muscles?

11. What are the two major angulations of the femur?

12. According to the usual coordination of femoropelvic rhythm, which pelvic action accompanies flexion of the thigh at the hip joint?

13. What joint actions are possible at the tibiofemoral joint?

14. What motions are limited by the medial and lateral collateral ligaments of the knee joint?

15. What is the major purpose of the patella?

16. What is abduction of the tibia (in the frontal plane) relative to the femur called?

17. What does the Q-angle of the knee joint measure?

18. Name the three tibiofemoral joints.

19. What defines a ray of the foot?

20. Name the three arches of the foot.

21. What is the function of the retinacula of the ankle joint?

22. What is the name of the ankle joint ligament that limits eversion?

23. What two oblique plane motions are allowed at the subtalar joint?

24. To what two bones does the spring ligament of the foot attach?

____

____

25. The transverse tarsal joint is composed of what two joints?

____

____

26. What two bones articulate at the 4th TMT joint?

____

____

27. Which ray is the central stable pillar of the foot?

____

____

28. Name the two ligaments that stabilize the intermetatarsal joints?

____

____

____

____

29. What position of the MTP joint increases the height of the arch and the rigidity of the foot (via the windlass mechanism)?

____

____

____

____

30. Where are plantar plates of the foot located?

____

____

____

Chapter 9

Joints of the Upper Extremity

CHAPTER OUTLINE

CHAPTER OBJECTIVES

After completing this chapter, the student should be able to perform the following:

❑ Explain why the term *shoulder joint complex* is a better term than *shoulder joint*, when describing movement of the shoulder.
❑ Describe why the term *shoulder corset* might be a better term than *shoulder girdle*.
❑ Describe the concepts of mobility and stability as they pertain to the glenohumeral joint, and explain why the glenohumeral joint is often called a *muscular joint*.
❑ Explain why the scapulocostal joint is considered to be a functional joint, not an anatomic joint.
❑ Explain why stabilization of the sternoclavicular joint is important toward proper functioning of the upper extremity.
❑ Describe why the sternoclavicular joint can be classified as either *biaxial* or *triaxial*.
❑ Describe the importance of acromioclavicular joint motion to motion of the shoulder girdle.
❑ Explain the concept of scapulohumeral rhythm, and give an example for each of the six cardinal ranges of motion of the arm at the shoulder joint.
❑ Describe the concept and importance of the carrying angle.
❑ Describe the component motions that occur at the proximal and distal radioulnar joints that create pronation and supination of the forearm.
❑ Describe the structure and function of the hand.
❑ Describe the structure and function of the wrist, and specifically, the carpal tunnel.
❑ Explain why the radiocarpal joint is the major articulation between the forearm and the carpus.
❑ Describe the importance of motion at the 4th and 5th carpometacarpal joints.
❑ Describe the importance of motion at the 1st carpometacarpal joint (i.e., saddle joint of the thumb).
❑ Describe the component actions of opposition and reposition of the thumb.
❑ Discuss the similarities and differences between the metacarpophalangeal joints and the interphalangeal joints.
❑ List the joints of the shoulder joint complex, the elbow joint complex, the wrist joint complex, and the hand.

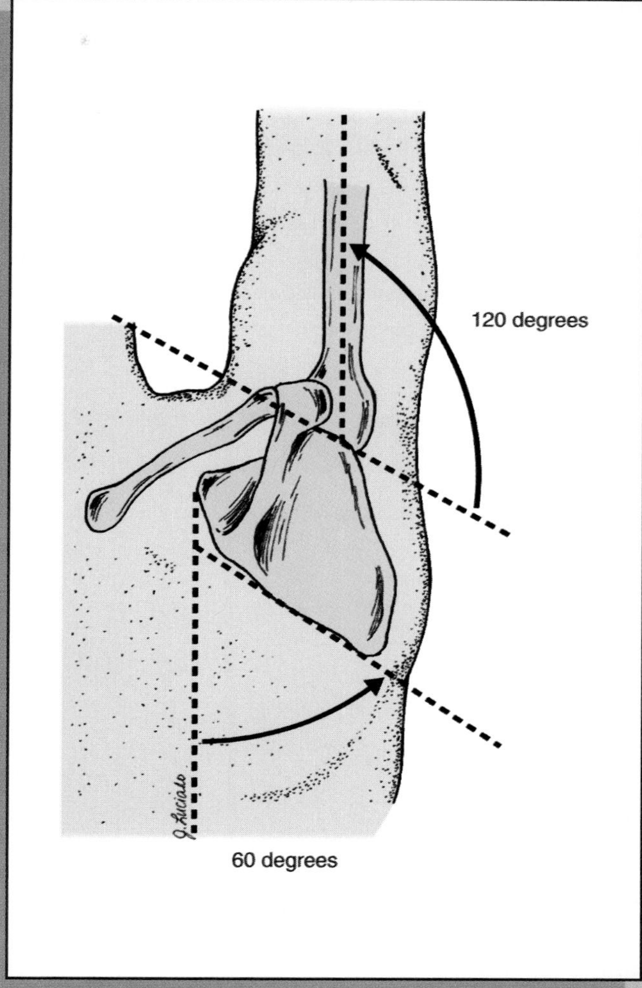

❑ Classify each joint covered in this chapter structurally and functionally.
❑ List the major ligaments and bursae of each joint covered in this chapter. Further, explain the major function of each ligament.
❑ State the closed-packed position of each joint covered in this chapter.
❑ List and describe the actions possible at each joint covered in this chapter.
❑ List and describe the reverse actions possible at each joint covered in this chapter.
❑ List the major muscles/muscle groups (and their joint actions) for each joint covered in this chapter.
❑ Define the key terms of this chapter.
❑ State the meanings of the word origins of this chapter.

OVERVIEW

While Chapters 5 and 6 laid the theoretical basis for the structure and function of joints, this chapter concludes our study of the regional approach of the structure and function of the joints of the body that began in chapters 7 and 8. This Chapter addresses the joints of the upper extremity. Whereas the lower extremity is primarily concerned with weight bearing and propulsion of the body through space, the major purpose of the upper extremity is to place the hand in desired positions, and move the hand as necessary to perform whatever tasks are required. Toward that end, the many joints of the upper extremity must work together to achieve these goals. Thus there is an intimate linkage between the joints of the shoulder complex, elbow/forearm, wrist, hand, and fingers. Sections 9.1 through 9.5 concern themselves with an examination of the joints of the shoulder joint complex; Section 9.6 then completes the study of the shoulder joint complex with an in-depth exploration of the concept of scapulohumeral rhythm. Sections 9.7 through 9.9 address the joints of the elbow complex and forearm joints. Sections 9.10 through 9.16 then complete our tour of the upper extremity by examining the joints of the wrist complex and hand.

KEY TERMS

Acromioclavicular joint (a-KROM-ee-o-kla-VIK-you-lar)
Acromioclavicular ligament
Anatomic joint (an-a-TOM-ik)
Annular ligament (AN-you-lar)
Anterior oblique ligament
Anterior sternoclavicular ligament (STERN-o-kla-VIK-you-lar)
Arches (of the hand)
Basilar arthritis (BAZE-i-lar)
Bone spurs
Carpal tunnel (CAR-pal)
Carpal tunnel syndrome
Carpometacarpal joints (CAR-po-MET-a-car-pal)
Carpometacarpal ligaments
Carpus (CAR-pus)
Carrying angle
Central pillar of the hand
Check-rein ligaments (CHEK-RAIN)
Conoid ligament (CONE-oyd)
Coracoacromial arch (kor-AK-o-a-KROM-ee-al)
Coracoacromial ligament
Coracoclavicular ligament (kor-AK-o-kla-VIK-you-lar)
Coracohumeral ligament (kor-AK-o-HUME-er-al)
Costoclavicular ligament (COST-o-kla-VIK-you-lar)
Coupled movement
Cubitus valgus (CUE-bi-tus VAL-gus)
Cubitus varus (VAR-us)
Deep transverse metacarpal ligaments (MET-a-CAR-pal)
Degenerative joint disease
Distal interphalangeal joint of the hand (IN-ter-FA-lan-GEE-al)
Distal radioulnar joint (RAY-dee-o-UL-nar)
Distal transverse arch
Dorsal carpometacarpal ligaments (CAR-po-MET-a-car-pal)
Dorsal digital expansion
Dorsal hood
Dorsal intercarpal ligament (IN-ter-CAR-pal)
Dorsal intermetacarpal ligaments (IN-ter-MET-a-CAR-pal)
Dorsal radiocarpal ligament (RAY-dee-o-CAR-pal)
Dorsal radioulnar ligament (RAY-dee-o-UL-nar)
Double-jointed
Extensor expansion
Extrinsic ligaments (of the wrist)
First (1st) intermetacarpal ligament (IN-ter-MET-a-CAR-pal)
Flexor retinaculum (of the wrist) (ret-i-NAK-you-lum)
Foramen of Weitbrecht (VITE-brecht)
Functional joint
Glenohumeral joint (GLEN-o-HUME-er-al)
Glenohumeral ligaments
Glenoid labrum (GLEN-oyd)
Golfer's elbow
Heberden's nodes (HE-ber-denz)
Humeroradial joint (HUME-er-o-RAY-dee-al)
Humeroulnar joint (HUME-er-o-UL-nar)
Inferior acromioclavicular ligament (a-KROM-ee-o-kla-VIK-you-lar)
Inferior glenohumeral ligament (GLEN-o-HUME-er-al)
Intercarpal joints (IN-ter-CAR-pal)
Interclavicular ligament (IN-ter-kla-VIK-you-lar)
Intermetacarpal joints (IN-ter-MET-a-CAR-pal)
Intermetacarpal ligaments
Interosseus carpometacarpal ligaments (IN-ter-OS-ee-us CAR-po-MET-a-CAR-pal)
Interosseus intermetacarpal ligaments (IN-ter-MET-a-CAR-pal)
Interosseus membrane (of the forearm) (IN-ter-OS-ee-us)
Interphalangeal joints (manus) (IN-ter-fa-lan-GEE-al)
Intertendinous connections (IN-ter-TEN-din-us)

Intrinsic ligaments (of the wrist)
Lateral collateral ligament (of the elbow joint)
Lateral epicondylitis (EP-ee-KON-di-LITE-us)
Longitudinal arch
Medial collateral ligament (of the elbow joint)
Medial epicondylitis (EP-ee-KON-di-LITE-us)
Metacarpal ligaments (MET-a-CAR-pal)
Metacarpophalangeal joints (MET-a-CAR-po-FA-lan-GEE-al)
Metacarpus (MET-a-CAR-pus)
Midcarpal joint (MID-CAR-pal)
Middle glenohumeral ligament (GLEN-o-HUME-er-al)
Middle radioulnar joint (RAY-dee-o-UL-nar)
Muscular joint
Oblique cord
Osteoarthritis (OST-ee-o-ar-THRI-tis)
Palm
Palmar carpometacarpal ligaments (CAR-po-MET-a-CAR-pal)
Palmar fascia (FASH-a)
Palmar intercarpal ligament (IN-ter-CAR-pal)
Palmar intermetacarpal ligaments (IN-ter-MET-a-CAR-pal)
Palmar plate
Palmar radiocarpal ligaments (RAY-dee-o-CAR-pal)
Palmar radioulnar ligament (RAY-dee-o-UL-nar)
Pectoral girdle (PEK-tor-al)
Posterior oblique ligament
Posterior sternoclavicular ligament (STERN-o-kla-VIK-you-lar)
Proximal interphalangeal joint (of the hand) (IN-ter-FA-lan-GEE-al)
Proximal radioulnar joint (RAY-dee-o-UL-nar)
Proximal transverse arch
Radial collateral ligament (of the elbow joint)
Radial collateral ligament (of the interphalangeal joints manus)
Radial collateral ligament (of the metacarpophalangeal joint)
Radial collateral ligament (of the thumb's saddle joint)
Radial collateral ligament (of the wrist joint)
Radiocapitate ligament (RAY-dee-o-KAP-i-tate)
Radiocapitular joint (RAY-dee-o-ka-PICH-you-lar)
Radiocarpal joint (RAY-dee-o-UL-nar)
Radiolunate ligament (RAY-dee-o-LOON-ate)
Radioscapholunate ligament (RAY-dee-o-SKAF-o-LOON-ate)
Radioulnar disc (RAY-dee-o-UL-nar)
Radioulnar joints
Ray
Rheumatoid arthritis (ROOM-a-toyd ar-THRI-tis)
Saddle joint (of the thumb)
Scapuloclaviculohumeral rhythm (SKAP-you-lo-kla-VIK-you-lo-HUME-er-al)
Scapulocostal joint (SKAP-you-lo-COST-al)
Scapulohumeral rhythm (SKAP-you-lo-HUME-er-al)
Scapulothoracic joint (SKAP-you-lo-thor-AS-ik)
Shoulder corset
Shoulder girdle
Shoulder joint complex
Sternoclavicular joint (STERN-o-kla-VIK-you-lar)
Sternoclavicular ligaments
Subacromial bursa (SUB-a-CHROME-ee-al)
Subdeltoid bursa (SUB-DELT-oyd)
Superior acromioclavicular ligament (a-KROM-ee-o-kla-VIK-you-lar)
Superior glenohumeral ligament (GLEN-o-HUME-er-al)
Tennis elbow
Transverse carpal ligament (CAR-pal)
Trapezoid ligament (TRAP-i-zoyd)
Triangular fibrocartilage (FI-bro-KAR-ti-lij)
Ulnar collateral ligament (of the elbow joint)
Ulnar collateral ligament (of the interphalangeal joints manus)
Ulnar collateral ligament (of the metacarpophalangeal joint)
Ulnar collateral ligament (of the thumb's saddle joint)
Ulnar collateral ligament (of the wrist joint)
Ulnocarpal complex (UL-no-CAR-pal)
Ulnocarpal joint
Ulnotrochlear joint (UL-no-TRO-klee-ar)
Volar plate (VO-lar)
Winging of the scapula
Wrist joint complex

WORD ORIGINS

Annular—From Latin *anulus,* meaning *ring*
Arthritis—From Greek *arthron,* meaning *a joint,* and *itis,* meaning *inflammation*
Carpus—From Greek *karpos,* meaning *wrist*
Cubitus—From Latin *cubitum,* meaning *elbow*
Digital—From Latin *digitus,* meaning *finger* (or *toe*)
Fore—From Old English *fore,* meaning *before, in front of*
Manus—From Latin *manus,* meaning *hand*
Osteoarthritis—From Greek *osteon,* meaning *bone,* and *itis,* meaning *inflammation*
Pollicis—From Latin *pollicis,* meaning *thumb*
Ray—From Latin *radius,* meaning *extending outward (radially) from a structure*
Rein—From Latin *retinere,* meaning *to restrain*
Rheumatoid—From Greek *rheuma,* meaning *discharge* or *flux,* and *eidos,* meaning *resembling, appearance*
Trochlea—From Latin *trochlea,* meaning *pulley*

☐ 9.1 SHOULDER JOINT COMPLEX

- When the term *shoulder joint* is used, it is usually used to describe movement of the arm relative to the scapula at the glenohumeral (GH) joint.
- However, most every movement of the arm at the GH joint also requires a **coupled movement** of the **shoulder girdle** (i.e., the scapula and clavicle).

BOX 9-1 SPOTLIGHT ON THE SHOULDER GIRDLE

A girdle is an article of clothing that encircles and thereby holds in and stabilizes the abdomen. Similarly, the scapulae and clavicles (along with the manubrium of the sternum) are called the *shoulder girdle,* because they perform a similar function. They encircle the upper trunk and act as a stable base from which the upper extremity may move. However, the shoulder girdle shows a greater similarity to a corset than a girdle. Although a girdle completely encircles the body, a corset is open in back and requires lacing to truly encircle the body.

In this regard, the shoulder girdle is also open in back, because the two scapulae do not articulate with each other. In fact, the musculature (i.e., middle trapezius and rhomboids) that attaches the medial borders of the scapulae to the spine can be viewed as the lacing of a corset. For this reason, the term **shoulder corset** might be more appropriate! Further, just as the stability of a corset is dependent on the tension of the lacing, the stability of the *shoulder corset* is dependent on the strength and integrity of the musculature that laces the two scapulae together.

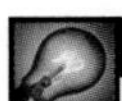

BOX 9-2

The shoulder girdle is also known as the **pectoral girdle**.

- The scapula and clavicle may move at the sternoclavicular (SC), acromioclavicular (AC), scapulocostal (ScC), and GH joints (Figure 9-1; Table 9-1).
- Because most movement patterns of the shoulder require motion to occur at a number of these joints, the term **shoulder joint complex** is a better term to employ when describing motion of the shoulder. From a "big picture" point of view, the sternoclavicular (SC) joint may be looked at as the master joint that orients the position of the scapula because motion of the clavicle at the SC joint results in motion of the scapula at

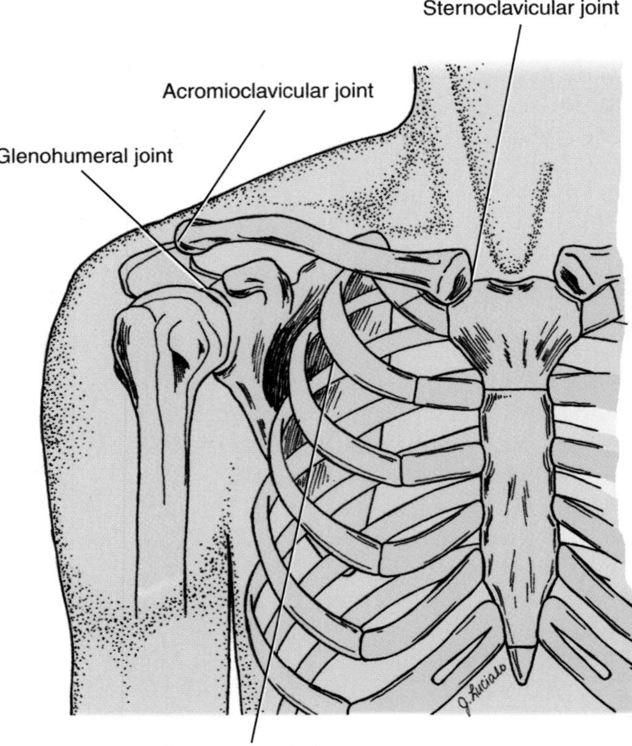

Figure 9-1 Anterior view illustrating the right shoulder joint complex. The shoulder joint complex is comprised of many joints. The glenohumeral (GH) joint, often referred to as the *shoulder joint,* is located between the head of the humerus and the glenoid fossa of the scapula. The scapulocostal (ScC) joint is located between the anterior surface of the scapula and the ribcage of the trunk. The acromioclavicular (AC) joint is located between the acromion process of the scapula and the lateral end of the clavicle; the sternoclavicular (SC) joint is located between the sternum and the medial end of the clavicle. (Courtesy Joseph E. Muscolino.)

TABLE 9-1

Average Ranges of Motion of the Entire Shoulder Joint Complex from Anatomic Position

Flexion	180 Degrees	Extension	150 Degrees
Abduction	180 Degrees	Adduction	0 Degrees*
Lateral rotation	90 Degrees	Medial rotation	90 Degrees

*Pure adduction from anatomic position is blocked because of the presence of the trunk. However, if the arm is first flexed or extended, further adduction is possible anterior or posterior to the trunk.

the scapulocostal joint. Fine tune adjustments and augmentation of scapular movement also occur at the acromioclavicular (AC) joint. The net result of SC and AC joint motion is to orient the scapula to the desired position. Position of the scapula is important to facilitate humeral motion at the glenohumeral joint. Thus, motion of the arm at the shoulder joint truly is dependent upon a complex of joints!

- This coupling of shoulder girdle movement with arm movement is called **scapulohumeral rhythm**. Given that motion of the clavicle is also required, perhaps a better term would be **scapuloclaviculohumeral rhythm**. (The concept of coupled movements [i.e., coupled actions] is addressed in Section 13.12. The coupled actions of the shoulder joint complex are described in detail in Section 9.6.)
- The shoulder girdle primarily moves as a unit. When this occurs, movement occurs between the clavicle of the shoulder girdle and the sternum at the SC joint, and between the scapula of the shoulder girdle and the ribcage at the ScC joint. Movement may also occur between the scapula of the shoulder girdle and the humerus at the GH joint.
- However, the scapula and clavicle of the shoulder girdle do not always move together as a fixed unit; the presence of the AC joint between these two bones allows for independent motion of the scapula and clavicle relative to each other within the shoulder girdle.

9.2 GLENOHUMERAL JOINT

- Generally when the context is not made otherwise clear, the term *shoulder joint* refers to the **glenohumeral (GH) joint.**

Bones:

- The GH joint is located between the scapula and the humerus.
  - More specifically, it is located between the glenoid fossa of the scapula and the head of the humerus.
- Joint Structure Classification: Synovial joint
  - Subtype: Ball-and-socket joint
- Joint Function Classification: Diarthrotic
  - Subtype: Triaxial

Major Motions Allowed:

- The GH joint allows flexion and extension (i.e., axial movements) in the sagittal plane around a mediolateral axis (Figure 9-2; Table 9-2).
- The GH joint allows abduction and adduction (i.e., axial movements) in the frontal plane around an anteroposterior axis (Figure 9-3; Box 9-3).

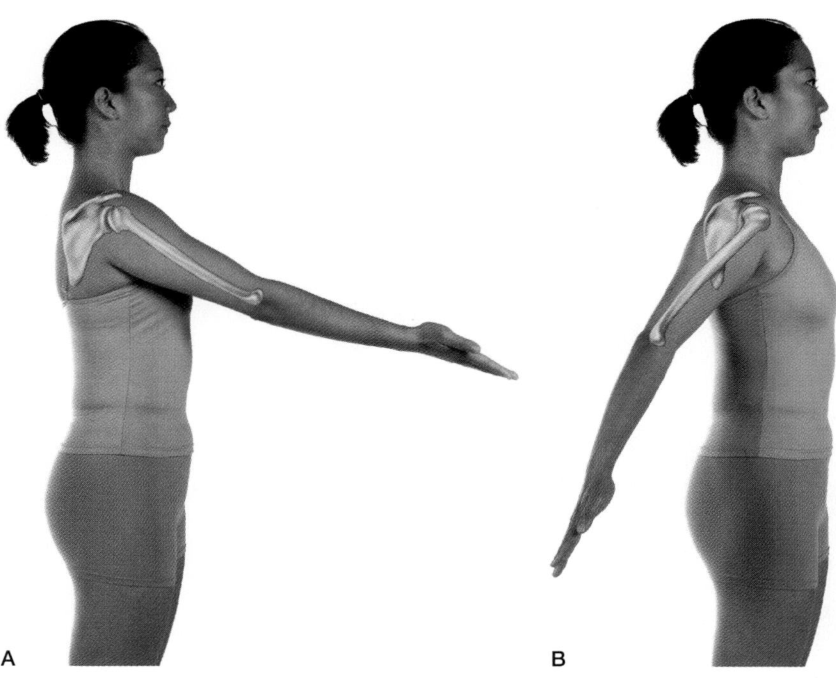

Figure 9-2 Sagittal plane actions of the arm at the shoulder joint. *A,* Flexion. *B,* Extension.

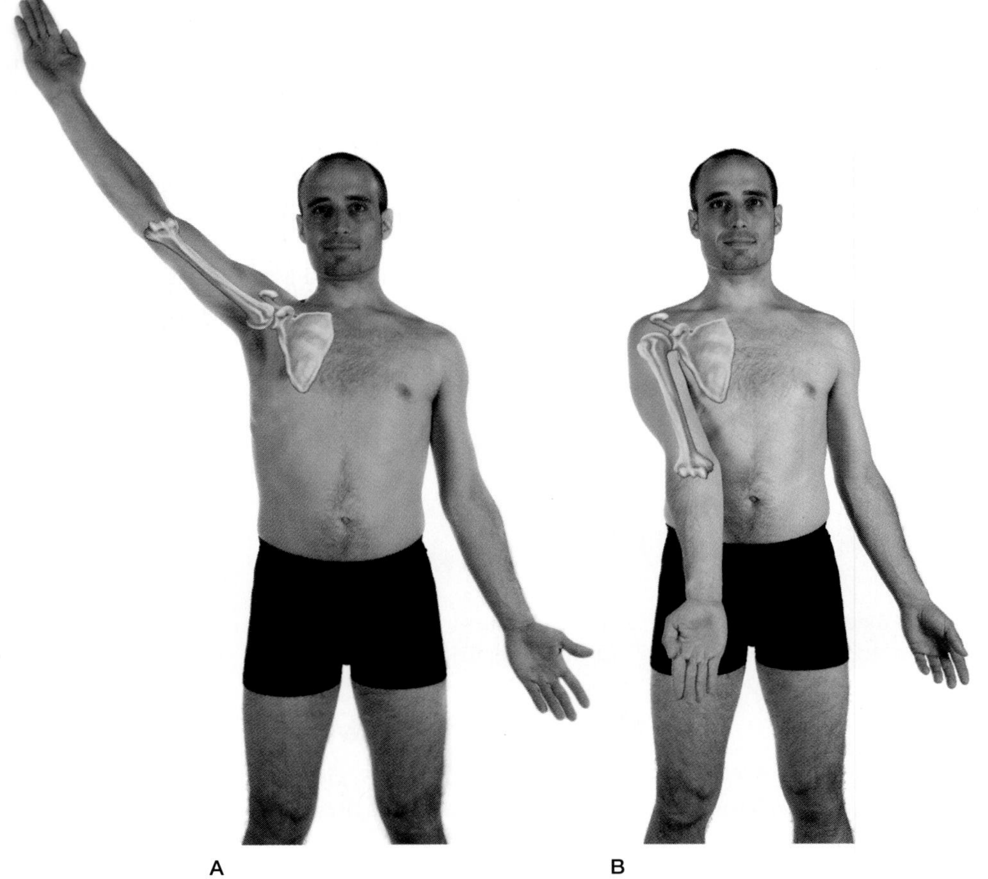

Figure 9-3 Frontal plane actions of the arm at the shoulder joint. *A,* Abduction. *B,* Adduction.

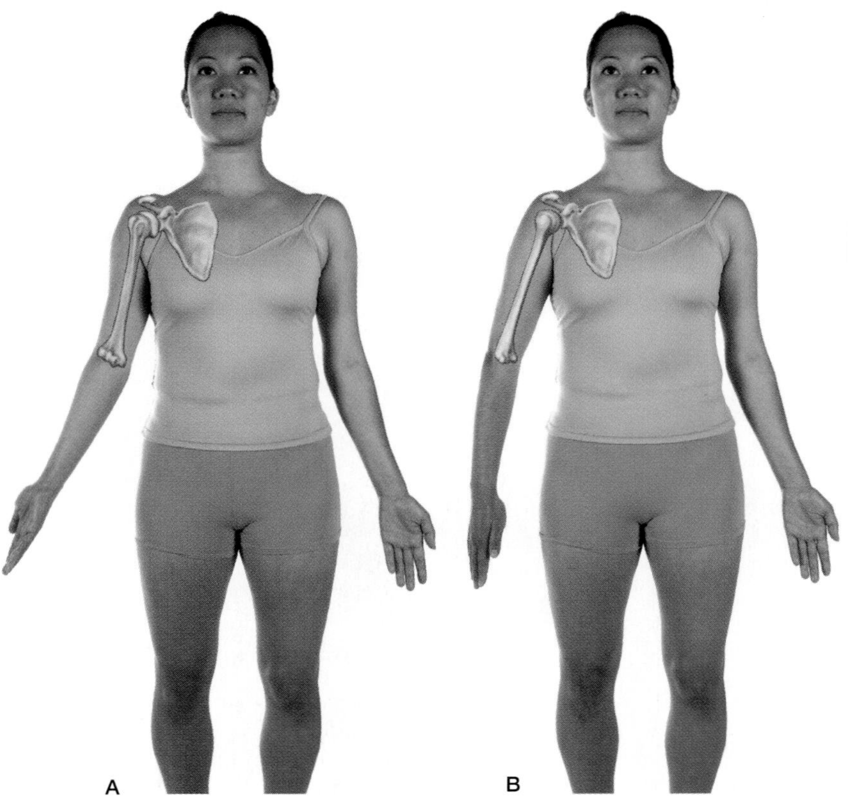

Figure 9-4 Transverse plane actions of the arm at the shoulder joint. *A,* Lateral rotation. *B,* Medial rotation.

TABLE 9-2

Average Ranges of Motion of the Arm at the Glenohumeral Joint from Anatomic Position

Flexion	100 Degrees	Extension	40 Degrees
Abduction	120 Degrees	Adduction	0 Degrees*
Lateral rotation	50 Degrees	Medial rotation	90 Degrees

*Pure adduction from anatomic position is blocked because of the presence of the trunk. However, if the arm is first flexed or extended, further adduction is possible anterior to or posterior to the trunk.

BOX 9-3

If the arm is in a neutral position or medially rotated, abduction of the arm at the glenohumeral (GH) joint will be restricted because the greater tubercle of the head of the humerus will bang into the acromion process above. If the arm is laterally rotated first, then abduction of the arm at the GH joint is much greater because the greater tubercle is moved out of the way of the acromion process.

- ❑ The GH joint allows lateral rotation and medial rotation (i.e., axial movements) in the transverse plane around a vertical axis (Figure 9-4).

Reverse Actions:

- ❑ The muscles of the GH joint are generally considered to move the more distal arm on the more proximal scapula. However, the scapula can move at the GH joint relative to the humerus; this is especially true if the arm is fixed such as when the hand is gripping an immovable object (i.e., during a closed-chain activity). (For an explanation of closed-chain activities, see Section 8.9.)
- ❑ The major reverse actions of the scapula at the GH joint are upward rotation and downward rotation.

BOX 9-4

An example of the reverse action of the scapula relative to the humerus at the glenohumeral (GH) joint occurs when the deltoid contracts to create abduction of the arm at the GH joint. If the scapula is not sufficiently stabilized (i.e., fixed), the pull of the deltoid's contraction can also create downward rotation of the scapula at the GH joint. (Note: When the reverse action of the scapula moving relative to the humerus at the GH joint occurs, the scapula may move relative to the ribcage as well. Therefore scapular actions at the GH joint can also be described as occurring at the scapulocostal [ScC] joint.)

Major Ligaments of the Glenohumeral Joint:

The GH joint has several major ligaments (Figures 9-5 and 9-6; Table 9-3):

BOX 9-5

LIGAMENTS OF THE GLENOHUMERAL JOINT

- Fibrous joint capsule
- Superior glenohumeral (GH) ligament
- Middle GH ligament
- Inferior GH ligament
- Coracohumeral ligament*

*The coracoacromial ligament is also involved with the GH joint.

Fibrous Joint Capsule:

- ❑ The capsule of the GH joint is extremely lax and permits a great deal of motion.

BOX 9-6

Note 1: The shoulder joint capsule is so lax that if the musculature of the shoulder joint is completely relaxed, the head of the humerus can be moved away (i.e., axially tractioned) from the glenoid fossa between 1 and 2 inches (2.5-5.0 cm).

Note 2: A small region of the anterior shoulder joint capsule called the **foramen of Weitbrecht** is located between the superior and middle glenohumeral (GH) ligaments. The foramen of Weitbrecht is a relatively weak region where the majority of shoulder dislocations occur.

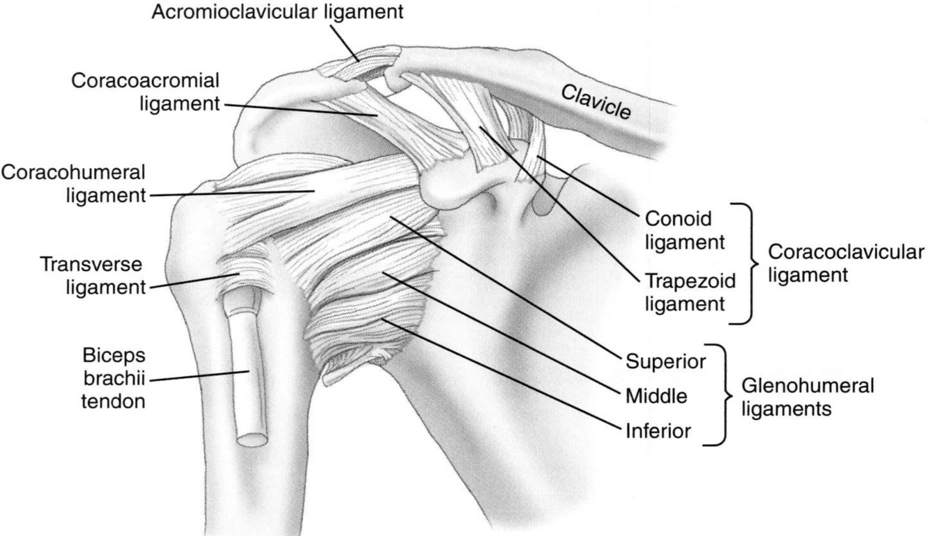

Figure 9-5 Anterior view of the ligaments that stabilize the right shoulder joint complex. The superior, middle, and inferior glenohumeral (GH) ligaments are thickenings of the anterior and inferior GH joint capsule. The coracohumeral ligament runs from the coracoid process of the scapula to the greater tubercle of the humerus. The coracoclavicular ligament runs from the coracoid process to the lateral clavicle; the coracoacromial ligament runs from the coracoid process to the acromion process; and the acromioclavicular (AC) ligament runs from the acromion process to the lateral clavicle. (Note: The transverse ligament that holds the long head of the biceps brachii tendon in the bicipital groove is also seen.)

- The GH joint capsule is thickened and strengthened by **glenohumeral (GH) ligaments**.
- Three GH ligaments exist: (1) the **superior glenohumeral ligament**, (2) the **middle glenohumeral ligament**, and (3) the **inferior glenohumeral ligament**.

Superior, Middle, and Inferior Glenohumeral Ligaments:

- These ligaments are thickenings of the anterior and inferior joint capsule (see Box 9-6, Note 2).
- Function: They prevent dislocation of the humeral head anteriorly and inferiorly.
- As a group, these three ligaments also limit the extremes of all GH joint motions.

Coracohumeral Ligament:

- Location: The coracohumeral ligament is located between the coracoid process of the scapula and the greater tubercle of the humerus.
- Function: It prevents dislocation of the humeral head anteriorly and inferiorly and limits extremes of flexion, extension, and lateral rotation.

Closed-Packed Position of the Glenohumeral Joint:

- Lateral rotation and abduction

Major Muscles of the Glenohumeral Joint:

- Flexors cross the GH joint anteriorly and are the anterior deltoid, pectoralis major, coracobrachialis, and biceps brachii.
- Extensors cross posteriorly and are the posterior deltoid, latissimus dorsi, teres major, and the long head of the triceps brachii.
- Abductors cross superiorly (over the top of the joint) and are the deltoid and supraspinatus.
- Adductors cross below the center of the joint from the trunk to the arm and are located both anteriorly and posteriorly. Some adductors are the pectoralis major, latissimus dorsi, and teres major.
- Lateral rotators such as the posterior deltoid, infraspinatus, and teres minor cross the GH joint and wrap around the humerus, ultimately attaching to the posterior side of the humerus.
- Medial rotators such as the anterior deltoid, latissimus dorsi, teres major, and subscapularis cross the GH joint and wrap around the humerus, ultimately attaching to the anterior side of the humerus.

Miscellaneous:

- A cartilaginous **glenoid labrum** forms a lip around the glenoid fossa (see Figure 9-6; Box 9-7, Note 1).

BOX 9-7

Note 1: The cartilaginous glenoid labrum is analogous to the acetabular labrum of the hip joint.

Note 2: The subacromial bursa is also known as the **subdeltoid bursa,** because it extends inferiorly and is also located between the deltoid muscle and the rotator cuff tendon. This bursa is the famous shoulder joint bursa that is so often blamed for soft tissue pain of the shoulder joint.

- ❑ The glenoid labrum deepens the glenoid fossa and cushions the joint.

❑ A bursa known as the **subacromial bursa** is located between the acromion process of the scapula and the rotator cuff tendon (see Figure 9-6b, and Box 9-7, Note 2).

- ❑ The subacromial bursa reduces friction between the rotator cuff tendon inferiorly and the acromion process and deltoid muscle superiorly.

BOX 9-8

Because the subacromial bursa actually adheres to the underlying rotator cuff tendon, irritation and injury to the rotator cuff tendon will usually result in irritation and injury to the subacromial bursa as well. Hence rotator cuff tendinitis and subacromial bursa problems usually occur together.

❑ The "roof" of the GH joint is formed by the **coracoacromial arch**.

- ❑ The coracoacromial arch is composed of the **coracoacromial ligament** and the acromion process of the scapula (see Figure 9-5; Box 9-9, Note 1).
- ❑ The coracoacromial arch functions to protect the superior structures of the GH joint (see Box 9-9, Note 2).

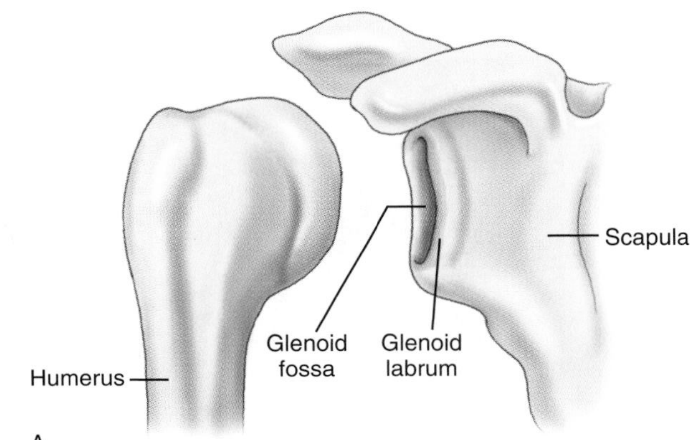

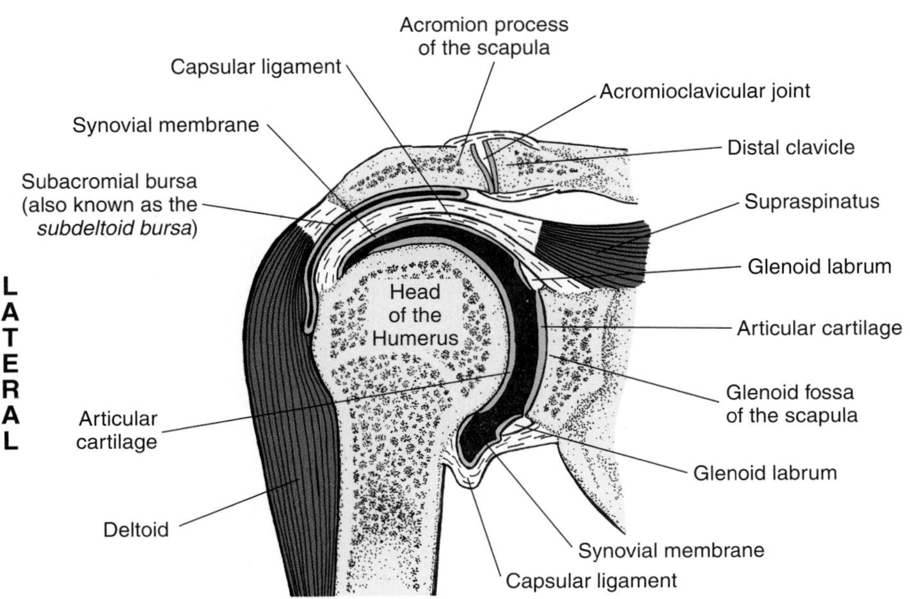

Figure 9-6 *A,* Anterior view of the right glenohumeral (GH) joint showing the glenoid labrum, which is a rim of cartilage that surrounds the glenoid fossa of the scapula. The glenoid labrum deepens and cushions the GH joint. *B,* Frontal (i.e., coronal) plane section through the GH joint. The subacromial bursa is visualized between the acromiom process of the scapula and the rotator cuff tendon of the supraspinatus muscle. (*B* from Muscolino JE: *The muscular system manual,* ed. 2. St Louis, 2005, Mosby.)

BOX 9-9

Note 1: The coracoacromial ligament is a bit unusual in that it attaches to two landmarks of the same bone—the coracoid process of the scapula to the acromion process of the scapula. Most often, musculoskeletal ligaments run from one bone to a different bone.

Note 2: Activities such as carrying a bag, purse, or laptop computer on the shoulder (let alone a traumatic fall on the top of the shoulder joint) might injure the superior structures of the glenohumeral (GH) joint if it were not for the protection of the coracoacromial arch. Ironically though, the superior structures of the GH joint (supraspinatus muscle and tendon, subacromial bursa, long head of the biceps brachii, and the superior aspect of the GH joint capsule) can become impinged as a result of being pinched between the head of the humerus and the coracoacromial arch; this often occurs with greater degrees of abduction and flexion of the arm at the shoulder joint. Therefore the presence of the coracoacromial arch can prove to be both a benefit and a problem.

- The long head of the biceps brachii is intra-articular (i.e., it runs through the joint cavity of the shoulder joint from the bicipital groove of the humerus to the supraglenoid tubercle of the scapula).
- The GH joint is the most mobile (and therefore the least stable) joint of the human body. This great mobility is due to the shallow nature of the glenoid fossa and the tremendous laxity of the joint capsule.
- The majority of stability this joint does have is provided by musculature, primarily the rotator cuff group of muscles.

BOX 9-10

Because the majority of the stability that the glenohumeral (GH) joint has is derived from musculature, the GH joint is often referred to as a **muscular joint**.

9.3 SCAPULOCOSTAL JOINT

- The **scapulocostal (ScC) joint** is also known as the **scapulothoracic joint**.

Bones:

- The scapula and the ribcage (Figure 9-7)
  - More specifically, the anterior surface of the scapula and the posterior surface of the ribcage
- In standing and seated positions, the scapula usually sits on the ribcage at the levels of the 2nd through 7th ribs. However, when a client is lying prone and the arms are hanging off the table, the location of the scapula relative to the ribcage changes as the scapula protracts and upwardly rotates.
- Joint type: Functional joint
  - The ScC joint is unusual in that it is not an **anatomic joint** because no actual union of the scapula and the ribcage is formed by connective tissue. (For a discussion of the anatomic structure of joints, see Section 6.1.) However, because it behaves like a joint in that movement of the scapula relative to the ribcage occurs, it is considered to be a **functional joint**.

Major Motions Allowed:

Major motions allowed are as follows (Figures 9-8 to 9-10; Table 9-3; Boxes 9-11 and 9-12):

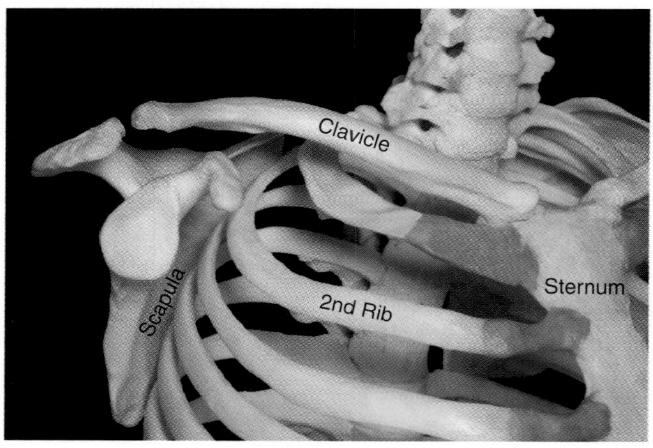

Figure 9-7 Anterolateral view of the upper trunk illustrating the right scapulocostal (ScC) joint located between the anterior (i.e., ventral) surface of the scapula and the posterior surface of the ribcage.

BOX 9-11

Of all the scapular actions possible, only elevation/depression and protraction/retraction can be primary movements, meaning that each one of these movements can be created separately by itself. The other scapular actions are secondary in that they must occur secondary to an action of the arm at the glenohumeral (GH) joint. (See Section 9.6 for more on this topic.)

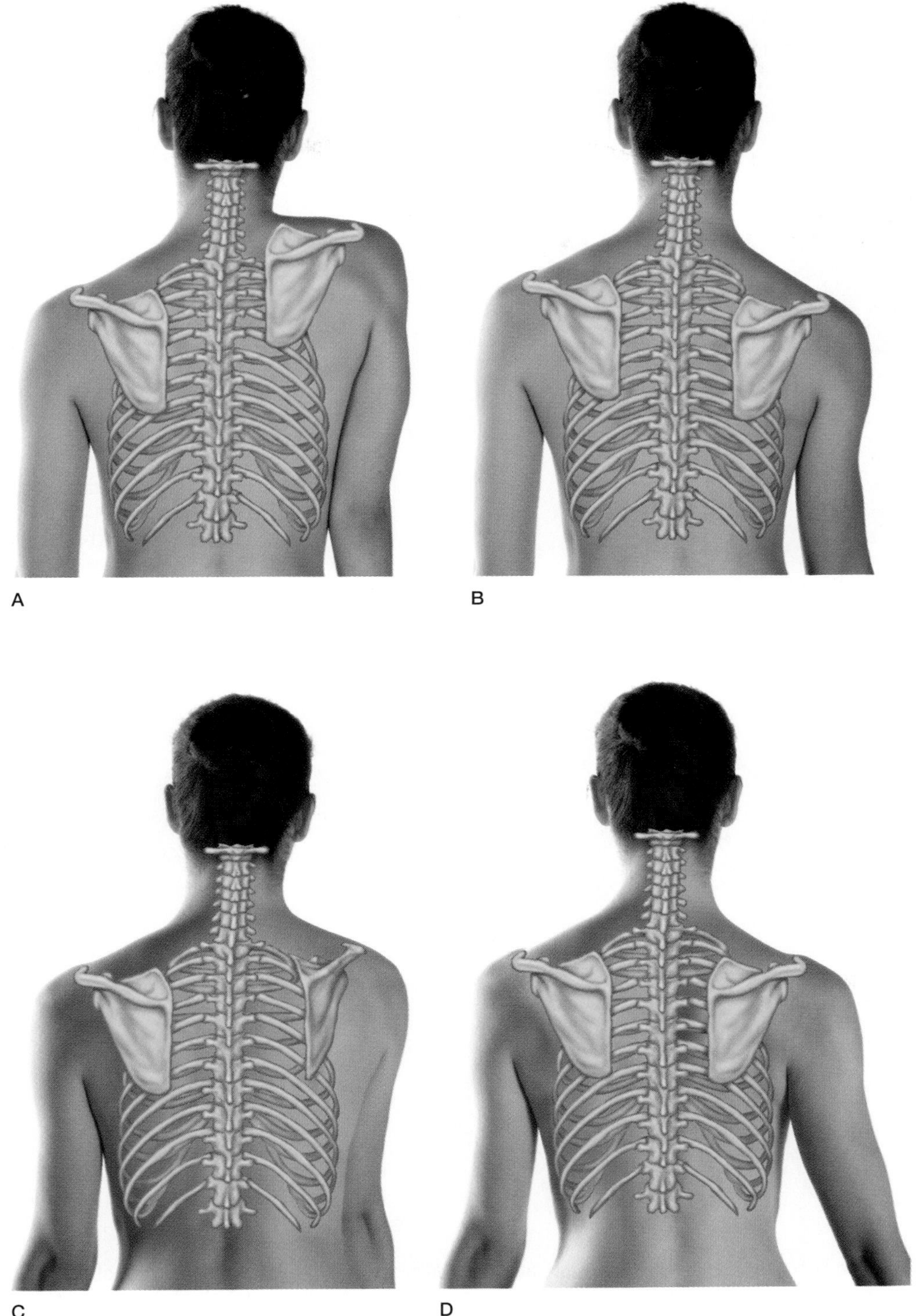

Figure 9-8 Nonaxial actions of elevation/depression and protraction/retraction of the scapula at the scapulocostal (ScC) joint. *A,* Elevation of the right scapula. *B,* Depression of the right scapula. *C,* Protraction of the right scapula. *D,* Retraction of the right scapula. The left scapula is in anatomic position in all figures. (Note: All views are posterior.)

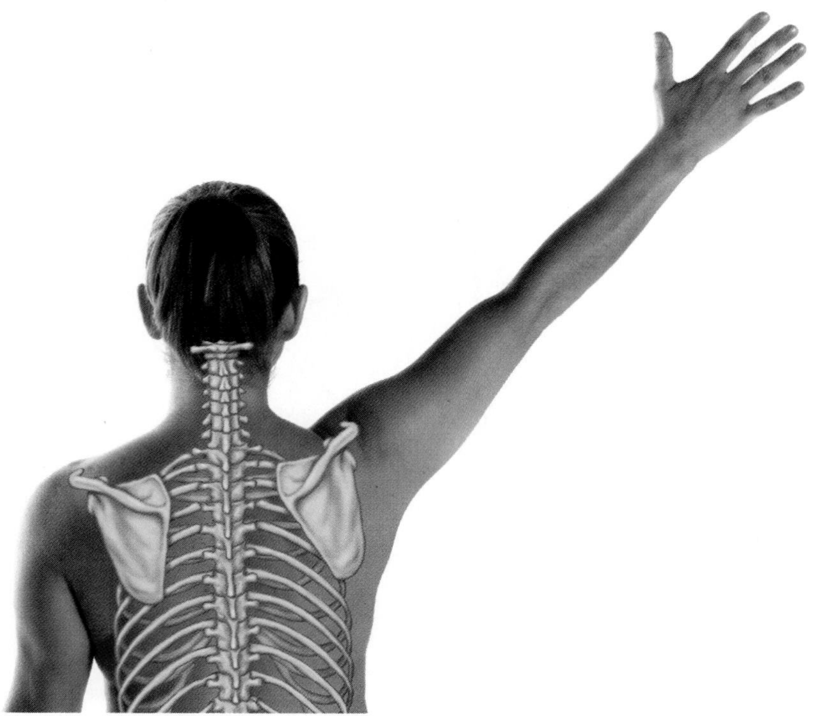

Figure 9-9 Upward rotation of the right scapula at the scapulocostal (ScC) joint. The left scapula is in anatomic position, which is full downward rotation. (Note: The scapular action of upward rotation cannot be isolated. It must accompany humeral motion. In this case, the humerus is abducted at the shoulder joint.)

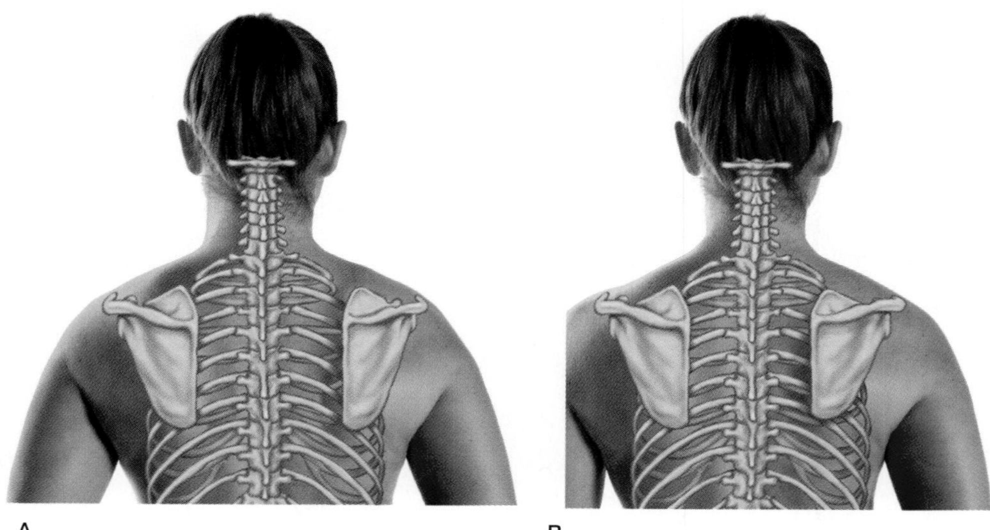

Figure 9-10 Tilt actions of the scapula at the scapulocostal (ScC) joint. *A,* Upward tilt of the right scapula; the left scapula is in anatomic position of downward tilt. *B,* Lateral tilt of the right scapula; the left scapula is in anatomic position of medial tilt. (Note: Both views are posterior.)

TABLE 9-3

Average Ranges of Upward Rotation and Downward Rotation Motion of the Scapula at the Scapulocostal Joint from Anatomic Position

Upward rotation	60 Degrees	Downward rotation	0 Degrees

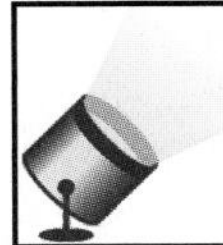

BOX 9-12 SPOTLIGHT ON SCAPULOCOSTAL JOINT MOTION

Motion of the scapula at the scapulocostal (ScC) joint cannot occur without motion also occurring at the sternoclavicular (SC) and/or acromioclavicular (AC) joint(s) as well. In other words, for the scapula to move relative to the ribcage at the ScC joint, it will also have to move relative to the clavicle at the AC joint, and/or move with the clavicle when the clavicle moves relative to the sternum at the SC joint.

Looking at this concept from another point of view, when the scapula moves relative to the clavicle at the AC joint, it also must move relative to the ribcage at the ScC joint. Interestingly, when the scapula moves relative to the arm at the glenohumeral (GH) joint (the reverse action of the GH joint), the scapula may also move relative to the ribcage at the ScC joint, or it may stay fixed to the ribcage at the ScC joint and the entire trunk may move with the scapula relative to the arm at the GH joint.

Therefore regarding whether scapular motion can be isolated at one joint or can or must occur at more than one of its joints, we see the following: (1) Motion of the scapula at the ScC joint must always be accompanied by motion of the scapula at another joint, and (2) the only joint at which scapular motion can be isolated is the GH joint; however, this can only occur if the scapula stays fixed to the ribcage and the trunk moves with the scapula relative to the arm.

- Protraction and retraction (i.e., nonaxial movements) of the scapula
- Elevation and depression (i.e., nonaxial movements) of the scapula
- Upward rotation and downward rotation (i.e., axial movements) of the scapula
  - Note: Upward rotation and downward rotation (i.e., axial movements) of the scapula occur within the frontal plane around an anteroposterior axis (these are approximations of the plane and axis, because the scapula is not situated perfectly within the frontal plane because of the shape of the posterior ribcage wall).

Accessory Movements:

Accessory movements include the following (Box 9-13, Note 1):

- Lateral tilt and medial tilt (i.e., axial movements) of the scapula.
- Upward tilt and downward tilt (i.e., axial movements) of the scapula

BOX 9-13

Note 1: The accessory motions of scapular tilting are defined differently by different sources. For our purposes, a healthy scapula in anatomic position is medially and downwardly tilted, and any lateral or upward tilt of the scapula involves the medial border or the inferior angle jutting away from the body wall, and is generally considered to be an unhealthy resting position of the scapulae. However, massage therapists and bodyworkers often use positions of lateral and upward tilt to gain access to the underside (i.e., anterior side) of the scapula, enabling them to work muscles that are deep to the scapula from the posterior side of the body.

Note 2: Lateral tilt of the scapula is usually referred to in lay terms as **winging of the scapula**.

Reverse Actions:

- The ribcage (i.e., the trunk) can move relative to the scapula.

BOX 9-14

One example of a reverse action at the scapulocostal (ScC) joint in which the ribcage (i.e., the trunk) moves relative to the scapula is when push-ups are done. The objective of a push-up is to exercise muscles by pushing the body up and away from the floor. At the very end of a push-up, after the upper extremities are perfectly vertical, a little more elevation of the trunk away from the floor is possible. This motion is caused by protractors of the scapula such as the serratus anterior contracting and pulling the trunk (which is more mobile) up toward the scapulae (which are fixed, because the hands are planted firmly on the floor).

Major Muscles of the Scapulocostal Joint:

- Elevators of the scapula attach from the scapula to a more superior structure; examples are the upper trapezius, levator scapulae, and the rhomboids.
- Depressors attach from the scapula to a more inferior structure; examples are the lower trapezius and the pectoralis minor.
- Protractors attach from the scapula to a more anterior structure; examples are the serratus anterior and the pectoralis minor.
- Retractors attach from the scapula to a more midline structure posteriorly; examples are the middle trapezius and the rhomboids.
- Upward rotators of the scapula include the serratus anterior and the upper and lower trapezius.
- Downward rotators include the pectoralis minor, rhomboids, and the levator scapulae.

Miscellaneous:

- The scapula articulates with the ribcage at the ScC joint, the clavicle at the AC joint, and the humerus at the GH joint. Therefore the scapula can move relative to any of these structures, and the motion could be described as occurring at the joint located between the scapula and any one of these three bones. Keep in mind that at times the scapula moves at only one of these joints; other times the scapula moves at more than one of these joints at the same time.

9.4 STERNOCLAVICULAR JOINT

- The **sternoclavicular joint** is also known as the SC joint.

Bones:

- The manubrium of the sternum and the medial end of the clavicle (Figure 9-11)
- Joint Structure Classification: Synovial joint
  - Subtype: Saddle
- Joint Function Classification: Diarthrotic
  - Subtype: Biaxial

BOX 9-15

The sternoclavicular (SC) joint actually permits motion in three planes about three axes; therefore it could also be classified as *triaxial.* However, because its rotation actions cannot be isolated, this joint is most often classified as being *biaxial.* In this regard, the SC joint is similar to the other more famous saddle joint of the human body, the saddle joint of the thumb (i.e., the carpometacarpal [CMC] joint of the thumb). (For information on the saddle joint of the thumb, see Section 9.13.)

Major Motions Allowed:

Major motions allowed are as follows (Figures 9-12 to 9-14; see Table 9-4):

- Protraction and retraction of the clavicle (i.e., axial movements): These motions occur within the transverse plane around a vertical axis.
- Elevation and depression of the clavicle (i.e., axial movements): These motions occur within the frontal plane around an anteroposterior axis.
  - Elevation and depression motions of the clavicle at the sternoclavicular joint are not oriented perfectly in the frontal plane. At rest, the clavicle is actually oriented approximately 20 degrees posterior to the frontal plane.
- Upward rotation and downward rotation of the clavicle (i.e., axial movements): These motions occur within the sagittal plane around a mediolateral axis (this axis runs through the length of the bone).

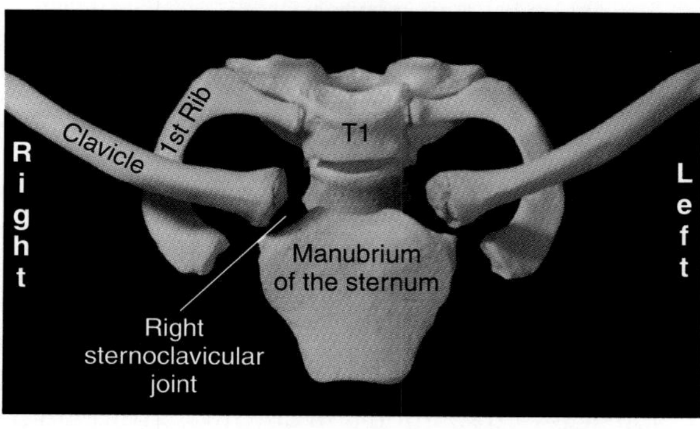

Figure 9-11 Anterior view of the upper trunk illustrating the sternoclavicular (SC) joints located between the manubrium of the sternum and the medial (i.e., proximal) ends of the clavicles.

TABLE 9-4

Average Ranges of Motion of the Clavicle at the Sternoclavicular Joint from Anatomic Position

Elevation	45 Degrees	Depression	10 Degrees
Protraction	30 Degrees	Retraction	30 Degrees
Upward rotation	45 Degrees	Downward rotation	0 Degrees

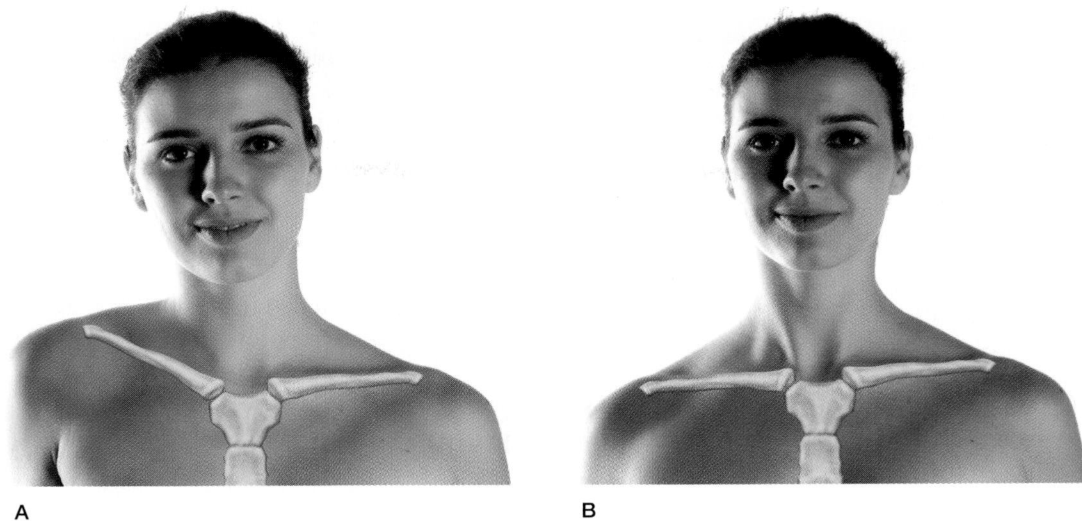

Figure 9-12 *A*, Elevation of the right clavicle at the sternoclavicular (SC) joint. *B*, Depression of the right clavicle. (Note: The left clavicle is in anatomic position. Both views are anterior.)

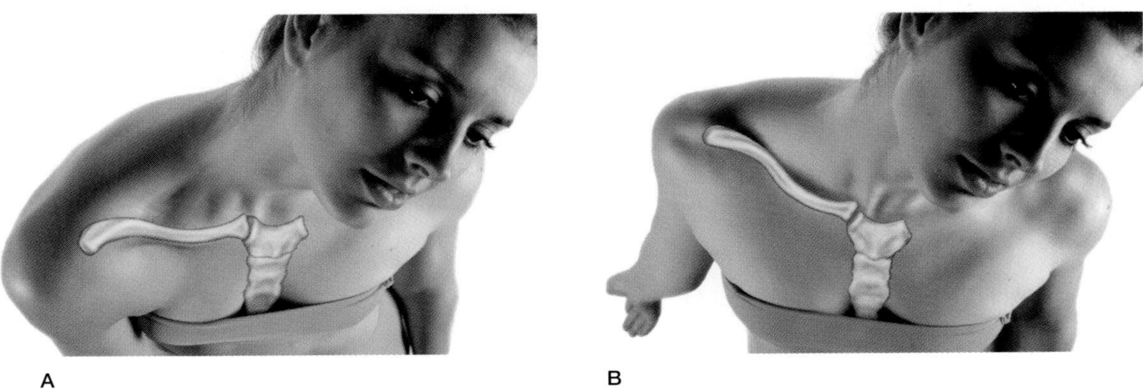

Figure 9-13 *A*, Protraction of the right clavicle at the sternoclavicular (SC) joint. *B*, Retraction of the right clavicle. (Note: Both views are anterior.)

Major Ligaments of the Sternoclavicular Joint:

The SC joint has several major ligaments (Figure 9-15; Boxes 9-16 and 9-17):

- The SC joint is the only osseous joint that connects the upper extremity (i.e., hand, forearm, arm, scapula, clavicle) to the axial skeleton. As such, it needs to be well stabilized.

BOX 9-16

LIGAMENTS OF THE STERNOCLAVICULAR JOINT

- Fibrous capsule
- Anterior sternoclavicular (SC) ligament
- Posterior SC ligament
- Interclavicular ligament
- Costoclavicular ligament

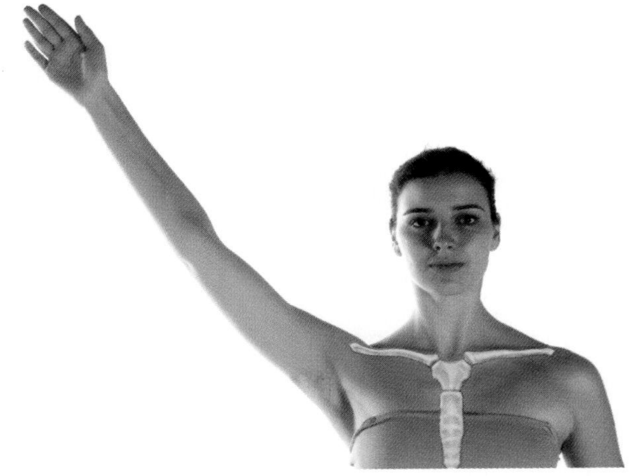

Figure 9-14 Anterior view that illustrates upward rotation of the right clavicle at the sternoclavicular (SC) joint; the left clavicle is in anatomic position, which is full downward rotation. (Note: Upward rotation of the clavicle cannot be isolated. In this figure the arm is abducted at the shoulder joint, resulting in the scapula upwardly rotating, which results in upward rotation of the clavicle.)

BOX 9-17

The sternoclavicular (SC) joint can be considered to be the basilar joint of the entire upper extremity. When the clavicle moves at the SC joint, the scapula is moved at the scapulocostal (ScC) joint. In fact, much if not most of the motion of the scapula at the ScC joint is driven by motion of the clavicle at the SC joint. In addition to ligamentous support, the sternoclavicular joint is also stabilized by the attachments of the sternocleidomastoid, sternohyoid, and sternothyroid muscles.

Fibrous Joint Capsule:

- The SC joint capsule is fairly strong and is also reinforced by **sternoclavicular ligaments**.
- Two SC ligaments exist: (1) the **anterior sternoclavicular ligament** and (2) the **posterior sternoclavicular ligament**.

Anterior and Posterior Sternoclavicular Ligaments:

- These are reinforcements of the joint capsule found anteriorly and posteriorly.

Interclavicular Ligament:

- The **interclavicular ligament** spans from one clavicle to the other clavicle.

Costoclavicular Ligament:

- The **costoclavicular ligament** runs from the 1st rib to the clavicle.
  - More specifically, it runs from the costal cartilage of the 1st rib to the costal tuberosity on the inferior surface of the medial (i.e., proximal) end of the clavicle.
- The costoclavicular ligament has anterior and posterior fibers.
- The costoclavicular ligament limits all motions of the clavicle except depression.

Closed-Packed Position of the Sternoclavicular Joint:

- Full upward rotation of the clavicle

Miscellaneous:

- A fibrocartilaginous articular disc is located within the SC joint.
- This disc helps to improve the congruence of the joint surfaces and also to absorb shock.

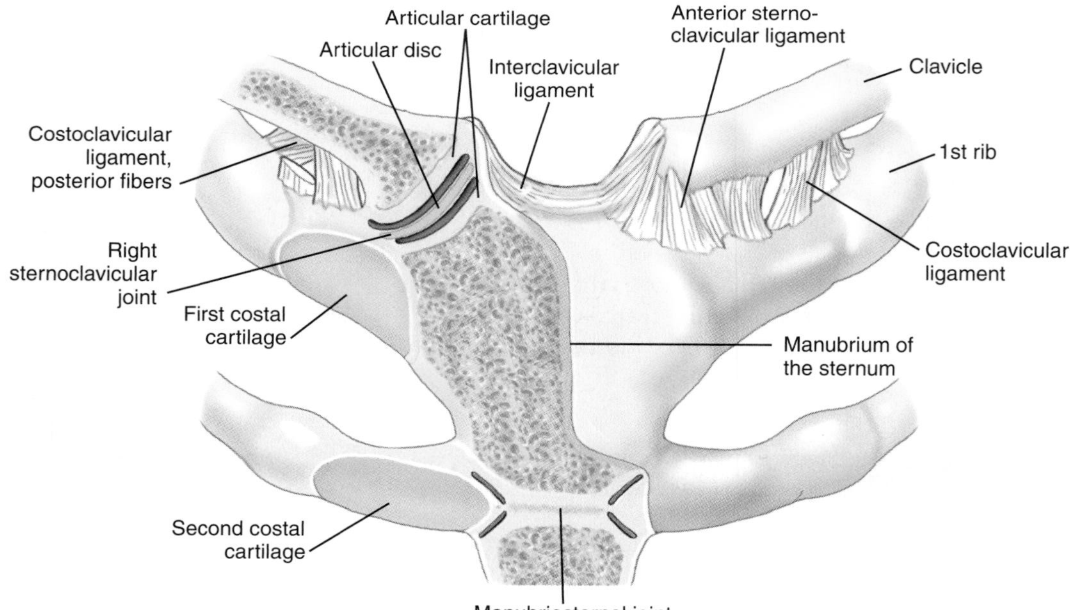

Figure 9-15 Anterior view of the sternoclavicular (SC) joints. The right joint is shown in a frontal (i.e., coronal) section; the left joint is left intact. The SC joint is stabilized by its fibrous capsule, anterior and posterior SC ligaments, the interclavicular ligament, and the costoclavicular ligament.

☐ 9.5 ACROMIOCLAVICULAR JOINT

❑ The **acromioclavicular** is also known as the AC joint.

Bones:

❑ The acromion process of the scapula and the lateral (i.e., distal) end of the clavicle (Figure 9-16)
❑ Joint Structure Classification: Synovial joint
  ❑ Subtype: Plane joint
❑ Joint Function Classification: Diarthrotic
  ❑ Subtype: Nonaxial

Motions Allowed:

❑ Upward rotation and downward rotation of the scapula (i.e., axial movements) relative to the clavicle.
❑ Without motion at the AC joint, the scapula and clavicle (i.e., the shoulder girdle) would be forced to always move as one fixed unit. The AC joint allows for independent motion between the scapula and clavicle. The major actions at the AC joint are movements of the scapula relative to the clavicle. These motions of the scapula allow greater overall motion of the shoulder joint complex, which translates into the ability to move and place the hand throughout a greater range of motion (Figure 9-17; Table 9-5).

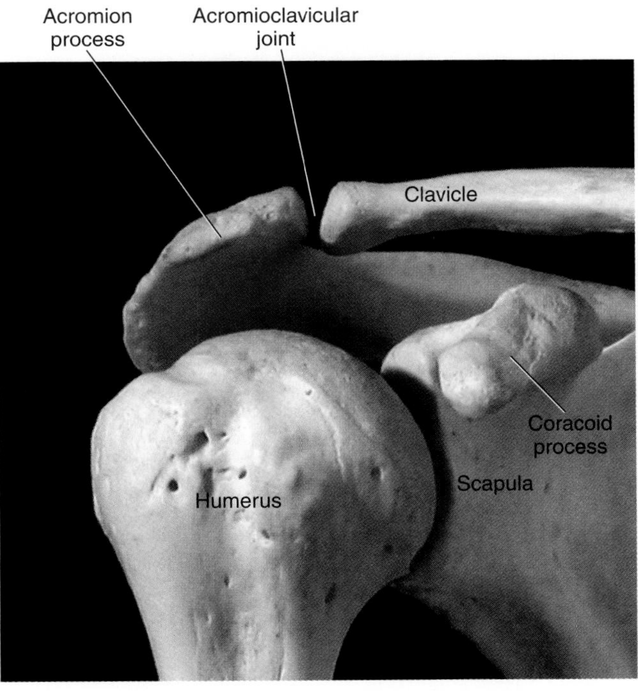

Figure 9-16 Anterior view of the right acromioclavicular (AC) joint formed by the union of the acromion process of the scapula and the lateral (i.e., distal) end of the clavicle.

Accessory Actions:

❑ Lateral tilt and medial tilt of the scapula (i.e., axial movements)
❑ Upward tilt and downward tilt of the scapula (i.e., axial movements)
❑ Note: The accessory tilt actions of the scapula are considered by many to be necessary to adjust the position of the scapula on the ribcage. Much of the motion of the scapula at the scapulocostal joint is actually driven by motion of the clavicle at the sternoclavicular joint. If there were no acromioclavicular joint, the scapula would have to follow the motion of the clavicle degree for degree. However, as the scapula moves along with the clavicle, its anterior surface may no longer remain snug against the ribcage. For this reason, fine tune adjustments of the scapula at the acromioclavicular joint are necessary to maintain the proper position of the scapula relative to the ribcage. For illustrations of scapular tilt actions, please see Section 9-3.

Reverse Actions:

❑ The clavicle can move relative to the scapula at the AC joint.

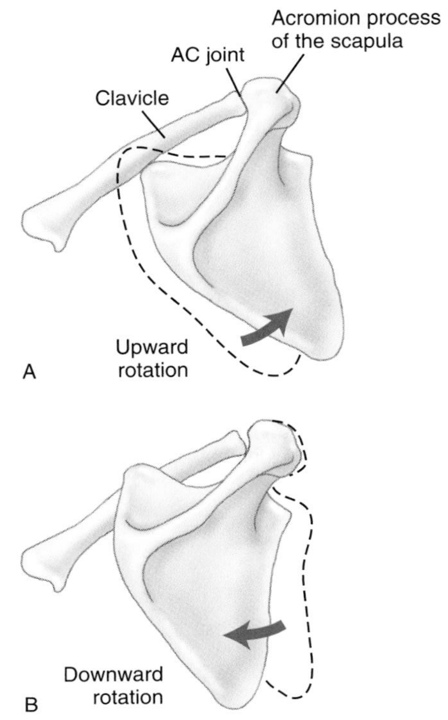

Figure 9-17 Motion of the scapula relative to the clavicle at the right acromioclavicular (AC) joint. *A*, Upward rotation. *B*, Downward rotation. (Note: Both views are posterior. When the scapula moves relative to the clavicle at the AC joint, it also moves relative to the ribcage at the scapulocostal [ScC] joint.)

TABLE 9-5

Average Ranges of Motion of the Scapula at the Acromioclavicular Joint from Anatomic Position

Upward rotation	30 Degrees	Downward rotation	0 Degrees

Note: Lateral/medial tilts and upward/downward tilts have been measured at between 10-30 degrees.

Major Ligaments of the Acromioclavicular Joint:

The AC joint has several major ligaments (Figure 9-18):

BOX 9-18

LIGAMENTS OF THE ACROMIOCLAVICULAR JOINT

- Fibrous capsule
- Acromioclavicular (AC) ligament
- Coracoclavicular ligament (trapezoid and conoid)

BOX 9-19

In addition to the ligamentous support, the acromioclavicular (AC) joint is also stabilized by the attachments of the trapezius and deltoid muscles.

Fibrous Joint Capsule:

- ❑ The joint capsule is weak and is reinforced by the **acromioclavicular ligament**.

Acromioclavicular Ligament:

- ❑ The AC ligament is a reinforcement of the AC joint capsule.
- ❑ The AC ligament is often divided into the **superior acromioclavicular ligament** and the **inferior acromioclavicular ligament**, which are reinforcements of the AC joint capsule found superiorly and inferiorly.

Coracoclavicular Ligament:

- ❑ The **coracoclavicular ligament** has two parts: (1) the **trapezoid ligament** and (2) the **conoid ligament**.
- ❑ Location: The coracoclavicular ligament attaches from the coracoid process of the scapula to the clavicle.
  - ❑ More specifically, it attaches to the lateral (i.e., distal) end of the clavicle on the inferior surface.
- ❑ The trapezoid ligament is more anterior in location and attaches from the superior surface of the coracoid

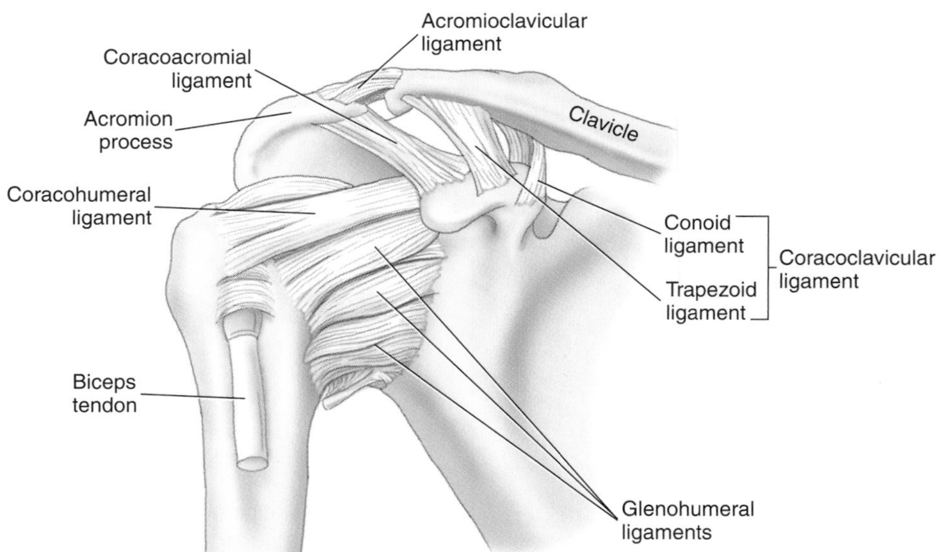

Figure 9-18 Anterior view of the right acromioclavicular (AC) joint. The AC joint is stabilized by its fibrous capsule, the AC ligament, and the coracoclavicular ligament. The coracoclavicular ligament has two parts: (1) the trapezoid and (2) conoid ligaments.

process to the trapezoid line of the clavicle (on the inferior surface at the lateral end of the clavicle).

- The conoid ligament is more posterior in location and attaches from the proximal base of the coracoid process of the scapula to the conoid tubercle of the clavicle (on the inferior surface at the lateral end of the clavicle).
- Function: The coracoclavicular ligament does not directly cross the AC joint itself, but it does cross from the scapula to the clavicle and therefore add stability to the AC joint.

Closed-Packed Position of the Acromioclavicular Joint:

- Full upward rotation of the scapula

Miscellaneous:

- Often a fibrocartilaginous disc is located within the AC joint.
- The AC joint is very susceptible to injury (e.g., a fall on an outstretched arm) and degeneration.

9.6 SCAPULOHUMERAL RHYTHM

- When a small degree of arm movement is needed, motion may occur solely at the glenohumeral (GH) joint. However, if any appreciable degree of arm motion is necessary, the entire complex of shoulder joints must become involved. The result is that arm motion requires coupled joint actions of the scapula and clavicle. (The concept of coupled actions is addressed in Section 13.12; see also Section 8.11 for coupled actions between the thigh and pelvis.) This pattern of coupled actions is called **scapulohumeral rhythm**; however, given the involvement of the clavicle, it might better be termed **scapuloclaviculohumeral rhythm**.
- The reason that shoulder girdle movement must accompany arm movement is that the GH joint, albeit the most mobile joint in the human body, does not allow sufficient movement of the arm to be able to place the hand in all desired locations. For example, if one wants to reach a book that is located high up on a shelf that is located to the side of the body, it is necessary to abduct the arm at the GH joint. However, the GH joint only allows 120 degrees of abduction, which is not sufficient. Therefore to reach higher, movement of the scapula and clavicle must occur to bring the hand up higher. When all motions of the shoulder joint complex have occurred, the arm appears to have abducted 180 degrees because the position of the arm relative to the trunk has changed 180 degrees. In reality, only 120 degrees of that motion occurred at the GH joint. The other 60 degrees (fully $^{1}/_{3}$ of the motion) was due to scapular motion relative to the ribcage at the ScC joint with the arm "going along for the ride" (this scapular motion at the ScC joint is dependent on motion of the clavicle at the SC joint and motion of the scapula relative to the clavicle at the AC joint). Therefore scapulohumeral rhythm is an important concept, and a full understanding of the motions at all the joints of the shoulder joint complex is important when assessing clients who have decreased range of motion of the arm.
- Following is a list of the scapular actions at the ScC joint that couple with motions of the arm at the GH joint. In each circumstance, keep in mind that the coupled action of the scapula facilitates further movement of the arm in the direction it is moving. Further, it should be noted that it is not that the arm first moves as much as it can, and then the scapula begins to move. Rather, the scapula will usually begin to move earlier on; from that point onward, motion will be a combination of arm and shoulder girdle movement.

BOX 9-20

The exact point at which scapular movement begins to couple with arm movement in scapulohumeral rhythm is approximately at 30 degrees of arm movement at the glenohumeral (GH) joint. However, this number is not fixed; rather, it varies from one individual to another based on a number of factors.

Sagittal Plane Actions:

- Flexion of the arm at the GH joint couples with protraction and upward rotation of the scapula at the ScC joint.
- Extension of the arm at the GH joint couples with retraction and downward rotation of the scapula at the ScC joint.
- Extension of the arm at the GH joint beyond neutral (i.e., extension beyond anatomic position) couples with upward tilt of the scapula at the ScC joint.

Frontal Plane Actions:

- Abduction of the arm at the GH joint couples with upward rotation of the scapula at the ScC joint (Figure 9-19). (For more details on scapulohumeral rhythm that occurs with abduction of the arm, see the *Spotlight on Scapulohumeral Rhythm of Arm Abduction* in Box 9-21.)
- Adduction of the arm at the GH joint couples with downward rotation of the scapula at the ScC joint.

BOX 9-21 SPOTLIGHT ON SCAPULOHUMERAL RHYTHM OF ARM ABDUCTION

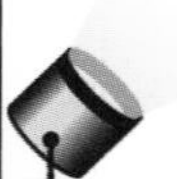

Scapulo(claviculo)humeral rhythm motion of the coupled joint actions of the shoulder joint complex that accompany frontal plane abduction of the arm at the glenohumeral (GH) joint has been extensively studied. Following is a summation of this complex of coupled actions (see Figure 9-19). (Note: The details that follow are not meant to overwhelm the reader; they are presented to manifest the beautiful complexity of scapulohumeral rhythm and illustrate the need for a larger more global assessment of shoulder joint motion in clients who have shoulder problems!)

- ❑ Full frontal plane abduction of the arm is considered to be 180 degrees of arm motion relative to the trunk. Of that motion, the arm abducts 120 degrees at the GH joint, and the scapula upwardly rotates 60 degrees at the scapulocostal (ScC) joint (with the arm going along for the ride); 120 degrees + 60 degrees equals 180 degrees total arm movement relative to the trunk. This total movement pattern can be divided into an early phase and a late phase, each one consisting of 90 degrees.

Early Phase (Initial 90 Degrees):

- ❑ During the early phase, the arm abducts 60 degrees at the GH joint and the scapula upwardly rotates 30 degrees at the ScC joint.
- ❑ This scapular upward rotation of 30 degrees relative to the ribcage is created by two motions:
    1. The clavicle elevates 25 degrees at the sternoclavicular (SC) joint and the scapula goes along for the ride, thus changing its position and upwardly rotating relative to the ribcage.
    2. The scapula upwardly rotates 5 degrees at the acromioclavicular (AC) joint relative to the clavicle; again, changing its position and upwardly rotating relative to the ribcage.

Late Phase (Final 90 Degrees):

- ❑ During the late phase, the arm abducts another 60 degrees at the GH joint and the scapula upwardly rotates another 30 degrees at the ScC joint.
- ❑ This scapular upward rotation of 30 degrees relative to the ribcage is created by two motions:
    1. The clavicle elevates another 5 degrees at the SC joint and the scapula goes along for the ride, again changing its position and upwardly rotating relative to the ribcage.
    2. The scapula upwardly rotates another 25 degrees at the AC joint relative to the clavicle; again, changing its position and upwardly rotating relative to the ribcage.

Summation of Early and Late Phases:

- ❑ The arm has abducted at the GH joint relative to the scapula 120 degrees.
- ❑ The scapula has upwardly rotated at the ScC joint relative to the ribcage 60 degrees.
- ❑ This scapular upward rotation relative to the ribcage is comprised of 30 degrees of elevation of the clavicle at the SC joint and 30 degrees of upward rotation of the scapula at the AC joint.

A Detailed Explanation of How and Why these Motions of the Scapula Occur:

- ❑ The scapula and clavicle are linked together as the shoulder girdle at the AC joint. Hence muscular contraction that pulls and moves one bone of the shoulder girdle tends to result in movement of the entire shoulder girdle. Therefore muscles that pull and cause upward rotation of the scapula tend to also pull the clavicle into elevation; conversely, muscles that pull the clavicle into elevation also result in the scapula upwardly rotating.

Early Phase:

- ❑ The force of muscular contraction (by scapular upward rotators and clavicular elevators) results in elevation of the clavicle at the SC joint relative to the sternum (25 degrees); by simply going along for the ride, the scapula succeeds in upwardly rotating relative to the ribcage (i.e., at the ScC joint). The clavicle elevates until it encounters resistance to this motion by the costoclavicular ligament becoming taut, which limits further motion.
- ❑ Once the costoclavicular ligament becomes taut, because the clavicle cannot elevate further, the force of the scapular upward rotation musculature continues to pull on the scapula and results in upward rotation of the scapula relative to the clavicle at the AC joint (5 degrees). The scapula upwardly rotates at the AC joint until the coracoclavicular ligament becomes taut, which limits further motion.
- ❑ The muscles of upward rotation of the scapula continue to pull on the scapula. However, the clavicle cannot elevate any further at the SC joint, and the scapula cannot upwardly rotate any further at the AC joint.

Late Phase:

- ❑ This continued pull of the scapular upward rotation musculature creates a pull on the scapula that creates tension on the coracoclavicular ligaments. This tension of the coracoclavicular ligaments then pulls on the clavicle in such a way that the clavicle is pulled into upward rotation at the SC joint (the clavicle upwardly rotates approximately 35 degrees).
- ❑ Once the clavicle is upwardly rotated at the SC joint, the clavicle can now elevate an additional 5 degrees at the SC joint and, more importantly, the scapula can now upwardly rotate at the AC joint another 25 degrees.

Conclusion:

- ❑ It can be seen that abduction of the arm in the frontal plane is strongly dependent on scapular movement; thus the importance of the term *scapulohumeral rhythm*. However, it is just as clear that the scapular motion of upward rotation is strongly dependent on clavicular motion; thus the importance of amending the term to *scapuloclaviculohumeral rhythm*! Therefore when assessing a client with limited frontal plane motion of the arm, it is crucially important to assess not just GH joint motion but also ScC joint motion; assessing ScC joint motion then necessitates assessment of SC and AC joint motion as well. Thus a case study of frontal plane arm abduction truly manifests the need for healthy coordinated functioning of all components of the shoulder joint complex!

Transverse Plane Actions:

- ❑ Medial rotation of the arm at the GH joint couples with protraction of the scapula at the ScC joint.
- ❑ Lateral rotation of the arm at the GH joint couples with retraction of the scapula at the ScC joint.

Other Coupled Actions of Scapulohumeral Rhythm:

In addition to the usual coupled actions of scapulohumeral rhythm, two other coupled actions should be mentioned:

- ❑ When the arm abducts at the GH joint above approximately 90 degrees, it also needs to rotate laterally at the GH joint. The reason for this is that when a medially rotated arm abducts, the greater tubercle of the head of the humerus bangs into the acromion process of the scapula. By laterally rotating the arm, the greater tubercle is moved out of the way and the arm can fully abduct.

BOX 9-22

If the head of the humerus bangs into the acromion process of the scapula, the tissues located between these two bones will be pinched. The rotator cuff tendon and subacromial bursa are located in this precarious position. Understanding this, imagine the possible health consequences to a client who has a chronic posture of rounded shoulders (i.e., protracted scapulae and medially rotated humeri). As this client perpetually raises the medially rotated arm into abduction, damage to these soft tissues will occur.

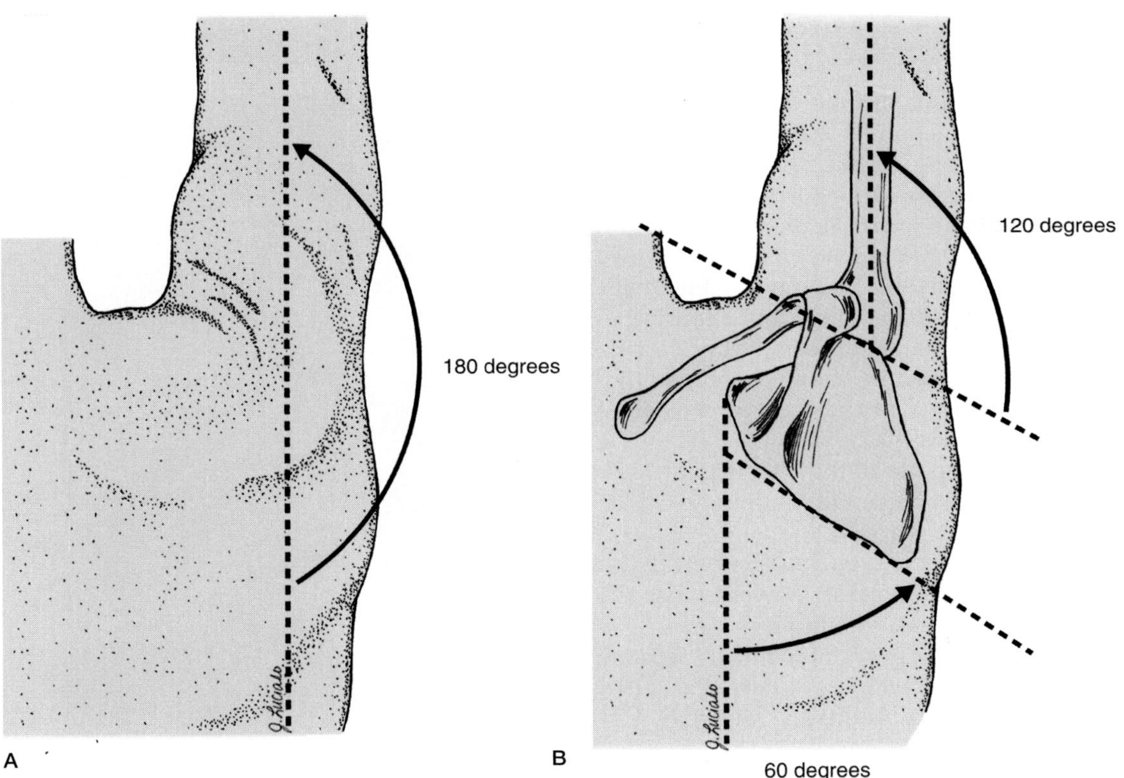

Figure 9-19 Concept of scapulohumeral rhythm. *A,* Right arm that has been abducted relative to the trunk 180 degrees. *B,* Of the 180 degrees of abduction of the arm relative to the trunk, only 120 degrees of that motion are the result of abduction of the arm at the glenohumeral (GH) joint; the remaining 60 degrees of motion are the result of upward rotation of the scapula at the scapulocostal (ScC) joint. Thus motion of the arm is intimately linked to motion of the scapula. (Note: Both views are posterior.) (Courtesy Joseph E. Muscolino.)

- When any motion occurs that causes the distal end of the humerus to elevate (i.e., flex, extend, abduct, or adduct) from anatomic position, the proximal end of the humerus (i.e., the head) must be held down into the glenoid fossa of the scapula. This is necessary because otherwise, whatever muscle *elevates* the distal end would also *pull* and *elevate* the head of the humerus into the acromion process, resulting in impingement and damage to the tissues of the GH joint. To prevent this from occurring, other muscles must contract isometrically to fix (i.e., stabilize) the head of the humerus in place. The rotator cuff musculature is usually credited with accomplishing this. The result is that the proximal end of the humerus stays fixed in place while the distal end elevates.

BOX 9-23

Flexion of the arm at the elbow joint is one of the classic reverse actions that is typically used to explain the concept of reverse actions. For example, a pull-up involves flexion of the arm at the elbow joint. (For more on the concept of reverse actions, see Section 5.29.)

9.7 ELBOW JOINT COMPLEX

- The elbow joint is unusual in that three articulations are enclosed within one joint capsule.
- These three articulations are the (1) **humeroulnar joint**, (2) the **humeroradial joint**, and (3) the **proximal radioulnar joint** (Figure 9-20).
- Because all three of these articulations are enclosed within one joint capsule and share one joint cavity, anatomically (i.e., structurally) they can be considered to be one joint, or one joint complex. However, because three separate articulations are involved, physiologically (i.e., functionally) they can be considered to be three separate joints.
- Classically, when one speaks of the "elbow joint," it is the humeroulnar and humeroradial joints to which one refers.
- Of these two joints, it is the humeroulnar joint that is functionally the most important. Movement at the humeroradial joint is of less significance.
- The proximal radioulnar joint is functionally separate from the elbow joint and will be considered as a part of the radioulnar joints (Section 9.9).

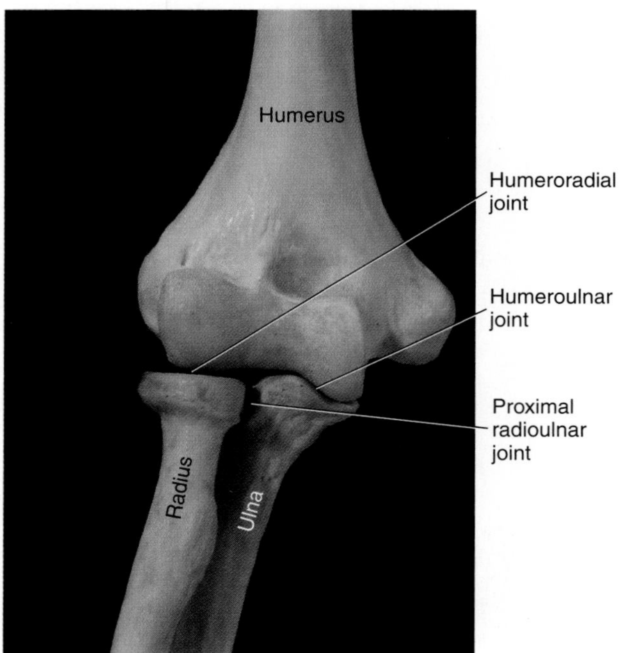

Figure 9-20 Anterior view of the right elbow joint complex. Three joints share the same joint capsule; these joints are the humeroulnar and humeroradial joints between the distal humerus and the ulna and radius, respectively, and the proximal radioulnar joint between the head of the radius and the proximal ulna. Of these, the humeroulnar joint is functionally the most important for elbow joint motion.

☐ 9.8 ELBOW JOINT

- ❑ The elbow joint is comprised of the humeroulnar and humeroradial joints (see Figure 9-21).
- ❑ The humeroulnar joint is also known as the **ulnotrochlear joint**.
- ❑ The humeroradial joint is also known as **radiocapitular joint**.

Bones:

- ❑ The humeroulnar joint is located between the distal end of the humerus and the proximal end of the ulna.
  - ❑ More specifically, the trochlea of the humerus articulates with the trochlear notch of the ulna.
- ❑ The humeroradial joint is located between the distal end of the humerus and the proximal end of the radius.
  - ❑ More specifically, the humeroradial joint is located between the capitulum of the humerus and the head of the radius.

Humeroulnar Joint:

- ❑ Joint structure classification: Synovial joint
  - ❑ Subtype: Hinge
- ❑ Joint function classification: Diarthrotic
  - ❑ Subtype: Uniaxial

Humeroradial Joint:

- ❑ Joint structure classification: Synovial joint
  - ❑ Subtype: Atypical ball-and-socket joint
- ❑ Joint function classification: Diarthrotic
  - ❑ Subtype: Biaxial

BOX 9-24

In addition to the movement that occurs at the humeroradial joint in the sagittal plane as the elbow joint flexes and extends, the head of the radius can also spin relative to the distal end of the humerus (in the transverse plane) as the radius pronates and supinates at the radioulnar joints.

Major Actions of the Elbow Joint:

- ❑ Flexion and extension of the forearm in the sagittal plane around a mediolateral axis (Figure 9-22; Table 9-6).

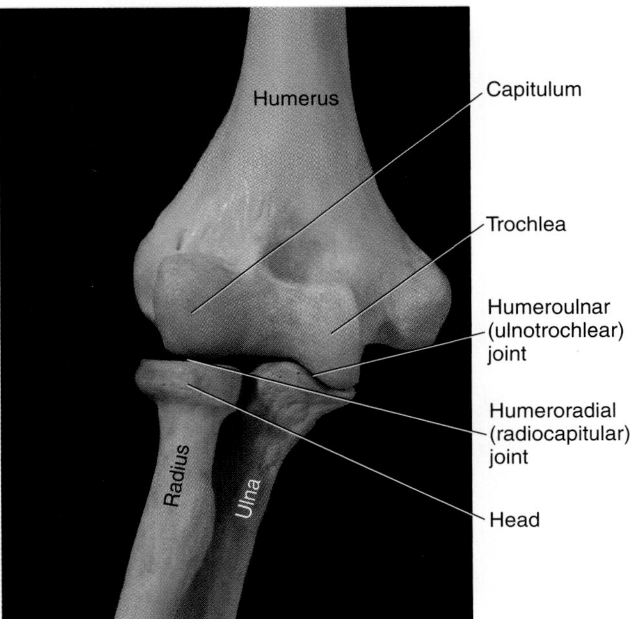

Figure 9-21 Anterior view of the right humeroulnar and humeroradial joints. When motion occurs at the elbow joint, it occurs at these two joints; the humeroulnar joint is functionally more important. The humeroulnar joint is also known as the *ulnotrochlear joint,* because the ulna articulates with the trochlea of the distal humerus. The humeroradial joint is also known as the *radiocapitular joint,* because the radius articulates with the capitulum of the distal humerus.

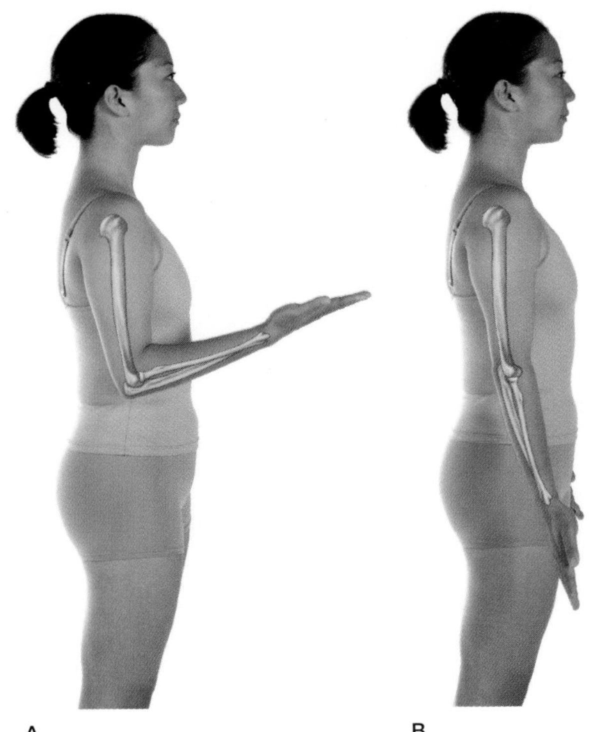

Figure 9-22 Motion at the elbow joint. The elbow joint is uniaxial and only allows flexion and extension in the sagittal plane. *A,* Flexion of the forearm at the elbow joint. *B,* Extension of the forearm at the elbow joint. (Note: Both views are lateral.)

TABLE 9-6

Average Ranges of Motion of the Forearm at the Elbow Joint from Anatomic Position

Flexion	145 Degrees	Extension	0 Degrees

Note: From anatomic position, usually 5 degrees of hyperextension of the forearm are possible at the elbow joint.

Reverse Actions:

- ❑ The arm can move relative to the forearm at the elbow joint (Box 9-23).

Major Ligaments of the Elbow Joint (Humeroulnar and Humeroradial Joints):

The elbow joint has several major ligaments (Figure 9-23; Box 9-25):

BOX 9-25

LIGAMENTS OF THE ELBOW JOINT

- Fibrous capsule
- Medial (i.e., ulnar) collateral ligament
- Lateral (i.e., radial) collateral ligament

Medial Collateral Ligament:

- ❑ The **medial collateral ligament** consists of three parts: (1) anterior, (2) posterior, and (3) transverse fibers.
- ❑ The majority of the fibers of the medial collateral ligament attaches from the medial epicondyle of the humerus to the ulna.
- ❑ The function is to stabilize the medial side of the elbow joint and to prevent abduction of the forearm at the elbow joint.
- ❑ The medial collateral ligament is also known as the **ulnar collateral ligament.**

Lateral Collateral Ligament:

- ❑ The **lateral collateral ligament** consists of two parts: (1) annular fibers and (2) ulnar fibers.

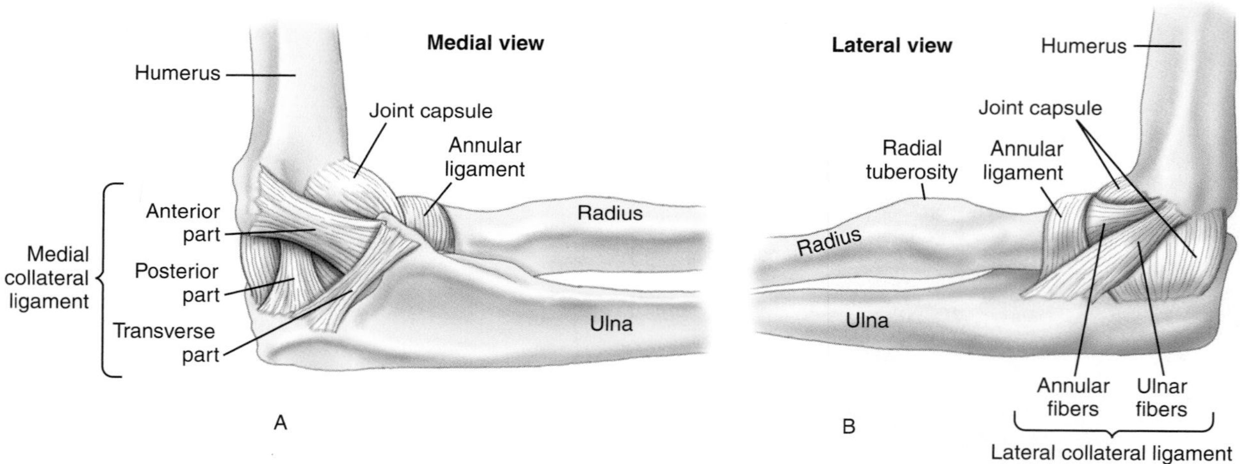

Figure 9-23 Ligaments of the left elbow joint. *A,* Medial view demonstrating the joint capsule and the medial collateral ligament. The medial collateral ligament has three parts: (1) anterior, (2) posterior, and (3) transverse. *B,* Lateral view demonstrating the joint capsule, lateral collateral ligament, and the annular ligament of the proximal radioulnar (RU) joint. The lateral collateral ligament has two parts: (1) annular fibers that blend into the annular ligament and (2) ulnar fibers that attach onto the ulna.

- The lateral collateral ligament attaches from the lateral epicondyle of the humerus to the annular ligament that lies over the radial head, and to the ulna.
- The function is to stabilize the lateral side of the elbow joint and to prevent adduction of the forearm at the elbow joint.
- The lateral collateral ligament is also known as the **radial collateral ligament.**

Closed-Packed Position of the Elbow Joint:

- Extension

Major Muscles of the Elbow Joint:

- Being a hinge joint, the actions of the elbow joint are restricted to flexion and extension. All muscles that cross the elbow joint anteriorly can do flexion, and all muscles that cross posteriorly can do extension.
  - The major flexors at the elbow joint are the brachialis, biceps brachii, brachioradialis, and pronator teres.
  - The major extensor of the elbow joint is the triceps brachii. The anconeus and extensor carpi ulnaris can also extend the elbow joint.
- Note: Two other groups of muscles (the wrist flexor group and wrist extensor group) have bellies that are located near the elbow joint and proximal tendons that originate and attach onto the humerus. The wrist flexor group attaches to the medial epicondyle of the humerus via the common flexor tendon; the wrist extensor group primarily attaches to the lateral epicondyle of the humerus via the common extensor tendon. Even though these muscles do cross the elbow joint and therefore can move the elbow joint, their primary actions (as their names imply) are at the wrist joint.

BOX 9-26

Tennis elbow and **golfer's elbow** are the names given to irritation and/or inflammation of the common extensor tendon and common flexor tendon, respectively (and/or their attachments onto the humerus). Technically, tennis elbow is called **lateral epicondylitis** and golfer's elbow is called **medial epicondylitis**. These conditions are considered to be tendinitis or tendinosis problems; they usually also involve hypertonicity of the involved muscles. (Note: tendinosis is distinguished from tendinitis by an absence of inflammation; *itis* means inflammation). Even though these conditions are named as elbow problems, they are not elbow joint problems; rather, they are functionally related to use of the hand at the wrist joint.

Miscellaneous:

- From the anterior perspective, it can be seen that the humerus and ulna are not aligned in a perfectly straight line within the frontal plane; rather, the ulna deviates laterally. This lateral deviation of the ulna relative to the humerus is known as the **carrying angle** (Figure 9-24).

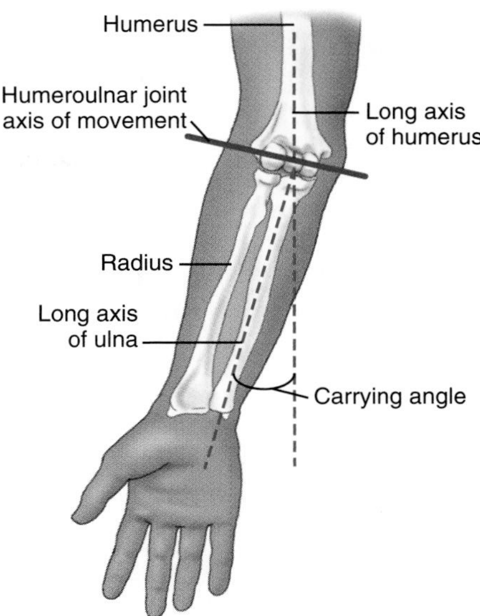

Figure 9-24 Carrying angle of the upper extremity. The carrying angle is formed by the intersection of two lines: one through the long axis of the humerus and the other through the long axis of the ulna. The usual carrying angle is between 5 and 15 degrees. The carrying angle is formed because of the axis of movement of the humeroulnar joint, which is not horizontal. Having a carrying angle allows for objects carried in the hand to be held away from the body.

BOX 9-27

Note 1: Given that women tend to have a wider pelvis, it stands to reason that the carrying angle would need to be greater!

Note 2: The term *valgus* refers to a lateral deviation of a body part; in this case the ulna. A carrying angle that is appreciably greater than 15 degrees is referred to as an *excessive cubitus valgus*, and a carrying angle appreciably less than 15 degrees is referred to as **cubitus varus**.

- The usual carrying angle is approximately 5-15 degrees. It is usually approximately 5-10 degrees in men and approximately 10-15 degrees in women (Box 9-27, Note 1).
- This carrying angle is also known as **cubitus valgus** (see Box 9-27, Note 2).
- The reason that the carrying angle exists is that the axis of movement at the elbow (i.e., humeroulnar) joint is not purely horizontal (see Figure 9-24). Rather, from medial to lateral, it is directed slightly superiorly, because the medial lip of the trochlea protrudes further than does the lateral lip of the trochlea (see Figure 4-64a).
- The advantage of a carrying angle is that objects carried in the hand are naturally held away from the body.

9.9 RADIOULNAR JOINTS

- When the radius moves relative to the ulna during pronation and supination, these actions occur at the **radioulnar (RU) joints**.
- Three radioulnar joints exist: (1) the **proximal radioulnar joint**, (2) the **middle radioulnar joint**, and (3) the **distal radioulnar joint** (see Figure 9-25).

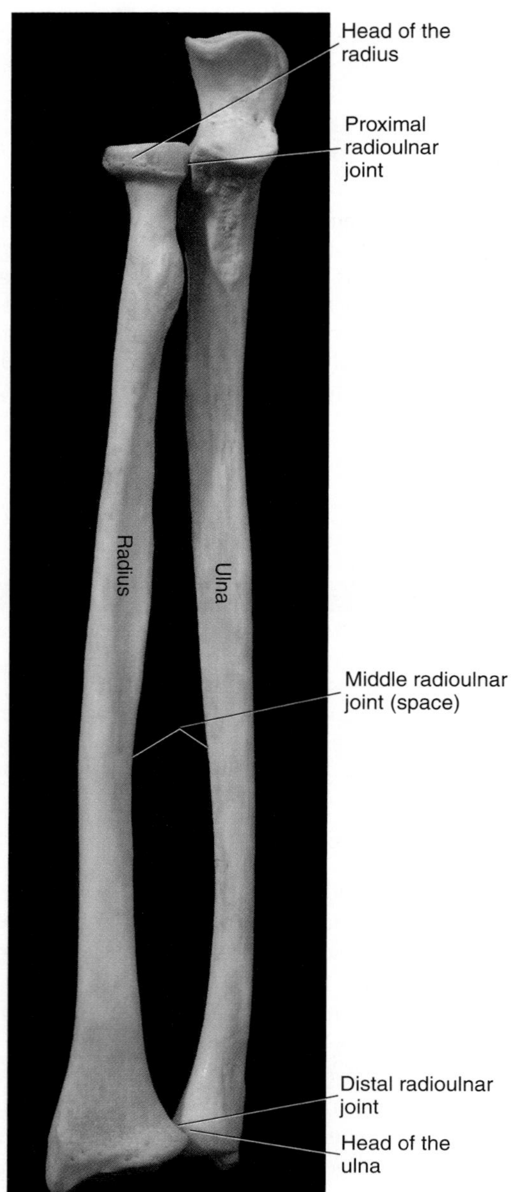

Figure 9-25 Anterior view that illustrates the three radioulnar (RU) joints of the right forearm. The proximal RU joint is located between the head of the radius and the radial notch of the ulna. The middle RU joint is located between the shafts of the radius and ulna. The distal RU joint is located between the head of the ulna and the ulnar notch of the radius.

- Although all three RU joints are functionally related in that their combined movements allow pronation and supination of the forearm, they are anatomically distinct from each other.
  - In fact, the proximal RU joint shares its joint capsule with the elbow joint, whereas the distal RU joint shares its joint capsule with the radiocarpal joint of the wrist joint complex.

Bones:

- The RU joints are located between the radius and ulna.
- The proximal RU joint is located between the proximal radius and the proximal ulna.
  - More specifically, the proximal RU joint is located between the head of the radius and the radial notch of the ulna.
- The middle RU joint is formed by the interosseus membrane that connects the shafts of the radius and ulna.
- The distal RU joint is located between the distal radius and the distal ulna.
  - More specifically, the distal RU joint is located between the ulnar notch of the radius and the head of the ulna.

Proximal Radioulnar Joint:

- Joint structure classification: Synovial joint
  - Subtype: Pivot
- Joint function classification: Diarthrotic
  - Subtype: Uniaxial

Middle Radioulnar Joint:

- Joint structure classification: Fibrous joint
  - Subtype: Syndesmosis
- Joint function classification: Amphiarthrotic
  - Subtype: Uniaxial

Distal Radioulnar Joint:

- Joint structure classification: Synovial joint
  - Subtype: Pivot
- Joint function classification: Diarthrotic
  - Subtype: Uniaxial

Major Actions of the Radioulnar Joints:

- The combined movements at the RU joints allow for pronation and supination of the forearm (Figure 9-26; Table 9-7 and Figures 4-68 and 4-70.)
- With pronation and supination, it is the radius that does the vast majority of the movement; in comparison, the ulna moves very little.

TABLE 9-7

Average Ranges of Motion of the Forearm at the Radioulnar Joints from Anatomic Position

Pronation	160 Degrees	Supination	0 Degrees

Forearm pronation and supination motions are often measured from a neutral "thumbs-up" position. From this neutral position, 85 degrees of forearm supination and 75 degrees of forearm pronation are possible.

BOX 9-28

During pronation and supination of the forearm, it is usually the radius that does the majority of the motion around a relatively fixed ulna. However, when the hand is fixed (i.e., closed-chain activity), the radius becomes fixed during pronation and supination motions and it is the ulna that does the majority of the motion (see Section 11.9, Figure 11-15).

- This action of the radius occurs around an axis that runs from the head of the radius to the head of the ulna; this axis in not purely vertical (see Section 5.18, Figure 5-18).
  - Movement at the proximal RU joint: The head of the radius medially rotates during pronation of the forearm; the head of the radius laterally rotates during supination of the forearm.
  - Movement at the distal RU joint: The distal radius swings around the distal ulna..

BOX 9-29 SPOTLIGHT ON MOTION AT THE DISTAL RADIOULNAR JOINT

The terms *pronation* and *supination* are used to describe motions of the radius, because the radius does not move in a typical manner for a long bone. During pronation of the radius, the head of the radius clearly medially rotates relative to the proximal ulna. This medial rotation involves the proximal radius spinning medially and remaining "in place." However, the distal radioulnar (RU) joint does not allow the distal radius to do pure medial rotation and stay in its same location in space (medial and lateral rotation of a long bone usually occur around an axis that runs through the shaft of the bone; consequently the bone spins *in place*). When the proximal radius medially rotates, the distal radius is forced to rotate and "swing around" the distal ulna.

This *rotating-and-swinging* motion can be described in terms of roll, spin, and glide (see Sections 5.7 and 5.8). In this case the distal radius rolls and glides in the same direction, as is usual for a concave bone moving relative to a convex bone. However, what is unusual about the roll/glide dynamics here is that the roll and glide occur in a line that is perpendicular to the long axis of the radius; roll and glide usually occur in the same line as the long axis of the bone.

Describing distal RU motion in the terminology system of flexion/extension, abduction/adduction, and medial rotation/lateral rotation, is even more awkward because it does not fit well into any one of these categories. If one were to try to place this motion into one of these categories of motion, the closest fit would be to say that the distal radius medially rotates, but that this rotation occurs around an axis that lies outside of the shaft of the radius. Because this axis runs through the distal ulna (see Section 5.18, Figure 5-18), pronation and supination of the radius at the distal RU joint involve the distal end of the radius actually rotating <u>and</u> "swinging" around the distal ulna.

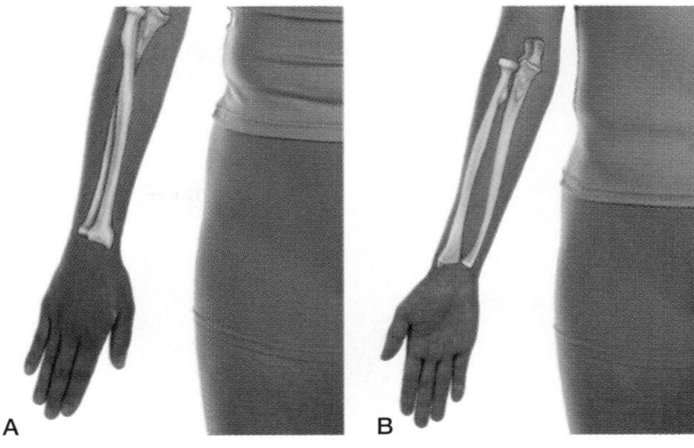

Figure 9-26 Pronation and supination of the right forearm at the radioulnar (RU) joints. *A,* Pronation. *B,* Supination, which is anatomic position for the forearm. Pronation and supination are joint actions created by a combination of motions at the proximal, middle, and distal RU joints. (Note: Both figures are an anterior view of the forearm.)

Major Ligaments of the Radioulnar Joints:

The proximal, middle, and distal RU joints have several major ligaments (Figure 9-27; Table 9-8):

Proximal Radioulnar Joint:

- Fibrous capsule
- Annular ligament
  - The **annular ligament** attaches to the anterior ulna, wraps around the head of the radius, and then attaches to the posterior ulna.
  - Function: It stabilizes the proximal RU joint and creates a cavity within which the head of the radius can rotate.

Middle Radioulnar Joint:

- Interosseus membrane of the forearm
  - The **interosseus membrane** is a fibrous sheet of tissue that unites the radius and ulna of the forearm, forming the middle RU joint.
  - Function: It stabilizes the middle RU joint by binding the radius and ulna together.

TABLE 9-8

Ligaments of the Radioulnar Joints

Proximal Radioulnar (RU) Joint:
- Fibrous joint capsule
- Annular ligament

Middle RU Joint:
- Interosseus membrane
- Oblique cord

Distal RU Joint:
- Fibrous joint capsule
- RU disc (triangular fibrocartilage)

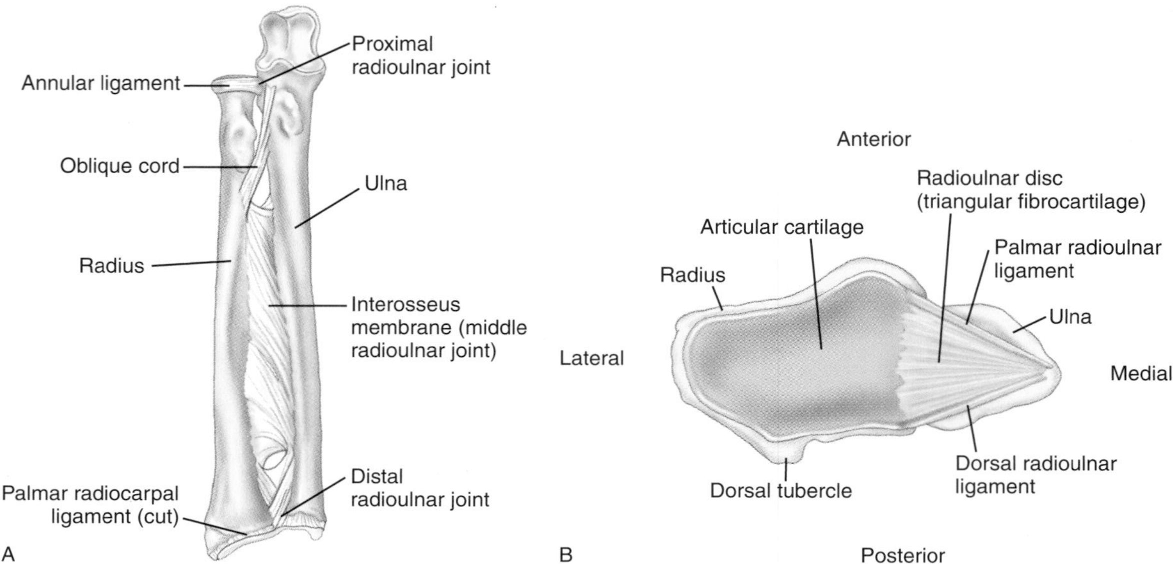

Figure 9-27 Ligamentous structures of the right radioulnar (RU) joints. *A,* Anterior view demonstrating the interosseus membrane and oblique cord, which form the middle RU joint, and the annular ligament of the proximal RU joint. The joint capsule of the distal RU joint (which it shares with the wrist joint) is also seen. *B,* View of the distal ends of the radius and ulna, depicting the RU disc of the distal RU joint. (Reader should note its triangular shape; hence its other name, the *triangular fibrocartilage.*)

BOX 9-30

The interosseus membrane, by binding the radius and ulna together, helps to stabilize the two bones of the forearm (i.e., the middle radioulnar [RU] joint). However, it also serves another important function. When compression forces travel up from the hand into the radius of the forearm (e.g., when doing an activity such as a push-up), these forces need to be transferred into the arm and from there into the trunk. However, the radius is not the principle bone of the elbow joint to be able to transfer this force to the humerus; it is the ulna that forms the major articulation at the elbow joint with the humerus. Therefore to transfer this force up to the arm, the radius must first transfer it to the ulna. This is accomplished by the interosseus membrane.

Because of the direction of the fibers of the interosseus membrane (see Figure 9-27), if an upward force travels through the radius, the interosseus membrane will transfer this force to the ulna by pulling upward on the ulna. This force can then be transferred across the humeroulnar (i.e., elbow) joint to the humerus. Similarly, a downward force that travels from the trunk and through the arm will cross the elbow joint into the ulna. The interosseus membrane will then transfer that force into the radius (given its fiber direction, a downward force on the ulna will create a downward pulling force on the radius), which can then be transferred across the radiocarpal (i.e., wrist) joint into the hand.

- **Oblique cord**
  - The oblique cord runs from the proximal ulna to the proximal radius. Its fibers are oriented perpendicular to the fibers of the interosseus membrane.
  - Function: It assists the interosseus membrane in stabilizing the middle RU joint.

Distal Radioulnar Joint:

- Fibrous capsule
  - The fibrous capsule is thickened on the dorsal and palmar sides.

BOX 9-31

The dorsal and palmar thickenings of the fibrous capsule of the distal radioulnar (RU) joint are called the **dorsal radioulnar ligament** and the **palmar radioulnar ligament** (see Figure 9-27b).

Radioulnar Disc:

- The RU disc runs from the distal radius to the distal ulna.
- It also blends into the capsular/ligamentous structure of the distal RU joint.
- Function: It stabilizes the distal RU joint.
- The RU disc is also known as the **triangular fibrocartilage**.

BOX 9-32

Because the distal radioulnar (RU) joint and the radiocarpal joint share the same joint capsule, the radioulnar (RU) disc, also known as the *triangular fibrocartilage*, is involved with both joints. It blends into the capsular/ligamentous structure of both the distal RU joint and the radiocarpal joint and adds to the stability of both these joints. (For more information on the RU disc, see Section 9.11; for information on the radiocarpal joint, see Sections 9.10 and 9.11.)

Miscellaneous:

- The proximal RU joint shares its joint capsule with the elbow joint.
- The distal RU joint shares its joint capsule with the radiocarpal joint of the wrist joint complex.

9.10 OVERVIEW OF THE WRIST/HAND REGION

- The wrist/hand region involves a number of bones and a number of joints. Generally the organization of the wrist/hand region is as follows (Figure 9-28):
- The two bones of the forearm, radius and ulna, articulate with the hand at the wrist joint.
- The hand is defined as everything distal to the radius and ulna.
  - The bones of the hand can be divided into carpals, metacarpals, and phalanges.
  - Just as the tarsal bones are the anklebones, the carpal bones are known as the *wrist bones*.
- The hand can be divided into three regions:
  1. The **carpus** is composed of the eight carpal bones.
  2. The **metacarpus**, also known as the *body of the hand*, contains the five metacarpal bones. The **palm** is the anterior region of the metacarpus of the hand.
  3. The fingers contain the phalanges.
- The term **ray** refers to a metacarpal and its associated phalanges; the hand has five rays:
  - The 1st ray is composed of the 1st metacarpal and the two phalanges of the thumb.
  - The 2nd ray is composed of the 2nd metacarpal and the three phalanges of the index finger (i.e., 2nd finger).
  - The 3rd ray is composed of the 3rd metacarpal and the three phalanges of the middle finger (i.e., 3rd finger).
  - The 4th ray is composed of the 4th metacarpal and the three phalanges of the ring finger (i.e., 4th finger).
  - The 5th ray is composed of the 5th metacarpal and the three phalanges of the little finger (i.e., 5th finger).

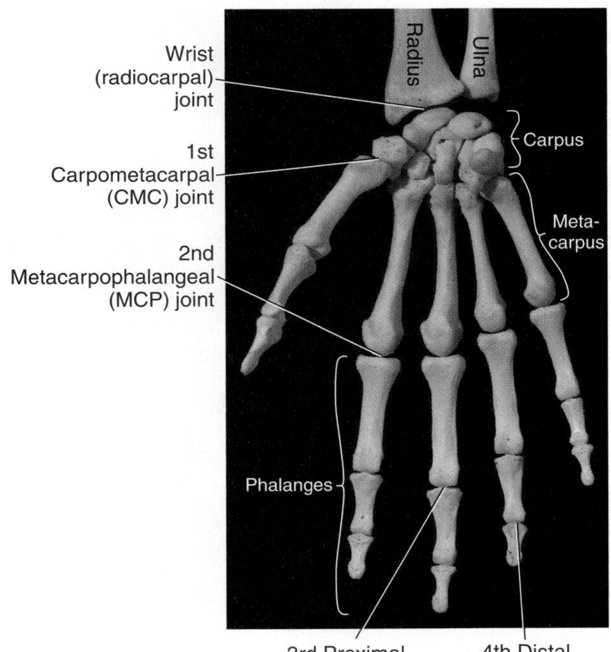

Figure 9-28 Anterior view of the skeletal structure of the right distal forearm and hand. The hand is located distal to the radius and ulna of the forearm. The hand can be divided into three parts: (1) the carpus, (2) metacarpus, and (3) phalanges. The carpus is composed of the carpal (i.e., wrist bones). The metacarpus, also known as the *body of the hand*, is composed of the metacarpals. The phalanges define the fingers.

Functions of the Hand:

- The human hand is an amazing structure. With the presence of an opposable thumb, the hand allows us to create, grasp, and use tools. The brain is usually credited as the distinguishing structure that has allowed human beings to advance and create civilization; however, some give equal credit to the hand. Although the brain conceptually designs civilization, the hand actually creates it. In this regard the hand may be viewed as the tool of expression of our brain!
- To free our hands for use, a bipedal stance on two legs instead of four is necessary. It is then up to the joints of the upper extremity to move our hand through space and place it in whatever location is necessary for the desired task. Because the upper extremity joints are freed from their weight-bearing responsibility, they have been able to trade off stability for the increased mobility necessary to place the hand in most any position in all three cardinal planes.

General Organization of the Joints of the Wrist/Hand Region:

Wrist Joint:

- The wrist joint is actually a complex of two joints: (1) the **radiocarpal joint** and (2) the **midcarpal joint**.
  - The radiocarpal joint is located between the distal end of the radius and the proximal row of carpal bones.
  - The midcarpal joint is located between the proximal row of carpal bones and the distal row of carpal bones.

Carpometacarpal Joints:

- The carpometacarpal (CMC) joints are located between the distal row of carpals and the metacarpal bones.
  - The 1st CMC joint (of the thumb) is a saddle joint that is specialized to allow a great degree of movement.

Intermetacarpal Joints:

- The intermetacarpal (IMC) joints are located between adjacent metacarpal bones.

Metacarpophalangeal Joints:

- The metacarpophalangeal (MCP) joints are located between the metacarpal bones and the phalanges.

Interphalangeal Joints (of the Hand):

- The interphalangeal (IP) joints are located between phalanges of a finger (see Figure 9-28).
  - Proximal interphalangeal (PIP) joints are located between the proximal and middle phalanges of fingers #2-5.
  - Distal interphalangeal (DIP) joints are located between the middle and distal phalanges of fingers #2-5.
  - The IP joint of the thumb is located between the proximal and middle phalanges of the thumb (i.e., finger #1).

Arches of the Hand:

- Although the foot is usually thought of when discussing arches, the hand also has arches. The arches of the hand create a concavity of the palm and a concavity of the fingers that helps the hand fit more securely around objects that are held, increasing the security of one's grasp (Figures 9-29 and 9-30).
- The hand has three arches:
  - **Proximal transverse arch**: The proximal transverse arch of the hand runs transversely (i.e., across the hand) and is formed by the two rows (proximal and distal) of carpal bones.

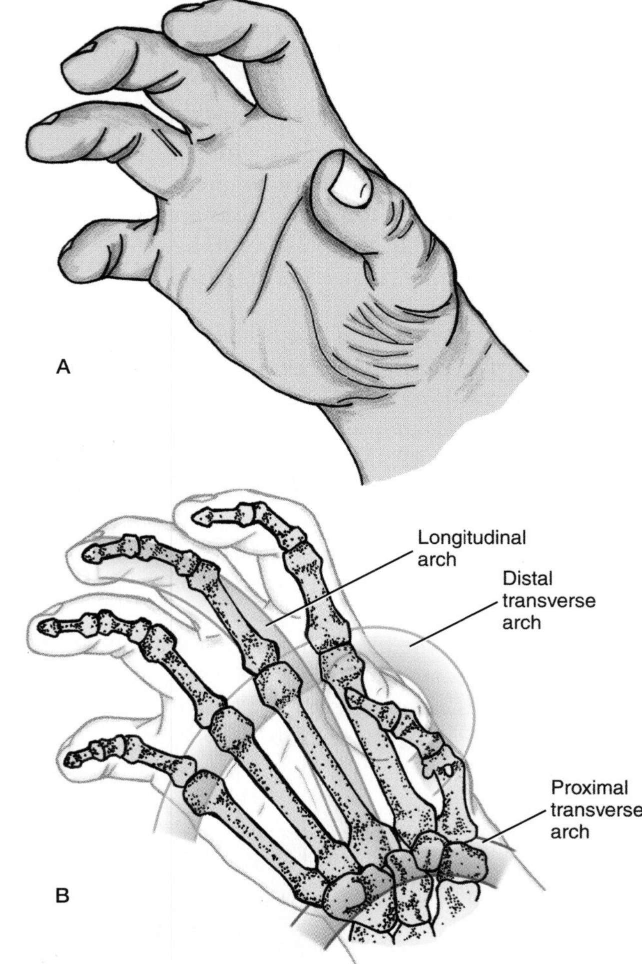

Figure 9-29 Arches of the hand. The hand has three arches: (1) a proximal transverse arch formed by the carpals, (2) a distal transverse arch formed at the metacarpophalangeal (MCP) joints, and (3) the longitudinal arch formed by the length of the metacarpals and phalanges. The arches of the hand better enable the hand to close in around the center of the hand, thereby providing a secure grasp of an object held in the hand. (Courtesy Joseph E. Muscolino.)

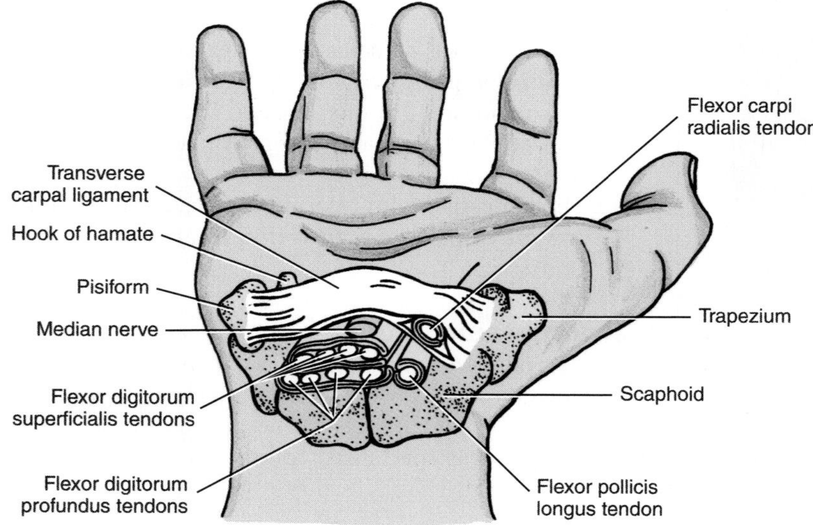

Figure 9-30 Illustration looking distally into the right hand. The tunnel formed by the carpal bones (i.e., the carpal tunnel) can be seen. The floor of the carpal tunnel is formed by the carpal bones; the roof is formed by the transverse carpal ligament. The transverse carpal ligament attaches to the pisiform and hook of the hamate on the ulnar side and to the tubercles of the scaphoid and trapezium on the radial side. The carpal tunnel contains the median nerve and nine extrinsic flexor tendons of the fingers. (Courtesy Joseph E. Muscolino.)

- **Distal transverse arch**: The distal transverse arch runs transversely (i.e., across the hand) and is located at the MCP joints.

BOX 9-33

Unlike the proximal transverse arch, which is fairly rigid, the distal transverse arch is quite mobile. When an object is held in the hand, the mobile 1st, 4th, and 5th metacarpals wrap around the stable 2nd and 3rd metacarpals.

- **Longitudinal arch**: The longitudinal arch runs the length of the hand and is formed by the shape of the metacarpals and fingers. The shape of the metacarpals is somewhat fixed, but flexion of the fingers increases the longitudinal arch of the hand.

Carpal Tunnel:

- The carpal tunnel is located anteriorly at the wrist and is a tunnel formed by the arrangement of the carpal bones (see Figure 9-30).
  - It is located between the archlike transverse concavity of the carpal bones and the **transverse carpal ligament** that spans across the top of the carpal bones.
  - The carpal tunnel provides a safe passageway for the median nerve and the distal tendons of the extrinsic finger flexor muscles of the forearm to enter the hand.
  - The distal tendons of the extrinsic finger flexor muscles located within the carpal tunnel are the four tendons of the flexor digitorum superficialis (FDS), four tendons of the flexor digitorum profundus (FDP), and the tendon of the flexor pollicis longus.
  - The radial (lateral) part of the transverse carpal ligament has a superficial part and a deep part. Running between these two parts is the distal tendon of the flexor carpi radialis. Technically, the distal tendon of the flexor carpi radialis is not located within the carpal tunnel.

BOX 9-34

Note 1: The transverse carpal ligament is also known as the **flexor retinaculum** (of the wrist), because it functions as a retinaculum to hold down the extrinsic finger flexor muscles that enter the hand from the forearm. It attaches to the pisiform and hook of the hamate on the ulnar side and to the tubercles of the trapezium and scaphoid on the radial side (see Figure 9-30).

Note 2: If the carpal tunnel is injured, the median nerve may be impinged, causing sensory and/or motor symptoms within the region of the hand that is innervated by the median nerve. This condition is known as **carpal tunnel syndrome**. Sensory symptoms may occur on the anterior side of the thumb, index, middle and radial $^1/_2$ of the ring finger, as well as the posterior side of the fingertips of the same fingers; motor symptoms may result in weakness of the intrinsic thenar muscles of the thumb that are innervated by the median nerve. Individuals who work with their hands, especially bodyworkers and trainers, are particularly susceptible to this condition. Placing excessive pressure through the wrist when doing massage, bodywork, and training should be avoided. Falls on outstretched hands and swelling within the wrist can also cause carpal tunnel syndrome.

Palmar Fascia:

- The hand has a thick layer of dense fibrous tissue on the palmar side known as the **palmar fascia**. Although not as significant as the plantar fascia of the foot, the palmar fascia does increase the structural stability of the hand.

Dorsal Digital Expansion:

- The **dorsal digital expansion** is a fibrous aponeurotic expansion of the distal attachment of the extensor digitorum muscle on the fingers (index, middle, ring, and little) (Figure 9-31).
  - The dorsal digital expansion serves as a movable hood of tissue when the fingers flex and extend.
  - The dorsal digital expansion begins on the dorsal, medial, and lateral sides of the proximal phalanx of each finger and ultimately attaches onto the dorsal side of the middle and distal phalanges.
  - The dorsal digital expansion serves as an attachment site for a number of muscles.
  - These muscles are the lumbricals manus, palmar interossei, dorsal interossei manus, and the abductor digiti minimi manus.

BOX 9-35

Because the dorsal digital expansion eventually attaches onto the dorsal side of the middle and distal phalanges, it crosses the proximal interphalangeal (PIP) joint and the distal interphalangeal (DIP) joint on the dorsal side. Consequently, when any muscle that attaches into the dorsal digital expansion contracts, the pull of its contraction is transferred across these interphalangeal (IP) joints. Therefore all muscles that attach into the dorsal digital expansion can do extension of the fingers at the PIP and DIP joints.

  - The dorsal digital expansion is also known as the **extensor expansion** or the **dorsal hood**.
  - A dorsal digital expansion of the thumb is formed by the distal tendon of the extensor pollicis longus.

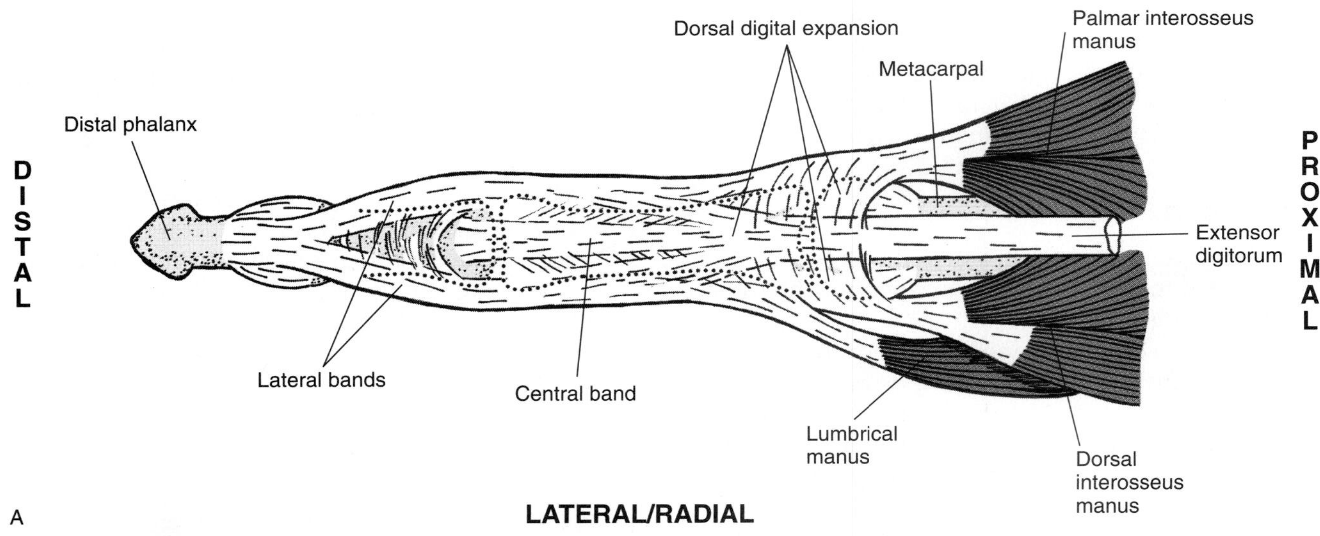

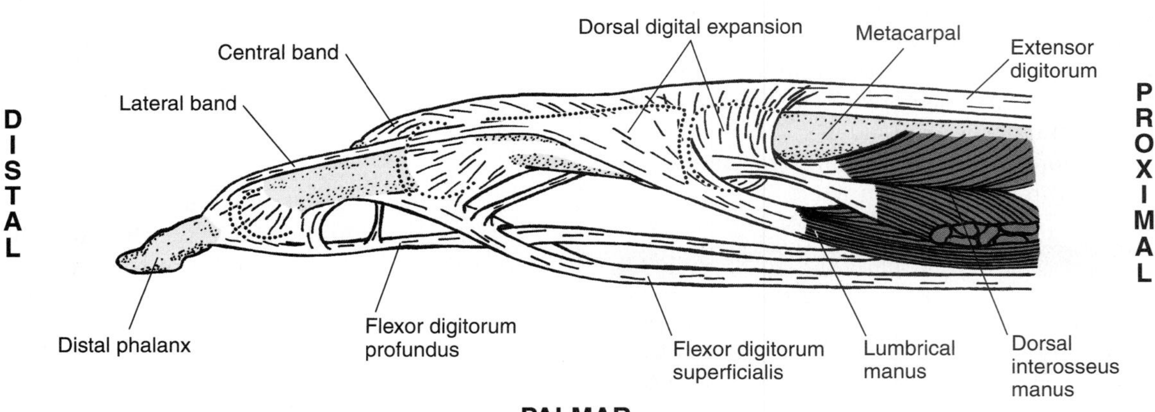

Figure 9-31 Dorsal digital expansion of the right hand. *A,* Dorsal view. *B,* Lateral view. The dorsal digital expansion is a fibrous expansion on fingers #2-5 of the distal tendons of the extensor digitorum muscle. The dorsal digital expansion serves as a movable hood of tissue as the fingers flex and extend; it also serves as an attachment site for a number of intrinsic muscles of the hand. (From Muscolino JE: *The muscular system manual: the skeletal muscles of the human body,* ed. 2. St Louis, 2005, Mosby.)

☐ 9.11 WRIST JOINT COMPLEX

❑ Movement at the wrist joint actually occurs at two joints: (1) the radiocarpal joint and (2) the midcarpal joint. For this reason, the wrist joint is better termed the **wrist joint complex** (Figure 9-32).

BOX 9-36

In addition to the radiocarpal and midcarpal joints, a great number of smaller **intercarpal joints** are located between the individual carpal bones of the wrist (e.g., the scapholunate joint is an intercarpal joint located between the scaphoid and lunate bones). However, these individual intercarpal joints do not contribute to movement of the hand relative to the forearm at the wrist joint.

Radiocarpal Joint:

Bones:

❑ The radiocarpal joint is located between the radius and the carpals.
   ❑ More specifically, the distal end of the radius articulates with the proximal row of carpal bones.
❑ The proximal row of carpals is made up of the scaphoid, lunate, and triquetrum.
❑ Because more than two bones are involved, the radiocarpal joint is a compound joint.
❑ The entire radiocarpal joint is enclosed within one joint cavity.

BOX 9-37

Note 1: The joint between the forearm and the carpal bones is called the *radiocarpal joint* because it is the radius that primarily articulates with the carpals. The ulna itself does not directly articulate with the carpal bones, because many soft tissue structures (of the ulnocarpal complex) are located between them. However, when looking at the wrist joint complex functionally, the **ulnocarpal joint** does transmit 20% of the load from the hand to the forearm when compression forces occur through the wrist (e.g., when doing a push-up). Therefore even though the radiocarpal joint is by far the more significant joint between the forearm and carpus, the ulnocarpal joint does have some functional significance.

Note 2: Even though the pisiform is in the proximal row of carpals, it does not participate in either the radiocarpal joint or the midcarpal joint. The pisiform is considered to be a sesamoid bone and functions to increase the contraction force of the flexor carpi ulnaris and also serve as an attachment site for the transverse carpal ligament that covers the carpal tunnel.

Note 3. The radiocarpal joint shares its joint cavity with the distal radioulnar (RU) joint. (For information on the distal RU joint, see Section 9-9.) Because the radiocarpal joint and the distal RU joint share the same joint capsule, the radioulnar disc (i.e., triangular fibrocartilage) located within this joint capsule is involved with both of these joints.

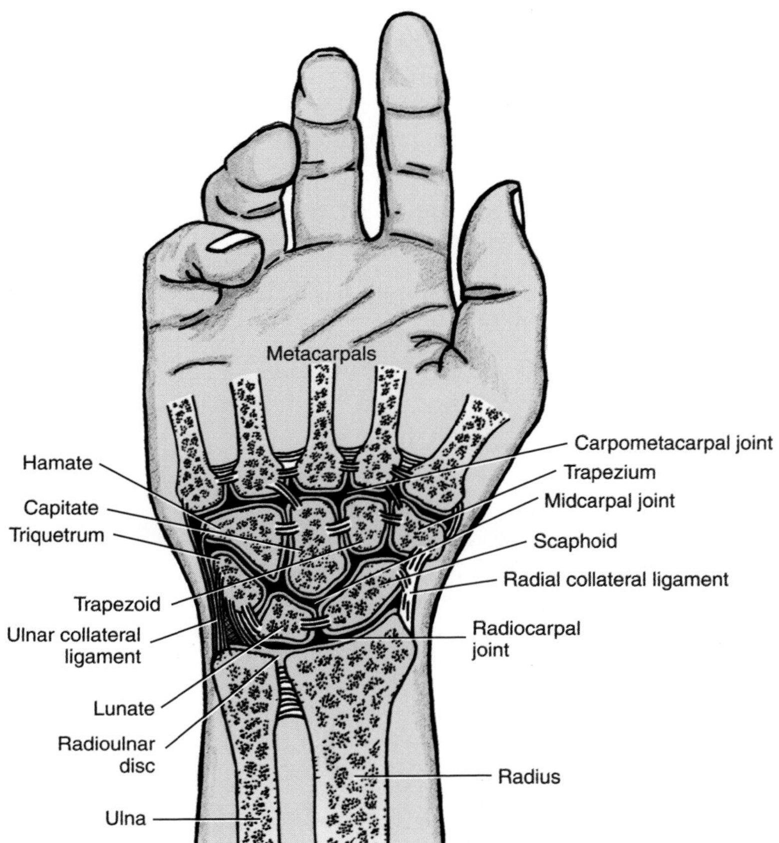

Figure 9-32 Anterior view of the wrist/hand region that illustrates the two major joints of the wrist joint complex. The more proximal joint is the radiocarpal joint; the more distal joint is the midcarpal joint. The radiocarpal joint is located between the distal radius and the proximal row of carpals; the midcarpal joint is located between the proximal row of carpals and the distal row of carpals. (Courtesy Joseph E. Muscolino.)

- In addition, an intra-articular disc is located with the radiocarpal joint.
  - This intra-articular disc is known as the *radioulnar disc* or the *triangular fibrocartilage*.

Midcarpal Joint:

Bones:

- The midcarpal joint is located between the proximal row of carpal bones and the distal row of carpal bones.
  - More specifically, the midcarpal joint is located between the scaphoid, lunate, and triquetrum proximally, and the trapezium, trapezoid, capitate, and hamate distally.
- Because more than two bones are involved, the midcarpal joint is a compound joint.
- The joint capsule of the midcarpal joint is anatomically separate from the joint capsule of the radiocarpal joint.
- The joint surfaces and capsule of the midcarpal joint are fairly irregular in shape and are continuous with the individual intercarpal joints of all the bones involved.

BOX 9-38

Because the midcarpal joint is so irregular in shape and the joint capsule is continuous with the joint spaces between the separate intercarpal joints involved, the midcarpal joint is often described as being more of a functional joint than an anatomic joint.

- The midcarpal joint is usually divided into a medial compartment and a lateral compartment.
  - The medial compartment is larger and its orientation is similar to the radiocarpal joint; its proximal surface is concave and its distal surface is convex. It is a compound joint formed between the proximal pole of the scaphoid, and the lunate and triquetrum proximally, and the capitate and hamate distally.
  - The lateral compartment is smaller and its orientation is opposite to the medial compartment; its proximal surface is convex and its distal surface is concave. It is a compound joint formed between the distal pole of the scaphoid proximally, and the trapezium and trapezoid distally.

Both Radiocarpal and Midcarpal Joints:

- Joint structure classification: Synovial joint
  - Subtype: Condyloid
- Joint function classification: Diarthrotic
  - Subtype: Biaxial

Major Motions Allowed:

- Flexion and extension of the hand (i.e., axial actions) in the sagittal plane around a mediolateral axis (Figure 9-33a-b; Table 9-9)
- Radial deviation and ulnar deviation (i.e., axial actions) of the hand in the frontal plane around an anteroposterior axis (Figure 9-33c-d)

BOX 9-39

From anatomic position, radial deviation (i.e., abduction) of the hand at the wrist joint is minimal as a result of the impingement of the carpus against the styloid process of the radius, which is located at the radial side of the radius. Ulnar deviation (i.e., adduction) is not as limited because the styloid process of the ulna is located posteriorly, not on the ulnar side of the ulna.

  - Note: Radial deviation is also known as *abduction*; ulnar deviation is also known as *adduction*.

Accessory Motions:

- The carpal bones permit a great deal of gliding motion.

Reverse Actions:

- The forearm can move relative to the hand at the wrist joint. This would occur when the hand is fixed (closed-chain activity), perhaps grasping an immovable object.

Major Ligaments of the Wrist Joint Complex:

The wrist joint complex has many ligaments (Figure 9-34; Box 9-40):

TABLE 9-9

Average Ranges of Motion of the Hand at the Wrist Joint from Anatomic Position

Flexion	80 Degrees	Extension	70 Degrees
Radial deviation	15 Degrees	Ulnar deviation	30 Degrees

The reader should keep two things in mind concerning the ranges of motion of the hand at the two compound joints of the wrist joint complex:
1. Flexion is greater at the radiocarpal joint and extension is greater at the midcarpal joint.
2. Radial deviation is greater at the midcarpal joint, and ulnar deviation occurs equally at the radiocarpal and midcarpal joints.

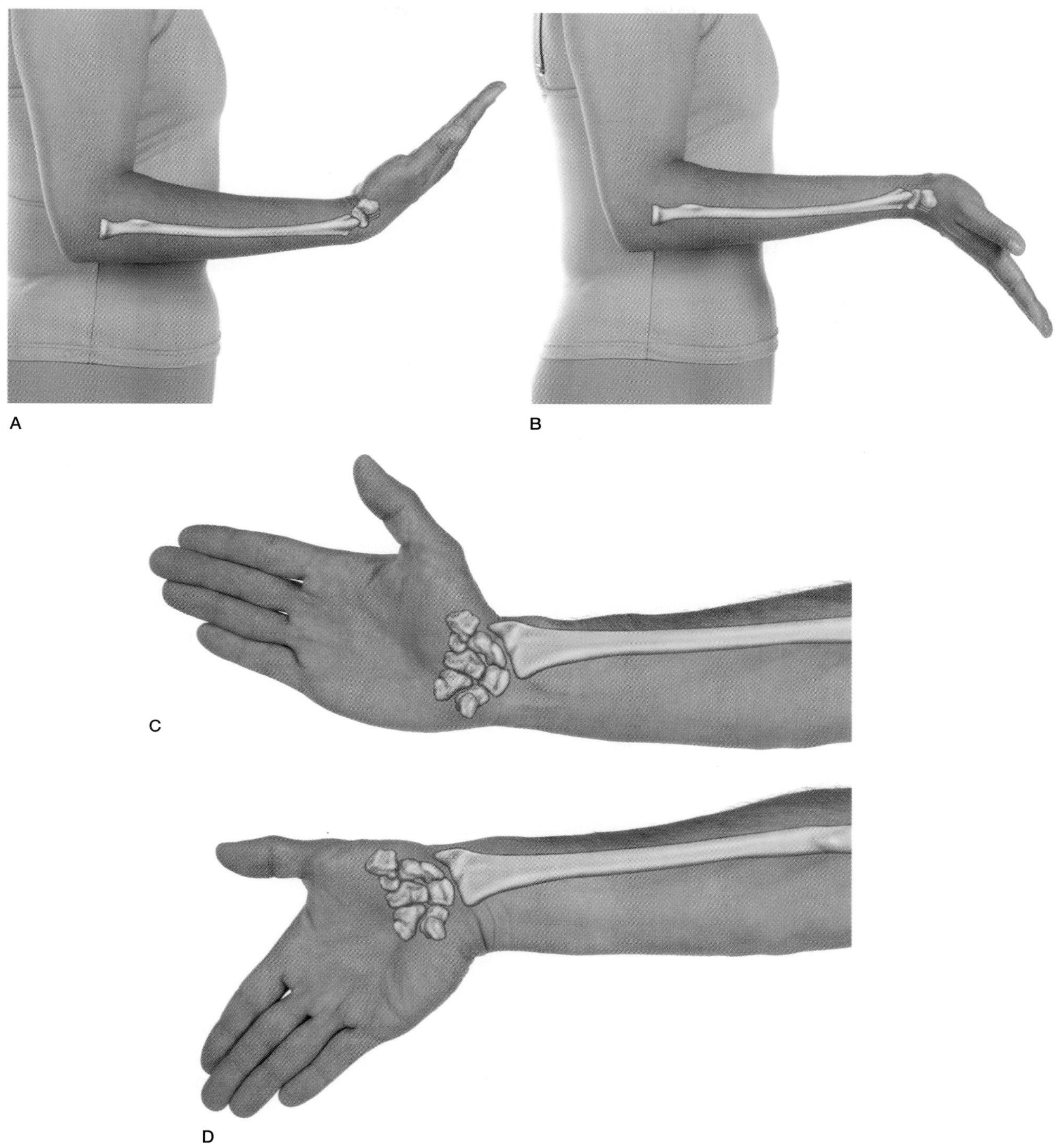

Figure 9-33 Motions of the hand at the wrist joint (radiocarpal and midcarpal joints). *A* and *B,* Lateral views illustrating flexion and extension of the hand, respectively. *C* and *D,* Anterior views illustrating radial deviation and ulnar deviation, respectively. Radial deviation of the hand is also known as *abduction*; ulnar deviation is also known as *adduction*.

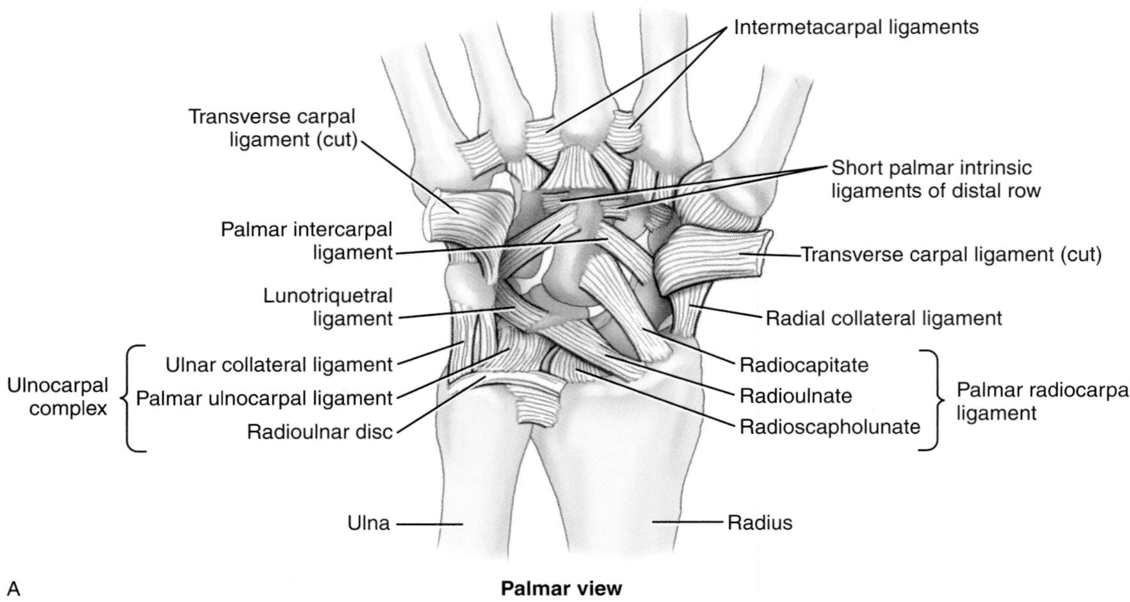

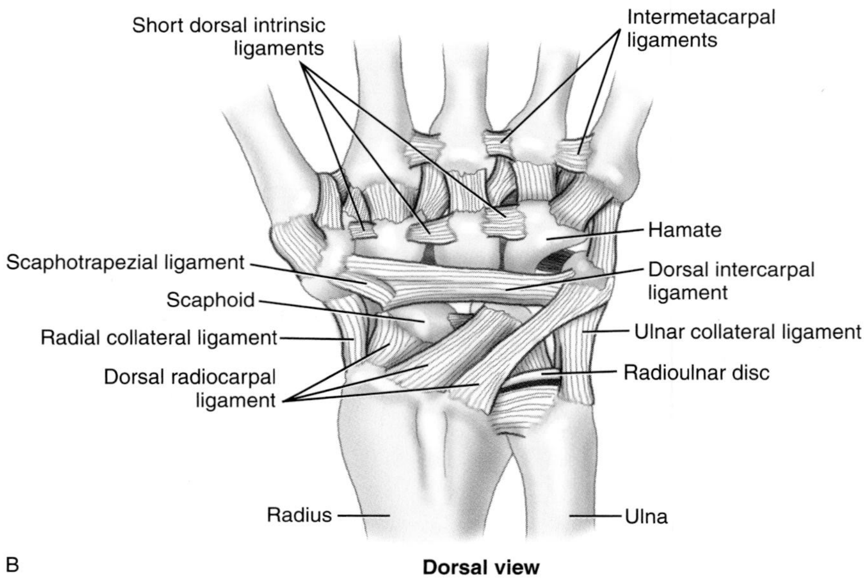

Figure 9-34 Ligaments of the right wrist joint complex region. *A,* Palmar (i.e., anterior) view. *B,* Dorsal (i.e., posterior) view. Most of the wrist joint complex ligaments are divided into two broad categories: (1) extrinsic ligaments that originate in the forearm and then attach onto the carpus and (2) intrinsic ligaments that originate and insert (i.e., are wholly located within) the carpus. The major extrinsic ligaments are the radial and ulnar collaterals and the dorsal and palmar radiocarpal ligaments. Intrinsic ligaments are divided into short, intermediate, and long ligaments. Two long intrinsic ligaments are the dorsal and palmar intercarpal ligaments. (Note: The intermetacarpal [IMC] ligaments of the proximal IMC joints are also seen.)

BOX 9-40

LIGAMENTS OF THE WRIST JOINT COMPLEX

- Fibrous capsule of the radiocarpal joint
- Radioulnar (RU) disc (i.e., triangular fibrocartilage)
- Fibrous capsule of the midcarpal joint
- Transverse carpal ligament

Extrinsic Ligaments
- Dorsal radiocarpal ligament
- Palmar radiocarpal ligaments
- Radial collateral ligament
- Ulnar collateral ligament

Intrinsic Ligaments
- Short
- Intermediate
- Long

Joint Capsule of the Radiocarpal Joint:

❑ The radiocarpal joint capsule is thickened and strengthened by the dorsal radiocarpal, palmar radiocarpal, radial collateral, and ulnar collateral ligaments.

Radioulnar Disc (Triangular Fibrocartilage):

❑ As its name indicates, the **radioulnar disc** is attached to the radius and ulna.

❑ It adds to the stability of the radiocarpal joint, because it blends into the capsular/ligamentous structure of the radiocarpal joint.

Joint Capsule of the Midcarpal Joint:

❑ Transverse carpal ligament: The transverse carpal ligament forms the roof of the carpal tunnel.
  - ❑ It attaches to the tubercles of the scaphoid and trapezium radially and to the pisiform and hook of hamate on the ulnar side.
  - ❑ Its function is to enclose and stabilize the carpal tunnel.
  - ❑ It also functions as a retinaculum for the extrinsic finger flexor muscles of the forearm that enter the hand.
  - ❑ The transverse carpal ligament is also known as the *flexor retinaculum of the wrist.*

❑ All other wrist joint ligaments are classified as *extrinsic* or *intrinsic*.
  - ❑ **Extrinsic ligaments** attach onto one or both of the forearm bones and then attach distally onto carpal bones. They stabilize the radiocarpal joint. If they cross the midcarpal joint, they add to the stability of that joint as well.
  - ❑ **Intrinsic ligaments** attach proximally and distally onto carpal bones, crossing and stabilizing the midcarpal joint.

Extrinsic Ligaments:

❑ Function: Extrinsic ligaments limit motion primarily at the radiocarpal joint.

Dorsal Radiocarpal Ligament:

❑ Location: The **dorsal radiocarpal ligament** is located on the dorsal (i.e., posterior) side from the radius to the carpal bones).

❑ Function: It limits full flexion.

BOX 9-41

Regarding the radiocarpal ligaments of the wrist joint complex, one dorsal radiocarpal ligament and three palmar radiocarpal ligaments exist. All radiocarpal ligaments attach the radius to carpal bones, as their names imply. The dorsal radiocarpal ligament attaches the radius to the capitate, lunate, and scaphoid bones. The three palmar radiocarpal ligaments are (1) the **radiocapitate ligament**, (2) the **radiolunate ligament**, and (3) the **radioscapholunate ligament**. These ligaments attach the radius to the bones stated within their names.

Palmar Radiocarpal Ligaments:

❑ Location: The **palmar radiocarpal ligaments** are located on the palmar (i.e., anterior) side from the radius to the carpal bones.

❑ Function: They limit full extension.

Radial Collateral Ligament:

❑ Location: The **radial collateral ligament** is located on the radial side, from the radius to the carpal bones.
  - ❑ More specifically, it is located from the styloid process of the radius to the scaphoid and trapezium.

❑ Function: It limits ulnar deviation (i.e., adduction).

Ulnar Collateral Ligament:

❑ Location: The **ulnar collateral ligament** is located on the ulnar side, from the ulna to the carpal bones.

BOX 9-42

Many sources describe the ligaments between the distal end of the ulna and the carpus on the ulnar side of the wrist as being the **ulnocarpal complex;** included in this complex are the ulnar collateral ligament, the palmar ulnocarpal ligament, and the radioulnar disc (triangular fibrocartilage).

  - ❑ More specifically, it is located from the styloid process of the ulna to the triquetrum.

❑ Function: It limits radial deviation (i.e., abduction).

Intrinsic Ligaments:

❑ Function: Intrinsic ligaments stabilize and limit motion between carpal bones.

❑ The intrinsic ligaments of the wrist are divided into short, intermediate, and long ligaments.
  - ❑ Short: Short intrinsic ligaments connect the distal row carpal bones to each other.
  - ❑ Intermediate: The intermediate ligaments primarily function to connect the bones of the proximal row together.

- Long: The long intrinsic ligaments connect the scaphoid, triquetrum, and capitate to each other.
- Note: Two long ligaments exist: (1) the **dorsal intercarpal ligament** and (2) the **palmar intercarpal ligament**.

Closed-Packed Position of the Wrist Joint:

- Extension and slight ulnar deviation

BOX 9-43

Having extension as the closed-packed position of the wrist joint complex allows for greater stability when doing such activities as crawling on hands and knees and performing pushups.

Major Muscles of the Wrist Joint:

- The muscles that cross the wrist joint may be divided into four major groups: those that cross on the anterior, posterior, radial, and/or on the ulnar side.
- The anterior muscles can all do flexion.
  - The major flexors are the flexor carpi radialis, palmaris longus, and flexor carpi ulnaris (collectively known as the *wrist flexor group*), as well as the finger flexors (flexors digitorum superficialis and profundus).
- The posterior muscles can all do extension.
  - The major extensors are the extensor carpi radialis longus, extensor carpi radialis brevis, and extensor carpi ulnaris (collectively known as the *wrist extensor group*), as well as the finger extensors (extensors digitorum and digiti minimi).
- The radial muscles all can do radial deviation (i.e., abduction).
  - The major radial deviators are the flexor carpi radialis and extensors carpi radialis longus and brevis.
- The ulnar muscles can all do ulnar deviation (i.e., adduction).
  - The major ulnar deviators are the flexor carpi ulnaris and extensor carpi ulnaris.
- Of course all other muscles that cross the wrist can also create motion at the wrist joint; the specific action would be determined by which side(s) of the wrist joint the muscle crosses.

☐ 9.12 CARPOMETACARPAL JOINTS

- The carpometacarpal (CMC) joints are located between the distal row of carpal bones and the metacarpal bones (Figure 9-35).
- Five CMC joints exist:
  1. The 1st CMC joint is located primarily between the trapezium and the base of the 1st metacarpal.
  2. The 2nd CMC joint is located primarily between the trapezoid and the base of the 2nd metacarpal.
  3. The 3rd CMC joint is located primarily between the capitate and the base of the 3rd metacarpal.
  4. The 4th CMC joint is located primarily between the hamate and the base of the 4th metacarpal.
  5. The 5th CMC joint is located primarily between the hamate and the base of the 5th metacarpal.
- Note: Each metacarpal and its associated phalanges make up a ray of the hand.

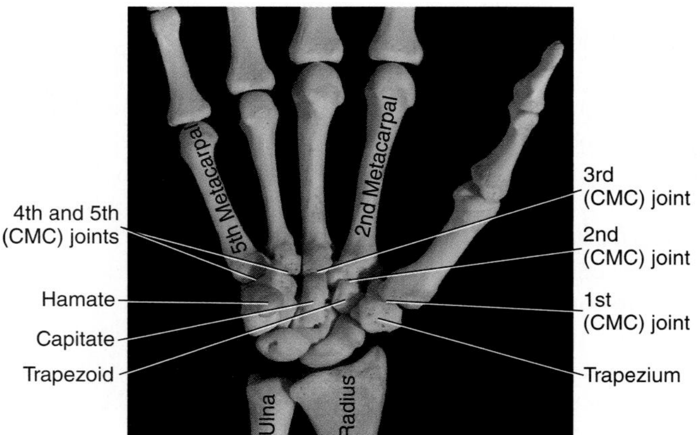

Figure 9-35 Anterior view of the carpometacarpal (CMC) joints. Five CMC joints are formed between the distal row of carpals and the metacarpal bones.

2nd and 3rd CMC Joints:

- Joint structure classification: Synovial joint
  - Subtype: Plane
- Joint function classification: Synarthrotic
  - Subtype: Nonaxial

1st, 5th, and 4th CMC Joints:

- Joint structure classification: Synovial joint
  - Subtype: Saddle
- Joint function classification: Diarthrotic
  - Subtype: Biaxial

CMC Joint Motion:

- The more peripheral CMC joints are more mobile, creating more mobile rays (Figure 9-36).
- The (1st) CMC saddle joint of the thumb is the most mobile, allowing the thumb to oppose the other fingers (i.e., move toward the center of the palm) (see Section 9.13, Figure 9-39, or Section 5.23, Figure 5.24). (For more details on the CMC joint of the thumb, see Section 9.13.)

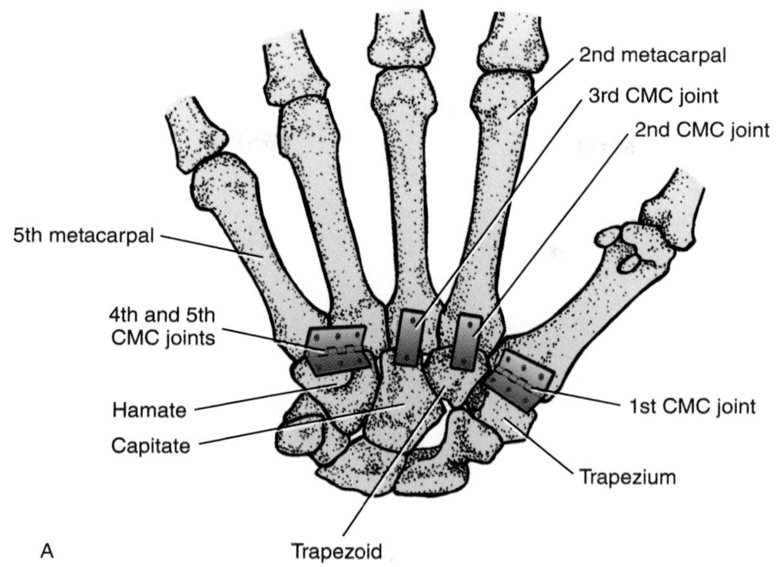

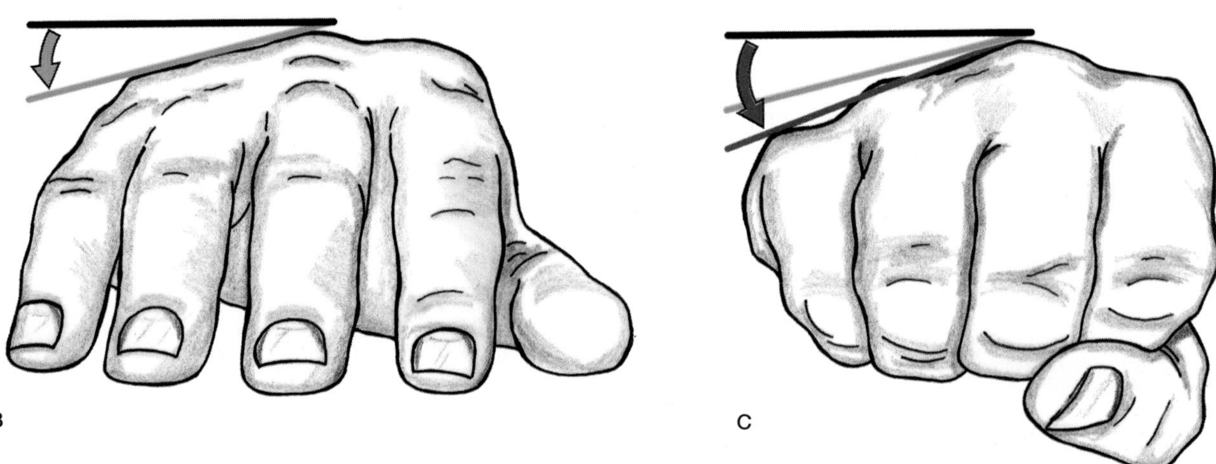

Figure 9-36 Motion of the carpometacarpal (CMC) joints of the hand. *A,* Anterior view of the right hand that depicts the concept of the relative mobility of the 1st, 5th, and 4th CMC joints and the relative rigidity/stability of the 2nd and 3rd CMC joints. The 2nd and 3rd rays form the stable central pillar of the hand. *B* and *C,* Two views of the hand that show the motion of the 4th and 5th CMC joints that is evident when the fingers flex. Motion of the CMC joints assists the 1st, 4th, and 5th rays of the hand to close around the central pillar of the hand, resulting in a firm grasp on objects held in the hand. (*A* modeled from Neumann DA: *Kinesiology of the musculoskeletal system: foundations for physical rehabilitation.* St Louis, 2002, Mosby; parts *B* and *C* courtesy Joseph E. Muscolino.)

- The 5th and 4th CMC joints are also fairly mobile, allowing the ulnar side of the hand (the 5th and 4th metacarpals) to fold toward the center of the palm (see Box 9-44).
- Therefore the 1st ray is the most mobile, followed by the 5th and then 4th ray.
- The 2nd and 3rd CMC joints are relatively rigid, forming a stable **central pillar of the hand**. When the hand grasps and closes in around an object, the central pillar of the hand stays fixed and the other rays close in around it.

BOX 9-44

The ability of the 4th, 5th, and 1st metacarpals to fold toward the center of the palm increases the distal transverse arch of the hand, creating a better grip on objects held.

Major Motions Allowed:

- The CMC joints primarily allow flexion/extension (see Figure 9-36; Table 9-10).
- The CMC joints are stabilized by their joint capsules, as well as **carpometacarpal (CMC) ligaments**.

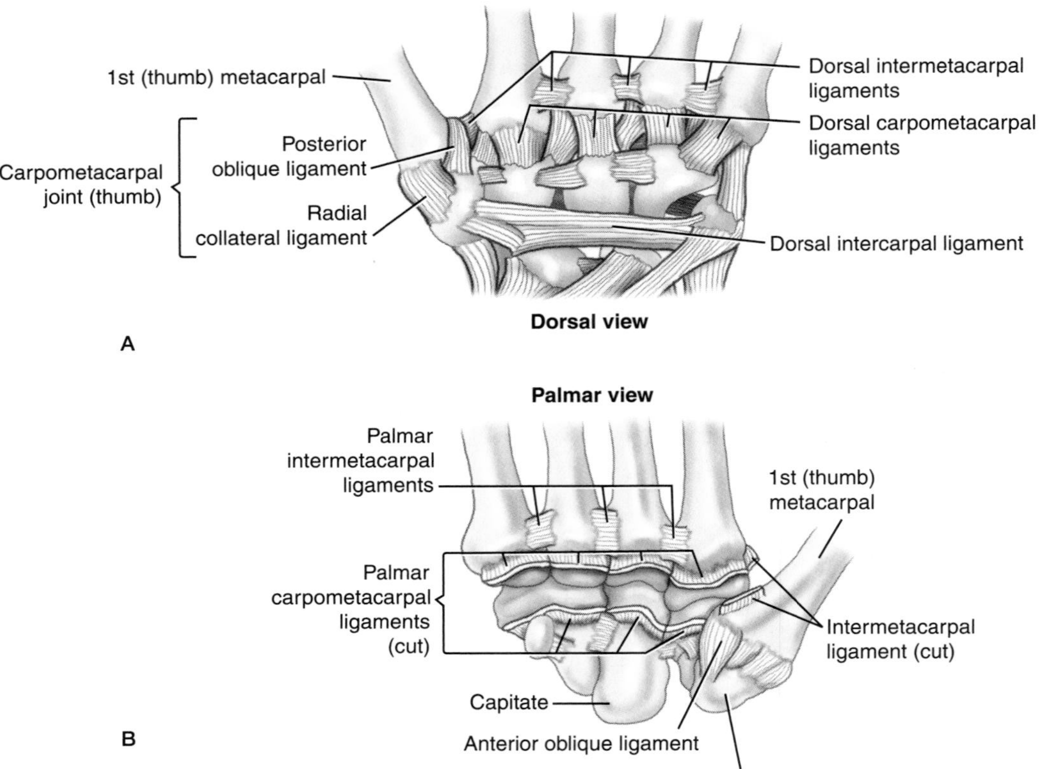

Figure 9-37 Dorsal and palmar carpometacarpal (CMC) ligaments of the CMC joints of fingers #2-5. *A,* Dorsal (i.e., posterior) view. *B,* Palmar (i.e., anterior) view with the carpometacarpal joints opened up. (Note: The CMC ligaments of the saddle joint of the thumb are also seen.) (Modeled from Neumann DA: *Kinesiology of the musculoskeletal system: foundations for physical rehabilitation.* St Louis, 2002, Mosby.)

TABLE 9-10

Average Ranges of Motion from Anatomic Position of the Metacarpals at the 2nd-5th Carpometacarpal (CMC) Joints*

	Flexion	Extension
5th CMC	20 Degrees	0 Degrees
4th CMC	10 Degrees	0 Degrees
3rd CMC	0 Degrees	0 Degrees
2nd CMC	0-2 Degrees	0 Degrees

Notes: 1. Some abduction/adduction occurs at the 4th and 5th CMC joints.
2. Some lateral rotation/medial rotation occurs at the 5th CMC joints.
3. The abduction/adduction and lateral/medial rotation motions of the 5th metacarpal at the 5th CMC joint allow for opposition/reposition of the little finger.

*Ranges of the motion of the metacarpal of the thumb at the 1st CMC joint are covered in Section 9-13, Table 9-11.

❑ The **CMC** ligaments are the **dorsal carpometacarpal ligaments,** the **palmar carpometacarpal ligaments,** and the **interosseus carpometacarpal ligaments** (Figure 9-37).

BOX 9-45

LIGAMENTS OF THE CARPOMETACARPAL (CMC) JOINTS

- Fibrous capsules

CMC ligaments:
- Dorsal CMC ligaments
- Plantar CMC ligaments
- Interosseus CMC ligaments

Miscellaneous:

❑ As stated, a metacarpal and its associated phalanges make up a ray. Therefore motion of a metacarpal at its CMC joint is functionally related to motion of the phalanges of that ray at the MCP and IP joints. In other words, metacarpal movement is related to finger movement.

❑ The word *pollicis* means *thumb.*

❑ The word *digital* refers to fingers #2-5 (or toes #2-5).

9.13 SADDLE (CARPOMETACARPAL) JOINT OF THE THUMB

- The saddle joint of the thumb is the 1st CMC joint (Figure 9-38).
- The **saddle joint of the thumb** is the classic example of a saddle joint in the human body. (See Section 6.11, for more information on saddle joints.)

Bones:

- The saddle joint of the thumb is located between the trapezium and the 1st metacarpal (the metacarpal of the thumb).
  - More specifically, the distal end of the trapezium articulates with the base of the 1st metacarpal.

BOX 9-46

Because of its tremendous use, degenerative arthritic changes are commonly found at the saddle joint of the thumb. This condition is called **basilar arthritis**, because the saddle joint of the thumb is the base joint of the entire thumb.

- Joint Structure Classification: Synovial
  - Subtype: Saddle
- Joint Function Classification: Diarthrotic
  - Subtype: Biaxial

BOX 9-47

The saddle joint of the thumb is usually classified as a *biaxial joint*. However, this joint actually permits motion in three planes about three axes; therefore it could also be classified as *triaxial*. However, its rotation actions in the transverse plane cannot be actively isolated. Because of the shape of the bones of the joint, medial rotation of the 1st metacarpal must accompany flexion of the 1st metacarpal, and lateral rotation must accompany extension. Because the third axial actions of rotation cannot be actively isolated, this joint is most often classified as being *biaxial*.

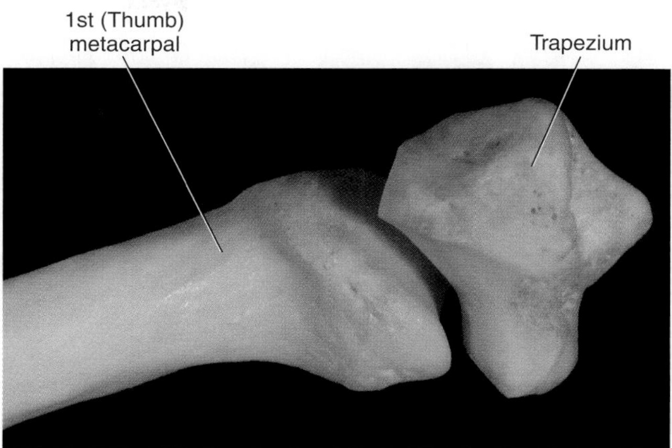

Figure 9-38 Palmar (i.e., anterior) view of the 1st carpometacarpal (CMC) (i.e., saddle) joint of the thumb of the right hand. The reason that this joint is called a *saddle joint* is evident. That is, each articular surface is concave in one direction and convex in the other; further, the convexity of one bone fits into the concavity of the other bone.

Major Motions Allowed:

The saddle joint of the thumb allows several major motions (Figure 9-39; Table 9-11):

BOX 9-48

It is usually stated that the thumb moves at the saddle (i.e., carpometacarpal [CMC]) joint. To be more specific, it can be stated that the 1st metacarpal (of the thumb) moves at the thumb's saddle joint. The thumb can also move at its metacarpophalangeal (MCP) and interphalangeal (IP) joints. The proximal phalanx moves at the MCP joint, and the distal phalanx moves at the IP joint.

TABLE 9-11

Average Ranges of Motion of the Metacarpal of the Thumb at the Thumb's Saddle Joint (1st Carpometacarpal [CMC] Joint) from Anatomic Position

Abduction	60 Degrees	Adduction	10 Degrees
Flexion	40 Degrees	Extension	10 Degrees
Medial rotation	45 Degrees	Lateral rotation	0 Degrees

Note: Anatomic position has the thumb in near full extension and adduction.

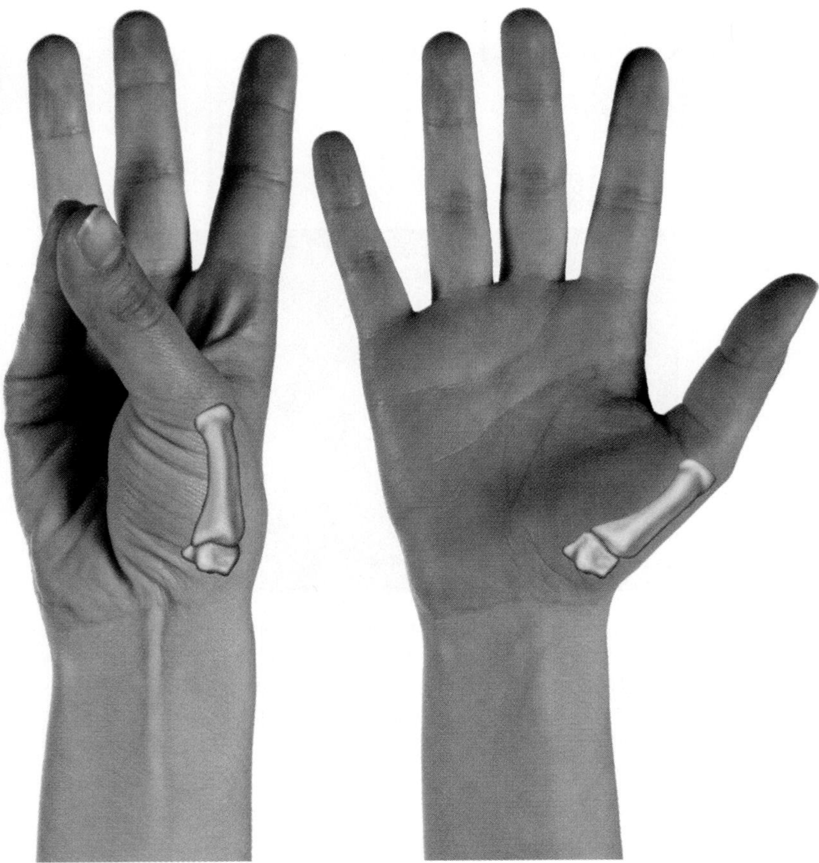

Figure 9-39 Actions of the thumb at the 1st carpometacarpal (CMC) joint (also known as the *saddle joint of the thumb*). *A* and *B,* Opposition and reposition of the thumb, respectively. Opposition and reposition are actually combinations of actions; the component actions of opposition and reposition are shown in *C* to *F. C* and *D,* Flexion and extension, respectively; these actions occur within the frontal plane. *E* and *F,* Abduction and adduction, respectively; these actions occur within the sagittal plane. Medial rotation and lateral rotation are not shown separately, because these actions cannot occur in isolation; they must occur in conjunction with flexion and extension. (Note: Flexion of the phalanges of the thumb and little finger at metacarpophalangeal joint is also seen in *A*; flexion of the thumb at the interphalangeal joint is also seen in *C.*)

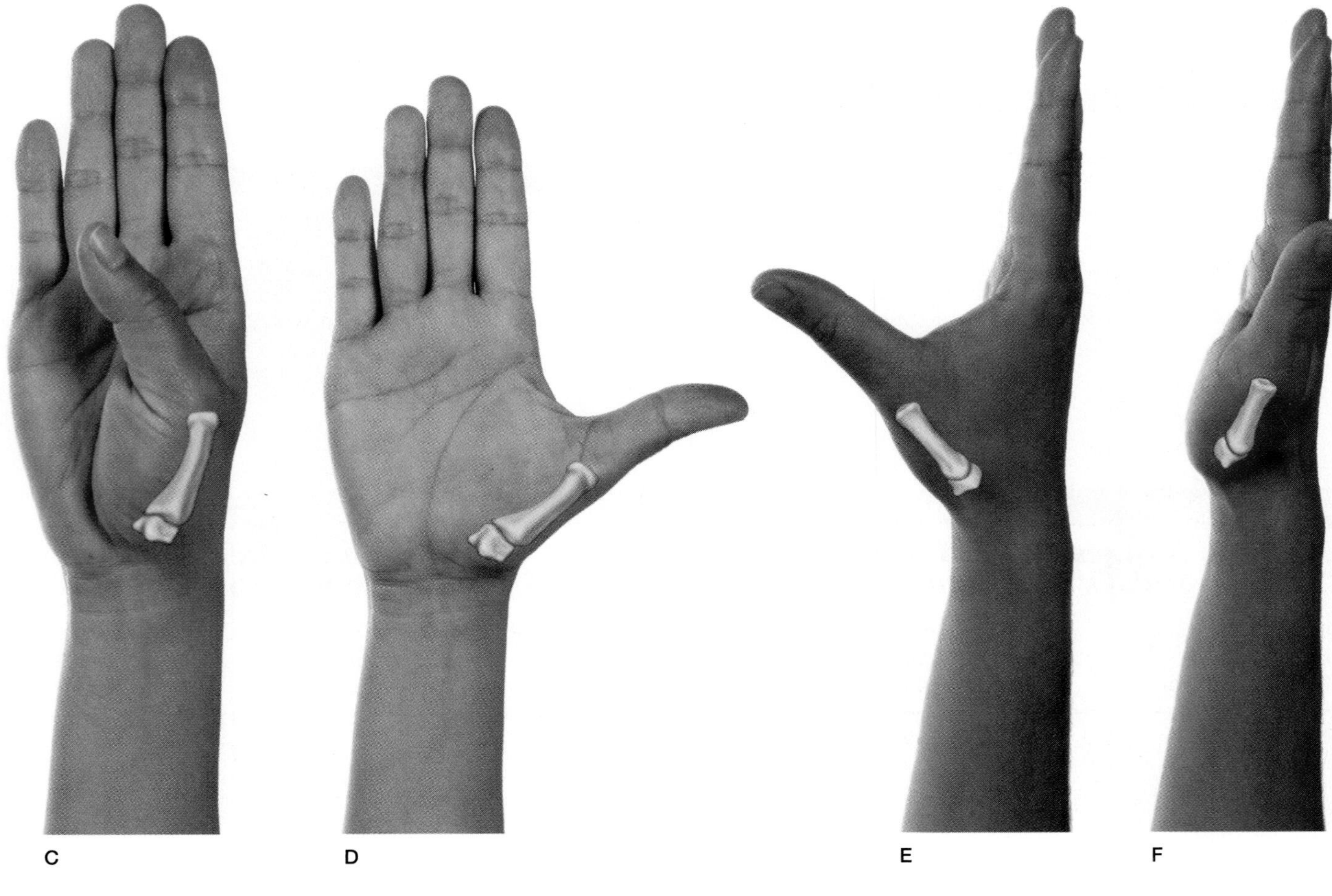

- Opposition and reposition of the thumb
  - Opposition and reposition of the thumb are not specific actions, they are combinations of actions.
  - Opposition is a combination of abduction, flexion, and medial rotation of the thumb's metacarpal; reposition is a combination of adduction, extension, and lateral rotation of the thumb's metacarpal. (For more on opposition/reposition, see Section 5.23.)
- Flexion and extension of the thumb in the frontal plane around an anteroposterior axis.
- Abduction and adduction of the thumb in the sagittal plane around a mediolateral axis.
- Medial rotation and lateral rotation of the thumb in the transverse plane around a vertical axis.

BOX 9-49

Because of the rotation of the thumb that occurs embryologically, flexion and extension occur within the frontal plane instead of the sagittal plane, and abduction and adduction occur within the sagittal plane instead of the frontal plane. (For more on opposition/reposition of the thumb, see Section 5.23.)

Reverse Actions:

- The trapezium of the wrist (along with the remainder of the hand) could move relative to the metacarpal of the thumb.

Major Ligaments of the Saddle Joint of the Thumb:

The saddle joint of the thumb has several major ligaments (Figure 9-40; Box 9-50):

- The CMC joint of the thumb is stabilized by its fibrous joint capsule and five major ligaments.
- The fibrous joint capsule of the thumb is loose, allowing large ranges of motion.
- Generally the ligaments of the thumb become taut in full opposition and/or full abduction or full extension.

Radial Collateral Ligament:

- Location: The **radial collateral ligament** is located on the radial side of the joint.
  - More specifically, it is located from the radial surface of the trapezium to the base of the metacarpal of the thumb.

Ulnar Collateral Ligament:

- Location: The **ulnar collateral ligament** is located on the ulnar side of the joint.
  - More specifically, it is located from the transverse carpal ligament to the base of the metacarpal of the thumb.

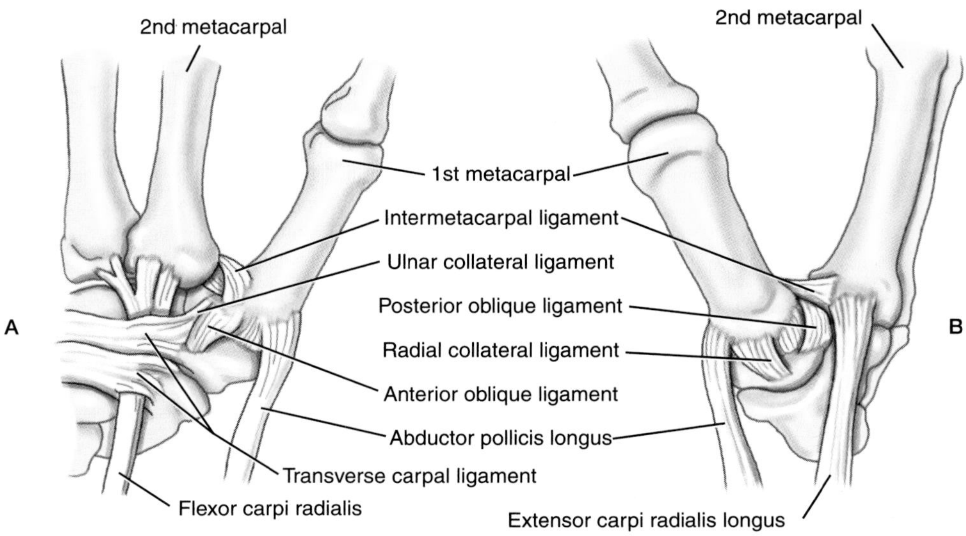

Figure 9-40 Ligaments of the 1st carpometacarpal (CMC) (i.e., saddle) joint of the right thumb. *A,* Palmar (i.e., anterior) view in which the ulnar collateral and anterior oblique ligaments are seen. *B,* Radial (i.e., lateral) view in which the radial collateral and posterior oblique ligaments are seen. (Note: The intermetacarpal [IMC] ligament between the thumb and index finger is also seen.) (Modeled from Neumann DA: *Kinesiology of the musculoskeletal system: foundations for physical rehabilitation.* St Louis, 2002, Mosby.)

Anterior Oblique Ligament:

- Location: The **anterior oblique ligament** is located on the anterior side of the joint.
  - More specifically, it is located from the tubercle of the trapezium to the base of the metacarpal of the thumb.

Posterior Oblique Ligament:

- Location: The **posterior oblique ligament** is located on the posterior side of the joint.
  - More specifically, it is located from the posterior surface of the trapezium to the palmar-ulnar surface of the base of the metacarpal of the thumb.

1st Intermetacarpal Ligament:

- Location: The **1st intermetacarpal ligament** is located between metacarpals of the thumb and index finger (i.e., the 1st and 2nd metacarpals).
  - More specifically, it is located from the base of the metacarpal of the index finger to the base of the metacarpal of the thumb.

BOX 9-50

LIGAMENTS OF THE SADDLE JOINT (CARPOMETACARPAL [CMC] JOINT) OF THE THUMB

- Fibrous capsule
- Radial collateral ligament
- Ulnar collateral ligament
- Anterior oblique ligament
- Posterior oblique ligament
- 1st Intermetacarpal (IMC) ligament

Closed-Packed Position of the Saddle Joint of the Thumb:

- Full opposition

Major Muscles of the Saddle Joint of the Thumb:

- The muscles of the saddle joint of the thumb can be divided into extrinsic muscles (that originate on the arm and/or forearm) and intrinsic muscles (wholly located within the hand).
  - The extrinsic muscles are the flexor pollicis longus, extensors pollicis longus and brevis, and abductor pollicis longus.
  - The intrinsic muscles of the thumb are the three muscles of the thenar eminence (i.e., the abductor and flexor pollicis brevis and the opponens pollicis) and the adductor pollicis.

BOX 9-51 SPOTLIGHT ON OPPOSITION OF THE THUMB

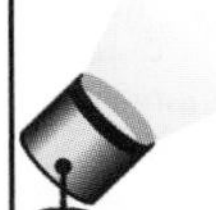

Opposition is usually defined simply as the pad of the thumb meeting the pad of another finger. Most textbooks will then state that opposition is a combination of three component actions: (1) abduction, (2) flexion, and (3) medial rotation of the thumb (more specifically, the metacarpal of the thumb at the carpometacarpal [CMC] joint [i.e., the saddle joint] of the thumb). However, the exact component motions and the degree of those component motions that are necessary to create opposition will vary based on three factors:

1. The starting position of the thumb: If the thumb begins opposition from anatomic position, more abduction is needed than if the thumb begins opposition from the *relaxed* position of the thumb wherein it is already in some degree of abduction.
2. The finger to which the thumb is being opposed: For example, it takes relatively more flexion to oppose the thumb to the little finger than it does to oppose the thumb to the index finger.
3. The position of the finger to which the thumb is being opposed: If the finger to which the thumb is being opposed is held fixed in or close to anatomic position (it does not move toward the thumb), then the thumb may have to adduct, depending on the position from which it began opposition. If instead the finger to which the thumb is being opposed is flexed toward the thumb, then the thumb would most likely not need to adduct.

Given this discussion, it should be clear that the opponens pollicis is not the only muscle that can help create opposition of the thumb. The degree to which each muscle contributes to opposition will vary based on the exact component motions of opposition in a particular situation.

9.14 INTERMETACARPAL JOINTS

Bones:

- **Intermetacarpal (IMC) joints** are located between the metacarpal bones of the hand (Figure 9-41a).
- Proximal IMC joints and distal IMC joints exist.
- All five metacarpals (#1-5) articulate with each other proximally at their bases; hence four proximal IMC joints exist.
- Only metacarpals #2-5 articulate with each other distally at their heads; hence three distal IMC joints exist.

IMC Motion:

- These IMC joints allow nonaxial gliding motion of one metacarpal relative to the adjacent metacarpal(s).
- Apart from the motion between the 1st and 2nd metacarpals, the joint between the 5th and 4th metacarpals allows the most motion.
- Motion between the metacarpals at the IMC joints increases the ability of the hand to close in around an object and grasp it securely. For this reason, the 1st and 5th metacarpals (i.e., the metacarpals on either side of the hand) are the most mobile.
- Joint structure classification: Synovial joint
  - Subtype: Plane
- Joint function classification: Amphiarthrotic
  - Subtype: Nonaxial

Intermetacarpal Ligaments:

- IMC joints are stabilized by their fibrous capsules and ligaments (Figure 9-41b).
- The proximal IMC joints are stabilized by the **intermetacarpal (IMC) ligaments** that connect the base of each of the five metacarpals to the base of the adjacent metacarpal(s).
- The distal IMC joints (between metacarpals #2-5) are stabilized by **deep transverse metacarpal ligaments** that connect the heads of metacarpals #2-5.

BOX 9-52

LIGAMENTS OF THE INTERMETACARPAL JOINTS

Proximal Intermetacarpal (IMC) Joints:
- Fibrous capsules
- IMC ligaments

Distal IMC Joints:
- Fibrous capsules
- Deep transverse metacarpal ligaments

BOX 9-53

Note 1: Three sets of intermetacarpal (IMC) ligaments stabilize the proximal IMC joints: (1) **dorsal intermetacarpal ligaments**, (2) **palmar intermetacarpal ligaments**, and (3) **interosseus intermetacarpal ligaments**. (Note: IMC ligaments of the proximal IMC joints are also known simply as **metacarpal ligaments**.)

Note 2: Stability of the proximal intermetacarpal joints indirectly helps to stabilize the associated carpometacarpal (CMC) joints of the hand.

Note 3: Although all five distal ends of the metatarsals in the foot are connected by deep intermetatarsal ligaments, the hand does not have a deep transverse metacarpal ligament connecting the distal ends of the metacarpals of the thumb and index finger. The absence of this ligament between the thumb and index finger is one aspect that allows the thumb much greater range of motion than the big toe of the foot. Therefore the hand is designed primarily for manipulation (i.e., fine motion), whereas the foot is designed primarily for weight bearing and propulsion. In theory, the only difference between the potential coordination of the hand and the foot is the ability to oppose digits.

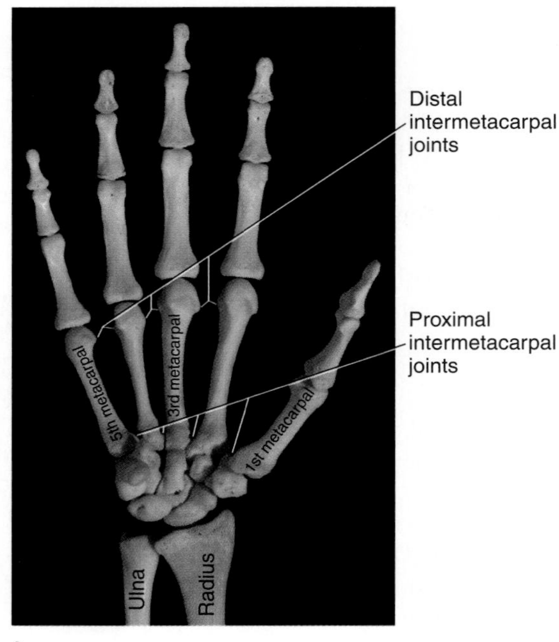

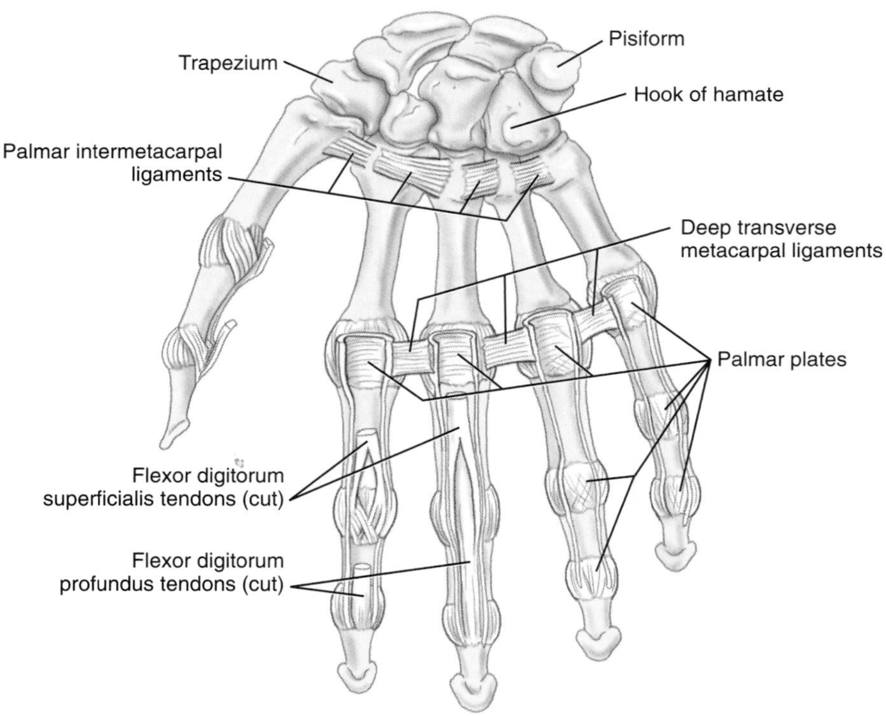

Figure 9-41 Intermetacarpal (IMC) joints of the hand. *A,* Anterior view shows the osseous joints. (Note: Three proximal IMC joints and four distal IMC joints exist.) *B,* Anterior view illustrates the ligaments of the proximal and distal IMC joints. Proximal IMC joints are stabilized by intermetacarpal ligaments. Distal IMC joints are stabilized by deep transverse metacarpal ligaments. (Note: Palmar plates of the metacarpophalangeal and interphalangeal joints are also seen.)

☐ 9.15 METACARPOPHALANGEAL JOINTS

Bones:

- The **metacarpophalangeal (MCP) joints** are located between the metacarpals of the palm and the phalanges of the fingers (Figure 9-42).
  - More specifically, they are located between the heads of the metacarpals and the bases of the proximal phalanges of the fingers.

BOX 9-54

Note 1: **Rheumatoid arthritis** (RA) is a progressive degenerative arthritic condition that weakens and destroys the capsular connective tissue of joints. Although this condition attacks many joints, the metacarpophalangeal joints (MCP) of the hand are particularly hard hit. Clients with RA will usually develop a characteristic ulnar deviation deformity of the proximal phalanges at the MCP joints. This occurs because the capsules of the MCP joints are no longer sufficiently stable to be able to resist the forces that push against the fingers in an ulnar direction when objects are held between the thumb and the other fingers (opposition of the thumb to another finger to grasp an object creates an ulnar force against that finger).

Note 2: When the fingers are numbered, the thumb is considered to be finger #1.

- Five MCP joints exist:
  - The 1st MCP joint is located between the 1st metacarpal and the proximal phalanx of the thumb (i.e., finger #1).
  - The 2nd MCP joint is located between the 2nd metacarpal and the proximal phalanx of the index finger (i.e., finger #2).
  - The 3rd MCP joint is located between the 3rd metacarpal and the proximal phalanx of the middle finger (i.e., finger #3).
  - The 4th MCP joint is located between the 4th metacarpal and the proximal phalanx of the ring finger (i.e., finger #4).
  - The 5th MCP joint is located between the 5th metacarpal and the proximal phalanx of the little finger (i.e., finger #5).
- Joint Structure Classification: Synovial
  - Subtype: Condyloid
- Joint Function Classification: Diarthrotic
  - Subtype: Biaxial

Major Motions Allowed:

The MCP joint allows several major motions (Figure 9-43; Tables 9-12 and 9-13):

- The MCP joint allows flexion and extension (i.e., axial movements) within the sagittal plane around a mediolateral axis (Box 9-55).

TABLE 9-12

Average Ranges of Motion of the Proximal Phalanx of Fingers #2-5 at a Metacarpophalangeal (MCP) Joint, from Anatomic Position*

Flexion	90-110 Degrees†	Extension	0-20 Degrees‡
Abduction	20 Degrees	Adduction	20 Degrees

*When people are described in lay terms as being **double-jointed**, they do not have double joints; rather, they have ligaments that are so lax that they permit a greater than normal passive range of motion. Passive extension beyond normal (i.e., hyperextension) of the fingers at the metacarpophalangeal (MCP) joints is a very common location for this type of ligament laxity that is described as double-jointed.

†Flexion is greatest at the little finger and least at the index finger.

‡From anatomic position, sources differ on how much active extension (hyperextension) is possible at the MCP joints. However, most sources agree that passive (hyper) extension of 30-40 degrees is possible.

TABLE 9-13

Average Ranges of Motion of the Proximal Phalanx of the Thumb at the 1st Metacarpophalangeal Joint, from Anatomic Position

Flexion	60 Degrees	Extension	0 Degrees

Notes:

Abduction/adduction are negligible and considered to be accessory motions.

Passive hyperextension of the thumb at the metacarpophalangeal (MCP) joint is minimal as compared with the MCP joints of fingers #2-5.

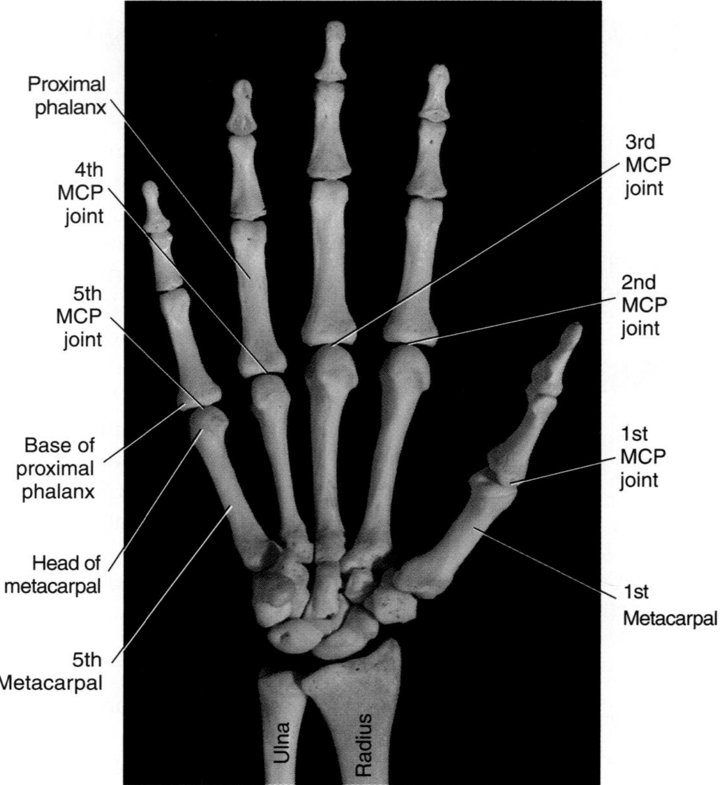

Figure 9-42 Metacarpophalangeal (MCP) joints of the hand. MCP joints are located between the heads of the metacarpals and the bases of the proximal phalanges of the fingers. They are numbered #1-5, starting on the radial (i.e., lateral) side with the thumb.

BOX 9-55 SPOTLIGHT ON THE EXTENSOR DIGITORUM'S TENDONS

The extensor digitorum is an extrinsic finger extensor muscle. Its belly, which is located in the posterior forearm, gradually transitions into four tendons. These four tendons attach onto the dorsal side of the middle and distal phalanges of fingers #2-5 (one tendon into each finger). However, these tendons do not remain fully separated from each other; they have what are called **intertendinous connections** (see illustration). As a result, extension of one finger can be influenced by the position of other fingers. If the hand is placed in the position shown in the accompanying photograph, the person will find that it is difficult if not impossible to raise the ring finger (i.e., extend the 4th finger at the metacarpophalangeal [MCP] joint). The reason is that maximally flexing the middle finger as shown pulls the tendon of the middle finger of the extensor digitorum distally. Because of the orientation of the intertendinous connection between the middle and ring fingers, when the distal tendon of the middle finger is pulled distally, the distal tendon of the ring finger is also pulled distally, resulting in it becoming slackened. Now, when the fibers of the extensor digitorum that would normally extend the ring finger contract, they cannot generate sufficient tension (i.e., a proximal pull on the ring finger's distal tendon) to overcome the slack that is present within the tendon to the ring finger. As a result, in this position it is difficult or impossible to extend the ring finger at the MCP joint. (Photo courtesy Joseph E. Muscolino.)

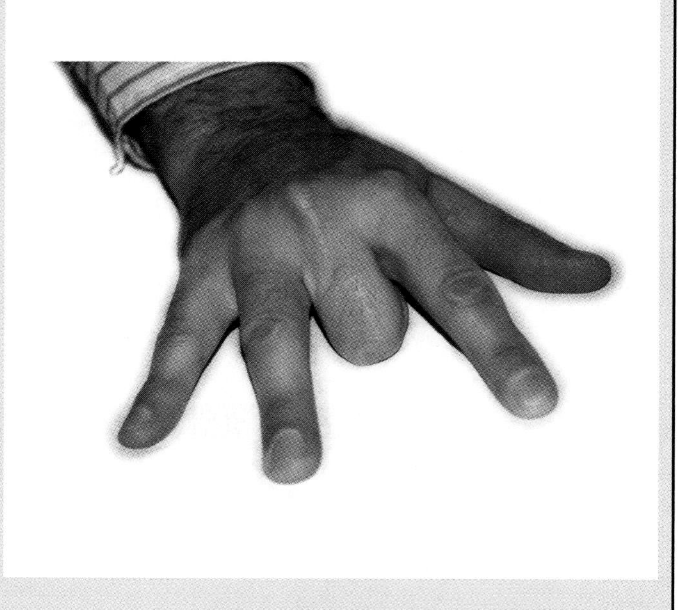

- The MCP joint allows abduction and adduction (i.e., axial movements) within the frontal plane around an anteroposterior axis.
- The reference for abduction/adduction of the fingers at the MCP joints is an imaginary line drawn through the middle finger when it is in anatomic position. Movement toward this imaginary line is adduction; movement away from this imaginary line is abduction. Because frontal plane movement of the middle finger in either direction is away from this imaginary line, both directions of movement are termed *abduction*. Lateral movement of the middle finger is termed *radial abduction*; medial movement of the middle finger is termed *ulnar abduction* (see Figure 9-43e–f).

Reverse Actions:

- The muscles of the MCP joints are generally considered to move the proximal phalanx of the finger (i.e., the more distal bone) toward a fixed metacarpal bone (i.e., the more proximal bone). However, a metacarpal of the palm of the hand can move toward the proximal phalanx of a finger instead.

Accessory Motions:

- The MCP joints allow a great deal of passive glide in all directions (i.e., anterior to posterior, medial to lateral, and axial distraction), as well as passive rotation. These accessory motions help the hand to better fit around objects that are being held, resulting in a firmer and more secure grasp.

Major Ligaments of the Metacarpophalangeal Joints:

- Each MCP joint is stabilized by a fibrous capsule and ligaments (Figure 9-44; Box 9-55).

BOX 9-56

LIGAMENTS OF THE METACARPOPHALANGEAL JOINTS

- Fibrous capsules
- Radial collateral ligaments
- Ulnar collateral ligaments
- Palmar plates

- The fibrous capsule of the MCP joint is lax when the joint is in extension and becomes somewhat taut when the joint is in flexion.
- Three ligaments of the MCP joint exist:
  - The **radial collateral ligament** is located on the radial side of the MCP joint.
  - The **ulnar collateral ligament** is located on the ulnar side of the MCP joint.
    - More specifically, both the radial and ulnar collateral ligaments attach proximally onto the head of the metacarpal and attach distally onto the base of the proximal phalanx (Box 9-57).

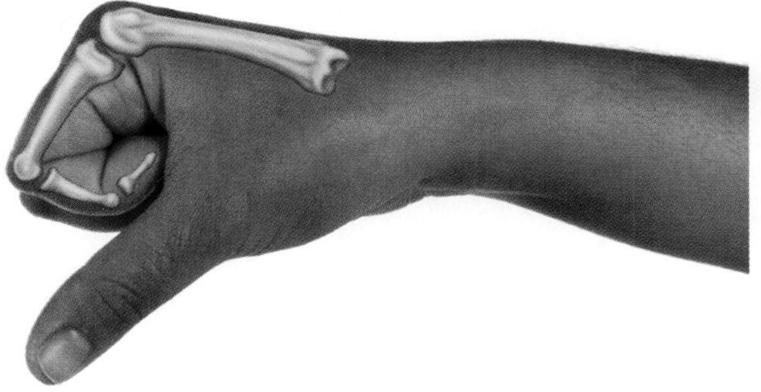

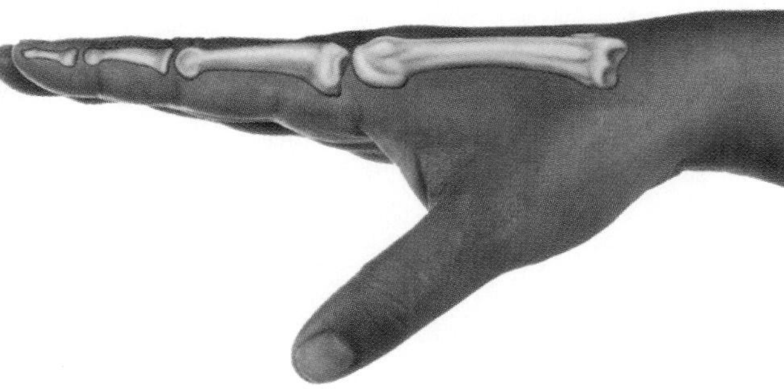

Figure 9-43 Actions of the fingers at the metacarpophalangeal (MCP) joints of the hand. An MCP joint is biaxial, allowing flexion and extension in the sagittal plane and abduction and adduction in the frontal plane. *A* and *B,* Radial (i.e., lateral) views illustrating flexion and extension, repectively, of fingers #2-5 at the MCP joints. (Note: Flexion of the fingers at the interphalangeal joints is also seen.)

Continued.

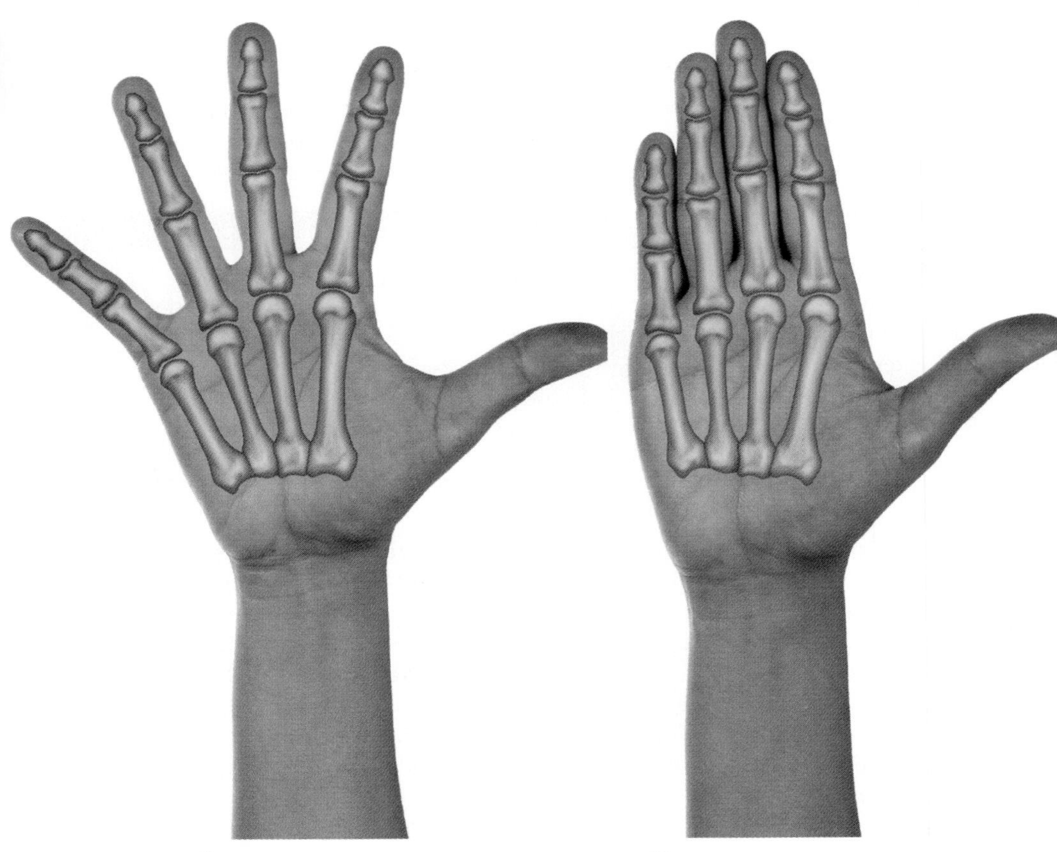

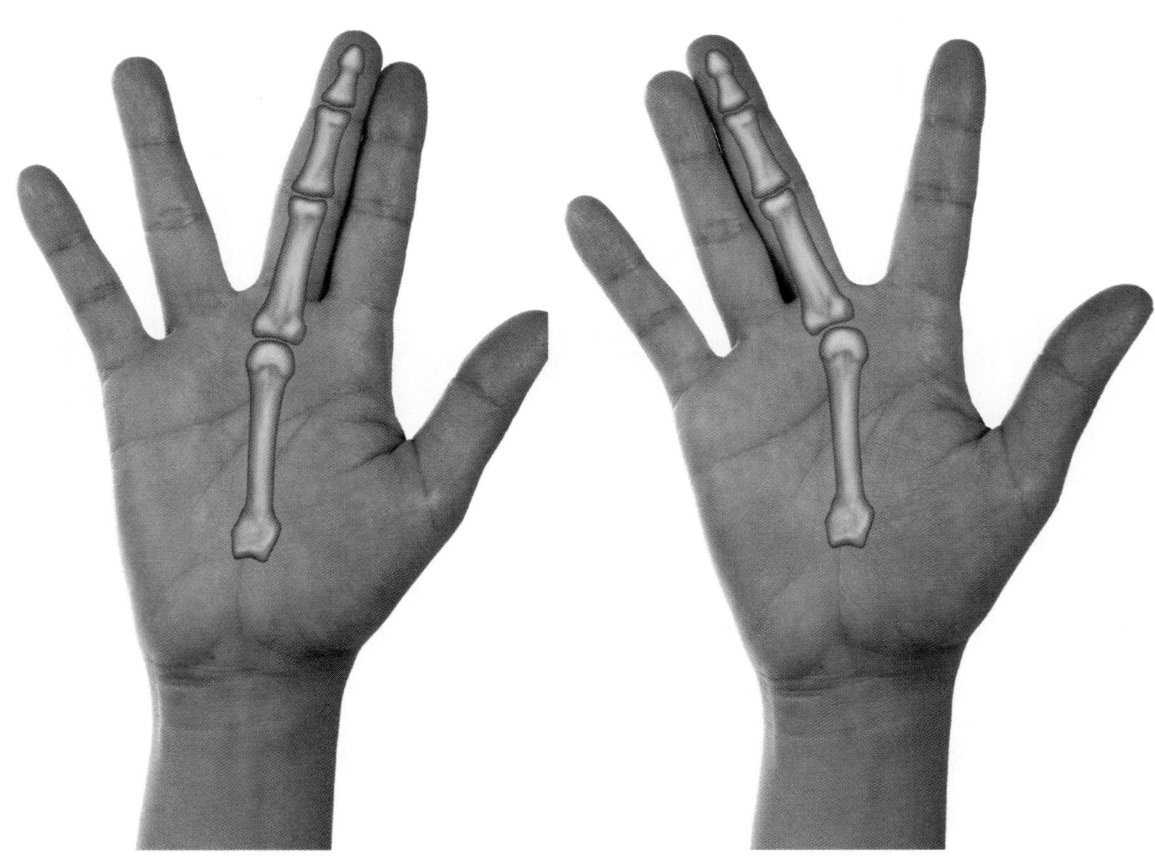

Figure 9-43, cont'd *C* and *D,* Abduction and adduction of fingers #2-5 at the MCP joints, respectively. (Note: The reference line for abduction/adduction of the fingers is an imaginary line through the center of the middle finger when in anatomic position.) *E* and *F,* Radial abduction and ulnar abduction of the middle finger at the 3rd MCP joint, respectively.

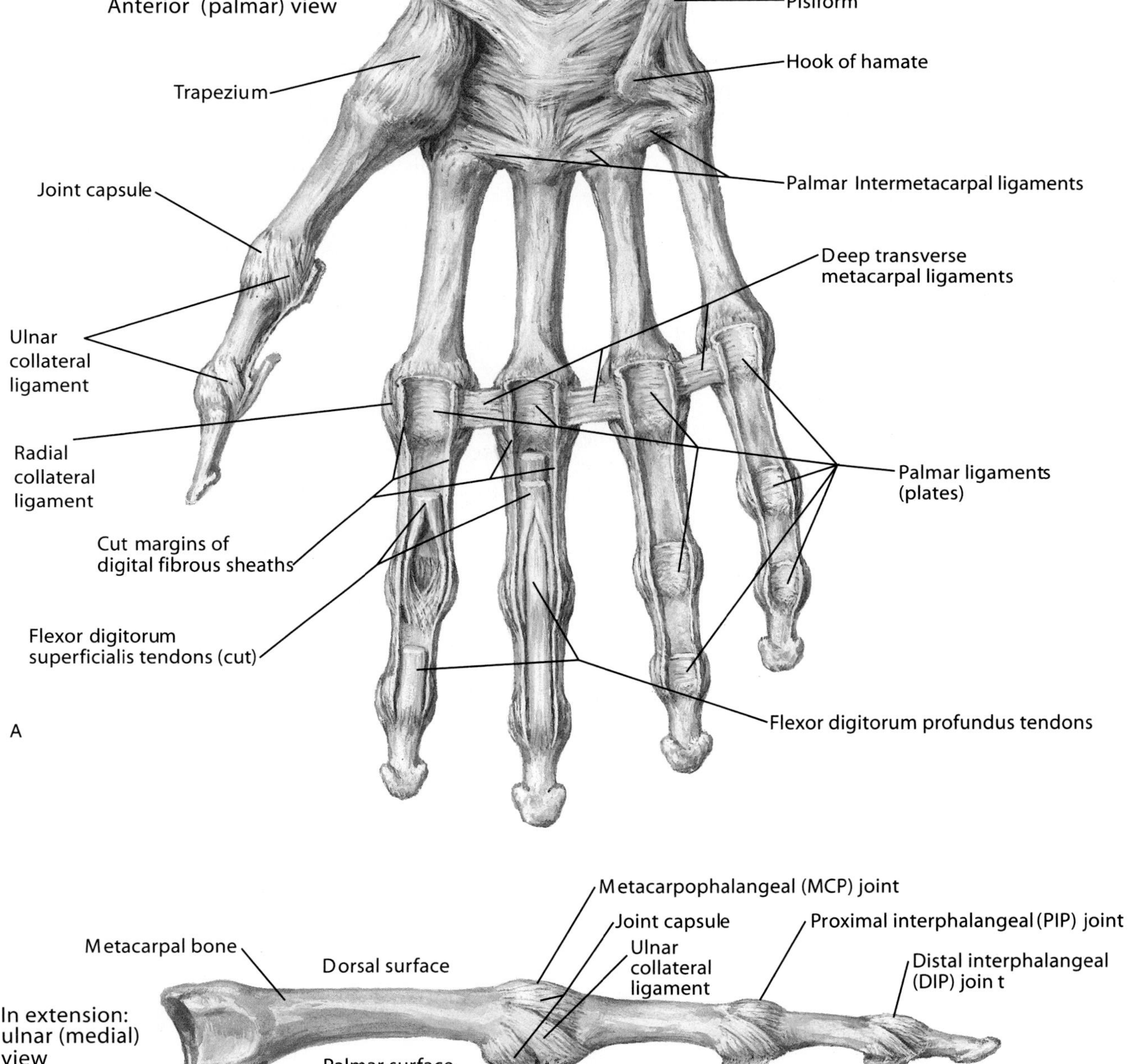

Figure 9-44 Ligaments of the metacarpophalangeal (MCP) joints of the hand. *A,* Anterior (palmar) view illustrating the fibrous capsules, collateral ligaments, and palmar plates of the MCP joints (and the palmar plates of the interphalangeal [IP] joints). *B,* Ulnar (i.e., medial) view of a finger illustrating the fibrous capsule, ulnar collateral ligament, and palmar plate of the MCP joint (and the palmar plate of the IP joint). (Netter illustrations used with permission of Elsevier Inc. All rights reserved.)

BOX 9-57

The radial and ulnar collateral ligaments of the metacarpophalangeal (MCP) joint are considered to have two parts: (1) the part that attaches onto the proximal phalanx is called the *cord* and (2) the part that attaches into the palmar plate is called the *accessory part*.

- ❑ The **palmar plate** is a ligamentous-like thick disc of fibrocartilage.
  - ❑ Location: It is located on the palmar side of the joint, superficial to the fibrous capsule.
    - ❑ More specifically, it is located from just proximal to the head of the metacarpal to the base of each proximal phalanx.
  - ❑ The purpose of the palmar plate is to stabilize the MCP joint and resist extension beyond anatomic position (i.e., resist hyperextension).
  - ❑ The palmar plate is also known as the **volar plate**.
  - ❑ Attaching between the palmar plates of the MCP joints are the deep transverse metacarpal ligaments of the distal intermetacarpal joints (see Section 9.14).
  - ❑ Attaching superficially to the anterior side of the palmar plates are fibrous sheaths that create tunnels for the extrinsic finger flexors (i.e., flexors digitorum superficialis and profundus) to travel to their attachment sites on the fingers (see Figure 9-44, *A*).

Closed-Packed Position:

- ❑ 70 degrees of flexion

Major Muscles of the MCP Joints:

- ❑ The muscles of the MCP joints move fingers and can be divided into extrinsic muscles (that originate on the arm and/or forearm) and intrinsic muscles (wholly located within the hand).
- ❑ The extrinsic muscles of fingers #2-5 are the flexors digitorum superficialis and profundus, extensor digitorum, extensor digiti minimi, and extensor indicis.
- ❑ The extrinsic muscles of the thumb are flexor pollicis longus and extensors pollicis longus and brevis.
- ❑ The intrinsic muscles of fingers #2-5 are abductor digiti minimi manus, flexor digiti minimi manus, opponens digiti minimi, lumbricals manus, palmar interossei, and dorsal interossei manus.
- ❑ The intrinsic muscles of the thumb are the abductor pollicis brevis, flexor pollicis brevis, opponens pollicis, and adductor pollicis (Box 9-57).

BOX 9-58

The frontal plane movements of abduction and adduction of the thumb at the metacarpophalangeal (MCP) joint are negligible and considered to be accessory motions. Abductor and adductor muscles that do cross the MCP joint of the thumb also cross the carpometacarpal (CMC) of the thumb and create abduction/adduction at that joint.

Miscellaneous:

- ❑ When the fingers are flexed at the MCP joints, the frontal plane movements of abduction and adduction are either greatly diminished or absent entirely.
  - ❑ This reduced frontal plane movement when in flexion is due to both the tension in the ligaments and to the shape of the bones of the joint.
  - ❑ Usually a pair of sesamoid bones is located on the palmar side of the MCP joint of the thumb.

☐ 9.16 INTERPHALANGEAL JOINTS OF THE HAND

- **Interphalangeal (IP) joints** of the hand are located between phalanges of the fingers (Figure 9-45).
  - More specifically, each IP joint is located between the head of a phalanx and the base of the phalanx distal to it.

BOX 9-59

Note 1: Interphalangeal (IP) joints are located in both the hand and the foot. To distinguish these joints from each other, the words *manus* (denoting hand) and *pedis* (denoting foot) are often used.

Note 2: **Osteoarthritis** (OA) is a progressive degenerative arthritic condition caused by increased physical stress to a joint. It weakens and destroys the articular cartilage of the joint and results in calcium deposition at the bony joint margins. Although this condition attacks many joints, the distal interphalangeal (DIP) joints of the hand are particularly hard hit. Clients with OA will usually develop characteristic increased bony formations, known as **bone spurs**, at the affected joints. Bone spurs at the DIP joints are particularly common and are called **Heberden's nodes**. OA is also known as **degenerative joint disease** (DJD).

Note 3: When motion occurs at an IP joint of the hand, we can say that a finger moves at the proximal or distal IP joint. To be more specific, we could say that the middle phalanx moves at the proximal interphalangeal (PIP) joint, and/or that the distal phalanx moves at the distal interphalangeal (DIP) joint.

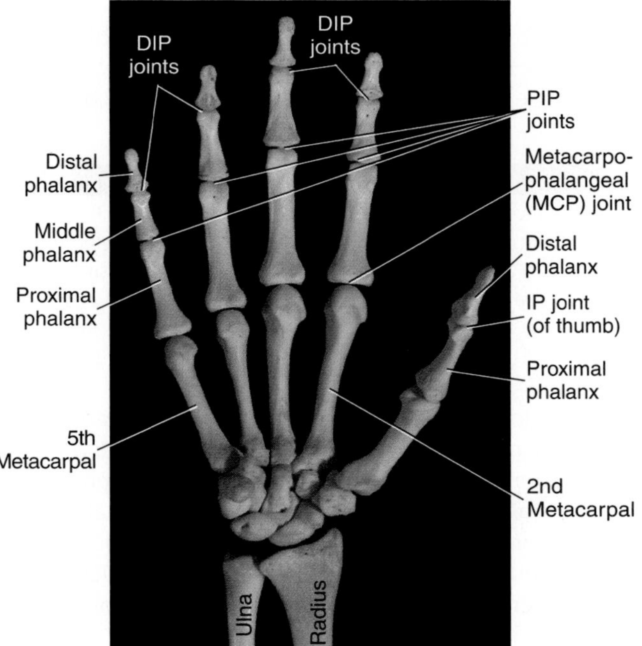

Figure 9-45 Anterior view that illustrates the interphalangeal (IP) joints of the hand. The thumb has one IP joint; each of the other four fingers has two IP joints: (1) a proximal interphalangeal (PIP) joint and (2) a distal interphalangeal (DIP) joint. IP joints are uniaxial hinge joints allowing only flexion and extension in the sagittal plane.

- One IP joint in the thumb exists. It is located between the proximal and distal phalanges of the thumb.
- Because each of fingers #2-5 has three phalanges, two IP joints exist in each of these fingers: (A) a **proximal interphalangeal (PIP) joint** and (B) a **distal interphalangeal (DIP) joint** (see Box 9-59, Note 3).
  - The IP joint located between the proximal and middle phalanges is called the *PIP joint (manus)*.
  - The IP joint located between the middle and distal phalanges is called the *DIP joint (manus)*.
- In total, nine IP joints are found in the hand (one IP, four PIPs, and four DIPs).
- Joint structure classification: Synovial joint
  - Subtype: Hinge
- Joint function classification: Diarthrotic
  - Subtype: Uniaxial

Major Motions Allowed:

The IP joints allow two major motions (Figure 9-46; Table 9-14):

- The IP joints allow flexion and extension (i.e., axial movements) within the sagittal plane about a mediolateral axis.

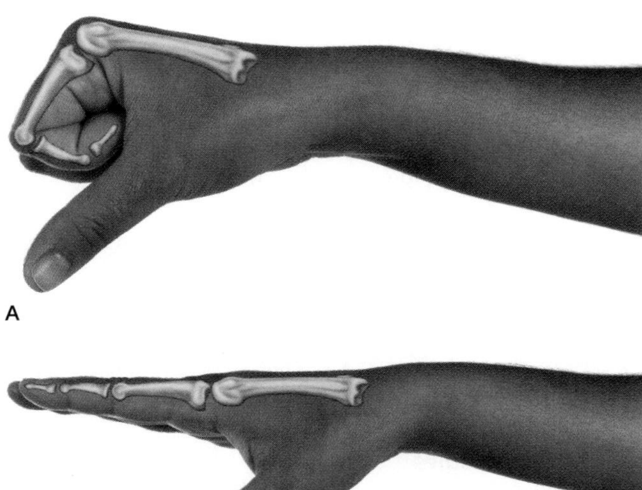

Figure 9-46 Flexion and extension of the fingers at the interphalangeal (IP) joints. (Note: All views are radial [i.e., lateral].) *A,* Flexion of the fingers at the proximal interphalangeal (PIP) and distal interphalangeal (DIP) joints. (Note: Flexion also seen at the metacarpophalangeal [MCP] joints. *B,* Extension of the fingers at the PIP and DIP joints. (Note: extension also seen at the MCP joints.)

TABLE 9-14

Average Ranges of Motion of the Fingers at the Interphalangeal Joints from Anatomic Position

Proximal Interphalangeal (PIP) Joints:			
Flexion	100-120 Degrees*	Extension:	0 Degrees
Distal Interphalangeal (DIP) Joints:			
Flexion	80-90 Degrees*	Extension	0 Degrees†
Interphalangeal (IP) Joint of the Thumb:			
Flexion	80 Degrees‡		

Note: The amount of passive extension beyond anatomic position (i.e., hyperextension) of the IP joint of the thumb is normally approximately 20 degrees. However, this amount often increases with use because of a loosening of the ligamentous structure of the joint. Massage therapists and other bodyworkers are prone to having this problem (i.e., thumbs that bend backwards) and must be careful not to overuse their thumbs, especially when doing deep work. When using the thumb for deep tissue work, it can be helpful to use a double contact (i.e., support your thumb that is in contact with the client with the thumb or fingers of the other hand). This will increase the stability of the IP joint of the thumb and lessen the deleterious effects of hyperextension forces.

*The amount of flexion at the PIP and DIP joints gradually increases from the radial side to the ulnar side fingers.

†From anatomic position, no further active extension is possible at the PIP and DIP joints; however, further passive extension (i.e., hyperextension) of approximately 30 degrees is possible at the DIP joints.

‡From anatomic position, no further active extension is possible at the IP joint of the thumb; however, further passive extension (i.e., hyperextension) of 20 degrees is possible.

Reverse Actions:

- ❑ The muscles of the IP joints are generally considered to move the more distal phalanx of a finger relative to the more proximal phalanx. However, it is possible to move the more proximal phalanx relative to the more distal one.

Major Ligaments of the Interphalangeal (IP) Joints:

- ❑ The ligament complex of the IP joints is very similar to that of the MCP joints (Figure 9-47).

BOX 9-60

LIGAMENTS OF THE INTERPHALANGEAL (PROXIMAL INTERPHALANGEAL [PIP] AND DISTAL INTERPHALANGEAL [DIP]) JOINTS

- Fibrous capsules
- Radial collateral ligaments
- Ulnar collateral ligaments
- Palmar plates
- Check-rein ligaments (DIP joint only)

- ❑ The PIP joint is stabilized by a fibrous capsule, two collateral ligaments (radial and ulnar), a palmar plate, and an additional structure called the *check-rein ligament*.
- ❑ The DIP joint is stabilized by a fibrous capsule, two collateral ligaments (radial and ulnar), and a palmar plate.
- ❑ The ligamentous structure of the IP joint of the thumb is similar to the DIP joint of fingers #2-5.

Radial and Ulnar Collateral Ligaments:

- ❑ The **radial collateral ligament** is on the radial side of the joint.
- ❑ The **ulnar collateral ligament** is on the ulnar side of the joint.
  - ❑ More specifically, both the radial and ulnar collateral ligaments attach proximally onto the head of the more proximal phalanx and distally onto the base of the phalanx that is located more distally.

BOX 9-61

The collateral ligaments of the interphalangeal (IP) joints are essentially identical to the collateral ligaments of the metacarpophalangeal (MCP) joint. The IP joint's collateral ligaments also have two parts: (1) a cord that attaches into the more distal bone of the joint and (2) an accessory part that attaches into the palmar plate.

- ❑ Function: The radial collateral ligament limits motion of the phalanx at that joint to the ulnar side; the ulnar collateral ligament limits motion of the phalanx at that joint to the radial side. Ulnar and radial motions are frontal plane motions that should not occur at the IP joints (aside from some passive joint play). These collateral ligaments help to restrict these frontal plane motions.

Palmar Plate:

- ❑ Each **palmar plate** is a ligamentous-like thick disc of fibrocartilage.
- ❑ Location: It is located on the palmar side of the joint, superficial to the fibrous capsule.

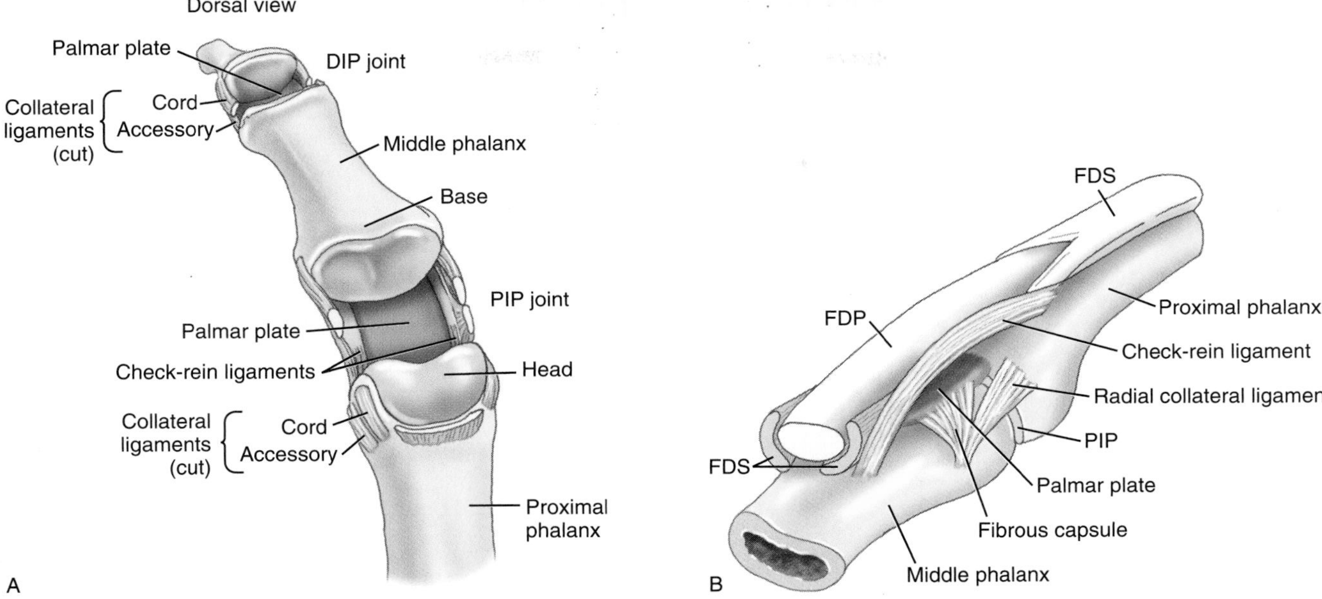

Figure 9-47 Ligaments of the interphalangeal (IP) joints (both the proximal interphalangeal [PIP] joints and the distal interphalangeal [DIP] joints). *A,* Dorsal (i.e., posterior) view with the IP joints opened up. The PIP joint is stabilized by a fibrous capsule, collateral ligaments, a palmar plate, and two check-rein ligaments. The DIP joint is stabilized by a fibrous capsule, collateral ligaments, and a palmar plate. (Note: The DIP joint has no check-rein ligaments.) *B,* A view of the palmar (i.e., anterior) surface of the PIP joint. In this view the relationship of the check-rein ligaments can be seen relative to the palmar plate and the tendons of the flexor digitorum superficialis (FDS) and the flexor digitorum profundus (FDP).

- ❑ More specifically, it is located from just proximal to the head of the more proximal phalanx to the base of the more distal phalanx.
- ❑ The purpose of the palmar plate is to stabilize the IP joint and resist extension beyond anatomic position (i.e., hyperextension).
- ❑ The palmar plate is also known as the **volar plate**.

Check-Rein Ligaments:

- ❑ The **check-rein ligaments** are located only at the PIP joint (not the DIP joint or the MCP joint).
- ❑ They are located immediately anterior to the palmar plate (and on either side of the long finger flexor muscles' tendons) (i.e., flexors digitorum superficialis and profundus).
- ❑ The check-rein ligaments strengthen the connection between the palmar plate and the bones of the joint. As with the palmar plate, the check-rein ligaments restrict hyperextension.

BOX 9-62

Passive hyperextension, which is possible at the metacarpophalangeal (MCP) and distal interphalangeal (DIP) joints, is not possible at the proximal interphalangeal (PIP) joint because of the presence of the check-rein ligaments.

Closed-Packed Position of the Interphalangeal Joints:

- ❑ Approximately full extension

Major Muscles of the Interphalangeal Joints:

- ❑ The IP joints are crossed by both extrinsic muscles (that originate on the arm and/or forearm) and intrinsic muscles (wholly located within the hand).
- ❑ Extrinsic flexors of fingers #2-5 are the flexor digitorum superficialis (FDS) (which only crosses the PIP joint) and the flexor digitorum profundus (FDP). The flexor pollicis longus is an extrinsic flexor of the thumb.
- ❑ No intrinsic flexors of the IP joints of the hand exist.
- ❑ Extrinsic extensors of fingers #2-5 are the extensor digitorum, extensor digiti minimi manus, and the extensor indicis. The extensor pollicis longus is an extrinsic extensor of the thumb.
- ❑ Intrinsic extensors of the IP joints of the hand include all intrinsics that attach into the dorsal digital expansion; they are the lumbricals manus, palmar interossei, dorsal interossei manus, and the abductor digiti minimi manus.

Miscellaneous:

- ❑ Other than the fact that fingers are quite a bit longer than toes, the IP joints of fingers #2-5 of the hand are essentially identical to the IP joints of toes #2-5 of the foot. However, most people do not learn the same fine-motor neural control of the toes of the foot that they have of the fingers of the hand.
- ❑ It is usually difficult to isolate finger flexion at the DIP joint.

REVIEW QUESTIONS

evolve Answers to the following review questions appear on the Evolve website accompanying this book.

1. Name the four joints of the shoulder joint complex.

2. What is the name of the term that describes the concept that scapular (and clavicular) movements accompany arm movements at the GH joint?

3. What are the names of the three ligaments that are thickenings of the anterior and inferior capsule of the GH joint?

4. Where do all extensors of the arm at the shoulder joint cross the shoulder joint?

5. Why is the ScC joint considered to be a functional joint and not an anatomic joint?

6. How many degrees of upward rotation of the scapula at the ScC joint are possible?

7. What is the only osseous articulation between the upper extremity and the axial skeleton?

8. What bones can move at the AC joint?

9. What are the two parts of the coracoclavicular ligament?

10. What scapular joint action couples with abduction of the arm at the shoulder joint?

11. What three articulations of the elbow joint complex share the same joint capsule?

12. What is the principle articulation at the elbow joint complex?

13. Where do all muscles that flex the forearm cross the elbow joint?

14. What is the reverse action of flexion of the forearm at the elbow joint?

15. Name the three RU joints.

16. What is the major ligament of the proximal RU joint?

17. What defines a ray of the hand?

18. Name the arches of the hand.

19. What structures are contained within the carpal tunnel?

20. What bones are involved in the radiocarpal joint?

21. Name the joint actions possible at the wrist joint?

22. Which wrist joint ligament limits radial deviation (i.e., abduction) of the hand at the wrist joint?

23. Other than the 1st CMC joint, which CMC joint is the most mobile?

24. What is the significance of the central pillar of the hand?

25. Around how many axes does the saddle joint of the thumb allow motion?

26. What are the component cardinal plane actions of opposition of the thumb at the 1st CMC joint?

27. What is the name of the ligament that stabilizes the distal IMC joint?

____

____

28. What is the functional classification of the MCP joint?

____

____

29. What are the names of the structures that stop passive extension beyond neutral (i.e., hyperextension) at the PIP joint?

____

____

____

30. What is the reference line for abduction/adduction of the fingers?

____

____

____

NOTES

Chapter 10

Anatomy and Physiology of Muscle Tissue

CHAPTER OUTLINE

CHAPTER OBJECTIVES

After completing this chapter, the student should be able to perform the following:

- ❑ List the three types of muscular tissue.
- ❑ Describe the characteristics and function of skeletal muscle tissue.
- ❑ Describe the structure and function of a skeletal muscle.
- ❑ Describe the structure and function of a skeletal muscle fiber.
- ❑ List the various types of muscular fascia.
- ❑ Describe the structure and function of muscular fascia.
- ❑ State the meaning of the term *myofascial unit.*
- ❑ Describe the structure of a sarcomere.
- ❑ Explain the sliding filament mechanism.
- ❑ Explain the relationship between the sliding filament mechanism and the bigger picture of muscle function.
- ❑ Describe how the energy needed for the sliding filament mechanism is supplied.
- ❑ Describe the structure of the neuromuscular junction.
- ❑ Explain how the nervous system controls and directs muscular contraction.
- ❑ Define a motor unit.
- ❑ Explain the importance of a motor unit, and explain the differences between motor units.
- ❑ Define the all-or-none response law, and explain to which structural levels of the muscular system it is applied.
- ❑ List and define the bands of skeletal muscle tissue.
- ❑ Describe the structural and functional characteristics of red slow-twitch and white fast-twitch fibers.
- ❑ Explain the concepts of myofascial meridian theory and tensegrity and how they apply to the body.
- ❑ Define the key terms of this chapter.
- ❑ State the meanings of the word origins of this chapter.

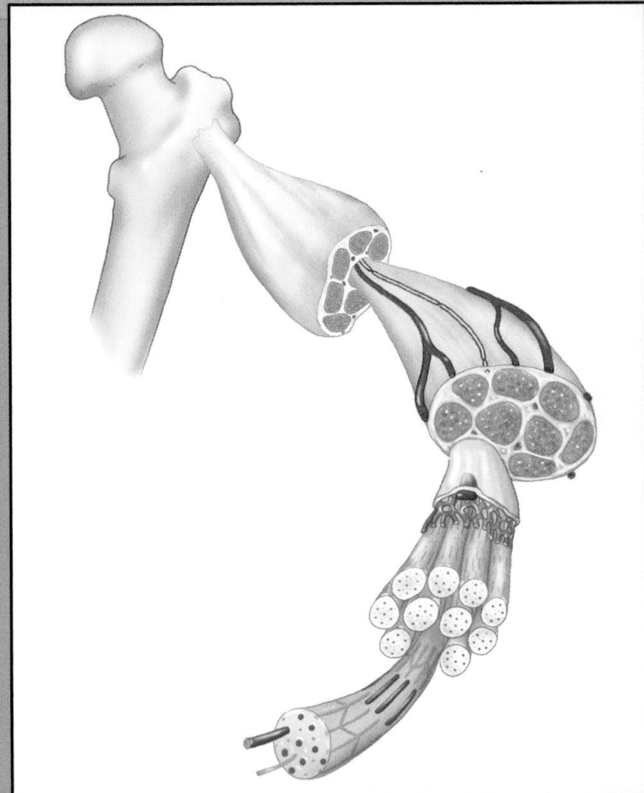

OVERVIEW

The anatomy and physiology of skeletal tissues were addressed in Chapter 3. Before examining the larger kinesiologic concepts of muscle function, this chapter focuses on the anatomy and physiology of a skeletal muscle. The two major tissue types, skeletal muscle tissue and muscular fascia are examined. Specifically, an understanding of the microanatomy of the sarcomere of a muscle fiber and the sliding filament mechanism are presented; the context of the sliding filament mechanism within the context of the bigger picture of muscle function is then given. Energy sources for muscle contraction and nervous system control of muscle contraction are also covered. The concepts of motor units, the all-or-none response law, and red slow-twitch versus white fast-twitch fibers are then presented, as well as two sections that offer an in-depth view of the structure of the sarcomere and the sliding filament mechanism. The chapter concludes with an exploration of the concepts of myofascial meridian theory and tensegrity.

KEY TERMS

A-band
Actin filament (AK-tin FIL-a-ment)
Actin filament active site
Actin filament binding site
Actin molecule
Acetylcholine (a-SEET-al-KOL-een)
Acetylcholinesterase (a-SEET-al-KOL-een-EST-er-ace)
Adenosine triphosphate (ATP)
All-or-none-response law
Anatomy train
Aponeurosis, pl. aponeuroses (AP-o-noo-RO-sis, AP-o-noo-RO-seez)
Cardiac muscle tissue
Cytoplasmic organelles (SI-to-PLAS-mik OR-gan-els)
Deep fascia (Fash-a)
Easily fatigued fibers
Endomysium, pl. endomysia (EN-do-MICE-ee-um, EN-do-MICE-ee-a)
Epimysium, pl. epimysia (EP-ee-MICE-ee-um, EP-ee-MICE-ee-a)
Fascicle (FAS-si-kul)
Fasciculus, pl. fasciculi (fas-IK-you-lus, fas-IK-you-lie)
Fast glycolytic (FG) fibers (GLIY-ko-LIT-ik)
Fatigue-resistant fibers
Glycolysis (gliy-KOL-i-sis)
Glycolytic fibers (GLIY-ko-lit-ik)
H-band
Heavy meromyosin (MER-o-MY-o-sin)
I-band
Innervation (IN-ner-VAY-shun)
Intermediate-twitch fibers
Lactic acid (LAK-tik)
Large fibers
Kreb's cycle (KREBS)
Langer's lines (LANG-ers)
Light meromyosin (MER-o-MY-o-sin)
M-band
M-line
Motor end plate
Motor unit
Muscle cell
Muscle fiber
Muscle memory
Muscular fascia (Fash-a)
Myofascial meridian (MY-o-FASH-al me-RID-ee-an)
Myofascial meridian theory
Myofascial unit (MY-o-FASH-al)
Myofibril (my-o-FIY-bril)
Myoglobin (my-o-GLOBE-in)
Myosin filament (MY-o-sin FIL-a-ment)
Myosin cross-bridge (MY-o-sin)
Myosin head (MY-o-sin)
Neuromuscular junction (noor-o-MUS-kyu-lar)
Neurotransmitters (noor-o-TRANS-mit-ers)
Organ
Oxidative fibers (oks-i-DATE-iv)
Oxygen debt
Perimysium, pl. perimysia (per-ee-MICE-ee-um, per-ee-MICE-ee-a)
Phasic fibers (FAZE-ik)
Ratchet theory
Red slow-twitch fibers
Respiration of glucose (res-pi-RAY-shun)
S1 fragment
S2 fragment
Sarcolemma (SAR-ko-lem-ma)
Sarcomere (SAR-ko-meer)
Sarcoplasm (SAR-ko-plazm)
Sarcoplasmic reticulum (SAR-ko-plaz-mik re-TIK-you-lum)
Skeletal muscle tissue (SKEL-i-tal)
Sliding filament mechanism (FIL-a-ment)
Slow oxidative (SO) fibers (oks-i-DATE-iv)
Small fibers
Smooth muscle tissue
Striated muscle (STRIY-ate-ed)
Synapse (SIN-aps)
Synaptic cleft (sin-AP-tik)
Synaptic gap
Tendon
Tensegrity (ten-SEG-ri-tee)
Tonic fibers
Transverse tubules (TOO-byools)
Tropomyosin molecule (tro-po-MY-o-sin)
Troponin molecule (TRO-po-nin)
T-tubules (TOO-byools)
Type I fibers
Type II fibers
White fast-twitch fibers
Z-band
Z-line

WORD ORIGINS

- ❑ Aer—From Latin *aer,* meaning *air*
- ❑ Cardiac—From Latin *cardiacus* meaning *heart*
- ❑ Elle—From Latin *ella,* meaning *little*
- ❑ Endo—From Greek *endon,* meaning *within, inner*
- ❑ Epi—From Greek *epi,* meaning *on, upon*
- ❑ Fasc—From Latin *fascia,* meaning *band, bandage*
- ❑ Fibrous—From Latin *fibra,* meaning *fiber*
- ❑ Glyco—From Greek *glykys,* meaning *sweet*
- ❑ Lysis—From Greek *lysis,* meaning *dissolution, loosening*
- ❑ Myo—From Greek *mys,* meaning *muscle*
- ❑ Mys—From Latin *mys,* meaning *muscle*
- ❑ Peri—From Greek *peri,* meaning *around*
- ❑ Sarco—From Greek *sarkos,* meaning *muscle, flesh*

10.1 SKELETAL MUSCLE

Muscle Tissue:

- Three types of muscle tissue exist in the human body:
  - **Cardiac muscle tissue**, located in the heart
  - **Smooth muscle tissue**, located in the walls of hollow visceral organs and blood vessels
  - **Skeletal muscle tissue**, located in skeletal muscles

This chapter, and indeed this entire book, deals with skeletal muscle tissue.

Characteristics of Skeletal Muscle:

- Because skeletal muscle tissue exhibits a striated (i.e., banded) appearance under a microscope, it is often called **striated muscle**.
- Skeletal muscle is under voluntary control.

BOX 10-1

Note 1: Skeletal muscle tissue and cardiac muscle tissue are both striated in appearance under a microscope; smooth muscle tissue is not.

Note 2: Smooth muscle and cardiac muscle tissues are not under voluntary control, at least not typical full voluntary control. Although it is possible via biofeedback to affect the tone of smooth and cardiac muscle, it is not the full voluntary control that we have over skeletal muscles.

Skeletal Muscle—The Big Picture:

- A skeletal muscle attaches onto two bones, thereby crossing the joint that is located between the two bones.

BOX 10-2

This describes a typical skeletal muscle, which has two attachments, each onto a bone. However, some skeletal muscles may have more than two bony attachments and some skeletal muscles attach into soft tissue instead of bone.

- The big picture of how a skeletal muscle works is that it can contract, attempting to shorten toward its center. (For a thorough explanation of the bigger picture of how skeletal muscles work, please see Chapter 11.)
- This contraction creates a pulling force on the bony attachments of the muscle.
- If this pulling force is sufficiently strong, one or both of the bones to which the muscle is attached will be pulled toward the center of the muscle.
- Because bones are located within body parts, movement of a bone results in movement of a body part (Figure 10-1).

To better understand the big picture of how muscles create movements of the body, it is necessary to explore and understand the microanatomy and microphysiology of skeletal muscle tissue.

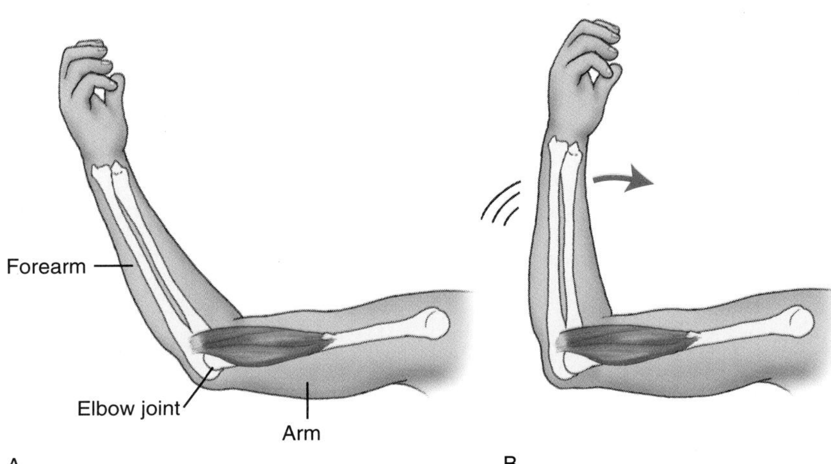

Figure 10-1 The "big picture" of muscle contraction. *A*, Muscle attaching from the humerus to the ulna and crossing the elbow joint located between these two bones. When the muscle contracts, it creates a pulling force on the two bones to which it is attached. *B*, This pulling force has resulted in movement of the forearm toward the arm.

10.2 TISSUE COMPONENTS OF A SKELETAL MUSCLE

- A skeletal muscle is an organ of the muscular system.

BOX 10-3

By definition, an **organ** is made up of two or more different tissues, all acting together for one function. In the case of a skeletal muscle, that function is to contract.

- As an organ, a skeletal muscle contains more than one type of tissue. The two major types of tissue found in a skeletal muscle are (1) skeletal muscle tissue and (2) fibrous fascia connective tissue (Figure 10-2).
- Skeletal muscle tissue itself is composed of skeletal muscle cells. These muscle cells are the major structural and functional units of a muscle.
  - They are the major structural units of a muscle in that the majority of a muscle is made up of muscle cells.
  - More importantly, they are the major functional units of a muscle in that they do the work of a muscle (i.e., the cells contract).
- The fibrous fascia of a muscle provides a structural framework for the muscle by enveloping the muscle tissue.
  - Fibrous fascia wraps around the entire muscle, groups of muscle cells within the muscle, and each individual muscle cell.
- This fibrous fascia also continues beyond the muscle at both ends to create the tendons that attach the muscle to its bony attachment sites.
- Skeletal muscles also contain nerves and blood vessels.
- The nerves carry both motor messages from the central nervous system to the muscle that instruct the muscle to contract, and sensory messages from the muscle to the central nervous system that inform the brain and spinal cord as to the state of the muscle.
- The blood vessels bring needed nutrients to the muscle tissue and drain away the waste products of the muscle's metabolism.

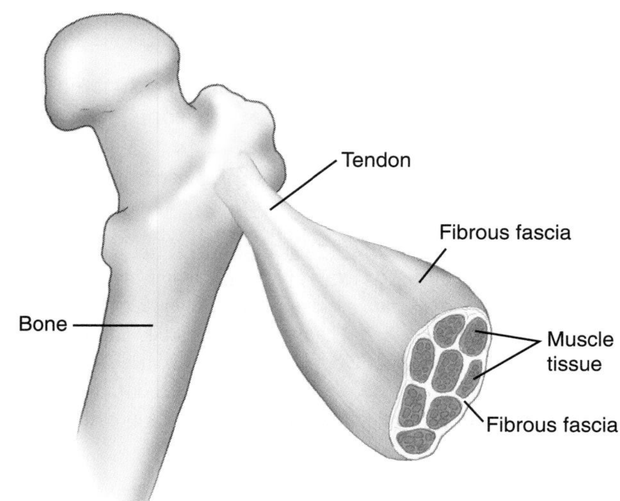

Figure 10-2 Cross-section of a muscle attached via its tendon to a bone. On cross-section, we see that the muscle is made up of skeletal muscle tissue and fibrous fascial tissue.

10.3 SKELETAL MUSCLE CELLS

As stated, the major structural and functional component of skeletal muscle tissue is the skeletal muscle cell (Figure 10-3).

- Because a skeletal muscle cell has an elongated cylindric shape, a muscle cell can also be called a *muscle fiber* (i.e., the terms **muscle cell** and **muscle fiber** are synonyms).
- Muscle fibers can vary from approximately $^1/_2$ inch to 20 inches (1-50 cm) in length.
- Essentially, a skeletal muscle is made up of many muscle fibers that run lengthwise within the muscle.

BOX 10-4

The exact manner in which the muscle fibers run within a muscle can vary and is described as the *architecture* of the muscle fibers. (For more details on muscle fiber architecture, please see Section 15.2.)

- It is rare for muscle fibers to run the entire length of a muscle. Usually they either lay end to end in series or lay parallel and overlap each other within the muscle (Figure 10-4).

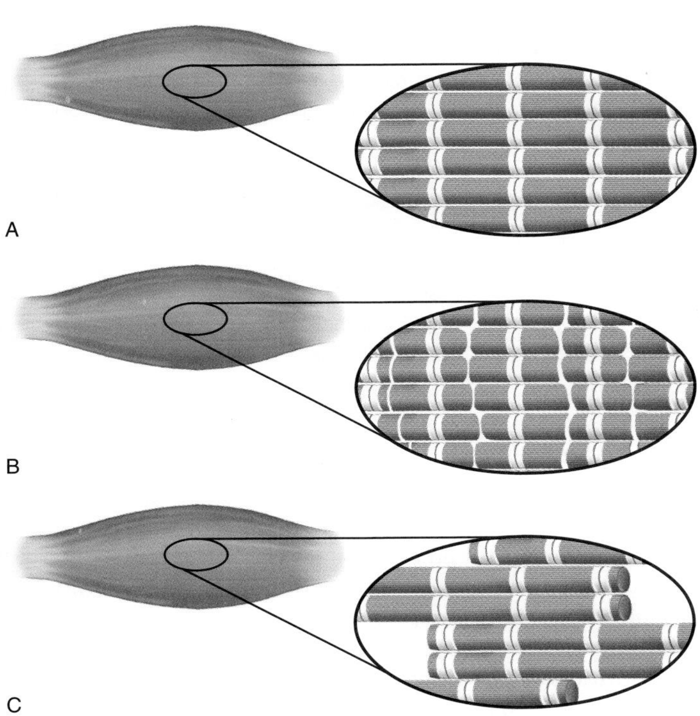

Figure 10-4 Various ways in which muscle fibers can be arranged within a muscle. *A,* Long muscle fibers lying parallel and running the length of the muscle. *B,* Shorter muscle fibers lying parallel and arranged end to end within the muscle. *C,* Muscle fibers lying parallel and overlapping.

- These muscle fibers are organized into a bundle known as a **fascicle**. A fascicle may contain as many as 200 muscle fibers.

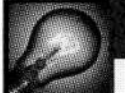

BOX 10-5

A synonym for fascicle is **fasciculus** (plural, fasciculi).

- A skeletal muscle is composed of a number of fascicles (Figure 10-5).

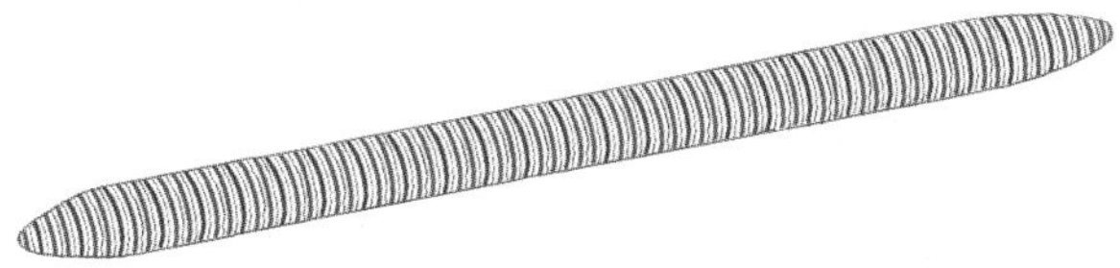

Figure 10-3 Individual skeletal muscle fiber. The striated appearance should be noted.

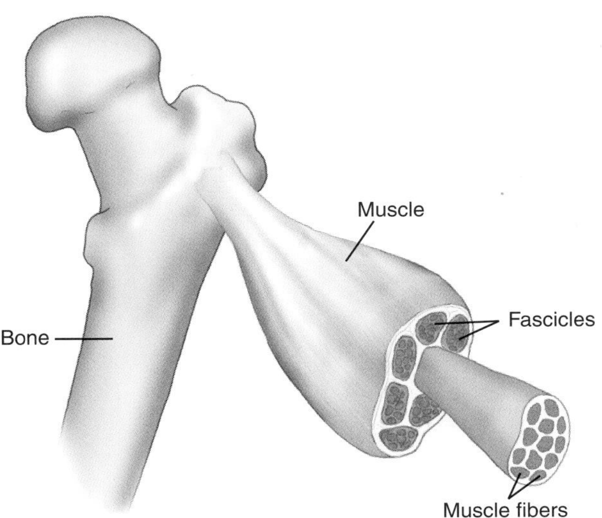

Figure 10-5 Cross-section of a muscle attached via its tendon to a bone. On cross-section, we see that the muscle is made up of a number of fascicles. One fascicle has been brought out further, and we can see that it is longitudinal in length. Each fascicle is bundle of muscle fibers.

☐ 10.4 MUSCULAR FASCIA

- The tissue that creates the structural organization of a muscle is the tough fibrous fascia connective tissue that is also known as **muscular fascia** or **deep fascia**.
- The major component of muscular fascia is collagen fibers.
- A small component of elastin fibers also exist in muscular fascia.

BOX 10-6

It is the fascia of a muscle that gives it its elasticity.

- Although all muscular fascia is uniform in its composition, it is given different names depending on its location (Figure 10-6).
- The fibrous fascia that surrounds each individual muscle fiber is called **endomysium**.
- The fibrous fascia that surrounds a group of muscle fibers, dividing the muscle into bundles known as *fascicles,* is called **perimysium**.
- The fibrous fascia that surrounds an entire muscle is called **epimysium**.

BOX 10-7

Mys, epi, peri, and *endo* are all Greek roots. *Mys* refers to muscle; *epi* means *upon*; *peri* means *around*; *endo* means *within.*

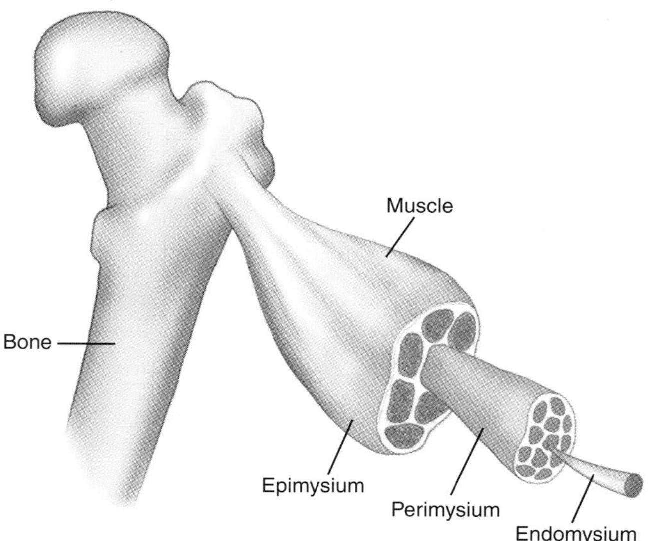

Figure 10-6 Organization of muscular fascia within a muscle. Each muscle fiber is surrounded by endomysium; perimysium surrounds a number of muscle fibers, creating groups of fibers known as *fascicles.* The entire muscle is surrounded by epimysium. All three of these fibrous fascial layers then meld together to create the tendons and/or aponeuroses that attach the muscle to its bony attachments.

- It is important to note that all three of these layers of fibrous fascia blend together and continue beyond the muscle to attach the muscle to a bone. The role of the fascial attachment is to transfer the force of the muscle contraction to the bone.
- If the muscular fascia that attaches the muscle to a bone is round and cordlike, it is called a **tendon**.
- If the muscular fascia is broad and flat, it is called an **aponeurosis**.

BOX 10-8

Regarding their tissue composition, tendons and aponeuroses are identical; they differ only in shape. It should also be emphasized that although skeletal muscles usually attach to bones of the skeleton, hence their name, they often attach to other soft tissues of the body as well. One reason to have a broad and flat aponeurosis instead of a cord-like tendon is that an aponeurosis can spread out the force of a muscle's pull on its attachment site; this can allow for the muscle to attach into soft tissue that otherwise would not be able to withstand the concentrated force of a tendon pulling on it.

- Hence the tendons and/or aponeuroses of a muscle are an integral part of the muscle and cannot be divorced from the muscle. Indeed, many texts now refer to a muscle as a **myofascial unit**—the *myo* referring to the muscular tissue component and the *fascial* referring to the fibrous fascial component.

BOX 10-9

There is an interesting application of this knowledge to massage and bodywork. Many techniques focus on their effect on the muscles; others purport to work solely on the fascial planes of muscles. It is impossible to do any type of bodywork and not affect both the muscular tissue and the fascial tissue of a muscle!

- In addition to the fact that muscular fascia extends beyond the muscles to become tendons and aponeuroses, it also creates thick intermuscular septa that separate muscles of the body and provide a site of attachment for adjacent muscles.
- Muscular fascia also creates even more expansive thin aponeurotic sheets of fascia that envelope large groups of muscles in the body (Box 10-10).
- Another function of these fascial planes of tissue is that they provide pathways for the nerves and blood vessels that innervate and feed nutrients to the muscle fibers (Figure 10-7).

BOX 10-10

The collagen fibers of aponeurotic sheets of deep fascia have a discernable direction. The directional lines of these fibers are called **Langer's lines** *(see accompanying illustration).* An application of this knowledge is that when a CORE myofascial therapist is doing spreading strokes, they are applied in accordance with Langer's lines.

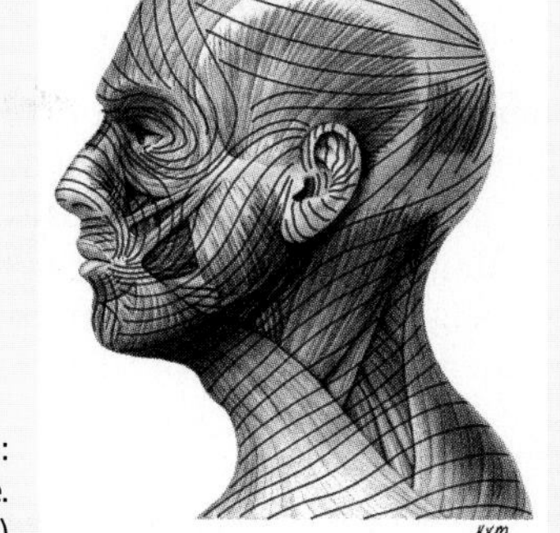

(From Standring S, ed: Gray's anatomy, 38th edition: the anatomical basis of clinical practice. Edinburgh, 2001, Churchill Livingstone.)

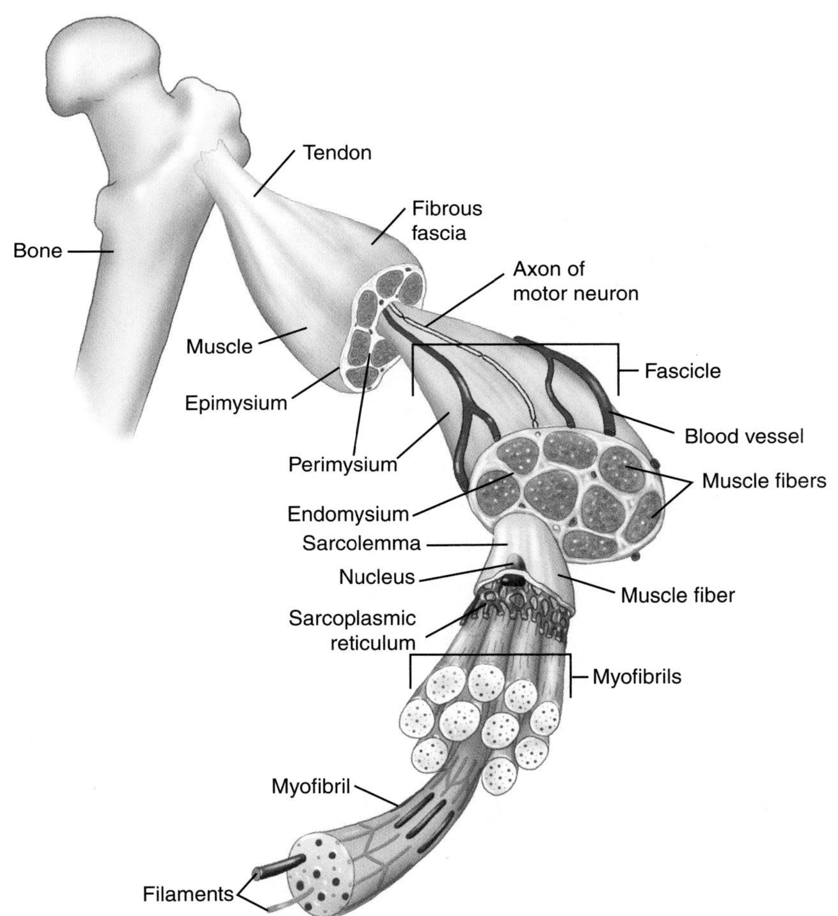

Figure 10-7 Interior of a muscle fiber (i.e., muscle cell). The large number of myofibrils that fill the sarcoplasm of the muscle fiber should be noted. These myofibrils run the entire length of the muscle fiber.

10.5 MICROANATOMY OF A MUSCLE FIBER/SARCOMERE STRUCTURE

- Like any other type of cell in the human body, skeletal muscle fibers are enveloped by a cell membrane and contain many **cytoplasmic organelles**.
- However, the names given to many of these cellular structures are slightly different from those given to most of the other types of cells of the body in that the root word *sarco* is often incorporated into the name.

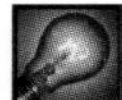

BOX 10-11

Sarco is the Greek root denoting flesh (i.e., muscle tissue).

- For example, the cytoplasm of a skeletal muscle fiber is called the **sarcoplasm**; the endoplasmic reticulum is called the **sarcoplasmic reticulum**; and the cell membrane is called the **sarcolemma**.
- Further, skeletal muscle fibers are unusual in that they are multinucleate (they contain many nuclei), they are rich in mitochondria, and they contain an oxygen-binding molecule called **myoglobin**.

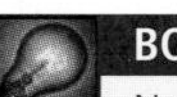

BOX 10-12

Note 1: A muscle fiber contains multiple nuclei because it developed from multiple stem cells grouping together.

Note 2: Mitochondria create adenosine triphosphate (ATP) molecules aerobically. Because muscle tissue contraction requires a great amount of energy expenditure, multiple mitochondria furnish this energy in the form of ATP molecules.

Note 3: Myoglobin is similar to hemoglobin of red blood cells, except that it has an even greater ability to bind oxygen.

- However, the most stunning structural characteristic of skeletal muscle fibers is their tremendous number of cytoplasmic organelles called *myofibrils*. Each **myofibril** is longitudinally oriented within the cytoplasm, running the entire length of the muscle fiber (see Figure 10-7).

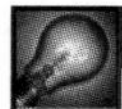

BOX 10-13

Approximately 1000 myofibrils exist in a muscle fiber.

- Myofibrils are composed of units called **sarcomeres** that are laid end to end from one end of the myofibril to the other end.

BOX 10-14

Sarcomeres are very short. On average, approximately 10,000 sarcomeres are found per linear inch (approximately 4000 per cm) of myofibril.

- The boundaries of each sarcomere are known as **Z-lines**.
- Within each sarcomere are protein filaments known as *actin* and *myosin*.
  - **Actin filaments** are thin, and **myosin filaments** are thick.
- These filaments are arranged in an orderly fashion. Actin filaments are attached to the Z-lines at both ends of a sarcomere; myosin filaments are not attached to the Z-lines, rather they are located in the center of the sarcomere.

BOX 10-15

Skeletal muscle tissue is said to be striated; this means that under a microscope it appears to have lines. It is the characteristic pattern of the overlapping of the actin and myosin filaments that creates this striation pattern that skeletal muscle tissue possesses.

- It is also important to note that myosin filaments have globular projections known as *heads*. Each **myosin head** sticks out toward the actin filaments (Figure 10-8).
- It is the sarcomere (of the myofibrils of muscle fibers) that is the actual functional unit of skeletal muscle tissue.
- That is, sarcomeres perform the essential physiologic function of contraction that makes muscle tissue unique from all other tissue types of the body.
- Therefore to truly understand the functioning of a muscle, we must examine the function of a sarcomere. If the function of a sarcomere is understood, then the larger picture of musculoskeletal function (i.e., the field of kinesiology) can be better understood.
- The name that is given to this physiologic process of a sarcomere is the *sliding filament mechanism*.

BOX 10-16

The knowledge of how the sliding filament mechanism works is essential to understanding the larger picture of how muscles function. Indeed, a clear understanding of concentric, eccentric, and isometric contractions, as well as the principles of trigger point genesis and active insufficiency (among other concepts), are dependent on a fundamental understanding of the sliding filament mechanism. Instead of being merely an abstract study of the microphysiology of muscle cells, the sliding filament mechanism creates the foundation for being able to truly understand (instead of having to memorize) the larger concepts needed to be an effective therapist/trainer in the musculoskeletal field.

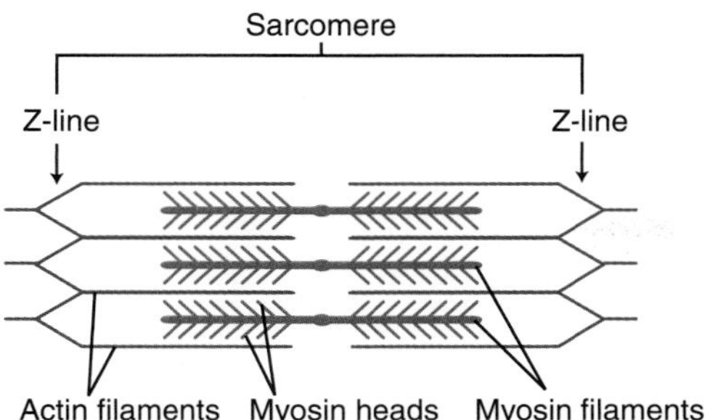

Figure 10-8 Structure of a sarcomere. A sarcomere spans from one Z-line to another Z-line. Sarcomeres contain two types of filaments: (1) actin and (2) myosin. Myosin filaments are the thicker filaments located in the center of the sarcomere. Actin filaments are the thinner filaments attached to the Z-lines. The armlike globular projections, called *heads of the myosin filaments,* should be noted.

10.6 SLIDING FILAMENT MECHANISM

- The mechanism that explains how sarcomeres shorten is called the **sliding filament mechanism,** because during shortening of a sarcomere, the actin and myosin filaments slide along each other.

BOX 10-17

The sliding filament mechanism is often termed the *sliding filament theory.* It should be noted that the word *theory* in the field of science is often misunderstood today. In everyday English, the word *theory* means *a guess or conjecture that remains to be proven*; it is a fairly weak term that connotes a fair amount of doubt as to whether or not it is true. However, in the field of science, the word *theory* is a much stronger term (indeed, the word *law,* which is even stronger, is rarely used). Little doubt exists as to the veracity of the mechanism of the sliding filament theory.

The sliding filament theory is also known as the **ratchet theory**. The name *ratchet theory* denotes the idea of how the myosin's cross-bridges pull on the actin filament in a ratchetlike manner. A ratchet wrench exerts tension on a nut, then lets go of this tension as you swing it back, then exerts tension once again; this cycle being repeated over and over. Similarly, a myosin cross-bridge pulls on the actin filament exerting tension; then it relaxes by letting go, exerts tension once again, and then relaxes again. This cycle is repeated many times.

- In essence, the mechanism of the sliding filament mechanism is as follows (Figure 10-9):

1. A message is sent from the nervous system that tells muscle fibers to contract.
2. This message causes the sarcoplasmic reticulum to release stored calcium into the sarcoplasm (cytoplasm).
3. These calcium ions attach onto the actin filaments, exposing **actin filament binding sites**.

BOX 10-18

Actin filament binding sites are often called **actin filament active sites**.

4. Myosin heads attach onto these exposed binding sites of the actin filaments, creating cross-bridges between the myosin filament and the actin filaments.
5. Each **myosin cross-bridge** then bends, creating a pulling force that pulls the actin filament in toward the center of the sarcomere.
6. These cross-bridges then break, reattach onto the next binding sites of the actin filaments, and bend, further pulling the actin filaments in toward the center of the sarcomere.

BOX 10-19

When an illustration of actin and myosin filaments is shown, it is common to simplify and show only one or a few cross-bridges. In reality, thousands of cross-bridges exist between a myosin and an actin filament. When some of these cross-bridges break, others remain attached so that the actin filament does not slip back.

7. This process occurs over and over again as long as the message to contract is given to the muscle by the nervous system.
8. Because the actin filaments are attached to the Z-lines of the sarcomere (i.e., the boundaries of the sarcomere), the Z-lines are pulled in toward the center of the sarcomere.
9. When Z-lines are pulled in toward the center of the sarcomere, the sarcomere shortens (Figure 10-10).
10. To relate this concept to the bigger picture of how a muscle works, it is important to realize that when all the sarcomeres of a myofibril shorten in this manner, the myofibril shortens; when all the myofibrils of a muscle fiber shorten, the muscle fiber shortens. When enough muscle fibers of a muscle shorten, the muscle shortens, exerting a pulling force on its bony attachments. If this pulling force is sufficiently strong, the bones are pulled toward each other, creating movement of the body parts within which the bones are located. Hence via the sliding filament mechanism, muscles can create movement of body parts!

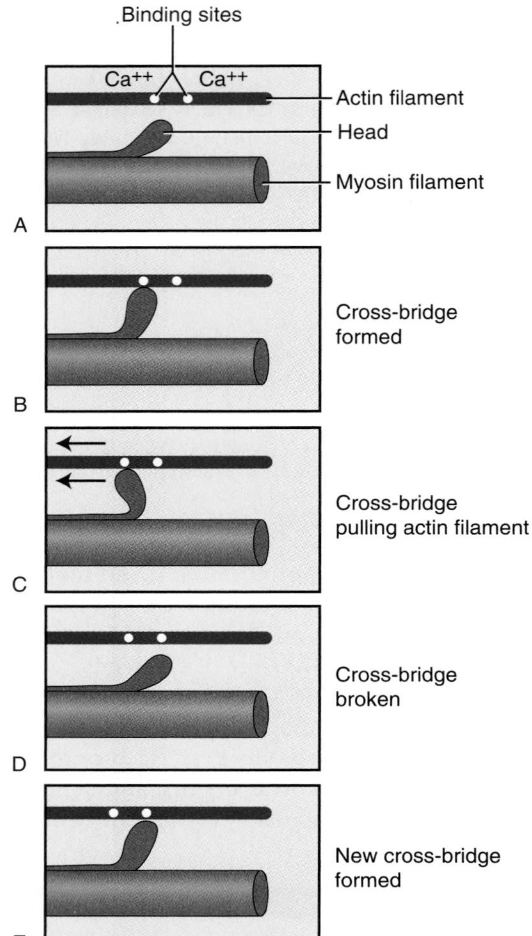

Figure 10-9 Steps of the sliding filament mechanism. *A,* Binding sites are exposed because of the presence of calcium ions that have been released by the sarcoplasmic reticulum. *B,* Myosin head forms a cross-bridge by attaching the actin binding site. *C,* Myosin head bends, pulling the actin filament toward the center of the sarcomere. *D,* Myosin cross-bridge breaks. *E,* Process begins again when the myosin head attaches to another actin binding site.

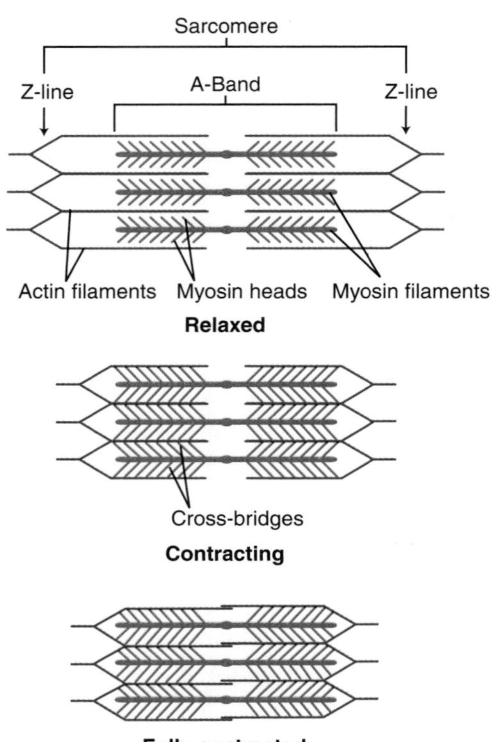

Figure 10-10 Illustration of how the sliding filament mechanism results in a change in length of the sarcomere. From the resting length of a sarcomere when it is relaxed, we see that as the sarcomere begins to contract, it begins to shorten toward its center. When the sarcomere is fully contracted, the sarcomere is at its shortest length.

10.7 ENERGY SOURCE FOR THE SLIDING FILAMENT MECHANISM

It is intuitively known that muscle contraction demands a great deal of energy expenditure by the body. We only need to exercise for a short period of time to realize how energy demanding muscle contraction is.

- The energy that drives the sliding filament mechanism comes from **adenosine triphosphate** (ATP) molecules.
- Two steps of the sliding filament mechanism require the expenditure of energy by ATP molecules:
  1. Energy must be furnished by ATP molecules for myosin-actin cross-bridges to form.
  2. The reuptake of calcium back into the sarcoplasmic reticulum when a muscle contraction is completed also requires energy to be provided by ATP molecules.

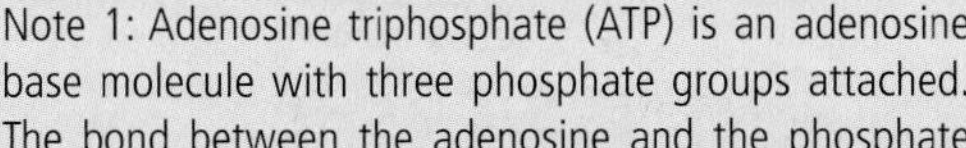

BOX 10-20 SPOTLIGHT ON ATP

Note 1: Adenosine triphosphate (ATP) is an adenosine base molecule with three phosphate groups attached. The bond between the adenosine and the phosphate groups contain energy and can be broken to liberate energy for use by the sliding filament mechanism. Once the bond has been broken, adenosine diphosphate and a free phosphate group results. The adenosine diphosphate can be converted back to ATP for use again by the body. Thus ATP molecules can be likened to rechargeable batteries that provide energy for the processes for metabolism.

Note 2: More specifically, energy provided by ATP is necessary for myosin-actin cross-bridges to first break; they then reform and bend. (For more detail, see Section 10.12.)

Note 3: It is because energy is required to break the myosin-actin cross-bridges that accounts for rigor mortis, which is the stiffness caused by muscle contractions that occurs shortly after a person dies. Two reasons for these contractions exist: (1) Some of the muscles were in a state of contraction when the person died, and (2) other muscle contractions occur after death because of calcium ions that leak out of the sarcoplasmic reticulum into the sarcoplasm, triggering myosin-actin cross-bridges to occur. However, because the person's metabolism stops after death, no further ATP molecules are created to break these cross-bridges of contraction. Rigor mortis continues until the tissue actually breaks down and the cross-bridges cease to exist.

Note 4: ATP expenditure for the reuptake of calcium back into the sarcoplasmic reticulum explains the current theory for how trigger points form and why they persist. Trigger points squeeze blood vessels, thereby diminishing blood flow. Loss of blood flow decreases the delivery of glucose to the muscle cells, resulting in a deficiency of ATP production. This energy shortage results in a decreased ability to both break the cross-bridges that exist and to reuptake the calcium from the sarcoplasm back into the sarcoplasmic reticulum; thus cross-bridges persist in that local area in the form of trigger points.

- Following is the order of the four steps in which ATP molecules are supplied to provide the energy needed for the sliding filament mechanism.
  1. Stored ATP
  2. Regeneration of ATP from stored creatine phosphate
  3. Regeneration of ATP from anaerobic breakdown of glucose
  4. Regeneration of ATP from aerobic breakdown of glucose
- First, stored ATP molecules within the muscle fiber are used. However, the supply of stored ATP molecules is very small and is soon depleted.
- Therefore the second step is to regenerate more ATP from creatine phosphate molecules that are present and stored in the muscle fiber.
- When the stored creatine phosphate supply is exhausted, ATP must be regenerated from another source, the breakdown of glucose.

BOX 10-21

Breakdown of glucose is more correctly termed **respiration of glucose**.

- Breakdown of glucose can occur in two ways: (1) aerobically or (2) anaerobically.
  - Regeneration of ATP from glucose first occurs anaerobically (without the presence of oxygen) within the sarcoplasm of the cell.

BOX 10-22

Anaerobic breakdown of glucose is known as **glycolysis** (*glyco* means *sugar*, *lysis* means *breakdown*). For each molecule of glucose broken down by the process of glycolysis, two adenosine triphosphate (ATP) molecules are formed and the waste product **lactic acid** is created.

  - If a continuing supply of energy is still needed, the muscle fiber gradually transitions to the breakdown of glucose aerobically within the mitochondria (Box 10-23, Note 1). Aerobic breakdown of glucose within the mitochondria requires oxygen (hence the name *aerobic*) and therefore requires circulation of blood to deliver this oxygen; this increased circulation places a demand on the heart to pump more blood and thereby exercises the heart (Box 10-23, Note 2).

BOX 10-23

Note 1: Aerobic breakdown of glucose is known as the *Kreb's cycle* (it is also known as the *citric acid cycle*). The Kreb's cycle creates approximately 36 molecules of adenosine triphosphate (ATP) for each molecule of glucose that is broken down; it is much more efficient than the process of glycolysis. The waste products of the Kreb's cycle are carbon dioxide and water. It is interesting to note that the role of oxygen in the Kreb's cycle is to bond to the carbon atoms that are created when a glucose molecule is broken down; this creates carbon dioxide, which is a gas that can be easily carried away in the bloodstream and eliminated from the body via the lungs. Thus oxygen's role in our bodies is to facilitate the elimination of the carbon atoms.

Note 2: People often speak of aerobic and anaerobic exercises, which actually refer to the method of the breakdown of glucose to generate ATP for energy for the sliding filament mechanism. Because the body turns to aerobic breakdown of glucose last, aerobic exercises must be, by necessity, exercises that are sustained. For example, a sprint is anaerobic and a marathon is aerobic. It actually takes only 1-2 minutes for the energy of an exercise to be primarily delivered via aerobic breakdown of glucose. Of course, once this threshold is reached, it must be sustained for a further period of time for cardiovascular benefits to be gained. Exactly how much longer is optimal is debated.

Oxygen Debt:

- If a person exercises and overcomes the ability of the cardiovascular system to deliver oxygen for the aerobic breakdown of glucose, then the muscle fibers must rely on anaerobic breakdown of glucose to a greater degree. Because anaerobic breakdown of glucose creates lactic acid as a waste product, lactic acid can build up in the muscle fibers. This lactic acid is usually transported to the liver where it can be converted back to glucose. However, this conversion requires oxygen, and the oxygen needed can be looked at as a debt that the body owes itself. For this reason, the term **oxygen debt** is used to describe this debt of oxygen that is needed to convert the buildup of lactic acid back to glucose. This oxygen debt explains why a person may continue to breathe deeply even after their exercise is completed.

10.8 NERVOUS SYSTEM CONTROL OF MUSCLE CONTRACTION

- A skeletal muscle fiber cannot contract on its own; it must be told to contract by the nervous system.
- Contraction of a skeletal muscle fiber is directed by a message from the central nervous system that travels within a motor neuron that is located within a peripheral nerve. The peripheral spinal nerve that goes out into the periphery and directs the muscle to contract is said to provide **innervation** to the muscle (Figure 10-11).

BOX 10-24

Regarding neurologic terms: the central nervous system is located in the center of the body; hence the name. It is comprised of the brain and the spinal cord. A neuron is a nerve cell; a motor neuron is a motor nerve cell (i.e., a nerve cell that tells muscles to contract). A peripheral nerve is located in the periphery of the body (i.e., not in the center or central nervous system). Spinal nerves that come from the spinal cord and cranial nerves that come from the brain are peripheral nerves. Each peripheral nerve contains many neurons.

- When the motor neuron reaches the muscle fiber, it does not physically attach or connect directly to the muscle fiber. Rather, a small space is located between them that is known as the **synaptic cleft**.

BOX 10-25

A synaptic cleft is also known as a **synaptic gap** or simply a **synapse**.

- The electrical message for contraction that the motor neuron carries causes the motor neuron to release molecules into the synapse. These molecules transmit the neural message for contraction to the muscle fiber; hence they are called **neurotransmitters**.

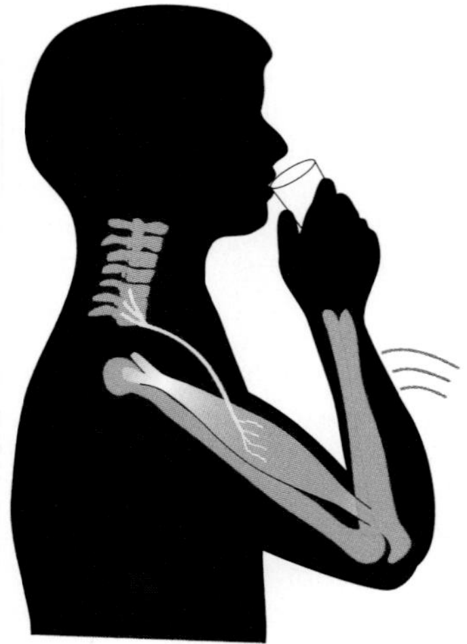

Figure 10-11 A person contracting an arm muscle to flex the forearm at the elbow joint to drink a glass of water. The order to contract this muscle occurs within the central nervous system and is then carried within a motor neuron that is located within a peripheral spinal nerve that exits the spinal cord in the cervical spine region. This peripheral spinal nerve is said to innervate this muscle.

BOX 10-26

Many neurotransmitters exist in the human body. The one that is released between motor neurons and skeletal muscle fibers is **acetylcholine**. When a motor neuron is no longer stimulated to secrete acetylcholine, the acetylcholine that was secreted and is present within the synaptic cleft is removed by the enzyme **acetylcholinesterase**. Once the neurotransmitter acetylcholine is no longer present, the muscle cell is no longer stimulated to contract and can relax.

- The location where the motor neuron and muscle fiber meet (i.e., junction) is known as the **neuromuscular junction** (Figure 10-12).
- At the neuromuscular junction, the sarcolemma (i.e., cell membrane) of the muscle fiber is specialized to receive the neurotransmitters of the motor neuron and is known as the **motor end plate**.
- These neurotransmitters float through the fluid of the synapse and bind to the motor end plate of the muscle fiber.
- The binding of the neurotransmitters to the motor end plate initiates an electrical impulse to travel along the sarcolemma of the entire muscle fiber. The electrical impulse is then transmitted into the interior of the muscle fiber via the **transverse tubules** (usually called **T tubules**) of the muscle fiber (Figure 10-13).
- Once this electrical message to contract has reached the interior of the muscle fiber, it triggers the sliding filament mechanism to begin by causing the release of stored calcium from the sarcoplasmic reticulum into the sarcoplasm. (See the discussion of the sliding filament mechanism in Section 10.6.)
- Motor neurons only carry a message for contraction of the muscle fiber. As long as the motor neuron is stimulating a muscle fiber, calcium will continue to be released from the sarcoplasmic reticulum into the sarcoplasm, which will continue the sliding filament mechanism for contraction, and the muscle fiber will remain in a contracted state.
- If the central nervous system desires a muscle fiber to relax, then a message for contraction is not sent to the muscle. In other words, in the absence of a neural message for contraction, a muscle fiber relaxes.

BOX 10-27

It is important to emphasize that a muscle fiber has no ability to contract on its own. Further, it has no stored pattern or memory of how or when to contract. The term **muscle memory**, used so prevalently in the fields of bodywork and exercise, describes the very important concept of the memory pattern of muscle contractions that exists in the body. However, muscle memory resides in the nervous system, not within the muscle tissue itself. A muscle that has lost its innervation loses its ability to contract completely (unless electricity is applied to it from an outside source, such as from physical therapy equipment).

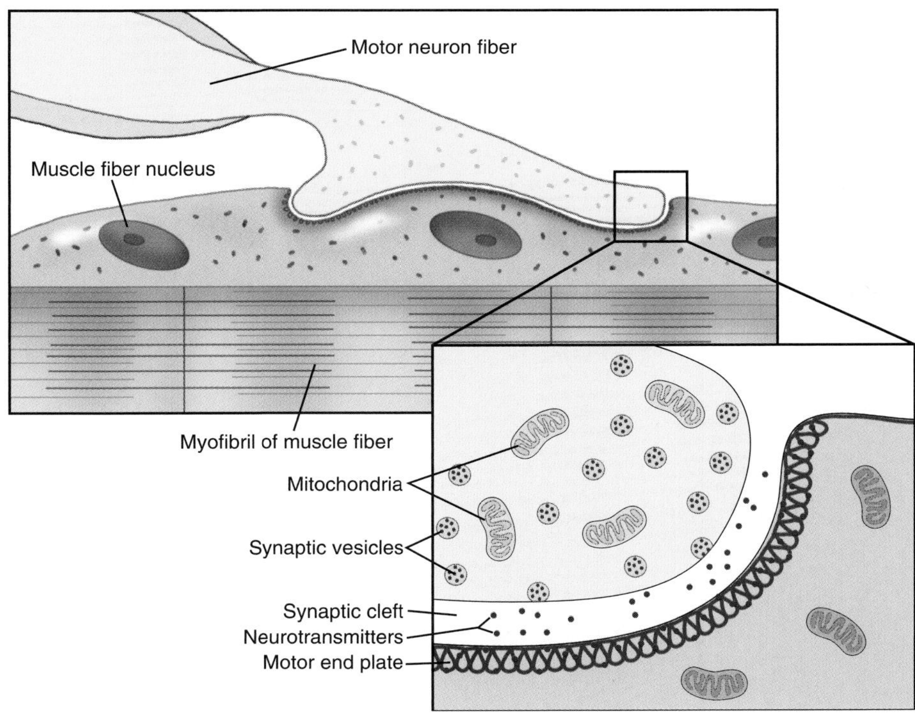

Figure 10-12 Neuromuscular junction. We see the synaptic vesicles containing neurotransmitter molecules in the distal end of the motor neuron. These neurotransmitters are released into the synaptic cleft and then bind to the motor end plate of the muscle fiber. (Note: The inset box provides an enlargement.)

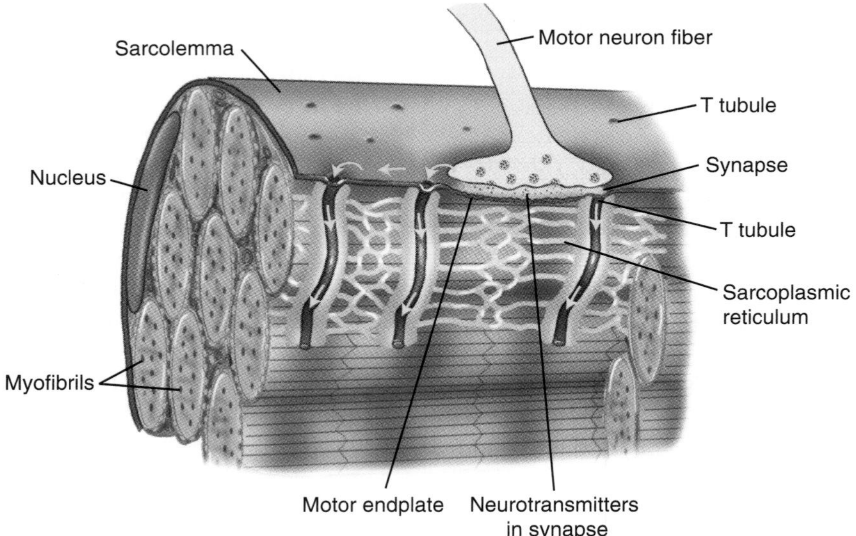

Figure 10-13 Binding of the neurotransmitters onto the motor end plate of the muscle fiber initiates an electrical impulse to travel along the sarcolemma of the entire muscle fiber. The electrical impulse is then transmitted into the interior of the muscle fiber via the transverse tubules (i.e., T tubules) of the muscle fiber.

- ❑ Once a muscle fiber is no longer stimulated to contract, the calcium ions that were released by the sarcoplasmic reticulum are reabsorbed back into the sarcoplasmic reticulum. Once the calcium is no longer present, the binding sites on actin are no longer available to the myosin heads; thus cross-bridges cannot be made, and the sliding filament mechanism can no longer occur. Therefore muscle fiber contraction ceases and the muscle fiber relaxes.

BOX 10-28

As previously stated in Section 10.7, reabsorption of calcium back into the sarcoplasmic reticulum necessary to stop the sliding filament mechanism requires energy expenditure by adenosine triphosphate (ATP).

10.9 MOTOR UNIT

- A **motor unit** is defined as "one motor neuron and all the muscle fibers that it controls" (i.e., with which it synapses).
- When a motor neuron reaches a muscle, it branches numerous times to synapse with a number of muscle fibers. In this manner, a motor neuron actually controls a number of muscle fibers.

BOX 10-29

It is interesting to note that one motor unit usually has muscle fibers that are located in a number of different fascicles; in other words, motor units have fibers that are somewhat spread throughout the muscle and are not restricted to fascicular organization.

- This branching is important because skeletal muscle fibers cannot pass the message to contract from one to another. Instead, each individual muscle fiber must be told to contract directly by the motor neuron.
- The distinguishing factor that determines the size of a motor unit is the number of branches, and therefore the number of muscle fibers that one motor neuron controls; this varies from as few as 2-3 to as many as 2000.

BOX 10-30

All motor units are similar in that they have one motor neuron. Motor units of different sizes vary in the number of muscle fibers that they contain. The number of muscle fibers varies from just a few to as many as 2000. The average number of fibers in a motor unit is between 100 and 200.

- The term *motor unit* is used to describe this concept (Figure 10-14).
- Smaller motor units create contraction of a smaller number of muscle fibers and therefore create smaller, finer, more precise actions.
  - Therefore smaller motor units exist where very fine and precise body movements are needed. The smallest motor units exist in the muscles that move the eyeball (i.e., extraoccular muscles).
- Larger motor units create a contraction of a greater number of muscle fibers and therefore create larger, grosser, more powerful actions.
- Therefore larger motor units tend to exist where larger movements are needed and finer precise movements are not necessary. Larger motor units exist in such muscles as the gluteus maximus and gastrocnemius. (For information on the types of muscle fibers that are found in smaller versus larger motor units, see Section 10.13. For more details on how and when motor units are recruited to contract, see Section 15.1.)
- Generally a muscle will have a mixture of motor units; some will be small and some will be large.

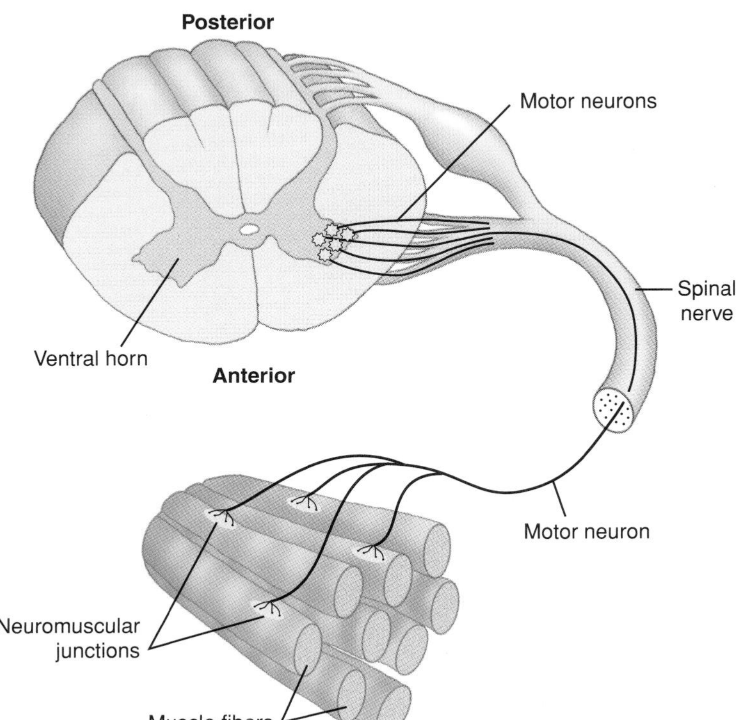

Figure 10-14 Small motor unit containing four muscle fibers. A motor neuron is shown exiting the spinal cord and traveling through a spinal nerve and innervating four muscle fibers of a muscle. One motor neuron and the muscle fibers that it controls are defined as a motor unit.

☐ 10.10 ALL-OR-NONE RESPONSE LAW

- When a message for contraction is sent from the nervous system to a muscle fiber, that message instructs the muscle fiber to contract completely (i.e., 100%). If no message is sent, then the muscle fiber relaxes completely (i.e., 0% contraction).
- Therefore a muscle fiber contraction is an all-or-nothing mechanism and this concept is called the **all-or-none response law**.
- If we understand how muscle tissue is innervated by the nervous system, then it is easy to apply the all-or-none response law to muscle tissue.
  - The all-or-none response law applies to the sarcomere, the myofibril, the muscle fiber, and the motor unit, because all these structural levels of muscle tissue are innervated by a single motor neuron that either carries the message to contract or does not carry the message to contract.
  - However, the all-or-none response law does not apply to an entire skeletal muscle. A skeletal muscle can have partial contractions.
  - A skeletal muscle has a number of motor units within it; some of these motor units may be told to contract by their motor neurons, whereas other motor units within the muscle may be relaxed because their motor neurons are not stimulating them to contract at that time.
  - Therefore an entire skeletal muscle can have partial contractions because the nervous system can order some motor units to contract while others are relaxed. In this manner, the nervous system can control the degree of contraction of a muscle. By having the ability to control the degree of contraction, a person can generate just the right amount of force as needed for each particular situation. For example, if a person wants to do a bicep curl and lift a 5-lb weight, a partial contraction of the biceps brachii muscle is needed. If however, the person wants to do a bicep curl and lift a 15-lb weight, a stronger partial contraction by the biceps brachii is needed. Again, a partial contraction of a muscle occurs by having some of the motor units of the muscle contract completely and other motor units of the muscle not contract at all (Figure 10-15). In other words, more motor units will contract to lift the 15-lb weight than the 5-lb weight.

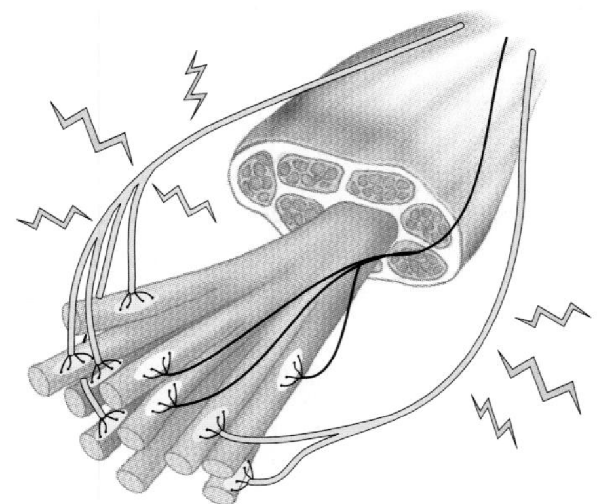

Figure 10-15 Illustration of the idea that a muscle contains multiple motor units and that some may contract while others are relaxed. In this figure, two motor units *(yellow)* are contracting, while the other motor unit *(black)* is relaxed.

10.11 SARCOMERE STRUCTURE IN MORE DETAIL

- A myofibril of a muscle fiber is made up of many sarcomeres that are arranged both next to each other and that also lay end to end along the length of the sarcomere.
- Each sarcomere is made up of actin and myosin filaments. These filaments are arranged in a hexangular fashion so that a myosin filament is located in the center of the sarcomere and six actin filaments are located around the myosin filament, partially overlapping it (Figure 10-16).
- This consistent pattern of overlapping filaments within the sarcomeres gives myofibrils a banded striated appearance. These bands are designated with letters (Figure 10-17a).
- The two main bands are the A-band and the I-band.

BOX 10-31

The letters *A* in A-band and *I* in I-band stand for *anisotropic* and *isotropic*, which are optical terms that describe how light is affected when viewing this tissue under a microscope.

  - The **A-band** is dark and is defined by the presence of myosin. Because myosin is in the center of a sarcomere, the A-band is located in the center of the sarcomere. Note: Within the A-band a region exists where only myosin is located and a region exists where myosin and actin are located.
  - The **I-band** is light and is defined by where only actin filaments are located. Note that the I-band is partially within one sarcomere and partially located within the adjacent sarcomere.
  - Again, these alternating dark and light bands give skeletal muscle its striated appearance (Figure 10-17b–c).
- Smaller bands are also located within these larger bands:
  - The **H-band** is the region of the A-band that contains only myosin.
  - The **M-band** (usually referred to as the **M-line**) is within the H-band (which in turn is located within the A-band) at the center of the myosin molecule.
  - The **Z-band**, usually referred to as the Z-line, is at the center of the I-band. Remember that the Z-line is the border between two adjacent sarcomeres.

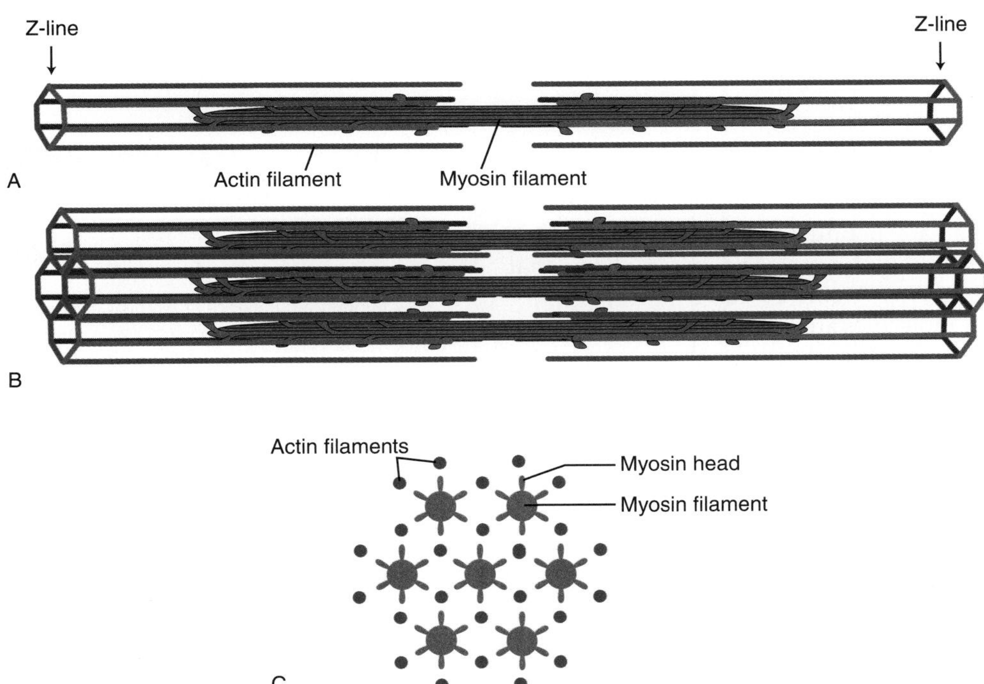

Figure 10-16 *A,* One myosin filament surrounded by six actin filaments. *B,* How multiple sarcomeres that lay next to each other are arranged. *C,* Cross-section of a sarcomere showing that each myosin is surrounded by six actin filaments. (Note: More than one myosin may form cross-bridges with the same actin filament.)

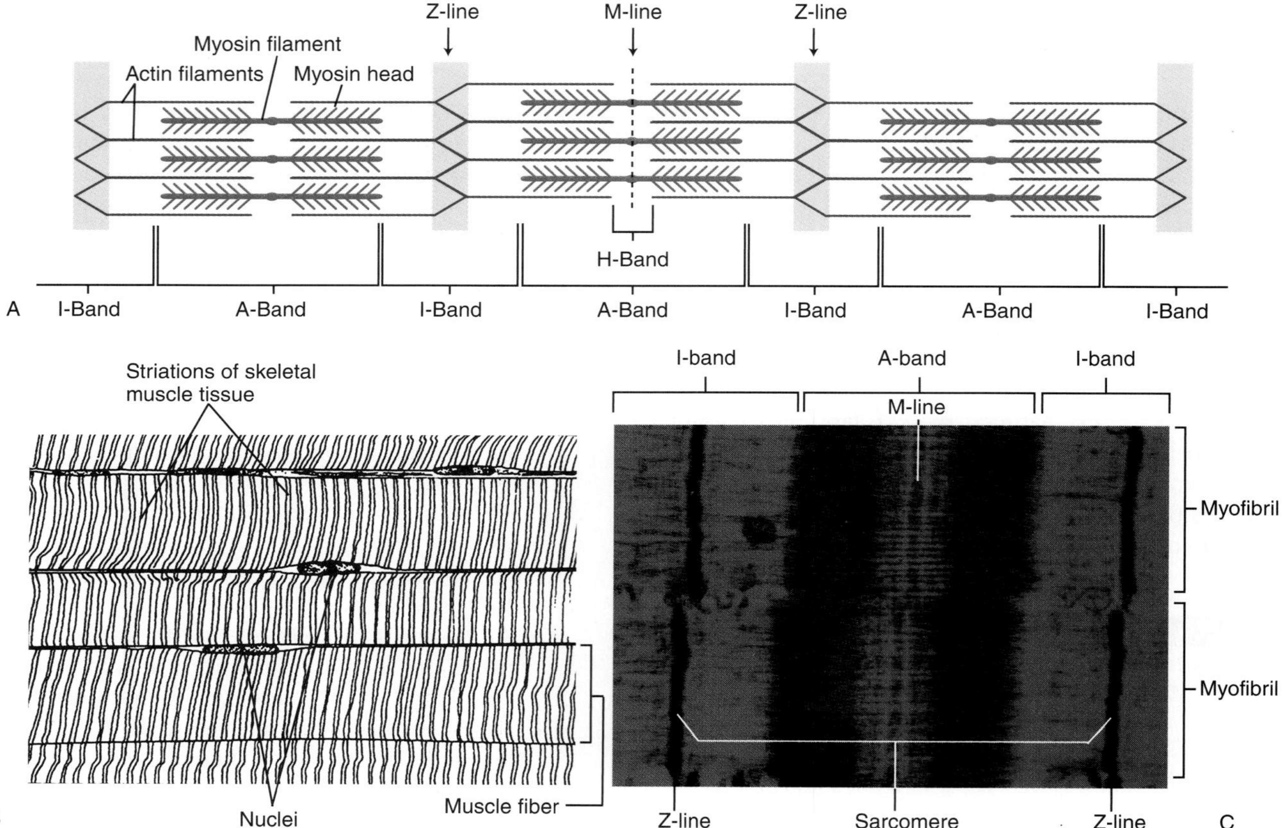

Figure 10-17 *A,* Three sarcomeres laid end to end. The consistent overlapping of actin and myosin filaments creates bands of striations that are named with letters. The two major bands are the A-band (where actin and myosin overlap) and the I-band (where only actin is present). *B,* Sketch of photomicrograph of skeletal muscle tissue that demonstrates the striated appearance. *C,* Same view as in *B* but at greater magnification in an electron micrograph. The A-band and I-bands are easily seen and identified. (*B* and *C* from Thibodeau GA, Patton KT: *Anatomy and physiology,* ed 5, St Louis, 2003, Mosby.)

Myosin Filament in More Detail:

- A myosin filament is actually made up of many myosin molecules that are bound together (Figure 10-18a). Each individual myosin molecule has a shape that resembles a golf club (Figure 10-18b).
- These myosin molecules are arranged such that half of them have their heads sticking out at one end of the sarcomere and the other half of them have their heads sticking out at the other end of the sarcomere.
- Each myosin molecule is composed of two main parts: (1) the **myosin tail** and (2) the myosin head.
- The tail is the main length of the myosin molecule.

BOX 10-32

The tail of a myosin molecule is called the **light meromyosin** component.

- The head is the part that sticks out to attach onto the actin filament, forming the actin-myosin cross-bridge.

BOX 10-33

The actin-myosin cross-bridge is called the **heavy meromyosin** component. It is actually composed of two subcomponents: (1) the head (also known as the **S1 fragment**) and (2) the neck (also known as the **S2 fragment**).

Although a number of differences exist between the different types of muscle fibers (see Section 10.13 for details), the largest difference seems to occur in the cross-bridge of myosin filaments.

Actin Filament in More Detail:

- An actin filament is made up of three separate protein molecules: (1) actin, (2) troponin, and (3) tropomyosin.
- The bulk of the actin filament is composed of many small spheric **actin molecules** that are strung together like beads, forming two strands that twist around each other (Figure 10-19a).
  - Each actin molecule is a binding site to which a myosin cross-bridge can attach. However, these binding sites are not normally *exposed.*

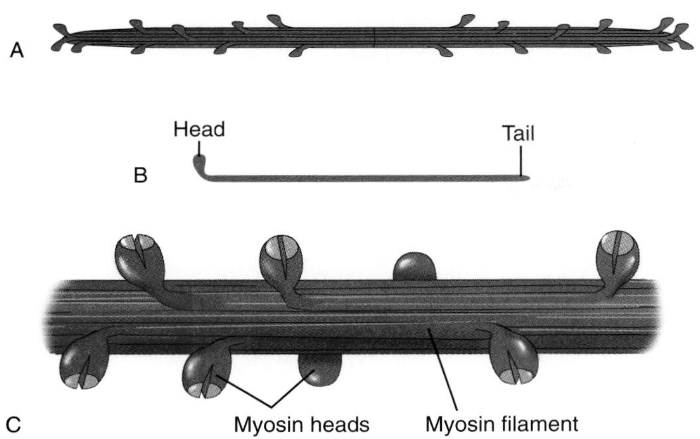

Figure 10-18 *A,* Myosin filament made up of many myosin molecules. *B,* One myosin molecule. *C,* Close-up of a myosin filament.

- Attached to these strands of actin molecules are troponin and tropomyosin molecules (Figure 10-19b).
  - **Tropomyosin molecules** normally block the binding sites of actin from being exposed (and bound to by myosin's heads).
  - **Troponin molecules** have the ability to move tropomyosin out of the way so that the binding sites of actin are exposed.

BOX 10-34

When calcium ions attach to the troponin molecules of the actin filament, the troponin molecules move the tropomyosin molecules out of the way so that the binding (active) sites of actin are exposed. This allows for the formation of cross-bridges (i.e., contraction).

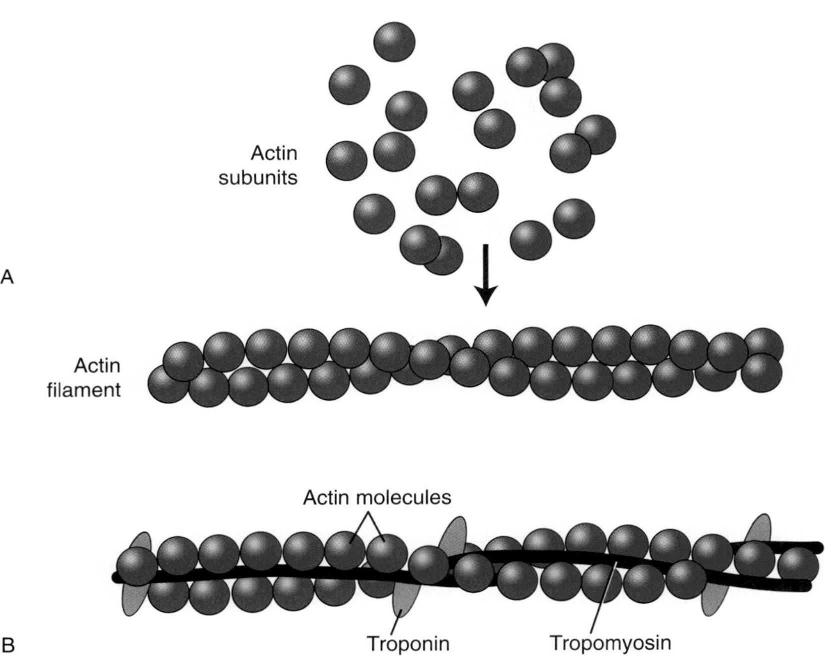

Figure 10-19 *A,* Actin molecules (i.e., subunits) form into two chains that twist together. *B,* Complete actin filament composed of actin molecules, tropomyosin, and troponin molecules.

10.12 SLIDING FILAMENT MECHANISM IN MORE DETAIL

- In more detail, the steps of the sliding filament mechanism occur as follows:
  1. When we will a contraction of a muscle, a message commanding this to occur originates in our brain. This message travels as an electrical impulse within our central nervous system.
  2. This electrical impulse then travels out into the periphery in a motor neuron of a peripheral nerve to go to the skeletal muscle.

BOX 10-35

The message may be carried in a cranial nerve or a spinal nerve, and this message may be carried in many motor neurons (i.e., one motor neuron for each motor unit that is directed to contract).

  3. When the impulse gets to the end of the motor neuron, the motor neuron secretes its neurotransmitters (i.e., acetylcholine) into the synaptic cleft at the neuromuscular junction.
  4. These neurotransmitters float across the synaptic cleft and bind to the motor end plate of the muscle fiber.
  5. The binding of these neurotransmitters onto the motor end plate causes an electrical impulse on the muscle fiber that travels along the muscle fiber's cell membrane.
  6. This electrical impulse is transmitted into the interior of the muscle fiber by the T tubules (i.e., transverse tubules).
  7. When this electrical impulse reaches the interior, it causes the sarcoplasmic reticulum of the muscle fiber to release stored calcium ions into the sarcoplasm.
  8. These calcium ions then bind onto troponin molecules of the actin filament.
  9. This causes a structural change, causing the tropomyosin molecules of the actin filament to move.
  10. When the tropomyosin molecules move, the binding sites of the actin filament (the actual actin molecules themselves) become exposed.
  11. Heads of the myosin filament attach onto the binding sites of the actin filament creating cross-bridges. These cross-bridges then bend, pulling the actin filament in toward the center of the sarcomere.
  12. If no ATP is present, this cross-bridge bond will stay in place and no further sliding of the filaments will occur.
  13. When ATP is present, the following sequence occurs: the cross-bridge between the myosin and actin breaks, the myosin head attaches onto the next binding site on the actin molecule, forming a new cross-bridge. This new cross-bridge bends and pulls the actin filament in toward the center of the sarcomere (Figure 10-20c, steps 1-4).
  14. This process in step 13 will continue to occur as long as ATP molecules are present to initiate the breakage, reattachment, and bending of the myosin cross-bridge.
  15. In this manner, the sarcomeres of the innervated muscle fibers will contract to 100% of their ability.
  16. When the nervous system message is no longer sent, neurotransmitters will no longer be released into the synapse. The neurotransmitters that were present are either broken down or are reabsorbed back into the motor neuron.
  17. Without the presence of neurotransmitters in the synapse, no impulse is sent into the interior of the muscle fiber, and calcium ions are no longer released from the sarcoplasmic reticulum.
  18. Calcium that was present in the sarcoplasm is reabsorbed into the sarcoplasmic reticulum by the expenditure of energy by ATP molecules.
  19. As the concentration of calcium drops, calcium will no longer be available to bind to troponin. Without calcium bound to it, troponin will no longer keep the tropomyosin from blocking the binding sites of the actin filament and the actin binding sites will be blocked once again. Therefore cross-bridges will no longer be made, and the sliding of filaments will no longer occur.

The big picture of the sliding filament mechanism must not be lost!

- The entire point of this process is that if actin filaments slide along myosin filaments in toward the center of the sarcomere, then the Z-lines that the actin filaments attach to will be pulled in toward the center of the sarcomere and the sarcomere will shorten.
- Because myofibrils are made up of sarcomeres laid end to end, when sarcomeres shorten, the myofibril shortens.
- Because a muscle fiber is made up of myofibrils, when myofibrils shorten, the muscle fiber shortens.
- Because a muscle is made up of many muscle fibers, when enough muscle fibers shorten, the muscle shortens in toward its center.
- Because the muscle is attached to two bones via its tendons, if this pulling force toward the center of the muscle is sufficient, the bones that the muscle attaches to will be pulled toward each other.
- Because bones are within body parts, movement of parts of our body can occur!
- In this manner, the sliding filament mechanism creates the force of a muscle contraction that creates movement of our body. The different types of muscle contractions (concentric, eccentric, and isometric) will be discussed in Chapter 12.

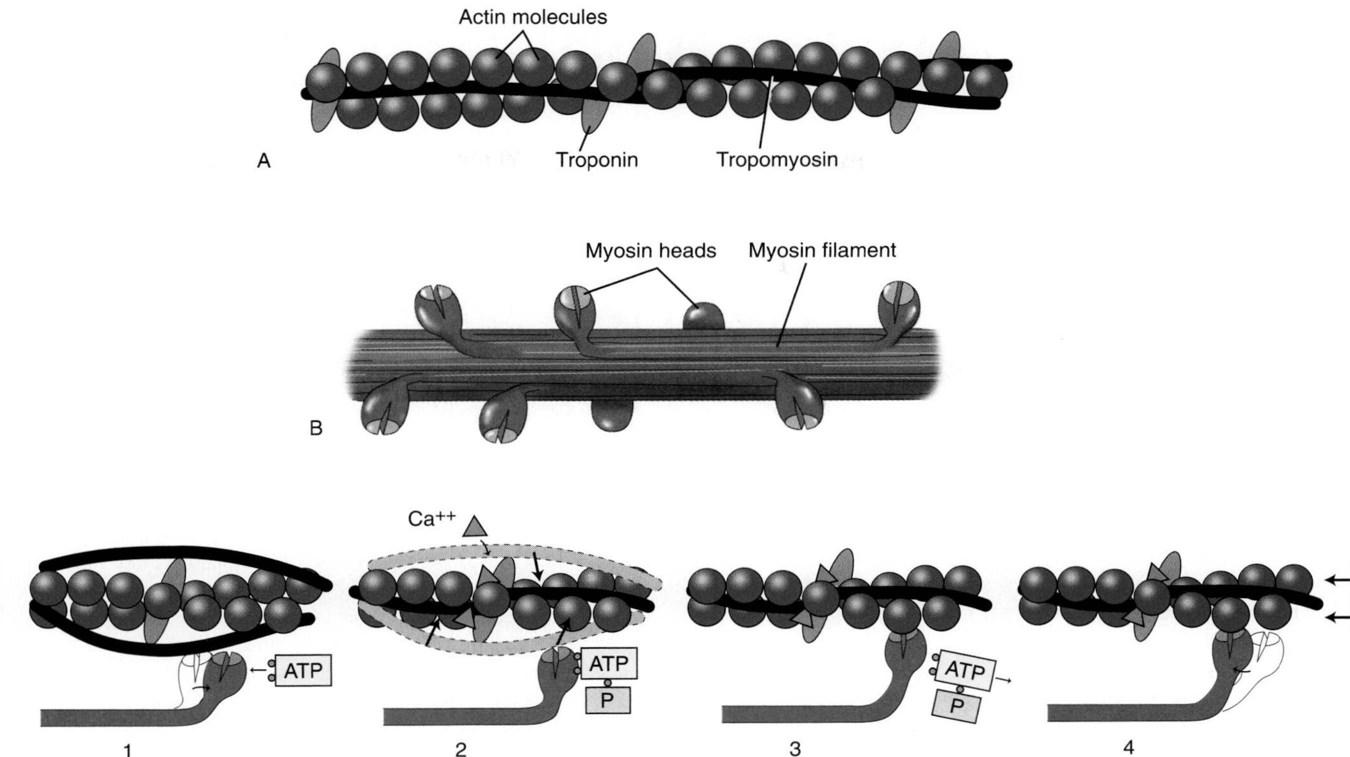

Figure 10-20 *A,* Structure of an actin filament; it is composed of actin, tropomyosin, and troponin molecules. *B,* Structure of a myosin filament. The heads stick out and can form cross-bridges by attaching to the binding sites of the actin filament when calcium is present. *C,* Steps of how the myosin-actin cross-bridges are formed and broken. In step 1, when an adenosine triphosphate (ATP) molecule attaches to the myosin head, the myosin head moves into its *resting position.* Step 2 shows calcium binding to the troponin molecule of the actin filament, causing the tropomyosin molecule to move out of the way and exposing the binding site of the actin filament. Step 3 shows the myosin head now attaching to the exposed binding site of the actin filament, forming the cross-bridge (and the ATP molecule is released from the myosin head). Step 4 shows the myosin head bend, pulling the actin filament in toward the center of the sarcomere (hence the sliding filament mechanism). (Note: The myosin head will remain bound to the actin filament in this position until another ATP binds to the myosin head, breaking the cross-bridge and causing the myosin head to move back to its resting position.)

10.13 RED AND WHITE MUSCLE FIBERS

Up until now, we have spoken about muscle fibers as if they are all identical. This is not true.

- Generally two types of muscle fibers exist: (1) red fibers and (2) white fibers.
  - Red fibers are also known as *red slow-twitch fibers;* white fibers are also known as *white fast-twitch fibers*.

BOX 10-36

Note 1: When dividing muscle fibers into categories, it is common to divide them into two categories: (1) red slow-twitch and (2) white fast-twitch. However, a 3rd intermediate category of fibers falls between the other two; the muscle fibers of this category are often termed **intermediate-twitch fibers**.

Note 2: Red and white fibers are analogous to dark and white meat in chicken or turkey. Dark meat of a chicken or turkey is muscle primarily composed of red fibers; white meat is muscle primarily composed of white fibers.

Note 3: Numerous terms describe the different types of muscle fibers. The names are based on describing different aspects of the fibers' anatomy or physiology. Beyond being described as red slow-twitch and white fast-twitch, these fibers are also described as being **Type I fibers** and **Type II fibers**, **oxidative fibers** and **glycolytic fibers**, **small fibers** and **large fibers**, **fatigue-resistant fibers** and **easily fatigued fibers**, and **tonic fibers** and **phasic fibers**, respectively. Furthermore, these terms are often combined together to create categories such as **slow oxidative (SO) fibers** and **fast glycolytic (FG) fibers**, among others. Unfortunately, all of these terms are used widely, so it is important that the student be at least somewhat familiar with them.

- **Red slow-twitch fibers** are so named because they are red and slow to contract.
  - The reason that red fibers are red is that they have a rich blood supply.
  - They are termed as *slow-twitch* because they are slow to contract from the instant that they receive the impulse to contract from the nervous system.
  - They take approximately $^1/_{10}$ of a second to reach maximum tension.
  - Red slow-twitch fibers are usually small in size.
- **White fast-twitch fibers** are so named because they are white and contract relatively fast.
  - The reason that white fibers are white is that they do not have a rich blood supply.
  - They are termed as *fast-twitch* because they contract quickly when they are directed to contract by the nervous system.
  - They take approximately $^1/_{20}$ of a second to reach maximum tension.
  - White fast-twitch fibers are usually large in size.

BOX 10-37 SPOTLIGHT ON MUSCLE TYPE AND BREAKDOWN OF GLUCOSE

The speed of contraction of a muscle fiber is primarily based on its method of adenosine triphosphate (ATP) formation from glucose. Red fibers rely primarily on the slower process of aerobic respiration of glucose via the Kreb's cycle in the mitochondria; thus the need for the greater blood supply to provide the oxygen needed for this pathway. Because aerobic respiration of glucose yields 36 ATPs per glucose molecule that is broken down, red slow-twitch fibers are ideally suited for endurance activities. White fibers rely primarily on the faster process of anaerobic respiration of glucose in the sarcoplasm via glycolysis; thus a lesser need for an oxygen-carrying blood supply. Because anaerobic respiration of glucose produces only two ATPs per glucose molecule that is broken down, white fast-twitch fibers are easily fatigued and are best suited for activities that require short bursts of maximal effort. Hence the relationship between red fibers and white fibers and aerobic and anaerobic activities stems from the blood supply and method of glucose breakdown. An analogy could be made between muscle fiber type and the classic story of the long-distance tortoise and the sprinter hare.

- Within a muscle, motor units are homogeneous, that is a motor unit has either all red slow-twitch fibers or all white fast-twitch fibers.
- Small motor units are composed of red slow-twitch fibers; large motor units are composed of white fast-twitch fibers.

BOX 10-38

Smaller motor units composed of red muscle fibers are innervated by smaller diameter motor neurons that carry the direction to contract at a slower rate from the central nervous system than the larger diameter motor neurons that innervate the larger motor units of composed of white fibers. This is another factor that accounts for the relative speed in which the different types of muscle fibers contract.

- Every muscle of the human body has a mixture of red and white fibers.
  - The percentage of this mixture will vary from one muscle to another muscle within one person's body.
  - Further, from one person to another person, the percentage of this mixture for the same muscle can also vary.

- Although some conversion seems possible, for the most part, the ratio of red and white fibers in our bodies is genetically determined.

BOX 10-39

Given that the percentage of red versus white fibers varies from individual to individual and the fact that these differences seem to be genetically determined, a natural conclusion is that although every person can improve at any sport with practice, based on our genetic differences of red/white muscle fiber concentrations, each person may have an inborn predisposition to excel at certain types of sports. For example, individuals with a greater concentration of red slow-twitch fibers are naturally suited for endurance activities such as long distance running, whereas individuals with a greater concentration of white fast-twitch fibers are naturally suited for sports that require short bursts of maximal energy such as sprinting.

- Generally red slow-twitch fibers contract slowly and do not create very powerful contractions, but they are able to hold their contraction for long periods of time. As a result, they are often more plentiful in muscles that must exhibit endurance and hold contractions for long periods of time, such as postural stabilization muscles.
- Generally white fast-twitch fibers are able to generate faster more powerful contractions, but they fatigue easily. Therefore they are usually more plentiful in muscles that need to create fast powerful movements but that do not have to hold that contraction for a long period of time, such as mobility muscles. (For more on postural stabilization versus mobility muscles, see Chapter 13, especially Section 13.6.)
  - For example, the soleus, which is more concerned with postural stabilization of the ankle joint generally contains approximately 67% red fibers and 33% white fibers; whereas the gastrocnemius, which is more concerned with creating movement at the ankle joint, generally contains approximately 50% red fibers and 50% white fibers.

10.14 MYOFASCIAL MERIDIANS AND TENSEGRITY

- When a student is first exposed to the study of kinesiology, it is customary to begin by learning the components of the musculoskeletal system separately. Thus we approach the study of kinesiology by first learning each of the individual bones and muscles of the human body as separate entities. We even separate the muscles from their fascial tissues, describing the muscle fibers as distinct from the endomysial, perimysial, and epimysial fascial wrappings, and separating the muscle belly from its fascial tendons/aponeuroses.
- Although this approach of breaking a whole into its parts may be useful and even necessary for the beginning student, it is crucially important that once the important job of learning these separate components has been accomplished, the student begins the even more important job of putting the pieces back together into the whole.
- After all, a muscle and its fascial tissues are one unit that cannot really be structurally or functionally separated. Indeed, the term *myofascial unit,* which describes this idea of the unity of a muscle and its fascial tissues, is gaining popularity. Further, even myofascial units (i.e., muscles) are not truly separate units that act in isolation from each other. Rather they belong to functional groups, the members of each group sharing a common joint action. These individual functional groups of muscles then coordinate together on an even larger stage to create body wide movement patterns. For more detail on functional groups of muscles, see Chapter 13.
- To this picture, fascial ligaments, joint capsules, bursae, tendon sheaths, and articular and fibrous cartilage must be added, creating a myofascial-skeletal system. In addition, because this system cannot function without direction from the nervous system, the nervous system must be included as well, creating a neuromyofascial-skeletal system that functions seamlessly.
- The concept of myofascial meridians is another way of looking at the structural and functional interconnectedness of this neuromyofascial-skeletal system. **Myofascial meridian theory** puts forth the concept that muscles operate within continuous lines of fascia that span across the body. Most notable for advancing this view is author Tom Myers. In his book, *Anatomy Trains,* Myers defines a **myofascial meridian** as a traceable continuum within the body of muscles embedded within fascial webbing. In effect, the muscles of a myofascial meridian are connected by the fibrous fascia connective tissue and act together synergistically, transmitting tension and movement through the meridian by means of their contractions. Myers has codified this interpretation of the myofascial system of the body into eleven major myofascial meridians or **anatomy trains**. Figure 10-21 illustrates the eleven major myofascial meridians (Box 10-40). (*Anatomy Trains* is published by Churchill Livingstone of Elsevier Science, 2002.)

BOX 10-40

The term *anatomy train* is synonymous with the term *myofascial meridian;* hence the name of Tom Myers's book, *Anatomy Trains.*

- The importance of myofascial meridian theory is manyfold:
  - First, it places muscles into larger structural and functional patterns that help to explain patterns of strain and movement within the body. Figure 10-22 illustrates an example of a line of strain/movement within the body. We see that when a monkey hangs from a branch, a continuum of muscles must synergistically work, beginning in the upper extremity and ending in the trunk. This myofascial continuum is an example of a structural and functional myofascial meridian. Thus myofascial meridian theory helps the kinesiologist understand the patterns of muscle contraction within the body.
  - Second, myofascial meridian theory creates a model that explains how forces placed on the body at one site can cause somewhat far-reaching effects in distant sites of the body. For example, in Figure 10-23 we see one of the myofascial meridians named the *superficial back line.* If tension develops at one point along this line, say in the gastrocnemius muscle, that tension could be transmitted up the line through the hamstrings to the ischial tuberosity attachment, through the sacrotuberous ligament to the sacrum, up through the thoracolumbar fascia and erector spinae musculature to the occiput, and from the occiput into the galea aponeurotica to the frontal region of the head. Therefore by the concept of strain moving along myofascial meridians, a person with excessive tightness in their gastrocnemius may experience an effect of that strain in the head, perhaps manifesting as a headache.
  - The repercussions of this are important for every therapist or trainer that works in a clinical or rehabilitative setting. The actual codification of eleven major myofascial meridians offers a blueprint with which the therapist/trainer can begin to address these patterns of strain and injury throughout the body.

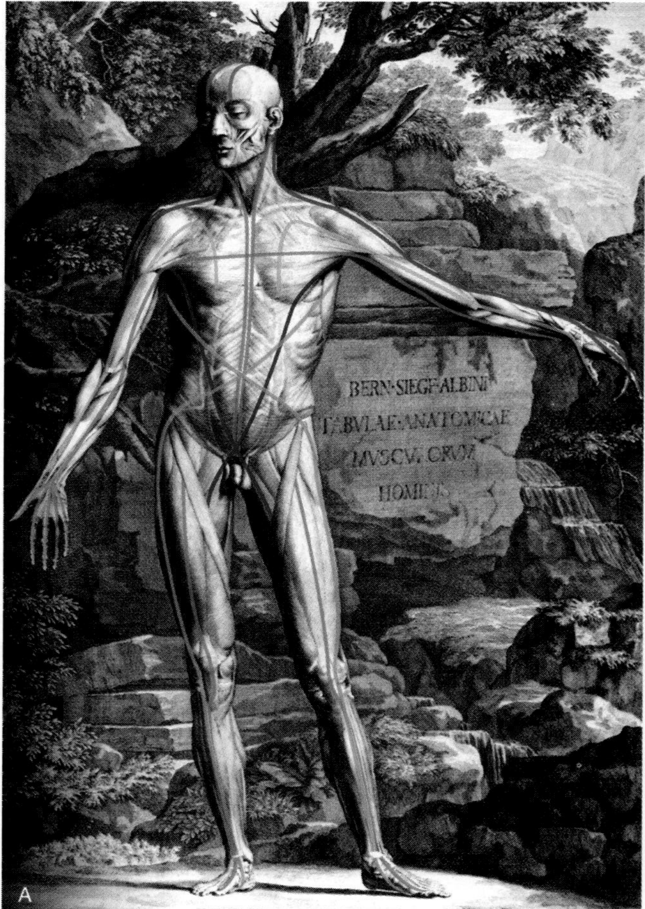

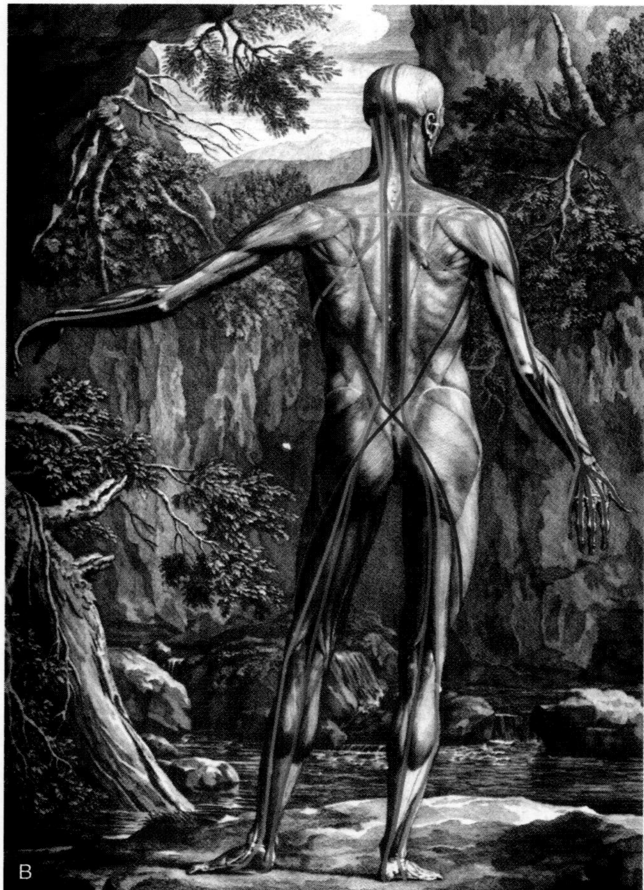

Figure 10-21 The 11 major myofascial meridians (i.e., anatomy trains) of the human body. (Courtesy Dover Publications, NY)

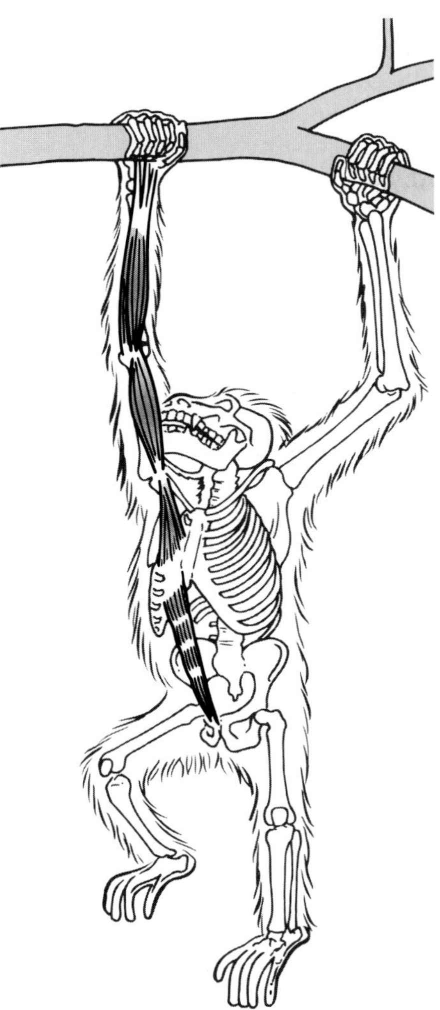

Figure 10-22 In this illustration we see that when a monkey is hanging from a branch, a chain of muscles must work in concert with each other and contract. This chain of muscles makes up a myofascial meridian. (From Myers TW: *Anatomy trains: myofascial meridians for manual and movement therapists,* Edinburgh, 2001, Churchill Livingstone.)

> **BOX 10-41**
>
> Given the *connective* nature of myofascial connective tissues, the concept of connectiveness and continuity of the myofascial tissues of the body cannot be disputed. Working with the myofascial meridians that Myers has mapped out, a force placed on any one point of a myofascial meridian will be transmitted along the myofascial meridian to distant sites in the body. However, it is likely that the magnitude of this transmitted force will lessen as the distance from the original site increases. Thus even though a strain/tension at the gastrocnemius can lead to this strain being transmitted to the hamstrings and erector spinae and on to the galea aponeurotica of the scalp, the intensity of the effects of this strain will lessen as we move along the myofascial meridian from the gastrocnemius toward the head. In other words, although myofascial meridian theory is of undeniable value to the field of bodywork, the actual clinical importance of the application of its conclusions should be evaluated on a case by case basis by the therapist.

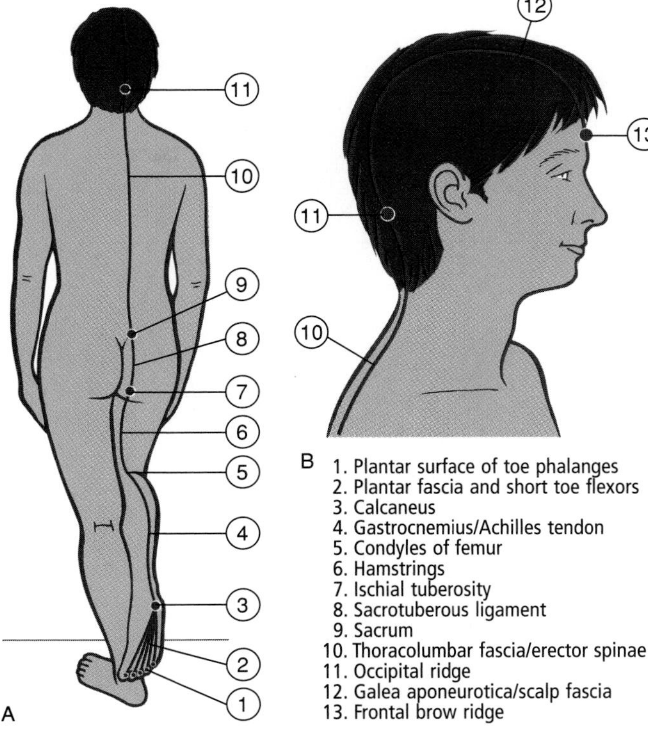

Figure 10-23 Illustration of the superficial back line myofascial meridian of the body. Conceptually, if a strain occurs at one point along this myofascial meridian, effects of that strain could be felt in distant locations along the myofascial meridian. Odd numbers indicate bony stations; even numbers are myofascial tracks. (Modified from Myers TW: *Anatomy trains: myofascial meridians for manual and movement therapists,* Edinburgh, 2001, Churchill Livingstone.)

- The third importance of the myofascial meridian theory relates to the concept of *tensegrity*.

Tensegrity:

- The concept of **tensegrity** relates to how the structural integrity and support of the body are created.
- The classic view of the body is that it is a compression structure made up of a number of parts, each one stacked on the other and bearing weight down through the body parts below. Thus the weight-bearing compression force of the head rests on the neck; the weight of the head and neck rests on the trunk; the weight of the head, neck, and trunk rests on the pelvis, and so forth, all the way down to the feet (Figure 10-24).
- Thus the structural integrity of the body is dependant on compression forces similar to a brick wall in which the structural integrity of the brick wall is dependent on the proper position of each brick on the brick below so that the weight of each brick can be transmitted through the bricks below.
- However, myofascial meridian theory, which views the musculoskeletal body as having continuous lines of pull created by muscles linked to each other in a web

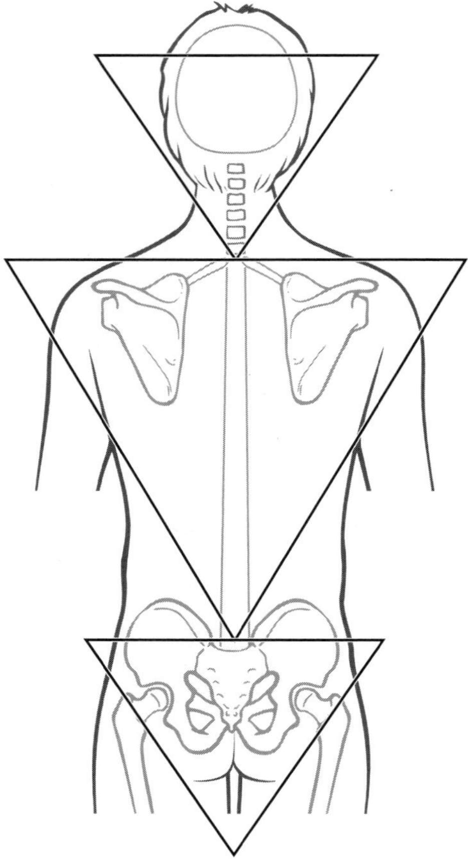

Figure 10-24 Typical view of the body as being a compression structure in which the structural integrity and support of the body are determined by the compressive weight-bearing forces transmitted through the body parts. (From Cailliet R: *Soft tissue pain and disability.* FA Davis, Philadelphia, 1997.)

or network of fascia offers another way to view the structural integrity of the body. Myofascial meridian theory looks at the lines of tension created by these myofascial meridians as being largely responsible for the structural integrity of the body. In this view, the proper posture and balancing of the bones of the skeleton are largely caused by the tensile forces created by muscles within myofascial meridians that act on the skeleton.

- The concept of structural integrity coming from tensile forces is termed *tensegrity*. The advantage of a tensegrity structure compared with a compression structure is that tensegrity structures are more resilient because stresses/forces that are applied to them are more efficiently transmitted throughout the structure, spreading out and diminishing their effect. Thus no one region of the skeleton bears the entire load of a stress. If a force is applied to a bone at any specific point along the skeleton, that force will be transmitted throughout the body along myofascial meridians, diminishing its effect at the local site of application.

BOX 10-42

The term *tensegrity* comes from the phrase *tension integrity* and was first used by designer R. Buckminster Fuller, an American engineer and inventor.

- For example, a force applied to any vertebral level of the lumbar spine, say L3, will have that force dissipated by tensile forces that will spread to the entire spine, head, arms, pelvis, and thighs via muscular attachments of such muscles as the erector spinae

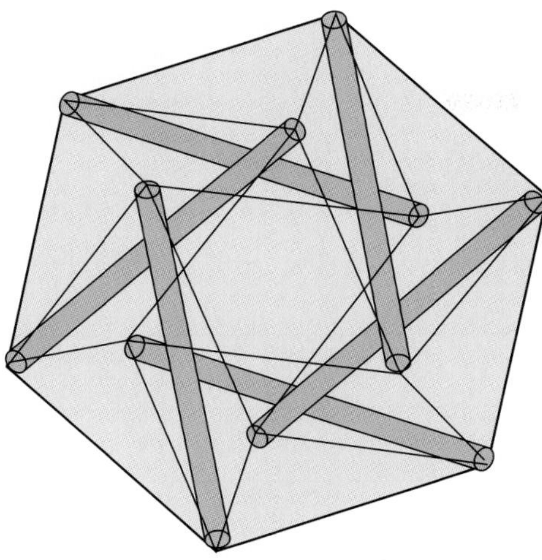

Figure 10-25 Classic tensegrity structure composed of dowels that are compression members suspended via rubber bands, which are the tension elements. The analogy to the human body is that our bones, which are compression elements, are largely suspended by our myofascial meridians of soft tissue, which are our tension elements. (From Fritz S: *Mosby's fundamentals of therapeutic massage,* ed 3, St. Louis, 2004, Mosby.)

group, transversospinalis group, psoas major, and latissimus dorsi muscles. Then the fascial attachments of these muscles to other muscles will then continue to spread the effects of the force to every other part of the body. The result will be that much of the force that was placed on L3 will be spread to other areas of the body, lessening the deleterious effect and likelihood of injury to L3.

- In reality, neither view is entirely exclusive of the other; the structural integrity of the body is dependent on both tensile and compressive forces.
  - The bones of the skeleton are compression members that do derive some of their structural stability from being stacked on one another and bearing weight down through the skeleton below.
  - However, much of the structural stability of the skeleton also comes from myofascial tensile forces attaching and spanning from one bone to every other bone of the body (Figure 10-25.
- Describing the body as having both compression integrity and tensile integrity (i.e., tensegrity), Myers describes the bones as being compression members that are like ". . . islands, floating in a sea of continuous tension." (Myers, *Anatomy Trains*, page 44).

REVIEW QUESTIONS

evolve Answers to the following review questions appear on the Evolve website accompanying this book.

1. Describe the big picture function of a muscle contraction.

2. What are the two major tissue types found in a skeletal muscle?

3. What is a synonym for the term *muscle cell*?

4. What is the term given to a bundle of muscle fibers?

5. What is the name given to the muscular fascia that surrounds an entire muscle?

6. What is the difference between a tendon and an aponeurosis?

7. What are myofibrils?

8. Describe the structure of a sarcomere.

9. Describe the steps of the sliding filament mechanism.

10. In order, what are the four sources of energy for the sliding filament mechanism within a muscle cell?

11. Regarding nervous system control of muscle contraction, what is the role of neurotransmitters?

12. Describe the concept of muscle memory.

13. Define motor unit.

14. Define and give and example of the all-or-none response law.

15. What is the A-band of skeletal muscle tissue?

16. What is the role of troponin molecules?

17. Describe the difference between red slow-twitch and white fast-twitch fibers.

18. Which type of muscle fibers predominate in postural stabilization muscles?

19. Define a myofascial meridian.

20. What is the difference between the concepts of tensegrity and compression integrity.

21. Apply the concepts of myofascial meridian theory and tensegrity to bodywork.

Chapter 11

How Muscles Function—The Big Picture

CHAPTER OUTLINE

CHAPTER OBJECTIVES

After completing this chapter, the student should be able to perform the following:

- ❑ Explain the "big picture" of how a muscle creates motion of a body part at a joint.
- ❑ Define and relate the terms *concentric contraction* and *mover* to the big picture of how a muscle creates joint motion.
- ❑ Explain why a muscle that contracts either succeeds or does not succeed in shortening toward the middle.
- ❑ Using the terms *fixed* and *mobile,* describe and give an example of each of the three scenarios that can occur when a muscle concentrically contracts (i.e., contracts and shortens).
- ❑ List what three things must be stated when fully describing a joint action.
- ❑ Describe and give an example of a *reverse action.*
- ❑ Explain what factors determine which attachment of a muscle moves when a muscle concentrically contracts.
- ❑ List and explain the importance of each of the steps of the five-step approach to learning muscles. Specifically, state the three questions that should be asked in step 3.
- ❑ Describe the importance of understanding the direction of fibers and/or the line of pull of a muscle relative to the joint that it crosses.
- ❑ Describe how to use the *rubber band exercise* to help learn the action(s) of a muscle.
- ❑ Explain the importance (relative to determining the possible actions of a muscle) of evaluating each of the three scenarios: (1) if a muscle with one line of pull has that one line of pull in a cardinal plane versus an oblique plane, (2) if a muscle has one line of pull or more than one line of pull, and (3) if a muscle is a one-joint muscle or a multijoint muscle.
- ❑ Explain how a muscle that has more than one action can contract, and yet only one or some of its actions occur.
- ❑ Explain how understanding functional mover groups of muscles can help one learn the actions of muscles.
- ❑ Describe the meanings of the terms *on-axis* and *off-axis,* and explain how the *off-axis attachment* method can be used to determine a muscle's rotation action. Further, state how one can determine the long axis of a bone.
- ❑ Give an example of and explain how a muscle can create an action at a joint that it does not cross.

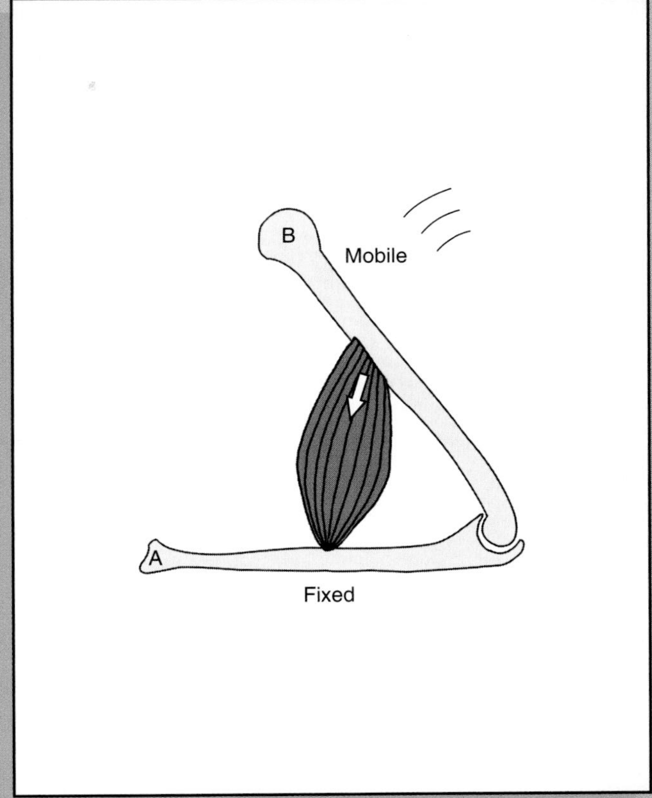

- ❑ Give an example of and explain how a muscle's action can change when the position of the body changes.
- ❑ Define the key terms of this chapter.
- ❑ State the meanings of the word origins of this chapter.

OVERVIEW

This chapter has two major thrusts: it explores the big picture of how muscles function concentrically (i.e., contracting and shortening) to create joint actions, and it offers easy methods that can be used by the student to learn muscles. Regarding muscle concentric contraction function, this chapter explores the idea of fixed versus mobile attachments of a muscle and introduces the concept of a muscle's reverse action(s). Included in this discussion is an exploration of the lines of pull of a muscle and how this affects the possible actions of the muscle. Other more advanced topics such as how a muscle can transfer the force of its contraction to another joint that it does not cross and how a muscle's actions can change with a change in joint position are also explored. Regarding learning muscles, a five-step approach to learning muscles is presented in this chapter. This five-step approach breaks the process of learning the attachments and actions of a muscle into five easy and logical steps. Particularly important is step 3, which shows how to figure out what the actions of a muscle are instead of having to memorize them. Specifically for the rotation actions of a muscle, the *off-axis attachment* method is explained. For kinesthetic learners, a *rubber band exercise* is given to further facilitate learning muscles. Continuing the process of learning muscles, a functional group approach is then given that greatly decreases the amount of time necessary to learn the actions of muscles.

KEY TERMS

Anatomic action
Concentric contraction (con-SEN-trik)
Fixator
Fixed attachment
Functional group
Functional mover group
Long axis
Mobile attachment
Mover
Multijoint muscle
Off-axis (AK-sis)
Off-axis attachment method
On-axis
One-joint muscle
Stabilizer

WORD ORIGINS

- ❑ Concentric—From Latin *con,* meaning *together* or *with,* and *centrum,* meaning *center*
- ❑ Fix—From Latin *fixus,* meaning *fastened*
- ❑ Mobile—From Latin *mobilis,* meaning *movable, mobile*
- ❑ Multi—From Latin *multus,* meaning *many, much*
- ❑ Stabilize—From Latin *stabilis,* meaning *not moving, fixed*

11.1 "BIG PICTURE" OF MUSCLE STRUCTURE AND FUNCTION

- A muscle attaches, via its tendons, from one bone to another bone. In so doing, a muscle crosses the joint that is located between the two bones (Figure 11-1).
- When a muscle contracts, it creates a pulling force on its attachments that attempts to pull them toward each other (i.e., this pulling force attempts to shorten the muscle toward its center). To understand how a muscle creates a pulling force, it is necessary to understand the sliding filament mechanism (see Sections 10.6 and 10.12).
- If the muscle is successful in shortening toward its center, then one or both of the bones to which it is attached will have to move (Figure 11-2).
- Because the bony attachments of the muscle are within body parts, if the muscle moves a bone, then the body part that the bone is within is moved. In this way, muscles can cause movement of parts of the body.
- When a muscle contracts and shortens as described here, this type of contraction is called a **concentric contraction** and the muscle that is concentrically contracting is called a **mover**.

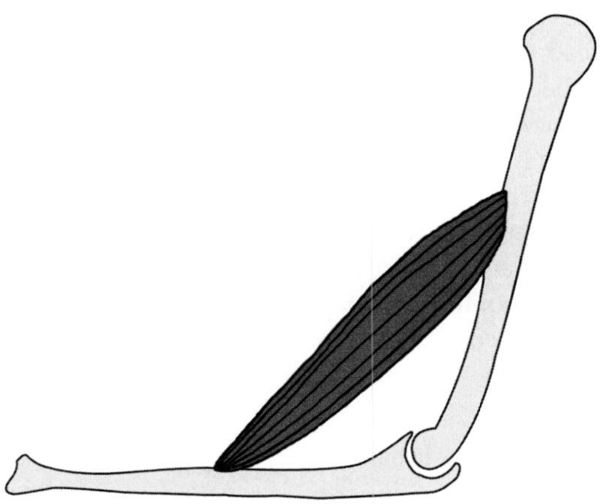

Figure 11-1 The location of a muscle is shown; it attaches from one bone to another bone and crosses the joint that is located between the two bones. (From Muscolino JE: *The muscular system manual: the skeletal muscles of the human body,* ed. 2, St Louis, 2005, Mosby.)

> **BOX 11-1**
>
> A muscle can contract and not shorten. A muscle contraction that does not result in shortening is called an *eccentric contraction* or *isometric contraction*. (For more information on eccentric and isometric contractions, see Chapter 12.)

- It is worth noting that whether or not a muscle is successful in shortening toward its center is determined by the strength of the pulling force of the muscle compared with the force necessary to actually move one or both body parts to which the muscle is attached.
- The force necessary to move a body part is usually the force necessary to move the weight of the body part. However, other forces may be involved.

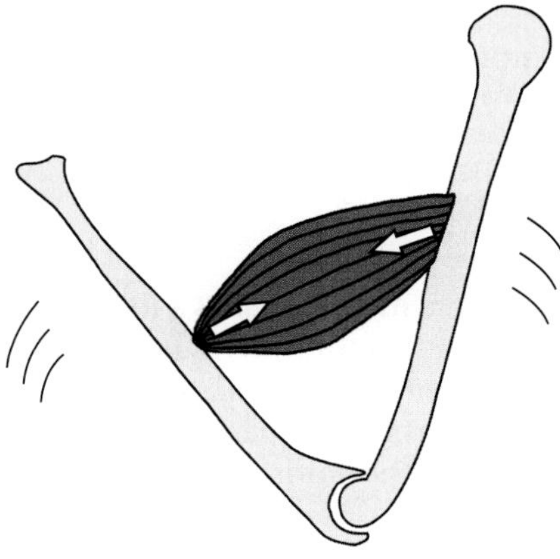

Figure 11-2 Muscle shown contracting and shortening (i.e., a concentric contraction). For a muscle to shorten, one or both of the bones that it is attached to must move toward each other. (From Muscolino JE: *The muscular system manual: the skeletal muscles of the human body,* ed. 2, St Louis, 2005, Mosby.)

☐ 11.2 WHAT HAPPENS WHEN A MUSCLE CONTRACTS AND SHORTENS?

- ❑ Assuming that a muscle contracts with sufficient strength to shorten toward its center (i.e., concentrically contract), it is helpful to look at the possible scenarios that can occur. (For more information on concentric contractions, see Sections 12.1-12.4.)
- ❑ If we call one of the attachments of the muscle *Bone A* and the other attachment of the muscle *Bone B,* then we see that three possible scenarios exist (Figure 11-3):
  1. *Bone A* will be pulled toward *Bone B.*
  2. *Bone B* will be pulled toward *Bone A.*
  3. Both *Bone A* and *Bone B* will be pulled toward each other.
- ❑ If an attachment of the muscle moves, it is said to be the **mobile attachment**. If an attachment of the muscle does not move, it is said to be the **fixed attachment**.

BOX 11-2

We usually think of a typical muscle as having two attachments and a typical muscle contraction as having one of its attachments fixed and its other attachment mobile. However, it is possible for a muscle to contract and have both of its attachments mobile as seen in Figure 11-3c. It is also possible for a muscle to contract and have both of its attachments fixed (as occurs during isometric contractions). (For more on this see Chapter 12.)

- ❑ In this manner, a muscle creates a joint action. To fully describe this joint action, we must state three things:
  1. The type of motion that has occurred
  2. The name of the body part that has moved
  3. The name of the joint where the movement has occurred

As an example to illustrate these concepts, it is helpful to look at the brachialis muscle. One attachment of the brachialis is onto the humerus of the arm, and the other attachment of the brachialis is onto the ulna of the forearm. In attaching to the arm and the forearm, the brachialis crosses the elbow joint that is located between these two body parts (Figure 11-4).

When the brachialis contracts, it attempts to shorten toward its center by exerting a pulling force on the forearm and the arm.

- ❑ Scenario 1: The usual result of the brachialis contracting is that the forearm will be pulled toward the arm. This is because the forearm is lighter than the arm and therefore would be likely to move before the arm would. (Additionally, if the arm were to move, the trunk would have to move as well, which makes it even less likely that the arm will be the attachment that will move.) To fully describe this action, we call it *flexion of the forearm at the elbow joint,* because the forearm is the body part that has moved and the elbow joint flexed (Figure 11-5a). In this scenario the arm is the attachment that is fixed and the forearm is the attachment that is mobile.
- ❑ Scenario 2: However, it is possible for the arm to move toward the forearm. If the forearm were to be fixed in place, perhaps because the hand is holding on to an immovable object, then the arm would have to move instead. This action is called *flexion of the arm at the elbow joint,* because the arm is the body part that has moved and the elbow joint flexed (Figure 11-5b). In this scenario the forearm is the attachment that is fixed and the arm is the attachment that is mobile. This scenario can be called a **reverse action**, because the attachment that is usually fixed, the arm, is now mobile, and the attachment that is usually mobile, the forearm, is now fixed. (Reverse actions are covered in more detail in Section 5.29.)

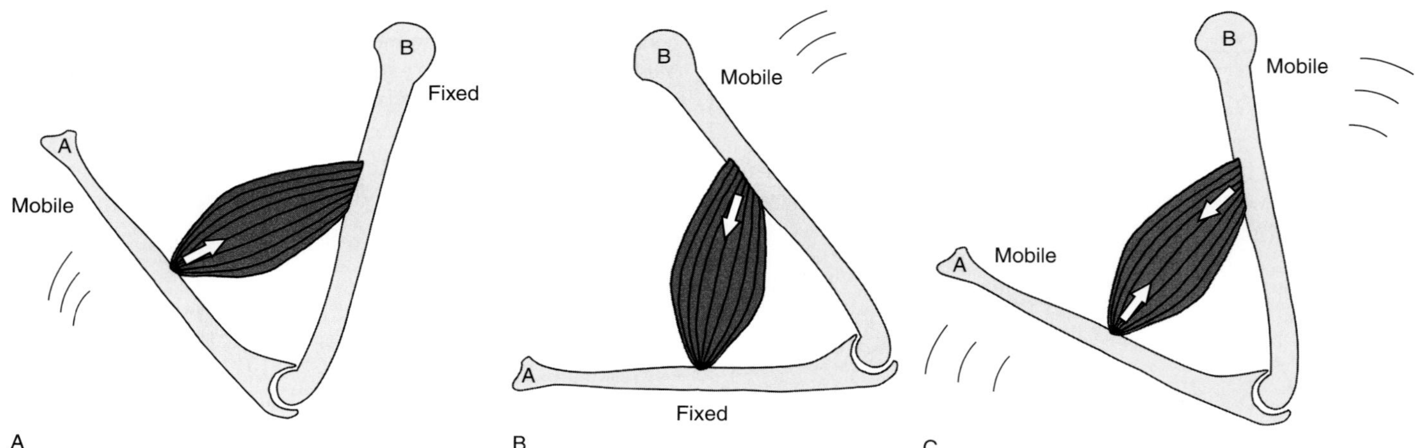

Figure 11-3 The three scenarios of a muscle contracting and shortening. If the attachment moves, it is said to be the mobile attachment; if the attachment does not move, it is said to be the fixed attachment. In *A, Bone A* moves toward *Bone B.* In *B, Bone B* moves toward *Bone A.* In *C, Bone A* and *Bone B* both move toward each other. (From Muscolino JE: *The muscular system manual: the skeletal muscles of the human body,* ed. 2, St Louis, 2005, Mosby.)

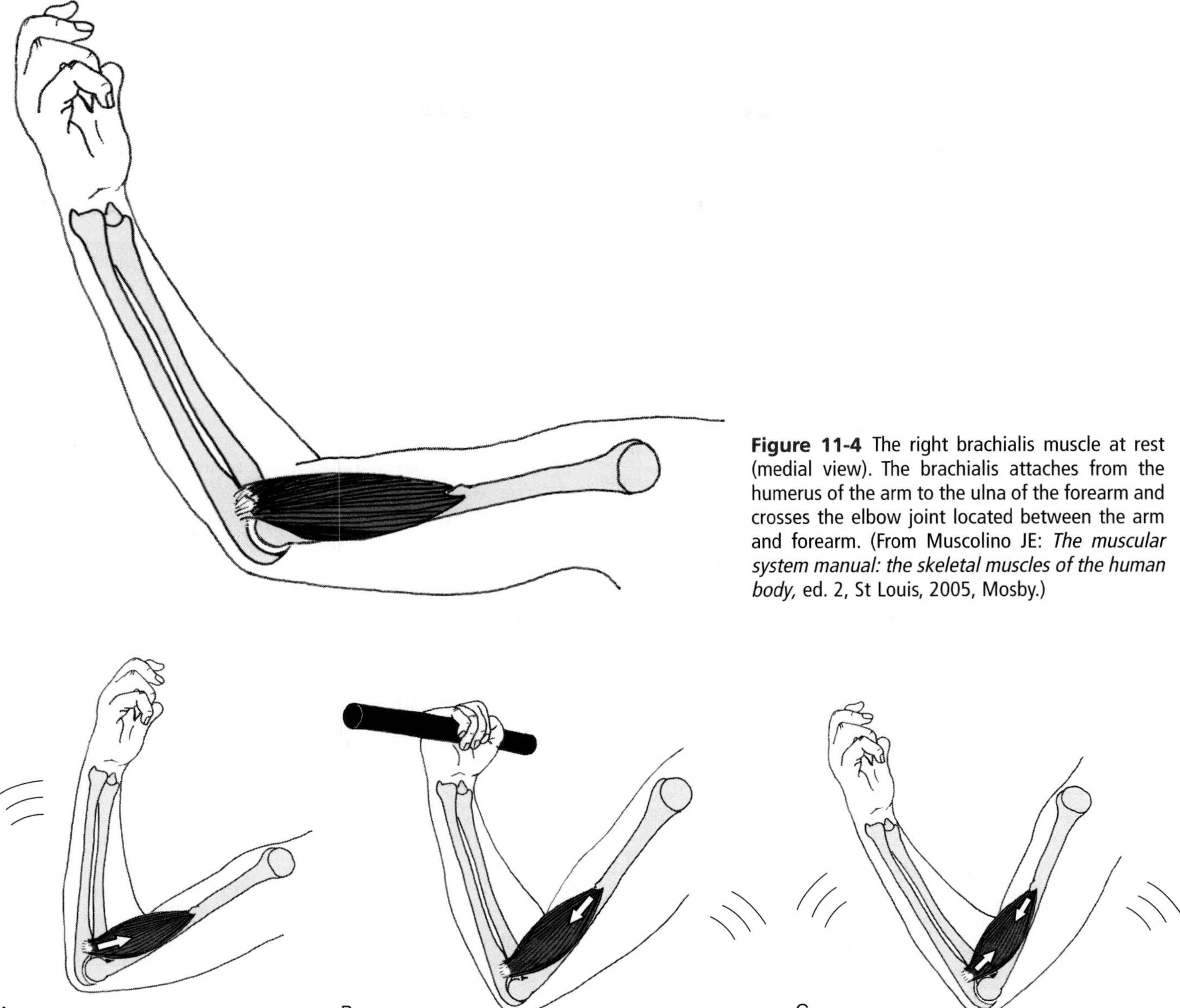

Figure 11-4 The right brachialis muscle at rest (medial view). The brachialis attaches from the humerus of the arm to the ulna of the forearm and crosses the elbow joint located between the arm and forearm. (From Muscolino JE: *The muscular system manual: the skeletal muscles of the human body,* ed. 2, St Louis, 2005, Mosby.)

Figure 11-5 The three scenarios that can result from a shortening (i.e., concentric) contraction of the brachialis muscle. *A,* Flexion of the forearm at the elbow joint. The arm is fixed, and the forearm is mobile, moving toward the arm. *B,* Flexion of the arm at the elbow joint. The forearm is fixed (the hand is holding onto an immovable bar). The arm is mobile, moving toward the forearm. *C,* Flexion of the forearm and the arm at the elbow joint. Neither attachment is fixed. Both attachments are mobile, moving toward each other. (From Muscolino JE: *The muscular system manual: the skeletal muscles of the human body,* ed. 2, St Louis, 2005, Mosby.)

- Scenario 3: Because the contraction of the brachialis exerts a pulling force on the forearm and the arm, it is possible for both of these bones to move. When this occurs, two actions take place: (1) flexion of the forearm at the elbow joint and (2) flexion of the arm at the elbow joint (Figure 11-5c). In this case both bones are mobile and neither one is fixed.
- It is important to realize that the brachialis does not intend or choose which attachment will move (or if both attachments will move).
- When a muscle contracts, it merely exerts a pulling force toward its center.
- Which attachment moves is determined by other factors.
- The relative weight of the body parts is the most common factor.
- However, another common determinant is when the central nervous system directs another muscle in the body to contract, which may stop or "fix" one of the attachments of the mover muscle. If this occurs, this second muscle that contracts to fix a body part would be called a **fixator** or **stabilizer** muscle. (For more information on fixator (stabilizer) muscles, see Section 13.5.)
- It follows that if a muscle does successfully shorten, and one attachment is fixed, then the other attachment must be mobile.

☐ 11.3 FIVE-STEP APPROACH TO LEARNING MUSCLES

- ❑ Essentially, when learning about muscles, two major aspects must be learned: (1) the attachments of the muscle and (2) the actions of the muscle.
- ❑ Generally speaking, the attachments of a muscle must be memorized. However, times exist when clues are given about the attachments of a muscle by the muscle's name.
  - ❑ For example, the name *coracobrachialis* tells us that the coracobrachialis muscle has one attachment on the coracoid process of the scapula and that its other attachment is on the brachium (i.e., the humerus).
  - ❑ Similarly, the name *zygomaticus major* tells us that this muscle attaches onto the zygomatic bone (and that it is bigger than another muscle called the *zygomaticus minor*).
- ❑ Unlike muscle attachments, muscle actions do not have to be memorized. Instead by understanding the simple concept that a muscle pulls at its attachments to move a body part, the action or actions of a muscle can be reasoned out.

Five-Step Approach to Learning Muscles:

When first confronted with having to study and learn about a muscle, the following five-step approach is recommended:

- ❑ Step 1: Look at the name of the muscle to see if it gives you any "free information" that saves you from having to memorize attachments or actions of the muscle.
- ❑ Step 2: Learn the general location of the muscle well enough to be able to visualize the muscle on your body. At this point, you need only know it well enough to know:
  - ❑ What joint it crosses
  - ❑ Where it crosses the joint
  - ❑ How it crosses the joint (i.e., the direction in which its fibers are running)
- ❑ Step 3: Use this general knowledge of the muscle's location (step 2) to figure out the actions of the muscle.
- ❑ Step 4: Go back and learn (memorize, if necessary) the specific attachments of the muscle.
- ❑ Step 5: Now look at the relationship of this muscle to other muscles (and other soft tissue structures) of the body. Look at the following: Is this muscle superficial or deep? In addition, what other muscles (and other soft tissue structures) are located near this muscle?

Figuring Out a Muscle's Actions (Step 3 in Detail):

- ❑ Once you have a general familiarity with a muscle's location on the body, then it is time to begin the process of reasoning out the actions of the muscle. The most important thing that you must look at is the following:
  - ❑ The direction of the muscle fibers relative to the joint that it crosses

  By doing this, you can see the following:
  - ❑ The line of pull of the muscle relative to the joint

BOX 11-3

When a muscle contracts, it creates a *pulling* force. It is this pulling force that can create motion (i.e., joint actions). (Note: Muscles never push, they *pull*!)

- ❑ This line of pull will determine the actions of the muscle (i.e., how the contraction of the muscle will cause the body parts to move at that joint).
- ❑ The best approach is to ask the following three questions:
  1. What joint does the muscle cross?
  2. Where does the muscle cross the joint?
  3. How does the muscle cross the joint?

Question 1—What Joint Does the Muscle Cross?

- ❑ The first question to ask and answer in figuring out the action(s) of a muscle is to simply know what joint it crosses.
- ❑ The following rule applies: If a muscle crosses a joint, then it can have an action at that joint. (Note: *This, of course, assumes that the joint is healthy and allows movement to occur.*)
  - ❑ For example, if we look at the coracobrachialis, knowing that it crosses the shoulder joint tells us that it must have an action at the shoulder joint.
  - ❑ We may not know what the exact action of the coracobrachialis is yet, but at least we now know at what joint it has its actions.
  - ❑ To figure out exactly what these actions are, we need to look at questions 2 and 3.
- ❑ Note: It is worth pointing out that the converse of the rule about a muscle having the ability to create movement (i.e., an action) at a joint that it crosses is also true. In other words, if a muscle does not cross a joint, then it cannot have an action at that joint.

BOX 11-4

The rule stating that if a muscle does not cross a joint, then it cannot have an action at that joint is not 100% accurate. Sometimes the force of a muscle can be transferred to another joint, even if the muscle does not cross that joint. (For more on this concept, see Section 11.9)

Questions 2 and 3—Where Does the Muscle Cross the Joint? How Does the Muscle Cross the Joint?

- These two questions must be looked at together.
- The *where* of a muscle crossing a joint is whether it crosses the joint anteriorly, posteriorly, medially, or laterally.
- It is helpful to place a muscle into one of these broad groups because the following general rules apply: muscles that cross a joint anteriorly will usually flex a body part at that joint, and muscles that cross a joint posteriorly will usually extend a body part at that joint; muscles that cross a joint laterally will usually abduct or laterally flex a body part at that joint, and muscles that cross a joint medially will usually adduct a body part at that joint.

BOX 11-5

Note 1: Flexion is nearly always an anterior movement of a body part, and extension is nearly always a posterior movement of a body part. However, from the knee joint and further distal, flexion is a posterior movement and extension is an anterior movement of the body part.

Note 2: Abduction occurs at joints of the appendicular skeleton; lateral flexion occurs at joints of the axial skeleton.

- The *how* of a muscle crossing a joint is whether it crosses the joint with its fibers running vertically or horizontally. This is also very important.
  - To illustrate this idea we will look at the pectoralis major muscle. The pectoralis major has two parts: (1) a clavicular head and (2) a sternocostal head. The *where* of these two heads of the pectoralis major crossing the shoulder joint is the same (i.e., they both cross the shoulder joint anteriorly). However, the *how* of these two heads crossing the shoulder joint is very different. The clavicular head crosses the shoulder joint with its fibers running primarily vertically; therefore it flexes the arm at the shoulder joint (because it pulls the arm upward in the sagittal plane, which is termed *flexion*). However, the sternocostal head crosses the shoulder joint with its fibers running horizontally, therefore it adducts the arm at the shoulder joint (because it pulls the arm from lateral to medial in the frontal plane, which is termed *adduction*).
- With a muscle that has a horizontal direction to its fibers, another factor must be considered when looking at *how* this muscle crosses the joint (i.e., whether the muscle attaches to the first place on the bone that it reaches, or whether the muscle wraps around the bone before attaching to it). Muscles that run horizontally (in the transverse plane) and wrap around the bone before attaching to it create a rotation action when they contract and pull on the attachment.
  - For example, the sternocostal head of the pectoralis major does not attach to the first point on the humerus that it reaches. Instead it continues to wrap around the shaft of the humerus to attach onto the lateral lip of the bicipital groove of the humerus. When the sternocostal head pulls, it medially rotates the arm at the shoulder joint (in addition to its other actions).
- In essence, by asking the three questions of Step 3 of the five-step approach to learning muscles (What joint does a muscle cross? Where does the muscle cross the joint? How does the muscle cross the joint?), we are trying to determine the direction of the muscle fibers relative to the joint. Determining this will give us the line of pull of the muscle relative to the joint, and that will give us the actions of the muscle—saving us the trouble of having to memorize this information!

☐ 11.4 RUBBER BAND EXERCISE

Visual and Kinesthetic Exercise for Learning a Muscle's Actions:

Rubber Band Exercise:

- ❑ An excellent method for learning the actions of a muscle is to place a large colorful rubber band (or large colorful shoelace or string) on your body, or the body of a partner, in the same location that the muscle you are studying is located.
- ❑ Hold one end of the rubber band at one of the attachment sites of the muscle, and hold the other end of the rubber band at the other attachment site of the muscle.
- ❑ Make sure that you have the rubber band running/oriented in the same direction as the direction of the fibers of the muscle. If it is not uncomfortable, you may even loop or tie the rubber band (or shoelace) around the body parts that are the attachments of the muscle.
- ❑ Once you have the rubber band in place, pull one of the ends of the rubber band toward the other attachment of the rubber band to see the action that the rubber band/muscle has on that body part's attachment. Once done, return the attachment of the rubber band to where it began and repeat this exercise for the other end of the rubber band to see the action that the rubber band/muscle has on the other attachment of the muscle (Box 11-6).
- ❑ By placing the rubber band on your body or your partner's body, you are simulating the direction of the muscle's fibers relative to the joint that it crosses.
- ❑ By pulling either end of the rubber band toward the center, you are simulating the line of pull of the muscle relative to the joint that it crosses. The resultant movements that occur are the actions that the muscle would have. This is an excellent exercise to both visually see the actions of a muscle and to kinesthetically experience the actions of a muscle.
- ❑ This exercise can be used to learn all muscle actions, and can be especially helpful for determining actions that may be a little more difficult to visualize, such as rotation actions.
- ❑ Note: The use of a large colorful rubber band is more helpful than a shoelace or string, because when you stretch out a rubber band and place it in the location that a muscle would be, the natural elasticity of a rubber band creates a pull on the attachment sites that nicely simulates the pull of a muscle on its attachments when it contracts.
- ❑ If you can, you should work with a partner to do this exercise. Have your partner hold one of the "attachments" of the rubber band while you hold the other "attachment." This leaves one of your hands free to pull the rubber band attachment sites toward the center.
- ❑ A further note of caution: If you are using a rubber band, be careful that you do not accidentally let go and have the rubber band hit you or your partner. For this reason, it would be preferable to use a shoelace or string instead of a rubber band when working near the face.

BOX 11-6

When doing the rubber band exercise it is extremely important that the attachment of the rubber band that you are pulling on is pulled exactly toward the other attachment and in no other direction. In other words, your line of pull should be exactly the same as the line of pull of the muscle (which is essentially determined by the direction of the fibers of the muscle).

When doing the rubber band exercise, the attachment of the muscle that you are pulling on would be the mobile attachment in that scenario; the end that you do not move is the fixed attachment in that scenario. Further, by doing this exercise twice (i.e., by then repeating it by reversing which attachment you hold fixed and which one you pull on and move), you are simulating the usual action and the reverse action of the muscle.

11.5 LINES OF PULL OF A MUSCLE

- Because the line of pull of a muscle relative to the joint it crosses determines the actions that it has, it is extremely important to fully understand the line or lines of pull of a muscle.
- It is helpful to examine four scenarios regarding a muscle and its line or lines of pull:
  - Scenario 1: A muscle with one line of pull in a cardinal plane
  - Scenario 2: A muscle with one line of pull in an oblique plane
  - Scenario 3: A muscle that has more than one line of pull
  - Scenario 4: A muscle that crosses more than one joint

BOX 11-7

For every scenario that is presented here with regard to a line of pull of a muscle and the resultant action that the muscle has, we are not considering the reverse action of a muscle. Given that a reverse action is always theoretically possible for every named *usual action* of a muscle, the complementary *reverse action* always exists.

Scenario 1—A Muscle with One Line of Pull in a Cardinal Plane:

- If a muscle has one line of pull and that line of pull lies perfectly in a cardinal plane, then that muscle will have one action.

BOX 11-8

Remember, for any action that a muscle has, the reverse action is always theoretically possible. Therefore given the existence of the reverse action, the muscle could actually be said to always have at least two actions.

  - A perfect example is the brachialis muscle. The brachialis crosses the elbow joint anteriorly with a vertical direction to its fibers. All of its fibers are essentially running parallel to each other and are oriented in the sagittal plane. Therefore the brachialis has one action, namely flexion of the forearm at the elbow joint (as well as its reverse action of flexion of the arm at the elbow joint). The brachialis's line of pull is in the sagittal plane; therefore the action that it creates must be in the sagittal plane, and that action is flexion (Figure 11-6).

Scenario 2—A Muscle with One Line of Pull in an Oblique Plane:

- If a muscle has one line of pull, but that line of pull is in an oblique plane, then the muscle will create movement in that oblique plane. However, when naming this movement, no name for oblique plane movement exists. Instead this movement has to be broken up into names for cardinal plane actions. (The concept of naming oblique plane motions is covered in Section 5.28.)
  - An excellent example is the coracobrachialis. The coracobrachialis has a line of pull that is in an oblique plane. That oblique plane is a combination of sagittal and frontal cardinal planes. When the coracobrachialis pulls, it pulls the arm diagonally in a direction that is both anterior and medial at the same time. However, no one name for this oblique plane motion exists. To name this one motion that would occur, we must break it up into its component cardinal plane actions of flexion in the sagittal plane and adduction in the frontal plane. Therefore even though the muscle actually creates only one movement in an oblique plane, we describe it as having two cardinal plane actions (Figure 11-7). (To understand how an oblique plane muscle can create only one of its cardinal plane actions, see Section 13.4.)
- For this reason, a muscle that has one line of pull can be said to have more than one cardinal plane action if that muscle's line of pull is oriented within an oblique plane. Of course, for each of its actions, a reverse action is theoretically possible.

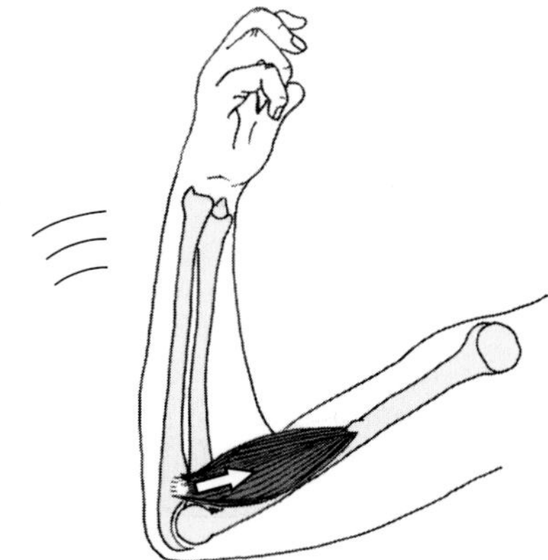

Figure 11-6 Demonstration of the fact that a muscle that has one line of pull and is located perfectly in a cardinal plane has one action. In this case the brachialis muscle has one line of pull to its fibers, and that line of pull is located within the sagittal plane; therefore the brachialis can flex the elbow joint. (Note: Flexion of the forearm at the elbow joint is its usual action; flexion of the arm at the elbow joint would be the complementary reverse action.) (From Muscolino JE: *The muscular system manual: the skeletal muscles of the human body,* ed. 2, St Louis, 2005, Mosby.)

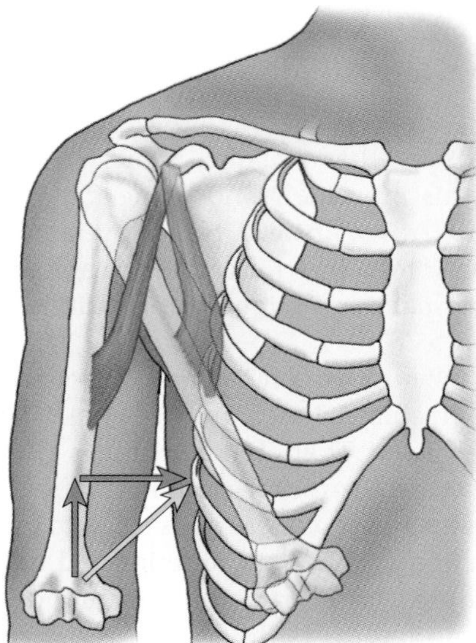

Figure 11-7 Illustration of the motion that is caused when the coracobrachialis contracts (with the scapula fixed and the humerus mobile). This one oblique plane motion (*yellow arrow*) must be broken down into its two cardinal plane actions (*green arrows*) when discussing the joint actions of the coracobrachialis. Hence the coracobrachialis can flex the arm in the sagittal plane and adduct the arm in the frontal plane (all at the shoulder joint).

Scenario 3—A Muscle That Has More Than One Line of Pull:

- If a muscle has more than one line of pull, then we apply the same logic that was used in scenarios #1 and #2 to this muscle.
- For each line of pull that is oriented perfectly in a cardinal plane, there will be one action possible (along with the corresponding reverse action).
- For each oblique plane line of pull, the movement that occurs in that oblique plane can be broken up into its separate cardinal plane components (with their corresponding reverse actions).
  - An example is the gluteus medius. The gluteus medius has posterior fibers, middle fibers, and anterior fibers, each with a different line of pull on the femur at the hip joint. The posterior fibers pull in an oblique plane; the cardinal plane components of this oblique plane are extension in the sagittal plane, abduction in the frontal plane, and lateral rotation in the transverse plane. The anterior fibers also pull in an oblique plane; their cardinal plane components are flexion in the sagittal plane, abduction in the frontal plane, and medial rotation in the transverse plane. However, the middle fibers are oriented perfectly in the frontal plane; therefore their action is only abduction in the frontal plane. In this example, the posterior and anterior fibers fit scenario #2 (one line of pull in an oblique plane), and the middle fibers fit scenario #1 (one line of pull in a cardinal plane) (Figure 11-8). (Note: The reverse actions of the gluteus medius are movements of the pelvis toward the thigh at the hip joint.)

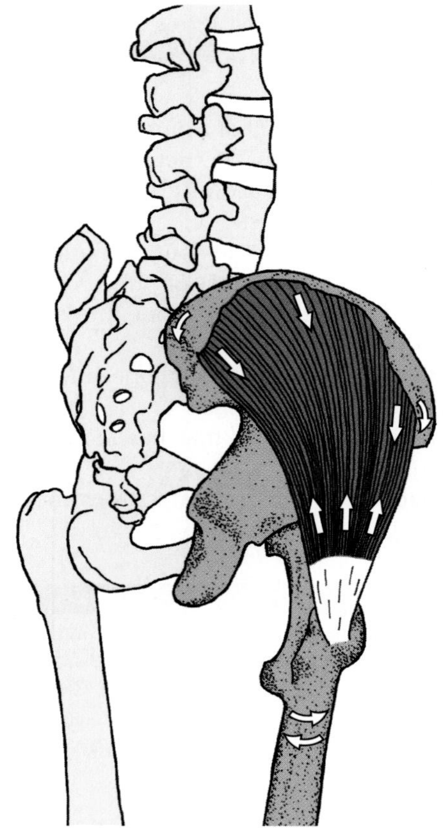

Figure 11-8 Gluteus medius muscle. The gluteus medius has posterior fibers and anterior fibers that are oriented in an oblique plane; therefore these fibers can be said to have an action in each of the cardinal planes that the oblique plane is within. The posterior and anterior fibers each have actions in the sagittal, frontal, and transverse planes. The middle fibers of the gluteus medius are oriented directly in a cardinal plane; hence it has only one action within that cardinal plane. (Of course, for any action that a muscle possesses, a reverse action is always theoretically possible. In the case of the gluteus medius, the reverse action would be movement of the pelvis toward the thigh at the hip joint instead of movement of the thigh toward the pelvis at the hip joint.) (From Muscolino JE: *The muscular system manual: the skeletal muscles of the human body,* ed. 2, St Louis, 2005, Mosby.)

Scenario 4—A Muscle that Crosses More Than One Joint:

- If a muscle crosses only one joint, it is termed a **one-joint muscle**; if a muscle crosses more than one joint, it is termed a **multijoint muscle**.
- If a muscle is a multijoint muscle, then the reasoning that is applied at one joint for each line of pull that the muscle has, is applied at each joint that the muscle crosses.
- Many multijoint muscles exist in the human body.

- Examples include the following:
  - The rectus femoris of the quadriceps femoris group crosses the knee and hip joints with one line of pull. Therefore it can extend the leg at the knee joint in the sagittal plane, and it can flex the thigh at the hip joint in the sagittal plane (as well as create the corresponding reverse actions) (Figure 11-9a).
  - The flexor carpi ulnaris crosses the elbow joint with one line of pull in a cardinal plane and crosses the wrist joint with one line of pull in an oblique plane. Therefore it can flex the forearm at the elbow joint in the sagittal plane, and it can flex and ulnar deviate (i.e., adduct) the hand at the wrist joint in the sagittal and frontal planes respectively (as well as create the corresponding reverse actions) (Figure 11-9b).

Can a Muscle Choose Which of its Actions Will Occur?

- No. Muscles are basically machines that contract when they are ordered to contract by the nervous system. If a muscle contracts, then whichever motor units are ordered to contract have every muscle fiber within them contract and attempt to shorten. (For more on this concept, see the All-or-None Response Law in Section 10.10.) Whatever line of pull these fibers lie within will have a pulling force created that will pull on the attachments of the muscle. When a muscle has only one line of pull, it must attempt to create every action that would occur from that one line of pull. Only muscles that have more than one line of pull can attempt to create certain actions and not other actions. This occurs when the central nervous system directs motor units that lie only within one line of pull of the muscle to contract (and not direct motor units to contract that lie within other lines of pull). An example is the trapezius. It has three parts: (1) upper, (2) middle, and (3) lower. Each part has its own line of pull. The upper trapezius can be ordered to contract without the middle or lower parts being ordered to contract. In this manner, a muscle with more than one line of pull can attempt to create some of its actions and not others.

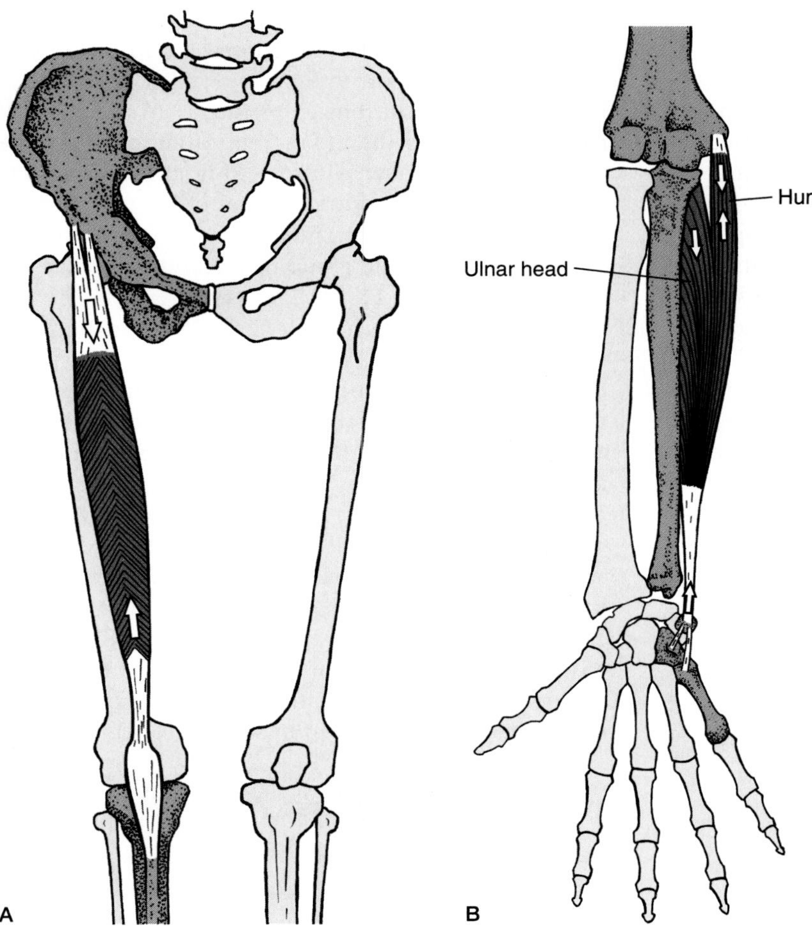

Figure 11-9 Whenever a muscle crosses more than one joint (i.e., is a multijoint muscle), it can create movement at each of the joints that it crosses. *A,* Rectus femoris (of the quadriceps femoris group), which crosses both the hip and knee joints. The rectus femoris can flex the thigh at the hip joint, and it can extend the leg at the knee joint (as well as create the corresponding reverse actions). *B,* Flexor carpi ulnaris, which crosses the elbow joint and also crosses the wrist joint. The flexor carpi ulnaris can flex the forearm at the elbow joint, and it can flex and ulnar deviate (i.e., adduct) the hand at the wrist joint (as well as create the corresponding reverse actions). (From Muscolino JE: *The muscular system manual: the skeletal muscles of the human body,* ed. 2, St Louis, 2005, Mosby.)

Other examples of muscles with more than one line of pull are the deltoid and gluteus medius.

Therefore we can state the following two rules:

- A muscle with one line of pull attempts to create every one of its actions when it contracts.
- A muscle with more than one line of pull does not necessarily attempt to create every one of its actions when it contracts. It may attempt to create the action(s) of one of its lines of pull but not the action(s) of another of its lines of pull.

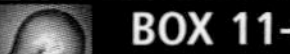

BOX 11-9

I spend most of my time reading about, studying, working on, teaching, and writing about muscles. As much as I love the muscular system, I often tell my students that muscles are *dumb machines.* They do not know what actions they are or are not creating; they do not intend anything. They simply contract when they are ordered to by the central nervous system. The movements that they make and the patterns of those movements are ultimately determined by the nervous system. Muscle contraction, muscle coordination, muscle patterning, muscle armoring, and muscle memory all reside in the nervous system. (For more information on how certain actions of muscles can occur and not others, see Section 13.4. For more on the nervous system control of the muscular system, see Chapter 16.)

11.6 FUNCTIONAL GROUP APPROACH TO LEARNING MUSCLE ACTIONS

- The best method for approaching and learning each action of a new muscle that you first encounter to learn is to use the reasoning of step 3 of the five-step approach. You have learned that for each aspect of the direction of fibers for a muscle, you apply the questions of *where* and *how* the muscle crosses the joint. This reasoning is solid and will lead you to reason out all actions of the muscle that is being studied.
- However, it can be very repetitive and time consuming as you apply this method to muscle after muscle after muscle that all cross the same joint in the same manner.
- Therefore once you are very comfortable with applying the questions of step 3 for learning the actions of each muscle individually, it is recommended that you begin to use your understanding of how muscles function and apply it on a larger scale.
- Instead of looking at each muscle individually and going through all of the questions of step 3 for that muscle, take a step back and look at the broad functional groups of muscles at each joint.

BOX 11-10

A muscle belongs to a **functional group** if it shares the same function (i.e., joint action) as the other members of the functional group. The type of functional group that is being referred to in this section is a **functional mover group** (i.e., all the muscles in a group create the same joint action when they concentrically contract). Muscles can also be functionally grouped in roles other than as movers of a joint action. (For more on the various roles of muscles, see Chapter 13.)

- For example, instead of individually using the questions of step 3 to learn that the brachialis flexes the forearm at the elbow joint, and then that the biceps brachii flexes the forearm at the elbow joint, and then that the pronator teres flexes the forearm at the elbow joint, and also the flexor carpi radialis, palmaris longus, and so forth, it is a simpler and more elegant approach to look at the functional group of muscles that all flex the elbow joint.
- In other words, the bigger picture is to see that *all muscles* that cross the elbow joint anteriorly flex the forearm at the elbow joint. Looking at the body this way, when you encounter yet another muscle that crosses the elbow joint anteriorly, you can automatically place it into the group of forearm flexors at the elbow joint (Figure 11-10).
- For each joint of the human body, look for the functional groups of movers. In the case of the elbow joint, because it is a pure hinge, uniaxial joint, it is very simple. Only two functional mover groups exist: (1) anterior muscles that flex and (2) posterior muscles that extend.
- Triaxial joints such as the shoulder or hip joint will have more functional mover groups (flexors, extensors, abductors, adductors, medial rotators, and lateral rotators), but the concept will always be the same. Once you clearly see this concept, learning the actions of muscles of the body can be greatly simplified and streamlined. (Guidelines to determine the functional group that a muscle belongs to are given in Section 11.7.)

Reminder About Reverse Actions:

Remember that the reverse actions of a muscle are always possible, even if they have not been specifically listed in this book! (For more information on reverse actions, see Section 5.29.)

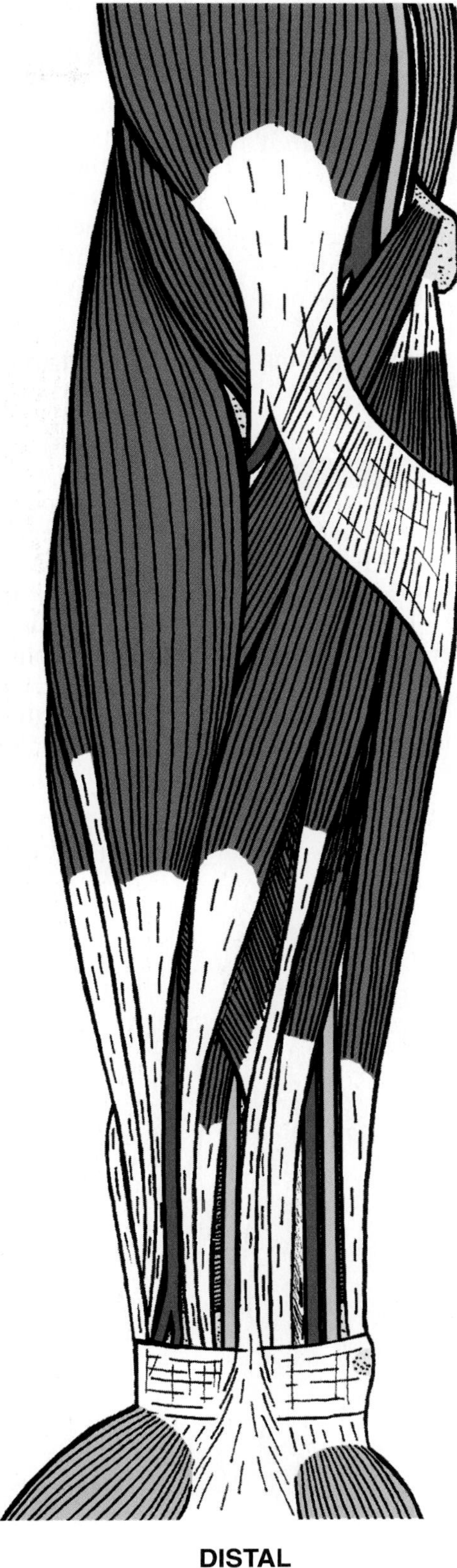

Figure 11-10 Anterior view of the elbow joint region. All muscles that cross the elbow joint anteriorly belong to the functional mover group of elbow joint flexors and have been colored red.

☐ 11.7 DETERMINING FUNCTIONAL GROUPS

Understanding actions of muscles from a functional group approach is the most efficient and elegant method to learn the actions of the muscles of the body.

- ❑ The muscles of a functional mover group are grouped together because they all share the same joint action. If their joint action is the same, then their line of pull relative to that joint must be the same. Therefore it stands to reason that a functional group can also be looked at as a structural group (i.e., the muscles of a functional group are located together).
- ❑ Generally certain guidelines can be stated regarding the location of functional groups of muscles.

BOX 11-11

The general rules presented for learning functional mover groups of muscles are not hard and fast. They are better looked at as guidelines, because exceptions to these rules exist. For example, across the ankle joint, frontal plane functional groups are named as *everters* and *inverters*, not *abductors* and *adductors*. Another example is the saddle joint of the thumb where flexion and extension occur in the frontal plane and abduction and adduction occur in the sagittal plane. Occasional exceptions aside, these general rules/guidelines are extremely valuable!

Sagittal Plane:

- ❑ All groups of muscles that cross a joint in the sagittal plane can either do flexion or extension (Figure 11-11).
  - ❑ If the muscles cross the joint anteriorly, they do flexion (except for the knee joint and further distal).
  - ❑ If the muscles cross the joint posteriorly, they do extension (except for the knee joint and further distal).

Frontal Plane:

- ❑ All groups of muscles that cross a joint in the frontal plane can either do right lateral flexion/left lateral flexion or abduction/adduction (Figure 11-12).
  - ❑ If the body part being moved is an axial body part, then the muscles do lateral flexion to the same side (i.e., muscles on the right side of the body do right lateral flexion; muscles on the left side of the body do left lateral flexion).
  - ❑ If the body part being moved is an appendicular body part, then the muscles do abduction if they cross on the lateral side of the joint, and the muscles do adduction if they cross on the medial side of the joint.

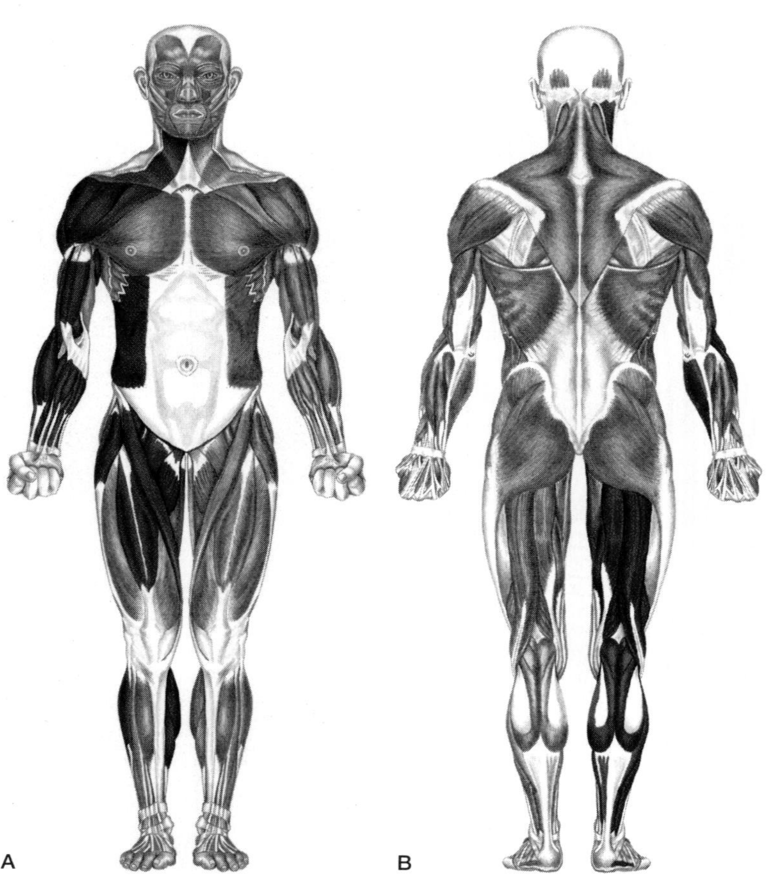

Figure 11-11 *A,* Anterior view of the musculature of the body. *B,* posterior view of the musculature of the body. The flexor functional mover groups are colored red on the right side of the body. (Note: The flexor muscles are generally located anteriorly [except for the knee joint and further distal].) (From Muscolino JE: *The muscular system manual: the skeletal muscles of the human body,* ed. 2, St Louis, 2005, Mosby.)

Transverse Plane:

- Transverse plane actions are slightly more difficult to determine because the muscles of a transverse plane functional mover group are not necessarily located together (as are the muscles of the sagittal and frontal planes functional mover groups).
  - For example, the right splenius capitis and the left sternocleidomastoid both do right rotation of the neck (and head) at the spinal joints. However, even though these two muscles share the same joint action and are therefore in the same functional group, they are not located together. The right splenius capitis is in the right side of the neck, and the left sternocleidomastoid is in the left side of the neck; further, the splenius capitis is located posteriorly, and the sternocleidomastoid is located primarily anteriorly.
- Functional groups of the transverse plane do rotation.
  - If the body part being moved is an axial body part, then the muscles do right rotation or left rotation.
  - If the body part being moved is an appendicular body part, then the muscles do lateral rotation or medial rotation.
- An easy method to determine the transverse plane rotation action of a muscle to place it into its functional mover group is to look at the manner in which the muscle *wraps around* the body part to which it attaches. (Another method to determine rotation actions that is technically more exacting is called the *off-axis attachment* method, presented in Section 11.8.)
  - For example, the right splenius capitis and the left sternocleidomastoid both have the same action of right rotation because they both wrap around the neck region in the same manner (Figure 11-13a).
  - The right pectoralis major and the right latissimus dorsi have the same action of the medial rotation of the right arm at the shoulder joint because they both wrap around the humerus in the same manner (Figure 11-13b).
- When trying to see the manner in which a muscle wraps, it is usually best to visualize the muscle from a superior (or proximal) perspective, as in Figures 11-13a–b.

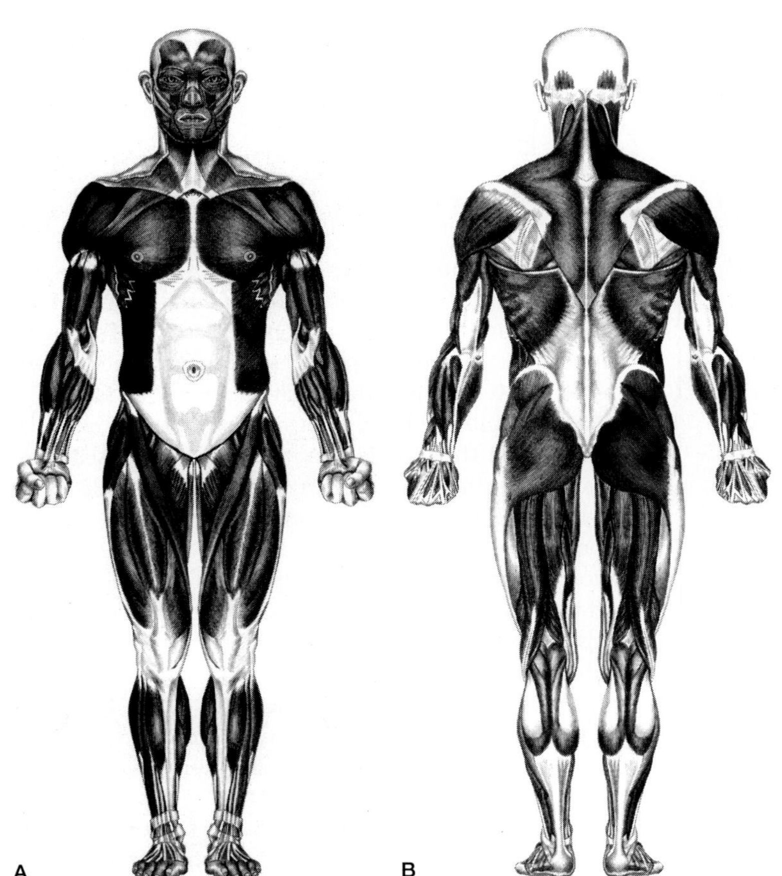

Figure 11-12 *A,* Anterior view of the musculature of the body. *B,* posterior view of the musculature of the body. The muscles of the lateral flexor functional mover groups (for axial body joints) are colored red, and the muscles of the abductor functional mover groups (for appendicular body joints) are colored green on the right side of the body. (Note: The muscles of these functional groups are generally located laterally.) (From Muscolino JE: *The muscular system manual: the skeletal muscles of the human body,* ed. 2, St Louis, 2005, Mosby.)

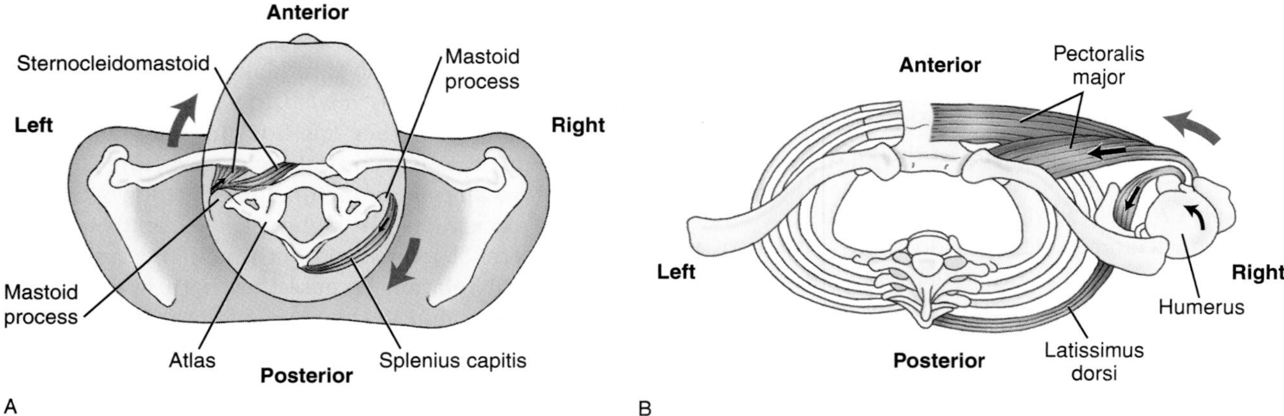

Figure 11-13 *A,* Superior view of the right splenius capitis and left sternocleidomastoid muscles. Even though one of these muscles is posterior and on the right side and the other is primarily anterior and on the left side, they both have the same action of right rotation of the neck and head at the spinal joints. This is because they both wrap around the neck/head in the same direction. *B,* Superior view of the right pectoralis major and right latissimus dorsi. Because they both wrap around the humerus in the same direction, they are both able to medially rotate the arm at the shoulder joint. As can be seen in these two examples, unlike other functional groups of movers, muscles of the same mover functional rotation group are often not located together.

☐ 11.8 OFF-AXIS ATTACHMENT METHOD FOR DETERMINING ROTATION ACTIONS

- ❑ Seeing how the direction of a muscle's fibers *wrap* around the bone to which it attaches is a convenient visual method for determining the transverse plane rotation action of a muscle.
- ❑ However, another method can be used to determine rotation actions that might be a little more difficult to visualize at first, but once it is seen and understood is a more accurate and elegant method to use. This method is called the **off-axis attachment method**.
- ❑ Figure 11-14a, illustrates a side view of a muscle that crosses from one bone (labeled *fixed*) to another bone (labeled *mobile*). It is fairly intuitive to see that this muscle will move the mobile bone toward the fixed bone. However, to determine whether this muscle can create a rotation motion requires that we see exactly where the muscle attaches onto this mobile bone; more specifically, we need to see whether the muscle attaches *on-axis* or *off-axis*.
- ❑ Figure 11-14b, is an oblique view that illustrates a hypothetical muscle that attaches onto the mobile bone **on-axis** (i.e., directly over the long axis of the mobile bone). When this muscle contracts long, even though the mobile bone will be moved toward the fixed bone, no rotation of the mobile bone will occur because the muscle attaches on-axis (i.e., it does not wrap around to attach onto the bone to the side of the axis). Figure 11-14c, is an oblique view of another hypothetical muscle that attaches onto the mobile bone; however, this muscle attaches **off-axis** (i.e., it wraps around the bone to attach off to the side of the long axis of the mobile bone). When this muscle contracts and shortens, it can move the mobile bone toward the fixed bone; it can also rotate the mobile bone as demonstrated by the red arrow. Figure 11-14d, shows a similar muscle attaching onto the mobile bone off-axis to the other side and shows the rotation that this muscle would produce when it contracts and shortens. (Note: The two muscles in Figure 11-14c–d, attach off-axis on the opposite sides of the long axis from one another; therefore they produce rotations actions that are opposite to each other.)
- ❑ Using the *off-axis attachment method* to determine the rotation action of a muscle necessitates that one visualize the long axis of a bone. If a muscle attaches onto the bone on-axis (i.e., such that its attachment is directly over the axis), it has no possible rotation action. However, if it attaches onto the bone off-axis (i.e., off the axis to either side), it can create a rotation action (Box 11-12).

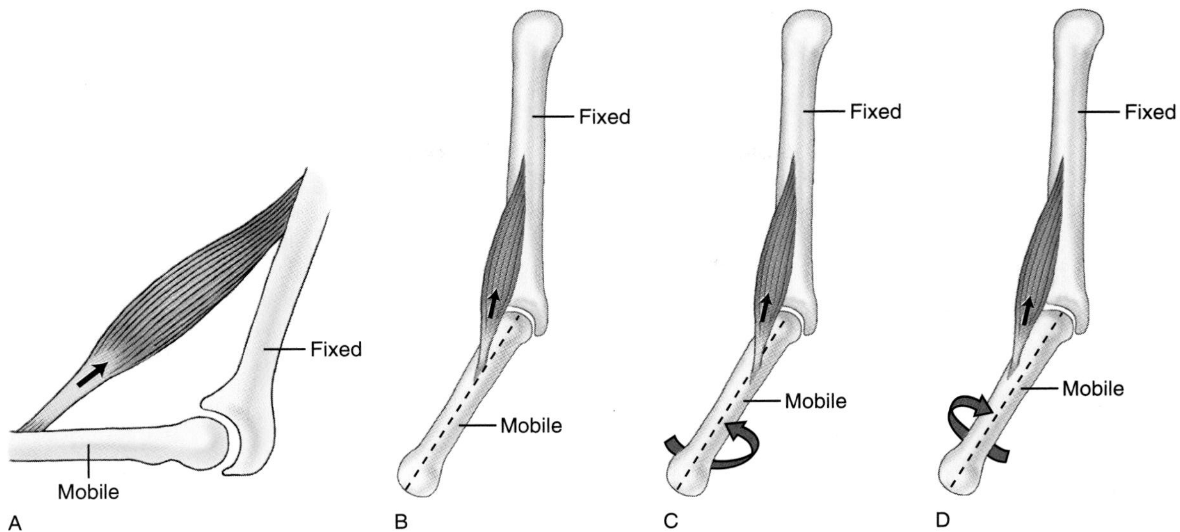

Figure 11-14 *A,* Side view of a muscle that attaches from one bone to another. When this muscle contracts and shortens, the mobile bone will be moved toward the fixed bone. *B* to *D,* Oblique views of muscles that cross from the same fixed bone to the same mobile bone. (Note: In all cases a dashed line indicates the long axis of the mobile bone.) The muscle in *B* attaches *on-axis*; therefore it produces no rotation action of the mobile bone. The muscles in *C* and *D* attach *off-axis*; therefore they can produce a rotation action of the mobile bone. The red arrows indicate these rotation actions. Any muscle that attaches onto a bone off-axis has the ability to create rotation of that bone at the joint that the muscle crosses. (Note: The muscles, bones, and joint illustrated in *A* to *D* are hypothetical; they are not meant to represent any specific structures of the body.)

BOX 11-12 SPOTLIGHT ON DETERMINING THE LONG AXIS OF A BONE

The axis of a bone that needs to be visualized to determine rotation actions of a muscle is the **long axis** (also known as the *longitudinal axis*) of the bone. The long axis of a bone is a straight line that runs from the center of the articular surface of the bone on one end to the center of the articular surface of the bone at the other end (i.e., from the center of the joint on one end to the center of the joint at the other end). This long axis usually runs through the shaft of the bone itself as seen in Figures 11-14b–d; however, depending on the shape of the bone, it may not. For example, the long axis of the femur is a straight line that connects the center of the hip and knee joints; as a result, its long axis lies outside the shaft of the femur (see accompanying figure). The location of this long axis is important in determining the rotation actions of muscles that attach onto the femur.

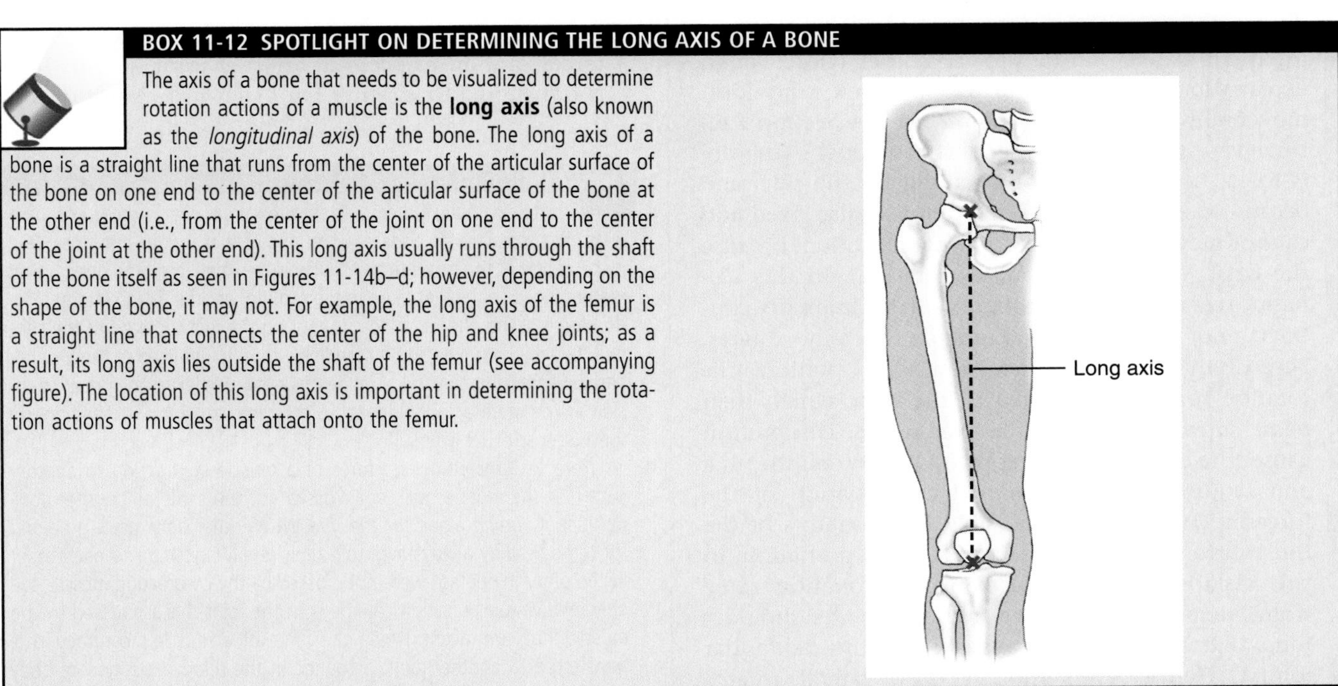

☐ 11.9 TRANSFERRING THE FORCE OF A MUSCLE'S CONTRACTION TO ANOTHER JOINT

In Section 11.3, we stated two rules about muscle contractions:

- ❑ Rule #1: If a muscle crosses a joint, it can have an action at that joint.
- ❑ Rule #2: If a muscle does not cross a joint, it cannot have an action at that joint.
- ❑ Although rule #1 is true, rule #2 is usually, but not always, true.

BOX 11-13

The rule that states that if a muscle crosses a joint, then it can have an action at that joint is always true . . . if the joint allows movement along the line of pull of the muscle.

- ❑ Sometimes the force of a muscle's contraction can be transferred to a joint that the muscle does not cross.
- ❑ An example of this is lateral rotation of the arm at the shoulder joint with the distal end of the upper extremity fixed. Usually when the lateral rotators of the arm contract, the humerus rotates laterally relative to the scapula at the shoulder joint, and the bones of the forearm and hand "go along for the ride," maintaining their relative positions to each other. (Note: For an explanation of the distinction between true joint movement and *going along for the ride,* see Section 1.6.) However, when the distal end of the upper extremity is fixed, the hand cannot go along for the ride; and because the hand is fixed, the radius is also fixed and cannot move (with regard to rotation motion, because the wrist joint does not allow rotation). In this scenario, when the lateral rotators of the humerus contract and shorten, the humerus laterally rotates. Because the elbow joint does not allow rotation, this rotation force is transferred to the ulna, which then *rotates laterally* relative to the fixed radius. This motion causes the ulna to cross over the radius. When the ulna and radius cross, it is defined as pronation of the forearm. Although it is possible for pronators of the forearm to create this action of forearm pronation, in this instance the force for forearm pronation came from lateral rotators of the humerus at the shoulder joint (whose force was transferred to the radioulnar joints). Hence, even though these lateral rotator muscles of the shoulder joint do not cross the radioulnar joints, they were able to create motion at the radioulnar joints because the force of their contraction was transferred to the radioulnar joints (Figure 11-15).

BOX 11-14

Whenever the distal end of an extremity is fixed, the activity is termed a *closed-chain* activity. An open-chain activity is one wherein the distal end of the extremity is free to move.

With pronation of the forearm, the radius is usually considered to move and cross over a fixed ulna. When the radius is fixed and the ulna is mobile, moving and crossing over the radius, it is still defined as pronation; however, it is an example of a reverse action in which the ulna moves instead of the radius (at the radioulnar joints).

- ❑ Another example of the force of a muscle being transferred to a joint that it does not cross is contraction of shoulder joint adductor muscles with the distal end of the upper extremity fixed. In this scenario movement of the humerus is transferred across the elbow joint to create extension of the forearm at the elbow joint (Figure 11-16).
- ❑ The force of a muscle's contraction is often transferred to another joint in the human body. This force transference usually occurs when the distal end of an extremity is fixed and does not allow for free motion of the distal body part to move. As a result, when the distal attachment of the contracting muscle moves, it forces motion to occur at another joint (i.e., its force is transferred to another joint that it does not cross).

BOX 11-15

Note 1: Many other scenarios exist in which the force of a muscle's contraction is transferred to a joint that it does not cross. One is the ability of the hamstrings to extend the knee joint in a person that is standing with the feet fixed to the ground; another is the lateral rotation force of the gluteus maximus causing the feet to invert at the subtalar tarsal joint if a person is standing with the feet fixed to the ground; and yet another is the ability of the ankle plantarflexors to create extension at the metatarsophalangeal joints when a person is standing. Try these scenarios for yourself.

Note 2: Transferring the force of a muscle contraction to another joint that the muscle does not cross is not the same as another body part simply *going along for the ride*. When other body parts go along for the ride, they always maintain their relative position to each other at the other joints that were not crossed by the contracting muscle; the only relative joint position change is at the joint that is crossed by the muscle that contracted. When the force of a muscle's contraction is transferred to another joint, a change in the relative position of body parts takes place at the other joint that is not crossed by the muscle that contracted. (To better visualize this, see Figures 11-15 and 11-16.)

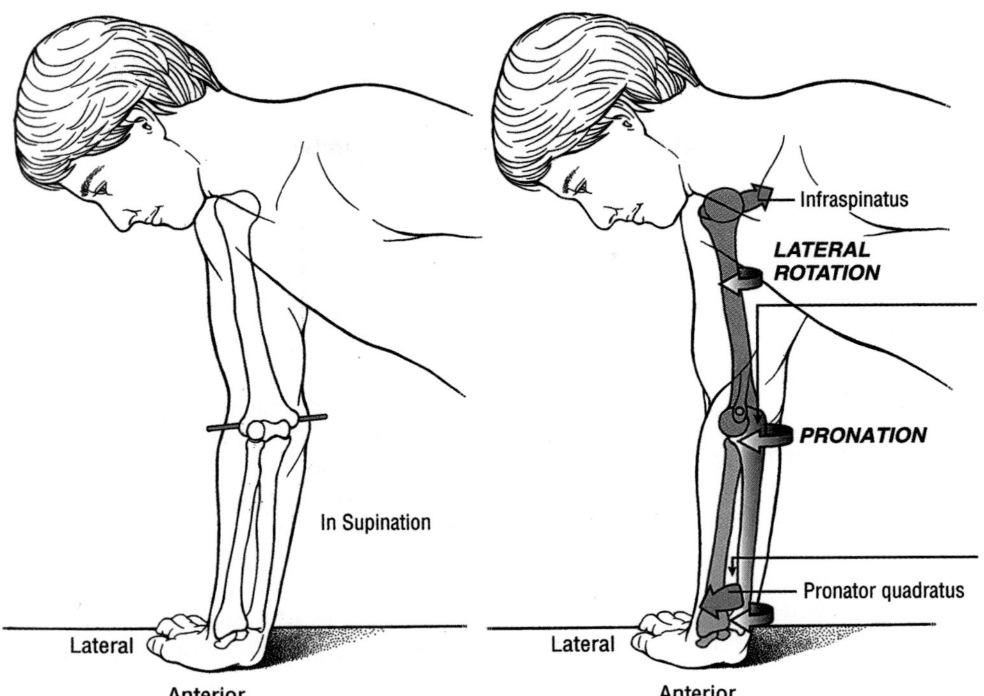

Figure 11-15 *A,* Person whose shoulder joint is medially rotated; forearm is supinated. (Note: The bones of the forearm are parallel to each other, and hand is fixed to a table top.) *B,* Person contracts the lateral rotator musculature of the shoulder joint (e.g., infraspinatus). When this occurs, the humerus laterally rotates At the shoulder joint relative to the scapula. Because the elbow joint does not allow rotation, the ulna moves along with the humerus and rotates laterally relative to the fixed radius. (Because the hand is fixed, the radius is unable to rotate because the wrist joint [i.e., the radiocarpal joint] does not allow rotation motions; therefore the radius is fixed relative to the hand.) This motion creates pronation at the radioulnar joints. In this scenario the force of shoulder lateral rotator muscles has been transferred to the radioulnar joints. This illustrates an example of a muscle that does not cross a joint but is able to create motion at that joint. (Note: This concept could work in the reverse manner. If pronation musculature [e.g., pronator quadratus] were to contract, the force would transfer across the elbow joint to the humerus, causing lateral rotation of the humerus at the shoulder joint. (From Neumann DA: *Kinesiology of the musculoskeletal system: foundations for physical rehabilitation,* St Louis, 2002, Mosby.)

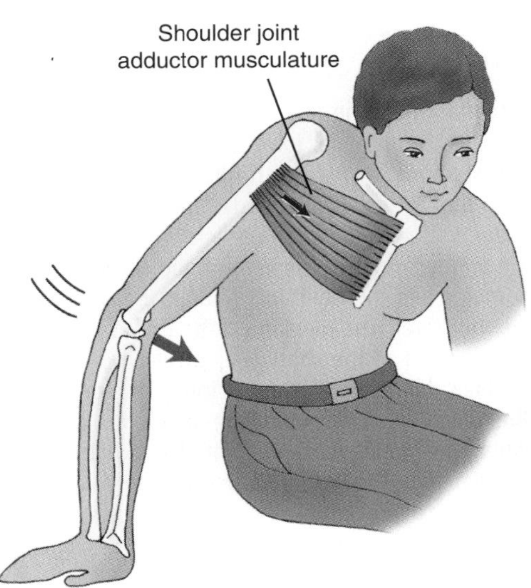

Figure 11-16 Person who is seated with the elbow joint partially flexed and the hand fixed to a tabletop. This person is contracting the shoulder joint adductor muscles. Because the hand is fixed, the distal forearm is also fixed and unable to move with the humerus. As a result, when the humerus is pulled into adduction by the shoulder adductor musculature, the proximal end of the forearm is pulled medially but the distal end of the forearm stays fixed. This results in elbow joint extension. This illustrates an example of musculature that does not cross a joint but is able to create motion at this joint because the force of its contraction is transferred to this other joint. (Modeled from Neumann DA: *Kinesiology of the musculoskeletal system: foundations for physical rehabilitation,* St Louis, 2002, Mosby.)

☐ 11.10 MUSCLE ACTIONS THAT CHANGE

Can a Muscle's Action Change?

- ❑ Yes. A muscle's action is dependent on its line of pull relative to the joint that it crosses; therefore if the relationship of the muscle's line of pull to the joint changes, the muscle's action changes. This relationship can change if the position of the joint changes.
- ❑ Example: Clavicular head of the pectoralis major:
  - ❑ The clavicular head of the pectoralis major is considered to be an adductor of the arm at the shoulder joint. This is because its line of pull is from medial to lateral, below the center of the shoulder joint.
  - ❑ However, if the arm is abducted to approximately 100 degrees or more, the orientation of the clavicular head of the pectoralis major relative to the shoulder joint changes from being below the center of the joint to be above the center of the joint (Figure 11-17). Like any muscle that crosses above the center of the shoulder joint (e.g., deltoid, supraspinatus), the clavicular head of the pectoralis major can now abduct the arm at the shoulder joint.
  - ❑ It stands to reason that if the line of pull relative to the joint changes, the action of the muscle changes. In anatomic position, the clavicular head of the pectoralis major is an adductor of the arm at the shoulder joint. However, with the arm abducted to 100 degrees or more, the clavicular head of the pectoralis major changes to become an abductor.

BOX 11-16

Some kinesiologists use the term **anatomic action** of a muscle to describe a muscle's action when the body is in anatomic position. This verbiage implicitly recognizes that a muscle's action on the body when the body is not in anatomic position may well be different from the action of the muscle when the body is in anatomic position.

- ❑ Note: This change in action becomes very useful. As the supraspinatus and deltoid muscles become functionally weaker with the arm in a great deal of abduction, the pectoralis major steps in to become an abductor to add strength to this joint action.
- ❑ Example: Adductor longus
  - ❑ The adductor longus is considered to be a flexor (in addition to being an adductor) of the thigh at the hip joint, because it passes anteriorly to the hip joint with a vertical direction to its fibers. All flexors of the thigh have their lines of pull anterior to the hip joint (Figure 11-18b). However, when the thigh is first flexed to approximately 60 degrees or more, the line of pull of the adductor longus lies posterior to the hip joint and the adductor longus becomes an extensor of the thigh at the hip joint (Figure 11-18a). Except for the adductor magnus, which is always an extensor at the hip joint, this change in action is true for the other adductors of the thigh at the hip joint. (Note: The *members of the adductors of the thigh group* are the pectineus, adductor longus, gracilis, adductor brevis, and adductor magnus.)
- ❑ Note: This change in action becomes very useful. While running, when we are in a position of extension, the adductors aid in flexing the thigh at the hip joint. However, when we are in a position of flexion, they aid in extending the thigh at the hip joint. This dual use may also explain why these muscles are so often injured.
- ❑ A muscle's action often changes when its line of pull relative to the joint changes (because of a change in the position of the joint).
- ❑ For this reason, a certain amount of flexibility is needed when learning the actions of muscles. If one

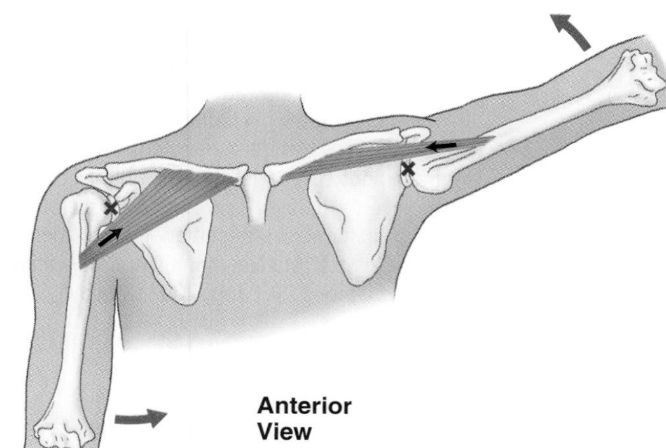

Figure 11-17 Orientation of the fibers of the clavicular head of the pectoralis major to the shoulder joint when the shoulder joint is in two different positions. *A,* Person's right arm is in anatomic position, and we see that the clavicular head of the pectoralis major is located below the center of the shoulder joint. In this position, given the direction of fibers relative to the joint, the clavicular head of the pectoralis major has the ability to adduct the arm at the shoulder joint. *B,* However, the person's left arm is abducted approximately 100 degrees at the shoulder joint. In this position, we see that the clavicular head of the pectoralis major is now located above the center of the shoulder joint. In this position, given the direction of fibers relative to the joint, the clavicular head of the pectoralis major has the ability to abduct the arm at the shoulder joint. Hence the action of a muscle can change when the position of the joint that it crosses changes. (Note: The center of the shoulder joint on both sides is indicated by an X.)

memorizes that a certain muscle does a certain action, it may or may not be true depending on the position of the joint. This is another reason why memorizing muscle actions is not recommended.

❑ Being able to reason a muscle's actions from its line of pull requires less brain memory, allows for a deeper and easier understanding of muscles' actions, and facilitates a better clinical application of this information!

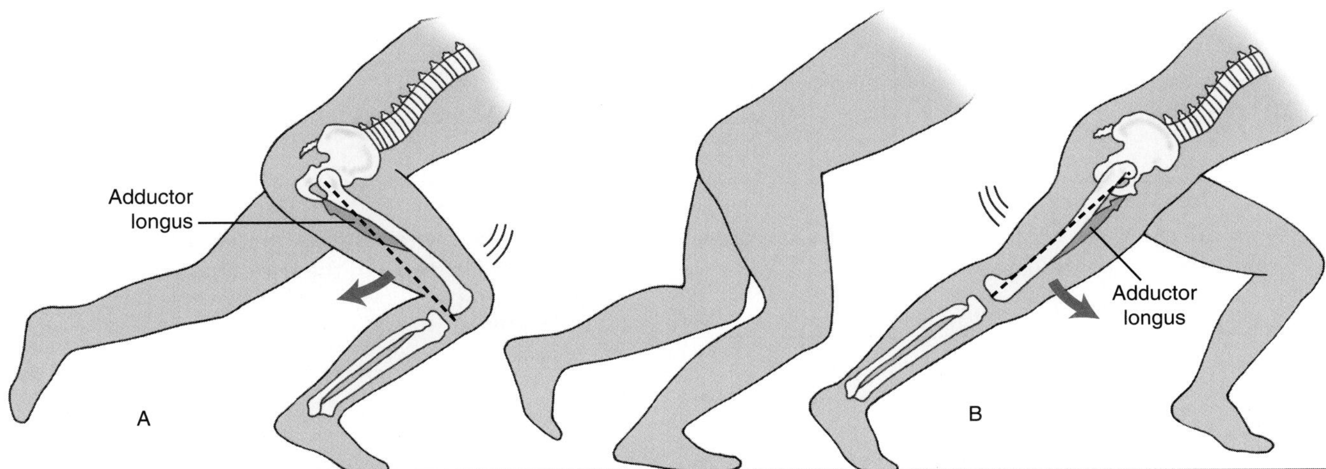

Figure 11-18 Illustration of a person that is running. *A,* Person's right thigh is in a position of flexion and is now being extended at the hip joint, helping to propel him forward. We see that the adductor longus assists in extending the thigh at the hip joint because in this position, the adductor longus is located posterior to the joint; therefore it can pull the femur posteriorly (i.e., do extension of the thigh at the hip joint). *B,* Person's right thigh is in a position of extension and is now beginning to flex at the hip joint. In this position the adductor longus in now located anterior to the joint, so it is able to assist in flexing the thigh at the hip joint. These figures illustrate the concept that a muscle, the adductor longus in this case, can change its action based on a change in the position of the joint that it crosses. (Note: In both figures the dashed line represents the axis for motion of the thigh at the hip joint.) (Modeled from Neumann DA: *Kinesiology of the musculoskeletal system: foundations for physical rehabilitation,* St Louis, 2002, Mosby.)

REVIEW QUESTIONS

evolve Answers to the following review questions appear on the Evolve website accompanying this book.

1. When a muscle contracts, does it always succeed in shortening?

2. What is the name given to a shortening contraction of a muscle?

3. What are the three possible scenarios that can occur when a muscle contracts and shortens?

4. What is the name given to the attachment of a muscle that moves and to the attachment of a muscle that does not move?

5. Describe and give an example of a *reverse action*.

6. What are the five steps of the five-step approach to learning muscles?

7. What are the questions that must be asked and answered in step 3 of the five-step approach to learning muscles?

8. What determines the action(s) of a muscle?

9. Other than the reverse action(s), how many actions will a muscle have if it is has one line of pull and that line of pull is oriented within a cardinal plane?

10. How does one determine the action(s) of a muscle that has its line of pull within an oblique plane?

11. Can a multijoint muscle create movement at every one of the joints that it crosses?

12. What is the importance of using the *functional group approach* to learning muscles?

13. Give an example of a muscle that has more than one line of pull.

14. Muscles that belong to flexor functional mover group are usually located in what plane?

15. Muscles that belong to an abductor functional mover group are usually located in what plane?

16. Muscles that belong to a rotation functional mover group are usually located in what plane?

17. How is the long axis of a bone determined?

18. Describe how the off-axis attachment method is used to determine the rotation action of a muscle.

19. Give an example of and explain how a muscle can create a joint action at a joint that it does not cross.

20. Give an example of and explain how a muscle can change its action at a joint based on a change in the position of that joint.

Chapter 12

Types of Muscle Contractions

CHAPTER OUTLINE

CHAPTER OBJECTIVES

After completing this chapter, the student should be able to perform the following:

- ❑ State and define the three types of muscle contractions (concentric, eccentric, and isometric).
- ❑ Give an example of each of the three types of muscle contractions.
- ❑ Describe the relationship between the terms *mover, antagonist, concentric contraction*, and *eccentric contraction.*
- ❑ Describe the relationship between the force of a muscle's contraction, the force of resistance to the muscle's contraction, and which type of muscle contraction results.
- ❑ Define and give an example of a resistance exercise.
- ❑ Relate the sliding filament mechanism to each of the three types of muscle contractions.
- ❑ Define the term *muscle contraction.*
- ❑ List and describe the three scenarios in which a concentric contraction occurs.
- ❑ List and describe the three scenarios in which an eccentric contraction occurs.
- ❑ List and describe the two scenarios in which an isometric contraction occurs.
- ❑ Describe the relationship between gravity, concentric, eccentric, and isometric contractions.
- ❑ Define the term *gravity neutral,* and describe its relationship to muscle contractions.
- ❑ State the most usual circumstance when an eccentric contraction occurs.
- ❑ Define, describe, and give an example of internal forces and external forces.
- ❑ Relate the analogy of the motor and brakes of a car to concentric and eccentric contractions.
- ❑ Explain how a muscle can create, modify, or stop movement.
- ❑ Describe the relationship between joint mobility and joint stability.
- ❑ Define the key terms of this chapter.
- ❑ State the meanings of the word origins of this chapter.

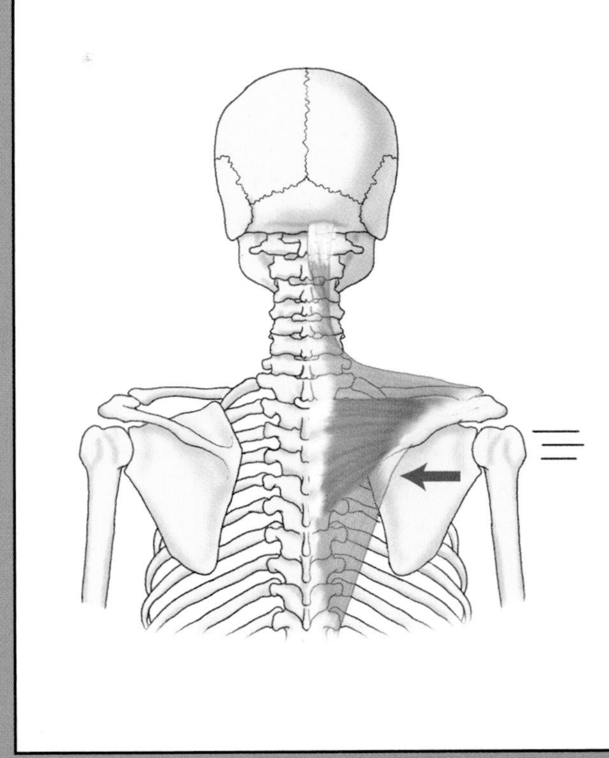

OVERVIEW

Most textbooks and classes that teach the actions of the muscles of the body teach the concentric actions of the muscles. That is, they teach the action(s) that a muscle will create if it contracts and shortens. Therefore when the student learns the actions of a particular muscle, the student learns the shortening concentric actions of that muscle. Nothing is inherently wrong with this approach to teaching muscles. Indeed, for beginning students, this simple and concrete approach to muscle contractions and actions is probably best. However, the one thing that must be kept in mind is that a muscle does not have to shorten when it contracts; in fact, the role of most muscle contractions in the human body is not to shorten and contract. This chapter examines concentric contractions and the other types of contractions that a muscle can have. Chapter 13 then continues to examine the various roles that muscles have in movement patterns when they contract in these ways.

KEY TERMS

Action in question
Antagonist (an-TAG-o-nist)
Aqua therapy (A-kwa)
Concentric contraction (con-SEN-trik)
Eccentric contraction (e-SEN-trik)
External force
Fix
Fixator (FIKS-ay-tor)
Gravity
Gravity neutral
Internal force
Isometric contraction (ICE-o-MET-rik)
Mover
Muscle contraction
Negative contraction
Resistance exercises
Resistance force
Stabilize
Stabilizer
Tension
Tone
Weight

WORD ORIGINS

- ❑ Antagonist—From Greek *anti,* meaning *against, opposite,* and *agon,* meaning *a fight, a contest*
- ❑ Concentric—From Latin *con,* meaning *together, with,* and *centrum,* meaning *center*
- ❑ Eccentric—From Greek *ek,* meaning *out of, away from,* and Greek *kentron* (or Latin *centrum*), meaning *center*
- ❑ Fix—From Latin *fixus,* meaning *fastened*
- ❑ Isometric—From Greek *isos,* meaning *equal,* and *metrikos,* meaning *measure*
- ❑ Stabilize—From Latin *stabilis,* meaning *not moving, fixed*
- ❑ Tension—From Latin *tensio,* meaning *to stretch*
- ❑ Tone—From Latin *tonus,* meaning *a stretching, tone*

☐ 12.1 OVERVIEW OF THE TYPES OF MUSCLE CONTRACTIONS

In Chapter 11 we went through a brief sketch of the big picture of learning how muscles function. It was explained that when a muscle is directed to contract by the nervous system, the muscle attempts to shorten toward its center.

- ❑ Whether or not a muscle is successful in shortening toward its center is determined by the strength of the pulling force of the muscle compared with the force necessary to actually move one or both body parts to which the muscle is attached.
- ❑ The force necessary to move a body part is usually the force necessary to move the weight of the body part. For example, when the brachialis muscle contracts, for it to be able to successfully shorten and flex the elbow joint, it will have to generate enough force to be able to move the weight of either the forearm or the arm. The weight of the forearm or the arm would be the force that is resistant to the brachialis contracting and successfully shortening.
- ❑ If the force of the muscle's contraction is greater than the resistance to the muscle's contraction, the muscle will successfully shorten.
- ❑ This type of contraction wherein a muscle contracts and shortens is called a **concentric contraction**. Further, because the concentrically contracting muscle generates the force that moves a body part to create the joint action that is occurring, it is termed the **mover**. Simply put, the mover creates the movement! Note: The joint action that is occurring is usually termed the **action in question**.

BOX 12-1

When analyzing muscle contractions, the joint action that is occurring is usually termed the action in question.

- ❑ The force that opposes this action of the mover is the **resistance force**. The resistance force in this scenario is an **antagonist** to the action that is occurring. The force of an antagonist is opposite to the action that is occurring (hence the term *antagonist*) (Figure 12-1; Box 12-2).
- ❑ If the force of the muscle's contraction is less than the resistance to the muscle's contraction (or put another way, if the force of the antagonist is greater than the force of the muscle), the muscle will lengthen instead of shorten.
- ❑ This type of contraction is called an *eccentric contraction*. An **eccentric contraction** occurs when a muscle contracts and lengthens (Figure 12-2, Box 12-2).
- ❑ When this situation occurs, the resistance force (i.e., the weight of the body part) creates the action that is occurring and is now termed *the mover*, and the muscle that is eccentrically lengthening is now called *the antagonist*.
- ❑ If the force of the muscle's contraction is exactly equal to the resistance force, then the muscle will neither shorten nor lengthen.
- ❑ This type of contraction is called an *isometric contraction*. An **isometric contraction** is one wherein the muscle contracts and stays the same length.
- ❑ In this case no movement of a body part at the joint occurs; therefore no joint action occurs (Figure 12-3).
- ❑ Because no joint action occurs, the muscle that is isometrically contracting is neither a mover nor an antagonist. (For more information on concentric, eccentric, and isometric contractions, see Sections 12.4-12.6. For more information on the roles of muscles as movers and antagonists, see Sections 13.1-13.2).

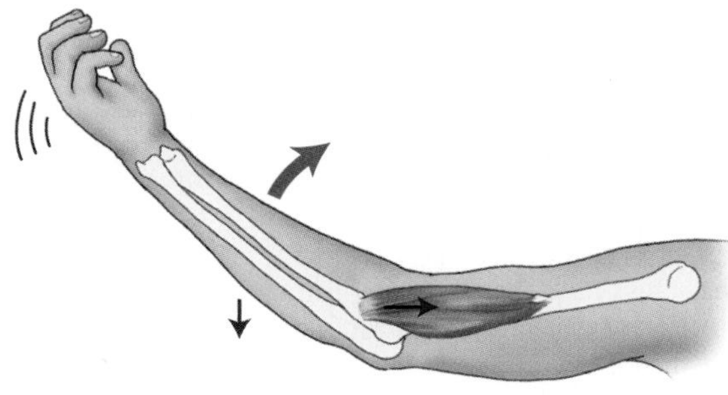

Figure 12-1 Medial view of the brachialis muscle. In this example, we are considering the arm to be fixed and the forearm to potentially be mobile. The arrow within the brachialis shows the line of pull of the muscle. For the brachialis to contract and successfully shorten, the force of its contraction would have to move the forearm up toward the arm. The red curved arrow above the forearm represents the strength and direction of pull of the brachialis acting upon the forearm; the straight brown arrow drawn downward from the forearm represents the strength and direction of pull of gravity (i.e., the weight of the forearm) acting upon the forearm, resisting the pull of the brachialis. When the force of the contraction of the brachialis is greater than the force of the weight of the forearm (i.e., the resistance force) as represented by the relative sizes of the arrows, the brachialis will successfully shorten and move the forearm toward the arm, as seen in this figure. In this scenario, the brachialis concentrically contracted and would be termed the *mover* of flexion of the forearm at the elbow joint. (Note: If the forearm had been fixed, the arm would have to have been moved for the brachialis to concentrically contract. Given the greater weight of the arm [compared to the forearm] and the fact that for the arm to move, the trunk would have to be pulled along with it, it is usually the forearm that moves when motion occurs at the elbow joint. If the brachialis were to contract and move the arm instead of the forearm in this instance, it would be termed a *reverse action*.)

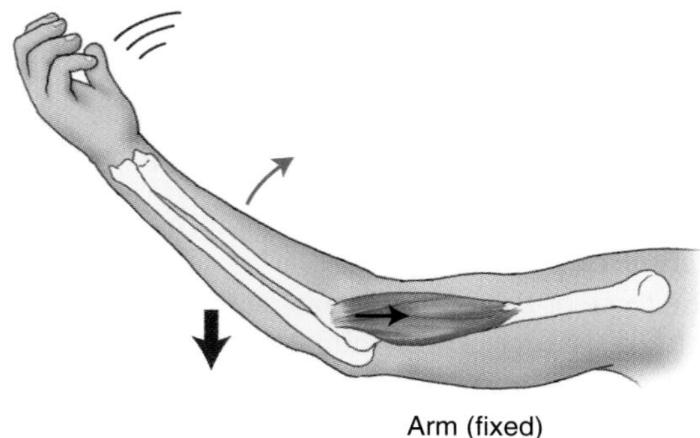

Figure 12-2 Medial view of the brachialis muscle pictured in Figure 12-1. However, in this scenario, the force of the contraction of the brachialis is less than the resistance force of the weight of the forearm. Because the force of the weight of the forearm is greater than the force of the brachialis' contraction, the forearm extends with gravity, causing the brachialis to lengthen. This scenario illustrates an eccentric contraction of the brachialis because it is contracting and lengthening. Further, because the weight of the forearm (caused by gravity) is creating the elbow extension, gravity is the mover; because the contraction of the brachialis creates a force that is opposite to the elbow joint extension that is occurring (i.e., the action in question), the brachialis is an antagonist in this scenario.

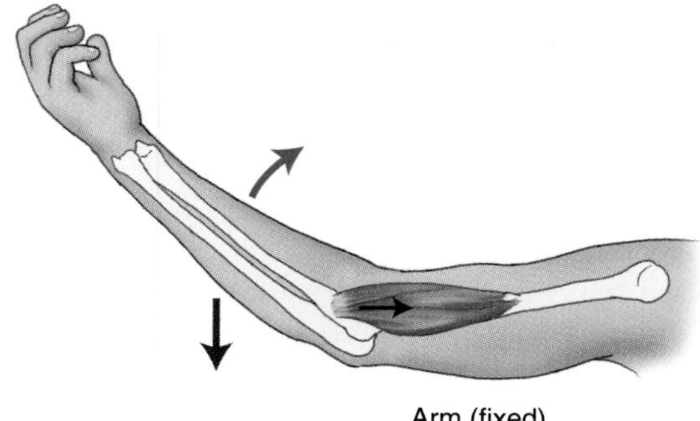

Figure 12-3 Medial view of the brachialis muscle pictured in Figures 12-1 and 12-2. In this scenario, the force of the contraction of the brachialis is exactly equal to the resistance force of the weight of the forearm. Since these two forces are exactly matched, the brachialis does not succeed in shortening and flexing the forearm, nor does gravity succeed in lengthening the brachialis and extending the forearm. This scenario illustrates an isometric contraction of the brachialis because it is contracting and staying the same length. Because no joint action takes place, no mover or antagonist exist.

BOX 12-2 SPOTLIGHT ON THE RESISTANCE TO A MUSCLE'S CONTRACTION

The force of resistance that a muscle must overcome to be able to contract and shorten is usually the result of the weight of the body part of one (or both) of the attachments of the muscle. However, when one body part moves, other body parts must often be moved with it. For example, for the brachialis muscle to contract, shorten, and move the forearm at the elbow joint, the hand must be moved as well. Therefore the contraction of the brachialis must be sufficiently strong to move the weight of the forearm and the hand together. If the brachialis is to create the reverse action and move the arm attachment instead of the forearm attachment at the elbow joint, then its contraction must be sufficiently strong to move not only the weight of the arm but also the weight of the entire trunk, because the arm cannot move without the trunk "going along for the ride."

Often, other factors affect the resistance to a muscle's contraction. When exercises are done with weights, the force of the muscle contraction must be strong enough to move the weight of the body part plus the weight that has been added. Additionally, certain exercises incorporate other forms of resistance. For example, the resistance of springs, rubber tubing, or large rubber bands is often used. In fact, these exercises are often called **resistance exercises**, because they add to the force of resistance that the contracting muscle must work against. Whether weights are used or other forms of additional resistance are used, if a muscle is to contract and successfully shorten when doing resistance exercises, the muscle must contract with greater force to overcome the greater resistance force that it encounters (Figure 12-4).

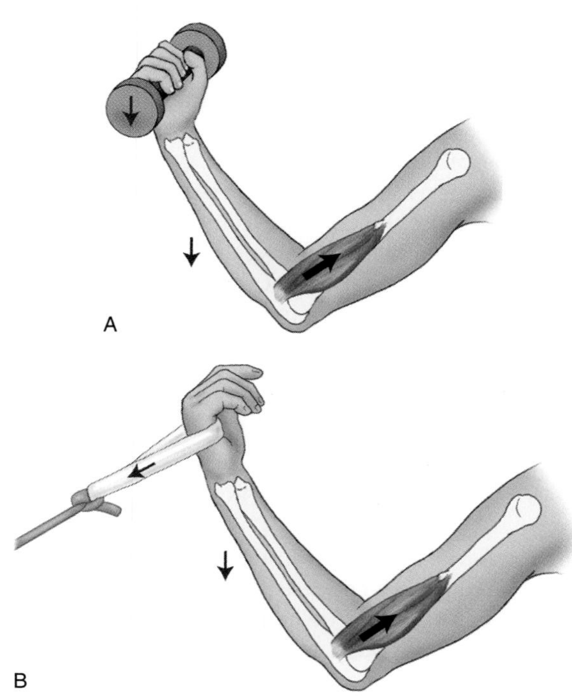

Figure 12-4 Two examples of resistance exercises. *A,* Added resistance to flexion of the forearm at the elbow joint is provided by a weight held in the person's hand. *B,* Added resistance is provided by the rubber tubing that must be stretched for the person to be able to flex the forearm at the elbow joint.

- There are times when it is desirable to reduce the force of resistance that a muscle must work against. For example, if exercises are done in water, the buoyancy of the water may support the body part being moved and would decrease the resistance force to the muscle's contraction. For this reason, exercise in pools (i.e., **aqua therapy**) is often recommended for clients who have recently sustained an injury and are beginning a rehabilitation program, because it provides a gentle way to begin strengthening exercises.

☐ 12.2 CONCENTRIC, ECCENTRIC, AND ISOMETRIC CONTRACTION EXAMPLES

Following are examples of concentric, eccentric, and isometric contractions.

- ❑ Figure 12-5 shows a person that is first abducting the arm at the shoulder joint, then adducting the arm at the shoulder joint, and then holding the arm in a static position of abduction at the shoulder joint.

In Figure 12-5a, he is abducting his arm at the shoulder joint. To accomplish this, he is concentrically shortening the abductor musculature of his shoulder joint. As this musculature shortens, the arm is lifted up into the air in the frontal plane (i.e., it abducts).

In Figure 12-5b, he is adducting his arm at the shoulder joint (from a *higher* position of abduction). To adduct the arm at the shoulder joint, the abductor musculature must lengthen. However, because gravity is adducting the arm, his abductor musculature contracts as it lengthens, creating an upward force of abduction of the arm that slows down the movement of adduction created by gravity. This slowing down of gravity is necessary to prevent gravity from slamming his arm/forearm/hand into the side of his body. The abduction force of his musculature must be less powerful than the force of gravity so that adduction of the arm continues to occur (but is slowed down). In this scenario the abductor musculature is lengthening as it contracts, therefore it is eccentrically contracting.

In Figure 12-5c, we see that he is holding his arm statically in a position of abduction. In this scenario his abductor musculature is contracting with exactly the same amount of upward force as the downward force of gravity. Therefore the arm neither moves up into further abduction nor falls down into adduction. Because no joint action is occurring, the musculature of the joint does not change in length. In this scenario the abductor musculature is staying the same length as it contracts; therefore it is isometrically contracting.

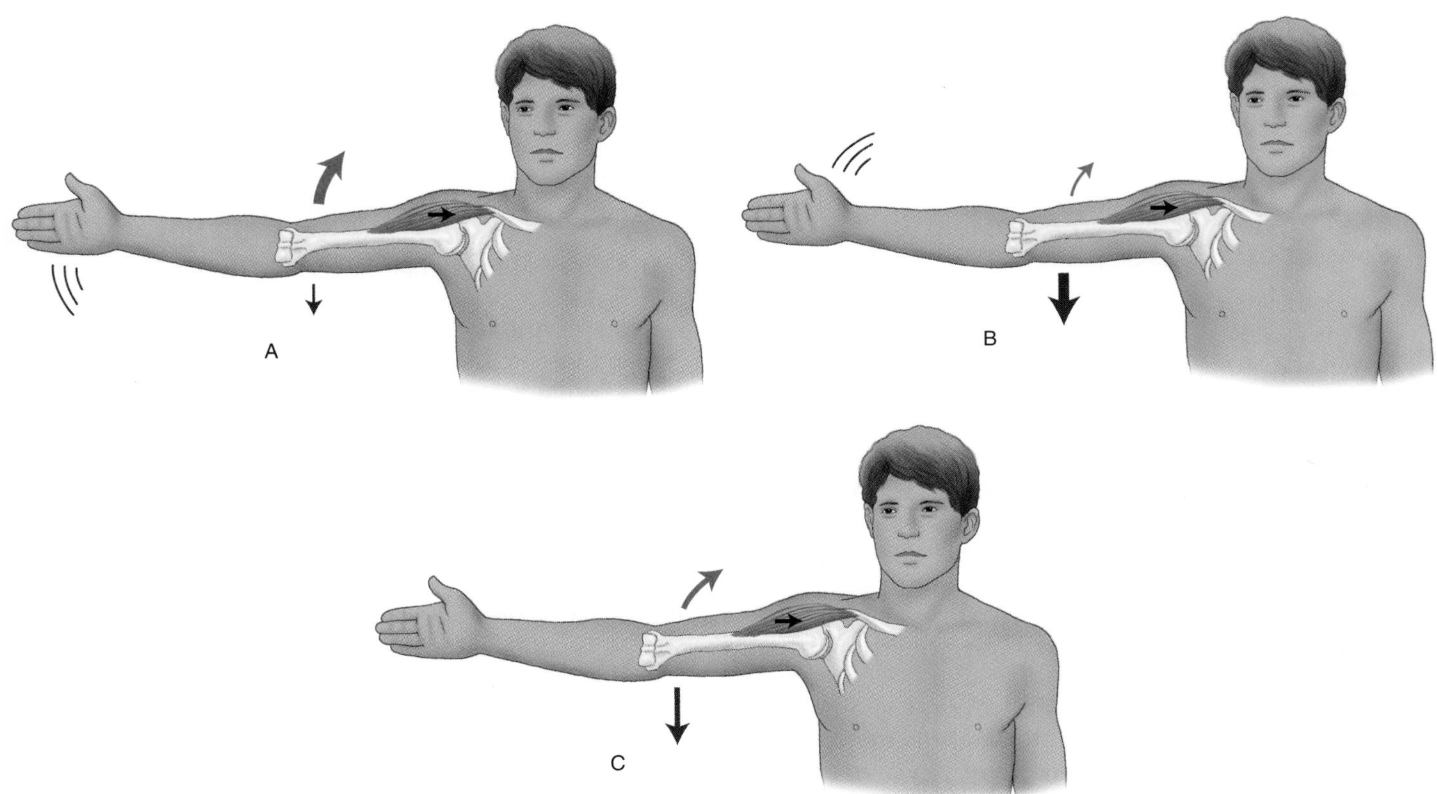

Figure 12-5 *A,* Person abducting the right arm at the shoulder joint against the force of gravity; this force of abduction is created by concentric contraction of the abductor musculature. *B,* Same person adducting the arm at the shoulder joint. In this case gravity is the mover force that creates adduction, but the abductor musculature is eccentrically contracting to slow down the force of gravity. *C,* Person statically holding the arm in a position of abduction. In this case the abductor musculature is isometrically contracting, equaling the force of gravity so that no motion occurs.

☐ 12.3 RELATING MUSCLE CONTRACTION AND THE SLIDING FILAMENT MECHANISM

Section 12.1 began with the assumption that when a muscle contracts, it attempts to shorten toward its center. To understand the concept of muscle contraction more fully, muscle structure and the sliding filament theory must be first understood. To accomplish this, a brief review of muscle structure, nervous system control, and the sliding filament mechanism is helpful.

Brief Review of Muscle Structure:

- ❑ A muscle is an organ that attaches from one bone to another (via its tendons), thereby crossing the joint that is located between the two bones.
- ❑ A muscle is composed of thousands of muscle fibers that generally run longitudinally within the muscle.
- ❑ Each muscle fiber is composed of many myofibrils that run longitudinally within the muscle fiber.
- ❑ Each myofibril is composed of thousands of sarcomeres laid end to end.
  - ❑ Each sarcomere is composed of actin and myosin filaments.
  - ❑ Each sarcomere has a myosin filament located at its center.
  - ❑ Actin filaments are located on both sides of the myosin filament and are attached to the Z-lines, which are the boundaries of the sarcomere.

Brief Review of Nervous System Control of a Muscle:

- ❑ A muscle is innervated by a motor nerve from the central nervous system.
- ❑ When a signal for contraction is sent to a muscle by the central nervous system, this signal is sent through neurons (i.e., nerve cells) located within a peripheral nerve.
- ❑ Each neuron that carries the message for contraction splits to innervate a number of muscle fibers.
- ❑ One motor neuron and all the muscle fibers that it controls are defined as a motor unit.
- ❑ A contraction message that is sent to any one muscle fiber of a motor unit is sent to every muscle fiber of that motor unit.
- ❑ At the muscle fiber, the message to contract from the neuron is carried into the interior of the muscle fiber and given to every sarcomere of every myofibril of the muscle fiber.
- ❑ The sliding filament mechanism explains how each sarcomere of a muscle fiber contracts.

Brief Review of the Sliding Filament Mechanism:

- ❑ As its name implies, the sliding filament mechanism explains how actin and myosin filaments slide along each other. (For more details on the sliding filament mechanism, see Sections 10.6 and 10.12.)
- ❑ When a muscle contraction is desired, the central nervous system sends a message for contraction to the muscle that is to be contracted.
  - ❑ When this message for contraction enters the interior of the muscle fiber, it causes calcium that is stored in the sarcoplasmic reticulum to be released into the sarcoplasm of the muscle fiber.
  - ❑ Calcium in the sarcoplasm binds to the actin filaments, causing a structural change in the actin that exposes its binding (active) sites.
  - ❑ When actins' binding sites are exposed, myosin heads attach to these binding sites of the actin filaments creating cross-bridges.
  - ❑ These cross-bridges bend, attempting to pull the actin filaments in toward the center of the sarcomere.
  - ❑ The attempted bending of the cross-bridges causes a pulling force on the actin filaments.
  - ❑ Because actin filaments are attached to Z-lines, this pulling force is transferred to the Z-lines.
  - ❑ Thus a pulling force toward the center of the sarcomere is exerted on the Z-lines of a sarcomere.
  - ❑ It is the formation of the cross-bridges between the myosin and actin filaments and the pulling force that they exert that defines a **muscle contraction**. In other words, when cross-bridges form and create a pulling force toward the center of the sarcomeres, the muscle is defined as contracting.
- ❑ What happens after this step determines the type of contraction that will occur.
- ❑ As we have seen, three types of contractions exist: (1) concentric, (2) eccentric, and (3) isometric.

Scenario One—Concentric Contraction:

- ❑ If the bending force of the myosin cross-bridges is successful in pulling the actin filaments in toward the center, the Z-lines are drawn toward the center of the sarcomere and the sarcomere shortens.
- ❑ Because this message for contraction is given to every sarcomere of the muscle fiber, if one sarcomere succeeds in shortening, every sarcomere will succeed in shortening and the entire muscle fiber will shorten (Box 12-3).

BOX 12-3

Picturing one sarcomere shortening is fairly simple. Both actins come in toward the center, bringing their Z-line attachments with them. However, some students have a difficult time picturing how two or more consecutive sarcomeres that are located next to each other can all shorten at the same time if the same Z-line is to be pulled in opposite directions. To picture this, we should look at a typical muscle contraction in which one attachment of the muscle stays fixed. The Z-line of the sarcomere located next to the fixed attachment is itself fixed and cannot move, so the other Z-line of that sarcomere must move toward the fixed Z-line. When this mobile Z-line moves toward the fixed one, the next sarcomere must move as a whole toward the fixed attachment. In addition, this sarcomere will also shorten toward its own center as it moves toward the fixed attachment of the muscle. In reality, what is happening is that the myosin filament on the fixed attachment side of each sarcomere is actually sliding toward the actin filament on that side. For this reason, the sliding filament mechanism is called the *sliding filament mechanism*, not the sliding *actin filament mechanism*. Either filament can slide along the other when the cross-bridges between the myosin and actin filaments bend.

- ❑ Because the message for contraction is given to every muscle fiber of a motor unit, every muscle fiber of that motor unit will shorten.
- ❑ If enough muscle fibers of a muscle shorten, the entire muscle shortens toward its center.
- ❑ When the entire muscle shortens toward its center, it pulls on its attachments such that one or both of its attachments will be pulled toward the center of the muscle.
- ❑ Because muscle attachments are on bones, and bones are within body parts, the body parts that the muscle attachments are within will be moved toward each other.
- ❑ This type of a contraction in which the muscle succeeds in shortening is called a *concentric contraction*. A concentric contraction is a shortening contraction.
- ❑ As explained in Section 11.2, a concentrically contracting muscle may shorten by moving either one or both of its attachments toward the center of the muscle (i.e., toward each other). (See Figure 12-5a, for an example of a concentric contraction.)
- ❑ Note: The foregoing explanation is how the concept of muscle contraction is usually explained. However, this scenario applies only to a shortening concentric contraction, and a muscle does not necessarily shorten when it contracts.

Scenario Two—Eccentric Contraction:

- ❑ If the force of resistance to the muscle shortening is greater than the force of the muscle contraction, then the myosin cross-bridges will not be successful in bending and pulling the actin filaments in toward the center, and the sarcomeres will not shorten. If the sarcomeres do not shorten, the muscle will not shorten. In fact, because the force of the resistance is greater than the muscle contraction force, the resistance force will actually pull the actin filaments away from the center of the sarcomere and each sarcomere will actually lengthen.
- ❑ If all of the sarcomeres (in the myofibrils of the muscle fibers of the motor unit) lengthen, the entire muscle will lengthen.
- ❑ A lengthening of the muscle results in the attachments of the muscle moving further from each other.
- ❑ Because muscle attachments are on bones, and bones are within body parts, the body parts that the muscle attachments are within will move further from each other.
- ❑ This type of a contraction in which the muscle lengthens is called an *eccentric contraction*. An eccentric contraction is a lengthening contraction. (See Figure 12-5b, for an example of an eccentric contraction.)

Scenario Three—Isometric Contraction:

- ❑ If the force of the muscle's contraction is exactly equal to the force of the resistance to the muscle contraction, then the myosin cross-bridges will not be able to bend and pull the actins in toward the center of the sarcomere; therefore the sarcomeres of the muscle will not shorten. However, the isometric contraction will generate enough strength to oppose any resistance force that would lengthen the sarcomeres. Therefore the sarcomeres neither shorten nor lengthen; rather they remain the same length.
- ❑ If the sarcomeres remain the same length, then the muscle will remain the same length and the attachments and body parts will not move.
- ❑ This type of a contraction in which the muscle stays the same length is called an *isometric contraction*. (See Figure 12-5c, for an example of an isometric contraction.)

Conclusion:

- ❑ What defines a muscle as contracting is the fact that myosin cross-bridges are grabbing actin filaments, *attempting* to bend and pull the actin filaments toward the center of the sarcomere. This creates the tension or pulling force toward the center of the sarcomere that defines contraction!
- ❑ Extrapolating this idea to an entire muscle, it can be stated that it is the tension or pulling force of the muscle toward its center that defines a muscle as contracting.

BOX 12-4

The term **tension** is defined as a pulling force; tensile forces are pulling forces. Because muscles only pull (they cannot push), muscles create tensile forces in the body.

In all three types of muscle contractions, what defines a muscle as contracting is not the length change of the muscle; when a muscle contracts, it may shorten, lengthen, or stay the same length. A muscle is defined as contracting when it generates a pulling force toward its center!

- The term **tone** is often used to describe when a muscle is contracting (i.e., when it is generating tension). Using the term *tone*, the following can be said:
  - A concentric contraction is when a muscle shortens with tone.
  - An eccentric contraction is when a muscle lengthens with tone.
  - An isometric contraction is when a muscle stays the same length with tone.

Hence three types of muscle contractions exist: (1) concentric, (2) eccentric, and (3) isometric.

BOX 12-5

The term *concentric* means *toward the center*; a concentric contraction is one in which the muscle moves toward its center. The term *eccentric* means *away from the center*; an eccentric contraction is one in which the muscle moves away from its center. The term *isometric* means *same length*; an isometric contraction is one in which the muscle stays the same length.

- A concentric contraction occurs when the force of the muscle's contraction is greater than the force of resistance to movement.
  - A concentric contraction is a shortening contraction.
- A lengthening eccentric contraction occurs when the force of the muscle's contraction is less than the force of resistance to movement.
  - An eccentric contraction is a lengthening contraction.
- An isometric contraction occurs when the force of the muscle's contraction is equal to the force of the resistance to movement.
  - An isometric contraction is one in which the muscle contracts and stays the same length.

12.4 CONCENTRIC CONTRACTIONS—MORE DETAIL

Concentric Contractions—Shortening Contractions:

- Concentric contractions are the type of contractions that are usually taught to beginning students of kinesiology when the actions of muscles are taught. Therefore it is usually not hard for students to understand concentric contractions and grasp when they occur in the body.
- A concentric contraction is defined as a shortening contraction (i.e., a muscle contracts and shortens).
- If the muscle shortens, then the attachments of the muscle must come closer together (i.e., the muscle shortens toward its center and pulls the attachments toward each other).
- As discussed in Section 11.1, either attachment can move toward the other, or both attachments can move toward each other.
- Usually the lighter (i.e., more mobile, less fixed) attachment does the moving because it is less resistant to moving.

When Do Concentric Contractions Occur?

- Concentric contractions occur in our body when the force of the concentric contraction is needed to move a body part. Because concentric contractions create movement, a muscle that concentrically contracts is called a *mover*. (For more information on the role of movers, see Section 13.1.)
- These concentric contractions can occur in three scenarios.

BOX 12-6

Another factor to consider when looking at the three scenarios of a concentric contraction is if another resistance force exists beyond the weight of the body part (i.e., beyond the force of gravity)? A resistance force may exist whether the movement is vertically upward, horizontal, or vertically downward. (For more on resistance forces, see Section 12.1) (see Figure 12-4).

Scenario 1—Against Gravity ("Vertically Up"):

- A concentric contraction is necessary whenever a body part is being lifted upward (i.e., when the motion is against gravity) (Figure 12-6a).
- Simply put, if gravity is not lifting our body part upward (which it cannot do, because gravity only pulls downward), then a muscle in our body must be generating the force that is creating this upward

movement. In this scenario the concentric contraction of the muscle is generating more upward force on the body part than the downward force that gravity is exerting on the body part (i.e., the weight of the body part).

BOX 12-7

Gravity is, by definition, a force that pulls downward. More specifically, gravity is the force caused by the mutual attraction between all physical matter (i.e., the mass of objects). Because the largest physical mass in the world is the earth itself, we feel the force of gravity pulling us toward the earth (i.e., downward). The force that gravity exerts on the mass of an object is then defined as the **weight** of that object.

When a concentric contraction creates a force to lift a body part up against gravity, it must lift the weight of the body part that is being moved; it must also move whatever other body part(s) is/are going along for the ride. For example, if the deltoid lifts the arm at the shoulder joint up into abduction, it must contract sufficiently to lift the arm *and* the forearm and hand, because these two body parts go along for the ride.

Scenario 2—Gravity Neutral ("Horizontal"):

- A concentric contraction is necessary whenever a body part is being moved horizontally (i.e., when the motion is **gravity neutral**). A gravity-neutral motion is one in which gravity neither resists the motion nor aids it (because the body part is not being lifted up or down) (Figure 12-6b).
  - Again, if gravity is not creating the movement, then our concentrically contracting muscle must be creating it. In this scenario because gravity is not opposing our muscle's movement of the body part, less force is usually required by our muscle's concentric contraction to move the body part.
- These horizontal gravity-neutral motions are often rotation movements, because rotations usually occur in the transverse plane, which is a horizontal plane.

BOX 12-8

Rotation actions are defined as occurring in the transverse plane in anatomic position. However, we do not always initiate all joint actions from anatomic position. Therefore not all rotation actions necessarily occur horizontal to the ground (i.e., gravity neutral).

Scenario 3—With Gravity ("Vertically Down"):

- A concentric contraction is necessary whenever a body part is moving downward and we want the body part to move *faster* than gravity would move it (Figure 12-6c).
  - Because gravity constantly supplies a downward force, whenever we want to move a body part downward, we can have a free ride and let gravity create this movement of the body part. Therefore no muscle contraction is necessary for the body part to move downward. However, if we want the body part to move downward *faster* than gravity would move it; then we have to concentrically contract muscles that add to the downward force of gravity.

BOX 12-9

The key aspect to understand when a muscle concentrically contracts to aid gravity's movement of a body part downward is to realize that we want to move the body part *faster* than gravity would move us. This is very common when strong exertions are desired such as in sports. For example, when bringing a golf club down to hit a golf ball, gravity alone would accomplish this task—but not with sufficient force to move the golf ball very far. Therefore we aid the force of gravity with concentric contractions of our musculature that move the golf club faster. (However, when we do not need a fast downward movement of a body part, we usually look to slow the force of gravity with eccentric muscular contractions that are antagonistic to the force of gravity.)

- In this discussion of a vertical downward movement (as in the other two scenarios), it was assumed that gravity was the only external force that existed. However, if other forces are present, the contraction of our musculature might change. For example, if another resistance force exists that resists the downward motion of the body part (and this force is greater than the force of gravity), then a concentric contraction would be necessary to move the body part downward (Figure 12-6d).

Analogy to Driving a Car:

- A good analogy to facilitate the understanding of why and when concentric contractions occur is to compare the motor of a car to a concentrically contracting muscle.
- Just as a concentrically contracting muscle creates a force to move a body part, the motor of a car creates a force to move the car. We can draw this analogy of a motor powering the movement of a car to the three scenarios that we just discussed for when concentric contractions occur.
  - Scenario 1: If we are driving a car uphill (i.e., against gravity), we step on the gas to make the motor of the car power the car up the hill (Figure 12-7a).
  - Scenario 2: If we are driving a car on a level surface (i.e., gravity neutral), we step on the gas make the motor of the car power the car to go forward (Figure 12-7b).
  - Scenario 3: If we are driving a car downhill (i.e., with gravity), and we want to drive *faster* than gravity

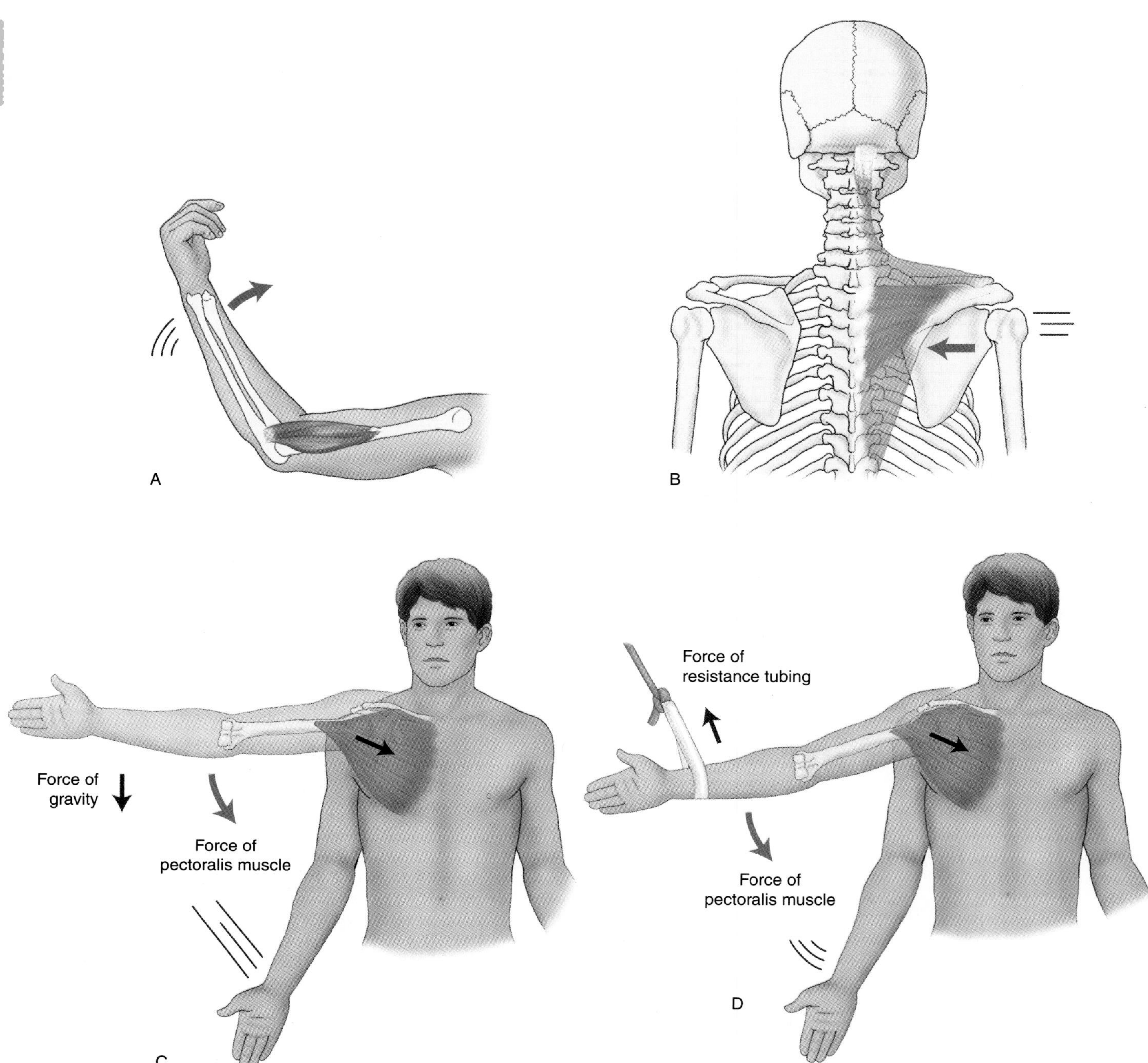

Figure 12-6 *A,* Forearm flexing at the elbow joint. This motion is vertically upward, against gravity; therefore the forearm flexor muscles must contract concentrically as movers to create this motion. The brachialis is seen contracting in this figure; however, any forearm flexor might concentrically contract to create this motion. *B,* Scapula retracting at the scapulocostal joint. This motion is horizontal and gravity neutral; therefore the muscles of scapular retraction must concentrically contract as movers to create this motion. The trapezius (and especially the middle trapezius) is seen contracting in this figure; however, any scapular retractor might concentrically contract to create this motion. *C,* The arm adducting at the shoulder joint. This motion is downward so gravity is the mover; therefore no muscles need to concentrically contract to create this motion. However, if we want to adduct the arm *faster* than would happen by gravity, shoulder adductors can contract concentrically as movers to add to the force of gravity and increase the speed of this action. The pectoralis major is seen contracting in this figure; however, any arm adductor might concentrically contract to create this motion. *D,* Same scenario as in *C,* but this time the person is adducting the arm against the resistance of rubber tubing. Therefore even though this motion is downward and aided by gravity, because of the resistance of the tubing, shoulder adductors must concentrically contract to overcome the resistance and adduct the arm at the shoulder joint.

would bring us down the hill, we step on the gas to make the motor power the car down the hill faster than coasting by gravity would provide (Figure 12-7c).

Conclusion:

- ❑ Concentric contractions occur to move a body part in three scenarios:
  - ❑ Scenario 1: Vertically upward (i.e., against gravity)
  - ❑ Scenario 2: Horizontally (i.e., gravity neutral)
  - ❑ Scenario 3: Vertically downward (i.e., to move faster than gravity would move us)

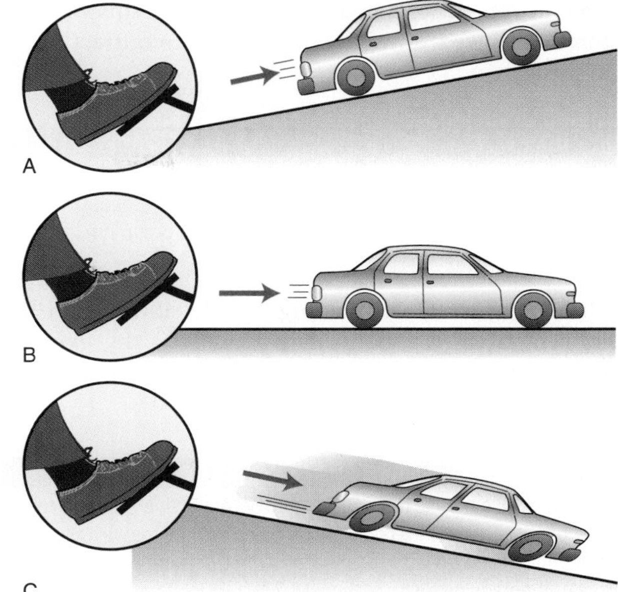

Figure 12-7 Illustration of the idea of the motor of a car being necessary to power the car in three scenarios. *A,* Car moving uphill. *B,* Car moving on level ground. *C,* Car moving downhill (*faster* than coasting with gravity). The concept of the motor powering the car to move in these three scenarios can be compared with a muscle concentrically contracting to move a body part and creating a joint action in three scenarios of movement: (1) vertically upward against gravity, (2) on level ground (i.e., gravity neutral), and (3) vertically downward, but faster than gravity would create.

❑ 12.5 ECCENTRIC CONTRACTIONS—MORE DETAIL

Eccentric Contractions—Lengthening Contractions:

- ❑ An eccentric contraction is defined as a lengthening contraction (i.e., a muscle contracts and lengthens).

BOX 12-10

Just because a muscle is lengthening, it does not mean that it is eccentrically contracting. A muscle can lengthen when it is relaxed (e.g., when a person stretches or does yoga). A muscle can also lengthen while it is contracting (i.e., when myosin's filament cross-bridges are grabbing actin filaments). Lengthening while contracting is defined as an eccentric contraction. It is important to distinguish between these two instances of a muscle lengthening!

- ❑ If a muscle is lengthening, then its attachments are moving away from each other.
- ❑ This movement of a muscle's attachments moving away from each other is usually not caused by muscle contractions within our body; rather, it is usually caused by an external force. An external force is a force that is generated external to (i.e., outside of) our body.

BOX 12-11 SPOTLIGHT ON INTERNAL AND EXTERNAL FORCES

An **internal force** is a force that originates inside our body; internal forces are created by our muscles. An **external force** is any force that originates outside our body. Gravity is the most common external force that acts on our body, but it is not the only one. By virtue of being an external force, it is not a force that we directly can control. When we move our body with muscular contractions (i.e., internal forces), we can speed up or slow down the movement by altering the command to the muscles from the nervous system. External forces however do not respond to our commands. For that reason, the movements that they create usually need to be modified or controlled by our muscular internal forces. These muscular internal forces modify/control the external forces acting on our body by opposing them; similar to how a brake controls the movement of a car that is caused by its motor. The muscles that do this braking and control eccentrically contract, allowing the motion by the external force to occur, but slowing it down as is necessary. Other examples of external forces that may act on the body are springs, rubber tubing (see Figure 12-4b), and bands that pull on the body during strengthening and rehabilitative exercising. Other examples include a strong wind, an ocean wave, wrestling with another person, or even the jostling of a subway train.

- The movement of a body part created by this external force is slowed down by an eccentric contraction of a muscle.

> **BOX 12-12**
>
> An eccentric contraction is sometimes called a **negative contraction**, perhaps because an eccentric contraction opposes (i.e., *negates* the force that is creating the action that is occurring).

- The eccentrically contracting muscle slows down the movement of the body part caused by the external force because it has an action that is opposite the action of the external force (Figure 12-8).

> **BOX 12-13**
>
> Because a muscle that is eccentrically contracting creates a force that is opposite the joint action that is occurring, an eccentrically contracting muscle always acts as an antagonist. (For more information on the role of antagonists, see Section 13.2.)

When Do Eccentric Contractions Occur?

- Eccentric contractions usually occur in our body when the force of the eccentric contraction is needed to slow down a movement caused by gravity or some other external force.
- These eccentric contractions can occur in three scenarios:

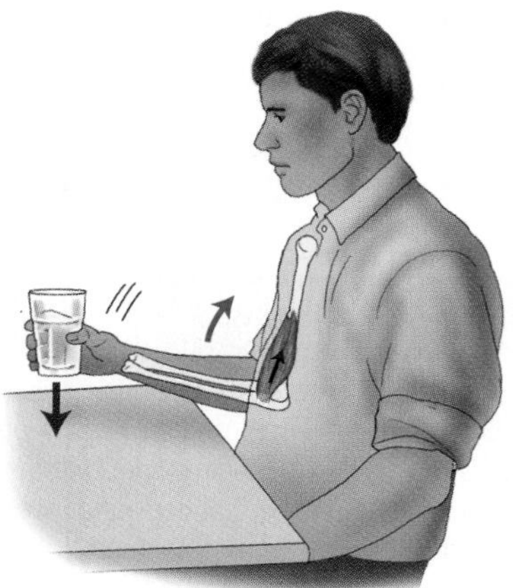

Figure 12-8 Person lowering a glass of water to a tabletop. The joint action that is occurring is extension of the forearm at the elbow joint and is caused by gravity (therefore gravity is the mover in this scenario). However, without control from our muscular system, gravity would cause the glass to come crashing down to the table and break. Therefore a flexor of the forearm must contract to oppose the elbow joint extension force that is being caused by gravity (the brachialis has been drawn in this illustration as our elbow joint flexor). The brachialis must contract with less force than gravity so that gravity in effect "wins" and succeeds in lowering the glass to the table; however, the brachialis acts as a brake on gravity, resulting in the glass being lowered more slowly. In this scenario the brachialis is contracting, but it is lengthening as it contracts. Therefore this is an example of an eccentric contraction. Further, because the brachialis opposes the joint action that is occurring, it is an antagonist.

> **BOX 12-14**
>
> Another factor to consider when looking at the possible ways that a muscle might eccentrically contract is the presence of other external resistance forces. A muscle often needs to contract to slow down other external forces that are acting on the body, whether the direction of movement that is being slowed is vertically upward, horizontal, or vertically downward. External forces providing resistance such as springs, rubber tubing, and bands are often used when exercising.

Scenario 1—"Slowing Gravity's Vertical Downward Motion":

- When gravity creates a downward movement of a body part, it is necessary for the eccentrically contracting muscle to create an upward force that is opposite the downward force of gravity, slowing gravity's movement of the body part.
- The reason to slow down the movement caused by gravity is that gravity only knows one speed; if it is not slowed down, then the body part would crash into whatever surface stops it, possibly causing injury (see Figure 12-8).

Scenario 2—"Slowing Momentum of a Horizontal Motion":

- Eccentric contractions also occur to slow down the movement of a body part when it is moving horizontally. Horizontal motion is gravity neutral (i.e., gravity neither adds to this motion nor resists this motion). In the case where a body part is moving horizontally because of a previous muscular contraction, if the muscle that initiated that movement were to relax, momentum would keep the body part moving further than we might want. If we want to slow it down, then we can eccentrically contract a muscle that does the opposite action of the horizontal movement of the body part that is occurring (Figure 12-9a).

Scenario 3—"Slowing Momentum of a Vertical Upward Motion":

- Eccentric contractions can also occur to slow down the movement of a body part when it is moving upward (i.e., against gravity). In the case where a body part is moving upward quickly because of a previous muscular contraction, if the muscle that initiated that movement were to relax, gravity would eventually slow down the upward movement of the body part. However, if we want to slow it down more rapidly than the force of gravity would, then we can eccentrically contract a muscle that does the opposite action of the upward movement of the body part that is occurring (Figure 12-9b).

Analogy to Driving a Car:

- A good analogy to facilitate the understanding of why and when eccentric contractions occur is to compare the brakes of a car to an eccentrically contracting muscle.
- Just as an eccentrically contracting muscle creates a force to slow down movement of a body part, the brakes of a car create a force to slow down the movement of a car. We can draw this analogy of the brakes of a car to the three scenarios that we just discussed for when eccentric contractions occur.
  - Scenario 1: If we are driving a car downhill (i.e., with gravity) and we do not want the car to gain too much speed because of the force of gravity, then we must step on the brakes to control the car's speed downhill (to slow the downward movement of the car) (Figure 12-10a).
  - Scenario 2: If we are driving a car on a level surface (i.e., gravity neutral) and the car has momentum because we have already pressed on the gas to go fast, then we can press on the brakes to slow the movement of the car (Figure 12-10b).
  - Scenario 3: If we are driving a car uphill (i.e., against gravity) and we need to slow down faster than we would if gravity were to slow us down, then we can press on the brakes to more quickly slow the movement of the car uphill (Figure 12-10c).

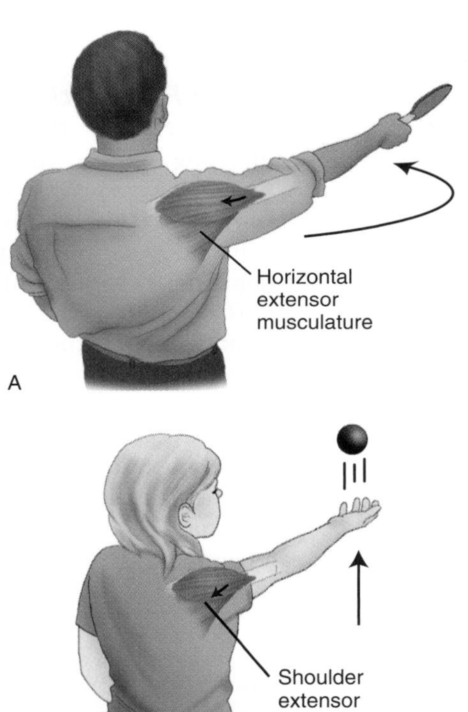

Figure 12-9 *A,* Person who has just hit a ping-pong ball with a forehand stroke by horizontally flexing the arm at the shoulder joint. After having initiated the stroke with muscular force, movement of the stroke continues with momentum. Toward the end of the stroke, the person eccentrically contracts muscles that do the opposite action of the stroke (i.e., horizontal extension) to slow down the motion of the arm, preventing it from moving too far. *B,* Girl that has just thrown a ball up into the air by flexing the arm at the shoulder joint. This motion was initiated by muscular contraction. After releasing the ball, this upward motion of flexion of the arm is slowed down by an eccentric contraction of muscles on the other side of the joint (i.e., the antagonistic shoulder extensors).

Conclusion:

- Eccentric contractions occur to slow movement of a body part in three scenarios:
  - Scenario 1: To slow vertically downward motion (i.e., to slow gravity's downward motion of the body part).
  - Scenario 2: To slow horizontal motion (i.e., gravity is neutral, but momentum must be slowed down).
  - Scenario 3: To slow vertically upward motion (i.e., to slow the upward motion of momentum more quickly than gravity alone would).

BOX 12-15

Of the possible ways in which a muscle eccentrically contracts, the most common example is to slow downward movement of a body part because of the force of gravity!

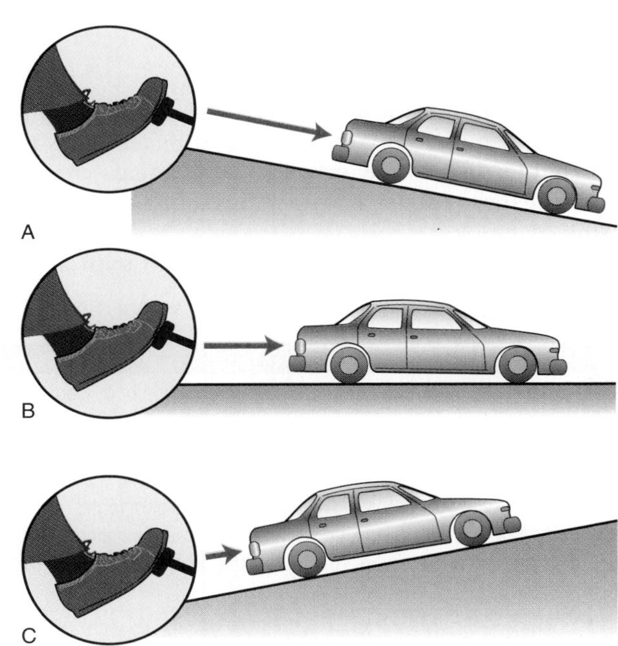

Figure 12-10 Illustration of the idea of the brakes of a car being necessary to slow down the movement of the car in three scenarios. *A,* Car moving downhill and slowing down. *B,* Car moving on level ground and slowing down. *C,* Car moving uphill and slowing down (slowing down more quickly than it would if just gravity were to slow it down). The concept of the brakes slowing the movement of a car in these three scenarios can be drawn to the concept of a muscle eccentrically contracting to slow the motion of a joint action that is occurring vertically downward with gravity, on level ground (i.e., gravity neutral), and vertically upward (but slowing the joint action more quickly than gravity alone would have done).

☐ 12.6 ISOMETRIC CONTRACTIONS—MORE DETAIL

Isometric Contractions—Same Length Contractions:

- ❑ An isometric contraction is defined as a contraction in which the muscle stays the same length (i.e., the muscle contracts and stays the same length).
- ❑ If a muscle contracts and stays the same length, then there must be an opposing force (of resistance) that is also acting on the body part that keeps the body part from moving and therefore stops the muscle from being able to shorten.
- ❑ This other force could be any external force such as gravity or could be an internal force created by another muscle in our own body.
- ❑ The force by our isometrically contracting muscle and the opposing force must be exactly the same strength (i.e., their forces balance each other out). Hence neither one succeeds in moving the body part.

BOX 12-16

A nice analogy to make to better see and understand isometric contractions is to think of a tug-of-war wherein both sides are pulling on the rope with exactly the same force and, as a result, no movement occurs (i.e., neither side is pulled toward the other).

- ❑ Isometric contractions are very easy to recognize because a muscle is contracting and its length is not changing; hence the muscles' attachments are not moving (i.e. whatever body part it is acting on is staying still).
- ❑ Because the body part is staying still, no joint action is occurring.

BOX 12-17

Because an isometric muscle contraction holds a body part still, it allows no joint movement. Because no joint movement occurs, when we start assigning roles to muscles, no mover or antagonist is named because these terms are defined relative to a movement of a body part at a joint. Instead, we simply have two equally strong forces acting on a body part to hold it still; these forces are usually called *fixator* (i.e., stabilizer) *forces.* (See Sections 13.5 and 13.6 for more on this muscle's role.)

BOX 12-18

There is an interesting example of isometric muscle contraction with joint motion. When a two-joint muscle (i.e., a muscle that crosses two joints) contracts, it can shorten across one joint that it crosses and lengthen across the other, the net result being that the muscle stays the same length overall but motion has occurred at both joints that it crosses. For example, the rectus femoris can shorten across the hip joint, causing flexion of the thigh at the hip joint, while at the same time lengthening across the knee joint, allowing the knee joint to flex (interestingly, at the same time, a hamstring muscle could have been shortening across the knee joint, causing flexion of the knee joint, while at the same time lengthening across the hip joint, allowing the hip joint to flex).

When Do Isometric Contractions Occur?

- ❑ Isometric contractions occur in our body when the force of the isometric contraction is needed to stop a body part from moving. When an isometric contraction acts to hold a body part in position, that body part is said to be *fixed* or *stabilized.* (For more information on these terms, see Sections 13.5 and 13.6.)
- ❑ These isometric contractions can be divided into two scenarios:

Scenario 1—Against Gravity ("Holding a Body Part Up"):

- ❑ The isometrically contracting muscle opposes gravity. This occurs whenever a body part is being held up against gravity (i.e. when the body part would fall because of gravity if the muscle were not isometrically contracting) (Figure 12-11a).

Scenario 2—Against Any Force Other Than Gravity ("Holding a Body Part in Position"):

- ❑ The isometrically contracting muscle opposes any force other than gravity. This occurs whenever a body part is being held in its position against any force other than gravity, (i.e. when the body part would move in some direction if our isometrically contracting muscle were not contracting). This other force could come from another muscle contracting within the body and acting on a body part. This other force could also be the result of an external force such as the springs/pulleys of an exercise machine or the elastic pulling force of a stretched rubber tubing or band used for exercising. Other examples of external forces might be another person acting on our body, a strong wind, or a wave in the ocean (Figure 12-11b).

Conclusion:

- ❑ Isometric contractions occur to hold still (i.e., fix or stabilize a body part). Isometric contractions can be divided into two scenarios:
  - ❑ Scenario 1: To statically hold a body part up in position against gravity
  - ❑ Scenario 2: To statically hold a body part in position against any force other than gravity

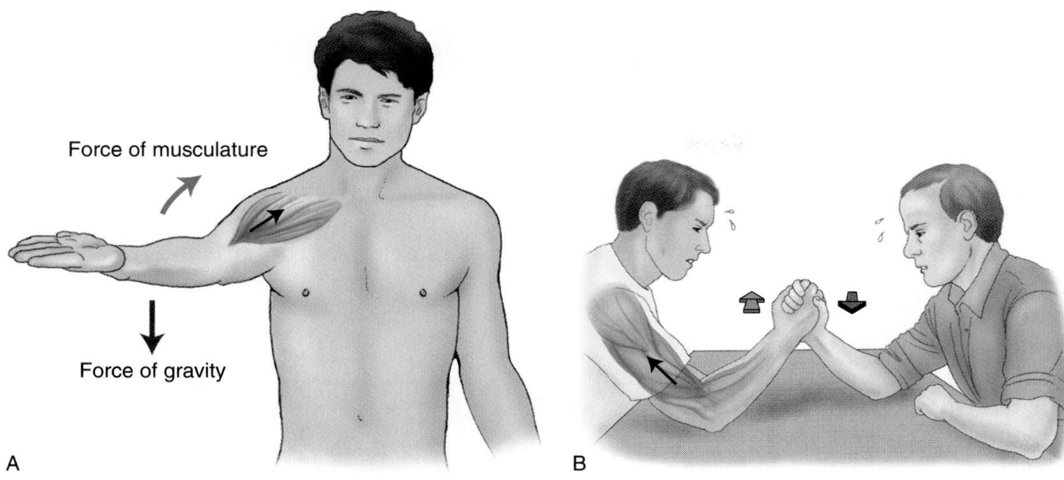

Figure 12-11 *A,* Person holding the arm in a position of flexion. To accomplish this, the shoulder joint flexor musculature must isometrically contract with enough force to equal the force of gravity (which is pulling the arm down toward extension). If the isometric force of shoulder joint flexion is exactly equal to the gravitational force of shoulder joint extension, the arm will be held statically still in this position. *B,* Person arm wrestling with another individual. In this case the force of the person's isometric contraction is exactly equal to the opposing force from the other individual; hence neither force is capable of moving a body part, and the part remains statically still. In both cases the person's musculature contracts and does not shorten (nor lengthen), but rather it remains the same length; therefore it is isometrically contracting.

☐ 12.7 MOVEMENT VERSUS STABILIZATION

- With a better understanding of the concept of muscle contraction, we see that what defines a muscle as contracting is not that it shortens but rather that it generates a pulling force (Box 12-19). Looking at the result of the muscle's contraction, we see the following:
  - A concentric contraction *creates movement*.
  - An eccentric contraction *modifies movement* that is being created by another force (often gravity).
  - An isometric contraction *stops movement* by creating a force that is equal to and therefore balances out an opposing force on a body part.
  - Although both concentric and eccentric contractions are involved with creating/modifying movement of a body part at a joint, isometric contractions are not. In fact, the purpose of an isometric contraction is to stop movement altogether.

BOX 12-19

When a muscle is said to contract, we can confidently state that it is generating a pulling force toward its center. However, we cannot state anything about its length unless we see the particular scenario to know all the other forces that are also acting on the body parts in question. A contracting muscle may successfully shorten, or it may lengthen, or it may stay the same length, depending on the interaction of the force of that muscle's contraction with the other forces, both internal and external, that are present.

- In Section 5.1, an overview of the roles of the parts of the musculoskeletal system was presented as the following:
  - Joints, being passive, allow movement.
  - Ligaments, holding bones together, limit movement at a joint.
  - Muscles (having the ability to contract and create a pulling force) can create movement.
- Although this overview is not wrong, we can see that it is a bit simplistic and incomplete because even though a muscle can create a force that can cause or modify movement of a body part at a joint, it can also create a force that can stop movement of a body part at a joint.
- Whenever a body part is stopped from moving and held still, it is said to be fixed or stabilized. Therefore a muscle that contracts to create a force that holds a body part in a static position is said to **fix** or **stabilize** that body part.

BOX 12-20

When a muscle acts to fix a body part in place (i.e., stabilize it), that muscle can be termed a **fixator** (i.e., **stabilizer**) muscle. (For more on fixator [i.e., stabilizer] muscles, see Section 13.5.)

- Isometric muscle contractions act to fix or stabilize body parts.
- The concept of joint stabilization is extremely important. Often, forces that act on body parts create joint movements that are undesired. Isometric contractions act to stop these undesired movements, thereby stabilizing the joint.
- Therefore when thinking of muscle contractions, we should keep in mind that they can act to create movement or they can act to create stability. For more on the concept of muscle contraction and stability, see Section 13.5 on the role of fixator (i.e., stabilizer) muscles, and Section 13.6 on core stability.
- Although joints exist to allow movement, they also must be sufficiently stable to remain healthy. An antagonistic relationship exists between joint mobility and joint stability: the more mobile a joint is, the less stable it is; the more stable a joint is, the less mobile it is. (For more on joint mobility/stability, see Section 6.2.)
  - Each joint of the body must find its balance between mobility and stability.
  - Muscles can create forces that both increase the mobility of a joint or increase the stability of a joint.

REVIEW QUESTIONS

evolve Answers to the following review questions appear on the Evolve website accompanying this book.

1. What are the three types of muscle contractions?

2. What is the name given to a muscle that concentrically contracts?

3. What is the name given to the force that a concentrically contracting muscle must work against?

4. What type of contraction occurs when a muscle contracts and shortens?

5. What type of contraction occurs when a muscle contracts and lengthens?

6. What type of contraction occurs when a muscle contracts and stays the same length?

7. Give an example of a resistance exercise.

8. What defines a muscle contraction?

9. What type of force is a tensile force?

10. Do muscles pull or push when they contract?

11. What does the term *gravity neutral* mean?

12. What type of muscle contraction is necessary for a person to flex the arm at the shoulder joint from anatomic position?

13. What type of muscle contraction is necessary for a person to slowly adduct the arm from a position of 90 degrees of abduction (at the shoulder joint) to anatomic position?

14. What type of muscle contraction is necessary for a person in anatomic position to rotate the neck to the right at the spinal joints?

______

______

15. What type of muscle contraction is necessary for a person (otherwise in anatomic position) to hold the left thigh in 30 degrees of abduction at the hip joint?

______

______

16. What is the most common scenario in which a muscle eccentrically contracts?

______

______

______

______

17. Why might a person contract mover muscles for a joint action that brings a body part downward?

______

______

______

______

18. Give an example of an internal force and an external force.

______

______

______

______

19. Which type of muscle contraction stops movement from occurring?

______

______

20. Which type of muscle contraction fixes (i.e., stabilizes) a body part in position?

______

______

21. What is the relationship between joint mobility and joint stability?

______

______

______

______

______

______

NOTES

Chapter 13

Roles of Muscles

CHAPTER OUTLINE

CHAPTER OBJECTIVES

After completing this chapter, the student should be able to perform the following:

- ❑ List and define the six major roles that a muscle may have when contracting.
- ❑ Describe the relationship between the role that a muscle plays and the action in question.
- ❑ Compare and contrast the roles of mover and antagonist.
- ❑ Describe the relationship between gravity and joint actions.
- ❑ Discuss the concept of cocontraction.
- ❑ Explain the application of tight antagonists to restricted joint motion.
- ❑ State the muscle that is working during the action in question.
- ❑ Describe the general concept of the relationship between fixators and neutralizers and the muscle that is working.
- ❑ Compare and contrast the roles of fixator and neutralizer.
- ❑ Give an example of a fixator and a neutralizer relative to a specific joint action (i.e., the action in question).
- ❑ State the step-by-step method for determining fixators and neutralizers relative to a specific joint action (i.e., the action in question).
- ❑ Describe the role of a support muscle.
- ❑ Explain the two ways in which a synergist can be defined.
- ❑ Compare and contrast synergists and antagonists for a given joint action.
- ❑ Explain the concept of coordination as it relates to the roles of muscles.
- ❑ Describe the possible clinical effects of isometric contractions.
- ❑ Define and give an example of a 2nd-order fixator.
- ❑ Explain why it is difficult to isolate a specific muscle contraction; further, explain and give an example of how muscle contractions tend to spread through the body.
- ❑ Discuss and give an example of the concept of coupled actions in the body.
- ❑ Define the key terms of this chapter.
- ❑ State the meanings of the word origins of this chapter.

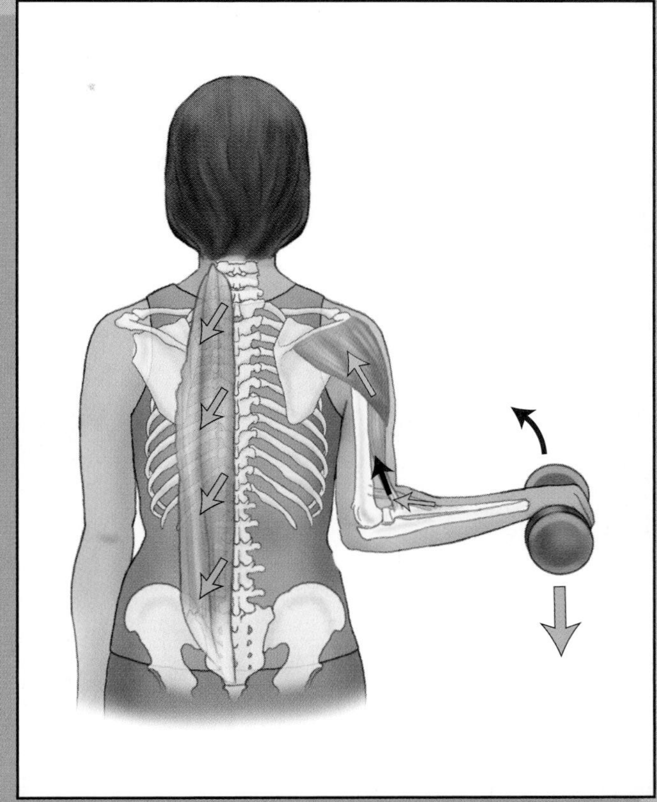

OVERVIEW

When muscles contract in our body to contribute to movements, these muscles may have different roles. The concepts of concentric contractions of movers and eccentric contractions of antagonists were briefly mentioned in Chapter 12. However, of all the muscle contractions that are occurring in the body at any given time, most muscles are not contracting concentrically as movers or eccentrically as antagonists but rather in other roles. The names of these roles are assigned relative to the specific joint action that is occurring. We term this joint action that is occurring, the *action in question*. Given that any muscle that contracts may be used, overused, and injured, it is critically important for manual and exercise therapists to understand the various roles in which a muscle may contract and potentially be injured.

Of course, most of the time as a part of larger movement patterns, we perform multiple joint actions at the same time. However, to simplify our ability to determine which muscles are working in which muscle roles, it is helpful to break more complicated movement patterns into specific joint actions and then determine the roles in which the muscles in our body are working relative to each specific action in question.

Muscles have six major roles when they contract:

1. Mover—A mover is a muscle (or other force) that can do the action in question.
2. Antagonist—An antagonist is a muscle (or other force) that can do the opposite action of the action in question.
3. Fixator (also known as *stabilizer*)—A fixator is a muscle (or other force) that can stop an unwanted action at the fixed attachment of the muscle that is working.
4. Neutralizer—A neutralizer is a muscle (or other force) that can stop an unwanted action at the mobile attachment of the muscle that is working.
5. Support—A support muscle is a muscle that can hold another part of the body in position while the action in question is occurring.
6. Synergist—A synergist is a muscle (or other force) that works with the muscle that is contracting.

KEY TERMS

Action in question
Agonist (AG-o-nist)
Antagonist (an-TAG-o-nist)
Assistant mover
Cocontraction
Contralateral muscle (CON-tra-LAT-er-al)
Coordination
Core stabilizers
Coupled action
Fixator (FIKS-ay-tor)
Ischemia (is-KEEM-ee-a)
Mobility muscles
Mover
Muscle role
Muscle that is working
Mutual neutralizers
Neutralizer
Phasic muscles (FAZE-ik)
Pilates method (pi-LAH-tees)
Postural stabilization muscles
Powerhouse
Prime antagonist (an-TAG-o-nist)
Prime mover
Prime mover group
Scapulohumeral rhythm (SKAP-you-lo-HUME-er-al)
Second (2nd)-order fixator (FIKS-ay-tor)
Stabilizer
Support muscle
Synergist (SIN-er-gist)
Tonic muscles (TON-ik)

WORD ORIGINS

- Agonist—From Greek *agon,* meaning *a contest*
- Antagonist—From Greek *anti,* meaning *against, opposite,* and Greek *agon,* meaning *a contest*
- Contralateral—From Latin *contra,* meaning *opposed, against,* and *latus,* meaning *side*
- Coordination—From Latin *co,* meaning *together,* and *ordinare,* meaning *to order, to arrange*
- Ischemia—From Greek *ischo,* meaning *to keep back,* and *haima,* meaning *blood*
- Prime—From Latin *primus,* meaning *first*
- Synergist—From Greek *syn,* meaning *together,* and *ergon,* meaning *to work*

13.1 MOVER MUSCLES

- A **mover** is a muscle (or other force) that can do the **action in question**.

BOX 13-1

The *action in question* is the term that is used to describe whatever specific joint action is occurring that we are examining. Assigning muscles the role of mover (and all other roles) is always done relative to the role that they play *relative to the action in question.*

- By definition, mover muscles shorten when the action in question occurs.
- A mover is called a *mover* because it can create the movement of the action in question (i.e., it can *move* the body part that is moving during this joint action). This movement occurs because when a mover contracts, it concentrically contracts, thereby shortening and causing one or both of its attachments to move. It is this movement of an attachment that is the action in question.

BOX 13-2

Students sometimes ask the following: What happens if the mover muscle contracts but does not concentrically contract? If a muscle contracts but does not concentrically contract, then it is not a mover. It is the shortening of the concentric contraction of a muscle that creates the movement and defines the muscle as the mover. If the muscle is eccentrically contracting, then another joint action is occurring and this muscle is not creating it; and it cannot be the mover if it does not create the movement. Similarly if the muscle is isometrically contracting instead of concentrically contracting, no joint action is occurring at all, because the muscle is not changing its length. Again, the muscle cannot be a mover (in this case because no movement is occurring). A contracting muscle must be concentrically contracting to be a mover. (For more information on concentric, eccentric, and isometric contractions, see Chapter 12.)

- A mover muscle can shorten in two ways:
  1. It can concentrically contract and shorten, generating the force that creates the action in question.
  2. It can be relaxed and shorten, in effect slackening because its attachments are brought closer together as the joint action is created by another mover force.
- For almost every joint action that is possible in the human body, a functional group of movers can contract to create this action. Just because a group of movers exists does not mean that every muscle of that group necessarily contracts every time the action in question occurs. It is entirely possible for one or a few muscles of a mover group to contract and create the action in question while the rest of the muscles of the mover group are relaxed when the action in question is occurring.

BOX 13-3

Two or more muscles can have lines of pull that are in different linear directions, yet create the same axial joint motion; these muscles form what is called a muscular **force-couple**. For example, the rectus abdominis pulls superiorly upon the pelvis and the biceps femoris of the hamstring group pulls inferiorly upon the pelvis; yet both muscles form a force-couple that creates posterior tilt of the pelvis. Another example is the right sternocleidomastoid pulls the anterior head/neck to the left and the left splenius capitis pulls the posterior head/neck to the right, yet they both form a force-couple that creates left rotation of the head and neck at the spinal joints. Therefore, even though the muscles of a force-couple may have different lines of pull, they are synergistic in that they are movers of the same joint action.

- If a mild force is needed to create the action in question, one or a few of the movers is/are recruited to contract; if a stronger force is needed, a greater number of movers are recruited to contract.
- Within each functional group of movers, there is usually one muscle is the most powerful at performing the action in question. This most powerful mover is called the **prime mover**.
- If a number of muscles are equally strong at performing the action in question, they are sometimes called the **prime mover group**.
- Some sources define any mover other than the prime mover (or muscles in the prime mover group) as an **assistant mover**.
- A mover is also known as an **agonist**.
- The role of mover is the most commonly known role of a contracting muscle. When students are first taught muscles, the actions that are taught for each muscle studied are its mover actions.

BOX 13-4

When we speak of learning the functional groups of muscles (as was discussed in Section 11.6), unless the context is made otherwise clear, it is usually assumed that we are speaking of learning the functional groups of mover muscles. However, muscles may act in roles other than mover; therefore other functional groups exist. This chapter examines these other functional groups of muscles.

- Although we usually think of actions occurring because of a muscle contraction, any force can cause the action in question to occur. For this reason, the definition of a mover is *a muscle (or other force) that can create the action in question*. The most common *other force* that can be a mover force is gravity.
  - Any joint action that moves downward is aided by gravity. Therefore in any downward movement, gravity is a mover.

- ❑ If gravity is the mover, then our muscle movers will usually be relaxed because another force is creating the joint action for them.

❑ Figure 13-1 demonstrates three examples of movers. In all three scenarios of Figure 13-1, whatever force can do the action in question is a mover. However, not every mover is necessarily working (see Figure 13-1).

Essential Facts:

- ❑ A mover is a muscle (or other force) that can do the action in question.
- ❑ By definition, during the action in question, mover muscles shorten.
- ❑ By definition, when a mover muscle contracts, it contracts concentrically.

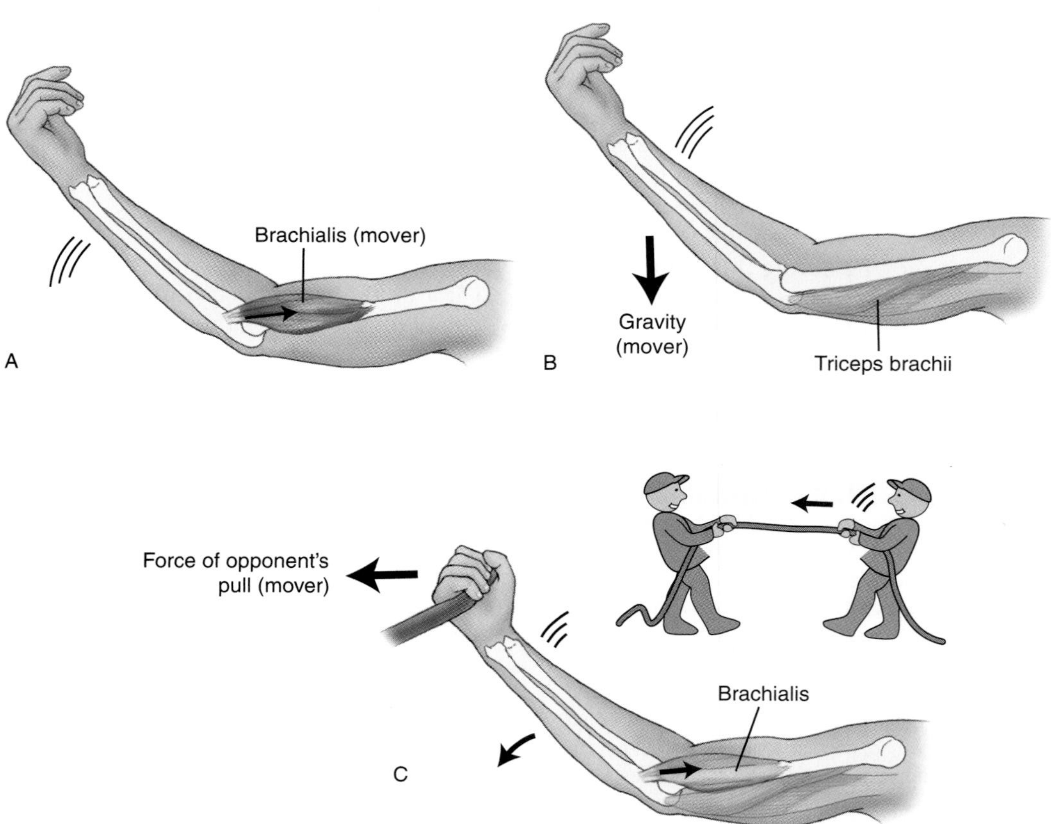

Figure 13-1 Three examples of movers. *A,* The forearm flexing at the elbow joint. Because this motion is upward, a muscle must generate the force to create this movement. In this scenario the brachialis is shown as the mover. However, any muscle that flexes the forearm at the elbow joint is a mover, because every muscle of this functional group can do this action. *B,* Forearm extending at the elbow joint. Because this motion is downward, gravity is capable of bringing the forearm downward; therefore no muscle needs to contract in this case. In this scenario, gravity is the mover. Any muscle that does extension of the forearm at the elbow joint, such as the triceps brachii, is also a mover, because it *can* do the action in question. In this scenario the triceps brachii is a mover, but it is not working; gravity is the mover force that is working. *C,* A person's forearm being pulled into extension at the elbow joint while playing tug-of-war. In this scenario the force of the opponent's pull is the mover force that is creating the action in question, namely extension of the forearm at the elbow joint. Again, any muscle that can extend the forearm at the elbow joint is a mover, even if it is not working.

13.2 ANTAGONIST MUSCLES

- An **antagonist** is a muscle (or other force) that can do the opposite action of the action in question.
- By definition, antagonists lengthen when the action in question occurs.
- An antagonist can lengthen in two ways:
  1. It can eccentrically contract and lengthen, generating a braking force on the action in question. (For more information on eccentric contractions, see Sections 12.1, 12.3, and 12.5.)
  2. It can be relaxed and lengthen, allowing the action in question to occur.
- When an antagonist lengthens, it lengthens because the joint action that is occurring (the action in question) is causing the two attachments of the antagonist muscle to move away from each other (either one or both attachments of the antagonist could be moving). If the attachments of the antagonist are moving away from each other, then the joint action that is occurring must be the opposite action from the joint action that the antagonist would perform if it were to shorten. Thus an antagonist can do the opposite action of the action in question.
  - For example, if the action that is occurring is protraction of the scapula at the scapulocostal (ScC) joint, then the scapula is moving anteriorly. An antagonist to this action is the rhomboids and as the scapula protracts, the attachments of the rhomboids are moving further from each other (i.e., the scapula is moving away from the spine). If the rhomboids were to concentrically contract, they would cause the opposite action of this action in question (i.e., they would cause retraction of the scapula at the ScC joint).
- Because an antagonist is usually located on the opposite side of the joint from the mover muscle(s) that can create the action in question, an antagonist is sometimes called a **contralateral muscle** (the term *contralateral* literally means *opposite side*).
- Usually for any joint action there will be a group of antagonists that can perform the opposite action of the action in question. Among the muscles of the antagonist group, the antagonist that is most powerful at opposing the action in question is called the **prime antagonist**.
- Although we usually think of antagonists as being muscles, any force can oppose the action in question. For this reason, the definition of an antagonist is *a muscle (or other force) that can do the opposite action of the action in question*. The most common *other force* that can be an antagonist is gravity.
  - Any joint action that moves upward is opposed by gravity. Therefore in any upward movement, gravity is an antagonist.
- When a mover contracts and shortens, creating a joint motion, the antagonist must lengthen. If this lengthening is sufficient, the antagonist will stretch. Like a rubber band that is stretched, a passive elastic recoil tension force will build up in the stretched antagonist. If the mover is relaxed and the antagonist is now contracted, the passive tension force that is built up within the antagonist will augment the force of the antagonist's active contraction, creating a stronger force by the muscle. Given the benefit of this passive tension force, this phenomenon has been termed **productive antagonism**.

BOX 13-5 SPOTLIGHT ON WHAT AN ANTAGONIST IS ANTAGONISTIC TO

The name *antagonist* literally means *anti*agonist (i.e., *anti*mover); therefore many people assume that the definition of an antagonist is that it performs the opposite action of the mover (i.e., it opposes the mover). Although the antagonist can oppose the action in question that is performed by the mover, the mover may have other actions that the antagonist cannot oppose. For this reason, it is always best to remember that an antagonist is defined as being able to do the opposite action of *the action in question*. For example, if the action in question is elevation of the scapula at the scapulocostal (ScC) joint and we choose to consider the upper trapezius as our mover (because it can do elevation of the scapula), then the lower trapezius would be an antagonist because it can do depression of the scapula at the ScC joint (i.e., the action that is opposite the action in question). Is the lower trapezius an antagonist to the upper trapezius? It is, only relative to the action of elevation of the scapula. The upper trapezius can also retract the scapula, as can the lower trapezius. With regard to the mover's action of retraction of the scapula, it should be noted that not only does the lower trapezius not do the opposite action of protraction, but it can actually help the upper trapezius do retraction. Therefore when we look at the action in question as being retraction of the scapula, the upper trapezius and lower trapezius are synergistic to each other (i.e., they perform the same action). For this reason, we do not say that a muscle is or is not an antagonist to another muscle; rather it is or is not an antagonist to a specific joint action (i.e., the action in question).

BOX 13-6

The term *productive antagonism* was coined by Don Neumann, PT, PhD. For more on this concept, please see his textbook, *Kinesiology of the Musculoskeletal System* (2002, Mosby).

Determining How an Antagonist Lengthens:

❑ It is critically important to realize that whenever a joint action occurs, the antagonist muscles must lengthen.

❑ However, as previously stated, an antagonist can lengthen in two manners:

1. It can eccentrically contract and lengthen, allowing the action in question to occur, but also creating a braking force on (i.e., slowing the action in question).
2. It can be relaxed and lengthen, allowing the action in question to occur.

❑ To determine how an antagonist lengthens (i.e., whether it is relaxed or eccentrically contracting), we need to look at whether the action in question needs to be slowed down in some manner.

❑ Generally when the mover force is gravity or any other external force that we cannot directly control, we need to slow the joint action to keep our body part from crashing to the ground (or crashing against some other surface).

- ❑ Therefore when gravity or some other external force is the mover, our antagonists usually eccentrically contract and lengthen.

BOX 13-7

By far, the most common scenario of a muscle being an antagonist is when it eccentrically contracts to slow a joint action that is caused by gravity (i.e., a joint action in which gravity is the mover).

❑ However, when one of our muscles provides the mover force (i.e., it is creating the action in question), no need exists to slow it down with our antagonistic muscles. If we feel our mover muscle is causing the action in question to occur too rapidly and that our body part that is moving will crash into something, we can simply command the mover muscle itself to not contract as hard, and the joint action will slow.

- ❑ Therefore when one of our muscles is the mover, our antagonists usually relax and lengthen.

❑ If the mover muscles and the antagonist muscles do contract at the same time, it is called **cocontraction**.

❑ Figure 13-2 demonstrates three examples of antagonists. In all three scenarios of Figure 13-2, whatever force can do the opposite action of the action in question is an antagonist.

❑ As with muscles of a mover group, it should be remembered that not every muscle of an antagonist group is necessarily working during a specific action in question.

BOX 13-8 SPOTLIGHT ON COCONTRACTION

Many new students of kinesiology assume that whenever a mover muscle concentrically contracts and shortens, the antagonist muscle eccentrically contracts and lengthens. This is not the case. Antagonists need to be relaxed and lengthen when mover muscles contract, otherwise the antagonists are fighting the movers. When both mover and antagonist muscles do contract at the same time, it is called *cocontraction*. Cocontraction is not generally considered to be healthy. An analogy would be to press on the gas and the brake of a car at the same time when driving (in this analogy, the mover muscles are the gas and the antagonist muscles are the brake). Just as this would wear out the engine and brakes of the car, cocontraction would fatigue and may eventually injure the mover and antagonist muscles of our body.

An interesting application of this principle to bodywork is when a new manual therapist is doing bodywork and is afraid of using too much pressure for fear of hurting the client. To deliver pressure, the therapist contracts the extensors of the elbow joint; however, at the same time the therapist is subconsciously contracting the flexors of the elbow joint to hold back from exerting too much pressure. This creates a situation in which the therapist is both ineffectual in delivering pressure to the client and is in danger of eventually hurting himself/herself.

Notes:

1. It should be emphasized that cocontraction is defined as the mover and antagonist muscles contracting *at the same time*. A contraction of the mover to initiate a contraction and then a contraction of the antagonist to slow down the momentum of that motion after the mover has relaxed is a sequence of muscle contractions that often occurs in the body and is not cocontraction.
2. If a cocontraction occurs in which the mover and antagonist muscles contract with the same force, then their forces will balance out and no joint action would occur. If no joint action occurs, then by definition these muscles are not defined as movers and antagonists. Rather, they are isometrically contracting opposed muscles.
3. Some kinesiologists believe that cocontraction is a necessary and natural occurrence when we are first learning a new sport or kinesthetic skill. They believe that as we refine and perfect this new skill, we gradually learn to lessen and eliminate the amount of our cocontraction. Therefore part of becoming more efficient, graceful, and coordinated is to learn to lessen the amount that we fight ourselves by cocontracting our muscles.
4. Although cocontraction is inefficient with regard to the production of movement, when stabilization of a body part is needed, cocontraction is desirable and often occurs (for more on stabilization, see Section 13.6).

Essential Facts:

❑ An antagonist is a muscle (or other force) that can do the opposite action of the action in question.

❑ By definition, during the action in question, antagonist muscles lengthen.

❑ By definition, when an antagonist muscle contracts, it contracts eccentrically.

❑ The most common scenario in which a muscle acts as an antagonist is when a muscle eccentrically contracts to slow down a joint action that is caused by gravity.

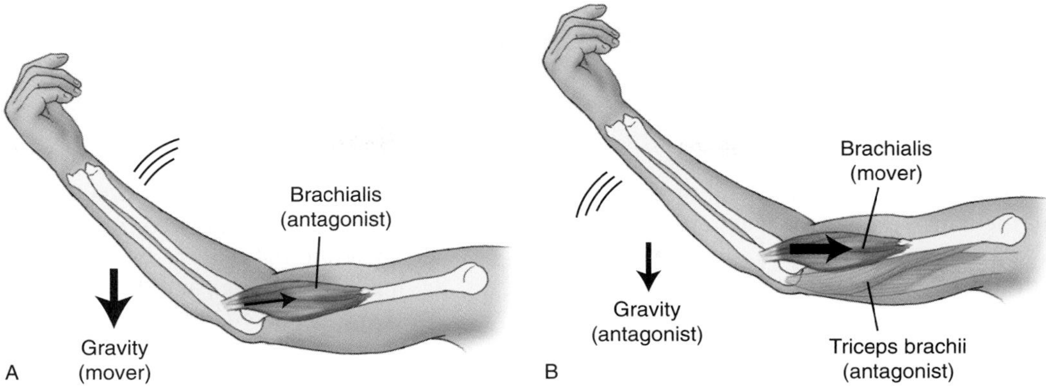

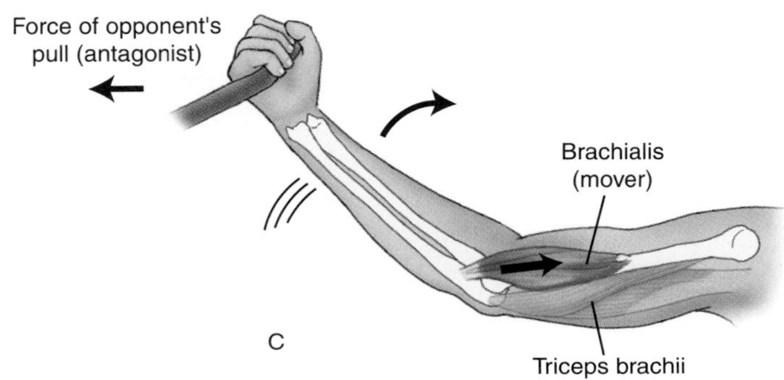

Figure 13-2 Three examples of antagonists. *A,* Forearm is extending at the elbow joint. Because this motion is downward, gravity is the mover that moves the forearm downward into extension. The brachialis (an elbow joint flexor) is shown eccentrically contracting to slow down the extension of the forearm; therefore the brachialis is an antagonist. (Every muscle that flexes the forearm at the elbow joint is an antagonist, because every elbow joint flexor opposes the action in question.) *B,* Forearm flexing at the elbow joint because of the contraction of the brachialis (i.e., the mover). Because this action is upward, gravity is an antagonist, because it exerts a force of extension of the forearm at the elbow joint. Elbow joint extensor muscles are also antagonists whether they are contracting or not, because they can do the opposite action to the action in question. *C,* Elbow joint of a person while playing tug-of-war. The force of the opponent's pull is the mover force that is pulling the person's forearm into extension at the elbow joint. In this case the person's brachialis is an antagonist, because it is opposing the action in question (which is extension of the forearm at the elbow joint) because it is a flexor of the elbow joint. Every flexor of the elbow joint is an antagonist, even if it is not working.

☐ 13.3 DETERMINING THE "MUSCLE THAT IS WORKING"

- ❏ As explained in Sections 13.1 and 13.2, mover muscles and antagonist muscles do not usually cocontract (contract at the same time) when a joint action is occurring.
  - ❏ If the movers are contracting, the antagonists are usually relaxing.
  - ❏ If the antagonists are contracting, the movers are usually relaxing.
- ❏ As a rule, either a mover *or* an antagonist contracts during the action in question (or if more force is necessary, a group of movers *or* a group of antagonists contract during the action in question).
- ❏ Whichever muscle does contract during the action in question is called the **muscle that is working**.
- ❏ To determine which functional group (i.e., movers or antagonists) is contracting (i.e., working), we need to look at what force is creating the action in question.

Role of Gravity in the Action in Question:

- ❏ Assuming that no other external forces are involved, the easiest way to determine what force is creating the action in question is to determine gravity's role with relation to the action in question.
- ❏ Gravity's force pulls downward.
- ❏ Therefore simply look at whether the action in question involves a downward, upward, or horizontal movement of a body part.
- ❏ Following are the three possible scenarios:
  1. Upward movement: If the joint action involves upward movement of a body part, then gravity cannot be causing it; therefore the mover muscles must be concentrically contracting to cause it.
     - ❏ Therefore the movers are concentrically contracting (i.e., working) in this scenario, and the antagonists are relaxed.
  2. Horizontal movement: If the joint action is neither up nor down (i.e., it is horizontal), then the force of gravity is neutral and is not involved. If gravity is not involved, then it cannot cause the action in question to occur; therefore the mover muscles must be concentrically contracting to cause it.
     - ❏ Therefore the movers are concentrically contracting (i.e., working), and the antagonists are relaxed.
  3. Downward movement: If the joint action involves downward movement of the body part, then gravity causes it and the mover muscles do not need to contract. They can relax and let gravity create the motion; in effect, they get a free ride.
     - ❏ However, to control the downward motion caused by gravity, the antagonist muscles most likely will eccentrically contract to slow the force of gravity.
     - ❏ Therefore the antagonists are eccentrically contracting (i.e., working) in this scenario, and the movers are relaxed.

Essential Facts:

- ❏ We can make the following three general rules for our muscle movers and antagonists:
  1. With upward movements, movers work and antagonists relax.
  2. With horizontal movements, movers work and antagonists relax.
  3. With downward movements, antagonists work and movers relax.
- ❏ Figure 13-3 illustrates the three general rules for when movers versus antagonists contract.
- ❏ Of course for every rule an exception exists: If we desire a downward movement that is faster than gravity alone would create, we can supplement the force of gravity with the contraction force of our muscle movers. The antagonists would not work, because we do not want to slow down the movement. Therefore in this scenario our muscle movers would be working and our antagonist muscles would be relaxed. An example is a downward golf swing.

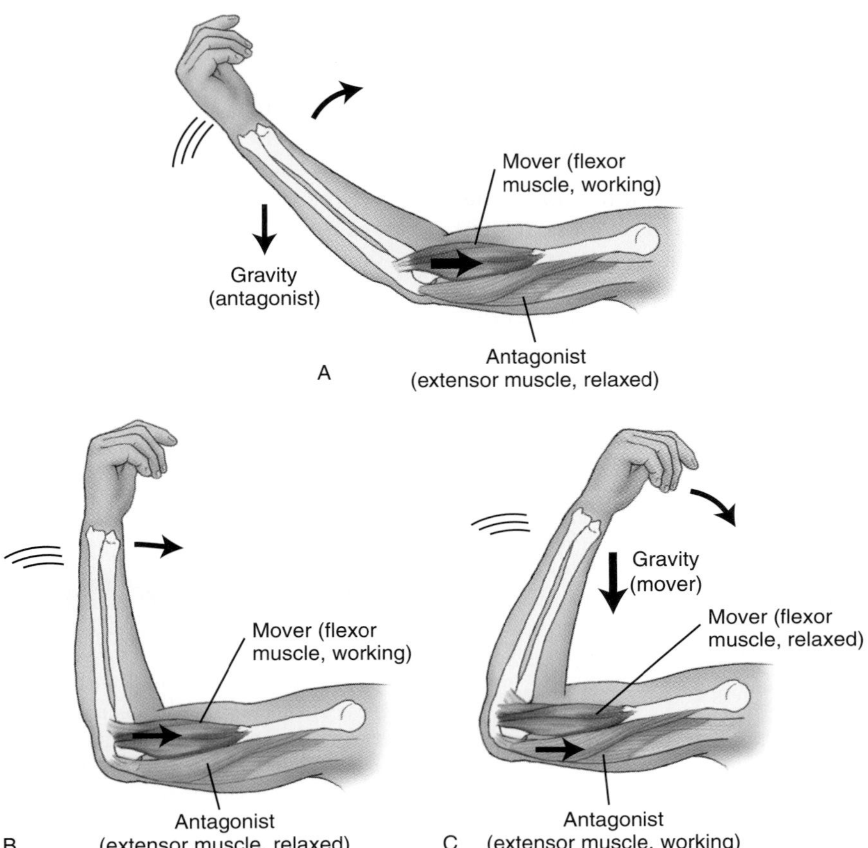

Figure 13-3 Three instances of a person flexing the forearm at the elbow joint. *A* and *B,* Forearm moves in an upward and horizontal direction, respectively. In both of these cases the movers of flexion at the elbow joint must work (i.e., concentrically contract) to create this action. In both of these cases the antagonists are relaxed, allowing the action to occur. (Note: In *A,* gravity is an antagonist; in *B,* gravity is neutral.) *C,* Forearm moves in a downward direction. In this instance, gravity is the mover of elbow joint flexion, so the muscular movers of flexion are relaxed; the extensors of the elbow joint are antagonists, working (i.e., eccentrically contracting) to slow the flexion of the forearm.

☐ 13.4 STOPPING UNWANTED ACTIONS OF THE "MUSCLE THAT IS WORKING"

❑ A muscle that is working is a muscle that is contracting when the action in question is occurring.

❑ In Section 13.3, we learned how to figure out whether it is the mover group or antagonist group that works.

❑ Now that we know which group is working, we must look at another factor. That is, are there any unwanted actions of the muscle that is working during an action in question that need to be canceled out?

Example of Stopping an Unwanted Action

❑ To understand this concept, it is helpful to look at the example of flexion of the fingers to make a fist. (Note: Flexion of fingers #2-5 occurs at the metacarpophalangeal [MCP] and interphalangeal [IP] joints.)

❑ If our upper extremity is in a position such that flexing the fingers is an upward motion, gravity cannot be the mover. This means we need a muscle mover to concentrically contract to do flexion of the fingers.

  ❑ Therefore movers are working (i.e., contracting), and antagonists are relaxed.

❑ Two movers can flex the fingers: (1) the flexor digitorum superficialis (FDS) and (2) the flexor digitorum profundus (FDP). We could choose either one, but for this example it will be helpful to consider the FDS.

  ❑ Therefore our action in question is flexion of the fingers, and our muscle that is working (i.e., the FDS) is the mover.

❑ As soon as the FDS flexes the fingers (the action in question), a fist is made. This means we are done, right?

❑ No, because if the only joint action that we want is flexion of the fingers, then we have a problem. This is because when the FDS contracts, it will attempt to create every one of its actions. (Note: The FDS has only one line of pull that crosses multiple joints. A muscle with one line of pull cannot intend only one of its actions to occur. When a muscle with one line of pull contracts, it attempts to create every action along that line of pull [see Section 11.5].)

❑ The FDS can also flex the hand at the wrist joint. Flexion of the hand at the wrist joint is an unwanted action of our muscle that is working (i.e., our contracting mover, the FDS).

❑ Whenever our *working* muscle has an unwanted action, then that unwanted action has to be stopped.

❑ In this scenario it is the job of an extensor of the hand at the wrist joint to contract and stop flexion of the hand at the wrist joint. Palpate the common extensor tendon region near the lateral epicondyle of the humerus while making a fist, and a contraction will clearly be felt to occur when flexing fingers to make a fist.

BOX 13-9

Theoretically, any extensor of the hand at the wrist joint could stop the flexor digitorum superficialis (FDS) from flexing the hand at the wrist joint. However, the extensor carpi radialis brevis is the wrist joint extensor that is usually chosen by the central nervous system for this task.

❑ How? When a wrist joint extensor contracts, it creates a force of extension of the hand at the wrist joint that stops the FDS from flexing the hand at the wrist joint. (Note: The FDS also crosses the elbow joint and could cause flexion of the forearm that the elbow joint. Theoretically this is another unwanted action that would have to be stopped.)

❑ What role does the wrist joint extensor play? It cannot create the action in question (i.e., flexion of the fingers); therefore it is not a mover. It cannot do the opposite action of the action in question (i.e., extension of the fingers); therefore it is not an antagonist.

  ❑ In this scenario the role in which the wrist joint extensor functions is as a fixator muscle.

BOX 13-10

In the scenario of flexing the fingers and making a fist, the extensor carpi radialis brevis acts as a fixator muscle. An interesting clinical application arises from this example. Tennis elbow (also known as *lateral epicondylitis*) is overuse/misuse of the muscles of the common extensor tendon. Although the cause of tennis elbow is usually blamed on overuse of the wrist extensor muscles as movers (e.g., the client is extending the hand at the wrist joint when poorly executing a backhand stroke while playing tennis), another major aggravating factor of tennis elbow is the contraction of wrist extensors as fixators every time that the finger flexor muscles contract to make a fist or hold something. This means that every moment that the person holds and grips the tennis racquet, or for that matter, grasps a doorknob to open a door, grips a steering wheel, or simply holds a pen, the condition of tennis elbow is aggravated!

❑ Two types of muscle roles serve to stop unwanted actions of the muscle that is working. One is fixator as exemplified in the previously discussed scenario; the other is neutralizer.

Fixators and Neutralizers:

❑ Fixators and neutralizers are similar in that they both stop unwanted actions of the muscle that is working. (Again, the muscle that is working is either a mover concentrically contracting or an antagonist eccentrically contracting.)

- Fixators and neutralizers are different in that the fixator stops an unwanted action at the *fixed attachment* of the muscle that is working; the neutralizer stops an unwanted action at the *mobile attachment* of the muscle that is working.

BOX 13-11

Not every contracting muscle has one fixed attachment and one mobile attachment. It is possible for a muscle to contract and move both of its attachments, in which case both attachments are mobile and no fixed attachment exists. It is also possible for a muscle to contract isometrically and have both attachments stay fixed, in which case no mobile attachment exists. Further, some muscles have more than two attachments. Viewing a muscle as having two attachments (with one attachment fixed and one attachment mobile when it contracts) is the typical scenario.

The roles of fixators and neutralizers are explored in more detail in the next two sections (13.5 and 13.6).

Muscle That Is Working:

- In our scenario of flexing fingers to make a fist, the muscle that is working is the concentrically contracting mover, the FDS.
- However, as we have learned, movers do not always contract. Sometimes they are relaxed, and it is the antagonist group that is working. Just like a mover that is working, when an antagonist is working, it can also create a pulling force that would create unwanted actions. When this occurs, unwanted actions of the antagonist would need to be stopped just as the unwanted actions of a mover would have to be stopped.
- Therefore the muscle that is working could either be a concentrically contracting mover or an eccentrically contracting antagonist.

Essential Facts:

- The muscle that is working is the muscle that is contracting. It is either a concentrically contracting mover or an eccentrically contracting antagonist.
- Fixators and neutralizers are similar in that they both stop unwanted actions that would occur because of the contraction of the muscle that is working.
- Fixators and neutralizers differ in that fixators stop unwanted actions that would occur at the *fixed* attachment of the muscle that is working; neutralizers stop unwanted actions that would occur at the *mobile* attachment of the muscle that is working.

13.5 FIXATOR MUSCLES

- A **fixator** is a muscle (or other force) that can stop an unwanted action at the fixed attachment of the muscle that is working.
- A fixator is also known as a **stabilizer**.
- We have seen that whether it is the mover or the antagonist that is contracting during our desired action in question, this muscle that is working can cause other joint actions to occur. These other joint actions may be unwanted, and therefore they need to be stopped.
- The role of a fixator is to stop these unwanted actions that occur at the *fixed attachment* of the muscle that is working.
- This is why the fixator is so named; it "fixes" one attachment in place so that it does not move.
- To determine which attachment of the working muscle is fixed, simply look at the action in question that is occurring. Whichever body part is named as moving is the mobile attachment; whichever body part is not moving is the fixed attachment.
  - For example, if the right levator scapulae is contracting and creating right lateral flexion of the neck at the spinal joints, then the mobile attachment is the neck (because it is moving) and the fixed attachment is the scapula (because it is not moving).
- Fixator muscles fix a body part by creating a contraction force that is equal in strength but opposite in direction to the force of the unwanted action of the muscle that is working. By doing this, the attachment that is being pulled on by both the muscle that is working and the fixator muscle cannot move in either direction. (Note: In the example of making a fist in Section 13.4, the muscle that did extension of the hand at the wrist created an extension force on the hand that was equal in strength [but opposite in direction] to the force of flexion of the hand at the wrist joint that the FDS created.)
- Because the attachment is fixed by the fixator muscle, the attachment does not move. If the attachment does not move, the fixator muscle does not change its length. Therefore fixator muscles isometrically contract when they fix body parts in place.

Figures 13-4 to 13-6 provide examples of fixators.

- In Figure 13-4, we see a posterior view of the right levator scapulae muscle. If the levator scapulae muscle is the only muscle that contracts, it will create a pulling force on both the scapula and the neck. If we want only the neck to move, the actions of the right levator scapulae on the scapula have to be cancelled out (i.e.,

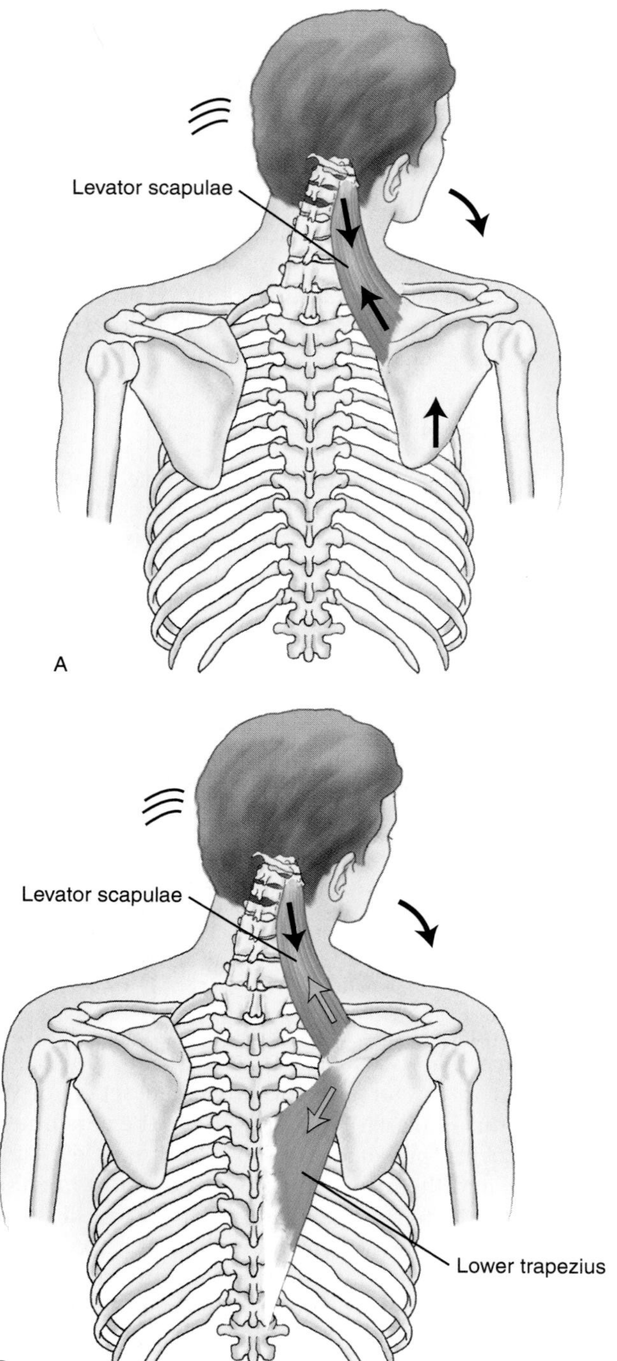

Figure 13-4 *A,* Right levator scapulae muscle contracts and creates a pulling force that moves both the scapula and the neck. *B,* Right lower trapezius is seen to contract as a fixator of the scapula by creating a force of depression on the scapula at the scapulocostal (ScC) joint that stops the levator scapulae from elevating the scapula. Because the right lower trapezius stops the scapula from moving (i.e., it fixes the scapula), the right lower trapezius is a fixator. (Note: The neck, which is the mobile attachment, is still free to move; fixators only work at the fixed attachment of the muscle that is working.)

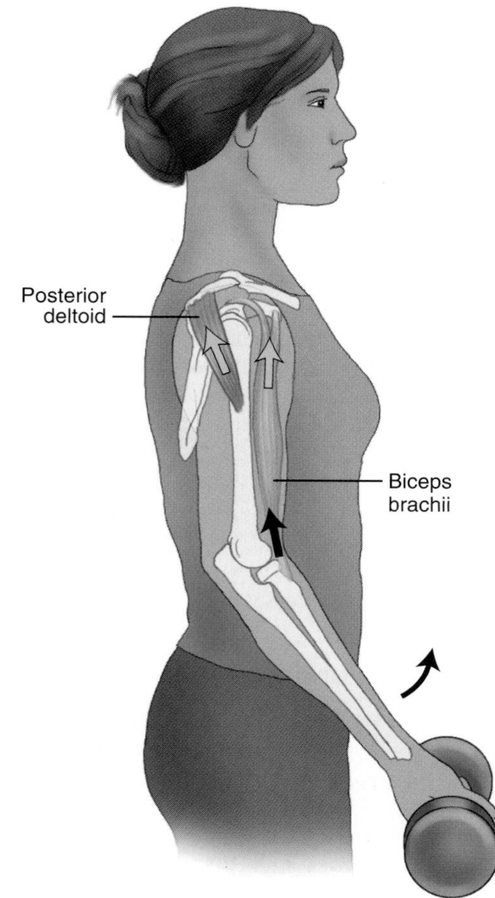

Figure 13-5 Right biceps brachii muscle contracts and creates a pulling force that could move both the forearm and the arm. The right posterior deltoid acts as a fixator of the arm by creating a force of extension on the arm at the shoulder joint that stops the biceps brachii from flexing the arm at the shoulder joint. Because the arm cannot move, it is fixed.

the scapula would have to be fixed so that it does not move). Figure 13-4a, shows the right levator scapulae elevating the scapula at the ScC joint and also moving the neck at the spinal joints (the neck is being right laterally flexed, extended, and rotated to the right); hence both attachments of the levator scapulae are mobile. Figure 13-4b, shows the right lower trapezius contracting at the same time. The lower trapezius creates a force of depression on the scapula at the ScC joint that stops the scapula from elevating; therefore the scapula is fixed in place and only the neck moves. In this scenario the right lower trapezius is a fixator that cancels out an unwanted action (i.e., elevation of the right scapula) at the fixed attachment of the right levator scapulae.

❑ Note: Any muscle that could do depression of the right scapula at the ScC joint would be a fixator in this scenario. The right lower trapezius shown in Figure 13-4 is simply the one chosen to illustrate this concept.

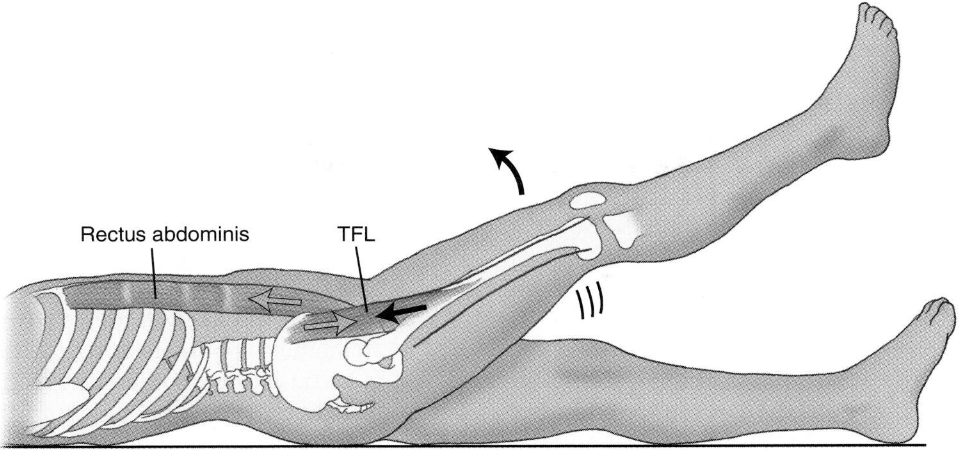

Figure 13-6 Right tensor fasciae latae (TFL) muscle contracts and creates a pulling force that could move both the thigh and the pelvis. The rectus abdominis acts as a fixator of the pelvis by creating a force of posterior tilt on the pelvis (at the lumbosacral joint) that stops the TFL from anteriorly tilting the pelvis (at the hip joint). Because the pelvis cannot move, it is fixed.

- Figure 13-5 is a lateral view of the right upper extremity with a weight in the hand. When the person does a bicep curl (i.e., flexes the forearm at the elbow joint) to lift the weight, the biceps brachii would also create a pulling force on the arm that would cause flexion of the arm at the shoulder joint. If we want just the forearm to move and not the arm, then the arm would have to be fixed from moving. The arm is fixed in place by a contraction of the posterior deltoid. In this scenario the posterior deltoid is a fixator, because it creates a force of extension of the arm at the shoulder joint that stops the biceps brachii from flexing the arm at the shoulder joint. (Note: Any muscle that does extension of the right arm at the shoulder joint would be a fixator in this scenario. The posterior deltoid is the muscle that we happened to show in Figure 13-5 to illustrate this concept.)
- If the person were to be lowering the weight (i.e., extending the forearm at the elbow joint), gravity would be the mover and the biceps brachii would become an eccentrically contracting antagonist that would still create a flexion force on the arm at the shoulder joint. In this scenario the posterior deltoid would still contract as a fixator to keep the arm fixed.
- Whether the muscle that is working (i.e., the biceps brachii) is working as a mover or as an antagonist, a fixator muscle functions to cancel out its unwanted action at the attachment that is fixed. (Note: The biceps brachii can create other joint actions that would also need to be fixed from occurring. They have not been considered here; they were omitted to simplify the example. The biceps brachii can also supinate the forearm at the radioulnar (RU) joints, abduct and adduct the arm at the shoulder joint, and also move the scapula at the shoulder and ScC joints (this scapular motion is a reverse action if the forearm and arm are held fixed and the biceps brachii concentrically contracts).

BOX 13-12

When we speak of a fixator working at the fixed attachment of the muscle that is working, we use the word *attachment* loosely. What is really being referred to is any *body part* that needs to be held fixed when the muscle contracts. For example, in Figure 13-5, the arm needs to be fixed when the biceps brachii contracts. However, the biceps brachii does not actually attach onto the humerus of the arm; it attaches to the scapula and the forearm. However, because the biceps brachii crosses the shoulder joint and would cause movement of the arm, the arm needs to be fixed.

- Figure 13-6 is a lateral view of the tensor fasciae latae muscle. When it contracts, it could potentially move both the thigh at the hip joint and the pelvis at the hip joint. If we want just the thigh to move, the pelvis must be fixed. To fix the pelvis from moving, we see that the rectus abdominis is contracting as a fixator. The rectus abdominis creates a force of posterior tilt of the pelvis (at the lumbosacral joint); this stops the tensor fasciae latae from anteriorly tilting the pelvis (at the hip joint).
- Any muscle that can do posterior tilt of the pelvis (at the either the lumbosacral joint, a hip joint unilaterally, or both hip joints bilaterally) would be a possible fixator in this scenario.
- In these examples of fixators, it is important to emphasize that similar to the idea that as many possible movers or antagonists can contract when a joint action

occurs, many possible fixators can contract to fix the fixed attachment of the muscle that is working. For example, in Figure 13-5, we showed the posterior deltoid as the fixator. Theoretically, we could have chosen any extensor of the arm at the shoulder joint, such as the latissimus dorsi, teres major, or the long head of the triceps brachii. However, cases exist in which a certain fixator might make more sense than another. For example, in Figure 13-5, contraction of the long head of the triceps brachii would not be an efficient fixator because it is also an antagonist to the action in question (i.e., it extends the forearm at the elbow joint that opposes flexion of the forearm to lift the weight). Therefore even though the long head of the triceps brachii would accomplish its fixation task, it would also oppose the action that we do want, namely flexion of the forearm at the elbow joint. It is more likely that the body would choose the posterior deltoid or the teres major instead.

- Just as movers and antagonists are not always muscles, fixator forces do not always need to be muscles. Any external force can be a fixator. In fact, the external force of gravity is an extremely common fixation force.
  - For example, when the brachialis contracts and the forearm flexes at the elbow joint instead of the reverse action of the arm flexing at the elbow joint, the reason the forearm tends to move instead of the arm is that the forearm is lighter than the arm (plus if the arm moved, the weight of the trunk would also have to be moved, because the trunk would have to move with the arm). Weight is a factor of the force of gravity. Therefore gravity acts as a fixator, fixing the arm so that the forearm moves instead.
- Figures 13-4 to 13-6 are three examples of fixators working. Given that a reverse action of a muscle is always theoretically possible; theoretically, a fixator force always exists in every instance of a *working* muscle that contracts; the fixator force is working to hold one attachment fixed and stop the reverse action from occurring. The examples that were chosen in Figures 13-4 to 13-6 were chosen because they are relatively a straightforward way to help the new student understand the concept of fixators. Seeing the fixator in some scenarios can be harder than seeing it in others.
  - The concept of the terminology system of naming the heavier more proximal attachment of a muscle as the *origin* and naming the lighter more distal attachment of a muscle as the *insertion* is primarily based on the heavier proximal attachment being relatively less likely to move than the lighter distal attachment. In other words, the force of gravity acts as a fixator force that tends to stop movement of the heavier proximal attachment of the muscle.
- In the terminology system of origin and insertion, fixator muscles work at the origin.

BOX 13-13

The use of the term *reverse action* is also based on the concept of the fixation force of gravity. A reverse action describes when the proximal attachment (which is less likely to move because of the fixation force of gravity) moves instead of the distal attachment (which would be more likely to move because less fixation force by gravity exists). When this occurs, a reverse action is said to occur and the origin and insertion of the muscle switch. That is, what is usually called the *origin* is now the *insertion* because it moves, and what is usually called the *insertion* is now the *origin* because it stays fixed. If the origin of a muscle is strictly defined as the attachment that does not move (whether it is the heavier proximal one or the lighter distal one), then we can say that fixators always work at the origin of a muscle.

Essential Facts:

- A fixator is a muscle (or other force) that can stop an unwanted action at the fixed attachment of the muscle that is working.
- Fixators are also known as *stabilizers*.
- By definition, when a fixator muscle contracts, it contracts isometrically.
- In the terminology system of origin/insertion, fixator muscles work at the origin.

☐ 13.6 CONCEPT OF FIXATION AND CORE STABILIZATION

- Muscles in the body are often divided into two general categories:
  1. Mobility muscles
  2. Postural stabilization muscles

Mobility Muscles

- **Mobility muscles** tend to be larger, longer, more superficial muscles.
- These muscles are important primarily for their ability to concentrically contract and create large joint movements.
- Therefore during any particular action in question, the mobility muscles would tend to be the movers of the joint action.

BOX 13-14

Although antagonists do not *create* motion, they do act to modify motion that is created by other mover forces such as gravity. In that role, antagonist muscles can also be considered to be mobility muscles.

- Mobility muscles tend to be composed of a greater percentage of white fiber fast-twitch motor units. This fiber type is best suited for motions that need to occur but are not held for long periods of time.
- Mobility muscles are often called **phasic muscles**.

Postural Stabilization Muscles

- **Postural stabilization muscles** tend to be smaller, deeper muscles that are located close to joints.
- These muscles are important primarily for their ability to isometrically contract and hold the posture of joints fixed while mobility muscles do their actions.
- Therefore during any particular action in question, the postural stabilization muscles would be the fixators (remember that the term *fixator* is synonymous with the term *stabilizer*), stopping unwanted movement of the fixed attachments of the muscles that are working.
- Postural stabilization muscles tend to be composed of a greater percentage of red fiber slow-twitch motor units. This fiber type is best suited for endurance contractions that need to occur to hold a muscle attachment fixed for longer periods of time.
- Because more proximal attachments usually need to stay fixed as more distal attachments are moved, postural stabilizers muscles are often referred to as **core stabilizers**; the term *core* referring to the proximal core of the body (i.e., the axial body and pelvis).
- When a number of muscles are ordered to contract for a particular joint motion, there is usually an order to the contraction of the muscles, some being ordered to contract slightly earlier than others. Generally, postural stabilization muscles tend to be engaged to contract slightly earlier than mobility muscles so that the joint is stabilized before powerful muscle contraction forces are placed upon it.
- Postural stabilization muscles are often termed **tonic muscles**.

BOX 13-15

Smaller, deeper postural stabilizer muscles have often been overlooked by people who exercise and work out. Perhaps one of the reasons is that they are smaller and deeper and do not directly show when a person tones the body. Further, because they do not directly contribute appreciable strength to the joint action that is occurring, it is easy to discount them. However, these underappreciated muscles may very well be more important to the health and efficiency of the body than the larger more visible mobility muscles. When exercising, it is important to work the smaller, deeper core stabilization muscles, as well the larger, more superficial mobility muscles.

- This concept of core stabilization is crucial to the functioning and health of the body for two reasons:
  1. Core stabilization creates stronger and more efficient movements.
  2. Core stabilization is important for the health of the spine.

BOX 13-16

The major tenet of the **Pilates method** of body conditioning (developed by Joseph Pilates) is to strengthen what they refer to as the **powerhouse** of the body. Essentially, the powerhouse equates to the core of the body. Through exercises that are primarily designed to isometrically tone the core powerhouse muscles and to create efficient coordination of these postural stabilization powerhouse muscles with mobility muscles, Pilates creates a stronger, healthier, more efficient body.

How Does Core Stabilization Create Stronger and More Efficient Movements of Our Body?

- Whenever a muscle concentrically contracts, it pulls toward its center and exerts a pulling force on both of its attachments. If we desire one of the attachments to move powerfully and efficiently, then the other attachment must stay fixed, because any part of the pulling force of the muscle that is allowed to move the attachment that is supposed to stay fixed will diminish the strength of the pulling force on the mobile attachment that we want to move. This will lessen the strength and efficiency of the joint movement. Because we often want to move our extremities relative to our axial body, it is essential that we stabilize our core axial body so that all the strength of the muscle's contraction goes toward moving the body parts of the upper and/or lower extremities, and is not lost on unwanted movement of our core.

- For example, if we contract hip flexor musculature with the intention of flexing the thigh at the hip joint while exercising. Any anterior tilt of the pelvis that is allowed to occur by this *hip flexor* musculature will decrease the strength with which our thigh can move into flexion. Therefore strong abdominals help to hold the pelvis posturally stabilized (i.e., fixed) so that the thigh may move more powerfully and efficiently. In this scenario, abdominals are acting as postural stabilizer muscles (Figure 13-7).

How Does Core Stabilization Create a Healthier Spine?

- Apart from the concept of strength and efficiency, core stabilization can help to maintain a healthier spine by diminishing unwanted excessive motions of the spine. Excessive use of a joint in time leads to overuse, misuse, and abuse; the result would be a degenerated osteoarthritic spine.
- For example, if we intend to move our arm into flexion or abduction, both of which require the coupled action of upward rotation of the scapula at the ScC joint, a pull will be exerted on the spine as the upper trapezius contracts (as an upward rotator of the scapula at the ScC joint). (Note: For information on the coupled actions of the arm and shoulder girdle, see Section 9.6) If the smaller deeper postural stabilizer muscles of the vertebrae of the spine do not contract to hold the position of the vertebrae fixed, the vertebrae will be moved with these movements of the arm. When we think of how often the arm is lifted forward and/or to the side (i.e., flexion and/or abduction) during activities of daily life, let alone sports activities, the accumulation of stress that would be placed on the spine by these repetitive motions would eventually create degenerative osteoarthritic changes. The smaller deeper spinal muscles such as the multifidus, rotatores, interspinales, and intertransversarii are crucial to posturally stabilizing (i.e., fixing) the core (i.e., the spine in scenarios such as this) (Figure 13-8).
- Although it can be helpful to examine the muscles of the body in their roles as mobility muscles and postural stabilizer muscles, it is important to keep in mind that these two groups of muscles must always work together. The proper coordination of these two roles is essential for efficient motion and stability of the body!

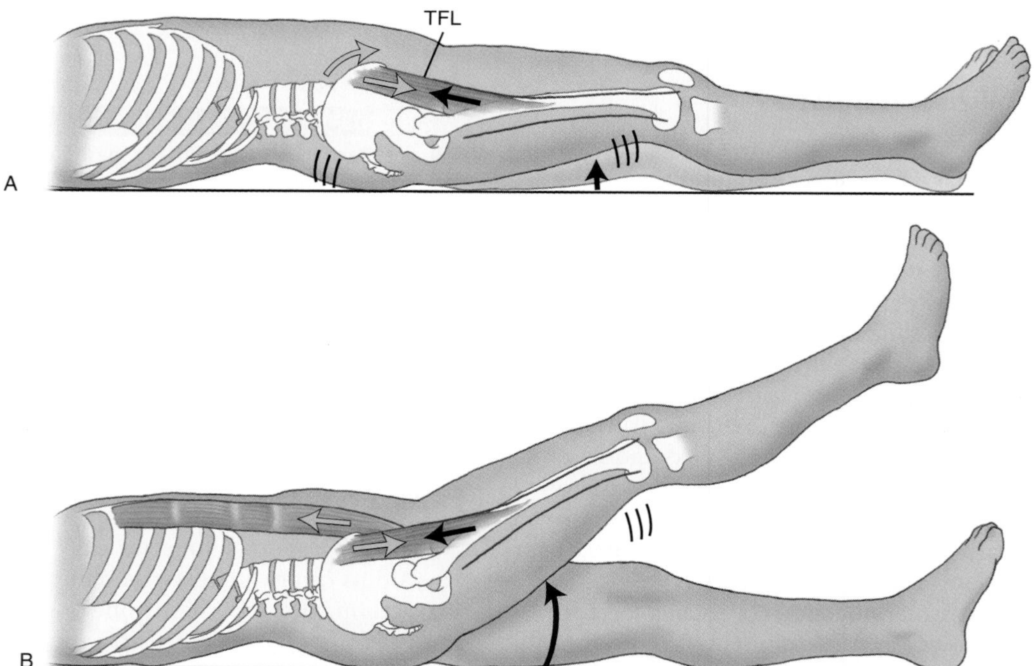

Figure 13-7 *A,* Tensor fasciae latae (TFL) contracting and creating both flexion of the thigh at the hip joint and anterior tilt of the pelvis at the hip joint. *B,* Pelvis is fixed by the rectus abdominis. Because some of the pulling force of the TFL's contraction went toward moving the pelvis in *A,* the thigh does not flex as much as it does in *B,* when all the pulling force went toward moving the thigh.

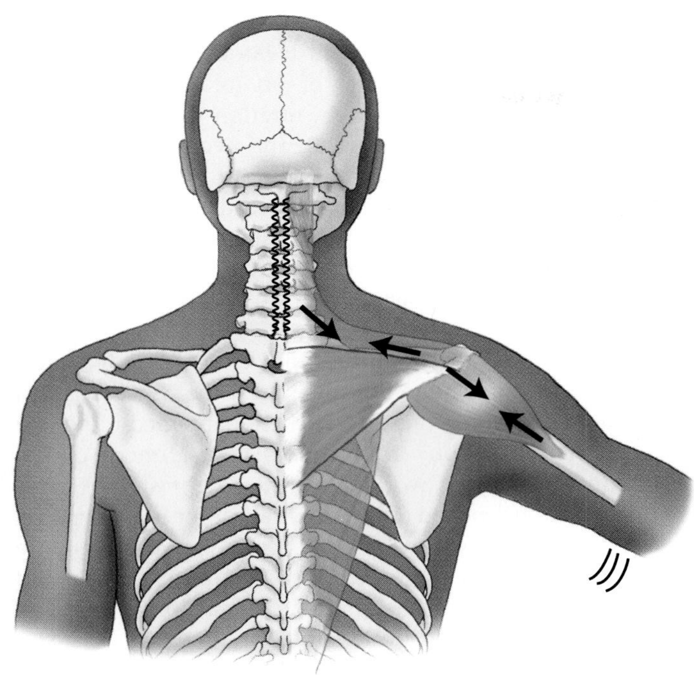

Figure 13-8 A person lifts the right arm up into abduction at the shoulder joint. This action requires the coupled action of upward rotation of the scapula at the scapulocostal (ScC) joint; the right upper trapezius is seen contracting to create this coupled action. We also see that the upper trapezius creates a pulling force on its spinal attachment. If the vertebrae are not well stabilized (i.e., fixed), then the vertebrae will be moved every time the arm abducts. These repetitive motions can lead to degenerative osteoarthritic changes of the spine over time.

13.7 NEUTRALIZER MUSCLES

- A **neutralizer** is a muscle (or other force) that can stop an unwanted action at the mobile attachment of the muscle that is working.
- We have seen that whether a mover or antagonist contracts during our desired action in question, it can cause other joint actions to occur. These other joint actions may be unwanted and therefore need to be stopped.
- The role of a neutralizer is to stop these unwanted actions that occur at the *mobile attachment* of the muscle that is working.
- To determine which attachment of the working muscle is mobile, simply look at the action in question that is occurring. Whichever body part is moving during the action in question is the mobile attachment.
  - For example, if the right levator scapulae is contracting and creating right lateral flexion of the neck at the spinal joints, then the mobile attachment is the neck, because it is moving (and the fixed attachment is the scapula, because it is not moving).
- When the muscle that is working contracts and creates a desired action of the mobile attachment, that desired action occurs within one of the three cardinal planes. However, the muscle that is contracting might also create an unwanted motion of the mobile attachment in another plane. It is the unwanted action that occurs in this other plane that is stopped by a neutralizer muscle.

BOX 13-17

Three cardinal planes (sagittal, frontal, and transverse) exist. Assuming that the *desired* action occurs in one of those three planes, then there could be one or two *unwanted* actions that would occur in one or both of the other two planes that a neutralizer muscle or neutralizer muscles would have to stop.

- Neutralizer muscles stop an unwanted action of a mobile body part by creating a contraction force that is equal in strength but opposite in direction to the force of the unwanted action of the muscle that is working. By doing this, the neutralizer muscle stops the mobile attachment's unwanted action within that plane.
- Because the mobile attachment does not move within that plane, the neutralizer muscle does not change its length within that plane; therefore some sources state that neutralizers isometrically contract. However, the neutralizer muscle may change its length within another plane; this means it does not necessarily stay the same length and therefore does not necessarily contract isometrically.

BOX 13-18

If a neutralizer muscle is neutralizing an unwanted action of a mover, the neutralizer would likely shorten overall; therefore even though it does not change its length in the plane of the action that it is stopping, it will shorten in the plane of the motion that is occurring at the mobile attachment of the mover. In this case the neutralizer concentrically contracts. If the neutralizer muscle is neutralizing an unwanted action of an antagonist instead (remember, the muscle that is working can be an antagonist), the same reasoning applies, except that now the neutralizer would be lengthening overall and therefore eccentrically contracting.

Figures 13-9 and 13-10 provide examples of neutralizers.

- ❑ In Figure 13-9a, we see a posterior view of the right levator scapulae muscle. In this illustration, the right levator scapulae is contracting and causing the neck to right laterally flex, extend, and rotate to the right (note: the scapula would also move if not fixed by a fixator, as was explained in Section 13-5, Figure 13-4). If we want the neck to only right laterally flex, then the other two actions of the right levator scapulae must be stopped. In Figure 13-9b, we see that the right sternocleidomastoid (SCM) is contracting as a neutralizer to stop these other two actions of the right levator scapulae that are undesired. The right SCM creates a force of flexion of the neck which cancels out the extension force of the right levator scapulae; and the right SCM creates a force of left rotation of the neck which cancels out the right rotation force of the right levator scapulae. As a result, the neck can only right laterally flex at the spinal joints. In this scenario, the right SCM is a neutralizer because it cancels out unwanted actions at the mobile attachment of the muscle that is contracting, the right levator scapulae. (Note: the right lower trapezius acting as a fixator is also seen.)
- ❑ Note: To be a neutralizer, a muscle need only cancel one unwanted action of the muscle that is working. In the example in Figure 13-9, there happened to be two unwanted actions at the mobile attachment of the muscle that was working and the right sternocleidomastoid happened to be a neutralizer for both of them. We could have chosen two separate neutralizers, one for each of these two actions. Any muscle that could do flexion of the neck at the spinal joints and any muscle that could do left rotation of the neck at the spinal joints would potentially be a neutralizer in this example.
- ❑ In Figure 13-10, we see an anteromedial view of the right biceps brachii muscle. In this illustration, the

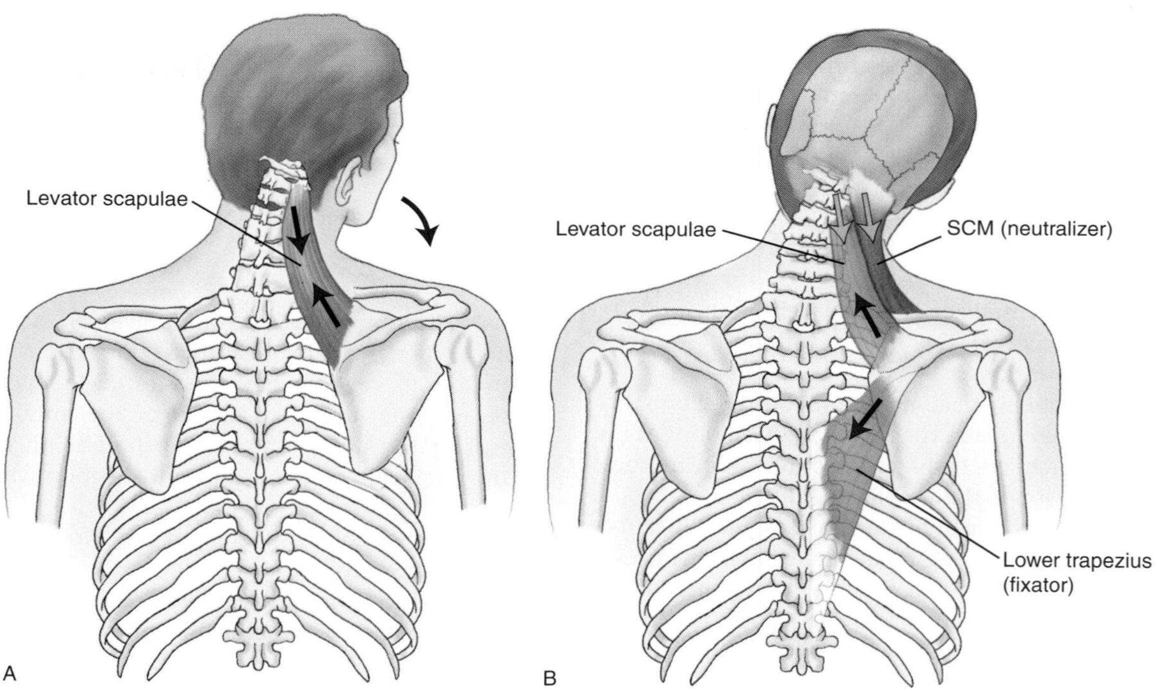

Figure 13-9 *A,* Right levator scapulae muscle is contracting and moving the neck into right lateral flexion, extension, and right rotation. *B,* Right sternocleidomastoid is also contracting. The right sternocleidomastoid is a neutralizer of the neck, because it creates a force of flexion on the neck at the spinal joints that stops the right levator scapulae from extending the neck, and it creates a force of left rotation of the neck at the spinal joints that stops the right levator scapulae from rotating the neck to the right. Because it cancels out unwanted actions of the right levator scapulae at the neck, the right sternocleidomastoid is a neutralizer. (Note: In *B,* the right lower trapezius is also seen contracting as a fixator.)

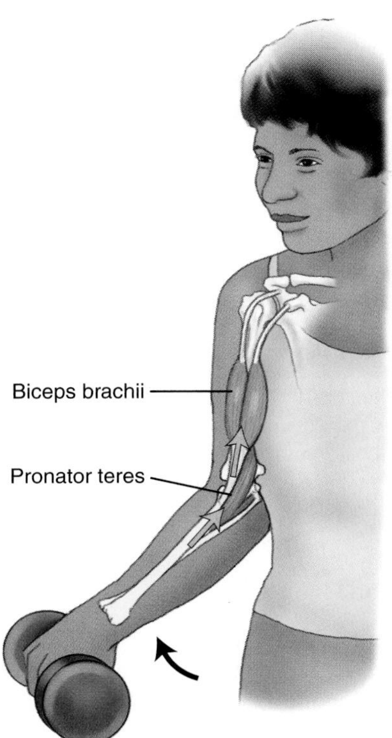

Figure 13-10 Biceps brachii is contracting as a mover of flexion of the forearm at the elbow joint; therefore the forearm is its mobile attachment. If we assume that the arm is fixed from moving at the shoulder joint by a fixator muscle, the biceps brachii should also supinate the forearm (at the radioulnar [RU] joints) because this is another one of its actions. In this illustration, the pronator teres is a neutralizer, because it creates a force of pronation of the forearm at the RU joints that cancels out supination of the forearm at the RU joints by the biceps brachii.

right biceps brachii is contracting, and the only joint action that is occurring is flexion of the forearm at the elbow joint. (Note: We are considering the arm to be fixed in this scenario; see Section 13.5, Figure 13-5.) However, the biceps brachii can also supinate the forearm (at the radioulnar [RU] joints), which is its mobile attachment. If supination is not canceled out (i.e., neutralized), it would occur. Although any pronator could do this, the pronator teres is seen in Figure 13-10 as the neutralizer. By creating a force of pronation of the forearm at the RU joints, the pronator teres stops the biceps brachii from supinating the forearm at the RU joints; therefore the pronator teres is a neutralizer.

- ❑ In Figure 13-11, the right upper trapezius and left upper trapezius muscles contract as movers to extend the neck and head at the spinal joints (in the sagittal plane). However, they would also create unwanted actions in the frontal and transverse planes as well. These unwanted actions do not occur because each upper trapezius cancels out these unwanted actions of the other upper trapezius. In the frontal plane the right lateral flexion of the right upper trapezius is neutralized by the left lateral flexion of the left upper trapezius, and the left lateral flexion of the left upper trapezius is neutralized by the right lateral flexion of the right upper trapezius. In the transverse plane, the left rotation of the right upper trapezius is neutralized by the right rotation of the left upper trapezius, and the right rotation of the left upper trapezius is neutralized by the left rotation of the right upper trapezius. Therefore these two movers act as neutralizers of each other's unwanted actions, and only the desired action of pure extension of the head and neck at the spinal joints results.

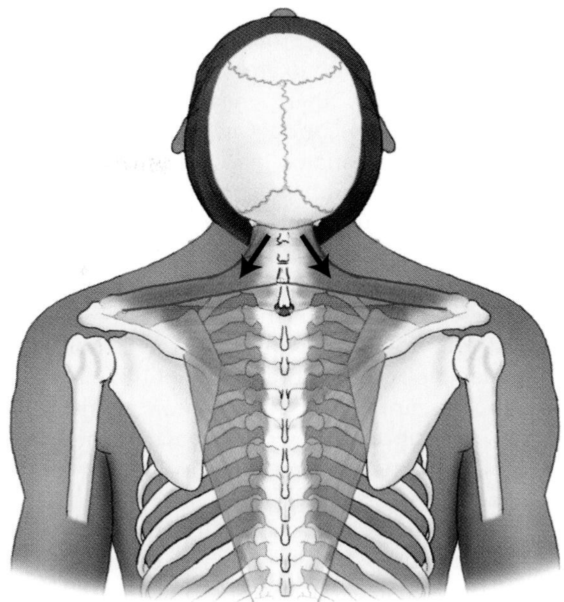

Figure 13-11 Right and left upper trapezius muscles are both contracting to cause the action in question (i.e., extension of the head and neck at the spinal joint); therefore they are both movers. They also both act as neutralizers, canceling out each other's frontal and transverse plane actions (i.e., lateral flexion and rotation actions) of the head and neck at the spinal joints.

BOX 13-19

Two muscles that are both movers (or both antagonists) of the action in question and neutralize each other's unwanted actions are called **mutual neutralizers**. Mutual neutralizers are actually very common. In every pair (right and left sided) of axial body muscles (e.g., right and left trapezius, right and left sternocleidomastoid, and so forth), the muscles act as mutual neutralizers to each other when they both contract. They cancel out whatever frontal and/or transverse plane motions they each have, and the result is a pure sagittal plane motion (either flexion or extension depending on the muscle). Although this is the most common example, a set of mutual neutralizers do not have to be the same pair of muscles. Another example is the TFL and sartorius. Although they are both movers of flexion of the thigh at the hip joint in the sagittal plane, they cancel out each other's transverse plane motions (the TFL is a medial rotator of the thigh at the hip joint, and the sartorius is a lateral rotator of the thigh at the hip joint).

- In these examples of neutralizers, it is important to emphasize that similar to the idea that many possible movers, antagonists, or fixators can contract when a joint action occurs, there may be many possible neutralizers that will contract as well. In Figure 13-9, we showed the pronator teres as the neutralizer. Theoretically, we could have chosen a different pronator of the forearm at the RU joints, such as the pronator quadratus.
- It should also be recognized that a neutralizer is not always present in every given scenario. If no undesired action at the mobile attachment of the muscle that is working takes place, then there will not be a neutralizer.
- Just as movers, antagonists, and fixators are not always muscles, neutralizer forces do not always need to be muscles. Any external force such as gravity can be a neutralizer.
    - For example, when a person is in anatomic position and the anterior deltoid contracts causing the arm to medially rotate at the shoulder joint but not abduct and/or flex (its other two actions), part of the reason is that to abduct or flex, the arm would have to be lifted up against the force of gravity. In this instance, with a weak contraction by the anterior deltoid, gravity would tend to stop (i.e., neutralize) these upward motions of the arm of abduction and flexion. Of course, if the contraction of the anterior deltoid were strong enough, enough force would be generated to move the arm upward into abduction and/or flexion; with this stronger contraction of the anterior deltoid, neutralizer muscles would then have to be recruited to fully stop these actions if they were unwanted.
- In the terminology system of origin and insertion, neutralizers work at the insertion.

BOX 13-20

If the insertion is strictly defined as the attachment of a muscle that does move (regardless of which attachment it is [i.e., the lighter distal one that usually does move or the heavier proximal one that usually does not move]), then we can say that neutralizers always work at the insertion of a muscle.

Essential Facts:

- A neutralizer is a muscle (or other force) that can stop an unwanted action at the mobile attachment of the muscle that is working.
- In the terminology system of origin/insertion, neutralizer muscles work at the insertion.

13.8 STEP-BY-STEP METHOD FOR DETERMINING FIXATORS AND NEUTRALIZERS

- Once the concept of how fixator and neutralizer muscles work in the body is fully understood, figuring out possible fixators and neutralizers can be reasoned out; however, like all aspects of knowledge, getting to the point of *full* understanding is a work in progress as we gradually see things in increasing layers of depth and clarity. For some students, determining fixators and neutralizers takes a little more time. For that reason, the following rubric is offered. This rubric gives a step-by-step method for determining the fixators and neutralizers in any given scenario.
- To demonstrate the steps of this rubric, it is helpful to look at the following scenario: The right levator scapulae is contracting, and only right lateral flexion of the neck at the spinal joints is occurring (Figure 13-12; Table 13-1).
- Based on the steps of the rubric, the right lower trapezius was chosen as a fixator and the right sternocleidomastoid was chosen as a neutralizer (as used as examples in Section 13.5, Figure 13-4, and Section 13.7, Figure 13-9, respectively). Again, it is important to emphasize that other possible fixators and neutralizers could have been chosen. In addition, the right sternocleidomastoid happened to work as a neutralizer for both undesired actions of the mover at the mobile attachment (we could have chosen two different neutralizers instead, as long as they opposed the actions that needed to be cancelled at the mobile attachment). The exact fixators and neutralizers that the body chooses will vary from individual to individual and will also vary based on the needed strength of the fixators and neutralizers.

TABLE 13-1

Following are the Steps of the Rubric to Determine Fixators and Neutralizers Using the Example Given in Figure 13-12:

Step 1: Determine the action in question:
- ❑ Right lateral flexion of the neck at the spinal joints

Step 2: Determine the muscle that is working and its role:
- ❑ Right levator scapulae; it is a mover

Step 3: Determine which attachment is the fixed attachment and which attachment is the mobile attachment (mobile attachment is whichever attachment is moving in the action in question):
- ❑ Fixed attachment: Scapula
- ❑ Mobile attachment: Neck

Step 4: List all actions of the muscle that is working (i.e., the right levator scapulae), and state whether each action is the desired action or an undesired action; further, state if the undesired actions occur at the fixed or mobile attachment and what muscle role stops each undesired action:
- ❑ Right lateral flexion of the neck at the spinal joints (desired action—do not stop)
- ❑ Elevation of the right scapula at the scapulocostal (ScC) joint (undesired action at the fixed attachment—stop with a fixator)
- ❑ Extension of the neck at the spinal joints (undesired action at the mobile attachment—stop with a neutralizer)
- ❑ Right rotation of the neck at the spinal joints (undesired action at the mobile attachment—stop with a neutralizer)

Step 5: Determine the action of each fixator at the fixed attachment (i.e., the scapula); it will be the opposite action of the undesired action at the fixed attachment:
- ❑ ~~Elevation~~ Depression of the right scapula at the ScC joint

Step 6: Choose a muscle that can do the action determined for each fixator:
- ❑ Right lower trapezius (any muscle that does depression of the right scapula is a fixator)

Step 7: Determine the action of each neutralizer at the mobile attachment (i.e., the neck). It will be the opposite action of the undesired action at the mobile attachment:
- ❑ ~~Extension~~ Flexion of the neck at the spinal joints
- ❑ ~~Right rotation~~ Left rotation of the neck at the spinal joints

Step 8: Choose a muscle that can do the action determined for each neutralizer:
- ❑ Right sternocleidomastoid (any muscle that does flexion of neck is a neutralizer)
- ❑ Right sternocleidomastoid (any muscle that does left rotation of neck is a neutralizer)

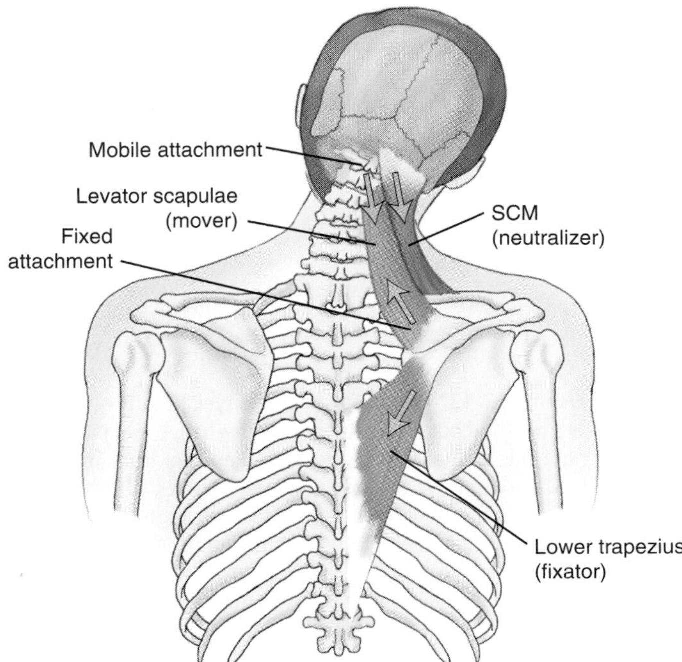

Figure 13-12 Right levator scapulae is contracting, and the only joint action that is occurring is right lateral flexion of the neck at the spinal joints. In this scenario the right lower trapezius is a fixator, stopping the right levator scapulae from elevating the right scapula at the scapulocostal (ScC) joint, and the right sternocleidomastoid is a neutralizer, stopping the right levator scapulae from flexing the neck and rotating it to the right at the spinal joints.

13.9 SUPPORT MUSCLES

- A **support muscle** is a muscle that can hold another part of the body in position while the action in question is occurring.
- Unlike movers, antagonists, fixators, and neutralizers, support muscles do not work directly at the site of the action in question.
- The role of a support muscle is to hold *another* body part in position while the action in question is occurring. Therefore support muscles often work far from the joint where the action in question is occurring.
- Support muscles usually work against gravity (i.e., they keep a body part from falling down).
- They do this by creating a contraction force that is equal in strength but opposite in direction to the force that gravity exerts on that body part. By doing this, the body part that is being pulled downward by gravity does not fall (and the support muscle does not contract so hard that the body part is moved upward either).
- Because the body part is held in place by the support muscle, it does not move. If the body part does not move, the support muscle does not change its length. Therefore support muscles isometrically contract when they hold body parts in place.

Figures 13-13 and 13-14 provide examples of support muscles.

- In Figure 13-13, we see a person holding a heavy weight in her right hand at the side of her body. The action in question is flexion of the right forearm at the elbow joint as she does a bicep curl. However, given the presence of this heavy weight on her right side, her trunk would be pulled to the right and fall into right lateral flexion of the trunk at the spinal joints if it were not for the isometric contraction of her left erector spinae group. The left erector spinae group creates a force of left lateral flexion that counters gravity's force of right lateral flexion on the trunk. The left erector spinae group supports and holds the trunk in position while the action in question (i.e., flexion of the right forearm) occurs elsewhere; therefore the left erector spinae group is a support muscle in this scenario.
- Figure 13-14 shows a person typing at a keyboard. The action in question is the motion of the fingers as they hit the keys. However, in this position, notice that the person has his arms abducted at the shoulder joints away from his body. This requires his arm abductor musculature to isometrically contract to hold this position of arm abduction so that his arms do not fall into adduction. These arm abductors are support muscles because they support the arms in position while the action in question (occurring at the fingers) is being carried out. (Note: This scenario illustrates an example of someone who has poor ergonomic posture and as a result stresses his musculature [in this case his muscles of arm abduction at the shoulder joint]. If this person were to relax and let his arms rest at his sides, his posture and health would be improved.)

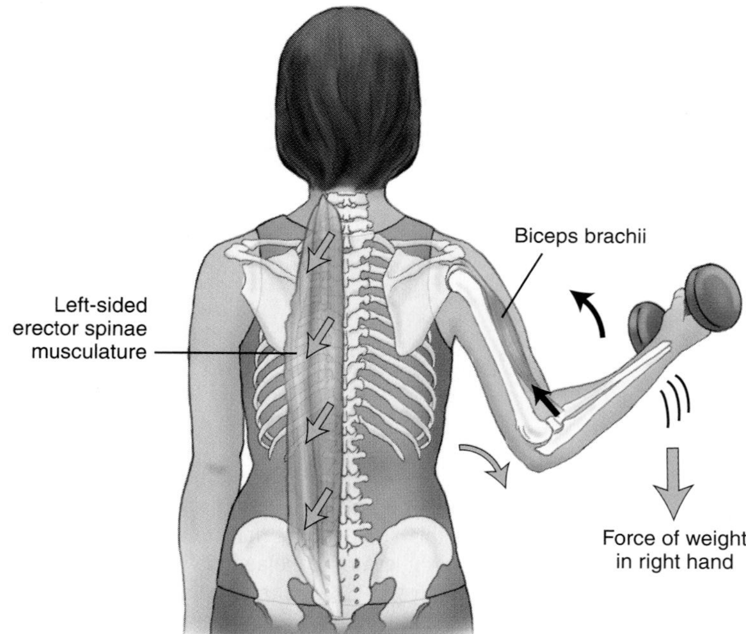

Figure 13-13 As this person lifts a weight out to the right side of the body, the presence of the heavy weight on her right side creates a force that would pull her trunk into right lateral flexion at the spinal joints. Muscles of left lateral flexion of the trunk (the left erector spinae group is shown) contract isometrically to hold the trunk in position so that it does not fall into right lateral flexion. These left lateral flexors are supports muscles, because they hold the trunk in position while the action in question (i.e., flexion of the right forearm at the elbow joint) is occurring elsewhere.

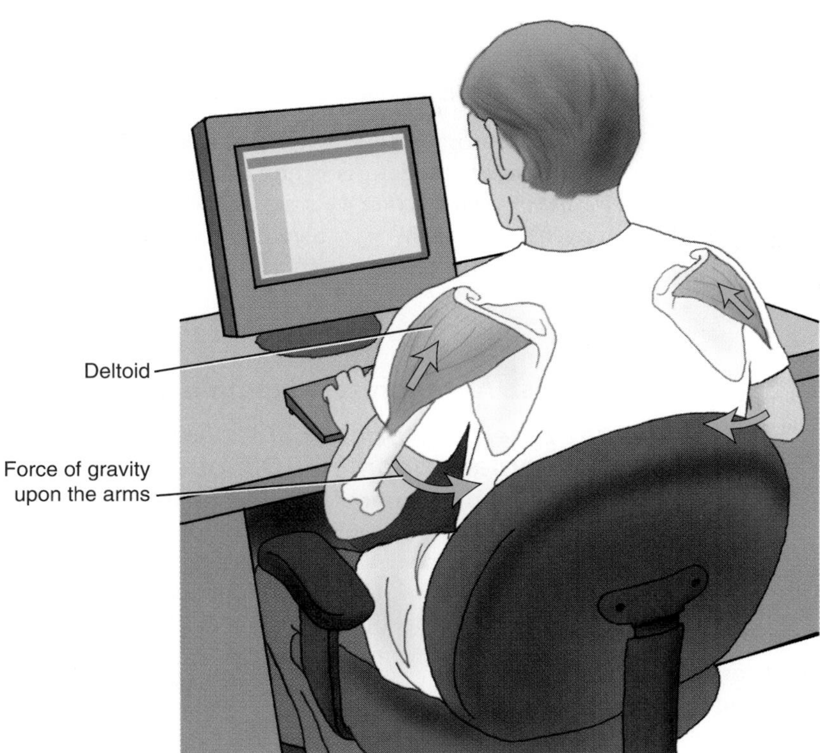

Figure 13-14 Person typing at a keyboard with the arms in a position of abduction. The abductor musculature of the shoulder joints are support muscles in this scenario, because they isometrically contract to support and hold the arms abducted against gravity as the action in question (i.e., finger motion on the keyboard) occurs elsewhere.

- ❑ In these examples of support muscles, it is important to note that similar to the idea that as many possible movers or antagonists can contract when a joint action occurs, many possible support muscles can contract to hold another body part in position. For example, in Figure 13-13, we showed the left erector spinae group as the support muscle. Theoretically, we could have chosen any left lateral flexor of the trunk at the spinal joints as the support muscle.
- ❑ Support muscles are often overlooked, because the focus of the activity is elsewhere. As a result, the client may have no idea that support muscles are being tremendously overworked and irritated.

BOX 13-21

Clinically, it is easy for the therapist to overlook an overused/abused support muscle. When we ask the client what activity he or she is engaging in that causes pain, unless we ask the client to actually show or explain the position of the *entire body* when the activity is done, we may miss the patterns of use of support muscles distant from the site of the activity itself. Clinically, support muscles usually stop body parts from letting gravity pull them down. This means that if one looks at the posture of the body with relation to gravity, any unbalanced body part that should fall because of gravity, yet is not falling, must be supported by muscular activity. The support musculature responsible for this should be evaluated. (See Sections 17.1-17.7 on posture for more on this topic.)

- ❑ Just as movers, antagonists, fixators, and neutralizers are not always muscles, support forces do not always need to be muscles. Any external force that helps to hold a body part in position could be termed a *support*.
  - ❑ For example, a male ballet dancer that holds a ballerina in position during a dance performance would be a support force. External objects may also act as a support. For example, the headrest of a car, which supports the head of the driver as he or she leans the head back against it, is a support.

Essential Facts:

- ❑ A support muscle is a muscle that can hold another part of the body in position while the action in question is occurring.
- ❑ Support muscles do not work directly at the joint where the action in question is occurring; they work on another body part at a distant joint.
- ❑ Support muscles usually oppose the force of gravity on a body part.
- ❑ By definition, when a support muscle contracts, it contracts isometrically.

☐ 13.10 SYNERGISTS

- A **synergist** is a muscle (or other force) that *works with* the muscle that is contracting.

BOX 13-22

The word *synergist* literally means to *work with*: *syn* means *with*; *erg* means *work*.

- The term *synergist* can be defined two different ways.
  1. Defined broadly, a synergist is any muscle other than the prime mover (or prime antagonist) that works (i.e., contracts) to help the joint action in question occur.
     - By this definition, a synergist could be any other mover or antagonist (whichever group is working), as well as any other fixator, neutralizer, or support muscle.
  2. Defined narrowly, a synergist is any mover that contracts other than the prime mover or any antagonist that contracts other than the prime antagonist.
     - For example, because the iliopsoas is the prime mover of flexion of the thigh at the hip joint, when the thigh is flexing at the hip joint, any other flexor of the thigh at the hip joint that contracts to help create this joint action (e.g., tensor fasciae latae, rectus femoris) would be a synergist.
- When determining that a muscle is a synergist, it is important to always keep in mind that this term, like all the other terms for muscle roles, is relative to a particular joint action (i.e., the action in question).
- Confusion often arises when people describe a muscle as being a synergist (i.e., synergistic) to another muscle. It is more accurate to say that these two muscles are synergistic with regard to a particular joint action.
- The same concept is true for the term *antagonist*. An antagonist is antagonistic to a specific joint action, not to another muscle generally. The following two examples illustrate this point.

Synergist/Antagonist—Example #1:

Biceps Brachii and Pronator Teres:

- Would the biceps brachii and the pronator teres be considered synergistic or antagonistic to each other (Figure 13-15a)?
- The biceps brachii and the pronator teres both flex the forearm at the elbow joint in the sagittal plane; therefore they are synergists. However, the biceps brachii supinates the forearm at the radioulnar (RU) joints in the transverse plane, whereas the pronator teres pronates the forearm at the RU joints in the transverse plane; therefore they are antagonists.
- For this reason, asking whether any two muscles are synergists or antagonists is not a valid question *unless we specify which action we are considering*. Two muscles may be synergistic with regard to one action in one plane, yet antagonistic with regard to another action in another plane.

Synergist/Antagonist—Example #2:

Right External Abdominal Oblique and Left Internal Abdominal Oblique:

- Would the right external abdominal oblique and the left internal abdominal oblique be considered synergistic or antagonistic to each other (Figure 13-15b)?
- The right external abdominal oblique and the left internal abdominal oblique both flex the trunk at the spinal joints in the sagittal plane; therefore with respect to sagittal plane motion, they are synergistic to each other.
- The right external abdominal oblique does right lateral flexion of the trunk in the frontal plane, whereas the left internal abdominal oblique does left lateral flexion of the trunk in the frontal plane. Therefore with respect to frontal plane motion, they are antagonistic to each other.
- The right external abdominal oblique, being a contralateral rotator, does left rotation of the trunk in the transverse plane; the left internal abdominal oblique, being an ipsilateral rotator, also does left rotation of the trunk in the transverse plane. Therefore with respect to transverse plane motion, these two muscles are synergistic to each other.
- As we can see, the right external abdominal oblique and the left internal abdominal oblique are neither inherently synergistic nor antagonistic to each other. Rather, they can only be considered to be synergistic or antagonistic to each other with respect to a specific joint action within a particular plane.
- As with all roles of muscles, the roles of synergist and antagonist are relative to the action in question.

Essential Facts:

- A synergist is a muscle (or other force) that *works with* the muscle that is contracting.
- Defined broadly, a synergist is any muscle other than the prime mover (or prime antagonist) that works (i.e., contracts) to help the joint action in question occur.
- Defined narrowly, a synergist is any mover that contracts other than the prime mover or any antagonist that contracts other than the prime antagonist.

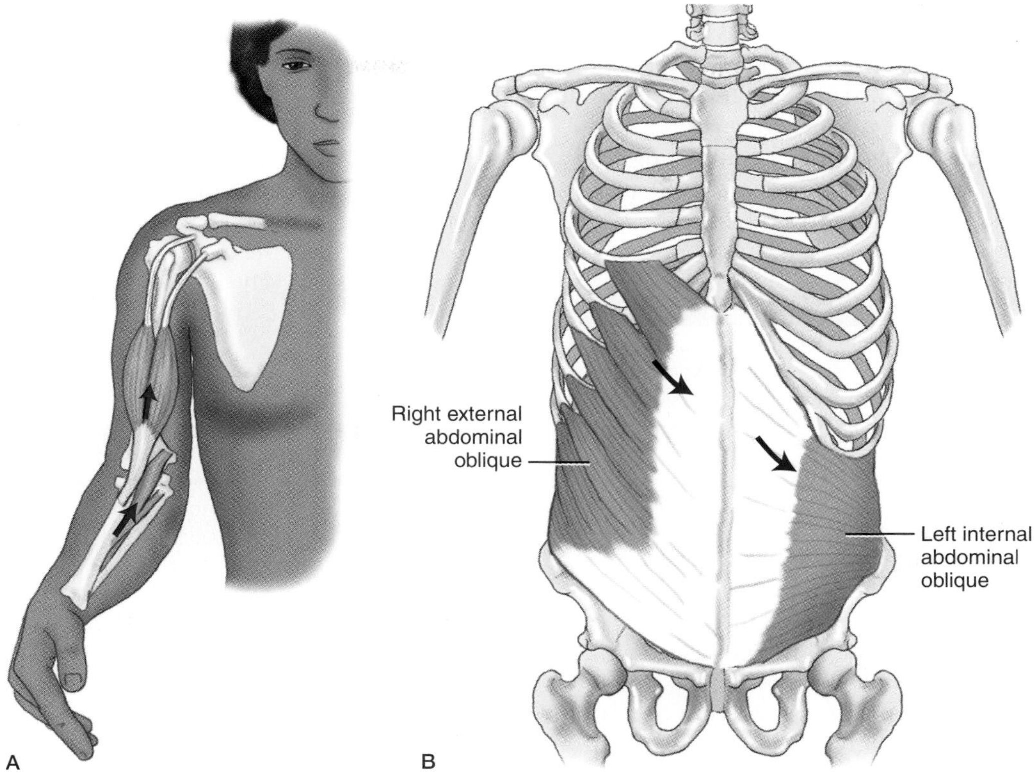

Figure 13-15 Illustration of the concept that two muscles are inherently neither synergistic nor antagonistic to each other. Being synergistic or antagonistic is determined relative to a specific plane of motion. *A,* Biceps brachii and pronator teres muscles. With respect to sagittal plane motion at the elbow joint, these two muscles are synergistic to each other, because they both flex the forearm at the elbow joint. However, with respect to transverse plane motion at the radioulnar (RU) joints, these two muscles are antagonistic to each other, because the biceps brachii does supination and the pronator teres does pronation (of the forearm at the RU joints). *B,* Right external abdominal oblique and left internal abdominal oblique muscles. With respect to sagittal and transverse plane motions at the spinal joints, these muscles are synergistic to each other, because they both flex and left rotate the trunk at the spinal joints. However, with respect to frontal plane motion at the spinal joints, these two muscles are antagonistic to each other, because the right external abdominal oblique does right lateral flexion and the left internal abdominal oblique does left lateral flexion of the trunk at the spinal joints.

13.11 COORDINATING MUSCLE ROLES

- Beginning kinesiology students often approach a joint action of the body with the question, What muscle does this action? This question presupposes that one specific muscle is responsible for each specific joint action that can occur in the body. Yet, as we can see, muscles rarely act in isolation.
- First, among a functional group of movers, a number of muscles may contract for any given joint action. Depending on the strength needed for the contraction, one or more of them may contract.
- If gravity or some other outside force is creating the action in question, then most likely the movers are not working, and it is the functional group of antagonists that is working to slow down and control the joint action. Depending on the antagonistic force needed, one or more antagonists will be ordered to contract.
- For either functional group that is working, movers or antagonists, it is likely that the other attachment of each and every one of the working muscles will need to be fixed for every unwanted action that would occur there. This will require functional groups of fixators to become involved and contract, and within each fixator group, a number of muscles can be ordered to contract.
- Additionally, for every unwanted action at the mobile attachment of every muscle that is working, functional groups of neutralizers would also have to be ordered

to contract, and many of these can be ordered to work.

- Beyond this, functional groups of support muscles are likely to be working elsewhere in the body to hold the posture of the body parts against gravity.
- Thus we have muscles potentially contracting in five major roles: (1) movers, (2) antagonists, (3) fixators, (4) neutralizers, and (5) support muscles.

BOX 13-23

A **muscle role** is defined as the role that the muscle plays relative to the action in question. The major roles of muscles are mover, antagonist, fixator, neutralizer, and support muscle. A sixth term to describe a muscle role is *synergist.* (For more information on synergists, see Section 13-10.)

- All of this is necessary for one simple joint action. When coupled actions or more complex movement patterns need to be executed simultaneously, the complexity of the co-ordering of all the muscles that must work seamlessly is multiplied many times.
  - It is the complexity of this co-ordering of muscles that defines coordination in the body. **Coordination** is defined as the co-ordering of muscles in the body in their various roles to create smooth and efficient movement.
  - It is for this reason that humans spend years and decades becoming coordinated. In addition, when we consider dance and athletic performances at a higher level, we can spend our entire lives learning to master the most efficient coordination of the muscles involved.
- A science exists to the kinesiology of our body, and this chapter should provide the understanding and tools to help determine what muscles might be contracting, as well as when and for what reasons. However, we should never lose sight of the fact that an art also exists to the kinesiology of our body. The exact co-ordering of muscles that may occur for any specific joint action or more complex movement pattern will vary from individual to individual. It is this diversity that accounts for the many ways that we may walk, talk, dance, run, play tennis, or create every other movement pattern that exists. Although certain patterns of coordination may be more efficient than others, no one exact pattern of coordinating muscles is right or wrong. Each person's coordination pattern is unique.
- From a clinical point of view, we must always remember that muscles that do the actions that we learned when we first learned muscle actions (i.e., concentric shortening contractions of movers) are not the only muscles that work in our body. Unfortunately, initially learning muscles' actions only as concentric contractions tends to foster the rigid idea that muscles only shorten as movers when they contract. In reality, many other functional groups other than movers work in our body when we are physically active. Every muscle that works, regardless of its role in the movement, is a muscle that contracts and is used. In addition, if this same muscle is overused, it can become unhealthy and injured. Only when we have the ability to see beyond mover actions of muscles and realize the many roles that muscles can play in movement patterns, will we be able to have the critical reasoning needed to be able to work effectively in clinical and rehabilitative settings with clients.

BOX 13-24 SPOTLIGHT ON THE CLINICAL EFFECTS OF ISOMETRIC CONTRACTIONS

When it comes to clinical importance, the isometric contractions of fixators and support muscles are often more important than the concentric and eccentric contractions of movers, antagonists, and neutralizers. This is because of the effect of muscle contractions on blood supply. The strength of the heart's contraction is responsible for arterial circulation of blood to bring nutrients out to the tissues of the body. However, the heart is not able to pump the venous blood containing the waste products of metabolism from the tissues back to the heart. Instead, veins are dependent on muscle contractions to propel their blood back toward the heart. For this purpose, veins have thin collapsible walls with unidirectional valves that help to propel blood toward the heart when muscle contractions collapse them. Therefore alternating contractions and relaxation that naturally occur with concentric and eccentric contractions are necessary and valuable for venous circulation to eliminate the waste products of metabolism from the tissues. However, isometric contractions, by virtue of being sustained, close off these collapsible veins and keep them closed off for the entire length of the time that the isometric contraction is held, resulting in an interruption of venous blood circulation. This results in a buildup of toxic waste products in the tissues. The presence of these substances irritates the nerves in the region, which often results in further tightening of the muscles of the region via the pain-spasm-pain cycle (see Section 16.10). Further, if the strength of the isometric contraction is great enough, even the arterial supply could be closed off, resulting in a loss of nutrients and further irritation to the tissue of the body that is fed by these arteries (loss of arterial blood supply is called **ischemia**). Therefore based on the irritation to the muscles and other local tissues caused by the waste products of metabolism, and the possible ischemia, the clinical effects of sustained isometric contractions tend to be more important than the clinical effects of concentric and eccentric contractions. This is one more reason to look beyond the contractions of movers and antagonists and see the contractions of muscles in their other roles!

Figures 13-16 and 13-17 provide examples of the co-ordination of the many roles that muscles play in a joint action.

- Figure 13-16 shows the example that has been used throughout this chapter of a person doing a bicep curl at the right elbow joint. In this scenario the action in question is flexion of the right forearm at the elbow joint, and we see an example of each of the five muscle roles relative to this joint action.

- ❑ Mover: The biceps brachii is contracting as a mover to create flexion of the forearm at the elbow joint.
- ❑ Antagonist: If the weight were being lowered (i.e., the action is extension of the forearm at the elbow joint), then gravity would be the mover and the biceps brachii would eccentrically contract as an antagonist.
- ❑ Fixator: The posterior deltoid acts as a fixator, creating a force of extension of the arm at the shoulder joint, which stops the biceps brachii from flexing the arm at the shoulder joint.
- ❑ Neutralizer: The pronator teres acts as a neutralizer, creating a force of pronation of the forearm at the RU joints, which stops the biceps brachii from supinating the forearm at the RU joints.
- ❑ Support: The left erector spinae group acts as a support muscle, creating a force of left lateral flexion of the trunk at the spinal joints, which stops the trunk from falling into right lateral flexion because of the weight being held in the right hand.

BOX 13-25 SPOTLIGHT ON 2nd-ORDER FIXATORS

Although a fixator stops the unwanted motion of the fixed attachment of a mover or antagonist (whichever one is working in that scenario), a **2nd-order fixator** is a fixator that contracts to fix an attachment of a *fixator* or *neutralizer* during a joint action.

Figure 13-16 illustrates muscles acting in all five roles relative to the action in question. However, even more muscles would be ordered to contract than what is shown in Figure 13-16. For example, because the right posterior deltoid contracts as a fixator to stop the unwanted flexion of the arm, the pull of the right posterior deltoid on the scapula would cause downward rotation of the scapula at the scapulocostal (ScC) joint. We do not want this to occur, so the scapula would have to be fixed by a muscle that does upward rotation; the muscle that does this is a fixator. However, because it is a fixator of a fixator, it is called a *2nd-order fixator*. To continue along this line of reasoning, if the upward rotator 2nd-order fixator chosen by the body to contract is the right upper trapezius, then its other attachment on the head and neck may have to be fixed from extending, right laterally flexing, and left rotating by other 2nd-order fixators. (Perhaps a better term would be *3rd-order fixator*!) If instead of the upper trapezius, the serratus anterior had contracted as the upward rotator 2nd-order fixator, then its action of protraction of the scapula may have had to be stopped from occurring by another 2nd-order fixator that in this case retracts the scapula. Further, when the right posterior deltoid contracts as our fixator, it would have also created a force of abduction and lateral rotation on the arm at the shoulder joint; 2nd-order fixators (that can do flexion and/or medial rotation of the arm) might have to contract to stop the arm from doing these actions.

To kinesthetically experience this yourself, place a heavy weight in your right hand and slowly palpate each of the muscles mentioned in the caption for Figure 13-16, as well as the muscles mentioned in this Spotlight; you will probably be able to feel their contractions. The domino effect of muscle contractions that occurs through the body can be truly amazing! It makes one realize how silly it can be when we hear people in the fields of health and sports training talk about *isolating* a muscle when exercising.

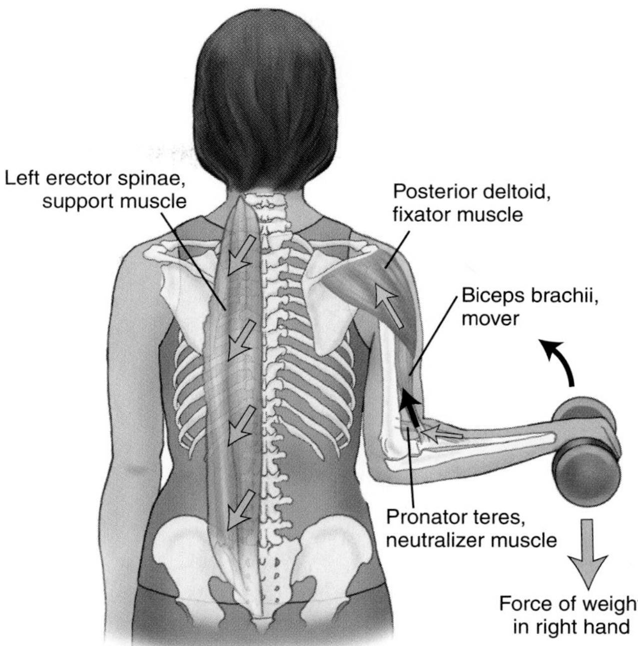

Figure 13-16 Person carrying out a simple joint action (i.e., flexion of the forearm at the elbow joint to do a bicep curl). The biceps brachii is seen as the mover of flexion of the forearm at the elbow joint (if the weight were being lowered, the biceps brachii would act as an antagonist instead). The posterior deltoid acts as a fixator of the arm at the shoulder joint. The pronator teres acts as a neutralizer of the forearm at the radioulnar (RU) joints. The left erector spinae group acts a support muscle, holding the trunk in place.

- ❑ Figure 13-17 shows a person kicking a soccer ball with her right foot. In this scenario the action in question is flexion of the right thigh at the hip joint.
  - ❑ Mover: The rectus femoris is contracting as a mover to create flexion of the thigh at the hip joint.
  - ❑ Fixator: The rectus abdominis acts as a fixator, creating a force of posterior tilt of the pelvis at the lumbosacral joint, which stops the rectus femoris from anteriorly tilting the pelvis at the hip joints.
  - ❑ Neutralizer: If the rectus femoris is the mover that contracts, there will be no neutralizer because the rectus femoris has no other action on the thigh at the hip joint. (Note: If a different mover such as the right iliopsoas or one of the right-sided adductors of the thigh at the hip joint contracts, then there would be other undesired actions of the thigh at the hip joint that would need to be neutralized.)
  - ❑ Support: The left quadriceps femoris group acts as a support muscle, creating a force of extension of the left knee joint, preventing the left knee joint from flexing and the person falling to the ground.
- ❑ As we can see from these examples, the contractions of muscles leapfrog through the body like the ripples of a stone thrown into a pond. Certainly as the

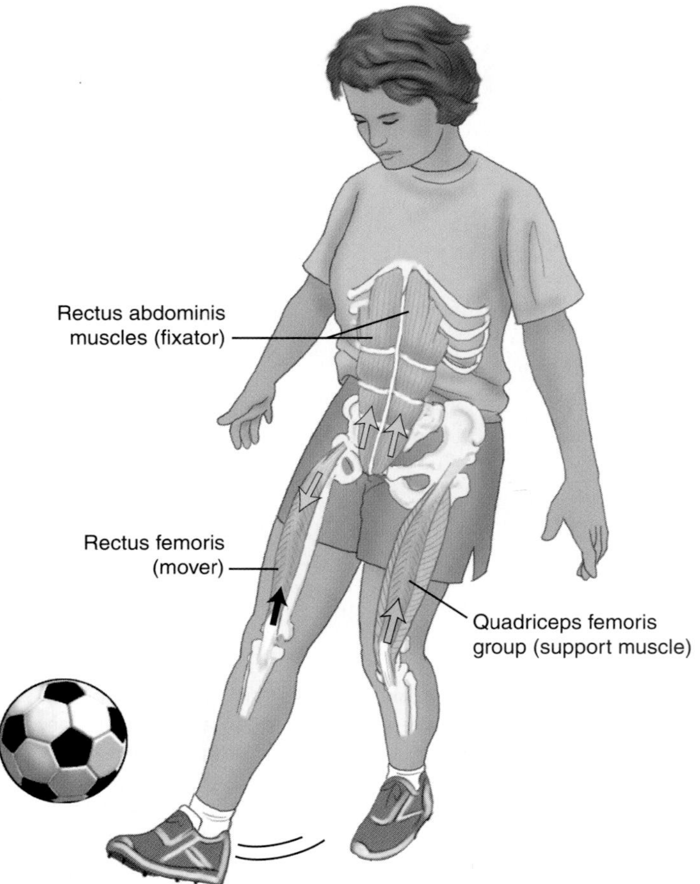

Figure 13-17 Person doing flexion of the right thigh at the hip joint to kick a soccer ball. The right rectus femoris of the quadriceps femoris group is seen as the mover of flexion of the right thigh at the hip joint. The rectus abdominis acts as a fixator of the pelvis. Because the rectus femoris has no undesired action on the thigh at the hip joint, no neutralizer exists. The left quadriceps femoris group acts as a support muscle, holding the left knee joint extended against the force of gravity that would otherwise flex it, causing the person to fall.

contractions become more distant from the original contraction of the concentrically contracting mover or eccentrically contracting antagonist (whichever is the muscle that is working), the strength of these contractions diminishes. However, they do occur and in injured clients may be functionally important to their health! To fully explore all the contractions that would occur, one must examine every line of pull in every plane of every muscle that is contracting!

- ❏ It must be emphasized that the particular set of muscles that contracts in any given movement pattern can vary greatly from one person to another and from one circumstance to another.
- ❏ Each person has his or her own coordination pattern that has been learned through his or her lifetime. The change of even one mover for a joint action can have ripple effects that change which fixators and neutralizers then have to contract, which then changes which 2nd-order fixators have to contract, and so forth.
- ❏ Further, the strength needed for a contraction and the position of the body during a joint action can alter muscle contraction patterns.
  - ❏ Depending on the force of contraction needed for a specific joint action, more or less movers (or antagonists) might need to contract. This would then affect the coordination pattern of fixators and neutralizers. For example, lifting a 10-lb weight instead to a 5-lb weight might trigger an entirely different pattern of coordinating muscles.
  - ❏ Further, if the body is in a different position while doing the joint action, the role of gravity might change, triggering a different pattern of coordinating muscles.

13.12 COUPLED ACTIONS

- Although we often choose to direct multiple specific joint actions to occur as part of more complex movement patterns, sometimes two joint actions *must* occur together (i.e., one joint action cannot occur unless the 2nd joint action also occurs at the same time).
- Two separate joint actions that must occur simultaneously are called **coupled actions**, because they exist as a couple.

> **BOX 13-26 SPOTLIGHT ON MOVEMENT PATTERNS**
>
> The concept of coupled actions points to the larger picture of how the muscular system works. When the brain directs muscular activity, it does not think in terms of directing specific joint actions to occur or even directing specific muscles to contract. Rather, the brain thinks in terms of movement patterns to achieve a desired position of the body. For example, if we want to reach a book that is up on a high shelf, the brain does not think of creating abduction of the arm at the shoulder joint or any other specific joint action. Instead, its only goal is create whatever coordinated movement pattern is necessary to bring the hand to this elevated position and whatever muscular contractions are necessary to create this will be directed to occur. Therefore, muscles that abduct the arm at the shoulder joint will be ordered to contract along with scapular and clavicular muscles that upwardly rotate the shoulder girdle to further the ability of the hand to reach this elevated position. Additionally, muscles of the elbow, wrist, and finger joints will also be ordered to contract. Beyond the upper extremity, muscular activity throughout the contralateral upper extremity, lower extremities, and axial body will also be recruited to aid in raising the hand higher. Ordering each of these specific muscular contractions is not consciously thought of, rather, they happen automatically as a part of the larger movement pattern with the intended goal of bringing the hand higher. Further, if for some reason one body part cannot be moved as a part of this set of movements (perhaps due to an injury), another body part will automatically be recruited by the brain to compensate for this loss. For example, if the arm cannot abduct, muscles that elevate the scapula and clavicle might be directed to contract in an attempt to raise the hand higher. In short, the essence of neural control of the muscular system is that the brain does not talk to specific muscles per se; rather it thinks in larger movement patterns and talks to motor units of multiple muscles throughout the body to achieve whatever larger movement patterns are desired!

- We do not consciously direct a coupled 2nd action; rather it is automatically ordered subconsciously by our nervous system when we order the 1st joint action to occur.
- Coupled actions are different from a muscle that has more than one action at a joint; they are also different from a multijoint muscle that has actions at more than one joint.
- Coupled actions are separate actions that are caused by separate movers.
- The best examples of coupled actions in the human body are the coupled actions of the arm and shoulder girdle. These actions couple together, because for full excursion of the humerus to occur, the shoulder girdle must move as well. The coupled actions of the arm and shoulder girdle are usually referred to as **scapulohumeral rhythm**, because a rhythm exists to the movement between the humerus and the scapula. (Note: For a more detailed exploration of scapulohumeral rhythm, see Section 9.6.) Coupled actions of the thigh and the pelvic girdle are also common. Just as the shoulder girdle must move to allow for a fuller excursion of the humerus, motion of the pelvic girdle must occur to allow for a fuller excursion of the femur. (For information on the coupled actions of the thigh and pelvic girdle, see Section 8.11.)
- The classic example of coupled actions that been most extensively studied involves abduction of the arm coupled with shoulder girdle actions.
- Figure 13-18a, illustrates an arm that is abducted 180 degrees *relative to the rest of the body.* Normally we assume that arm abduction occurs relative to the scapula at the shoulder (glenohumeral [GH]) joint. However, in Figure 13-18a, we see that of these 180 degrees of arm abduction, only 120 degrees were movement of the humerus relative to the scapula at the GH joint; the remaining 60 degrees were the result of upward rotation of the scapula relative to the ribcage at the ScC joint (Box 13-27). This scapular action is coupled with the humeral action of abduction, because otherwise the head of the humerus would bang into the acromion process of the scapula, both limiting overall humeral range of motion and causing impingement of the rotator cuff tendon and shoulder joint bursa. Figure 13-18b, illustrates the mover muscles that work in this circumstance: The deltoid is the mover of abduction the arm at the shoulder joint, and the upper trapezius and lower trapezius are movers of upward rotation the scapula at the ScC joint. We do not consciously choose to contract the trapezius in this circumstance; its contraction is automatically ordered by the nervous system to couple with the deltoid's action of abduction of the arm at the shoulder joint. (Note: Only these movers of arm abduction and scapula upward rotation have been shown; the various fixators and neutralizers as well as other possible movers that would need to contract during this coordination pattern are not shown.)

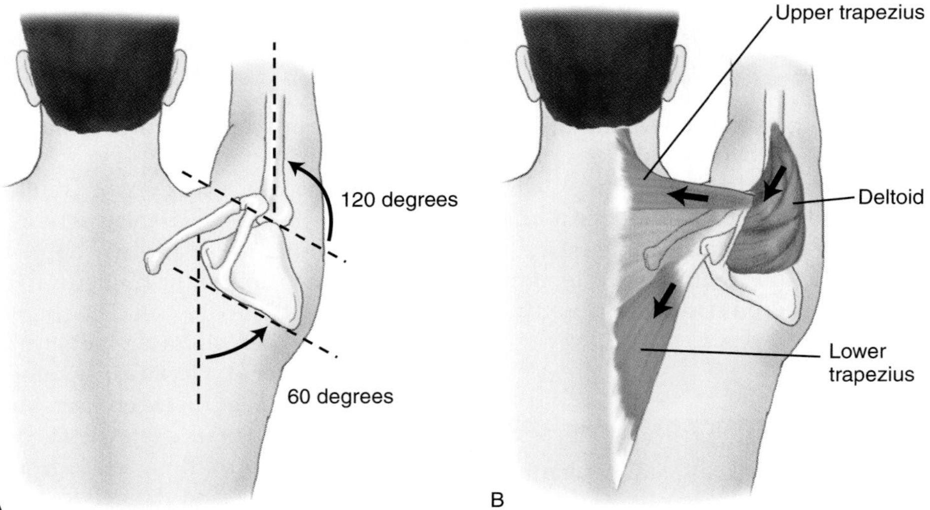

Figure 13-18 Illustration of the concept of coupled actions in the body. *A,* 180 degrees of abduction of the arm relative to the trunk is actually made up of two separate coupled joint actions: (1) humeral motion at the shoulder (i.e., glenohumeral [GH]) joint and (2) scapular motion at the scapulocostal (ScC) joint. B, Two separate movers must independently contract to create these two coupled actions: (1) the deltoid is the mover of abduction of the arm at the shoulder joint, and (2) the upper trapezius and lower trapezius are the movers of upward rotation of the scapula at the ScC joint.

BOX 13-27

The scapular upward rotation that couples with humeral abduction also involves coupled actions of clavicular elevation and upward rotation. Overall, for the arm to abduct, coupled actions of the humerus, scapula, and clavicle must occur at the glenohumeral, scapulocostal, sternoclavicular, and acromioclavicular joints! See Section 9.6 for more information on the coupled actions of the arm and shoulder girdle.

Essential Facts:

- ❑ Two separate joint actions that must occur simultaneously are called *coupled actions*.
- ❑ Coupled actions are separate joint actions that are caused by separate movers.

REVIEW QUESTIONS

evolve Answers to the following review questions appear on the Evolve website accompanying this book.

1. What are the six major roles in which a muscle can contract during a joint action?

2. What is the definition of a mover?

3. When a joint action occurs, what happens to the length of a mover?

4. Do mover muscles always contract when a joint action occurs?

5. What is the definition of an antagonist?

6. When a joint action occurs, what happens to the length of an antagonist?

7. Do antagonist muscles always contract when a joint action occurs?

8. What is the most common external force that can be a mover or an antagonist?

9. Define cocontraction.

10. What is the definition of a fixator?

11. What is the definition of a neutralizer?

12. What do fixators and neutralizers have in common? What is the difference between a fixator and a neutralizer?

13. What is the importance of core stabilization, and what effect does it have on our health?

14. What is the difference between postural stabilization muscles and mobility muscles?

15. What is the definition of a support muscle?

16. What are two ways in which a synergist can be defined?

17. Define the term *coordination,* and describe its application to the concept of muscle roles.

18. Explain why isometric contractions are more likely to diminish venous return of blood to the heart and also cause ischemia of tissues.

19. State a specific joint action (and the position that the body is in when performing this action), and give an example of a mover, antagonist, fixator, neutralizer, and support muscle for this action; further, state whether it is the mover group or the antagonist group that is working in this scenario.

20. What is the difference between a regular fixator (i.e., 1st-order fixator) and a 2nd-order fixator?

21. Give an example of a coupled action in the human body.

NOTES

Chapter 14

Types of Joint Motion and Musculoskeletal Assessment

CHAPTER OUTLINE

CHAPTER OBJECTIVES

After completing this chapter, the student should be able to perform the following:

- ❑ Define, discuss, and give an example of passive and active range of motion of joints.
- ❑ Define and discuss the relationship of joint play and joint adjustments.
- ❑ Define and discuss ballistic motion and explain why ballistic motions occur in the body.
- ❑ Define, discuss, and give an example of resisted motion in the body.
- ❑ Explain how active range of motion, passive range of motion, and resisted motion can be used as test procedures to assess musculoskeletal soft tissue conditions.
- ❑ List the five major guidelines, as well as the additional guidelines to palpating muscles; further, be able to explain the importance of each of these guidelines and apply them to a muscle palpation.
- ❑ Explain the importance of assessing and treating tight antagonists of a joint motion.
- ❑ Define the terms *signs* and *symptoms*.
- ❑ Discuss the importance of signs and symptoms when assessing and treating a client.
- ❑ Be able to make and explain an analogy between the concept of signs/symptoms and a glass of water that overflows.
- ❑ Define the key terms of this chapter.
- ❑ State the meanings of the word origins of this chapter.

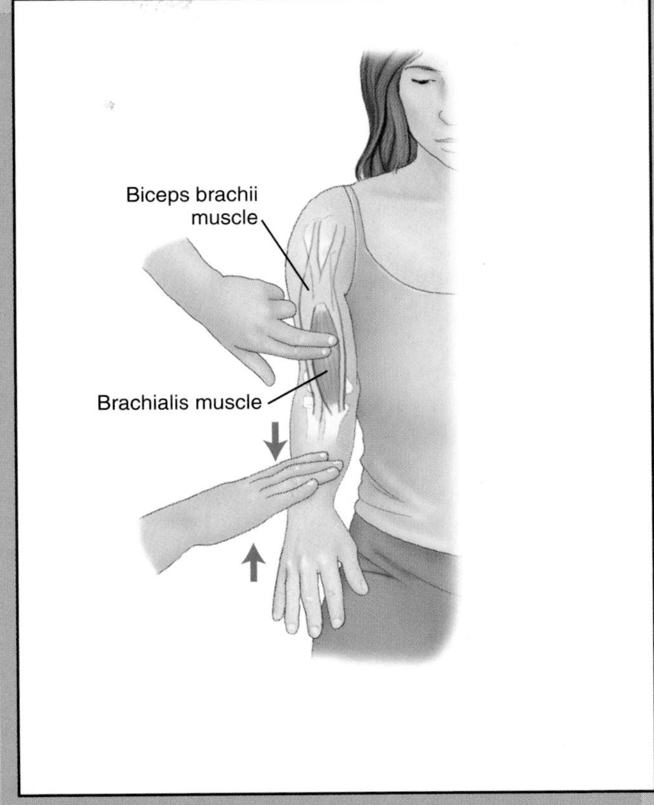

O V E R V I E W

The last few chapters have explored the various ways in which muscles can contract, and the various roles that muscles have when a joint action is occurring. We will now begin to investigate the different types of motion that can occur (i.e., active versus passive) when a joint action occurs. We will then use the understanding of these types of motion, along with resisted isometric contraction, to learn how to assess musculoskeletal soft tissue injuries. Continuing with assessment techniques, methods of muscle palpation are given. Finally, this chapter finishes with a discussion of the types of problems that manual and exercise therapists most commonly treat.

KEY TERMS

Active range of motion
Assessment
Ballistic motion
Diagnosis (DYE-ag-NO-sis)
False negative
False positive
Joint mobilization
Joint play
Orthopedic test procedures
Passive range of motion
Resisted motion
Signs
Sprain
Strain
Symptoms
Target muscle
Tendinitis
Test procedure

WORD ORIGINS

- ❑ Act—From Latin *actus,* meaning *to do*
- ❑ Assess—From Latin *assideo,* meaning *to assist in judging*
- ❑ Ballistic—From Greek *ballein,* meaning *to throw*
- ❑ Diagnosis—From Greek *diagnosis,* meaning *a decision, discernment*
- ❑ Orthopedic—From Greek *orthos,* meaning *correct,* and *paid,* meaning *child*
- ❑ Passive—From Latin *passivus,* meaning *permits, endures*
- ❑ Sign—From Latin *signum,* meaning *a sign, mark, warning*
- ❑ Sprain—From Old French *espraindre,* meaning *to twist*
- ❑ Strain—From Latin *stringere* meaning *to draw tight*
- ❑ Symptom—From Greek *symptoma,* meaning *an occurrence*

☐ 14.1 ACTIVE VERSUS PASSIVE RANGE OF MOTION

- ❑ Two types of range of motion (ROM) can occur at a joint (Figure 14-1):
  1. **Active range of motion** is defined as joint motion that is created by the mover muscles of that joint.
  2. **Passive range of motion** is defined as joint motion that is created by a force other than the mover muscles of that joint.
- ❑ The therapist does not have a role in performing active range of motion of the client.
  - ❑ Because active motion is created by the mover muscles of the client's joint that is moving, active range of motion must be done by the client. Figure 14-2 illustrates an example of active joint motion.

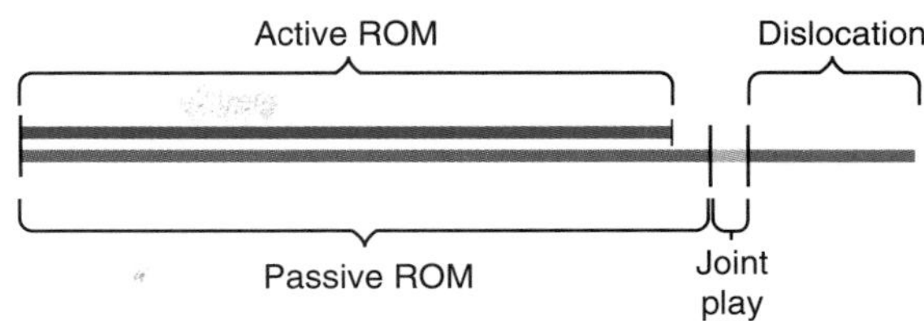

Figure 14-1 Schematic illustration of the relationship of the ranges of motion (ROM) of a typical healthy joint. The reader should note that passive range of motion is slightly greater than active range of motion and that a small amount of joint play is seen directly after the end of passive range of motion. Beyond joint play is dislocation.

BOX 14-1 SPOTLIGHT ON "JOINT PLAY"

In addition to active and passive range of motion, one other type of motion occurs at a joint; it is called *joint play.* **Joint play** is the small amount of gliding motion that is permissible at a joint at the end of a joint's passive range of motion. Two types of manipulations are possible within the realm of joint play. One type is a low velocity, long-lever arm stretching of the joint and is usually called joint play or joint mobilization (see photo below, left). The other type is a high velocity short-lever arm manipulation that is called an *adjustment* and is used by chiropractic and osteopathic physicians. Depending on the scope of license in the state, manual therapists may be permitted to do joint play. However, adjustments are usually only used by physicians (see photo below, right).

When a chiropractic/osteopathic adjustment is performed, a popping sound often occurs. During an adjustment, the bones of the joint are not "cracked" together as is commonly thought. What occurs is that the bones of the joint are distracted away from each other. This causes an increase in the space within the joint capsule, resulting in a lower pressure within the joint. This causes the gases that are dissolved within the synovial fluid to come out of solution and become gaseous. This change in the state of the gases of the joint fluid causes the characteristic popping sound that is associated with osseous adjustments. An analogy can be made between the popping sound of an osseous adjustment and the popping sound that occurs when a champagne bottle is opened. When a champagne cork is first removed from the bottle, a popping sound occurs; if the cork is then immediately placed back in the bottle and immediately removed again, no popping sound occurs the second time it is removed. However, if the cork is placed back in the bottle, left there for 20 minutes or so, and then removed again, the popping sound will occur once again because the gases had sufficient time to go back into solution. Similarly, if a joint is adjusted two times in a row quickly, there will be no popping sound the second time because the gases within the joint cavity, like the gases within the champagne bottle, did not have sufficient time to go back into solution. Keep in mind that the point of an adjustment is not to make the popping sound, but rather to increase the range of motion of the joint by stretching the joint capsule/ligaments of the joint. The popping sound is often just a good indicator that this objective was successfully achieved.

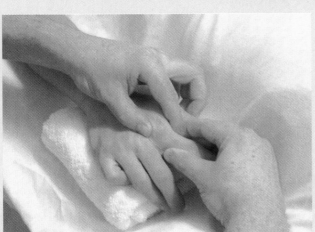

Dixon M: *Joint play the right Way for the peripheral skeleton: the training manual,* ed. 2. Port Moody, British Columbia, 2003, Arthrokinetic Publishing.

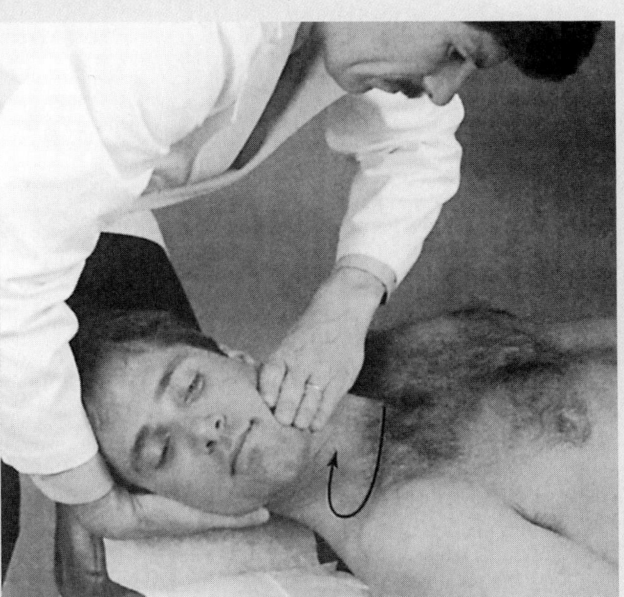

(From Peterson DH, Bergmann TF: *Chiropractic technique: principles and procedures,* ed 2, St Louis, 2002, Mosby.)

- The therapist can have a role in performing passive range of motion of the client.
  - Because the mover muscles of the joint that is being moved are not creating the joint motion, another force must do this; the force to move the joint in passive motion can be created by the therapist.
  - However, it is important to realize that passive range of motion of a client's joint can be done without the assistance of a therapist or trainer; a client can do passive range of motion by himself or herself. This can be accomplished by the client using muscles of one part of the body to create passive motion at another joint of the body. Because the mover muscles of the joint that is being moved are relaxed and passive, this motion is defined as passive range of motion. Figure 14-3 illustrates two examples of passive joint motion: one in which the therapist performs the passive motion of the client's joint and another in which the client performs passive range of motion alone.

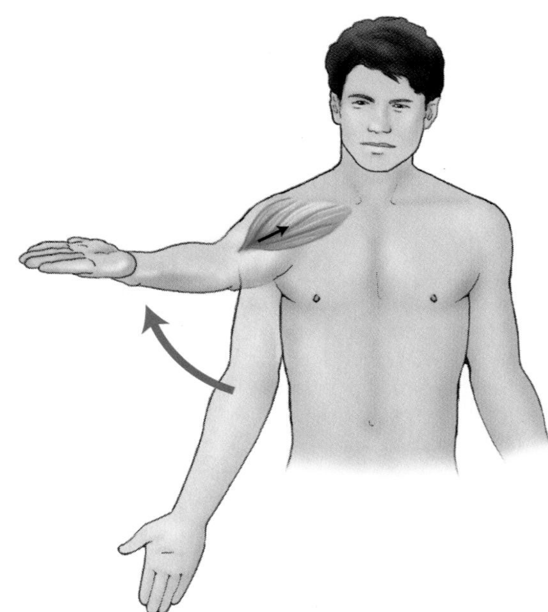

Figure 14-2 Active joint motion in which a person is actively flexing the right arm at the shoulder joint. This motion is defined as active, because the mover muscles of that joint (i.e., flexors of the right arm at the shoulder joint) are creating it.

- Knowledge of active and passive motion can be helpful when assessing and treating clients. (For more details on using active and passive range of motion to assess and treat clients, see Section 14.3.)

Ballistic Motion:

- Whenever a joint motion is begun actively by the client and then is completed passively by momentum, that motion is called a **ballistic motion**.

BOX 14-2

Most motions of the body are ballistic because ballistic motions are very efficient. A ballistic motion allows the muscles that actively contracted to initiate the joint motion to relax while momentum completes the motion. The normal swing of our lower and upper extremities when walking is a good example of ballistic motion. If these motions are not done in a ballistic manner, then our muscles would have to actively contract during the entire range of motion of the lower and upper extremities (the Nazi *goosestep* march of the 1930s and 1940s was done in this manner). Another good example of a ballistic motion is the swing of a tennis racquet or a golf club. A strong active contraction of the muscles of the joint is necessary to begin the motion; natural passive momentum then completes the swing, allowing our muscles to relax.

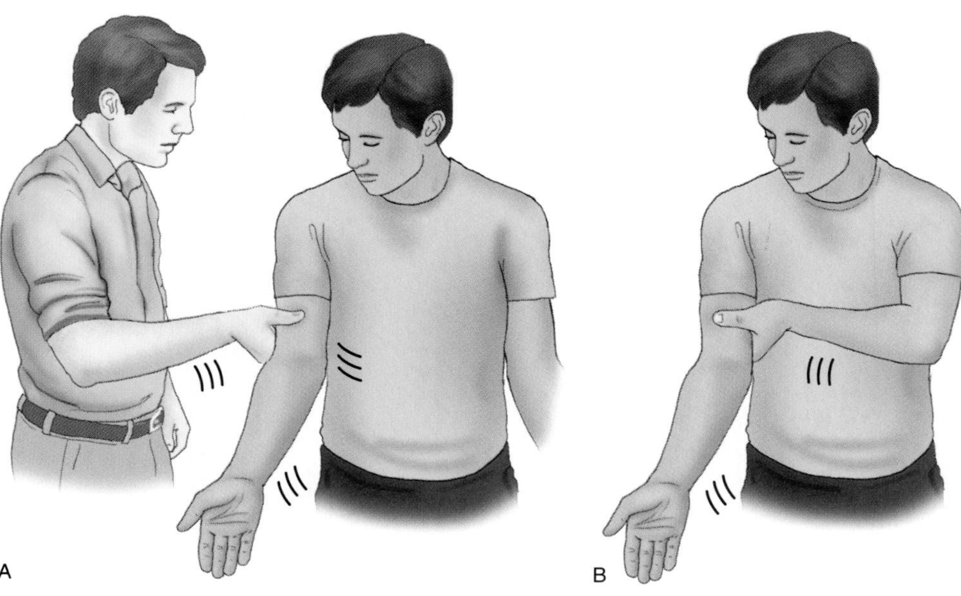

Figure 14-3 Two examples of passive joint motion. *A,* A therapist is flexing the client's right arm at the shoulder joint. *B,* Client is using the left upper extremity to flex the right arm at the shoulder joint. Both cases illustrate passive motion because the mover muscles of flexion of the right arm at the shoulder joint are relaxed and another force is creating the motion. In *A,* the force that creates the motion comes from the therapist. In *B,* the force comes from the client's left upper extremity.

☐ 14.2 RESISTED MOTION

- **Resisted motion** occurs when a resistance force stops the contraction of the muscles of the joint from being able to create motion at that joint.
  - Therefore resisted motion results in an isometric contraction of the muscles of the joint with no actual joint motion occurring.
- This force of resistance that stops motion from occurring can be provided by a therapist or trainer, an object, or even the client alone. Figure 14-4 illustrates examples of resisted motion.

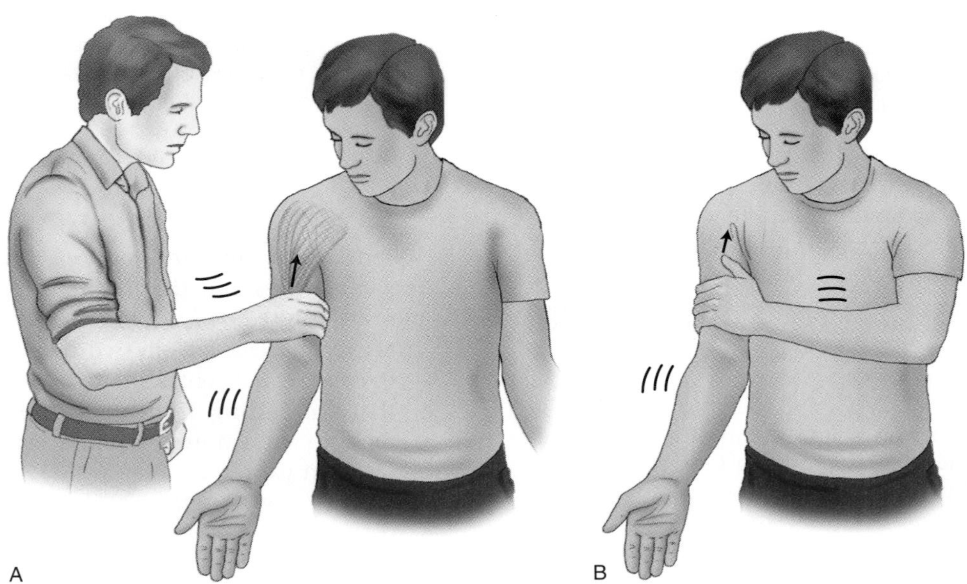

Figure 14-4 Two examples of resisted motion. In both cases flexion of the right arm at the shoulder joint is being resisted from occurring by another force. In *A*, the force resisting and stopping motion is coming from a therapist. In *B*, the client is using the left upper extremity to provide resistance to the motion. (Resistance could also have been provided by the presence of some immovable object such as a heavy table or wall.)

☐ 14.3 MUSCULOSKELETAL ASSESSMENT: MUSCLE OR JOINT?

❑ Most musculoskeletal conditions are either injury to the musculature (and the associated tendons) of a joint or to the ligament/joint capsule complex of a joint.

BOX 14-3

If a muscle is injured and torn, it is defined as a **strain**; an injured tendon that is inflamed is defined as **tendinitis** (also spelled *tendonitis*). If a ligament or joint capsule is injured and torn, it is defined as a **sprain**. Musculoskeletal injuries are often termed as either *muscular* in origin (i.e., muscle strain, tendinitis) or *joint* in origin (i.e., ligamentous/joint capsule in origin).

❑ Knowledge of active range of motion, passive range of motion, and resisted motion can be valuable in assessing these musculoskeletal conditions.

BOX 14-4

There can be a fine line between diagnosis and assessment. A **diagnosis** may be defined as the assigning of a name or label to a group of signs and/or symptoms by a qualified health care professional, whereas an **assessment** may be defined as a systematic method of gathering information to make informed decisions about treatment. The information provided in this section is to assist massage therapists, trainers, and other bodyworkers in assessing their clients' musculoskeletal conditions, not making diagnoses. An excellent text written for the world of bodywork that deals with the assessment of musculoskeletal conditions is *Functional Assessment* by Whitney Lowe, published by OMERI.

❑ Assessment requires critical thinking, and critical thinking requires a fundamental understanding of how the various parts of the musculoskeletal system function.

❑ The basis of an assessment **test procedure** is that it challenges a structure by placing a stress on it. If the structure is healthy, then it will be able to meet this stress in a symptom-free (e.g. pain-free) manner and the test procedure is declared negative. However, if the structure is injured in some way, symptoms (e.g. pain) will most likely result and the test procedure is declared positive. An injured muscle that is asked to contract (or is stretched) will usually cause pain, as will an injured ligament or joint capsule that is stretched or compressed in some manner.

❑ Active range or motion, passive range of motion, and resisted motion are valuable test procedures that can be used when assessing musculoskeletal soft tissue conditions.

❑ When assessing musculoskeletal soft tissue injuries, it is helpful to divide the soft tissues of the body into two major categories: (1) mover muscles and (2) the ligament/joint capsule complex. We can then look at the stresses placed on these soft tissues with active range of motion, passive range of motion, and resisted motion.

BOX 14-5

When assessing a musculoskeletal soft tissue injury, it is customary to divide the soft tissues into two categories: (1) mover muscles and (2) the ligament/joint capsule complex. However, a 3rd and very important category of soft tissue exists and should not be ignored. This 3rd category is the antagonist muscles (see *Spotlight on Orthopedic Assessment and Antagonist Muscles,* Box 14-8).

Active Range of Motion:

❑ When active range of motion is performed, both mover muscles and the ligament/joint capsule complex are stressed.

- ❑ Mover muscles are stressed because they are asked to contract concentrically to create the joint motion that is occurring. If the mover muscles and/or their tendons are injured in some way, this will likely result in pain.
- ❑ The ligament/joint capsule complex is stressed because the joint is moved, causing stretching and/or compression to various parts of the capsule and ligaments of the joint. If these structures are injured, pain will likely result.

❑ Therefore active range of motion would be expected to generate pain in most any musculoskeletal injury of mover musculature or ligament/joint capsule tissue. For this reason, active range of motion is useful as an initial screening procedure to determine if any type of soft tissue injury or dysfunction is present.

Passive Range of Motion:

❑ When passive range of motion is done, only the ligament/joint capsule complex is stressed.

- ❑ The ligament/joint capsule complex is stressed because the joint is being moved, causing stretching and/or compression to various parts of the capsule and ligaments of the joint. If these structures are injured, pain will likely result.

❑ However, mover muscles are not stressed because they are passive (i.e., relaxed as another force creates the joint action).

Resisted Motion:

❑ When resisted motion is done, only the mover musculature is stressed.

- ❑ Mover muscles are stressed because they are asked to contract isometrically in an attempt to create joint motion. This motion does not actually occur because the resistance force stops the mover muscle from being able to shorten and actually move the joint; however, the mover muscle still works by isometrically contracting. Therefore if it or its tendons are injured in some way, pain will likely result.
- ❑ The ligaments and joint capsule are not stressed because the joint does not actually move in any way. Therefore no force is placed on them; they are neither stretched nor compressed in any way.

❑ By doing these procedures on a client with musculoskeletal pain, the origin of the pain can usually be determined.

BOX 14-6

Following is the order of steps to be followed when assessing a client with musculoskeletal soft tissue pain:

1. Begin with active range of motion. A client that is positive for pain with active range of motion is confirmed as having either mover muscular *and/or* ligament/joint capsule complex injury.
2. Next do passive range of motion. If passive range of motion results in pain, the client's ligament/joint capsule complex is injured.
3. Then do resisted motion. If resisted motion results in pain, then the mover musculature is injured.

Note: Every test procedure has a certain degree of sensitivity and accuracy. Sometimes a **false negative** occurs wherein the client has a negative test (i.e., the client does not report pain [or does not exhibit whatever sign or symptom is indicative for that test procedure]) on performing the procedure, yet he or she actually does have the musculoskeletal condition. In other words, the negative result is incorrect (i.e., false). A **false positive** would be defined as a test procedure wherein the client does report pain (or whatever sign or symptom is indicative for that test procedure) on performing the procedure but does not actually have the musculoskeletal condition. In other words, the positive result is incorrect (i.e., false). These physical test procedures that deal with the musculoskeletal system are often called **orthopedic test procedures**. It should always be kept in mind that test procedures such as these are not 100% accurate.

❑ It is important to remember that a client may have injury to more than one type of tissue (e.g., mover muscles and the ligament/joint capsule complex can be injured). If you find that one type of tissue is injured, continue to assess the other tissue.

❑ In fact, given the concept of compensation, whenever one tissue of the body is dysfunctional, other tissues try to compensate for the functional weakness. Therefore the presence of one condition usually, in time, creates the presence of other conditions.

BOX 14-7

Too often we look to pigeonhole a client's condition into a neat little box, either assessing the client as having a strain to muscular tissue or a sprain to ligamentous/joint capsular tissue. In reality, clients who have had a traumatic accident of some sort rarely suffer from a pure strain or a pure sprain because any traumatic injury that causes damage to one of these tissues often causes damage to the other. Of course, the extent of damage to each tissue is not necessarily the same. Although a strain and sprain may both be present, the relative proportion of each one may vary. Determining the proportion of each one can be done with the same active, passive, and resisted motion test procedures, but it usually requires more experience and judgment to make finer distinctions. This is because it is not only important to note whether the client feels pain or not but also to note at what point pain begins and what degree of pain exists during the procedures. Although massage therapists, trainers, and other bodyworkers can address ligamentous/joint capsule problems with joint range of motion and other test procedures, muscular problems are usually the primary concern. For that reason, particular attention should be paid to the muscular elements of injury.

❑ Figure 14-5 demonstrates a flow chart for using these test procedures for musculoskeletal assessment.

BOX 14-8 SPOTLIGHT ON ORTHOPEDIC ASSESSMENT AND ANTAGONIST MUSCLES

The entire preceding discussion was aimed at discerning between injury to the ligament/joint capsule complex and the mover muscles. However, what about the antagonists muscles of a joint movement? If they are injured or they spasm, could they cause pain with active, passive, or resisted motion?

- ❑ Active range of motion and passive range of motion would both cause pain if the antagonist musculature is injured and/or tight, because any motion of the joint requires the antagonist muscles to lengthen and stretch, and an injured or tight antagonist muscle will be resistant to stretch, most likely resulting in pain.
- ❑ Resisted motion would not cause pain in the antagonist musculature on the other side of the joint to the *mover* musculature that is isometrically contracting and attempting to shorten. (In reality, the terms *mover musculature* and *antagonist musculature* do not even apply here, because no joint motion actually occurs and movers and antagonists are defined by their role relative to an actual joint motion.) Because no motion occurs, the muscles on the other side of the joint (i.e., antagonist musculature) are not lengthened and stretched, and are therefore not stressed.
- ❑ Understanding this, we realize that painful passive range of motion can indeed indicate muscular injury, but only of the antagonist muscles on the other side of the joint. If this is the case the client can usually localize the pain to the other side of the joint; localization of pain there indicates to the therapist that the pain is in antagonist musculature. To confirm this, resisted motion can be done to *these* muscles. If they are unhealthy, causing them to isometrically contract by resisting their contraction should elicit pain.

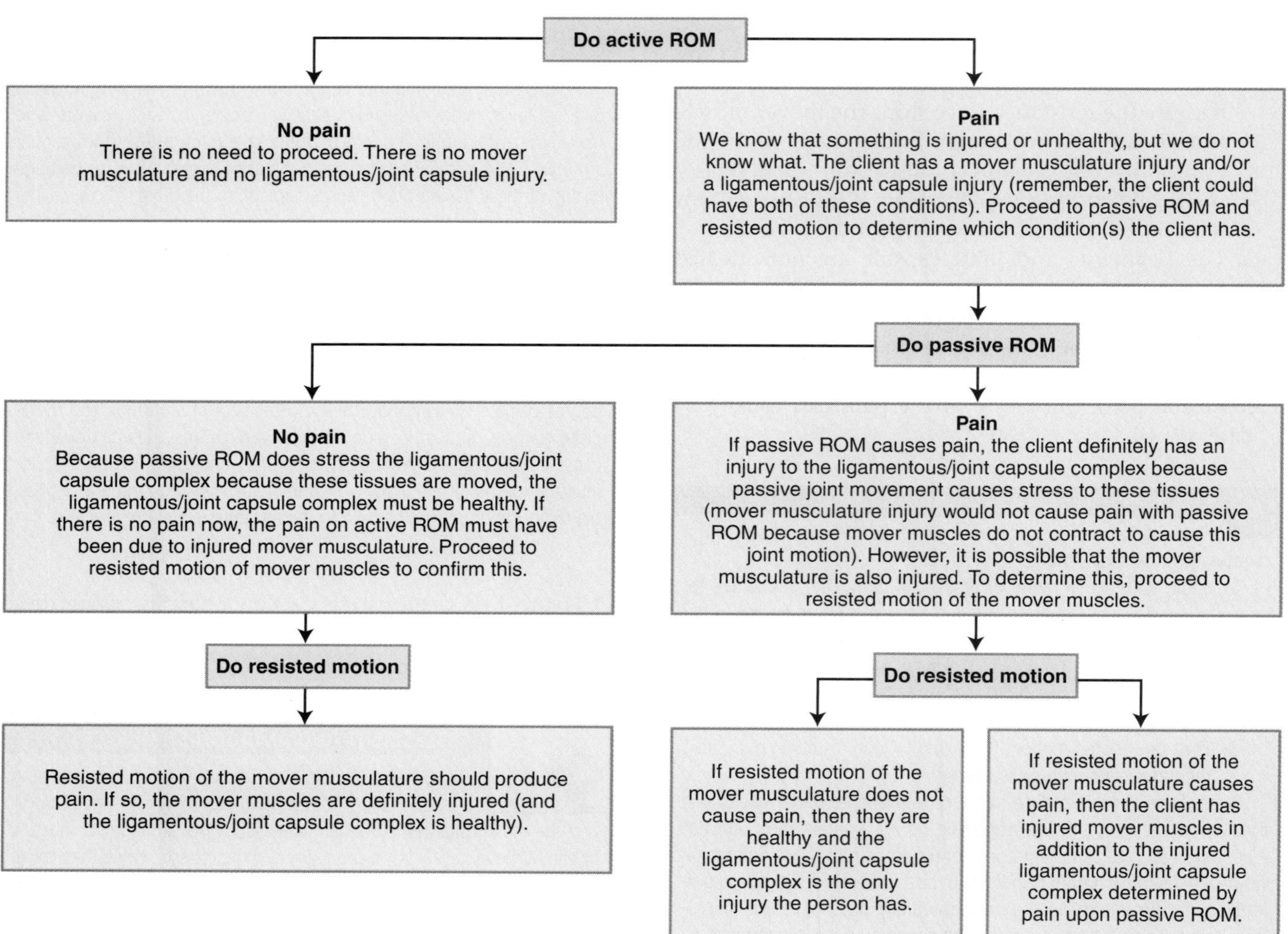

Figure 14-5 Flow chart demonstrates the proper sequence to follow when use the orthopedic test procedures of active range of motion, passive range of motion, and resisted motion to assess a musculoskeletal soft tissue injury. *ROM,* Range of motion.

14.4 MUSCLE PALPATION

- Regarding musculoskeletal assessment, perhaps no skill is more important or more valuable than assessment of resting muscle tone by muscle palpation. For this reason, it is extremely important for bodyworkers to have a solid foundation in how to palpate the skeletal muscles of the body.
- Most every textbook on muscles offers a method to palpate each skeletal muscle of the human body. Although providing these palpation directions can be helpful, memorization of them on the part of the student should not be necessary. If a student knows the attachments and actions of the muscles, palpation can be figured out. The best way to become a better palpator is to spend more time palpating. Beyond that, if the student has extra time, that time should be spent reinforcing the knowledge of the attachments and actions of a muscle, not spent trying to memorize palpation directions.

BOX 14-9

The student does not need to memorize the actions of a muscle—only the attachments need to be memorized. By following the five-step approach to learning muscles presented in Section 11.3, once the attachments are known, the line of pull of the muscle relative to the joint is known. Knowledge of this allows the actions to be figured out. Essentially the only muscle knowledge that needs to be memorized is the attachment information. Less memorization and more understanding eases the stress of being a student and allows for better critical thought and clinical application!

Five-Step Muscle Palpation Guideline:

- Following are the five basic guidelines to follow when looking to palpate the **target muscle** (i.e., the muscle that you desire to palpate) (Figure 14-6):

1. Know the attachments of the target muscle so that you know where to place your palpating fingers.

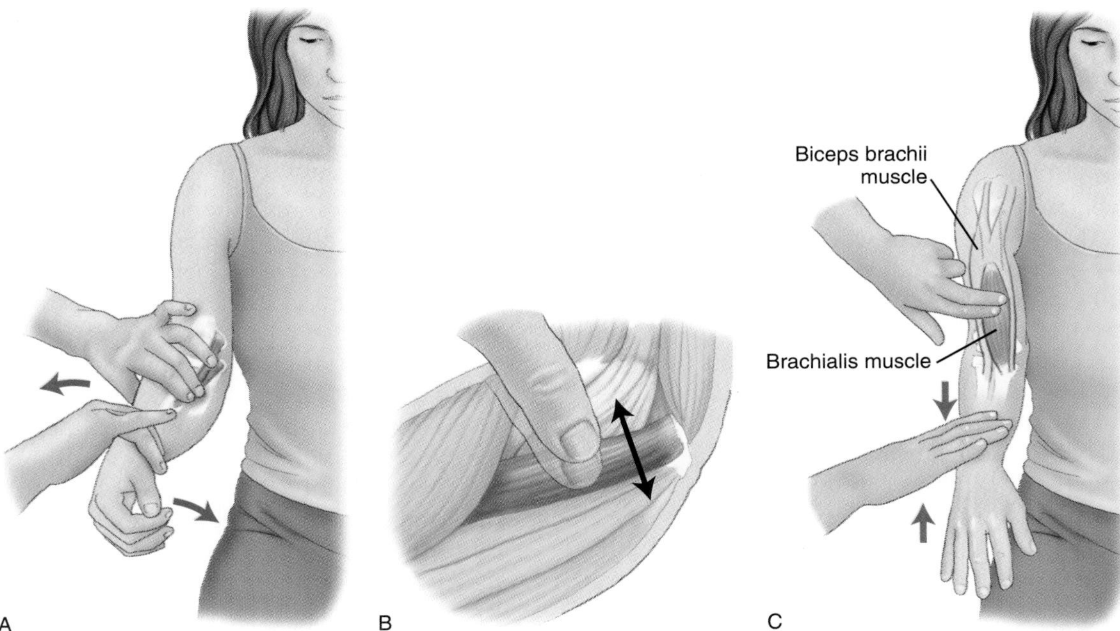

Figure 14-6 Five basic guidelines for palpating a muscle. *A,* Person palpating the pronator teres muscle while the client attempts to pronate the forearm at the radioulnar (RU) joints against resistance. Placement of the palpating fingers is determined by knowing the attachments of the pronator teres (palpation guideline #1). Asking the client to contract the muscle, attempting to pronate the forearm, makes the muscle become firmer and therefore more palpably discernible (palpation guideline #2). Resisting the client from performed pronation will increase the contraction of the pronator teres, making it even more discernibly palpable (palpation guideline #3). *B,* Close-up of the palpating fingers strumming perpendicular to the fiber direction of the pronator teres (palpation guideline #4). *C,* Palpation of the brachialis muscle through the biceps brachii using the neurologic reflex, reciprocal inhibition, to relax the biceps brachii (palpation guideline #5). Reciprocal inhibition is achieved in this case by having the client pronate the forearm at the RU joints, which is an action that is opposite to the action of supination of the forearm by the biceps brachii; therefore the biceps brachii relaxes, allowing the therapist to palpate the brachialis through it. Note: In *C,* the client is flexing her forearm (against gentle resistance by the therapist) to bring out the brachialis so it can be more easily palpated.

2. Know the actions of the target muscle so that you can ask the client to contract it. A contracted muscle is palpably firmer and easier to feel and discern from the adjacent soft tissue.

BOX 14-10

Assessment of a muscle is usually done to determine the resting tone of the muscle. Asking a client to contract a muscle is only done to help us find and locate the muscle. Once located, it is important to then ask the client to relax the muscle so that we can assess the resting tone of the muscle.

3. Add resistance—For a target muscle that is deep and more difficult to discern from adjacent musculature, it is often helpful to resist the client's contraction of the target muscle. Adding resistance causes the client to generate a forceful isometric contraction of the target muscle, making it even more palpable and discernable from adjacent muscles. When adding resistance, it is important that you do not place your hand that gives resistance beyond any joint other than the joint where the muscle is contracting. Otherwise, other muscles may contract that will cloud your ability to discern the target muscle (see Figure 14-6a).
4. Strum across the muscle—Once a muscle is contracted and taut, it can more easily be felt by strumming across the muscle. Whatever the direction of the fibers is, palpate (i.e., strum) the muscle perpendicular to that direction (see Figure 14-6b).
5. Use reciprocal inhibition—The idea of making a target muscle contract is to make it stand out from adjacent muscles. Therefore we ask the client to do an action of the target muscle that is different from the actions of the nearby muscles. However, sometimes the action (or actions) of the target muscle is the same as the action (or actions) of the adjacent muscles. In these instances, if we ask the client to do the action of the target muscle, then the adjacent muscle will also contract and it will be difficult to discern and feel the target muscle. This is especially true when the target muscle is deep to the adjacent muscle and contraction of this adjacent muscle would completely block our ability to palpate the deeper target muscle. In these instances, knowledge of the neurologic principle of reciprocal inhibition can be extremely valuable. (Note: For more information on the principle of reciprocal inhibition, see Section 16.3.) Reciprocal inhibition can be used by asking the client to do an action that is antagonistic to another action of the adjacent muscle that we want to relax. Doing this will cause this adjacent muscle to relax so that we can better palpate the target muscle (see Figure 14-6c).

BOX 14-11

Using reciprocal inhibition can be extremely valuable when trying to relax an adjacent or superficial muscle that blocks our ability to palpate the target muscle. However, even though reciprocal inhibition tends to relax this other muscle, if the client contracts the target muscle too forcefully, the nervous system will override the neurologic reflex of reciprocal inhibition and direct the muscle (that we wanted to relax) to contract. In this situation, reciprocal inhibition is overridden because the nervous system feels that it is more important to contract all muscles that can add to the strength of the joint action that the client is being asked to do, including contracting the muscle that was otherwise being reciprocally inhibited. For this reason, whenever using the principle of reciprocal inhibition, the client should not be asked to contract the target muscle too forcefully. In other words, only gentle resistance should be given to the contraction of the target muscle!

❑ Following are additional palpation guidelines that may prove useful:

1. Begin by palpating the target muscle in the easiest place possible. Once the target muscle has been palpated, it is usually easier to continue following it, even if it is deep to other muscles. For this reason, you must begin by finding and palpating the target muscle in the easiest location possible; then follow it to its attachments.
2. It is usually best to palpate with the pads of the fingers because they are the most sensitive.
3. Use appropriate pressure! Less can be more regarding palpatory pressure. Deeper pressure can be uncomfortable for the client and lessen your palpatory sensitivity. Having said that, many therapists press too lightly to feel deeper structures. Ideal palpatory pressure is *gentle but firm* and will also vary based on the depth of the muscle that is being palpated.
4. When you ask the client to actively contract a muscle so that you can palpate it (whether you resist the contraction or not), do not have the client sustain the isometric contraction for too long, because it may cause fatigue or injury to the client.
5. It is often helpful to ask the client to alternately contract and relax the target muscle. By doing this, you can better feel the changes in tissue texture when the muscle contracts and relaxes.
6. If a client is ticklish, have the client place his or her hand over your palpating hand. This will often lessen or eliminate the ticklishness. Being ticklish is oversensitivity as a result of a sense of intrusion on one's space (you cannot tickle yourself). By having the client's hand over your hand, that sense of intrusion is eliminated or diminished.

14.5 DO WE TREAT MOVERS OR ANTAGONISTS?

- When it comes to musculoskeletal treatment, treatment of muscles is usually the primary focus for most massage therapists, trainers, and other bodyworkers. However, a question arises: Which muscles do we treat?
- We have learned that muscles may act in many roles. Muscles may contract as movers, antagonists, fixators (i.e., stabilizers), neutralizers, and support muscles.
- When a client comes to the office and states that he or she has tightness/pain when turning the head to the right (i.e., right rotation of the head and neck at the spinal joints), what muscles come to mind to be assessed and treated?
  - When this question is asked of beginning students of kinesiology, 80% to 90% of the answers are muscles such as left upper trapezius, left sternocleidomastoid, right splenius capitis or cervicis, and so forth. In other words, most students immediately focus on the movers of the action of right rotation. Given that *mover actions* is the vehicle that we use to teach and learn muscles, this reaction should probably be expected. However, on further thought, why would we look to assess and treat movers of the action? Are the movers injured and not able to create their mover actions without pain? Perhaps this is the case; however, the most likely culprits are the antagonists.
- The most common problem that clients have causing restricted range of motion is tight muscles. Which muscles, if they are tight, would cause pain with right rotation? Right rotators? No. The left rotators that must lengthen and stretch when right rotation occurs are the muscles that will generate pain if they are tight. In other words, it will usually be tight antagonists that will be generating pain when a client performs a joint motion that is restricted and painful.
- This does not mean that we will not treat many clients with muscles that create pain when they perform their mover actions or muscles that are painful when they act as fixators, neutralizers, or support muscles. It simply means that more often it will be tight antagonists on the other side of the joint that will create pain when they are lengthened and stretched by a joint action.
- When a client has joint stiffness and pain, it is most prudent to assess every muscle and soft tissue that is stressed in any way during the joint actions. In fact, it may be a number of muscles or muscle groups that are involved in causing the pain. However, among all the possible muscles that are involved, the possibility that tight antagonists to joint motions are the most likely source of pain should be foremost in our thoughts for assessment and possible treatment.

14.6 DO WE TREAT SIGNS OR SYMPTOMS?

- When assessing a client's musculoskeletal condition, it is important to distinguish between signs and symptoms.
- **Signs** are objective (i.e., they are observable and measurable by someone other than the client). An example is a person's temperature. The client does not need to tell us that he or she has a fever; it is observable by palpation and measurable with a thermometer. Another example is the tone/tension level of a client's muscle. We do not need a client to tell us that he or she has a tight muscle; it can be objectively felt by the therapist.
- **Symptoms** are subjective (i.e., only the client can report them). An example is a client *feeling* feverish. No one but the client can report if the client feels feverish; that is a subjective statement only the client can report. Another example is a client's pain as a result of tight musculature. Only the client can experience and report the client's pain; no other person can tell a client what his or her pain level is.

BOX 14-12

Perhaps the best definition of pain comes from Margo McCaffery, a nurse in private practice. Her definition of pain is, ". . . whatever the experiencing person says it is, existing whenever he says it does."* The beauty of this definition is that it squarely recognizes that pain is a subjective symptom and must be defined by the client; it is not within the realm of a therapist or physician to define the client's pain! Therapists and physicians define signs, not symptoms. Symptoms must be reported by the client.

*From Porth CM: *Pathophysiology, concepts of altered health states,* ed 3, Philadelphia, 1990, JB Lippincott Co.

- It is crucially important to consider *both* the subjective symptoms that a client reports and the objective signs that we as therapists can determine. If a therapist bases all treatment on a client's subjective report of pain, the ability to accurately assess and effectively treat the cause of a client's condition is greatly diminished.

- Further, relying solely on a client's subjective pain to determine when treatment is appropriate and necessary can be dangerous for the health of the client. The experience of subjective symptoms usually lags far behind the presence of objective signs.
  - A mildly or moderately tight muscle is usually not felt by a client; the muscle usually has to get markedly tight before the client even experiences pain because of the tight muscle. Unfortunately, by that time the problem is larger, more chronically patterned into the client's body, and more difficult to improve with treatment.
- An analogy often made to clients to help them understand this concept is to explain that a cavity in a tooth begins forming long before the toothache appears. Waiting for muscle pain to appear before having massage, bodywork, or beginning a program of stretching and exercise, is similar to waiting for a toothache to appear before deciding to brush one's teeth.
- It is in the clients' best interest to encourage them to proactively approach their health. As therapists and trainers it is our job to educate clients about their musculoskeletal health and to treat signs, not just symptoms.

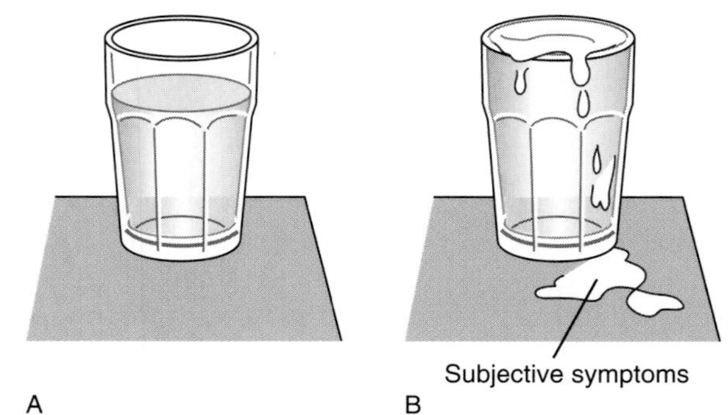

Figure 14-7 Analogy to a glass of water and a client's objective and subjective ill health/dysfunction. Amount of water in the glass *A* represents the degree of objective ill health of the client. However, as long as the glass contains the water, no subjective symptoms exist (i.e., the client feels fine). As soon as the level of dysfunction increases to the point that water spills out of the glass *B*, the water that spills out represents the subjective symptoms of the client (i.e., the client now feels the problem and knows that it is present). The point of this analogy is that objective dysfunction can build up for a long time before the client has symptoms and knows about the problem. A simple analogy such as this can help a client better see how to proactively approach his or her health care.

BOX 14-13

Although it is often in the best interest of the client to have massage, bodywork, or begin a physical exercise regimen of stretching and strengthening even when they are not experiencing pain or other symptoms, we must be careful that we always keep the client's best interest at heart when recommending a plan of care. It is highly unethical to recommend care to our clients that we know is unnecessary or inappropriate. Further, it is also unethical to push our clients into having care that they do not want to have, whether we feel it is in their best interest or not. Our role is to educate and encourage the client about his or her musculoskeletal health and offer options for care; it is up to client to accept or decline that advice and care.

- Another analogy used when explaining the value of massage, exercise, and other bodywork to a client who is focusing only on the level of his or her pain and other symptoms is to liken a person's condition and symptoms to a glass of water (Figure 14-7). In this analogy, water in the glass represents an accumulation of bad health on the part of the client (it would be a measure of the objective degree of the problem). The more water in the glass, the unhealthier the client. However, as long as the water is contained in the glass, the client experiences no symptoms because of the condition. However, once the glass is unable to contain the water and some of it spills out onto the counter, the client feels pain. In this analogy, the amount of water on the counter is equivalent to the degree of subjective pain experienced by the client. However, the water on the counter *and* the water that fills the glass is a more accurate representation of the objective degree of the client's actual condition. If we treat the client only long enough to eliminate the water that has spilled onto the counter, then even though the person now feels fine, the glass is full to the top and the slightest additional stress to the system will cause water to spill over again and create pain once again. At this point it is likely that an uneducated client will say that massage, exercise, and bodywork are nice, but their effects do not last. This type of approach does not help the health of the client and does not help the reputation of our work. Although we cannot fully empty the client's glass and return the client back to the health they had as a child or teenager, we should at least endeavor to do more than just stop the glass from spilling over. Instead we should try to somewhat lessen the water level below the top of the glass. By doing this, the client will have some leeway to encounter stress without every little stressor recreating the pain pattern. A reasonable approach like this is what is ultimately in the best interest of the client.
- Treating symptoms is analogous to only mopping up the water that has spilled on the counter. Treating signs is equivalent to treating the client to lessen the level of water in the glass and improve the client's condition now and into the future. What do you treat? Symptoms or signs?

REVIEW QUESTIONS

evolve Answers to the following review questions appear on the Evolve website accompanying this book.

1. What is the difference between active and passive range of motion.

2. Give an example of active range of motion; give an example of passive range of motion.

3. What type of joint motion is possible at the end of passive joint motion?

4. What is the difference between joint play and an osseous adjustment?

5. Give an example of a ballistic motion.

6. Resisted motion results in what type of muscular contraction?

7. What is an orthopedic test procedure?

8. Describe how active range of motion, passive range of motion, and resisted motion can be used to assess musculoskeletal soft tissue injuries.

9. What is the difference between a sprain and a strain?

10. What is the difference between an assessment and a diagnosis?

11. What are the five major guidelines to palpating a muscle?

12. Describe and give an example of reciprocal inhibition when palpating a muscle.

13. Explain why tight/injured antagonists are more likely the cause of a problem than tight/injured mover muscles.

14. If a client arrives at your office with decreased flexion of the right thigh at the hip joint, what musculature would most likely need to be treated (i.e., what musculature would you first look to assess and treat)?

15. What is the difference between signs and symptoms?

16. Describe how signs and symptoms are used in assessing a client's condition.

NOTES

Chapter 15

Determining the Force of a Muscle Contraction

CHAPTER OUTLINE

CHAPTER OBJECTIVES

After completing this chapter, the student should be able to perform the following:

- ❑ Describe how a muscle can have a partial contraction, and explain the meaning of the Henneman size principle.
- ❑ Explain the difference between the intrinsic strength of a muscle and the extrinsic strength of a muscle.
- ❑ Describe the various types of muscle fiber architecture, and explain the advantages/disadvantages of longitudinal versus pennate muscles.
- ❑ Describe active tension and passive tension of a muscle.
- ❑ Explain the relationship between the sliding filament mechanism and shortened active insufficiency and lengthened active insufficiency.
- ❑ Give an example of shortened active insufficiency and lengthened active insufficiency.
- ❑ Interpret the length-tension relationship curve for active tension, passive tension, and total tension of a muscle.
- ❑ Explain the meaning of the active, passive, and total tension curves of the length-tension relationship curve.
- ❑ Describe the relationship between the concepts of the sliding filament mechanism, active length-tension relationship curve, and active insufficiency.
- ❑ Explain the relationship between leverage and the extrinsic strength of a muscle.
- ❑ Describe the advantage and disadvantage of a muscle with greater leverage.
- ❑ Define the terms *internal force* and *external force,* and give an example of each.
- ❑ Explain why a muscle with an attachment that has a less than optimal angle of pull loses extrinsic strength.
- ❑ Explain how to determine the lever arm of a muscle.
- ❑ List the three classes of levers, and give a mechanical object and muscular example of each one.
- ❑ Define the resistance force to a muscle's contraction, and give two examples of a resistance force.
- ❑ Sketch the region of the body where a muscle is contracting, and draw in the arrows that represent the force of the muscle contraction and the resistance force that opposes the muscle contraction.
- ❑ Define the key terms of this chapter.
- ❑ State the meanings of the word origins of this chapter.

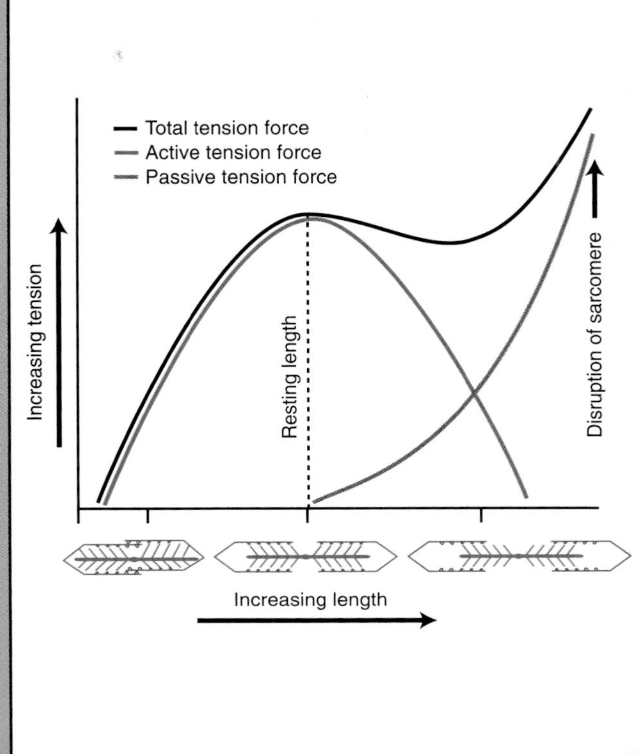

OVERVIEW

The all-or-none response law states that a muscle fiber either contracts all the way or not at all. Therefore a muscle fiber cannot have a partial contraction. The all-or-none response law also applies to motor units, because if any one muscle fiber of the motor unit is instructed to contract, then every muscle fiber of that motor unit will contract. Therefore a motor unit cannot have a partial contraction either. However, the all-or-none response law does not apply to an entire muscle. A muscle is an organ made up of many motor units, some of which may be ordered to contract and others not. Therefore a muscle can have a partial contraction. How strong a muscle's contraction will be is dependent on many factors. It is the focus of this chapter to examine the factors that affect the strength of a muscle's contraction, whether it is a partial or full contraction. Some of these factors are trinsic to the muscle, such as the active tension and ıssive tension of the muscle. A number of factors are trinsic to the muscle, such as the leverage of the ıscle's pulling force, including the angle at which the ıscle pulls on its bony attachment. Gravity must also be considered when evaluating the ability of a muscle contraction to create movement of the body. This chapter explores these intrinsic and extrinsic factors that determine the pulling force (i.e., the strength of a muscle's contraction).

EY TERMS

tive insufficiency
tive tension
is of motion (AK-sis)
ennate muscle (buy-PEN-nate)
ort arm
ternal forces
trinsic strength (ek-STRINS-ik)
ı-shaped muscle
st (1st)-class lever
rce-velocity relationship curve
siform-shaped muscle (FUSE-i-form)
nneman size principle (HEN-i-man)
ernal forces
rinsic strength (in-TRINS-ik)
ıgthened active insufficiency
ıgth-tension relationship curve
ver
ver arm
verage
ıgitudinal muscle
chanical advantage
chanical disadvantage
Moment arm
Multipennate muscle (MUL-tee-PEN-nate)
Muscle fiber architecture
Optimal angle of pull
Passive tension
Pennate muscle (PEN-nate)
Pennation angle (pen-NAY-shun)
Rectangular-shaped muscle
Resistance to movement
Rhomboidal-shaped muscle (rom-BOYD-al)
Second (2nd)-class lever
Shortened active insufficiency
Sphincter muscle (SFINGK-ter)
Spindle-shaped muscle
Spiral muscle
Squat bend
Stoop bend
Strap muscle
Third (3rd)-class lever
Triangular-shaped muscle
Unipennate muscle (YOU-nee-PEN-nate)

ORD ORIGINS

- ctive—From Latin *activus,* meaning *doing, driving*
- i—From Latin *bis,* meaning *two, twice*
- xtrinsic—From Latin *extrinsecus,* meaning *from without*
- ntrinsic—From Latin *intrinsecus,* meaning *on the inside*
- ever/leverage—From Latin *levis,* meaning *light, not heavy*
- ❑ Longitudinal—From Latin *longitudo,* meaning *length*
- ❑ Motor—From Latin *moveo,* meaning *a mover*
- ❑ Multi—From Latin *multus,* meaning *many, much*
- ❑ Passiv—From Latin *passives,* meaning *permit, endures*
- ❑ Pennate—From Latin *penna,* meaning *feather*
- ❑ Tension—From Latin *tensio,* meaning *to stretch*
- ❑ Uni—From Latin *unis,* meaning *one*

15.1 PARTIAL CONTRACTION OF A MUSCLE

- A muscle is an organ composed of many muscle fibers that are grouped into motor units. According to the all-or-none response law, a muscle fiber either contracts all the way, or not at all. Because whatever instruction is given to one muscle fiber is given to all muscle fibers of a motor unit, the all-or-none law also applies to a motor unit (i.e., all muscle fibers of a motor unit either contract all the way or they do not contract at all). (Note: For more information on motor units and the all-or-none response law, see Sections 10.9 and 10.10.)
- When looking at the contraction of motor units, a hierarchy of motor unit recruitment exists.
  - Generally when a muscle needs a weak contraction, a smaller motor unit is recruited to contract.
  - If the muscle then needs a stronger contraction, the muscle recruits a larger motor unit *in addition to* the smaller one that is already contracting.

BOX 15-1

Physiologists who study muscle function often like to say that when it comes to ordering musculature of the body to contract, the brain thinks in motor units, not muscles. Although this might be a strong statement, a certain truth to it exists. Neurons do not control muscles per se; they control the contraction of motor units. In that sense, it is the coordination of motor units of the body, not muscles, that creates the movement patterns of the body!

  - By starting with small motor units and then incrementally adding on increasingly larger motor units, a smooth transition occurs as a muscle begins its contraction and then increases the strength of its contraction.
  - This hierarchy of how motor units are recruited to contract is called the **Henneman size principle**.

BOX 15-2

A relationship exists between the size of a motor neuron, the size of a motor unit, and the type of muscle fibers that are within that motor unit. Generally, smaller motor units are innervated by smaller motor neurons and contain red, slow-twitch muscle fibers, which are more adapted toward creating joint stabilization, whereas larger motor units are innervated by larger motor neurons and contain white, fast-twitch muscle fibers, which are more adapted toward creating joint movement. Therefore when a joint action is ordered by the central nervous system (CNS), the smaller motor units that initially contract are meant to create stabilization of the joint before larger motor units are recruited to create the larger motion at that joint. (For more on joint stabilization, see Sections 13.5 and 13.6.)

- Although muscle fibers and motor units obey the all-or-none response law, muscles can have partial contractions.
- A number of factors should be considered when examining the intrinsic strength of a muscle's contraction:

BOX 15-3 SPOTLIGHT ON INTRINSIC VERSUS EXTRINSIC STRENGTH OF A MUSCLE

The strength of a muscle can be defined as the strength of its pulling force on its bony attachment(s). The overall strength of a muscle is a combination of two aspects: (1) the muscle's intrinsic strength and (2) the muscle's extrinsic strength. The **intrinsic strength** of a muscle is defined as the strength that the muscle generates within itself (i.e., intrinsically). It is a result of the strength that the muscle generates internally because of the sliding filament mechanism (i.e., active tension) and the elastic recoil property of the tissues of the muscle (i.e., passive tension). The intrinsic strength of a muscle is independent of the external surroundings. However, the intrinsic strength of a muscle is not the totality of the strength that a muscle displays when it contracts and pulls on its attachments. To complete the picture, the extrinsic strength of the muscle must also be taken into account. The **extrinsic strength** of a muscle takes into account all the factors outside of the muscle itself. These factors include such things as the leverage that the muscle has on its attachments, as well as the angle of the muscle's pull relative to the joint where the movement is occurring. Only when considering intrinsic and extrinsic factors can the sum total of a muscle's effect on its attachments (i.e., its strength) be understood. (Factors that affect the intrinsic strength of a muscle are covered in Sections 15.1 through 15.5; extrinsic factors that affect the muscle's strength are covered in Sections 15.6 through 15.9.)

- The most obvious factor regarding the strength or degree of a muscle's contraction is simply how many motor units are ordered to contract by the nervous system.
- If every motor unit of a muscle contracts, then the muscle will contract at 100% of its maximum strength (i.e., the muscle will have a full contraction).
- If only some motor units are ordered to contract, then the muscle will have a partial contraction.
- The degree of this partial contraction is not only determined by the number of motor units that contract but also by the number of muscle fibers in these motor units.
  - If, for example, a muscle has a total of 1000 fibers and three of its motor units contract, and if these three motor units each have 50, 100, and 250 muscle fibers in them respectively, then a total of 400 muscle fibers out of 1000 muscle fibers are contracting, yielding a 40% contraction of the muscle.
  - If instead, a muscle with a total of 1000 fibers has three motor units contract with 100, 200, and 300

fibers each, then that muscle has 600 muscle fibers contract out of 1000 muscle fibers and has a 60% contraction of the muscle.

- ❑ In both cases three motor units contracted, but the degree of strength of the contraction was determined by the number of muscle fibers that contracted, not the number of motor units.

❑ Therefore, a better determination of the strength of a muscle's contraction would be to count the number of muscle fibers that contract.

❑ However, not all muscle fibers are the same. For example, when a person does strengthening exercises and builds up the muscles, the number of muscle fibers does not change; what changes is the size of each fiber. With exercise, the number of sarcomeres and the number of contractile proteins (i.e., actin, myosin) increases. As a result, some muscle fibers are larger and stronger than others.

- ❑ Therefore the very best determinant of the strength of a muscle's contraction is the number of cross-bridges that are made between myosin and actin. A muscle is really nothing more than a great number of sarcomeres with cross-bridges that create a pulling force!

BOX 15-4

When looking at the strength of a muscle's contraction, even the number of myosin-actin cross-bridges is not the final determinant. Another factor must be considered (i.e., the orientation of the pull of the cross-bridges relative to the line of pull of the muscle itself). The orientation of the pull of the cross-bridges is determined by the orientation of the pull of the muscle fibers (i.e., the architecture of the muscle fibers relative to the muscle). (For more on the architecture of muscle fibers, see Section 15.2.)

❑ 15.2 MUSCLE FIBER ARCHITECTURE

❑ The orientation, in other words the arrangement of muscle fibers within a muscle, is called **muscle fiber architecture**.

❑ Muscles have two general architectural types in which their fibers are arranged: (1) longitudinal and (2) pennate.

Longitudinal Muscles:

❑ A **longitudinal muscle** has its fibers running longitudinally (i.e., along the length of the muscle). Most fibers of a longitudinal muscle run the full length of a muscle from attachment to attachment. (For more information on how muscles fibers are arranged within a muscle, see Section 10.3.)

- ❑ Therefore the force of the contraction of the fibers is in the same direction as the length of the muscle.

❑ Longitudinal muscles can be divided into various categories based on the shape. The following are the most common types of longitudinal muscles (Figure 15-1):

- ❑ **Fusiform** (also known as **spindle**)
- ❑ **Strap**
- ❑ **Rectangular**
- ❑ **Rhomboidal**
- ❑ **Triangular** (also known as **fan shaped**)

❑ Note: Other types of muscles such as a **sphincter muscle** [circular muscle; example: the orbicularis oculi] and a **spiral muscle** [muscle with a twist; example: the latissimus dorsi] may also be placed into the category of longitudinal muscles.

Pennate Muscles:

❑ A **pennate muscle** has its fibers arranged in a featherlike manner. The fibers are not arranged along the length of the muscle; rather, a central fibrous tendon runs along the length of the muscle. The muscle fibers themselves are arranged obliquely (i.e., at an angle) to the central tendon of the muscle.

- ❑ Therefore the force of the contraction of the fibers is not in the same direction as length of the muscle!

❑ Pennate muscles are divided into three types: (1) unipennate, (2) bipennate, and (3) multipennate (Figure 15-2).

BOX 15-5

The word *pennate* means *featherlike*. The word *pen* has the same origin, because pens were originally made from quills (i.e., feathers).

- ❑ A **unipennate muscle** has a central tendon within the muscle, and the fibers are oriented diagonally off one side of the tendon. An example of a unipennate muscle is the vastus lateralis muscle of the quadriceps femoris group.
- ❑ A **bipennate muscle** has a central tendon within the muscle, and the fibers are oriented diagonally off both sides of the tendon. An example of a bipennate muscle is the rectus femoris muscle of the quadriceps femoris group.
- ❑ A **multipennate muscle** has more than one central tendon with fibers oriented diagonally either

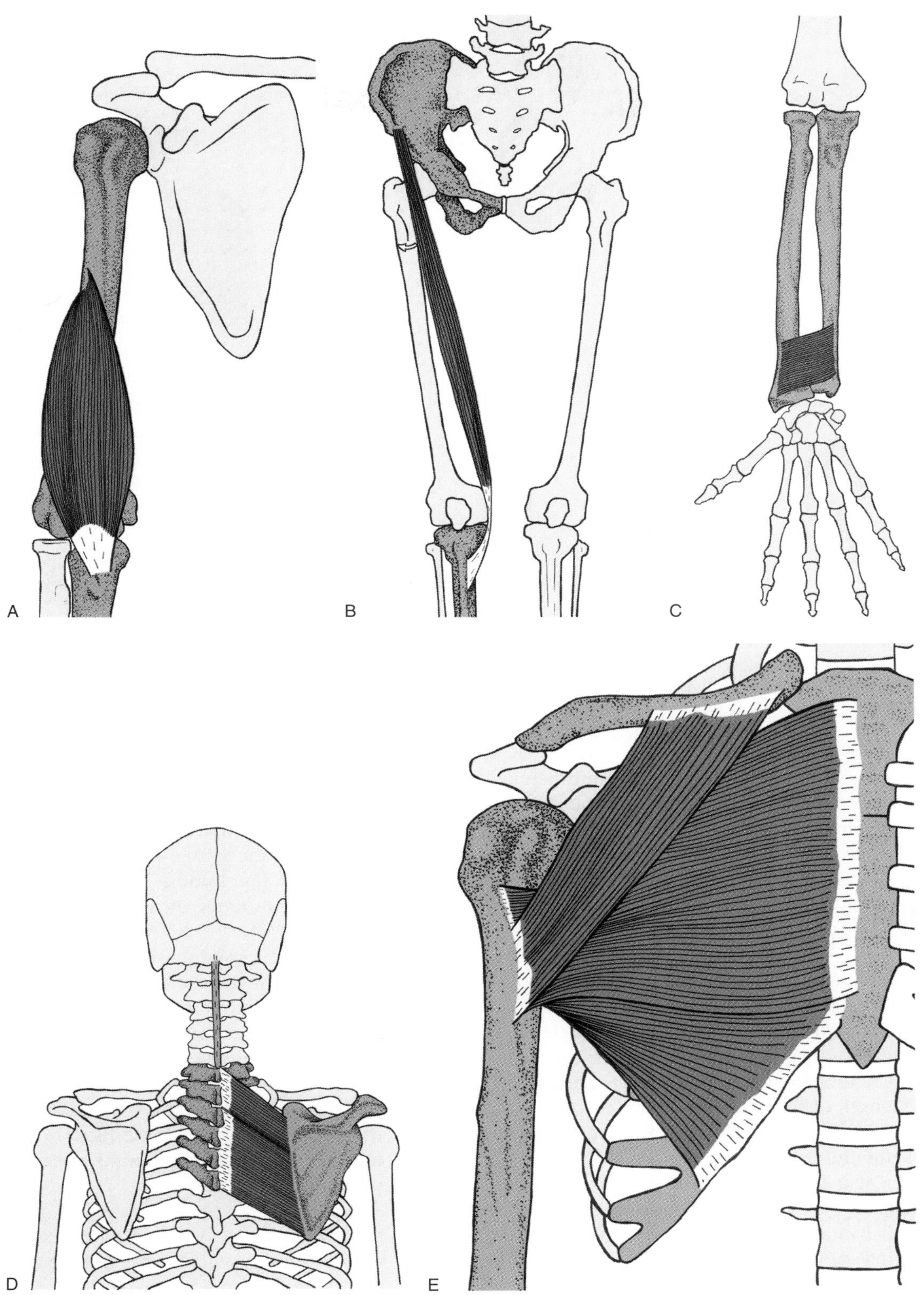

Figure 15-1 Various architectural types of longitudinal muscles. *A,* Brachialis demonstrates a fusiform-shaped (also known as *spindle shaped*) muscle. *B,* Sartorius demonstrates a strap muscle. *C,* Pronator quadratus demonstrates a rectangular-shaped muscle. *D,* Rhomboid muscles demonstrate rhomboidal-shaped muscles. *E,* Pectoralis major demonstrates a triangular-shaped (also known as *fan shaped*) muscle. (From Muscolino JE: *The muscular system manual: the skeletal muscles of the human body,* ed 2, St Louis, 2005, Mosby.)

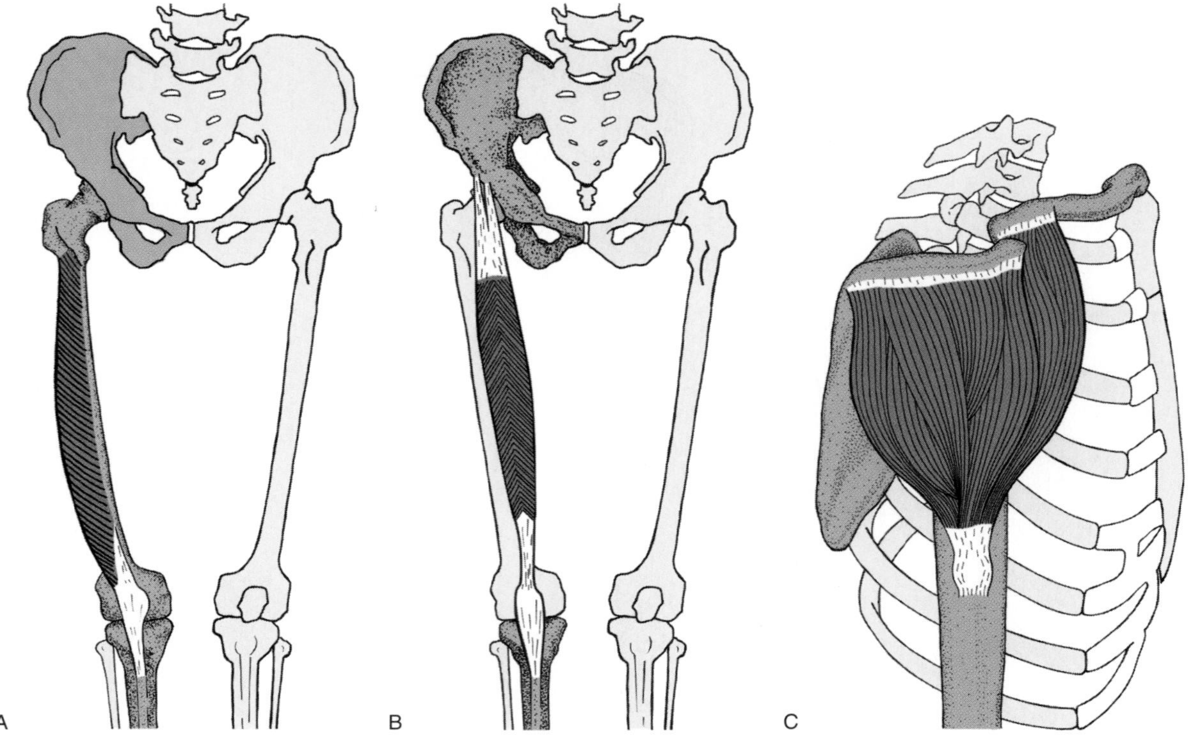

Figure 15-2 The three architectural types of pennate muscles. Pennate muscles have one or more central tendons running along the length of the muscle from which the muscle fibers come off at an oblique angle. *A,* Vastus lateralis is a unipennate muscle. (Note: Central tendon is not visible in the anterior view.) *B,* Rectus femoris is a bipennate muscle. *C,* Deltoid is a multipennate muscle. (From Muscolino JE: *The muscular system manual: the skeletal muscles of the human body,* ed 2, St Louis, 2005, Mosby.)

to one and/or both sides. In effect, a multipennate muscle has combinations of unipennate and bipennate arrangements. An example of a multipennate muscle is the deltoid muscle.

Longitudinal and Pennate Muscles Compared:

- ❑ A longitudinal muscle has long muscle fibers; a pennate muscle has short muscle fibers.
  - ❑ However, a pennate muscle has more muscle fibers than a longitudinal muscle.
- ❑ Further, the fibers of a longitudinal muscle are oriented along the length of the muscle, whereas the fibers of a pennate muscle are oriented at an oblique angle to the length of the muscle.
  - ❑ However, if a longitudinal muscle and a pennate muscle of the same overall size are compared, they will both contain the same mass of muscle tissue. Hence they will both contain the same number of sarcomeres and therefore the same number of myosin-actin cross-bridges.
- ❑ Because a muscle fiber can shorten to approximately $^1/_2$ of its resting length when it maximally concentrically contracts, longitudinal muscles, having longer fibers, shorten more than pennate muscles.
  - ❑ Therefore a longitudinal muscle is ideally suited to create a large range of motion of a body part at a joint.
- ❑ Pennate muscles have shorter fibers but have a greater number of them than longitudinal muscles.
  - ❑ Given that a pennate muscle has the same number of sarcomeres generating strength as a same-sized longitudinal muscle, but that same strength is concentrated over a shorter range of motion (because of the shorter fibers arranged at an oblique angle to the direction of the muscle [Box 15-6]), a pennate muscle exhibits greater strength over a shorter range of motion.
  - ❑ Therefore a longitudinal muscle is generally better suited for a greater range of motion contraction but with less force; whereas a pennate muscle is generally better suited for greater strength contraction over a shorter range of motion.

BOX 15-6 SPOTLIGHT ON THE PENNATION ANGLE

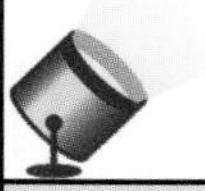

When determining the strength of a muscle, especially pennate muscles, one other factor needs to be taken into consideration, that is, the **pennation angle**. The pennation angle is the angle of the muscle fiber relative to the central tendon of the muscle. If a muscle fiber is parallel to its tendon (i.e., running along the length of the muscle as in longitudinal muscles), then its pennation angle is zero degrees and all of its pulling force pulls along the length of the tendon, pulling the attachments of the muscle toward the center of the muscle. However, as the angle of the muscle fiber becomes more oblique (as in pennate muscles), the pennation angle increases, the pull of the fiber is less in line with the tendon, and less of its contraction force contributes to the pull on the attachments. For this reason, as much as pennate muscles are designed to generate a greater force over a relatively small range of motion, some of the strength is lost because of the greater pennation angle (see figures).

In other words, the greater the pennation angle, the more fibers can be fit in the same mass and the greater relative strength over a shorter range of motion; however, some of the intrinsic strength of the muscle fibers is lost because they are not pulling along the length of the muscle! To determine the effect of the pennation angle on the strength of the muscle, trigonometry is used. A trigonometric formula can be used to determine what percentage of a pennate fiber's contraction contributes to the pulling force that occurs along the length of the muscle, because it is this force that effectively pulls the muscle's attachments toward the center of the muscle. For example, a fiber with a pennation angle of 30 degrees contributes 86% of its force to pulling the attachments toward the center, and a fiber with a pennation angle of 60 degrees contributes 50% of its force to pulling the attachments toward the center.

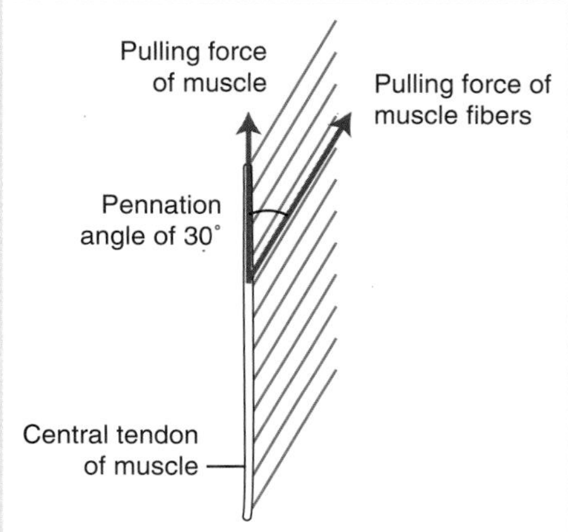

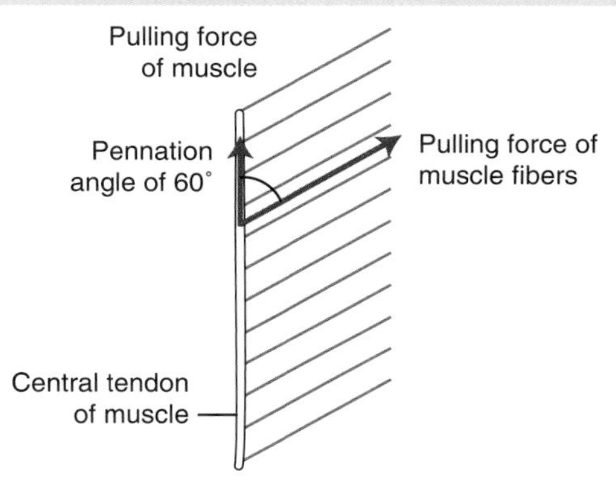

☐ 15.3 ACTIVE TENSION VERSUS PASSIVE TENSION

- When we talk about a muscle generating a forceful contraction, it is important to remember that a muscle can generate two types of forces: (1) an active force and (2) a passive force.
- The term *tension* is used to describe the pulling force that a muscle generates.

BOX 15-7

Interestingly, the word *tension,* which is used to describe pulling forces and therefore the degree of a muscle's contraction (i.e., its pulling force), actually means *stretch.* Perhaps the derivation of its use is that when something is being pulled on, it is stretched.

  - Therefore a muscle may pull on its attachments with active tension and with passive tension.

Active Tension:

- **Active tension** of a muscle is generated by the sliding filament mechanism (i.e., its contraction). This tension is termed *active,* because the muscle is actively creating this force (i.e., the muscle is expending energy in the form of adenosine triphosphate [ATP] to generate a contraction via actins being pulled by the cross-bridges of myosins toward the center of the sarcomere).
  - Hence this aspect of a muscle's pulling force is called *active tension.*

Passive Tension:

- A muscle can also generate a **passive tension** force that can contribute to its active tension pulling force.
- This passive force is created primarily by the fascia of the muscle.
- When a muscle is stretched beyond its resting length, the fascia of the muscle is stretched longer. Because the muscular fascia is elastic in nature, the stretched fascia will try to elastically bounce back to its resting length, creating a pulling force back toward its center.
- An analogy can be made to a rubber/elastic band. When an elastic band is stretched, its natural elasticity creates a pulling force that would pull on whatever is holding the elastic band in this stretched position. In a similar manner, all soft tissue, and especially muscular fascia, is elastic.
  - Therefore a stretched muscle would have an elastic pulling force that would pull the muscle's attachments toward the center of the muscle.
- This pulling force adds to the tension that a muscle generates on its attachments.

BOX 15-8

Most sports have a backswing before the actual stroke is performed; examples include the backswing in tennis, golf, or baseball. One reason for a backswing is that it first stretches the muscle that will be performing the stroke. This adds the passive elastic recoil force to the active contraction force of the muscle when it performs the stroke. The net result is a more powerful pulling force by the muscle!

- This elastic tension force is termed *passive tension,* because a muscle does not actively generate it (i.e., the muscle expends no energy to create it; it is inherent in the natural elasticity of the tissue).

Total Tension

- Hence the active tension of a muscle is generated by its contractile actin and myosin proteins, and the passive tension of a muscle is due to the natural elasticity of the fascia of the muscle.
- Therefore the total tension of a muscle, both its active and passive tension, must be measured when determining the force of a muscle's contraction.

☐ 15.4 ACTIVE INSUFFICIENCY

❑ Active tension describes the tension or force of contraction that a muscle can actively generate via the sliding filament mechanism.

❑ We have already said that the active strength of a muscle's contraction is based on the number of cross-bridges that exist between myosin and actin filaments.

  ❑ Therefore if the number of cross-bridges were to decrease, the strength of the muscle's contraction would decrease.

❑ If the strength of a muscle's contraction decreases sufficiently, the muscle could be said to be insufficient in strength.

  ❑ Hence an actively insufficient muscle is a muscle that cannot generate sufficient strength actively via the sliding filament mechanism.

  ❑ Therefore **active insufficiency** is the term used to describe a muscle that is weak because of a decrease in the number of myosin-actin cross-bridges during the sliding filament mechanism.

❑ Two states of active insufficiency exist: (1) shortened active insufficiency and (2) lengthened active insufficiency.

Shortened Active Insufficiency:

❑ **Shortened active insufficiency** of a muscle occurs when a muscle is shorter than its resting length and weak because of a decrease in myosin-actin cross-bridges.

❑ To understand why this situation occurs, we will compare a sarcomere at resting length with a sarcomere that is shortened (Figure 15-3).

❑ Figure 15-3b, shows a sarcomere at rest. At rest, we see that every myosin head is able to form cross-bridges by binding to the adjacent actin filaments. Given this maximal number of cross-bridge formation, the sarcomere at rest can generate maximal pulling force and is therefore strong.

❑ In Figure 15-3a, we see a sarcomere that is shortened. In a shortened sarcomere, the actin filaments overlap each other in such as way that some of the binding (active) sites on one of the actin filaments are blocked by the other actin filament (and some of the binding sites of the actin filament that is overlapping the other are too close toward the center and also not accessible by the myosin heads). Therefore the myosin heads that would normally form cross-bridges by attaching to those binding sites are unable to do so. This results in fewer cross-bridges. A sarcomere that forms fewer cross-bridges cannot generate as much pulling force, and its strength is diminished. Because a shortened muscle is composed of shortened sarcomeres, a shortened muscle exhibits shortened active insufficiency and is weaker because it forms fewer myosin-actin cross-bridges!

Lengthened Active Insufficiency:

❑ **Lengthened active insufficiency** of a muscle occurs when a muscle is longer than its resting length and weak because of a decrease in myosin-actin cross-bridges.

❑ To understand why this situation occurs, compare a sarcomere at resting length with a sarcomere that is lengthened (see Figure 15-3).

❑ Again, Figure 15-3b, shows a sarcomere at rest in which every myosin head is able to form cross-bridges by binding to the adjacent actin filaments. Given this maximal number of cross-bridge formation, the sarcomere at rest can generate maximal pulling force and is therefore strong.

❑ In Figure 15-3c, we see a sarcomere that is lengthened. In a lengthened sarcomere, the actin filaments are pulled so far from the center of the sarcomere that many of the myosin heads cannot reach the actin filaments to form cross-bridges. Therefore many of the

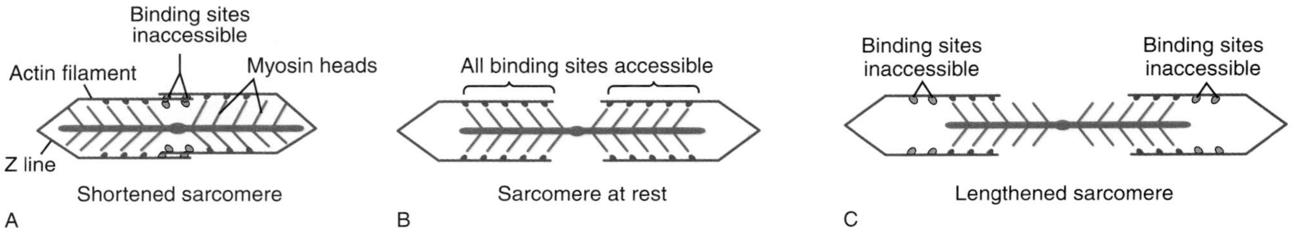

Figure 15-3 Sarcomere at three different lengths. *A,* Shortened sarcomere. *B,* Same sarcomere at resting length. *C,* Same sarcomere lengthened. (Note: The sarcomere at resting length can produce the greatest number of myosin-actin cross-bridges and therefore can produce the strongest contraction.) Fewer possible cross-bridges formed when the sarcomere is shorter or longer results in weakness of the muscle, called *active insufficiency* (i.e., shortened active insufficiency in *A*; lengthened active insufficiency in *C*).

myosin heads that would normally form cross-bridges are unable to do so. This results in fewer cross-bridges. A sarcomere that forms fewer cross-bridges cannot generate as much pulling force and its strength is diminished. Because a lengthened muscle is composed of lengthened sarcomeres, a lengthened muscle exhibits lengthened active insufficiency and is weaker because it forms fewer myosin-actin cross-bridges!

- An excellent example of both shortened active insufficiency and lengthened active insufficiency are shown in Figure 15-4. When a person makes a fist, the muscles that make a fist are the flexors of the fingers and thumb, and the specific muscles responsible for this action are primarily the extrinsic flexors that attach proximally in the arm/forearm (flexor digitorum superficialis, flexor digitorum profundus, flexor pollicis longus). These extrinsic flexors cross the wrist joint anteriorly to enter the hand; then they cross the metacarpophalangeal (MCP) and interphalangeal (IP) joints to enter the fingers.
- If the wrist joint is flexed as in Figure 15-4a, these extrinsic muscles would shorten across the wrist joint, and because of shortened active insufficiency, would be unable to generate sufficient strength to move the fingers and make a strong fist.

BOX 15-9

Another classic example that demonstrates shortened active insufficiency is abdominal curl-ups (i.e., crunches). A number of years ago, when people did sit-ups, they were done with the hip and knee joints straight. However, that style sit-up was found to excessively strengthen and most likely tighten the iliopsoas muscle, which could then have deleterious effects on the posture of the spine. Now it is routinely taught to bend the hip and knee joints when doing a sit-up (now termed a *curl-up* or *crunch*). The reason for bending the hip joint is to shorten the iliopsoas by bringing its attachments closer together (flexing the thigh at the hip joint brings the lesser trochanter closer to the pelvis and spine). By doing this, the iliopsoas becomes shortened and actively insufficient; therefore is not as readily recruited during the curl-up and is not strengthened as much. It should be noted that it is often recommended to not go past 30 degrees with a curl-up because at that point the iliopsoas will be recruited despite being actively insufficient.

- If the wrist joint is extended instead (as in Figure 15-4c), these muscles would be stretched longer across the wrist joint and, because of lengthened active insufficiency, would be unable to generate sufficient strength to move the fingers and make a strong fist. Compare your ability to make a fist when your wrist joint is flexed or extended with your ability to make a fist when your wrist joint is in a neutral position (see Figure 15-4b).

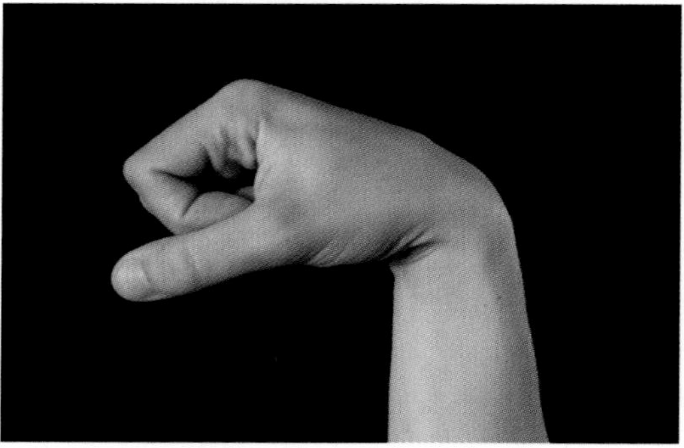

A

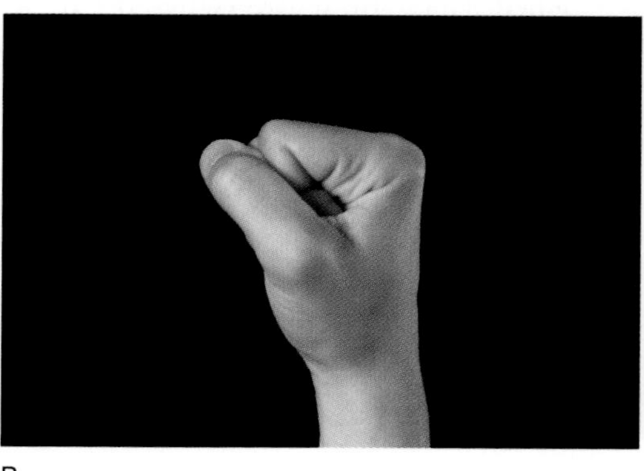

B

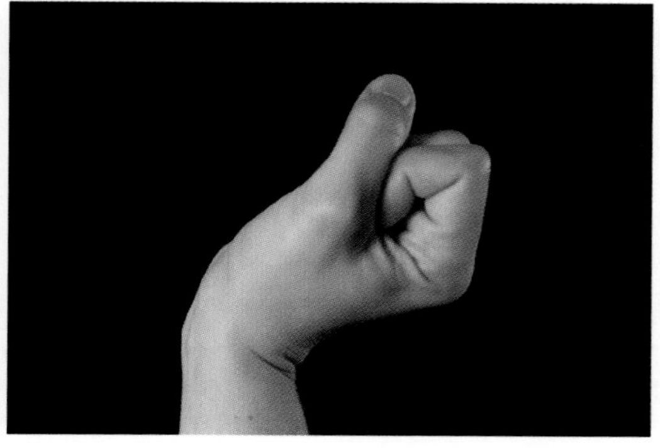

C

Figure 15-4 Concept of active insufficiency of the extrinsic finger flexor muscles that attach proximally in the arm/forearm. When these muscles contract to make a fist with the hand flexed at the wrist joint, these muscles become shortened and actively insufficient, resulting in a fist that is weak *(A)*. When these muscles contract to make a fist with the hand extended at the wrist joint, these muscles become lengthened and actively insufficient, also resulting in a fist that is weak *(C)*. However, when a fist is made with the hand in neutral position at the wrist joint, the strength of the fist is optimal *(B)*. (Courtesy Joseph E. Muscolino.)

15.5 LENGTH-TENSION RELATIONSHIP CURVE

- Given the concepts of passive tension and shortened and lengthened active insufficiency, it is clear that the length of a muscle has an effect on the tension that it can generate (i.e., the strength of its pulling force).
- The relationship between the length of a muscle and the active tension that a muscle can generate is related to the length of the sarcomeres and the tension that the sarcomeres can generate as has been explained in earlier sections of this chapter. This relationship can be depicted on a graph called the **length-tension relationship curve** (Figure 15-5).
- The length-tension relationship curve is a graph that compares the length of a sarcomere with the percentage of maximal contraction that the sarcomere can generate. Because a muscle is effectively composed of many sarcomeres, the relationship between the length and tension of a sarcomere can be extrapolated to the relationship between the length and tension of an entire muscle. (Note: The active length-tension relationship curve depicted in Figure 15-5 was created by measuring the contractile force of an isometric contraction for the continuum of lengths displayed. Some researchers caution that the values derived may not be able to be 100% correlated to concentric and eccentric contractions.)

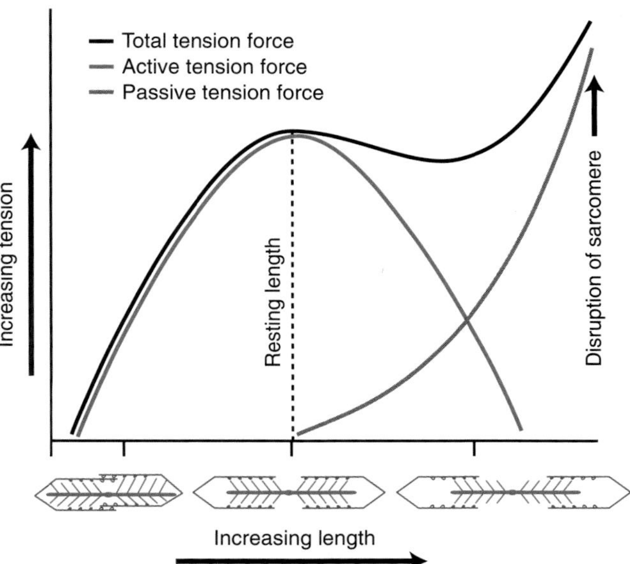

Figure 15-5 Three sarcomere length-tension relationship curves. These curves depict the relationship between the length of a sarcomere and the tension that it generates (i.e., its pulling force) at that length. Whatever information is given in these curves is helpful because it can be applied to the concept of the tension of the muscle itself. The red line represents the active tension force that a sarcomere can generate when it contracts via the sliding filament mechanism. (Note: The strength of the sarcomere's contraction is strongest at resting length where the maximal number of myosin-actin cross-bridges can form and weakest when the sarcomere is shortest and longest [i.e., where the sarcomere is actively insufficient because of fewer cross-bridges].) The brown line represents the passive tension force that the sarcomere generates when it is stretched. (Note: Passive tension force is zero at resting length and increases as the sarcomere is stretched longer [at the end of the passive tension curve would be tearing and disruption of the sarcomere].). The black line represents the sum total of the active tension curve and the passive tension curve; therefore it represents the total pulling force of the sarcomere.

BOX 15-10

There is another relationship curve for muscles called the **force-velocity relationship curve;** it states that the faster a muscle contracts, the weaker its contraction force becomes.

Extrapolating these values for an entire muscle, we see the following:

- The red line in Figure 15-5 considers only the active tension as the length of a muscle changes. The shape of this curve is a bell curve wherein the greatest tension is clearly when the muscle is at resting length. When the length of the muscle changes in either direction (i.e., gets longer or shorter), the active tension that the muscle can generate decreases.
  - Lessened active tension when a muscle is shortened is called *shortened active insufficiency*.
  - Lessened active tension when a muscle is lengthened is called *lengthened active insufficiency*.
- The brown line in Figure 15-5 considers only the passive tension as the length of the muscle changes. We see that passive tension is nonexistent when the muscle is shortened. However, as the muscle lengthens beyond resting length, the passive tension of the muscle increases.
  - This increased passive tension of a muscle as it lengthens is called *passive tension* and is due to the natural elasticity of the tissue.
- The black line in Figure 15-5 considers both the active tension and the passive tension of a muscle as its length changes.
  - We see that the overall tension (i.e., pulling force of the muscle) increases from a shortened length to resting length. The tension force in this range of the muscle's length is due to increasing active tension.
  - The pulling force then stays fairly high beyond resting length for quite some time. Most of the tension in this range of the muscle's length is due to increasing passive tension.
  - It is important to note that (as the graph shows) even though the total tension/pulling force of a muscle is greatest when it is longest, working a muscle at a much lengthened state is very dangerous, because at the end of this curve is tearing/disruption of the muscle tissue!

15.6 LEVERAGE OF A MUSCLE

Up until now we have been discussing factors that affect the intrinsic strength of a muscle. However, extrinsic factors also affect the strength with which the muscle can move a body part.

- A major extrinsic factor is the leverage of the muscle.
  - Leverage is another factor that affects the force that a muscle can generate when moving a body part.
  - **Leverage** is a term that describes the mechanical advantage that a force can have when moving an object.

BOX 15-11

When we study motion of the body, it is useful to realize that any movement that occurs will always be the sum total of all forces that act on that body part. Therefore it is important to have a sense of every force that is at work in a given situation. All forces can be divided into one of two categories: (1) internal forces or (2) external forces. **Internal forces** are generated internally, inside the body; muscles create internal forces. **External forces** are created externally, outside the body. Gravity is the most common external force, and no study of the kinesiology would be complete without a strong understanding of the force that gravity plays on the motion of the body. However, many other examples of external forces exist: using springs, resistance tubing, and therabands when exercising. In addition, other people acting on us provide external forces; even wind and the waves of the ocean are examples of external forces.

Levers:

To understand the idea of the mechanical advantage of leverage, one should consider the concept of levers.

- A **lever** is a rigid bar that can move (Figure 15-6).
- Movement of a lever occurs at a point that can be called the **axis of motion**.
- This movement occurs because of a force that acts on the lever.
- The distance from the axis of motion to the point of application of force on the lever is defined as the **lever arm**. (Note: Technically, the definition of a lever arm is the distance from the axis of motion to the point of application of force on the lever, only if the application of the force is perpendicular to the lever. When the application of force is not perpendicular, the definition of a lever arm is slightly different.) (See Section 15.7 for more information.)
  - A lever arm is also referred to as a **moment arm** or an **effort arm**.

Leverage:

- The longer the lever arm is, the less effort it takes to move the lever. This less effortful movement of a longer lever is called *leverage*. Thus the longer the lever arm is, the greater is the leverage.
- Leverage can be used to move a weight. When we want to move a weight that is otherwise too heavy to move, or we simply want to move a weight with less effort, we can use the concept of leverage to our advantage. In fact, the term **mechanical advantage** is used to describe the advantage of being able to move heavy objects with less effort.

BOX 15-12

Nothing is totally free; even the mechanical advantage of a longer lever arm comes with a price. Although a longer lever arm makes it easier to move an object that might otherwise be too difficult to move, the disadvantage is that the lever arm must be moved a great distance to move the object a short distance. No work or effort is actually saved. In effect, increased leverage simply spreads what would be a large effort into a smaller effort over a greater distance!

- A seesaw is as an example of the mechanical advantage of leverage. A seesaw is a lever. On a seesaw, the further from the axis of motion that a person sits, the more force the person exerts on the seesaw due to increased leverage. If two people sit on opposite sides of a seesaw and one person weighs $^{1}/_{2}$ the weight of the other person, the lighter person would be able to balance the heavier person by sitting further (i.e., twice as far) from the axis of motion of the seesaw. In this

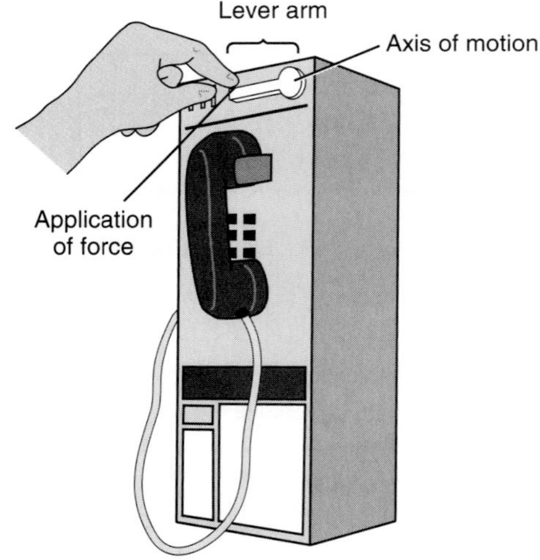

Figure 15-6 Illustration of a simple lever (i.e., a coin return on a pay phone). The lever is the rigid bar that someone pushes on to have the coins returned; the movement of the lever is created when someone pushes on it. The distance from the axis of motion of the lever to where the person pushes on the lever is called the *lever arm*.

example, the lighter person gains the mechanical advantage of greater leverage by increasing the lever arm on his side of the seesaw by sitting further from the center of the seesaw (i.e., the axis of motion) (Figure 15-7).

BOX 15-13

An everyday example of the concept of leverage is the location of a doorknob on a door. The doorknob on a door is nearly always located as far from the hinges (i.e., the axis of motion) as possible. This increased leverage (i.e., having a longer lever arm) provides increased mechanical leverage when opening or closing the door. In the same manner, when a muscle attaches further from a joint, it gains mechanical advantage or leverage because the lever arm is longer.

Leverage in the Human Body:

- ❑ Leverage is an important concept when it comes to the biomechanics of the musculoskeletal system.
- ❑ In the human body, bones are levers, muscles create the forces that move these levers, and the axis of motion is located at the joint.
- ❑ The mechanical advantage or leverage of a muscle increases as its attachment site on the bone is located further from the joint.
- ❑ As an example, consider two muscles that are the same size and therefore have the same intrinsic strength. Both of these muscles attach to the same bone and move it at the same joint. If muscle *B* were to attach twice as far from the joint as muscle *A*, muscle *B* would generate twice the force for movement on its attachment as muscle *A*, even though both muscles have the same intrinsic strength.
    - ❑ Therefore the location of the attachment of a muscle, although not changing the muscle's intrinsic strength, does change the force for movement that the muscle exerts on its attachment (i.e., its leverage) (Figure 15-8). Leverage is an example of an extrinsic factor that affects the force that a muscle exerts on its attachment(s).
- ❑ The disadvantage to the greater leverage of muscle *B* is that muscle *B* must contract a greater distance to move the bone the same amount that muscle *A* can move it with a shorter distance of contraction. Thus although muscle *B* can double the strength of its force by being twice as far from the joint as muscle *A*, muscle *B* must contract twice as far to move the bone the same amount that muscle *A* does. The consequence of having to contract a greater distance is that it is difficult to generate great speed of the body part that is being moved, because the muscle must contract a great amount in exchange for a small amount of movement.

BOX 15-14

Regarding the advantages and disadvantages of the leverage of muscle attachments, the following two rules can be stated:

1. Muscles with good leverage can generate greater extrinsic strength of contraction compared with muscles with poor leverage.
2. Muscles with poor leverage can generate greater speed of movement of the body part compared with muscles with good leverage.

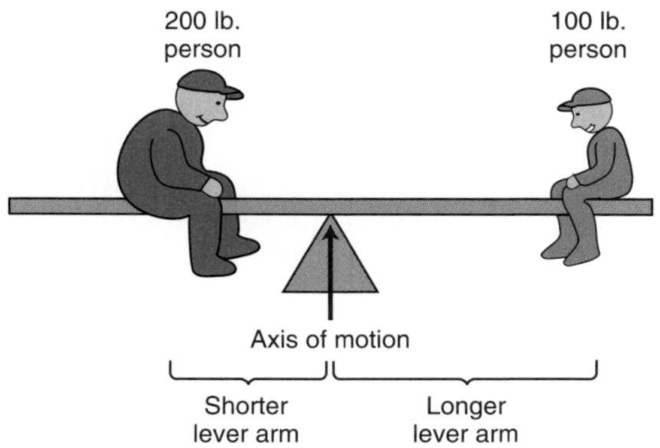

Figure 15-7 Illustration of the mechanical advantage of leverage. Two people are sitting on opposite sides of a seesaw. The lighter person on the right side is able to create a force that balances the heavier person on the left by the increased leverage of sitting further away from the center of the seesaw.

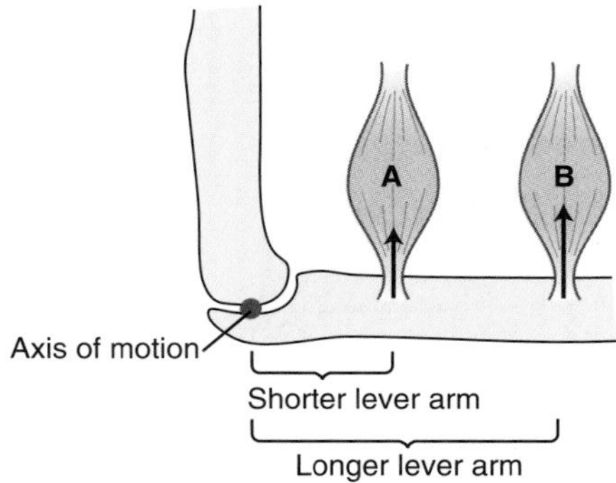

Figure 15-8 Illustration of the increased force that a muscle can generate by attaching further from the joint. Two muscles of the same size and intrinsic strength are crossing the same joint and attaching to the same bone. However, muscle *B* attaches onto the bone twice as far from the joint as muscle *A*. This gives muscle *B* greater leverage and therefore greater force to move the bone at the joint crossed. The axis of motion is located at the joint. The distance from the joint to the attachment of each muscle is its lever arm.

☐ 15.7 LEVERAGE OF A MUSCLE—MORE DETAIL

- ❑ Another factor must be considered when evaluating the strength of a muscle based on its leverage—the angle of pull of the muscle at its bony attachment.
- ❑ Technically, a lever arm is defined based on the application of force to move the lever as being perpendicular to the lever (i.e., the pull of the muscle on its attachment should be perpendicular to the bone to which it attaches). However, the pull of a muscle on a bone is rarely ever perfectly perpendicular. Therefore to evaluate the leverage of a muscle, we must consider the angle of the pull of the muscle on the bone.

Angle of Pull of the Muscle:

- ❑ The angle of pull that a muscle has relative to the bone to which it attaches is quite important. The effective strength of a muscle to move a body part at a joint is based on its ability to move the bone in the direction of the motion that is to occur. If the angle of pull is directly in line with that motion, then all of the force of muscle's contraction will contribute to moving the bone in that direction.
- ❑ The term **optimum angle of pull** is used to describe the optimal angle of pull that a muscle has on the bone to which it attaches. As a rule, the optimum angle of pull is perpendicular to the long axis of the bone (Figure 15-9a).

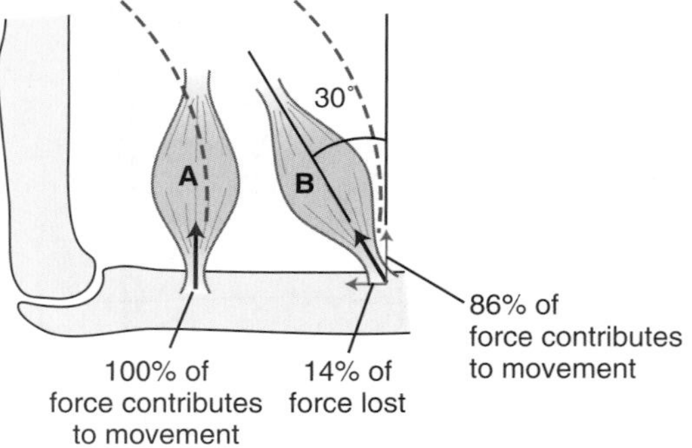

Figure 15-9 Illustration of the effect of the angle of pull of a muscle on its bony attachment. The efficiency of the pulling force toward creating movement of the bone at the joint crossed is best when the muscle's angle of pull is perpendicular to the bone. Any change from that angle will result in a weaker force placed on the bone. Muscle *A* has an optimal angle of pull; it attaches into the bone at exactly 90 degrees (i.e., perpendicular); therefore 100% of the strength of its contraction force goes toward moving the bone. Muscle *B* attaches into the bone at an oblique angle of 30 degrees. By using trigonometry, the percentage of its contraction force that contributes to motion at the joint is 86%; therefore with regard to creating movement, 14% of its contraction force is lost.

- ❑ If instead the muscle's line of pull is at an oblique angle to the bone, not all the force of the muscle will go toward moving the bone in the direction of the motion. (Note: This is similar to the discussion of the pennation angle of muscle fibers of pennate muscles; see Section 15.2.) The greater the obliquity of the muscle's attachment, the less of the force of the muscle contraction contributes to the motion at the joint (see Figure 15-9b). Simple trigonometry is used to figure out what percentage of a muscle's pulling force contributes to the motion that is occurring.

BOX 15-15

The optimum angle of pull of a muscle is defined as the angle of attachment of that muscle onto its bony attachment so that the muscle most efficiently moves the bone at the joint crossed. Generally the optimum angle of pull is perpendicular to the long axis of the bone. Any obliquity in the angle of the muscle's pull will result in a decrease of efficiency of movement when the muscle contracts. However, the advantage of an increased obliquity (i.e., a less-than-optimal angle of pull) is that a greater portion of the force of the muscle's contraction goes into stabilizing the joint. This is because any deviation from perpendicular increases the angle of pull of the muscle along the long axis of the bone toward the joint. This results in a portion of the muscle's contraction pulling the bone in toward the joint. This compression force of the bone in toward the joint increases the stability of the joint.

Lever Arm Definition Refined:

- ❑ In Section 15.6, it was stated that the definition of a lever arm is the distance along a lever from the axis of motion for the lever to the point of application of force on the lever. Applying this definition to the musculoskeletal system, a lever arm would be defined as the distance from the center of the joint (i.e., the axis of motion) to the point of attachment of the muscle (i.e., the point of application of force) onto the bone. However, this definition of a lever arm does not take into account the angle of the muscle's pull. To account for the change in leverage force of a muscle when its angle of pull is other than perpendicular to the bone, the definition of a lever arm must be slightly refined.
  - ❑ A more accurate definition of a musculoskeletal lever arm is the shortest distance from the center of the joint to the line of pull of the muscle.
- ❑ Figure 15-10a, illustrates the precise definition of a lever arm. We see a line drawn that is the shortest distance from the center of the joint to the line of pull of the muscle. Note that this lever arm is less than what it would be if it were measured from the center of the joint to the point of attachment of the muscle. Therefore using the line of pull of the muscle as the

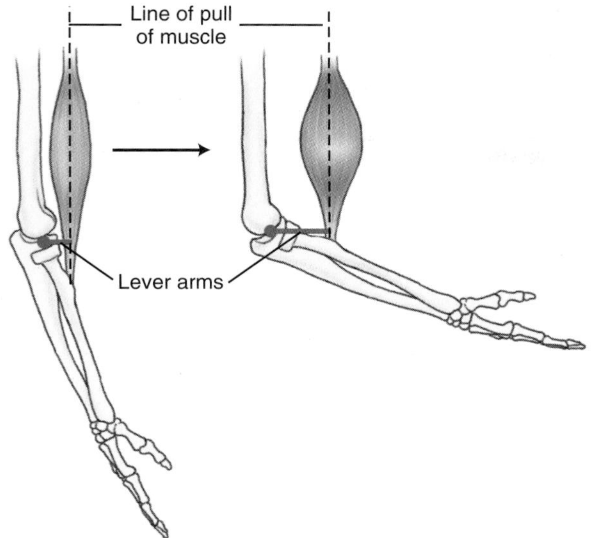

Figure 15-10 The precise definition of a musculoskeletal lever arm is the shortest distance from the center of the joint (i.e., the axis of motion) to the line of pull of the muscle. *A* and *B* illustrate the lever arms of the same muscle when the joint is in two different positions. (Note: The lever arm is greater in *B* than in *A*.)

defining distance for the definition of leverage changes the determination of leverage force. By amending the definition of a lever arm in this manner, the angle of the muscle's attachment into the bone is taken into consideration (and trigonometric formulas can be avoided).

- Figure 15-10b, shows the same muscle when the joint is in a different position. Note that the lever arm has changed. Therefore the leverage of the muscle changes from one joint position to the other. It must be noted and emphasized that as a bone moves through its range of motion at a joint, although the attachments of a muscle remain constant, the angle of pull of the muscle relative to the bone constantly changes. This means that the lever arm and therefore the leverage of the muscle's force changes.
  - Therefore the effective extrinsic strength of the muscle's contraction constantly changes as the joint position changes during a muscle's contraction!

15.8 CLASSES OF LEVERS

- Levers are divided into three classes.
  - These classes are called *1st-class, 2nd-class,* and *3rd-class levers*.
  - The difference between the three classes of levers is the relative location of the application of force to cause movement (F) and the force of **resistance to movement** (R) relative to the axis of motion (A) (Figure 15-11).
- Relating this to the musculoskeletal system, it can be said that the difference between the three classes of levers is the relative location of the line of pull of the muscle (F) and the weight of the body part (R) relative to the center of the joint (A).
  - The resistance to movement would be whatever force resists the motion from occurring. In the musculoskeletal system, apart from additional forces that might enter the picture, the resistance to motion would be the weight of the body part that has to be moved (or the body parts that have to be moved). For example, if a muscle attaches onto the hand and moves the hand at the wrist joint, the resistance to movement is the weight of the hand. However, if the muscle attaches onto the forearm and moves the forearm at the elbow joint, the resistance to movement is the weight of the forearm, as well as the weight of the hand (which must also be moved along with the forearm).

BOX 15-16

When evaluating the relative leverage within the musculoskeletal system of the force of a muscle contraction to the resistance it meets in trying to move the body part to which it attaches, we usually think of the resistance to movement as being the weight of whatever body part(s) that have to be moved. However, it is possible for other forces to come into play. For example, if a muscle must contract and move the upper extremity, the resistance force increases if the hand is holding a weight. Another example is if an exercise is being done in which springs or therabands are used to increase the resistance of the exercise.

1st-, 2nd-, and 3rd-Class Levers:

- A **1st-class lever** has the force that causes motion and the force of resistance to motion on opposite sides of the axis of motion.

BOX 15-17

The definition of a 1st-class lever is that the force creating movement (F) and force resisting movement (R) are on opposite sides of the axis of motion (A). However, which force is further from the axis of motion, and hence which force has greater leverage and therefore mechanical advantage for power, is not specified (whereas 2nd- and 3rd-class levers are defined based on which force [F or R] is greater). Therefore knowing that a muscle is a 1st-class lever does not immediately tell us about its relative leverage force compared with the leverage force of the resistance (i.e., it does not tell us if the muscle has a relative leverage advantage or leverage disadvantage). Each 1st-class lever muscle must be individually looked at to determine its relative leverage advantage/disadvantage. (Note: Leverage of the resistance force is covered in Section 15.9.)

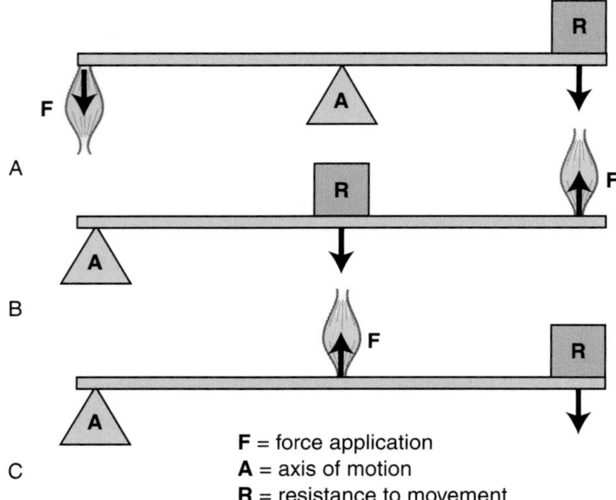

Figure 15-11 Illustration of the concept of the three classes of levers. These classes are based on the relative positions along the lever of the application of force, the resistance to movement, and the axis of motion. *A* is a 1st-class lever, *B* is a 2nd-class lever, and *C* is a 3rd-class lever.

- A **2nd-class lever** has the force that causes motion and the force of resistance to motion on the same side of the axis of motion, and the force that causes motion is further from the axis than the force of resistance.
  - Therefore 2nd-class levers inherently have greater leverage for strength of pulling force.
- A **3rd-class lever** has the force that causes motion and the force of resistance to motion on the same side of the axis of motion, and the force that causes motion is closer to the axis than the force of resistance.
  - Therefore 3rd-class levers inherently have less leverage for strength of pulling force.

1st-Class Levers:

- The typical example of a 1st-class lever is a seesaw (Figure 15-12a).
- With a seesaw, the axis of motion is located between the force for motion and the resistance to motion.
- An example of musculature in the human body that is a 1st-class lever is the extensor musculature that attaches to the back of the head (Figure 15-12b).

2nd-Class Levers:

- The typical example of a 2nd-class lever is a wheelbarrow (Figure 15-13a).
- With a wheelbarrow, both the force that causes motion and the force of resistance to the motion are on the same side of the axis of motion, and the force that causes the motion (i.e., the person lifting up on the handles) is further from the axis than the resistance force (i.e., weight of the loaded wheelbarrow). Because the force that causes motion is further from the axis of

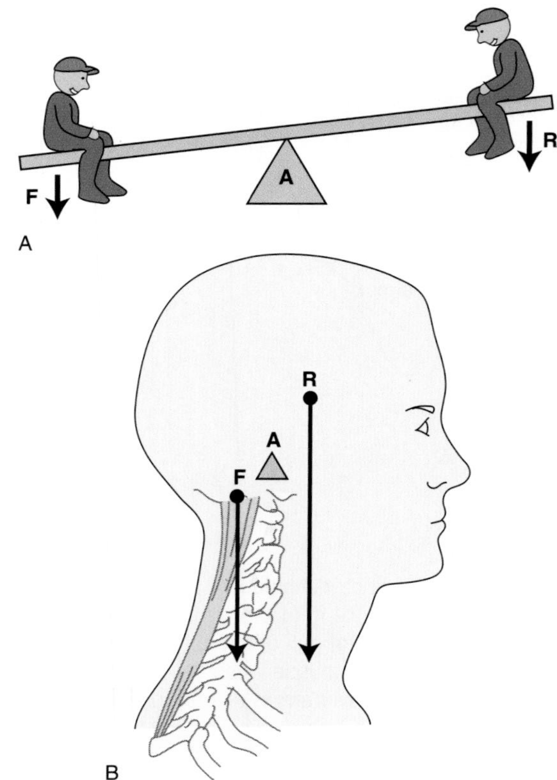

Figure 15-12 Two examples of a 1st-class lever. A 1st-class lever is one in which the force applied to the lever (F) and the resistance to movement of the lever (R) are on opposite sides of the axis of motion of the lever (A). *A* is a seesaw; *B* is the extensor musculature acting on the head.

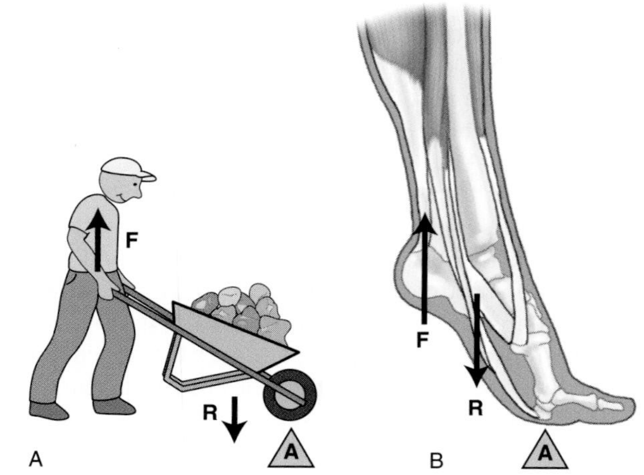

Figure 15-13 Two examples of a 2nd-class lever. A 2nd-class lever is one in which both the force applied to the lever (F) and the resistance to movement of the lever (R) are on the same side of the axis of motion of the lever (A); however, the force causing motion (F) is further from the axis than is the resistance (R). *A,* Wheelbarrow. (The mechanical advantage of a wheelbarrow should be noted; by virtue of being a 2nd-class lever, it allows us to lift and move objects that might otherwise be too heavy for us.) *B,* Plantarflexor musculature of the lower extremity acting on the foot. Its mechanical advantage allows it to lift the entire body (i.e., a heavy weight) relative to the toes at the metatarsophalangeal joints!

motion than the resistance force, wheelbarrows have a great amount of leverage and therefore allow us to lift and move heavy loads with relative ease.

- An example of musculature in the human body that is a 2nd-class lever is the plantarflexor musculature of the lower extremity that attaches into the calcaneus. When the plantarflexor musculature contracts with the foot on the ground, its contraction lifts the entire body relative to the toes at the metatarsophalangeal joints of the foot (Figure 15-13b).
- Attaching further from the axis of motion on the foot than the location of the force of resistance to contraction (i.e., the point of center of weight of the body) affords the plantarflexor musculature a great deal of leverage force to lift the entire weight of the body.
- Note: The disadvantage of this muscle (as well as every 2nd-class lever muscle) is that it must concentrically contract a great distance to create a small range of motion; therefore its ability to move the body quickly is less.

3rd-Class Levers:

- A typical example of a 3rd-class lever is a pair of tweezers (Figure 15-14a).
- With a pair of tweezers, both the force that causes motion and the force of resistance to the motion are on the same side of the axis of motion, and the force that causes the resistance (i.e., the resistance of the object being held) is further from the axis than the force that causes motion (i.e., the person squeezing the tweezers).
- An example of a muscle in the human body that is a 3rd-class lever is the brachialis that attaches to the proximal end of the forearm (Figure 15-14b).
- Attaching so far proximally on the forearm does not give the brachialis much leverage for strength of contraction, but as with all muscles that are 3rd-class levers, it means that a small amount of brachialis contraction will move the forearm through a large range of motion. Therefore the mechanical advantage the brachialis gives up in leverage for lifting heavy weights, it gains in speed of motion of the forearm.

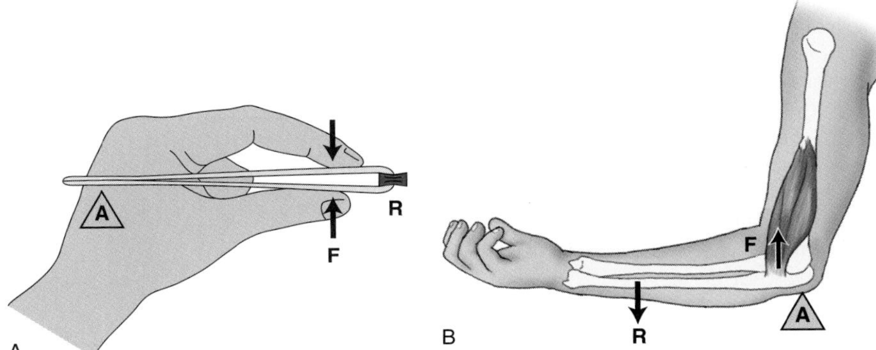

Figure 15-14 Two examples of a 3rd-class lever. A 3rd-class lever is one in which both the force applied to the lever (F) and the resistance to movement of the lever (R) are on the same side of the axis of motion of the lever (A). *A,* Pair of tweezers. *B,* Medial view of the brachialis muscle of the upper extremity. As a 3rd-class lever, the brachialis loses leverage for strength of contraction, but by virtue of being a 3rd-class lever, it gains the ability to quickly move the forearm through its range of motion!

15.9 LEVERAGE OF RESISTANCE FORCES

- Up until now we have spoken about leverage only from the point of view of the leverage of a muscle that is creating a force to move or stabilize the body. However, the force of resistance to our muscle's force may have greater leverage than our muscle does. When this occurs, whether our muscle's role is to move the body part against the resistance force or to hold the body part stable against the resistance force, our muscle is often at a **mechanical disadvantage** when working against a force with greater leverage.
  - Therefore just as it was important to understand the leverage of our muscle's force, it is equally important to look at and understand the leverage of the resistance force that our muscle must work against.

BOX 15-18

The term *mechanical disadvantage* describes the situation in which a muscle is at a mechanical disadvantage relative to the resistance force that opposes it. By definition, this situation occurs with 2nd-class levers, because 2nd-class levers are defined as having the resistance force further from the joint than the muscular attachment. It may also occur with 1st-class levers if the resistance force is located further from the joint than the muscular attachment. When the role of the muscle is to isometrically contract and stabilize the joint (to prevent movement), the muscle needs to contract forcefully enough to meet the strength of the resistance force; when the role of the muscle is to concentrically contract and move the joint, the muscle needs to contract more forcefully than the strength of the resistance force. Needing to generate contraction strength when the muscle is at a mechanical disadvantage increases the risk of a muscular strain.

- Figure 15-15a, depicts a muscle that is flexing the forearm at the elbow joint. When the forearm is in a position of 90 degrees of flexion, the resistance force (i.e., the weight of the forearm and hand) has a large lever arm that increases the resistance force that our forearm flexor muscle must overcome to be able to move the forearm. Figure 15-15b, depicts the same scenario after our muscle has succeeded in flexing the forearm at the elbow joint to a position that is near full flexion. In this position, the lever arm of the resistance force of the weight of the forearm and hand has greatly decreased. This decreased lever arm means that the resistance force of the weight of the forearm and hand has greatly decreased. Therefore the forearm flexor muscle does not need as powerful a contraction to move the forearm further into flexion. However, it should be noted that the lever arm (and therefore the leverage) of the muscle has also decreased in the position in Figure 15-15b, as compared with the position in Figure 15-15a.

BOX 15-19 SPOTLIGHT ON LEVERAGE AND HOLDING AN OBJECT

If a person is carrying a weight in the hand and the weight is being held in front of the body, the extra weight in front of the body would tend to make the trunk fall forward into flexion (at the spinal joints). If this weight is held further away from the body, the lever arm of the weight of the object increases and its force on our body increases. To keep the trunk from falling forward into flexion, the back extensors must contract to equal the force that the weight of the object is creating on the body. The further the weight is held away from the body, the greater the force on the body, and the greater the back extensors must contract. For example, a 10-lb weight that is held against the front of the body magnifies its force approximately seven times to 70 lbs if it is held away from the body at arm's length. For this reason, holding a heavy object far away from us is extremely stressful to our back muscles. To feel this, hold this book close to your body with one hand and palpate your erector spinae musculature with your other hand. Continue palpating your erector spinae musculature as you bring the book further away from your body. You should clearly feel the erector spinae's increased contraction as the book is moved further from the body. Knowledge of this principle allows us to better understand and examine the habits and work practices of our clients and better advise them how to lift and carry in a manner that is less stressful and healthier. The application of this concept is also extremely important when evaluating the physical stress on the body of a client when performing exercises with weights.

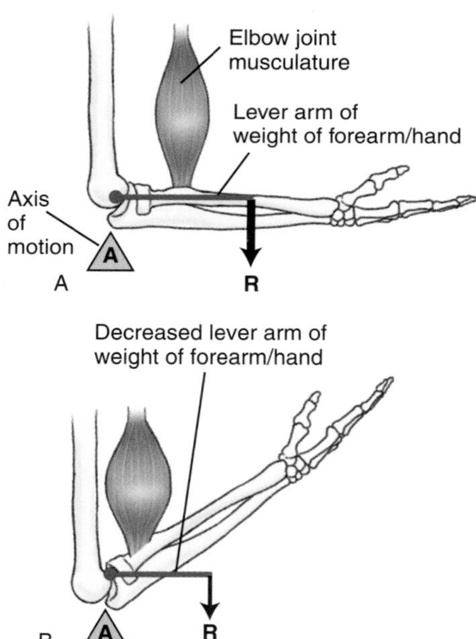

Figure 15-15 Illustration of the changing leverage of the force of gravity as a result of the weight of the forearm and hand when the angle of the elbow joint changes. The weight of the forearm and hand creates a resistance force (R) to flexor musculature of the elbow joint (also pictured). *B,* Lesser leverage of this resistance force than *A* because of the decreased lever arm when the elbow joint is in a position of greater flexion.

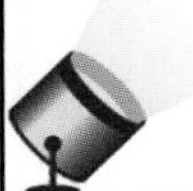

BOX 15-20 SPOTLIGHT ON LEVERAGE AND BENDING OVER

It is very common for a client to report that he or she bent over to pick up something and the back "went out." Often what occurs in these scenarios is that the extensor musculature in the back is strained and/or spasms. The client often cannot understand why this occurred, because whatever object was being picked up was not that heavy. Many times nothing was even being picked up; perhaps the client was just bending over to tie a shoelace. What is often not understood is that bending over in and of itself is stressful, because the back extensor musculature must eccentrically contract to slow down the descent of the trunk into flexion. If the client then comes back up from the bent over position, extensor muscles of the trunk must concentrically contract to lift the weight of the upper body (i.e., trunk, neck, head, and both upper extremities) back into extension.

When these actions occur, the muscles of the back are actually lifting quite a heavy weight. Even if nothing was picked up in the hands, they are lifting the weight of the body! Figure 1 depicts a typical **stoop bend** in which the back bends (i.e., the spine flexes); Figure 2 depicts a straight back **squat bend** in which the back has stayed straight and more vertical. Notice the large lever arm for the weight of the upper body of the person with the stoop bend; the extensor muscles of the back must contract forcefully to counter this force. It is no wonder that so many people strain and injure their backs when stooping over, regardless of whether a heavy object was being picked up or not. Compare the stoop bend with the decreased lever arm of the upper body weight when the person does a squat bend. For this reason, squat bending in which the knees and hips are bent is the safer way to bend over (see Note 1). If a heavy object is being lifted in the hands, it only magnifies the importance of this concept.

It should also be noted that many people are aware that the safe way to bend over is to bend the knees and hips and keep the back straight. However, they do not realize that it is also important to keep the back not only straight, but as vertical as possible. If the back is straight, but inclined forward (i.e., the pelvis is anteriorly tilted at the hip joints) as in Figure 2, then the lever arm for the weight of the upper body still increases. Although healthier than the stoop lift, this inclined squat lift is not as healthy as the vertical back squat lift depicted in Figure 3 (see Note 2).

Note 1. Squat bending in which the spinal joints are extended (i.e., the back is straight) is healthier than *stoop bending* in which the spinal joints are flexed (i.e., the back is hunched forward) for two reasons:

1. The squat bend tends to decrease the leverage of the body weight by keeping the trunk more vertical. If the leverage of the body weight is less, then the extensor muscles of the trunk do not need to contract as forcefully and the likelihood of a strain of the extensor musculature is low.
2. In the squat bend, the spinal joints are extended and therefore in the more stable closed-packed position. Therefore it is less likely that the spinal joints will be sprained with a squat bend.

Note 2. For all the cautioning that is done to encourage people to bend (and/or lift) in a healthy manner with a vertical back squat lift, it is amazing how few people actually bend in this manner on a regular basis. It turns out that many people resist this healthier method of bending for two good reasons:

1. Squat lifting places more pressure on the knee joints.
2. It actually takes more energy to squat bend than it does to stoop bend; so to save a few calories of energy, many people keep stoop bending and putting their backs in peril.

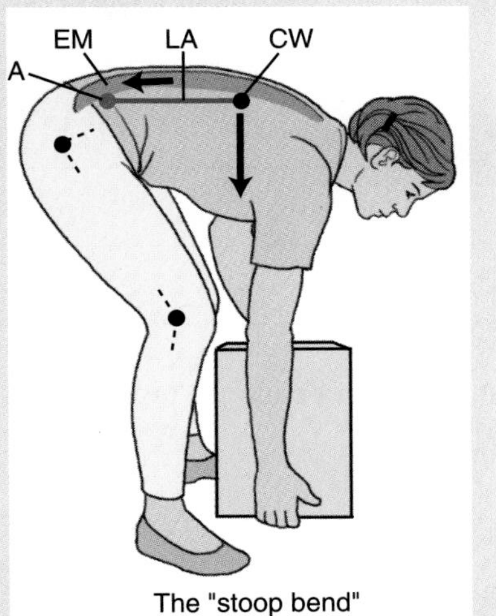

Figure 1

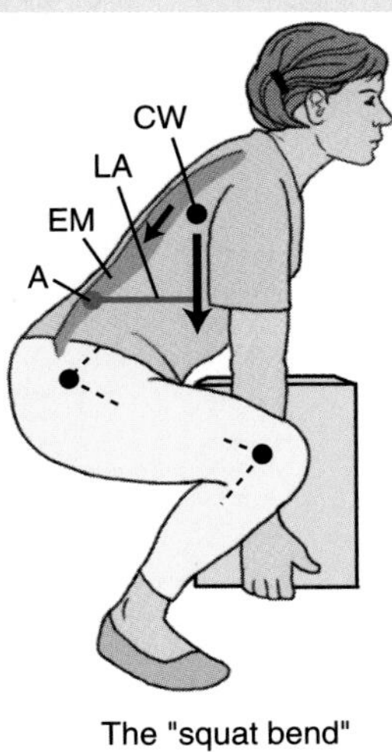

Figure 2

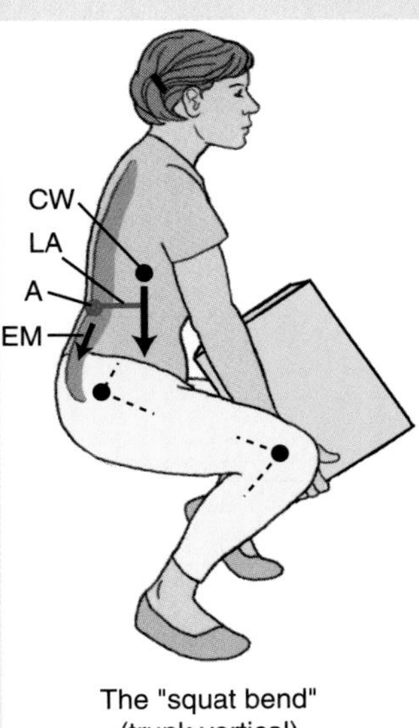

Figure 3

This figure illustrates the differences between the squat bend and the stoop bend. In *1*, the person is performing a *stoop bend* in which she bends her back forward. this creates a long lever arm for the force of the weight of the trunk and upper body; this in turn requires a forceful contraction of the extensor muscles of the spine, which increases the chance of a back strain. In *2*, the person is performing a *squat bend* in which she keeps her back straight. This decreases the lever arm of the weight of the trunk and upper body, decreasing the chance of a back strain. *C* illustrates a squat bend in which the trunk is kept totally vertical. The reader should note how the lever arm of the weight of the trunk and upper body in *3* is even less than in *2*. (*LA*, Lever arm; *CW*, center of weight of the trunk and upper body; *EM*, extensor musculature of the spine; *A*, axis of motion). (Note: The spine has multiple joints; therefore multiple axes of motion exist. To simplify this, the lumbosacaral joint has been used in all cases as the axis of motion to determine the relative lever arms.)

REVIEW QUESTIONS

evolve Answers to the following review questions appear on the Evolve website accompanying this book.

1. How can a muscle have a partial contraction?

2. What is the Henneman size principle?

3. What factor determines the intrinsic strength of a muscular contraction?

4. What factors determine the extrinsic strength of a muscular contraction?

5. Name two types of longitudinal muscle fiber architecture and three types of pennate muscle fiber architecture.

6. What is a pennation angle?

7. What is the difference between active tension and passive tension of a muscle?

8. What is the term used to describe the fact that a muscle's contraction is weakened when it is lengthened beyond resting length?

9. Why is the strength of a muscular contraction weakened when it is shortened beyond resting length?

10. What do the three length-tension relationship curves describe?

11. What is a lever? What is a lever arm?

12. What is the definition of leverage?

13. What advantage does a muscle gain by having greater leverage?

14. What disadvantage does a muscle have if it has greater leverage?

15. What is the optimum angle of pull for a muscle?

16. What is the definition of a 1st-class lever?

17. What is the similarity between a 2nd-class lever and a 3rd-class lever?

18. Name a muscle that acts as part of a 3rd-class lever system.

19. What is the importance of the resistance force to movement?

20. What is the resistance force to a person's anterior hip joint musculature flexing the thigh at the hip joint from anatomic position?

Chapter 16

The Neuromuscular System

CHAPTER OUTLINE

CHAPTER OBJECTIVES

After completing this chapter, the student should be able to perform the following:

- ❑ Compare and contrast sensory, integrative, and motor neurons.
- ❑ Describe the structural and functional classifications of the nervous system.
- ❑ Compare and contrast the neuronal pathways for the initiation of voluntary movement and a spinal cord reflex.
- ❑ Describe the difference between true reflexive behavior and learned/patterned behavior.
- ❑ Describe the relationship between neural facilitation and resting muscle tone.
- ❑ Describe the neuronal pathways for and the purpose of reciprocal inhibition.
- ❑ Describe how reciprocal inhibition can be used to aid muscle palpation and muscle stretching.
- ❑ Define and discuss proprioception.
- ❑ List the three major categories of proprioceptors and the specific proprioceptors found in each major category.
- ❑ Compare and contrast the function of Pacini's corpuscles and Ruffini's endings.
- ❑ Compare and contrast the neuronal pathway mechanism and the function of muscle spindles and Golgi tendon organs.
- ❑ Discuss the relationship between muscle spindles, Golgi tendon organs, and muscle stretching.
- ❑ Discuss the concept of muscle facilitation and muscle inhibition.
- ❑ Discuss the differences (including implications for treatment) between trigger points and global tightening of a muscle.
- ❑ Describe the mechanisms and functions of inner ear proprioceptors.
- ❑ Describe the relationship between inner ear proprioceptors and neck proprioceptors and the implications for bodywork and/or exercise.
- ❑ Describe the mechanism and purpose of the flexor withdrawal, crossed extensor, tonic neck, righting, and cutaneous reflexes.
- ❑ Discuss the mechanism and importance of bodywork and exercise to the pain-spasm-pain cycle.
- ❑ Describe the function of muscle splinting and body armoring.
- ❑ Describe the mechanism of the gate theory, including the implications for bodywork and exercise.

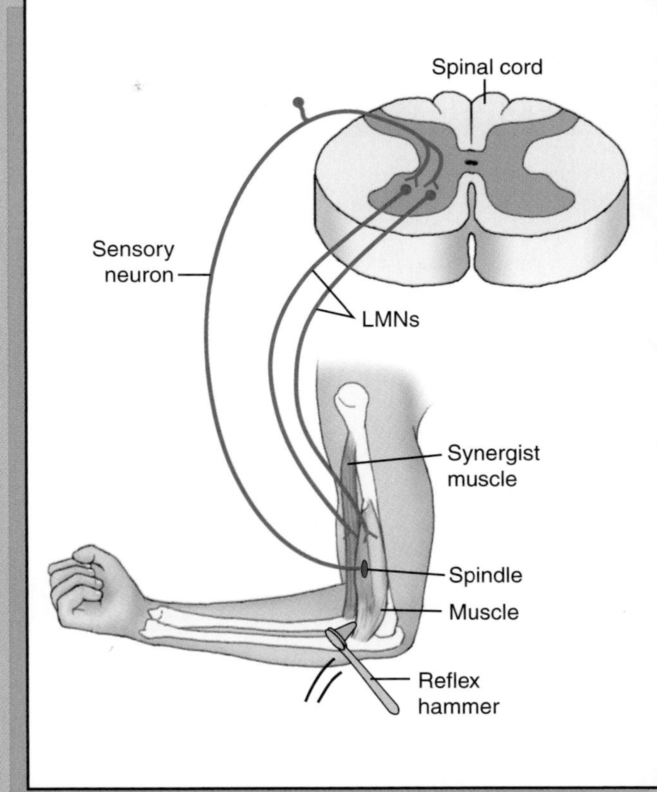

- ❑ Define the key terms of this chapter.
- ❑ State the meanings of the word origins of this chapter.

OVERVIEW

We have now studied the bones and joints of the skeletal system and the muscles of the muscular system. Bones provide rigid levers and come together to form the joints of the body; muscles attach to the bones and create movement at the joints. In this manner, the bones, joints, and muscles function together as the musculoskeletal system. However, this system cannot function in a harmonious fashion on its own. Indeed, its elements can be likened to the members of a symphony orchestra who are missing their conductor. Just as a conductor is needed to direct and coordinate the musicians of an orchestra, a conductor is needed to direct and coordinate the muscles of the musculoskeletal system. The conductor of the musculoskeletal system is the nervous system. It is the purpose of this chapter to examine the role that the nervous system plays in directing movement of the body. Indeed, a fine appreciation of the biomechanical functioning of the human body cannot exist without an understanding of the integrated role of the nervous system. In short, this chapter explores the functioning of the neuromusculoskeletal system.

KEY TERMS

Active isolated stretching
Afferent neuron (A-fair-ent NUR-on)
Alpha motor neurons (AL-fa NUR-onz)
Ampulla (am-POOL-a, am-PYUL-a)
Ascending pathways
Body armoring
Central nervous system
Cerebral motor cortex (se-REE-bral, KOR-tex)
CNS
Cocontraction
Contract-relax stretching
Counter irritant theory
CR stretching
Crista ampullaris (KRIS-ta AM-pyul-AR-is)
Crossed extensor reflex
Cutaneous reflex (cue-TANE-ee-us)
Descending pathways
Dizziness
Efferent neuron (E-fair-ent NUR-on)
Electrical muscle stimulation
Endogenous morphine (en-DAHJ-en-us)
Endorphins (en-DOOR-fins)
Equilibrium
Extrafusal fibers (EX-tra-FUSE-al)
Fascial/joint proprioceptors (PRO-pree-o-SEP-torz)
Feldenkrais technique (FEL-den-krise)
Flexor withdrawal reflex
Free nerve endings
Gamma motor neurons (GAM-ma, NUR-onz)
Gamma motor system
Gate theory
Global tightening
Golgi end organs (GOAL-gee)
Golgi tendon organ reflex
Golgi tendon organs
Inner ear proprioceptors (PRO-pree-o-SEP-torz)
Integrative neuron (NUR-on)
Interstitial myofascial receptors (IN-ter-STISH-al MY-o-fash-al)
Intrafusal fibers (IN-tra-FUSE-al)
Inverse myotatic reflex (MY-o-TAT-ik)
Joint proprioceptors (PRO-pree-o-SEP-torz)
Krause's end bulbs (KRAUS-es)
Labyrinthine proprioceptors (LAB-i-rinth-EEN PRO-pree-o-SEP-torz)
Labyrinthine righting reflex (LAB-i-rinth-EEN)
Learned behavior
Learned reflex
LMN
Lower crossed syndrome
Lower motor neuron (NUR-on)
Macula (MACK-you-la)
Mechanoreceptors (mi-KAN-o-ree-SEP-torz)
Meissner's corpuscles (MIZE-nerz CORE-pus-als)
Merkel's discs (MERK-elz)
Motor neuron (NUR-on)
Muscle facilitation
Muscle inhibition
Muscle proprioceptors (PRO-pree-o-SEP-torz)
Muscle spindle reflex
Muscle spindles
Muscle splinting
Myotatic reflex (MY-o-TAT-ik)
Nerve impulse
Neural facilitation (NUR-al)
Neuron (NUR-on)
Otoliths (O-to-liths)
Pacini's corpuscles (pa-SEEN-eez CORE-pus-als)
Pain-spasm-pain cycle
Patterned behavior
Peripheral nervous system
PIR stretching
Plyometric training (ply-o-MET-rik)
PNF stretching
PNS
Postisometric relaxation stretching
Proprioception (PRO-pree-o-SEP-shun)
Proprioceptive neuromuscular facilitation stretching (PRO-pree-o-SEP-tiv)
Reciprocal inhibition
Reflex arc
Resting tone
Righting reflex
Ruffini's endings (ru-FEEN-eez)
Semicircular canals
Sensory neuron
Stretch reflex
Target muscle
Tendon reflex
Tonic neck reflex (TON-ik)
Trigger points
UMN
Upper crossed syndrome
Upper motor neuron
Vestibule (VEST-i-byul)

WORD ORIGINS

- ❑ Ampullaris—From Latin *ampulla,* meaning *a two-handed bottle*
- ❑ Cortex—From Latin *cortex,* meaning *outer portion of an organ, bark of a tree*
- ❑ Crista—From Latin *crista,* meaning *crest*
- ❑ Endogenous—From Greek *endon,* meaning *within,* and *gen,* meaning *production*
- ❑ Equilibrium—From Latin *aequus,* meaning *equal,* and *libra,* meaning *a balance*
- ❑ Exogenous—From Greek *exo,* meaning *outside,* and *gen,* meaning *production*
- ❑ Facilitation—From Latin *facilitas,* meaning *easy*
- ❑ Inhibition—From Latin *in-hibeo,* meaning *to keep back* (from Latin *habeo,* meaning *to have*)
- ❑ Interstitial—From Latin *inter,* meaning *between,* and *sisto,* meaning *to stand* (*Interstitial* means *to stand between* or *to be located between.*)
- ❑ Macula—From Latin *macula,* meaning *a spot*
- ❑ Proprioception—From Latin *proprius,* meaning *one's own,* and *capio,* meaning *to take*

☐ 16.1 OVERVIEW OF THE NERVOUS SYSTEM

The following overview of the nervous system is not meant to be comprehensive; it is meant to overview only the aspects of the nervous system pertinent to muscle contraction.

- ❑ The nervous system is made up of nerve cells, also known as neurons (Figure 16-1a).
- ❑ A **neuron** is specialized to carry an electrical signal known as a **nerve impulse**.
- ❑ The typical neuron is composed of dendrites, a cell body, and an axon.
  - ❑ The dendrites carry the nerve impulse toward the cell body; the axon carries the nerve impulse away from the cell body.
- ❑ Functionally, a neuron can either be sensory, integrative, or motor.
  - ❑ A **sensory neuron** carries a sensory stimulus.
  - ❑ An **integrative neuron** integrates/processes the sensory stimuli received from the sensory neurons.
  - ❑ A **motor neuron** carries a message that directs a muscle to contract.

> **BOX 16-1**
>
> Sensory neurons are also known as **afferent neurons**; motor neurons are also known as **efferent neurons**.

- ❑ On a large scale, the nervous system can be structurally organized into the **central nervous system** (CNS) and the **peripheral nervous system** (PNS) (Figure 16-2).

Central Nervous System Structure:

- ❑ The central nervous system (CNS) is located in the center of the body (hence the name *central*) and is composed of the brain and spinal cord.
- ❑ The brain and spinal cord contain sensory, integrative, and motor neurons.

Brain:

- ❑ The brain is composed of three major parts: (1) the cerebrum, (2) brainstem, and (3) cerebellum.
  - ❑ The cerebrum is the largest part of the brain. The outer aspect of the cerebrum is called the *cortex* and is composed of gray matter. The inner aspect of the cerebrum is primarily made up of white matter, with some isolated clusters of gray matter called *nuclei* or *ganglia*.

> **BOX 16-2**
>
> White matter of the nervous system is white because of the presence of myelin. When myelin is present, it wraps around neuronal axons, insulating them and helping to speed the conduction of nerve impulses (see Figure 16-1). Gray matter is made up of dendrites, cell bodies, and unmyelinated axons of neurons. It is in the gray matter regions that connections and processing occur. Decisions made in these gray matter regions are then carried via white myelinated neurons to distant sites within the body. Gray matter regions may be likened to think tanks where questions are pondered and answered; white matter tracts are then analogous to the highways that carry these answers to other locations.

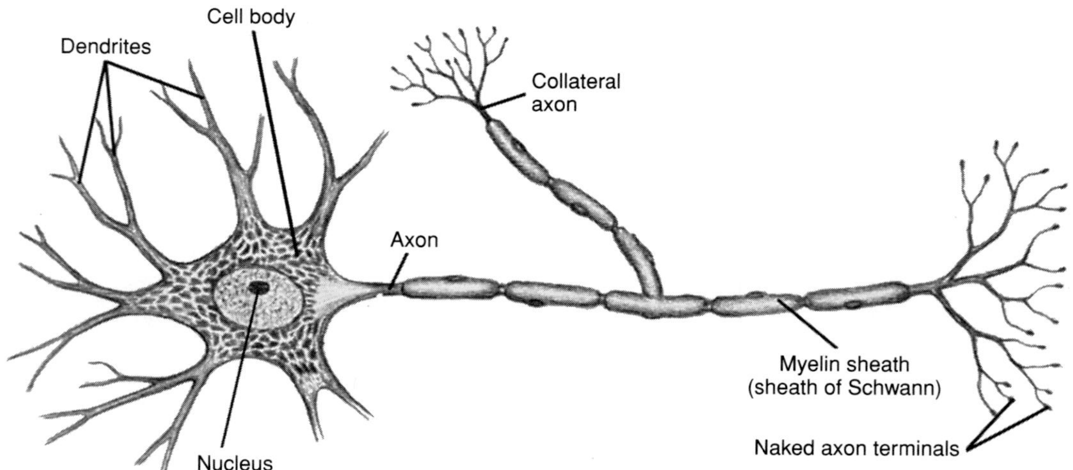

Figure 16-1 A nerve cell (also known as a *neuron*). A neuron is a type of cell that is specialized to carry a nerve impulse. The typical neuron has dendrites that carry the nerve impulse to the cell body and an axon that carries the nerve impulse away from the cell body. (From Thompson JM, McFarland GK, Hirsch JE, Tucker SM: Mosby's clinical nursing, ed 5. St Louis, 2002, Mosby.)

Spinal Cord:

- The spinal cord is composed of an outer area of white matter and an inner area of gray matter.
- The gray matter is where the connections occur.
- The outer white matter region of the spinal cord is made up of white matter tracts.
  - These white matter tracts are composed of ascending and descending pathways of information. The **ascending pathways** carry sensory information. The **descending pathways** carry motor information.
  - The ascending white matter tracts carry sensory information up from lower levels of the spinal cord to higher levels of the spinal cord and/or the brain. The descending tracts carry motor information down from the brain to the spinal cord or from higher levels of the spinal cord to lower levels of the spinal cord.

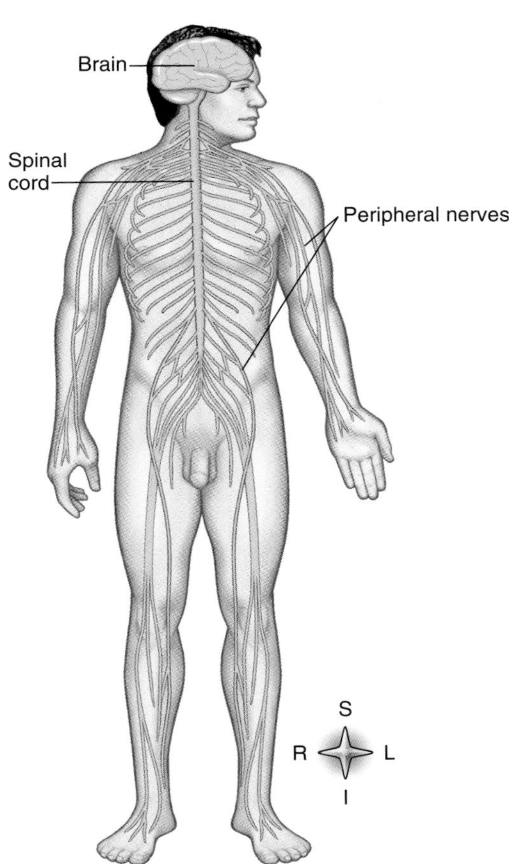

Figure 16-2 The two major structural divisions of the nervous system: (1) the central nervous system (CNS) and (2) the peripheral nervous system (PNS). The CNS is located in the center of the body and is composed of the brain and spinal cord. The PNS is located peripheral to the CNS and is composed of 31 pairs of spinal nerves and 12 pairs of cranial nerves. (Note: The cranial nerves are not shown.) (From Thibodeau GA, Patton KT: *Anatomy and physiology,* ed 5. St Louis, 2003, Mosby.)

Peripheral Nervous System Structure:

- The peripheral nervous system (PNS) is located peripherally and is composed of peripheral spinal and cranial nerves.
  - Entering and exiting the CNS are 31 pairs of spinal nerves and 12 pairs of cranial nerves.

BOX 16-3

A nerve of the peripheral nervous system (PNS) is technically an organ because it contains two different tissues organized for a common purpose, transmission of information via nerve impulses. It is also similar in organization to a muscle. A muscle is composed of bundles of muscle cells and is separated and enveloped by connective tissue coverings that surround each individual muscle cell (i.e., endomysium), each bundle of muscle cells (i.e., perimysium), and the entire muscle (i.e., epimysium). A nerve is composed of bundles of neurons (i.e., nerve cells) and is separated and enveloped by connective tissue coverings; each neuron is covered by endoneurium; each bundle of neurons is covered by perineurium; and the entire nerve is covered by epineurium.

- The PNS contains sensory and motor neurons.
- A peripheral nerve can contain all sensory neurons, in which case it is said to be a *sensory nerve*, or it can contain all motor neurons, in which case it is said to be a *motor nerve*. It can also contain both sensory and motor neurons, in which case it is said to be a *mixed nerve*.

Function of the Nervous System:

Generally the flow of information within the nervous system proceeds in the following order (Figure 16-3):

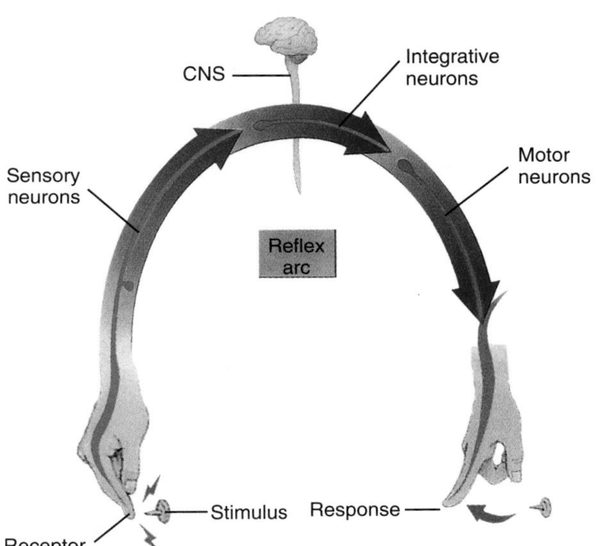

Figure 16-3 Illustration of the functional flow of information within the nervous system. Receptors attached to sensory neurons of a peripheral nerve detect a stimulus; this information is then relayed to central nervous system (CNS) via the sensory neurons of the peripheral nerve. Within the CNS, integrative neurons process the sensory stimuli. The response to the sensory stimuli is sent out to a muscle via motor neurons of a peripheral nerve. (Modified from Thibodeau GA, Patton KT: *Anatomy and physiology,* ed 5. St Louis, 2003, Mosby.)

- Sensory neurons located within peripheral nerves of the PNS carry sensory information (i.e., stimuli) from the periphery of the body into the CNS.
- The CNS then processes that sensory input via its integrative neurons.
- A motor response is carried back out from the CNS to the periphery within motor neurons of a peripheral nerve of the PNS. This motor response directs contraction of musculature.
- How much integration occurs with the CNS varies tremendously, depending on whether the movement being directed is a voluntary movement or a reflex movement.

16.2 VOLUNTARY MOVEMENT VERSUS REFLEX MOVEMENT

The nervous system can direct two types of movement: (1) voluntary movement and (2) reflex movement.

Initiation of Voluntary Movement:

- All voluntary motor control of movement originates in the outer portion of the cerebrum called the *cerebral cortex* (Figure 16-4a).
- When the integration and processing of sensory stimuli within the brain result in the determination that a joint action will be made, this decision is passed along to the **cerebral motor cortex** of the brain. The cerebral motor cortex then sends a directive down through the spinal cord within descending white matter tract pathways.

BOX 16-4

Most but not all voluntary movements are directed by the brain via the spinal cord to peripheral spinal nerves. The directions for some movements leave the brain directly via peripheral cranial nerves.

- The neurons within a descending white matter tract are motor neurons. More specifically, a motor neuron that travels down in a descending white matter tract is called an **upper motor neuron** (**UMN**).
  - Lower areas of the brain, such as the basal ganglia and the cerebellum, also feed into these pathways and influence the production of the movement of the body.

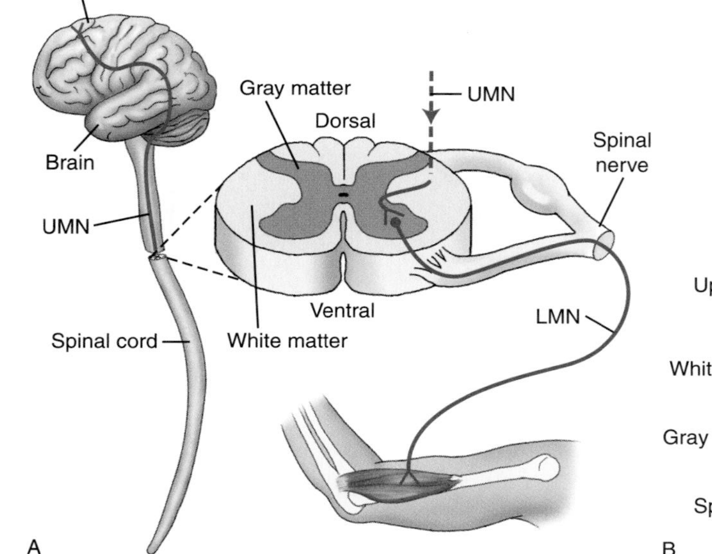

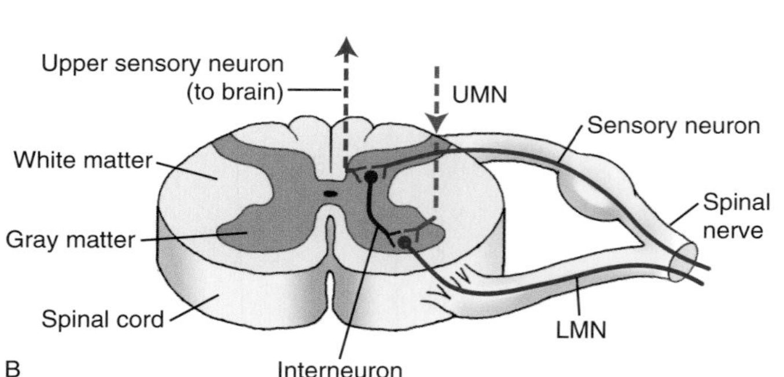

Figure 16-4 *A,* Pathways within the nervous system for initiation of voluntary movement. An upper motor neuron (UMN) originates within the motor cortex of the cerebrum and travels down through a descending white matter tract of the spinal cord where it then enters the gray matter of the spinal cord and synapses with a lower motor neuron (LMN). The LMN then exits the spinal cord and travels within a peripheral spinal nerve to connect with a muscle. *B,* Simple reflex arc that consists of a sensory neuron, interneuron, and LMN. Awareness of a reflex occurs via connections that travel up to the brain to alert the brain to what has just happened. The brain can influence a spinal cord reflex via UMNs that travel down through descending white matter tracts of the spinal cord. (Note: Connections to the brain through ascending and descending white matter tracts are not technically part of the reflex arc.)

- ❑ The UMN ends in the gray matter of the spinal cord.
- ❑ The UMN synapses (i.e., connects with) with the **lower motor neuron (LMN)** within the gray matter of the spinal cord.
- ❑ The LMN travels out of the gray matter of the spinal cord in a peripheral nerve.
- ❑ These LMNs then end at the neuromuscular junctions of the fibers of a muscle, where the muscle fibers are directed to contract. (Note: For the details of the neuromuscular junction and how the LMN creates the contraction of the muscle fibers to which it is attached, see Section 10.8.)

Initiation of Reflex Movement:

- ❑ Reflex movement is much simpler than voluntary movement (see Figure 16-4b).
- ❑ A sensory stimulus enters the spinal cord via a sensory neuron.
- ❑ The sensory neuron either synapses directly with a LMN within the spinal cord, or it synapses with a short interneuron that then synapses with a LMN within the spinal cord.
- ❑ This LMN is the same LMN involved in voluntary movement (mentioned previously).
- ❑ The LMN then travels out of the spinal cord to end at the neuromuscular junctions of the fibers of a muscle, where the muscle fibers are directed to contract.
- ❑ Because of the arclike shape of the sensory neuron into the spinal cord and the motor neuron out of the spinal cord, the pathway of a reflex is often called a **reflex arc**.
- ❑ Reflexes are "hardwired" in the body (i.e., they are innate [inborn]).

BOX 16-5 SPOTLIGHT ON LEARNED BEHAVIOR AND NEURAL FACILITATION

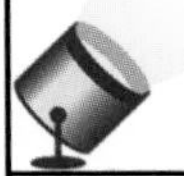

Sometimes the term **learned reflex** is used. Technically, this term is incorrect because reflexes are not learned; all reflexes are innate. The correct term that should be used is **learned behavior** or **patterned behavior**. A learned/patterned behavior describes an activity that is learned and so well patterned that it is carried out in what appears to be a "reflexive" manner. However, this learned/patterned behavior does not involve a reflex arc. The patterning of a learned behavior initially involves association within the brain between a certain stimulus and a certain response. After many repetitions, the association becomes so well patterned that our response becomes automatic without the necessity of conscious thought. A classic example of learned behavior is Pavlov's dog salivating after hearing a bell because the dog has learned to associate the sound of the bell with being fed. Many if not most of our daily activities are carried out in a learned behavior pattern. We rarely think of the muscles that we need to contract to walk across the room, tie our shoes, speak, or to drive a car along a route that we have taken many times before. In fact, it is likely that we may be driving our car while drinking a café latte and having a conversation at the same time, and we may realize halfway home that we have not even thought about which turns we have taken. If asked, we may not even know which road we are on; the body has been carrying out a series of learned behaviors as if it were operating on autopilot, with little or no conscious awareness!

The explanation that is given for how all associations are made, as well as why learned behaviors become so rooted in our nervous system, is the process of **neural facilitation**. Functionally, neural facilitation patterning that is made between a certain stimulus and a certain response becomes easier and easier to make as the association becomes reinforced through intensity or repetition. Structurally, neural facilitation is due to actual physical changes in the pathways of neurons that lower their threshold to form a certain pattern of connections (see figure). The result is a pattern of thinking and a pattern of behaving that becomes learned. The more this pattern is reinforced, the more entrenched this pattern becomes.

A number of crucially important applications of the concept of learned behavior (i.e., neural facilitation) are found in the health field. One application is to the field of massage and bodywork. Just as certain tasks and movement patterns are learned and patterned, the **resting tone** of our musculature can be learned and patterned. Normally, the resting tone of all our musculature should be relaxed. However, for many reasons, the resting tone of a client's muscle may increase when certain stressful circumstances occur. If the relationship of this muscle tightening is not addressed, the pattern of this muscle tightening because of certain stimuli such as being stressed psychologically can become entrenched. As a result, each time in the future when the client becomes psychologically stressed, it will be a triggering stimulus that will more easily cause the muscle to tighten up. In time, the stimulus/tight muscle response can become a learned behavior that occurs without us having any realization of the link between the two. As therapists working on the musculoskeletal system, changing this pattern of muscle tightness involves more than just working on the muscle itself; it involves working

Continued

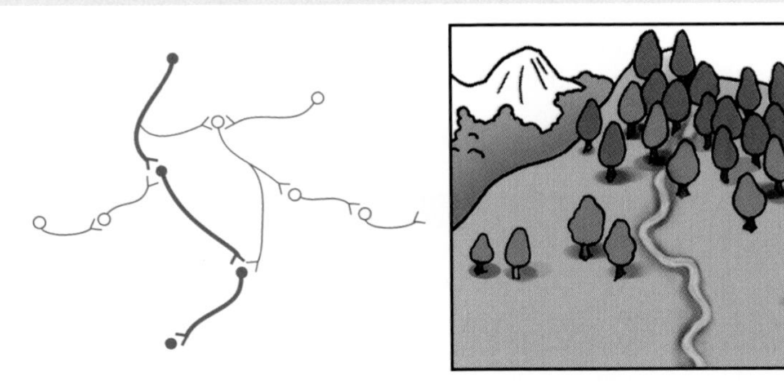

A pattern of neuronal synaptic connections being made via neural facilitation is analogous to water etching a deeper and deeper pathway into the side of a mountain over a period of time.

BOX 16-5 SPOTLIGHT ON LEARNED BEHAVIOR AND NEURAL FACILITATION—cont'd

with the nervous system to retrain its responses. In effect, we have to help the client's nervous system unlearn a certain pattern of response and relearn a new and healthier pattern of response.

An equally important application of neural facilitation to exercise exists. The pattern of co-ordering muscles (i.e., coordination) is also a learned/patterned behavior. When working with a client who exhibits poor technique when doing an exercise, this poor technique pattern is most likely entrenched via neural facilitation. To correct this faulty technique pattern, the client must create a new pattern that is healthy and proper to replace the old unhealthy pattern. In this regard, repetition is essential toward creating a new healthy neural facilitation pattern.

The concept of learned behavior/neural facilitation can also be applied to movement patterns and movement therapies. Often our movements are learned patterns that have become ingrained without conscious realization. As a result, poor movement patterns may be adopted that are inefficient, unhealthy, and functionally limiting. It is important to realize that these patterns exist within the nervous system, not within the musculoskeletal system. Therefore correction of these faulty patterns may be most efficiently accomplished by addressing the nervous system directly. **Feldenkrais technique** is a movement therapy that seeks to create client awareness of their movements including their faulty patterns of movement. Once aware, if the client desires to change his or her movement patterns, new patterns that are healthier and functionally freer may be learned.

- These reflexes are meant to be protective in nature. Before a child can know from experience which circumstances are safe and which are not, reflexes give automatic responses that are meant to protect the child from possible danger. For example, the startle reflex causes the child to turn toward the source of any loud noise. This brings attention to a potentially dangerous stimulus.
- Conscious awareness of a reflex is not part of the reflex arc itself. However, we do know that we have performed a reflex after it has happened. This knowledge occurs because of connections between the reflex arc and the brain that travel upward within ascending white matter tracts of the spinal cord to the brain; connections within the brain then bring the information to the cerebral cortex. These connections give us conscious awareness of what reflex has just occurred. (Note: Again, these connections are technically not part of the reflex arc itself.)
- In addition, descending connections exist from the brain to the reflex arc via the UMNs. These connections have the ability to modify the action of the reflex. This modification may increase the response of a reflex or it may inhibit it. If the inhibition is strong enough, the reflex may be entirely overridden.
- Using the example of the loud noise that caused the startle reflex mentioned earlier, as we age, we may find that certain loud noises are not a threat. Therefore experience teaches us when it is safe to override the startle reflex with descending influence from the brain. As we get older, we depend more and more on this descending influence to determine our actions instead of pure reflexive behavior.

16.3 RECIPROCAL INHIBITION

- **Reciprocal inhibition** is the name given to the neurologic reflex that causes the antagonist to a joint action to relax when the mover of that joint action is directed to contract.
- Muscles that are on the opposite sides of a joint have opposite actions at that joint (i.e., their actions are antagonistic to each other).
- If one of these muscles contracts to move the joint, it is termed the *mover*; the muscle on the opposite side is then termed the *antagonist*. (Note: For more information on movers and antagonists, see Sections 13.1 and 13.2.)
- If the mover contracts and shortens, the antagonist on the opposite side of the joint must relax and lengthen to allow that joint action to occur; otherwise the mover will not be able to efficiently move the joint.
- When the mover and antagonist both contract at the same time, it is called **cocontraction**.
- Cocontraction is by definition unwanted if a joint action is to occur, because the antagonist will fight the mover and lessen or stop the joint action from occurring.
- For this reason, whenever the nervous system desires a joint action to occur, it not only sends facilitory impulses to the LMN that control the mover(s) of that action but also sends inhibitory impulses to LMNs that control the antagonist(s) of that action.

BOX 16-6

Generally all nerve impulses can be considered to be either facilitory or inhibitory. Facilitory impulses facilitate the muscle contraction to occur (i.e., they send a signal to the muscle asking it to contract); inhibitory impulses inhibit the muscle contraction from occurring (i.e., they send a signal to relax the muscle so that it does not contract).

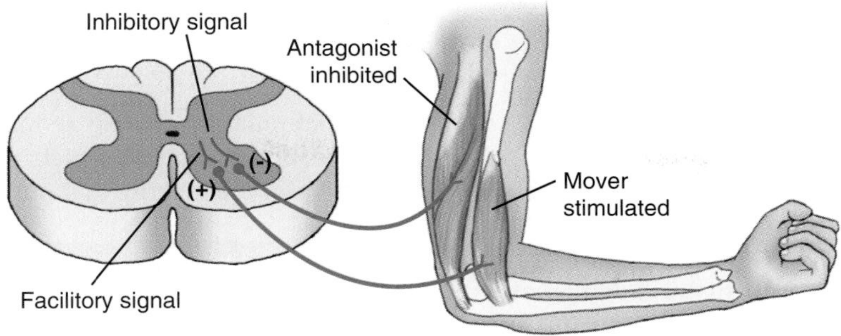

Figure 16-5 Neurologic reflex of reciprocal inhibition. When the lower motor neurons (LMNs) that control a mover muscle are facilitated to direct the mover to contract, the LMNs that control the antagonist muscle of that joint action are inhibited from sending an impulse to contract to the antagonist muscle. The result is that the antagonist muscles are inhibited from contracting and therefore relax. This relaxation allows the antagonist muscles to lengthen and stretch, thereby allowing the mover muscles to create their joint action without opposition.

- These inhibitory impulses cause the antagonist muscles of that joint action to relax so that they cannot contract and fight the mover muscles.
- This neurologic reflex that sends inhibitory impulses to the antagonists is called *reciprocal inhibition*.
- Therefore reciprocal inhibition helps to create joint actions that are strong and efficient. Figure 16-5 demonstrates an example of reciprocal inhibition.

BOX 16-7 SPOTLIGHT ON RECIPROCAL INHIBITION

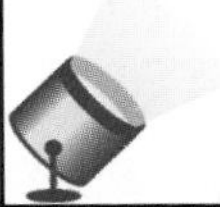

Reciprocal Inhibition and Muscle Palpation:
The neurologic reflex of reciprocal inhibition can be very usefully applied to muscle palpation. When trying to palpate and locate a **target muscle** (i.e., the particular muscle that you want to palpate), it is helpful to make the target muscle contract so that it stands out and can be easily felt and discerned from adjacent muscles. To do this, we need to have the client perform a joint action of the target muscle that the adjacent muscles cannot do. However, sometimes it is not possible to find a joint action that only the target muscle does (i.e., the other muscles that are adjacent to it all do the same action and will contract when the target muscle contracts). This makes it extremely hard to discern the target muscle. In these cases reciprocal inhibition can be used to stop the other adjacent muscles from contracting so that only the target muscle contracts; this allows for easier identification and palpation of the target muscle.

For example, if we want to palpate the brachialis, we ask the client to flex the forearm at the elbow joint so that the brachialis contracts and is more palpable. However, flexion of the forearm at the elbow joint also causes the biceps brachii to contract. Because the biceps brachii is superficial to most of the brachialis, its contraction blocks our ability to palpate the majority of the brachialis. In this case we need the brachialis to contract but the biceps brachii to stay relaxed. This can be accomplished by using reciprocal inhibition. Ask the client to flex the forearm at the elbow joint while the forearm is fully pronated at the radioulnar (RU) joints. Because the biceps brachii is a supinator of the forearm, having the client pronate the forearm reciprocally inhibits all supinators, including the biceps brachii. This allows us not only to better discern the brachialis lateral and medial to the biceps brachii where it is superficial but also to palpate the brachialis through the biceps brachii (see Figure 14-6c on page 537).

One cautionary note when using reciprocal inhibition to aid muscle palpation: Any reflex can be overridden, including reciprocal inhibition. If the client forcefully contracts, most or all movers of that joint action will be recruited to contract, including ones that are otherwise being reciprocally inhibited. Generally when using the principle of reciprocal inhibition, do not allow the client to contract forcefully.

Reciprocal Inhibition and Stretching:
Reciprocal inhibition can also be used to increase the effectiveness of a stretch. Stretches are often done in a passive manner. That is, the joint that is being stretched is moved passively in one direction, causing a stretch of the muscles on the other side of the joint (i.e., the antagonists). However, reciprocal inhibition can be used to increase the effectiveness of this stretch. Instead of having the client stretch passively, have the client actively contract the mover (i.e., agonist) muscles during the stretching maneuver. Actively contracting the movers will reflexly create a reciprocal inhibition to the antagonist muscles on the other side of the joint (which are the muscles that we are trying to stretch), causing them to relax, thus increasing the effectiveness of the stretch. This type of stretching is sometimes called *agonist contract* and is the basis for Aaron Mattes' method of **active isolated stretching** (for more on the use of reciprocal inhibition and stretching, see Section 17.10).

16.4 OVERVIEW OF PROPRIOCEPTION

- The word *proprioception* literally means *the body's sense of itself.*
- **Proprioception** is the ability of the nervous system to know the body's position in space and the body's movement through space.
- When we are young, we are usually taught that five senses exist: (1) sight, (2) hearing, (3) taste, (4) smell, and (5) touch. Another sense is called *proprioception.* As important as proprioception is, most people take this vital sense for granted.
- The sense of proprioception gives us awareness of the body's position in space and the body's movement through space.
- A proprioceptor is a receptor cell that is sensitive to a stimulus. When this stimulus occurs, the proprioceptor is stimulated, causing an impulse to travel through the sensory neuron to which it is attached. This sensory neuron then carries that impulse into the CNS.

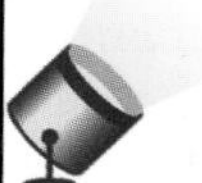

BOX 16-8

Each sensory receptor cell of the body is sensitive to a particular type of stimulus. For example, visual receptors (i.e., rods and cones) in the retina of the eye are sensitive to light; taste bud receptors on the tongue are sensitive to dissolved chemicals in the saliva. Most proprioceptor receptors are called **mechanoreceptors** because they are sensitive to mechanical pressure stimuli.

- Many types of proprioceptors are found in the human body. Generally they can be divided into three major categories:

BOX 16-9 SPOTLIGHT ON OTHER PROPRIOCEPTORS

Although three major categories of receptors are considered to be proprioceptors, any receptor that aids in the awareness of the body's position and movement can be considered to be proprioceptive in nature, even if its primary function is to provide us with another sense. Examples of these receptors that also have a proprioceptive function are vision, pain, and touch.

The sense of sight, although crucially important toward allowing us to know the objects in our surroundings, is also important toward giving us our own body's orientation in space. If a person is suspected of driving under the influence of alcohol, the police will often administer a sobriety test in which the person is asked to touch a finger to the nose. The ability to do this requires the proprioceptive awareness of the positions of the finger and nose, as well as the proprioceptive awareness of the movement of the upper extremity as the finger is moved toward the nose. Because alcohol particularly impairs centers of proprioception in the brain, this is a valuable test to determine a person's sobriety. However, when this test is administered, the person is instructed to close the eyes because vision would otherwise help guide the finger to the nose, destroying the test's

Continued

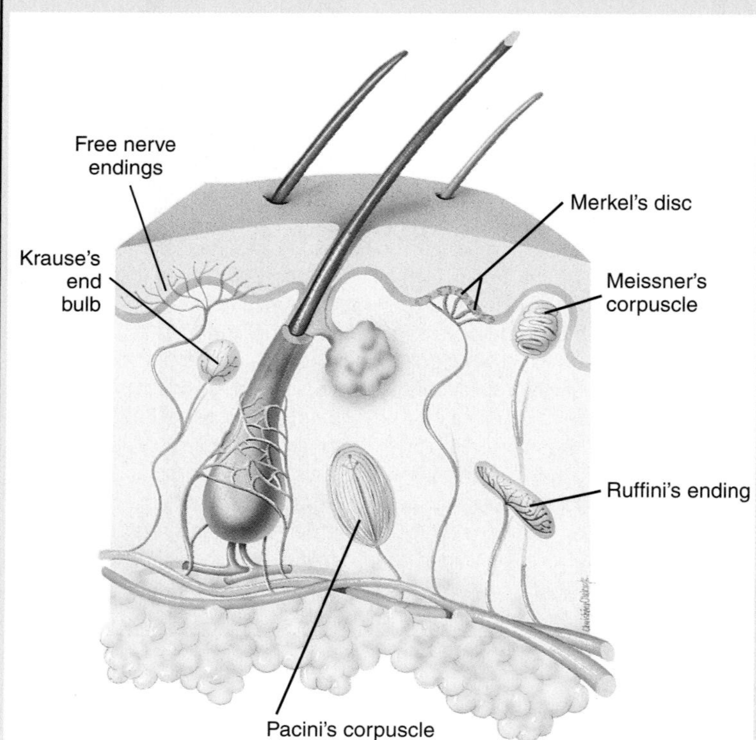

Modified from Thibodeau GA, Patton KT: *Anatomy and physiology,* ed 5. St Louis, 2003, Mosby.

BOX 16-9 SPOTLIGHT ON OTHER PROPRIOCEPTORS—cont'd

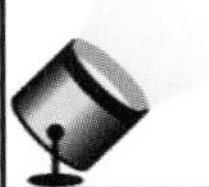

accuracy. Although not technically considered to be proprioceptive by some sources, vision certainly aids in our proprioceptive awareness.

The sense of pain can also aid our ability to sense the position and/or movement of the body. Using the sobriety test again as an example; try the sobriety test on yourself in two ways: (1) do it as described previously, and (2) try it after squeezing your nose hard enough to be painful. The presence of pain impulses coming from the nose will help someone to locate the nose with a finger. Although the primary function of pain is to alert our nervous system to possible tissue damage in the body, it should come as no surprise that pain in a body part also increases our awareness of that body part.

Touch receptors may also be proprioceptive in nature. Although touch is usually considered important toward alerting us to the physical presence of objects that are close to the body, touch that is sensed in a body part, similar to pain, also increases the nervous system's awareness of that body part. Interestingly, two major mechanoreceptors of touch located fairly deeply in the skin are Pacini's corpuscles and Ruffini's endings. These are the same receptors that are located within joint capsules and considered to be joint proprioceptors (see Section 16.5). Other touch mechanoreceptors located more superficially in the skin are **Meissner's corpuscles**, **Merkel's discs**, **Krause's end bulbs**, and **free nerve endings** (see figure).

1. **Fascial/joint proprioceptors**
2. **Muscle proprioceptors**
3. **Inner ear proprioceptors**

- Fascial/joint proprioceptors are located in and around the capsules of joints and provide information about the joint's static position and its dynamic movement. This information is used to give us conscious awareness of the positions and movements of the parts of the body.
  - They are also located in all other types of deep fibrous fascia of the body.
  - The two major types of fascial/joint proprioceptors are **Pacini's corpuscles** and **Ruffini's endings**.
- Muscle proprioceptors are located within the muscles of the body and not only provide proprioceptive awareness about the position and movement of the body but also function to create proprioceptive reflexes that protect muscles and tendons from injury.
  - Two major types of muscle proprioceptors exist: (1) **muscle spindles** and (2) **Golgi tendon organs**.
- Inner ear proprioceptors provide information about the static position and dynamic movement of the head.
  - Proprioceptive sensation from the inner ear (both static and dynamic) is often referred to as the sense of **equilibrium**.
  - The inner ear static proprioceptors for head position are located in the vestibule of the inner ear.
  - The inner ear dynamic proprioceptors for movement are located in the semicircular canals of the inner ear.

16.5 FASCIAL/JOINT PROPRIOCEPTORS

- Fascial/joint proprioceptors are located deeper in the body within dense fascia, both in and around joint capsules, as well as within deep muscular fascia. They are often referred to simply as *joint proprioceptors*.

Joint Proprioceptors:

- **Joint proprioceptors** are mechanoreceptors located in and around the capsules of joints.
- When the position of a joint changes, the soft tissues around the joint are compressed on one side of the joint and stretched on the other side of the joint.
- When this compression and stretching occurs, it creates a mechanical force on the joint proprioceptors that deforms them. Because they are mechanoreceptors, they are sensitive to this mechanical deformation and this stimulus causes the joint proprioceptors to fire, sending their signal into the central nervous system (CNS) (Figure 16-6).
- Based on which side(s) of the joint has proprioceptors stimulated and in what pattern this stimulation occurs, the CNS is able to determine which position the joint is in.
- For example, if the hip joint flexes (whether the thigh flexes toward the pelvis or the pelvis anteriorly tilts toward the thigh), the joint proprioceptors located on the anterior and posterior sides of the hip joint are deformed and stimulated, causing signals to be sent into the CNS. Knowing that it is the anterior and posterior proprioceptors that fired, and knowing the pattern of how this firing occurred, the CNS knows that the joint is flexed. If the joint action had been extended instead, the pattern of anterior and posterior receptors would have been different and the CNS would have interpreted the position as extension. Similarly, impulses from lateral and medial proprioceptors would signal abduction/adduction movements. Medial and lateral rotations would be indicated by the

characteristic pattern of compression that they would create. This concept can be applied to any joint of the body.

- Two types of joint proprioceptors exist: (1) **Pacini's corpuscles** and (2) **Ruffini's endings** (see the figure in Box 16-9, pp. 576-577.

BOX 16-10

A 3rd group of mechanoreceptors (i.e., proprioceptors) are found within joint capsules; they are known as **interstitial myofascial receptors**. Interstitial receptors are actually the most numerous receptor found within deep dense fascia. They are small receptors that are believed to be involved in pain reception and proprioception. Some are fast adapting and some are slow adapting.

- Both Pacini's corpuscles and Ruffini's endings are sensitive to mechanical force as described previously. The difference between them lies in how quickly they adapt to the application of the mechanical force.
- Pacini's corpuscles adapt quickly to mechanical force. This means that as they are being deformed, they send impulses into the CNS apprising it of the movement that is causing the deformation. However, as soon as the movement ceases, the Pacini's corpuscles adapt to this new level of deformation and stop sending impulses into the CNS. As a result, Pacini's corpuscles are only sensitive to and stimulated by changes in position (i.e., movement).

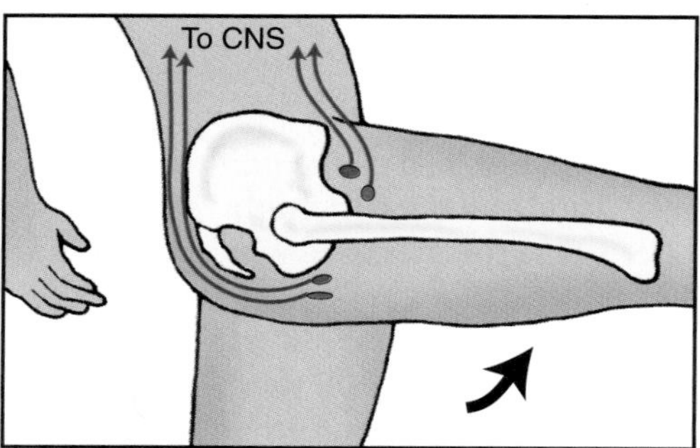

Figure 16-6 Flexion of the hip joint, which deforms the proprioceptors (i.e., Pacini's corpuscles, Ruffini's endings) located around the joint by compressing those located anteriorly and stretching those that are located posteriorly. Deformation of the proprioceptors stimulates them, which causes nerve impulses to travel to the central nervous system (CNS). The pattern of proprioceptive signals sent to the CNS is interpreted by the brain and informs us of the position and movement of the hip joint.

- Ruffini's endings are slow to adapt. This means that as they are being deformed, they send impulses into the CNS, apprising it of the movement that is causing the deformation. However, when the movement ceases and the change in deformation stops, the Ruffini's endings continue to send impulses into the CNS. As a result, Ruffini's endings are sensitive to and stimulated by a change in position (i.e., movement) and the static position of the joint.

BOX 16-11

Even Ruffini's endings have a limit to how long they will continue to be stimulated before adapting to the new position of the joint. If you have ever stayed very still in one position for an extended period of time (perhaps 15-20 minutes), you may have experienced a loss of Ruffini's ending proprioception from a joint; this results in an inability to feel the position of the body part(s) of that joint. If you cannot see the body part, it literally feels as if the body part is missing. The proprioceptive feel of the region can be immediately regained if you move the joint even a slight amount because this movement stimulates the Pacini's corpuscles and Ruffini's endings of the joint once again. (Note: This phenomenon is not the same as when a body part "falls asleep," which occurs when the blood supply to a body part such as the foot is lost, resulting in the nerves of the foot losing their blood supply. Having lost their blood supply, the nerves are no longer able to send any signals, including proprioceptive signals, into the central nervous system [CNS]. When this occurs, loss of sensation may also occur, but the return of sensation takes much longer and usually feels like "pins and needles" as the blood supply gradually returns and the nerves "reawaken.")

Essential Facts:

- Pacini's corpuscles give us proprioceptive information only about the movement of our joints.
- Ruffini's endings give us proprioceptive information about the movement of our joints and the static position of our joints.

Other Fascial Proprioceptor Locations:

- Aside from their location within joint capsules, all types of proprioceptors that are located within joint capsules are also located in all other types of deep fibrous fascia (i.e., ligaments, muscular fascia, tendons, aponeuroses, and intermuscular septa).
- Pressure applied to these fascial/joint proprioceptors has been found to have direct reflex effects, causing an increase in circulation of blood to the local area, a decrease in the tone of the muscles in the local area, and a decrease in sympathetic nervous system output. This pressure reflex has been found to occur during the application of bodywork and movement therapies, as well as exercise.

16.6 MUSCLE SPINDLES

- A **muscle spindle** is a type of muscle proprioceptor that is located within a muscle and is sensitive to a stretch (i.e., lengthening of the muscle).
  - Muscle spindle cells are located within the belly of a muscle and lie parallel to the fibers of the muscle.

BOX 16-12

The number of muscle spindles that a muscle contains varies from one muscle to another in the body. The muscles with the greatest proportion of muscle spindles are the muscles of the suboccipital group. Other muscles with a very high concentration of muscle spindles are the intertransversarii and the rotatores. Some sources state that because small deep muscles such as these contain such a high number of muscle spindles, their primary importance is to act as proprioceptive organs, not to contract and move or stabilize body parts.

  - Muscle spindle cells contain fibers that are known as **intrafusal fibers**. In contrast, regular muscle fibers are known as **extrafusal fibers**.
  - These intrafusal fibers of the muscle spindle are contractile like extrafusal fibers (i.e., they are able to contract and shorten).
- A muscle spindle is sensitive to the stretch (i.e. the lengthening) of the muscle within which it is located. More specifically, it is sensitive to two aspects of the stretch:
  1. The amount of stretch of the muscle.
  2. The rate (i.e., speed) of the stretch of the muscle.
- When the muscle is stretched sufficiently, the muscle spindle is also stretched and becomes stimulated, creating an impulse in a sensory neuron that enters the spinal cord to alert the CNS that the muscle has just been stretched.
- Because a stretched muscle may be overly stretched and torn, this impulse in the spinal cord causes a reflex contraction of the muscle (Figure 16-7). By contracting and shortening, the muscle stops any excessive stretching that might tear the muscle (Box 16-13, Note 1).
- This reflex is called the **muscle spindle reflex** or the **stretch reflex** (Box 16-13, Note 2).
  - The muscle spindle reflex is also known as the **myotatic reflex**.
- Therefore a muscle spindle and its stretch reflex are protective in nature. They prevent a muscle from being overly stretched and torn (Box 16-13, Note 2).

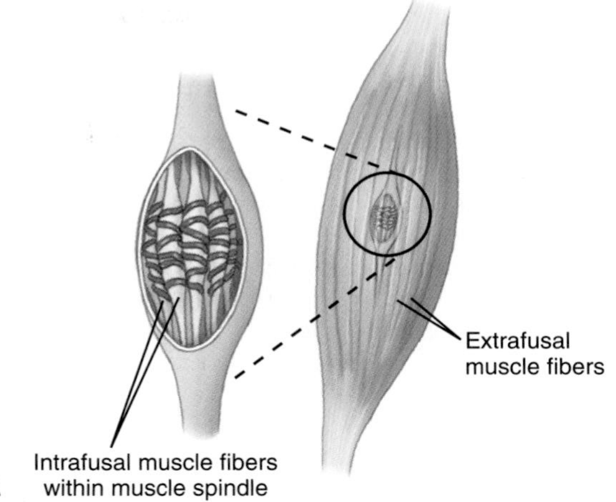

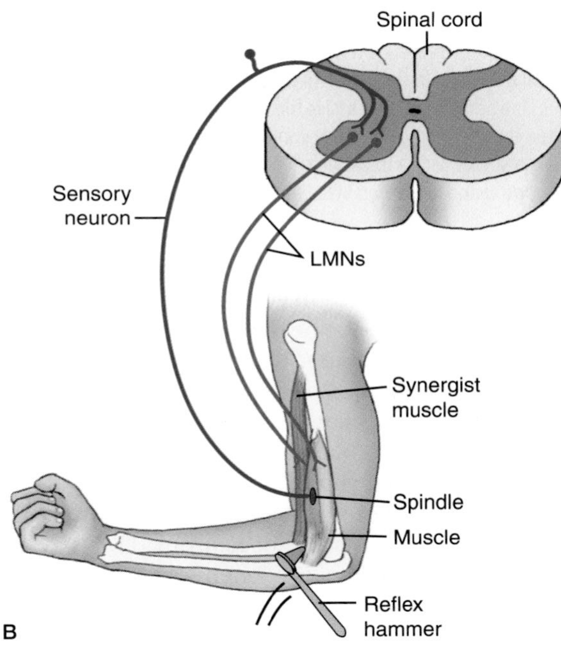

Figure 16-7 *A,* Illustration of how a muscle spindle is located within the belly of a muscle and runs parallel to the extrafusal muscle fibers of the muscle. *B,* Muscle spindle reflex. When the tendon of the muscle is tapped with the reflex hammer, the tendon elongates and creates a pulling force on the muscle belly. This in turn stretches the muscle spindles located within the belly, triggering a stretch reflex. The stretch reflex occurs when a sensory neuron from the muscle spindle carries a nerve impulse into the spinal cord where it synapses with the lower motor neuron (LMN) that returns to the muscle and causes it to contract (as well as causing synergistic muscles that do the same action to contract as shown). Any strong or fast stretch of a muscle may result in the stretch reflex causing the muscle to contract.

BOX 16-13

Note 1. Because of the presence of the muscle spindle stretch reflex, stretches done must be done slowly and in a fairly gentle manner; they cannot be forced. Heavy-handed and/or fast stretches will by definition result in tightening of the muscles involved. Further, although it was done for many years, it is now known that bouncing when you stretch is unhealthy. The reason for this is that bouncing quickly lengthens the muscle that is being stretched. Unfortunately, a quick lengthening of the muscle activates the muscle spindle reflex, which results in a contraction and tightening of the muscle. Although the purpose for the bouncing stretch is to relax and lengthen the muscle, this purpose is defeated because the muscle ends up being tighter.

Note 2. Although muscle spindle stretch reflexes are protective in nature, they also serve another purpose (i.e., to increase the strength of a muscle contraction immediately after it has been quickly stretched). If you observe any sport that involves throwing, kicking, or swinging, you will notice that the athlete uses a backswing before the actual throw, kick, or swing. For example, before serving a tennis ball, the tennis player quickly brings the racquet back. The purpose of this fast backswing immediately before the forward swing to actually hit the ball is to trigger the stretch reflex so that the power of the forward swing will be augmented by the reflex contraction of the stretch reflex. **Plyometric training** uses this concept and involves exercises that rapidly stretch a muscle and then immediately follows the stretch with contraction of the same muscle. (Note: The addition of the passive force of elastic recoil created by stretching the muscle during the backswing is a further benefit gained by preceding a stroke with a backswing. This phenomenon is called *productive antagonism* and is covered in Section 13.2.)

- Because muscles are less likely to be torn when they are relaxed and more likely to be torn when they are tight, muscle spindles need to be able to adapt to these different circumstances. Therefore it is important that the sensitivity of a muscle spindle to the stretch of the muscle can be regulated.
- The sensitivity of a muscle spindle is set by the **gamma motor system**.
  - The gamma motor system has upper motor neurons (UMNs) and lower motor neurons (LMNs). Gamma UMNs travel from the brain down to the spinal cord, where they synapse with gamma LMNs in the gray matter of the spinal cord. Gamma LMNs then travel from the spinal cord out to the muscle spindle (Box 16-14, Note 1).
  - The gamma LMN is responsible for directly setting the sensitivity of the muscle spindle (Figure 16-8). It does this by contracting and shortening the intrafusal fibers of the muscle spindle so that they are tauter. The shorter and tauter a muscle spindle is, the more sensitive it is to a stretch of the muscle (Box 16-14, Note 2).
  - However, the ultimate control of the gamma LMN rests with the UMNs of the gamma motor system. These gamma UMNs reside in the brain. The degree of sensitivity that these UMNs exert on the LMNs is based on subconscious processing of many factors within the brain. Some of these factors include previous and present physical traumas to the region of the body where the muscle is located, the need for stability in the region, and general emotional and physical stress levels (Box 16-15).

BOX 16-14

Note 1. Motor neurons that are directly concerned with controlling muscle contraction are called **alpha motor neurons**. This is done to differentiate them from the **gamma motor neurons** of the gamma motor system. Therefore alpha upper motor neurons (UMNs) and alpha lower motor neurons (LMNs), as well as gamma UMNs and gamma LMNs, exist. The alpha system directs muscle contraction by directing the regular extrafusal fibers of the muscle to contract. The gamma motor system directs muscle spindle contraction by contracting the intrafusal fibers of the muscle spindle to contract.

Note 2. A muscle spindle has a spindlelike or fusiform shape. The two ends of the muscle spindle are contractile (i.e., they can contract and shorten when stimulated by the gamma LMN). The central section houses the sensitive receptor portion of the spindle and is noncontractile. The sensitivity of a muscle spindle to stretch is caused by the gamma LMN causing a contraction at both ends of the spindle cell. This in turn stretches the noncontractile central portion from both ends, making it tauter and more sensitive and therefore more likely that a stretch of the muscle will cause the muscle spindle to trigger its stretch reflex.

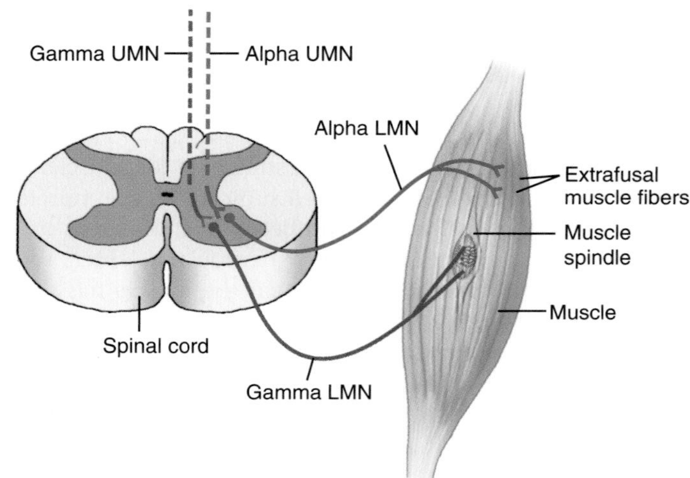

Figure 16-8 Innervation of a muscle spindle by the gamma motor system. A gamma lower motor neuron (LMN) travels from the spinal cord and synapses with the intrafusal fibers of a muscle spindle. The gamma LMN can contract the muscle spindle, making it tauter and therefore more sensitive to stretch. The more sensitive a muscle spindle is, the more likely it is to trigger a stretch reflex when it is stretched. (Note: The LMN that travels from the spinal cord and synapses with the regular extrafusal fibers of the muscle is called an *alpha LMN* to distinguish it from the gamma LMN. Just as alpha LMNs are controlled by alpha UMNs, gamma LMNs are controlled by gamma UMNs.)

BOX 16-15 SPOTLIGHT ON MUSCLE SPINDLES AND MUSCLE FACILITATION

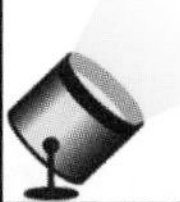

As bodyworkers and trainers, a major concern (perhaps *the* major concern) is working on our clients' tight muscles. A muscle that is tight when it is being directed to contract and work to move the body is not a concern. We are concerned with the muscles of our clients that are tight when they should be relaxed (i.e., when they are at rest). In other words, our concern is when the resting tone of a muscle is too tight. At rest, muscles are rarely totally relaxed. Some degree of contraction is usually present to maintain the proper posture of the joints of the body. This resting tone of our muscles is set by the gamma motor system that resides in the brainstem and works without our conscious control. However, the resting tone of muscles often gets too tight. Whether this is due to injury to the area, chronically bad posture, or any other reason, the gamma upper motor neurons (UMNs) of the brain order the gamma lower motor neurons (LMNs) to tighten the muscle spindles within the musculature. When the muscle spindles are tauter, they more readily trigger the stretch reflex, resulting in alpha LMNs that direct the muscle fibers of the muscle to tighten. Therefore it is actually the gamma motor system's control of the muscle spindle that sets the resting tone of a muscle (indirectly by setting the sensitivity of the muscle spindles to the stretch reflex). Whatever tone the gamma motor system sets for the spindles will shortly thereafter become the tone for the muscle itself. In this manner, the gamma motor system may create **muscle facilitation** or **muscle inhibition**. If the tone of the muscle's spindles (and therefore the tone of the muscle itself) is set high, the muscle is said to be *facilitated*. If the tone of the muscle's spindles (and therefore the tone of the muscle itself) is set low, the muscle is said to be *inhibited*.

When a muscle is facilitated, it is poised to be able to respond to any stimulus and contract more quickly than if it was not facilitated. The downside of muscle facilitation is that the muscle may tighten more easily; massage therapists and other manual therapists and bodyworkers are very sensitive to this condition of their clients. However, the upside of muscle facilitation is that the muscle is more responsive to the surrounding environment and can react more quickly and efficiently; this is extremely important during sporting events and exercise in general; trainers are very sensitive to this aspect of their client's muscle tone. On the other hand, when a muscle's spindles are lax and therefore not set as sensitive, the muscle is said to be *inhibited*. An inhibited muscle is most likely more relaxed (i.e., less tight); however, it is also less able to respond to stimuli and tighten quickly and efficiently when the need arises. The balance between facilitation and inhibition of a muscle is important. In a healthy individual, the relative proportion of this balance should be flexible and able to shift between greater or lesser facilitation or greater or lesser inhibition as the circumstances change and the need arises.

Interestingly, it seems that there are certain patterns of resting tone dysfunction within the body. Sources have divided most muscles of the body into two groups: those that tend toward becoming facilitated/tight, and those that tend toward becoming inhibited/weak. While this division should not be taken as absolute, these patterns do seem to generally be true. Examples of muscles that tend toward being overly facilitated are: neck extensors, pectoralis major and minor, subscapularis, lumbar erector spinae, hip flexors and adductors, hamstrings, and foot plantarflexors. Examples of muscles that tend toward being overly inhibited are: longus colli and capitis, lower trapezius and rhomboids, infraspinatus and teres minor, thoracic erector spinae, rectus abdominis, gluteus maximus, vastus lateralis and medialis, and foot dorsiflexors. As a general rule, it seems that flexors and medial rotators needed to achieve fetal position tend to be overly facilitated, while extensors and lateral rotators tend to be overly inhibited! An application of the asymmetry of this facilitation/inhibition pattern is that it predisposes the human body to two well known postural distortion patterns known as the **upper crossed syndrome** and the **lower crossed syndrome** (see accompanying illustration).

As bodyworkers, it is important to make a distinction between the two general types of muscle tightness that may be encountered: (1) local small areas of hypertonicity (i.e., **trigger points**) and (2) **global tightening** of the entire muscle. Although trigger points are created locally and require specific local work to remedy, a muscle that is globally tight is not really a local problem. The true cause is the sensitivity setting of the spindles by the gamma motor system of the brain (i.e., the muscle is overly facilitated). Therefore even though we may address this problem locally by treatment to the muscle itself, we must be aware that the root cause lies within the central nervous system (CNS). Whatever attention can be given to encourage the gamma motor portion of the nervous system to relax its activity (i.e., its facilitation of the muscle) may ultimately prove to be the most valuable aspect of our treatment. While being careful to not overstep the boundaries of one's profession, when looking at gamma motor system facilitation, many parameters of the client's health must be considered. These parameters include both physical and emotional/psychologic factors. The subconsciously perceived fragility and vulnerability of the region of the body where the muscle is located are particularly important. Also of importance is the chronicity of neural facilitation patterning of how the client's body responds to stressors of all types, or put more simply, where he or she tends to hold stress.

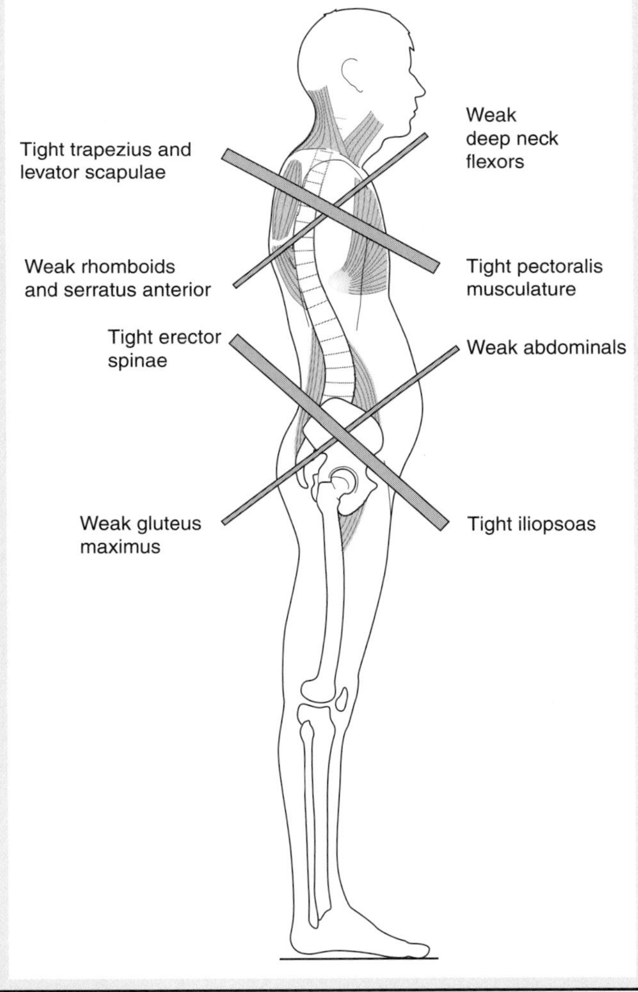

16.7 GOLGI TENDON ORGANS

- A **Golgi tendon organ** is a type of muscle proprioceptor that is located within a tendon of a muscle and is sensitive to a pulling force that is placed on the tendon.
- Pulling forces on a tendon primarily occur when the tendon's muscle belly contracts; therefore Golgi tendon organs sense contraction of the muscle belly.
- Golgi tendon organs are located within the tendon of a muscle near the musculotendinous junction.

BOX 16-16

Golgi receptors are also located within joint capsules and ligaments; they are referred to as **Golgi end organs**.

- They are attached in series (end to end) to a number of muscle fibers.
- When these muscle fibers contract and shorten, they create a pulling force on the Golgi tendon organ.
- A Golgi tendon organ is sensitive to the pulling force of the muscle fibers to which it is attached.
- When the muscle contracts and shortens sufficiently, the Golgi tendon organ is stretched, becomes stimulated, and creates an impulse in a sensory neuron that enters the spinal cord to alert the CNS that the muscle has just contracted and shortened, pulling on its tendon(s).
- Because a pulling force on a tendon may stretch and tear it, this impulse in the spinal cord causes a reflex relaxation of the muscle (Figure 16-9). By relaxing the muscle, the muscle no longer creates a pulling force that might tear the tendon.
- This reflex is called the **Golgi tendon organ reflex** or simply the **tendon reflex**.

BOX 16-17

Because the Golgi tendon organ reflex has the opposite effect of the *myotatic reflex* of the muscle spindle, it is also referred to as the **inverse myotatic reflex**.

- The relaxation of the muscle is accomplished by the sensory neuron from the Golgi tendon organ synapsing with an interneuron that inhibits the alpha LMN to the muscle. If the alpha motor neuron to the muscle is inhibited from carrying an impulse, the muscle will be inhibited from contracting and will therefore relax.
  - Therefore a Golgi tendon organ and its tendon reflex are protective in nature. They prevent a tendon from being overly stretched and torn by a muscle that otherwise might contract too forcefully.

BOX 16-18

The Golgi tendon organ reflex is often used as a part of the physical therapy treatment called **electrical muscle stimulation** (EMS) (also referred to as *E-stim*). An EMS machine puts an electrical current into the client's muscle that is similar to the electrical current that would come from the alpha lower motor neuron (LMN); this causes the muscle to contract. The therapy is kept on for 5-10 minutes, keeping the muscle in a sustained isometric contraction. In response to this contraction, the Golgi tendon organ reflex is triggered, resulting in relaxation of the muscle.

Essential Facts:

- Muscle spindles and Golgi tendon organs are similar in that they are both protective in nature.
- They differ regarding which structure they each protect and the result of their reflexes.
  - The muscle spindle reflex results in contraction of a muscle and acts to prevent a muscle from being overly stretched and torn.
  - The Golgi tendon organ reflex results in relaxation of a muscle and acts to prevent the tendon from being overly stretched and torn (by an overly contracting muscle) (Box 16-19).

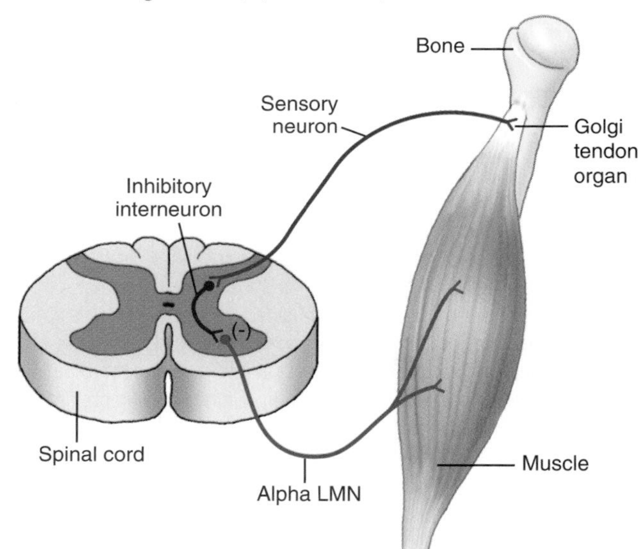

Figure 16-9 Illustration of the neural pathways of the Golgi tendon organ reflex. A Golgi tendon organ is located within a muscle's tendon (as its name implies) and is sensitive to a stretch placed upon the tendon. An overly contracting muscle pulls on its tendons and may excessively stretch a tendon, resulting in a tear or complete rupture of the tendon. The Golgi tendon organ reflex protects the tendon from this potential injury. When a Golgi tendon organ is stimulated by a stretch upon the tendon of the muscle in which it is located, it causes a relaxation of the muscle, thereby eliminating the excessive stretch from being placed upon the tendon. This reflex is accomplished by the sensory neuron from the Golgi tendon organ synapsing with and stimulating an interneuron, which in turn inhibits the alpha lower motor neurons (LMNs) that control the muscle fibers. Inhibition of a muscle's alpha LMNs results in a relaxation of the muscle.

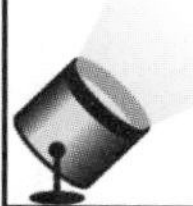

BOX 16-19 SPOTLIGHT ON THE GOLGI TENDON ORGAN REFLEX AND STRETCHING

Using the Golgi tendon organ reflex can be a powerful tool to increase the effectiveness of a stretch with your client. When doing a stretch in this manner, have the client actively isometrically contract the muscle that you want to stretch against your resistance. After the isometric contraction, ask the client to relax the muscle; you can then stretch the muscle further than you would have been able to otherwise because of the reflex inhibition of the muscle by the Golgi tendon organ reflex.

This type of stretching is known as **CR stretching** or **PIR stretching**. CR stands for **contract-relax stretching** because the client contracts and then relaxes; PIR stands for post-isometric relaxation stretching, because the client isometrically contracts and then relaxes. It is also commonly referred to as **PNF stretching**; PNF stands for proprioceptive neuromuscular facilitation because a **proprioceptive neuromuscular** reflex (the Golgi tendon organ reflex) is used to facilitate the stretch.

Although the exact manner in which this type of stretching is carried out varies from therapist to therapist, it is customary to have the client hold the isometric contraction for approximately 5-8 seconds each time before the relaxation/stretch is done; this can be repeated approximately three times, usually with a stronger isometric contraction each time. Although the hamstrings are usually the muscles used when demonstrating CR stretching (and are shown here in the accompanying figure), this type of stretching is extremely effective and can be used for any muscle of the body.

An interesting footnote to CR stretching is that when done on one side of the body, it can help the same muscles on the other side of the body relax, even though the muscles on that side were not directly touched and stretched. To try this using the hamstrings as an example again, evaluate the maximum passive range of motion of the client's hamstrings muscles bilaterally. Then do the CR stretch technique three times as described here on only one side of the body. After completing the stretch on one side, check the range of motion of the untouched side and its passive range of motion should have increased! The reason for this is that the effect of stretching one side of the body affects the sensitivity of the gamma motor system in the brain. Therefore the upper motor neurons (UMNs) of the gamma motor system relax the muscle spindles bilaterally for that muscle group (i.e., the hamstrings on both sides of the body will have the sensitivity of the muscle spindles relaxed, resulting in a greater passive range of motion on both sides).

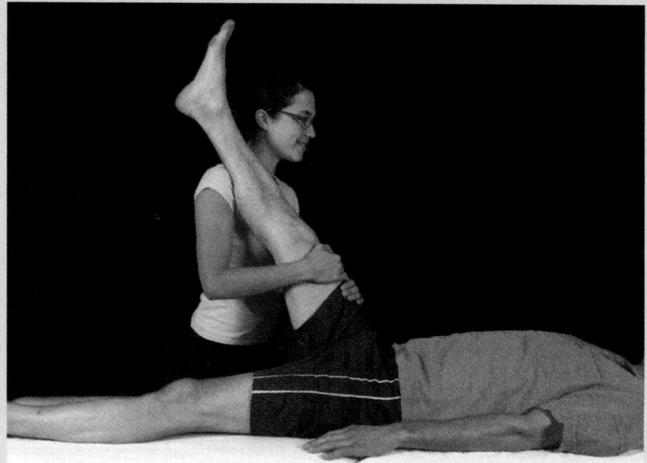

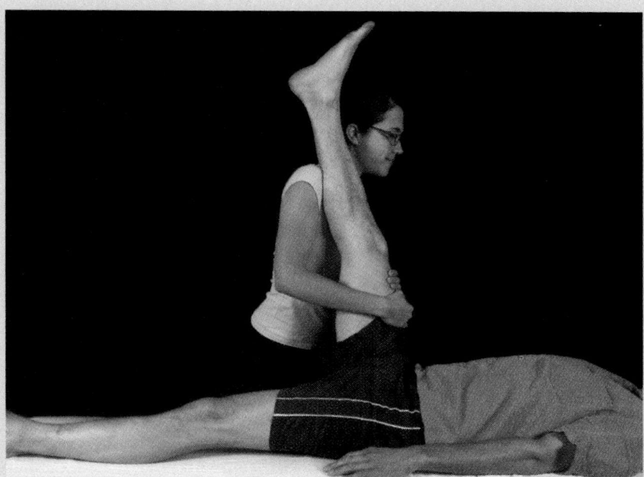

Contract-relax (CR) stretching is demonstrated in these two photos. The 1st photo illustrates the 1st step of CR stretching in which the therapist asks the client to take in a deep breath and hold it in while isometrically contracting the hamstrings against resistance for 5-8 seconds. The 2nd photo illustrates the 2nd step in which the client relaxes and exhales while the therapist gently stretches the client's hamstrings. This two-step process should be repeated approximately three times. Each time, the client should gradually increase the force of the isometric contraction, and the therapist should be able to gently increase the range of motion of the stretch. (Courtesy Joseph E. Muscolino.)

16.8 INNER EAR PROPRIOCEPTORS

- Inner ear proprioceptors provide information as to the static position and dynamic movement of the head.
- Inner ear proprioception is often referred to as the *sense of equilibrium*.

BOX 16-20

The term **equilibrium** is used to describe our ability to maintain our balance both during statically held positions and during dynamic movements. Although the inner ear is usually credited with giving us the sensory information to have this ability, all proprioceptors are involved in maintaining equilibrium.

- Two types of proprioceptive organs are located in the inner ear (Figure 16-10):
  1. The **macula**, which provides static proprioception informing the brain of the static position of the head (Figure 16-11)
  2. The **crista ampullaris**, which provides dynamic proprioception informing the brain of the movement of the head (Figure 16-12)

BOX 16-21

The inner ear is often called the *labyrinth*. For this reason, the inner ear proprioceptors are often referred to as the **labyrinthine proprioceptors**. Information from the labyrinthine proprioceptors of the inner ear, as well as the sense of hearing from the cochlea of the inner ear, travel in cranial nerve (CN) VIII, which is named the *vestibulocochlear nerve*.

Static Proprioception:

- Two maculae are located within the **vestibule** of the inner ear.
- A macula consists primarily of a mass of gelatinous substance. Within the gelatinous substance are hair cells that are attached to sensory neurons, and crystals called **otoliths**. The purpose of the otoliths is to increase the weight of the gelatinous substance, making it more responsive to changes in position (see Figure 16-11a).
- When the position of the head changes, such as when the head tilts (i.e., flexes) forward, the otoliths fall with gravity, dragging the gelatinous substance with them. The movement of the gelatinous substance causes the hairs to bend, resulting in impulses being sent through sensory neurons that travel to the brain (see Figure 16-11b).
- Based on which hair cells are bent and how they are bent (i.e., based on the pattern of nerve impulses received from the macula), the brain can determine the position of the head relative to gravity.
- It is important to emphasize that the macula can only detect the static position of the head itself, not the position of the trunk or any other body part.

Dynamic Proprioception:

- Three crista ampullaris structures are located within the **semicircular canals** of the inner ear (one is located in each of the three semicircular canals) (see Figure 16-12a).
- One semicircular canal is located in each of the three cardinal planes (sagittal, frontal, and transverse).
- A semicircular canal is a fluid-filled canal that is semicircular in shape. It has an expanded end that is called the **ampulla**, where the crista ampullaris is located.
- A crista ampullaris is a structure that has hair cells attached to sensory neurons.

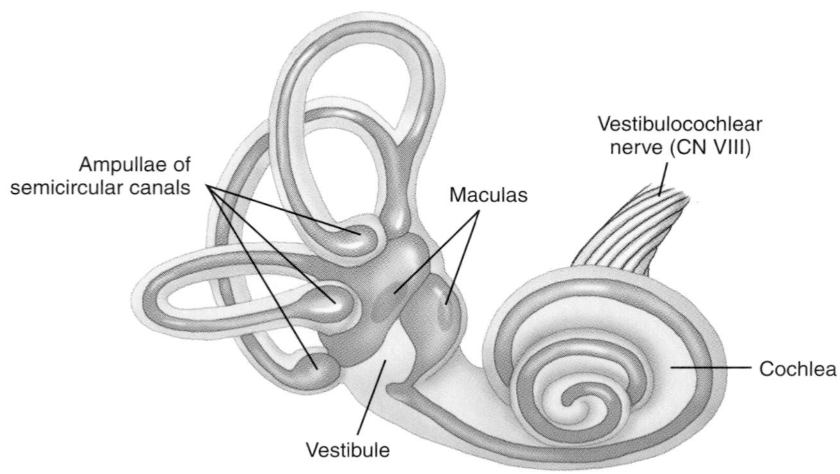

Figure 16-10 Structure of the inner ear, which includes the three semicircular canals, the vestibule, and the cochlea. The vestibule houses the maculae, which detect static equilibrium. Each semicircular canal houses a crista ampullaris (within an ampulla), which detects dynamic equilibrium. (Note: The cochlea is the part of the inner ear that is involved with the sense of hearing.)

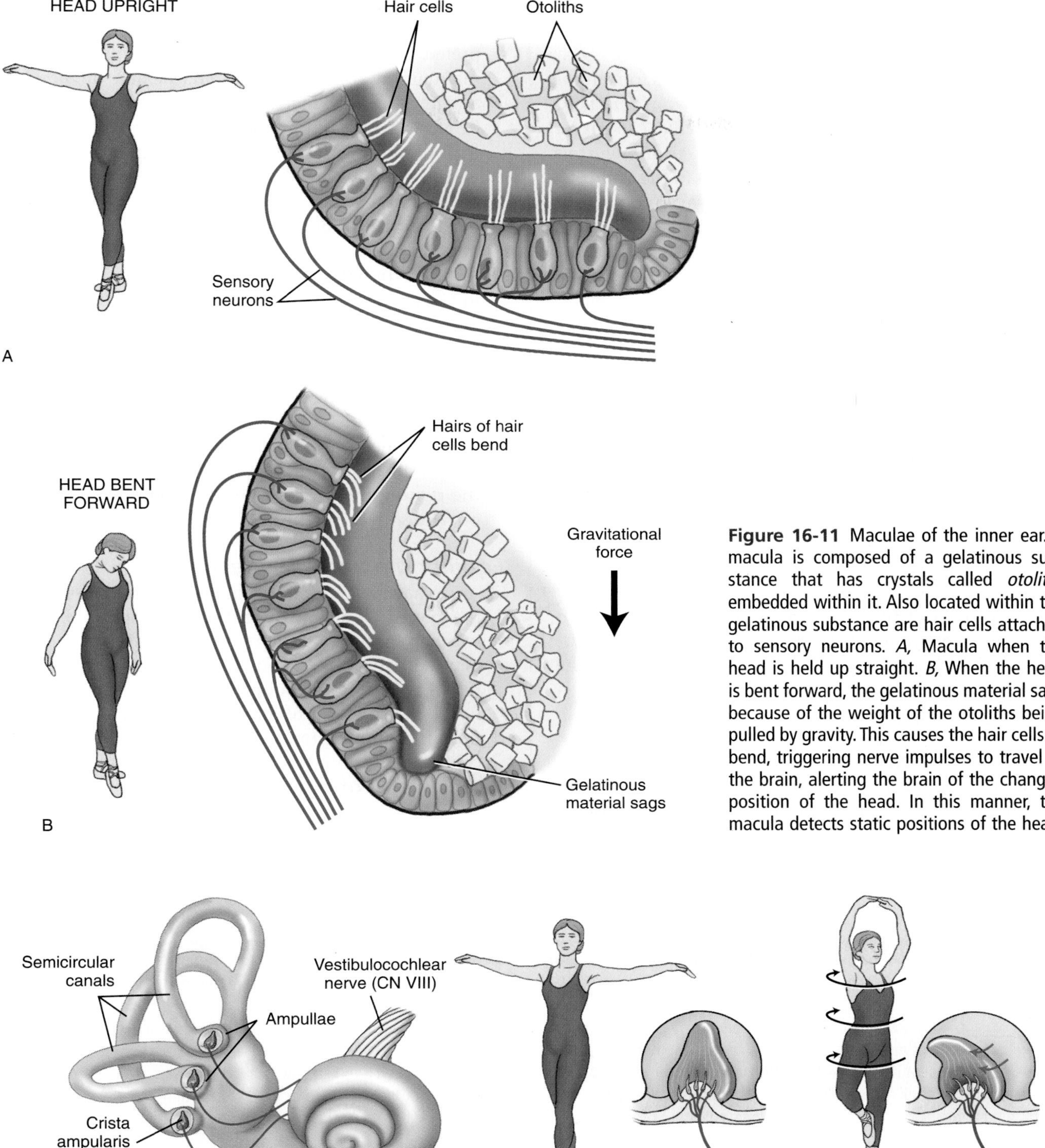

Figure 16-11 Maculae of the inner ear. A macula is composed of a gelatinous substance that has crystals called *otoliths* embedded within it. Also located within the gelatinous substance are hair cells attached to sensory neurons. *A,* Macula when the head is held up straight. *B,* When the head is bent forward, the gelatinous material sags because of the weight of the otoliths being pulled by gravity. This causes the hair cells to bend, triggering nerve impulses to travel to the brain, alerting the brain of the changed position of the head. In this manner, the macula detects static positions of the head.

Figure 16-12 *A,* Crista ampullaris of the semicircular canals of the inner ear. Three semicircular canals exist, one in each of the three cardinal planes (sagittal, frontal, and transverse). A crista ampullaris is composed of hair cells and is located within the ampulla of a semicircular canal. Also located within the semicircular canal is fluid. When a person moves the head within a cardinal plane, the fluid within the canal that is oriented within that cardinal plane is set in motion, causing the hair cells of the crista ampullaris to be bent (as can be seen in *C* in which the ballerina spins within the transverse plane). This triggers the neurons attached to the hair cells to send this information to the brain, alerting the brain to the movement of the head. In this manner, the crista ampullaris detects motion of the head.

- When the head moves, depending on the direction of movement, fluid is set in motion within one or more of the semicircular canals (see Figure 16-12b–c).
  - For example, if the motion of the head is forward or backward (i.e., within the sagittal plane), the fluid within the sagittally oriented semicircular canal is set in motion, and impulses from the sensory neurons from that semicircular canal are sent to the brain.
  - If the motion of the head is sideways (i.e., within the frontal plane), impulses are sent to the brain from the frontally oriented semicircular canal.
  - If the motion of the head is rotary (i.e., within the transverse plane), impulses are sent to the brain from the transversely oriented semicircular canal.
- Any oblique plane movement of the head results in a pattern of impulses from two or three semicircular canals that the brain can decipher and interpret as that particular oblique direction of motion.
- It is important to emphasize that the crista ampullaris structures of the semicircular canals can only detect motion of the head itself; they cannot detect motion of the trunk or any other body part.

Essential Facts:

- The macula of the inner ear provides the brain with proprioception about the static position of the head.
- The crista ampullaris of the inner ear provides the brain with proprioception about the dynamic movement of the head.

Righting Reflex:

- Proper proprioceptive information from the inner ears and the eyes is crucially important for the sense of proprioception (i.e., for interpreting position and movement). This proprioceptive input is best interpreted when the head is level. (Note: To prove this, try maintaining a position of lateral flexion of the head and neck for an extended period of time. It will quickly be felt to be uncomfortable to sense proprioception in this position.) Hence a reflex called the **righting reflex** acts to keep the head level. (Note: For more on the righting reflex, see Section 16.9.) Whenever the head becomes unlevel, the righting reflex directs the muscles of the body to alter the position of the joints to bring the head back to a level position. The righting reflex can be very important posturally. One example of this is the effect of the righting reflex caused by a collapsed arch in the foot. A collapsed arch in the foot creates one lower extremity that is shorter than the other; the result of this is that the body would lean toward the lower side, resulting in the head being unlevel. The righting reflex will create a compensation so that the head returns to being level. In this instance, the righting reflex will cause the spine to curve scoliotically so that the head is level (see Figure 17-5).

Equilibrium and Dizziness:

- As we have seen, proprioceptive information regarding the position and movement of the body is provided by many sources. Whenever a disagreement exists between what the various proprioceptors of the body report regarding the position and/or movement of the head (perhaps as a result of injury or malfunction of certain proprioceptors), the brain experiences proprioceptive confusion. We feel and describe proprioceptive confusion as **dizziness**.

BOX 16-22 SPOTLIGHT ON THE INNER EAR AND NECK PROPRIOCEPTORS

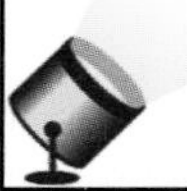

The inner ear proprioceptors are located within the head. Consequently, they can only report to the brain what the position and movement are of the *head.* They cannot know the position or movement of the trunk (or of any other body part). However, it is imperative for the brain to know what the position and movement of the trunk are as well, because the trunk is the heaviest body part, and maintaining proper static and dynamic posture of the trunk is important so that we do not fall. How then does the brain know about trunk posture? The critical link to know trunk posture is provided by the joint and muscular proprioceptors of the neck. These proprioceptors report the posture of the neck (i.e., whether it is straight or bent). If the brain knows the position of the head from the inner ear receptors, and it then knows whether the neck is straight or bent (and if it is bent, in what position it is bent), then the brain can determine the position of the trunk.

For example, if the inner ear proprioceptors report that the head is inclined forward, the brain needs to know whether or not the trunk is also inclined forward. If the neck proprioceptors report that the neck is straight, then the brain knows that the trunk must also be inclined forward; therefore the brain would have to order back extensor muscles to contract to keep the trunk from falling into flexion. However, if the neck proprioceptors instead report that the neck is flexed, then the brain can determine that the trunk is vertical and no postural muscles would have to be activated to keep the trunk from falling.

This role of the neck proprioceptors is critically important and has an important clinical application to bodywork. If the neck has been injured (e.g., as the result of a whiplash accident or an asymmetric muscle spasm in the neck), incorrect proprioceptive signals may be sent from the neck proprioceptors to the brain. Because these incorrect proprioceptive signals will contradict other proprioceptive signals (e.g., signals from the eyes), proprioceptive confusion will most likely result. Because proprioceptive confusion is experienced as dizziness, the client may become dizzy. In other words, not all dizziness comes from inner ear infections as is often believed. When dizziness does result from a neck that is unhealthy musculoskeletally, bodyworkers are empowered to work on the necks of these clients and may possibly relieve them of the dizziness that they are experiencing!

☐ 16.9 OTHER MUSCULOSKELETAL REFLEXES

Other than reciprocal inhibition, muscle spindle, and Golgi tendon organ reflexes, a number of other musculoskeletal reflexes occur in the human body. Following are some such reflexes that are applicable to movement (i.e., to the study of kinesiology):

Flexor Withdrawal Reflex:

- ❑ The **flexor withdrawal reflex** involves a flexion withdrawal movement of a body part when that body part experiences pain. Like most reflexes, the flexor withdrawal reflex is mediated by the spinal cord. Any conscious knowledge that we have flexed and withdrawn a body part in response to pain occurs after the reflex has occurred (by information that goes up through ascending white matter tracts of the spinal cord to the brain). Figure 16-13 illustrates the flexor withdrawal reflex.
  - ❑ The flexor withdrawal reflex is a protective reflex meant to prevent injury to the body by removing the body part from possible injury.
- ❑ Note that reciprocal inhibition is a necessary component of the flexor reflex. As the flexor muscles are ordered to contract, the extensor muscles on the same side of the body are inhibited from contracting (i.e., ordered to relax), otherwise flexion away from the pain-causing object would not be efficiently possible. (Note: The reciprocal inhibition component of the flexor withdrawal reflex has not been shown in Figure 16-13.)

Crossed Extensor Reflex:

- ❑ The **crossed extensor reflex** is a reflex that works in conjunction with the flexor withdrawal reflex. As the body part that experiences pain flexes and withdraws, the extensor muscles of the contralateral (i.e., opposite side) extremity contract to move that extremity into extension. Figure 16-14 illustrates the crossed extensor reflex.
  - ❑ The crossed extensor reflex is so named because this reflex crosses to the other side of the spinal cord to create a contraction in the contralateral extensor muscles.
  - ❑ The purpose of the crossed extensor reflex is to create a balanced posture of the body when one side flexes and withdraws. For example, if one lower extremity flexes and withdraws, the contralateral lower extremity must go into extension to support the body from falling; if one upper extremity flexes and withdraws, then extension of the contralateral upper extremity helps to create a more balanced posture.
- ❑ Note that reciprocal inhibition is a part of the crossed extensor reflex. As the extensor muscles are ordered to contract, the flexor muscles on that side of the body are inhibited from contracting (i.e., ordered to relax), otherwise extension of the contralateral extremity would not be efficiently possible. (Note: The reciprocal inhibition component of the crossed extensor reflex has not been shown in Figure 16-14.)

Tonic Neck Reflex:

- ❑ The **tonic neck reflex** orders contraction of the muscles of the arms based on the change in position of the neck. For example, if the neck rotates to the right, extensor muscles of the right arm are ordered to contract and flexor muscles of the left arm are ordered to contract (of course, reciprocal inhibition inhibits the flexors on the right and the extensors on the left). Figure 16-15 demonstrates the tonic neck reflex.

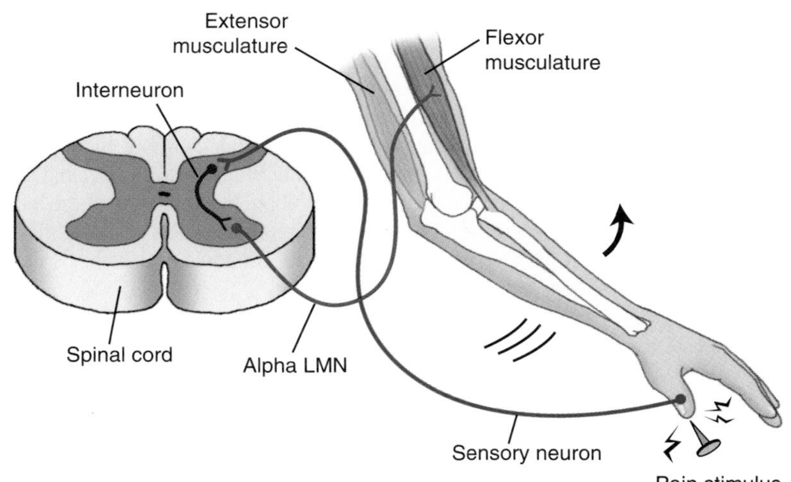

Figure 16-13 Illustration of the flexor withdrawal reflex, which is reflex mediated by the spinal cord. When a painful stimulus has occurred, it travels via a sensory neuron into the spinal cord where it synapses with an interneuron, which then synapses with an alpha lower motor neuron (LMN). The alpha LMN then directs the flexor musculature in that region of the body to contract so that the body part is flexed and withdrawn from the cause of the painful stimulus.

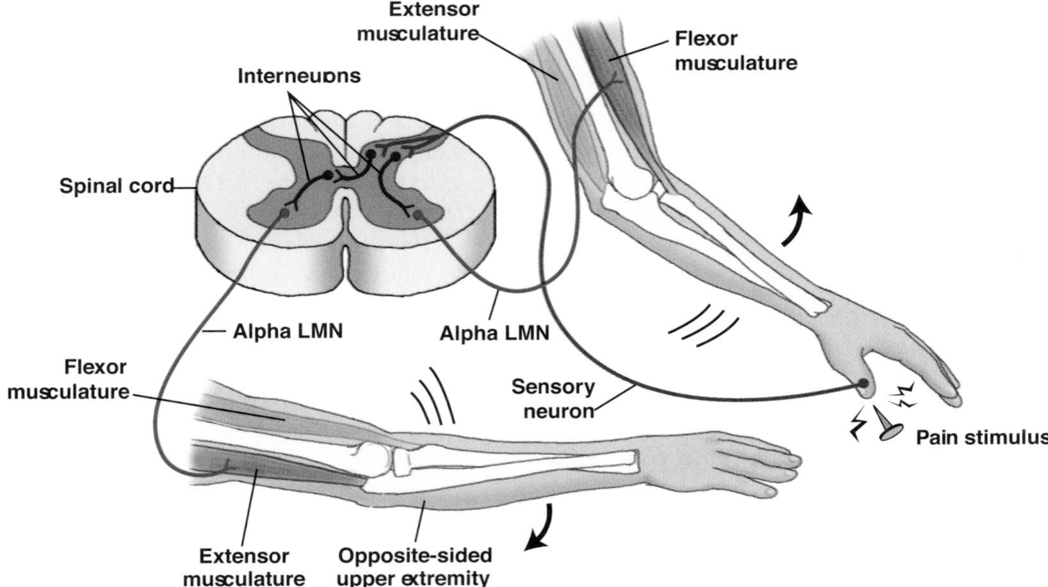

Figure 16-14 Illustration of the crossed extensor reflex and the flexor withdrawal reflex. When the flexor withdrawal reflex causes flexion and withdrawal of the extremity on the same side as the painful stimulus, the information that enters the spinal cord also crosses over to the other side of the cord and synapses with alpha lower motor neurons (LMNs), which direct the extensor musculature of the opposite sided extremity to contract. This additional reflex component that crosses to the other side of the cord and directs extensor contraction is called the *crossed extensor reflex*.

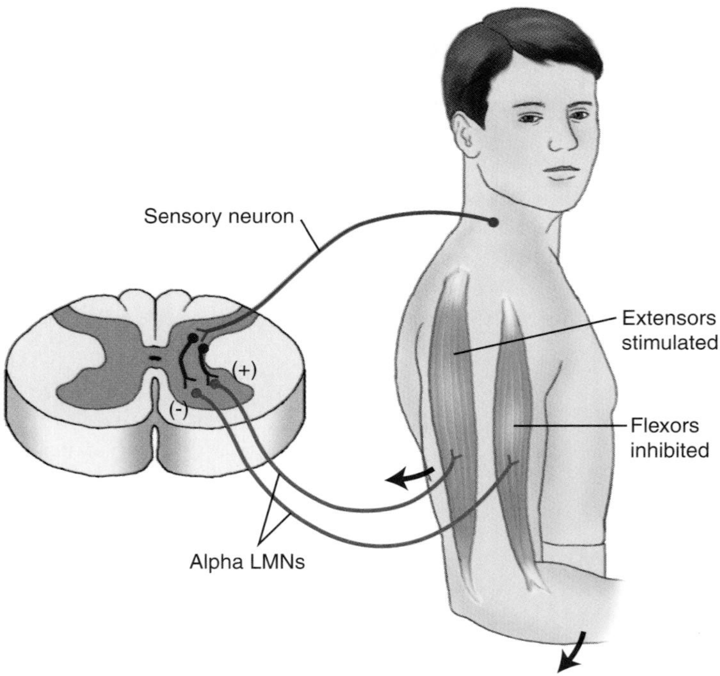

Figure 16-15 Illustration of the tonic neck reflex, which orders contraction of extremity muscles when the neck moves. The purpose of this reflex is to orient the body in the same direction as the head is facing. In this illustration, when the neck rotates to the right, the extensors of the right upper extremity are reflexly ordered to contract (and via reciprocal inhibition, the flexors are inhibited and therefore relax). The flexors of the left upper extremity would also be ordered to contract (and via reciprocal inhibition, the extensors of the left upper extremity would be inhibited and relax). (Note: The left upper extremity component of the tonic neck reflex is not shown in this figure.)

❑ The purpose of the tonic neck reflex is to help orient the body in the direction to which the head is oriented (i.e., where we are faced and looking).

Righting Reflex:

❑ The **righting reflex** is meant to keep us upright in a balanced position. If the inner ear perceives that our posture is such that we might fall, then that information is sent into the brain, which then sends signals down through the spinal cord to many levels, ordering muscle contractions to try to keep us upright. One example of the righting reflex is when a person attempts to do a back dive into a pool. As soon as the head inclines backward, reflex contraction of the flexor musculature of the trunk and arms occurs to try to bring the person back into an upright posture (Figure 16-16). Allowing this reflex to occur would result in a failed and most likely painful back dive. Having to override this reflex is one reason why a back dive seems so difficult for a beginner.

❑ The righting reflex is also known as the **labyrinthine righting reflex**.

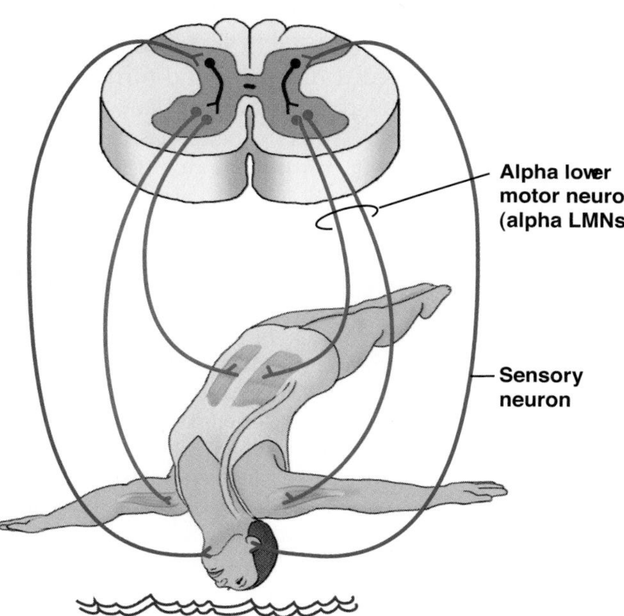

Figure 16-16 Illustration of the righting reflex. In this illustration, when a person attempts a back dive into a swimming pool, the head is no longer vertical. As a result, the righting reflex orders flexor musculature of the trunk and upper extremities to contract in an attempt to "right" the orientation of the head, bringing it back to a vertical orientation. A successful back dive requires the righting reflex to be overridden, because if the righting reflex is successful, the person's trunk will flex, and the trunk, neck, and head will return to a vertical position, resulting in an uncomfortable entry into the water.

Cutaneous Reflex:

❑ The **cutaneous reflex** causes relaxation in musculature after receiving either massage and/or an application of heat (Figure 16-17).

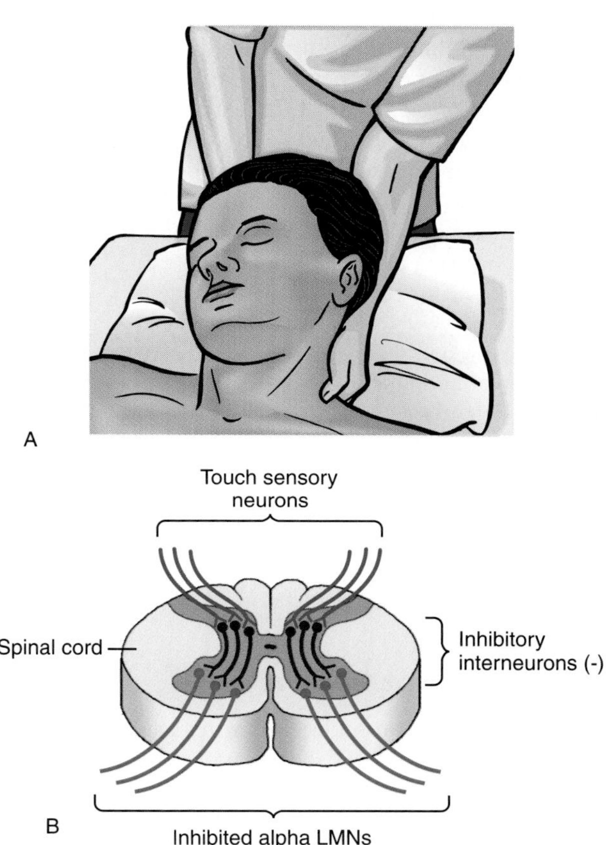

Figure 16-17 Illustration of the cutaneous reflex, which results in relaxation of musculature in response to touch and/or heat applied to the skin. Stimulation from touch travels into the spinal cord within sensory neurons. Within the cord, these sensory neurons synapse with inhibitory interneurons that inhibit alpha lower motor neurons (LMNs) from carrying nerve impulses. When alpha LMNs are inhibited, the musculature controlled by them relaxes. (A, From Fritz S: *Mosby's fundamentals of therapeutic massage,* ed 3. St Louis, 2004, Mosby.)

16.10 PAIN-SPASM-PAIN CYCLE

- The **pain-spasm-pain cycle** describes the vicious cycle of pain causing muscular spasm, which causes further pain, which causes further spasming and so forth.

Pain Causes Spasm:

- From an evolutionary standpoint, pain in the body was often caused by physical trauma such as a broken bone and/or a bleeding wound. If movement of a physically damaged body part such as this were to occur, the broken bone and bleeding wound would never have the opportunity to heal. For this reason, **muscle splinting** often occurs in the region of the injury. Muscle splinting is caused by the nervous system directing the musculature of the region to contract (i.e., spasm). In effect, by spasming the surrounding muscles, the area is splinted and cannot move, affording the injury a chance to heal.

BOX 16-23

Body armoring is a term used to describe when a person armors the body by splinting/spasming muscles in a region of the body for emotional or psychologic reasons. An example often given is if a person has a "broken heart," he or she may tighten the muscles of the pectoral region to "armor" the heart. Whether the root cause of muscle splinting/spasming is physical or emotional/psychological, once long-standing isometric tightening of musculature occurs, it is likely to lead into the pain-spasm-pain cycle.

Spasm Does Not Go Away:

- The presence of muscular spasm (caused by the pain) affords the damaged body part a chance to heal. However, with the physical lifestyle that people generally had before modern civilized society, some physicality of the body was required to survive. Perhaps water had to be gotten from the stream or well, or food had to be gathered from the woods or picked from the garden. There was no indoor plumbing, and it was not possible to call in sick to work or have meals delivered. As much as it seemed that the body was telling us to not use the body part, it simply was not possible to stop all physical activity. As a result of gradually having to use the body in a physical manner, the muscle spasms that were initially created to splint the injured body part and give it chance to heal were gradually worked free, and the area was gradually coaxed into loosening up. However, in our modern nonphysical lifestyle, physicality is often not required of us and, as a result, these muscle spasms, once begun, tend to continue.

Continued Spasm Causes Further Pain:

- As muscle spasming continues, pain increases because of two factors:
  1. The spasmed muscle itself—Because of the strong pull of its own contraction, the spasmed muscle causes pain by pulling on its attachments. In addition, most any movement that asks the spasmed muscle to stretch creates further pain because it is spasmed and resistant to stretch.
  2. Compromised blood flow—Continued muscle spasm closes off venous return of blood back to the heart. As venous return is blocked, waste products of metabolism build up in the body tissues distal to the site of the spasming. These waste products of metabolism contain acidic substances that irritate the nerves of the region, causing pain. If the spasming is sufficiently strong, even arterial supply can be closed off, resulting in **ischemia**, depriving body cells of needed nutrients, and further irritating nerves. All of this further irritation of nerves creates further pain. Thus the pain-spasm-pain cycle is complete and will continue to viciously cycle and worsen.

BOX 16-24 SPOTLIGHT ON ISOMETRIC MUSCLE SPASM AND VENOUS CIRCULATION

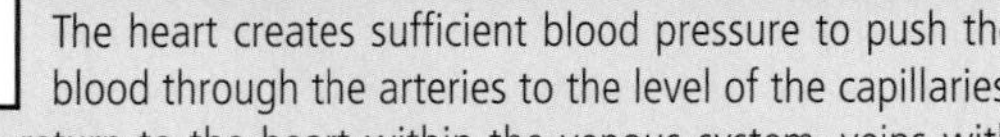

The heart creates sufficient blood pressure to push the blood through the arteries to the level of the capillaries. For blood to return to the heart within the venous system, veins with unidirectional valves and thin walls depend on skeletal muscular contractions to collapse the walls of the veins and push the blood back in the direction of the heart. Each muscle contraction collapses and pushes blood located in the vein; each subsequent relaxation of the muscle then allows the vein to fill up again with intercellular tissue fluid containing waste products of metabolism. The next contraction then recollapses the vein and pushes this blood toward the heart. Thus the venous system relies on alternating contractions and relaxations of the adjacent skeletal musculature. However, long-standing (i.e., isometric) muscle spasming causes a collapse and blockage of the veins that compromises or entirely stops local venous circulation for the duration of the muscle spasm. As a result, waste products of metabolism are allowed to build up. Many of these waste products are acidic and irritate the local tissues, resulting in further pain.

- With the pain-spasm-pain cycle, both pain and spasming are root causes that perpetuate the other.
- The role of the bodyworker or trainer in this scenario is to try to break this cycle. Addressing either of these factors (i.e., the pain or the spasm) directly or indirectly can help to achieve this. By working on these factors, bodyworkers and trainers can be a powerful part of the healing process for the client experiencing the pain-spasm-pain cycle.

- The trainer has the tools to guide the client through exercises that will gradually stretch and loosen the musculature and also facilitate venous return of blood. Further, exercise has been shown to increase the release of **endorphins**, which help to block pain.

BOX 16-25

The term *endorphin* comes from **endogenous morphine**, which literally means morphine produced within the body (*endogenous* means *formed within*). Morphine is a powerful pain-killing substance that is produced from plants and therefore comes from outside the body; therefore it is exogenous (*exogenous* literally means *formed outside*). When scientists saw that the human body already had receptors to this *exogenous* morphine from plants, they reasoned that there must be an internal chemical of the body for which these receptors were present. Based on this, they went searching for a substance produced within the body that would bind to these receptors and alleviate pain as morphine did. When they found this substance, they named it *endogenous morphine* or *endorphin* for short.

- The bodyworker may work directly on the spasmed muscles by using soft tissue techniques such as massage and stretching to relax the musculature. Bodyworkers can also do massage and joint range of motion techniques that are focused directly at increasing venous circulation.

16.11 GATE THEORY

- The **gate theory** proposes that a "gating mechanism" is present in the nervous system that blocks the perception of pain when faster signals of movement or pressure occur at the same time (Box 16-26).

BOX 16-26

Neurons do not all carry their impulses at the same speed. Larger and/or myelinated neurons conduct their impulses faster than smaller and/or nonmyelinated neurons. The sense of pain is carried in slow neurons; the senses of movement and pressure are carried in fast neurons.

- It is believed that this gating mechanism exists in the spinal cord.
- The name of this mechanism and how it works can be explained by making an analogy to a horse race in which a gate at the end of the race only allows the winner (i.e., the fastest horse) to enter. Once the fastest horse enters, the gate closes and blocks the entrance of the other slower horses.
- Relating this analogy to our nervous system, a similar gating mechanism is believed to exist in the spinal cord. When a number of sensory signals from the periphery enter the spinal cord at the same time, this gate allows the passage of impulses from the neurons that conduct their impulses the fastest, and it blocks transmission of the impulses of the slower neurons. Because pain is carried in slower neurons, the transmission of pain signals can be blocked by movement and/or pressure impulses carried in faster neurons. In effect, the sensation of pressure and/or movement can close the gate and block transmission of pain signals (Figure 16-18). Everyday examples that illustrate the gate theory are abundant. Two examples follow.

BOX 16-27

From an evolutionary point of view, the gate theory can be seen to be very valuable and protective in nature. Hundreds/thousands of years ago, physical encounters often involved fighting or taking flight from a dangerous, potentially life-threatening situation (e.g., battle with a wild animal or another person). During the actual battle, it was imperative that we could efficiently fight or take flight (a sympathetic nervous system–mediated response), or we would die; being distracted by pain caused by our wounds would have only hampered our ability to fight or take flight in that circumstance. After the activity was completed and we were no longer in a potentially dangerous circumstance, then we could safely experience our pain and "lick our wounds." In present times we are less often placed in actual life-threatening physical situations where the gate theory is necessary to save our lives. However, the gate theory still exists within the body and helps protect us in any situation in which a danger is perceived by our more primitive nervous system.

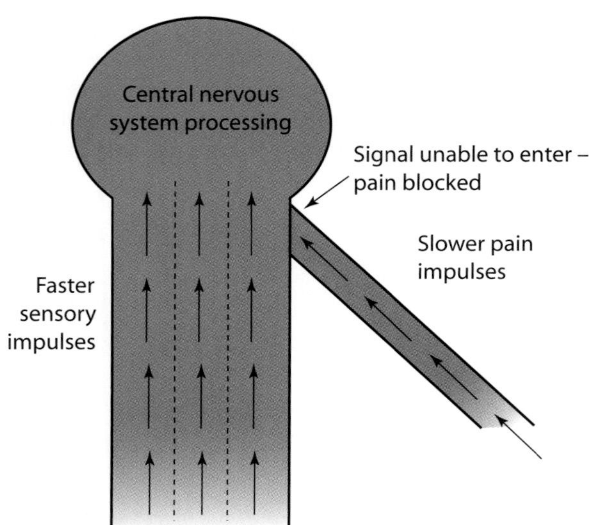

Figure 16-18 Illustration of the concept of the gate theory using an analogy to roads. Because of the presence of traffic in the faster lanes of the expressway, traffic from the smaller local road is blocked from entering the expressway and reaching its destination. In this analogy, the expressway carries the faster sensations of pressure and/or movement, and the local road carries the slower sensation of pain. Thus via the gate theory, the sensation of pain in the CNS can be blocked from reaching the brain because of the simultaneous presence of pressure and/or movement. (Modified from Fritz S: *Mosby's essential sciences for therapeutic massage: anatomy, physiology, biomechanics, and pathology,* ed 2. St Louis, 2004, Mosby.)

- Example 1: If a person burns or cuts the finger and pain is felt, it is common to see the person shake the injured hand or squeeze the hand near the wound. While doing either of these activities, the pain is blocked because the shaking causes movement signals to enter the spinal cord and/or the squeezing causes pressure signals to enter the spinal cord at the same time as the pain. Because movement and pressure signals both travel faster than pain signals, either one would help to block the sensation of the pain via the gate theory.
- Example 2: When a person exercises more than usual when working out or playing a sport, very often no pain is felt during the actual exercise. To some degree, this is due to the gate theory. While exercising, the constant input of movement and pressure sensory signals helps to block the pain signals at the gate. It is only later that evening or perhaps the next morning that the person realizes that he or she overdid it and was hurt.

Understanding the gate theory leads us to two very important clinical applications:

1. Clinical application 1: It is an age-old maxim in the world of alternative health that we should be in touch with the body and listen to what it tells us. However, understanding the gate theory, we realize that we are not always able to perceive all that is happening in the body. When we are very physically active, we may be causing physical damage yet not know it because our pain signals are being blocked by the gate theory. In cases like these, when giving advice to clients as to what they may safely do regarding physical exercise/exertion, it is important to caution them that they may not know that they are overdoing it during the actual physical activity and should judge more by how they feel after the exercise (anywhere from the remainder of that day until when they wake up the next morning).
2. Clinical application 2: We go to school and continuing education seminars to learn how best to apply treatment techniques, and we know that properly applied techniques are more beneficial than improperly applied ones. However, to some degree no matter what touch, exercise, or movement therapy we apply to the client (as long as it is not injurious), the client's pain will tend to be blocked due to the gate theory. In addition, of course, any blockage of pain may help to break the pain-spasm-pain cycle. (Note: For information on the pain-spasm-pain cycle, see Section 16.10.)

BOX 16-28

Another interesting clinical application of the gate theory to bodywork and training is the use of pain relief topical balms containing such substances as menthol, oil of wintergreen, and eucalyptus. Almost all of these balms work on the principle of the gate theory (i.e., they irritate the skin and distract the body from the pain). The term **counter irritant theory** is often used to describe the mechanism by which these balms function to relieve pain. Because their true function is to indirectly relieve pain by the counter irritant theory, in effect, they all have the same intrinsic value (apart from the strength of the formula and therefore the intensity of the *irritation* that they cause). Therefore using the one that the client finds the most pleasing is recommended!

REVIEW QUESTIONS

evolve Answers to the following review questions appear on the Evolve website accompanying this book.

1. What is the function of a sensory neuron, and what is the function of a motor neuron?

2. List the neurons involved in a spinal cord reflex arc.

3. List the neurons involved in initiation of voluntary movement.

4. What is the difference between patterned behavior and true reflexive behavior?

5. Give an example of an application of neural facilitation to bodywork and/or exercise.

6. What is the definition of reciprocal inhibition?

7. How can reciprocal inhibition be used to aid muscle stretching?

8. What is the definition of proprioception?

9. List the three major categories of proprioceptors.

10. Which fascial/joint proprioceptor detects static joint position?

11. What is the effect of a muscle spindle reflex?

12. What is the effect of a Golgi tendon organ reflex?

13. Bouncing when stretching activates which proprioceptive reflex?

14. CR stretching uses which proprioceptive reflex?

15. Which inner ear proprioceptor detects motion of the head?

16. Which proprioceptor (along with inner ear proprioceptors) is particularly important toward determining the posture of the trunk?

17. Which reflex is responsible for pulling the left foot away if it steps on a tack?

18. Which reflex is responsible for tightening the quadriceps femoris muscles of the right lower extremity in question #17?

19. Why does the pain-spasm-pain cycle perpetuate itself?

20. According to the gate theory, what sensations can help block pain?

NOTES

Chapter 17

Posture, Exercise, and the Gait Cycle

CHAPTER OUTLINE

CHAPTER OBJECTIVES

After completing this chapter, the student should be able to perform the following:

- ❑ Define good and bad posture, and give examples of the effects of bad posture.
- ❑ Define stress and discuss the positive and negative effects of stress on the body.
- ❑ Discuss the value of plumb line postural assessment, and list the landmarks for posterior and lateral plumb line assessments.
- ❑ Give and discuss an example of a postural distortion in each of the three cardinal planes (sagittal, frontal, and transverse).
- ❑ Explain the concept of center of weight, and discuss its application to postural analysis.
- ❑ Explain the relationship between a primary postural distortion, secondary postural distortion, and a postural distortion pattern.
- ❑ Compare and contrast consequential secondary postural distortions and compensatory secondary postural distortions.
- ❑ Give an example of a consequential secondary postural distortion, a compensatory secondary postural distortion, and a postural distortion pattern.
- ❑ Discuss and give examples of three general principles of compensation within the body.
- ❑ Discuss the possible effects on the body of the following postural distortions: protracted head, rounded shoulders, rounded back, swayback, scoliosis, elevated shoulder, and dropped arch.
- ❑ Discuss the possible effects on the body of wearing high-heeled shoes.
- ❑ Discuss the limitations of using a plumb line for postural analysis.
- ❑ List the two major types of exercises, and explain the benefit to the body of each type.
- ❑ Compare and contrast the concepts of power and endurance and aerobic and anaerobic exercises.
- ❑ List and give an example of each of the major strengthening exercise modalities; further, explain the major advantages and disadvantages of each one.
- ❑ Explain the concept of core stabilization exercises.
- ❑ List and describe each of the major stretching exercise methods.
- ❑ List the four stages of a healthy exercise routine, and explain why this order is recommended.
- ❑ Describe the major phases and landmarks of the gait cycle.

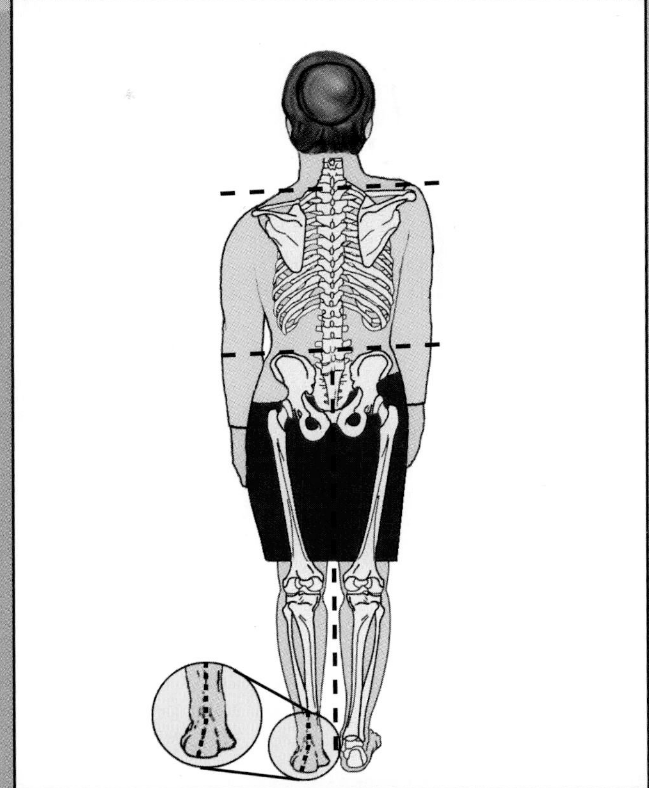

- ❑ Describe the relative rigidity/flexibility of the foot and its relation to the gait cycle.
- ❑ State when each of the major muscles of the lower extremity contracts during the gait cycle (i.e., relate the timing of its contraction to the landmarks of the gait cycle).
- ❑ Define the key terms of this chapter.
- ❑ State the meanings of the word origins of this chapter.

OVERVIEW

This chapter covers the three topics of posture, exercise, and gait. The word *posture* means *position*. Because the human body can be placed in an infinite number of possible positions, it can assume an infinite number of postures. When we examine a client's posture, we look to see how balanced and efficient it is. Based on balance and efficiency, we often describe the client as having good posture or bad posture. In addition to assessing a client's static postures, it is also important to consider the balance and efficiency of the human body in movement. In contrast to the term *posture*, which describes the static position of the body, the term *acture* is sometimes used to describe the balance and efficiency of the body during movement. Segueing from a discussion of static posture to movement, we then address the concept of exercise. Two major types of exercises exist: (1) strengthening and (2) stretching exercises. The various modalities/approaches of strengthening and stretching exercises are discussed, citing the relative advantages and disadvantages of each. Finally, the gait cycle is explained and discussed. Included in this discussion is an analysis of the timing of engagement of the major muscles of the lower extremity during the gait cycle.

KEY TERMS

AC stretching
Active isolated stretching
Active static stretching
Acture (AK-cher)
Adaptive shortening
Aerobic exercise (air-O-bik)
Agonist/antagonist pair (AG-o-nist/an-TAG-o-nist)
Agonist contract stretching
AIS stretching
Anaerobic exercise (AN-air-O-bik)
Bad posture
Ballistic stretching
Center of weight
Compensatory secondary postural distortion
Consequential secondary postural distortion
Contract-relax agonist contract stretching (AG-o-nist)
Contract-relax stretching
Core stabilization exercise
Counterbalance (COUNT-er-BAL-ans)
CR stretching
CRAC stretching
Double-limb support
Dropped arch
Dynamic posture
Dynamic stretching
Electromyography (e-LEK-tro-my-OG-ra-fee)
EMG
Endurance
Early swing
Exercise
Foot-flat
Foot slap
Gait (GATE)
Gait cycle
Good posture
Heel-off
Heel-strike
Idiopathic scoliosis (ID-ee-o-PATH-ik SKO-lee-os-is)
Isokinetic (EYE-so-kin-ET-ik)
Isometric exercise (EYE-so-MET-rik)
Isotonic exercise (EYE-so-TON-ik)
Joint dysfunction (dis-FUNK-shun)
Late swing
Midswing
Midstance
Military neck
Misalignment (MIS-a-LINE-ment)
Mobilization
Muscle hypertrophy (hi-PER-tro-fee)
Passive static stretching
PIR stretching
Planting and cutting
Plumb line (PLUM)
PNF stretching
Postisometric relaxation stretching (POST-EYE-so-MET-rik)
Postural distortion pattern
Posture
Power
Primary postural distortion
Proprioceptive neuromuscular facilitation stretching (PRO-pree-o-SEP-tiv)
Protracted head (PRO-tract-ed)
Reps
Rounded back
Rounded shoulders
Secondary postural distortion
Short leg
Stance phase
Step
Step angulation
Step length
Step width
Strength
Strengthening exercises
Stretching exercises
Stress
Stressors
Stride
Subluxation (SUB-luks-A-shun)
Swayback
Swing phase
Toe-off
Variable resistance exercise

WORD ORIGINS

- ❏ Acture—From Latin *actus,* meaning *to act*
- ❏ Aerobic—From Latin *aer,* meaning *air,* and Greek *bios,* meaning *life*
- ❏ Anaerobic—From Latin *a,* meaning *not, without;* and *aer,* meaning *air;* and Greek *bios,* meaning *life*
- ❏ Ballistic—From Greek *ballein,* meaning *to throw*
- ❏ Counterbalance—From Latin *contra,* meaning *against;* and *bi,* meaning *two;* and *lanx,* meaning *dish*
- ❏ Dynamic—From Greek *dynamis,* meaning *power*
- ❏ Dysfunction—From Greek *dys,* meaning *bad,* and Latin *functio,* meaning *to perform*
- ❏ Electromyography—From Greek *electron,* meaning *amber* (origin: static electricity can be generated by friction against amber); and *mys,* meaning *muscle;* and *grapho,* meaning *to write*
- ❏ Exercise—From Latin *exercitium,* meaning *to train, to drill*
- ❏ Hypertrophy—From Greek *hyper,* meaning *above, over;* and *trophe,* meaning *nourishment*
- ❏ Idiopathic—From Greek *idios,* meaning *private,* denoting *unknown;* and *pathos,* meaning *feeling, suffering*
- ❏ Isokinetic—From Greek *isos,* meaning *equal,* and *kinesis,* meaning *motion*
- ❏ Isometric—From Greek *isos,* meaning *equal,* and *metrikos,* meaning *measure*
- ❏ Isotonic—From Greek *isos,* meaning *equal,* and from Latin *tonus,* meaning *a stretching, tone*
- ❏ Misalignment—From Old English *mis,* meaning *bad,* and Latin *linea,* meaning *line*
- ❏ Plumb—From Latin *plumbum,* meaning *lead*
- ❏ Post—From Latin *post,* meaning *behind, after*
- ❏ Posture—From Latin *positura,* meaning *to place*
- ❏ Primary—From Latin *primaries,* meaning *1st*
- ❏ Secondary—From Latin *secundus,* meaning *2nd in order of rank*
- ❏ Stress—From Latin *stringere,* meaning *to draw tight*
- ❏ Subluxation—From Latin *sub,* meaning *under,* and *luxus,* meaning *dislocation*

☐ 17.1 IMPORTANCE OF GOOD POSTURE

- **Posture** means *position*.
- The position that a person's body is in is important because holding the body statically in a position places stresses on the tissues of the body.
  - Muscles may have to work causing them to be stressed.
  - Ligaments, joint capsules, and other soft tissues of the body may have pulling forces placed on them causing stress to these tissues.
  - Articular surfaces of bones may be compressed causing stress to them.
- It is impossible to entirely eliminate muscles from working, soft tissues from being pulled, and compression forces from existing in the body. However, when these stresses become excessive, injury and damage to tissues of the body may occur.

BOX 17-1

The term *stress* is often misused and misunderstood. **Stress** is caused by stressors, and a **stressor** is defined simply as anything that requires the body to change. Stressors may be physical or psychological/emotional. Because any change is potentially dangerous, stressors are viewed by the body as alarming and generally handled by the sympathetic branch of the autonomic nervous system. Having excessive stress is deleterious to the body, because the body is constantly keying up for possible dangers. However, to have no stress is not only equally unhealthy but also essentially impossible. Being alive implies change and growth, and it is the presence of stressors that challenges us to change and grow. An absence of all stress means a total absence of growth. Having a healthy amount of stress gives us the challenges we need to grow. In short, it is not stress that should be avoided; it is excessive stress that should be avoided.

- When we examine a client's posture to see if it is good or bad, we are looking to see how the position of the client's body may create stresses to the tissues of the body.
- **Good posture** is healthy because it is balanced and efficient; therefore it does not place excessive stresses on the tissues of the body.
- **Bad posture** is unhealthy because it is not balanced and not efficient; therefore it does place excessive stresses on the tissues of the body.

BOX 17-2

Bad, unhealthy postures place excessive stresses on the tissues of the body. Most commonly, muscles, ligaments, and/or bones are stressed by unhealthy postures.

17.2 IDEAL STANDING PLUMB LINE POSTURE

- When posture is analyzed, most often it is standing posture that is examined (Box 17-3, Note 1).
- Standing posture is usually analyzed by comparing the symmetry of the body against a perfectly vertical line that is created by a plumb line (see Box 17-3, Note 2).

BOX 17-3

Note 1: Most postural analyses are made of the client's standing posture. Although this does yield some important information, its value can be limited. The analysis of any posture is only valuable if the client spends time in that posture. Therefore if a client spends the bulk of the day sitting at a desk or computer, it would be much more valuable to assess the healthiness of that posture of the client. Further, most everyone sleeps at least 6-8 hours a night; that translates to literally $^1/_4$ to $^1/_3$ of our lives! If sleeping posture is unhealthy, that will also have a great influence on the health of the client, most likely a greater influence than standing posture does. Although this textbook does not examine each of these other postures, the fundamental principles addressed for standing posture can be extrapolated to apply to most other postures. In short, for every posture of the client, look for the stresses that would result to the tissues of the body.

Note 2: The word *plumb* of "plumb line" comes from the Latin word for lead. A **plumb line** is created by attaching a small heavy weight (originally made of lead) to a string. The weight pulls the string down, creating a straight vertical line that one can use to analyze the symmetry of the body in standing posture. Although one can buy fancy plumb line devices made for postural analysis, a string and a weight bought very inexpensively from a hardware store and attached to the ceiling create a perfectly good postural plumb line.

- When looking at the body in plumb line posterior and lateral views, we look for symmetry and balance of the parts of the body (Figure 17-1).

Frontal Plane Postural Examination (Posterior Plumb Line):

- A posterior postural examination yields information about postural distortions that exist in the frontal plane (see Figure 17-1a).
- When looking at the posterior view plumb line posture, are the left and right sides of the body symmetric and balanced in the frontal plane?
- The ideal posterior plumb line posture is to have the line travel straight down the center of the body, evenly dividing the body into two equal left and right halves.
- Look to see if left and right sides are equal in position.
- During a posterior postural exam, the following are fundamental things to check:
  - Are the shoulder heights equal, or is one side higher than the other?
  - Are the iliac crest heights equal, or is one side higher than the other?
  - Are the knee joints straight or does the client have genu valgum or genu varum? (Note: Genu valgum and genu varum are covered in Section 8.15.)
  - Does the client collapse over one or both of the arches (excessive pronation of the foot at the subtalar joint), resulting in an iliac crest height that is lower than the other?

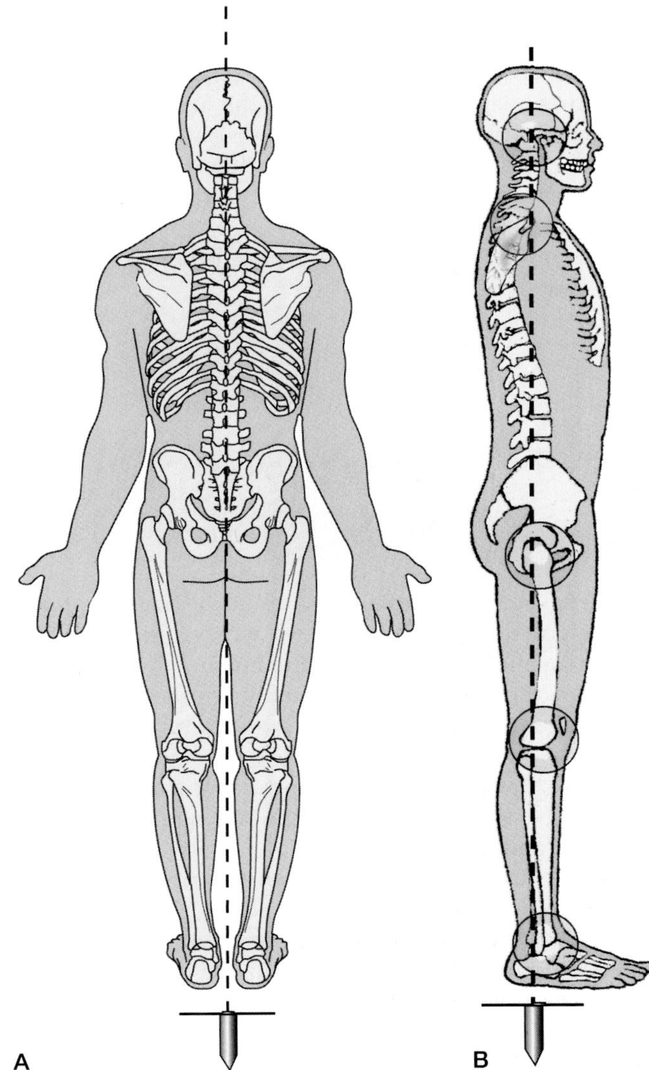

Figure 17-1 Plumb line postural assessments of posture. *A,* Posterior view. *B,* Lateral view. With ideal posture from the posterior view, the plumb line should bisect the body into equal right and left halves. With ideal posture from the lateral view, the plumb line should descend through the ear (i.e., external auditory meatus), acromion process of the scapula, greater trochanter of the femur, knee joint, and the lateral malleolus of the fibula.

Sagittal Plane Postural Examination (Lateral Plumb Line):

- ❑ A lateral postural examination yields information about postural distortions that exist in the sagittal plane (see Figure 17-1b).
- ❑ When looking at the lateral view plumb line posture, are the anterior and posterior sides of the body symmetric and balanced in the sagittal plane?
- ❑ The ideal lateral plumb line posture is to have the line travel straight down through the ear (i.e., external auditory meatus), the acromion process of the scapula, the greater trochanter of the femur, the knee joint, and the lateral malleolus of the fibula.
- ❑ Look to see if each body part is balanced over the body part that is below it. Are joints excessively flexed or extended? Are the curves of the spine normal?
- ❑ During a lateral postural exam, the following are fundamental things to check:
  - ❑ Are the spinal curves increased or decreased?
  - ❑ Is the head balanced over the trunk, or is it anteriorly held?
  - ❑ Is the trunk balanced over the pelvis, or is there a swayback?
  - ❑ Does the pelvis have excessive anterior or posterior tilt?
  - ❑ Are the knee or hip joints hyperextended?

Transverse Plane Postural Examination:

- ❑ Postural distortions that exist in the transverse plane are rotational distortions and are perhaps the most difficult to see and assess. (Note: Some common examples of transverse plane rotational postural distortions include scoliosis, medially rotated arms at the shoulder joints, and medially or laterally rotated thighs at the hip joints.) This is because a vertical plumb line cannot be used to assess a transverse plane distortion, because the transverse plane is horizontal.
- ❑ Ideally, the best view from which to see a transverse plane postural distortion is superior. From above, any transverse plane rotation distortion would show as an asymmetry. However, short of positioning yourself above a client by standing on a ladder, this is logistically difficult. For this reason, special attention must be paid when looking for transverse plane rotation distortions from the front, back, or sides!

❑ 17.3 ANALYZING PLUMB LINE POSTURAL DISTORTIONS

- ❑ We have said that when we look at the body in plumb line posterior and lateral views, we look for symmetry and balance of the parts of the body.
- ❑ When the body is not posturally symmetric and balanced, we can say that one or more postural distortions exist.
- ❑ As we have stated, each postural distortion places excessive stress on tissues of the body and may lead to injury and damage.
- ❑ When analyzing posture, two things should be determined:
  - ❑ What stressful effects will the client's postural distortion place on the tissues of the body? Knowing the stressful effects will allow us to relate the posture of the client to the symptoms that the client is experiencing.
  - ❑ What is causing this postural distortion (i.e., what activities and habit patterns of the client are causing the postural distortion[s])? Knowing the activities and habit patterns that the client engages in allows us to understand how this postural distortion occurred in the first place. This allows us to give postural lifestyle advice to help prevent these postural distortions from occurring or worsening in the future.

Frontal and Sagittal Plane Distortions:

- ❑ Any deviation from ideal posture in the posterior view means that the client has a postural distortion within the frontal plane.
- ❑ Any deviation from ideal posture in the lateral view means that the client has a postural distortion within the sagittal plane.

Examples of Postural Distortions:

Two common postural distortions, one in the frontal plane and one in the sagittal plane, are shown in Figures 17-2 and 17-3.

- ❑ Figure 17-2 is a posterior view that illustrates the frontal plane postural distortion of a person with the right shoulder higher than the left. We begin by looking at the stresses this posture places on the tissues of the body. To hold the right shoulder high means that the baseline resting tone of the musculature of elevation of the right shoulder girdle (i.e., elevators of the right scapula at the scapulocostal [ScC] joint) must be tighter on the right than on the left. Long-standing isometric contraction of elevators of

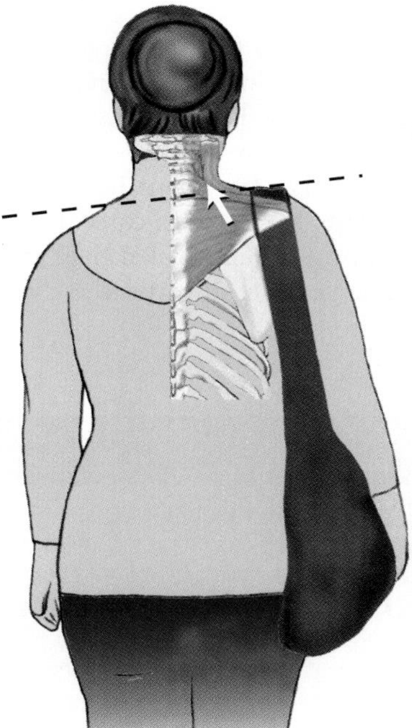

Figure 17-2 Person who on postural assessment is found to have a frontal plane postural distortion; her right shoulder girdle is higher than the left. Long-term carrying of a purse on the right side has led to chronic hypertonicity of her right-sided scapular elevator musculature. This musculature has tightened to elevate the right shoulder girdle so that the purse does not fall off; it has now become a chronic postural pattern.

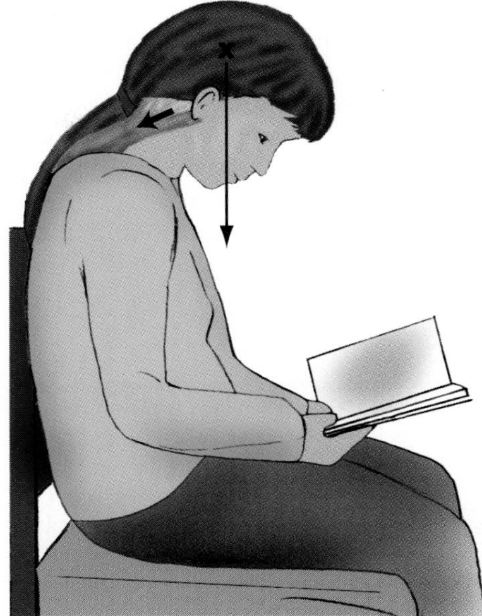

Figure 17-3 Person with a sagittal plane postural distortion; her head is held anteriorly. This results in the center of weight of the head no longer being balanced over the trunk. Long-term reading with a book down in her lap has led to chronic hypertonicity of her posterior extensor head/neck musculature. This musculature has tightened to prevent the head and neck from falling forward into flexion; it has now become a chronic postural pattern. (Note: The *X* indicates the center of weight of the head, which falls anterior to the trunk.)

the right scapula such as upper trapezius and levator scapulae can lead to trigger points and pain in these muscles. To then understand why the client has this postural distortion, it is important to do a thorough history to look for the activities and habit patterns the client has that might create it. It might be determined that the client habitually carries a purse on the right side. In this case constant elevation of the right shoulder girdle to hold a purse from falling off the shoulder has lead over the years to this frontal plane postural distortion.

BOX 17-4

When assessing the cause of a client's postural problem, it is easy to try to blame the problem on just one factor. Although this does sometimes happen, it is rare for a person's condition to be caused by just one thing. The cause for most conditions is multifactorial, meaning that many factors contribute to the condition. When you have found one cause for a problem, do not stop searching for others. It is in the client's interest for you to be thorough so that you can give better advice as to how to change all the pertinent habit patterns that contribute to the problem; this will help the client to be healthier in the future. Usually many *straws weigh down the camel's back*; all blame should not be placed on one straw that is found. Look to find all or at least most of the straws that contribute to the problem!

BOX 17-5 SPOTLIGHT ON CARRYING A SHOULDER BAG

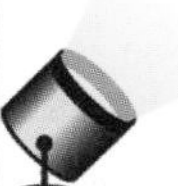

Carrying a purse or any type of shoulder bag is an extremely common habit that can lead to postural distortion. Although the weight of the bag is important because that weight bears down through the strap into the musculature of the shoulder girdle, the weight is not the most important aspect. Even carrying an empty shoulder bag will create the postural distortion of spasmed muscles that do elevation of the shoulder girdle. The reason is that the natural slope of the shoulder is such that a bag would fall off. To prevent that from occurring, the person isometrically contracts musculature to elevate the scapula to prevent this. This long-standing isometric contraction eventually leads to the chronic postural problem, regardless of the weight of the bag (although greater weight means that the muscles will have to contract more forcefully). Wearing a bag that has a strap that goes over the opposite shoulder and across the body is healthier, because it eliminates the necessity of having to isometrically contract musculature to change the slope of the shoulder.

- ❑ Figure 17-3 illustrates a lateral view that illustrates the sagittal plane postural distortion of a person with a protracted (i.e., anteriorly held) head. We begin by looking at the stresses this posture places on the tissues of the body. To hold the head anteriorly means that the center of weight of the head is no longer over the trunk; it is over thin air. Therefore the head and neck should fall into flexion resulting in the chin landing against the chest. The only reason this does not occur is that musculature of the posterior neck (that does extension of the neck and head) must be isometrically contracting, creating a counterforce to gravity, preventing the head and neck from falling into flexion. Long-standing isometric contraction of the muscles of the posterior neck such as the upper trapezius and semispinalis capitis can lead to trigger points and pain in these muscles. To then understand why the client has this postural distortion, it is important to do a thorough history to look for the activities and habit patterns the client has that might create this. It might be determined that the client habitually reads with a book in the lap. In this case a constant habit of reading with a book in the lap has led over the years to this sagittal plane postural distortion.

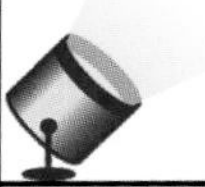

BOX 17-6 SPOTLIGHT ON CENTER OF WEIGHT

The concept of the **center of weight** is critical to the idea of a balanced posture. The center of weight of an object is an imaginary point where all the weight of the object could be considered to be located. If the center of weight of an object is over the object below, then the object on top will be balanced on the object below it. If instead the center of weight of the upper object is not over the object below, then the upper object is not balanced and would fall unless some force holds it there (see accompanying illustration). This concept applies to the major parts of the human body. The head should be balanced by having its center of weight over the trunk, the trunk should be balanced by having its center of weight over the pelvis, and so forth. If the head's center of weight is not over the trunk (e.g., it is protracted and anterior to the trunk), then extensor muscles must be in a constant isometric contraction to hold the head (and neck) in position so that it does not fall into flexion.

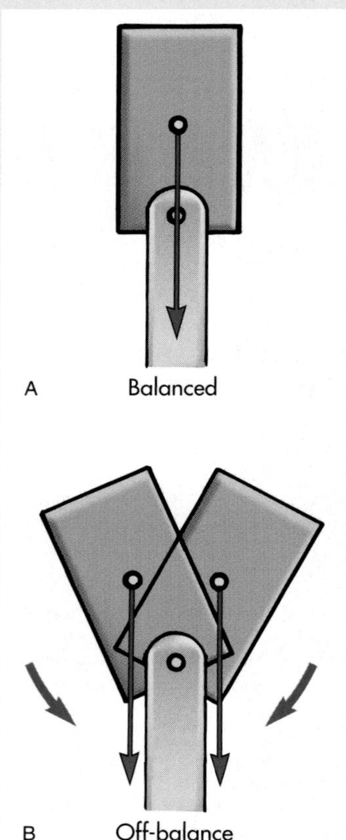

Modifed from Fritz S: *Mosby's fundamentals of therapeutic massage*, ed 3. St Louis, 2004, Mosby.

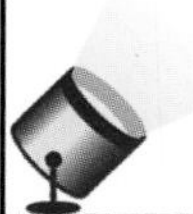

BOX 17-7 SPOTLIGHT ON PROTRACTED HEAD POSTURE

A **protracted head** (i.e., anteriorly held head) is one of the most common postural distortion patterns. Most every activity that we do is down and in front of us. From the day that a child is given crayons and a coloring book, through the years of sitting at a desk to read and write in elementary, middle, high school, and/or college, we tend to hold the head anteriorly to read, write, and study. Further, activities such as desk jobs, crafts such as sewing or needlepoint done in the lap, caring for children who are being held in parents' arms, preparing and cutting food while cooking, and working at a computer with a monitor that is too low all tend to place the head in an anteriorly held posture. It is no wonder that so many people have an anteriorly held head posture and the muscles of their posterior necks are so commonly tight. Use of a bookstand or an inclined desk, such as those used by architects and engineers, are easy ways to prevent this problem! (See Section 17-6 for more on the posture of a protracted head.)

17.4 SECONDARY POSTURAL DISTORTIONS AND POSTURAL DISTORTION PATTERNS

- A **primary postural distortion** of the body is a postural distortion that is due to a problem in that area of the body.
- A **secondary postural distortion** is a postural distortion that is due to a problem in another area of the body (i.e., it occurs secondary to this other problem).
- A **postural distortion pattern** is a set of interrelated postural distortions located in the body, including both the primary postural distortion and the secondary postural distortion(s).
- Not every postural distortion is primary. Sometimes a postural distortion pattern is created secondary to another postural distortion that already exists.
- Understanding when a postural distortion is primary versus secondary is important for bodyworkers and trainers, because massage, bodywork, or exercise of the muscles of a secondary postural distortion, no matter how good it feels to the client, will never eliminate the problem. This is because the cause of the problem lies elsewhere.
- A secondary postural distortion may exist as a consequence of the primary postural distortion, in which case it is called a **consequential secondary postural distortion**. Alternatively, it may be specifically created by the body as a compensation for the primary postural distortion, in which case it is called a **compensatory secondary postural distortion**.

Consequential Secondary Postural Distortions:

- Figure 17-4 is a posterior view of a person with a high right shoulder similar to the person in Figure 17-2. However, in this case the high right shoulder is not a primary postural distortion because of the musculature of the right shoulder girdle; rather it is due to the person's collapsed left arch, which has dropped the entire left side of the client. Because the left side is lower, the right shoulder is seen as higher. In this case the person's right-sided musculature of scapular elevation is not the reason for the elevated right shoulder girdle. Even if bodywork into these muscles feels good, the postural distortion of the high right shoulder will never be changed by working this region, because it is not the cause of the problem. The high right shoulder is a consequential secondary postural distortion and is simply the consequence of another (primary) postural distortion that has not been compensated for, the collapsed left arch. In this case correcting the collapsed left arch of the person's foot must be addressed to correct the high right shoulder.
- As Figure 17-4 illustrates, sometimes a secondary postural distortion is merely the consequence of another postural distortion that is primary. However, sometimes a secondary postural distortion is purposely created by the body as a compensation for a primary postural distortion.

Compensatory Secondary Postural Distortions:

- Sometimes the body creates a secondary postural distortion as a compensation mechanism for another primary postural distortion. These compensatory secondary postural distortions are meant to correct or prevent consequential secondary postural distortions that might otherwise occur.

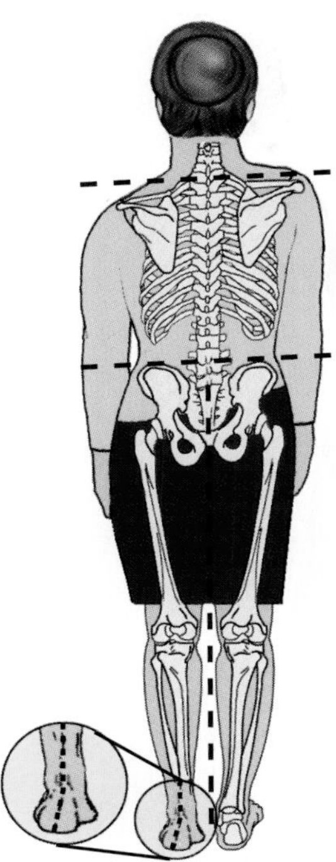

Figure 17-4 Person who on postural assessment is found to have a frontal plane postural distortion seemingly identical to what was found in Figure 17-2 (i.e., her right shoulder girdle is higher than the left). However, in this case the high right shoulder is not the result of a local problem of the right shoulder girdle region (i.e., it is not a primary postural distortion). Rather, it is a consequential secondary postural distortion that is the result of another primary postural distortion elsewhere. In this case it is due to a collapsed arch (i.e., overpronation of the subtalar joint) of the left foot. Loss of the left-sided arch has caused the entire left side to drop, making the right shoulder girdle relatively higher.

❑ Figure 17-5 illustrates a person with a collapsed arch of the left foot, which is a primary postural distortion. We have seen that an uncompensated dropped left arch would cause the entire left side of the person's body to drop (as shown in Figure 17-4), resulting in a low left shoulder girdle and relatively a high right shoulder girdle. However, in this person's case the spine has developed a scoliotic curve to compensate for the low left side. By curving the spine, the shoulder heights have been brought to level. Therefore this scoliosis is a compensatory secondary postural distortion that has been created as a compensation for the dropped left arch. Although work done on the scoliosis may feel good and be beneficial, it will never correct the scoliotic curve, because the cause is elsewhere. Correction of the dropped left arch is necessary to correct the scoliosis.

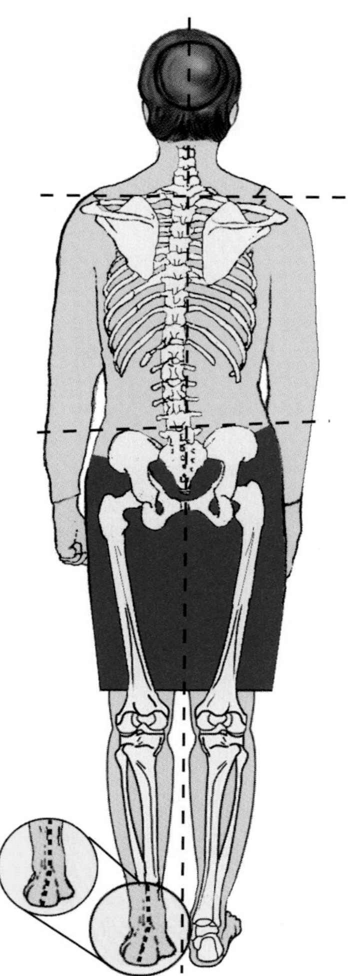

Figure 17-5 Same person as in Figure 17-4 with a collapsed left arch, which is a primary postural distortion. The only difference is that now the person's spine has compensated for the dropped arch in the left foot by having a (left thoracolumbar) scoliotic curve. This scoliosis is a compensatory secondary postural distortion that brings the left shoulder girdle back to being the same height as the right shoulder girdle.

Postural Distortion Patterns:

❑ Whether a person's secondary postural distortion is simply a consequence of an uncompensated primary postural distortion as in Figure 17-4 or is a compensation for a primary postural distortion as in Figure 17-5, we still see that once a primary postural distortion exists in the body, secondary postural distortions are likely to develop. In other words, a local primary postural distortion tends to create a larger postural distortion pattern that may spread throughout the body.

❑ These larger global distortion patterns mean that many local distortions will be present when examining a client's posture. By possessing a fundamental understanding of the musculoskeletal structure and function of the body and by critically thinking, it is usually possible to determine which postural distortion is the causative primary distortion (Box 17-8, Note 1). Although work on all postural distortions, including secondary distortions, feels good and may be beneficial, it is only through the correction of the primary postural distortion that a client's entire postural distortion pattern can be corrected (Box 17-8, Note 2).

BOX 17-8

Note 1: When analyzing posture, although a primary postural distortion at one level may travel inferiorly and create secondary postural distortions lower down in the body, it is more common for a lower primary postural distortion to create secondary postural distortions higher up in the body. To draw an analogy to the structure of a building, a building's foundation that is improper is more likely to crack the plaster on the 3rd floor than is a problem on the 3rd floor likely to create a problem with the building's foundation. Generally when putting together the various clues that one sees when analyzing a client's posture, it is best to think from the bottom up.

Note 2: It is true that a secondary postural distortion is functionally caused by another "primary" postural distortion and that the secondary postural distortion cannot be corrected unless the primary one is first eliminated. Unfortunately, not every secondary postural distortion will automatically disappear when the primary distortion is eliminated. If a secondary postural distortion has been present long enough, the soft tissues of the body will have most likely structurally changed to adapt to this postural distortion. To correct these structural changes, it may be necessary to work directly on them. In effect, the functional secondary postural distortion in time becomes its own structural primary postural distortion. This is one reason why the longer a client waits to address a problem, the more difficult it usually becomes to resolve it.

☐ 17.5 GENERAL PRINCIPLES OF COMPENSATION WITHIN THE BODY

- Understanding and being able to apply the principle of postural compensation throughout the body is an important skill for any therapist or trainer that works clinically. Following are some of the general principles of how postural compensation occurs in the body.

Counterbalancing Body Parts:

- When a body part is deviated to one side, the body part above it will usually be deviated to the opposite side to **counterbalance** the weight of the body.
  - One example of this is when a person is very heavy and has a large abdomen. The weight of the abdomen throws the center of weight of the lower trunk anteriorly. To compensate for this, the upper trunk will usually be deviated posteriorly to counterbalance the anteriorly deviated lower trunk. As a result, the center of weight of the trunk as a whole is centered and balanced.

Hypomobility/Hypermobility of Joints:

- When a joint of the body becomes hypomobile (i.e., its movement becomes restricted), other joints often compensate by becoming hypermobile.
  - An example of this is a spinal joint that has lost mobility (i.e., is hypomobile). For full range of motion of that region of the spine to occur, an adjacent spinal joint must compensate by increasing its mobility (i.e., becoming hypermobile). Another example is if one shoulder joint is painful and cannot be moved (thus hypomobile), the other shoulder joint will be used more and in time will likely become hypermobile.

BOX 17-9

An interesting addendum exists to a hypermobility that is caused as a compensation for a hypomobility. In time, the excessive motion and use of the hypermobile joint will often result in overuse and pain. The consequence of this will likely be muscle spasm to prevent the painful use. This muscle spasm will then decrease movement of that joint, resulting in another hypomobile joint. Now two hypomobile joints exist, which will then create another hypermobility, which by the same process will likely result in a 3rd hypomobile joint. Like dominoes falling, once one hypomobile joint exists, it sets a compensation pattern in motion that tends to spread throughout the body!

Tightened Antagonist Muscles:

- Opposing muscles on opposite sides of a joint usually need to balance their pull on the bone to which they attach. Indeed, the proper posture of the body part involved depends on a balanced pull of these muscles. If the tone of one of these muscles changes, it will usually cause a compensatory change in the tone of the muscles on the other side of the joint. For example, if a muscle on one side of a joint becomes tighter and therefore shortens, the opposing muscle on the other side of the joint will often become tighter in an attempt to even out the pulling force on their common attachment. Otherwise, the attachment would be unevenly pulled in one direction and a postural distortion would result.

BOX 17-10

Opposing muscles located on opposite sides of a joint are often called an **agonist/antagonist pair**. The muscles of an agonist/antagonist pair should usually be balanced in tone. If an agonist becomes excessively shortened and tightened (i.e., facilitated), two things may happen to the antagonist:

1. It can become lengthened and weakened (i.e., inhibited), allowing the tight agonist to excessively pull on the common attachment and resulting in a postural distortion of the body part involved.
2. It can tighten as a compensation to try to even out the pull of the agonist to prevent the postural distortion; this results in tight muscles on both sides of the joint!

  - One common example of this scenario is tightness of the muscles of the neck. For example, if the musculature of the left side of the neck becomes tight, the musculature of the right side of the neck will often become tight in an attempt to prevent the head and neck from being pulled to the left.

17.6 COMMON POSTURAL DISTORTION PATTERNS OF THE HUMAN BODY

The ability of bodyworkers and trainers to work with and improve the client's postural distortions is extremely important. As stated, a fundamental knowledge of anatomy and a fundamental understanding of the principles of physiology/kinesiology are crucial when critically assessing what the proper treatment for a client should be. Following are a few of the more common postural distortion patterns that occur. (See *Spotlight on Muscle Spindles and Muscle Facilitation* in Section 16.6 for an illustration of two common postural distortion patterns not covered in this section, the upper and lower crossed syndromes.) As you read through these postural distortion patterns, note how one distortion pattern often leads to other distortion patterns.

Note: One postural distortion pattern can lead to other postural distortion patterns.

BOX 17-11

It should be noted that most postural distortions are a factor of letting the posture of a region of the body fall with gravity. It can almost be likened to a war that the body wages with gravity through the years. The problem is that gravity never tires and usually wins out. Look at the posture of most senior citizens, and it can be seen that most exhibit postures in which a part of the body or many parts of the body have given in to gravity and are slumped forward. Much of the answer to winning the war with gravity is to keep the muscles that oppose gravity strong and healthy. Of course, keeping the antagonists to these muscles loose is also important so that these antagonists do not help gravity pull us down.

Protracted Head:

- A **protracted head** (i.e., anteriorly held head) is a sagittal plane postural distortion and is usually the result of an altered cervical spinal curve in which the lower cervical curve is straighter than usual (i.e., hypolordotic), projecting the head anteriorly. The upper cervical curve then increases (i.e., becomes hyperlordotic) to bring the eyes to a level posture to see forward. The result is that the head is held anteriorly and no longer balanced over the trunk. As covered in Section 17.3, a protracted head commonly occurs as the result of a multitude of postures that require the head/neck to flex forward to see and work with something that is down and in front of the body. Because the head is held anteriorly, increased stress occurs to a number of tissues of the body (Figure 17-6).

BOX 17-12

A hypolordotic cervical spinal curve (i.e., a straight neck) is also known as a **military neck**.

Muscles:

- With a protracted head, the center of the weight of the head is over thin air (instead of being located over the trunk). As a result, the head and neck should fall into flexion. The only reason that this does not happen is that the posterior neck musculature isometrically con-

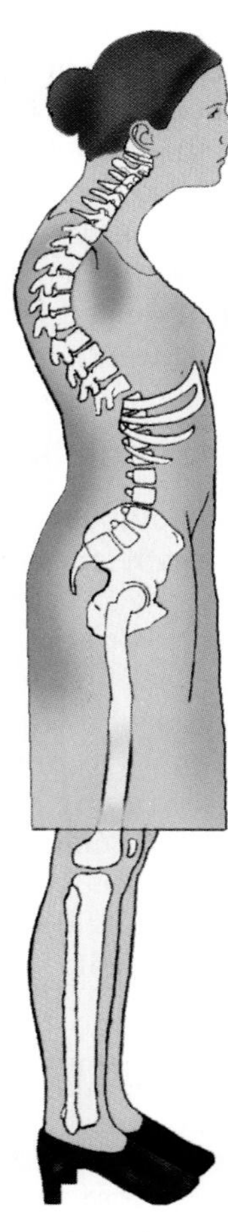

Figure 17-6 Body-wide sagittal plane postural distortion pattern. The person is wearing high-heeled shoes, which tend to throw her body weight anteriorly. To compensate for this, she has increased the curve in the lumbar spine (i.e., hyperlordotic lumbar spine, also known as *swayback*) to counterbalance and bring her weight posteriorly. As a result of her lumbar spine having an increased curve, her thoracic spinal curve increases as well (i.e., hyperkyphotic thoracic spine, also known as *rounded back*). This then tends to slump her shoulders forward (i.e., rounded shoulders) and throws her neck and head anteriorly (i.e., anteriorly held head). Like dominoes, a primary postural distortion pattern often leads to secondary postural distortion patterns, especially when it begins at the foundation of the body, the feet!

tracts, creating a force of extension that stops the head and neck from falling into flexion. This constant isometric postural contraction of the posterior neck musculature places a greatly increased stress on these muscles to constantly work. Hence they become overly facilitated and usually end up becoming tight. This postural deviation is very common and one reason why the muscles of the posterior neck region are so commonly tight. These tight neck muscles that attach onto the skull may then trigger tension headaches. Many people assert that the altered posture of the neck can also lead to increased stress on the temporomandibular (TMJ) joints, possibly leading to a TMJ disorder.

Ligamentous Complex:

- ❑ Because of the decreased curve of the cervical spine in an anteriorly held posture of the head, the ligaments of the posterior neck are pulled on and stressed. This results in posterior ligaments and joint capsules that have been lengthened out and become lax and less able to hold the proper posture of the cervical spine.

Bones/Joints:

- ❑ The loss of the normal lordotic curvature of the lower cervical spine results in a neck that is less able to absorb shock. As a result of the increased shock, in time the cervical spine is more likely to have degenerative changes (commonly called *osteoarthritis* [OA]). Further, if the muscles of the neck stay tight long enough, the cervical spinal joints will become hypomobile; this decreased mobility of the spinal joints is known as **joint dysfunction**.

BOX 17-13

The meaning of the term *joint dysfunction* is actually broader and covers any poor functioning of a joint. The prefix *dys* literally means *bad*; hence *dysfunction* means *bad function*. Given that the function of a joint is to allow movement, any altered motion of a joint, whether it is hypomobility or hypermobility, can be defined as joint dysfunction. This term is used widely in the field of chiropractic. The terms **subluxation** and **misalignment** are also used. Although their meanings are not identical, they are often used synonymously.

Rounded Shoulders:

- ❑ **Rounded shoulders** are an extremely common sagittal plane postural distortion pattern of the body that involves protraction of the scapulae at the ScC joints and medial rotation of the humeri at the shoulder (glenohumeral [GH]) joints. Rounded shoulders often accompany a protracted head posture and result from activities in which a person works in front of the body, but instead of holding the scapulae back into retraction, the shoulder girdles fall into protraction. Although most any activity that occurs in front of the body may cause rounded shoulders, deskwork and working at a computer are particularly common culprits.
- ❑ Rounded shoulders result in shortening and tightening of the protractors of the scapulae and medial rotators of the humeri, as well as lengthening and weakening of the retractors of the scapulae and lateral rotators of the humeri.
- ❑ A postural distortion of medial rotation of the arm (i.e., humerus) at the shoulder joint also leads to a decreased ability to abduct the arm at the shoulder joint and a decreased ability to take in a deep breath. (Note: For the relationship between rotation and abduction of the arm at the shoulder joint, see Section 9.6.)
- ❑ Rounded shoulders are often accompanied by an increased thoracic spinal curve (i.e., hyperkyphosis) as the person also slumps forward with the spine.

Hyperkyphotic Thoracic Spine (Rounded Back):

- ❑ A hyperkyphotic thoracic spine is a sagittal plane postural distortion. The normal curve of the thoracic spine is kyphotic. When the normal degree of thoracic curvature increases, it is called a *hyperkyphotic thoracic spine* or a **rounded back**. As with a protracted head posture and rounded shoulders, a hyperkyphotic thoracic spine usually results from working in front of the body and allowing gravity to pull the trunk/spine down into flexion (see Figure 17-6).
- ❑ The effects of a hyperkyphotic thoracic spine are increased compression on the anterior bodies of the vertebrae; this can result in greater stress on the vertebral bodies leading to degenerative osteoarthritic changes. Slumping into the increased flexion of an excessive kyphosis also closes in on the thoracic cavity, decreasing the ability of the lungs to freely expand when taking in a deep breath.
- ❑ The presence of a hyperkyphotic thoracic spinal curve also predisposes the person to having rounded shoulders and a hypolordotic lower cervical spine with a hyperlordotic upper cervical spine (i.e., a protracted head posture [covered previously]).

Hyperlordotic Lumbar Spine (Swayback):

- ❑ A hyperlordotic lumbar spine is a sagittal plane postural distortion. When the normal lordotic curve of the lumbar spine is increased, it is known in lay terms as a **swayback** or, more technically, as a *hyperlordotic lumbar spine*. Swayback is often the consequence of an anteriorly tilted pelvis, which in turn is often the consequence of an imbalance of anterior/posterior tilt muscles of the pelvis (a relative weakness of the posterior tilters in comparison to the anterior tilters) (see Figure 17-6) (For more on the relationship between pelvic posture and spinal posture, see Section 8.8.)

- A swayback shifts the weight-bearing function of the spine further posteriorly so that more weight is borne through the facet joints instead of the disc joints. This can result in greater stress on the facet joints leading to degenerative osteoarthritic changes.
- Swayback often leads to the postural distortions of an increased thoracic kyphosis, rounded shoulders, and a protracted head posture.

Wearing High-Heeled Shoes:

- Wearing high-heeled shoes creates many sagittal plane distortions and is perhaps one of the worst offenders to posture, because high-heeled shoes begin their effects at the very foundation of the body; the sequelae then occur all the way up the body (see Figure 17-6).
- High-heeled shoes place the foot into plantarflexion, which is an unstable position for the ankle and subtalar joints, increasing the chance of sprain.
- By elevating the heels, more body weight is shifted anteriorly on the foot. The ability of the transverse arch of the foot to absorb this weight bearing is overcome and the arch weakens and splays out, resulting in a widening of the forefoot. If the shoe is too tight, this then pushes the proximal phalanx of the big toe laterally, resulting in a bunion (i.e., hallux valgus).
- Further, because of the position of plantarflexion, the plantarflexor musculature becomes shortened and tightened, and the dorsiflexor musculature becomes lengthened and weakened. This often results in spasms in the gastrocnemius and soleus muscles. Ironically, because of the plantarflexor shortening, women that wear high-heel shoes often complain of pain when they do wear flat shoes because the plantarflexors are so tight, that they cannot stretch sufficiently when the person in is flats. As a result, many of these people continue to wear high-heeled shoes, erroneously believing that high-heeled shoes are better for their body than flats because the flats cause immediate pain! The remedy is to gradually switch the client from wearing higher-heeled shoes to less high-heeled shoes, and eventually to flats over a period of months, if not a year or more.
- Moving up the body, when high-heeled shoes are worn, the body weight is thrown forward because wearing high-heeled shoes is effectively like standing on a surface that is a steep downgrade. As a result, the trunk will fall into flexion if the body weight is not brought back to be balanced over the lower extremities. This is often accomplished by increasing the anterior tilt of the pelvis, which results in an increased lordotic curve of the low back. Now the person has a swayback, which then leads to the formation of other secondary postural distortions! Thus wearing high-heeled shoes often results in foot problems, swayback, rounded back, rounded shoulders, and a protracted head posture, as well as headaches and possibly TMJ dysfunction.

BOX 17-14

Many women who wear high-heeled shoes compensate for the imbalance of standing on the unlevel surface of the high-heeled shoes by anteriorly tilting the pelvis and increasing the curve (i.e., lordosis) of the lumbar spine; this serves to throw the center of weight of the upper body posteriorly as a counterbalance so that the person does not fall forward. However, an increased lumbar lordosis is an unhealthy posture for the low back and causes secondary postural distortions superiorly in the body. A healthier way to compensate for high-heeled shoes is to bring the body weight backward by posteriorly tilting the pelvis. This avoids the increased lumbar lordosis with all of the unhealthy effects that would follow.

Elevated Shoulder:

- An elevated shoulder girdle is a frontal plane postural distortion. This problem may be a primary problem because of tight musculature of the area. If so, many things can cause an elevated shoulder girdle, including carrying a bag or purse on the shoulder (regardless of the weight of the bag), crimping a phone between the shoulder and head, and improper desk height that requires the shoulders to be raised when working and typing. The upper shoulder girdle region is also a common region in which people hold psychologic stress (see Figure 17-4).
- When a high shoulder girdle is a primary muscular problem, the major effects are local tightness of the musculature. Because these muscles have their other attachments in the neck, pain will usually spread into the neck. If the neck muscles stay tight long enough, cervical spinal joint dysfunction and headaches may also occur.
- When a high shoulder girdle is secondary to another postural distortion, the muscles of the shoulder region may not be tight. However, any postural distortion that is allowed to exist long enough will gradually cause adaptive shortening of the muscles that are held in a shortened posture. Therefore if this condition is chronic, beyond finding and taking care of the primary cause, work into the musculature of the high shoulder girdle may also be necessary.

BOX 17-15

Adaptive shortening is the term that describes the concept that when a soft tissue is kept in a shortened position for a long period of time, it adapts to that shortened position and loses its ability to lengthen without injury. Adaptive shortening most likely occurs because of the buildup of fascial adhesions. Applying this concept to musculature, if a muscle is kept in a shortened state for an extended period of time, even if it is relaxed and slackened in this shortened state, it will become tighter and less flexible. One very common example of this in the human body is the hip joint flexor musculature; spending prolonged periods of time sitting with the hip joints in a position of flexion often results in adaptive shortening of the hip flexor musculature.

Scoliosis:

- A scoliosis is a frontal plane postural distortion of the spine in which the spine has curves when viewed from posterior to anterior (or anterior to posterior). Like most every postural distortion of the body, a scoliosis can be a primary problem or a secondary problem (see Figure 17-7).
- Whether a scoliosis is a primary or secondary problem, it causes shortening and eventual tightening of the muscles that are in the concavity of the curve and lengthening and eventual weakening of the muscles that are on the convex side of the curve. Clearly by virtue of its existence, a scoliosis involves structural changes to the shape of the spine. If this structural distortion is in existence for a number of years, the functioning of the spine (i.e., its mobility) will be affected and motion will decrease. Doing soft tissue work into the tight concave-side musculature, joint range of motion to keep the spinal joints mobile, and strengthening the weakened convex-side muscles can all be helpful.
- If a scoliosis is secondary to another problem such as a short lower extremity, then the primary cause must be addressed or the scoliosis will continue. In fact, in the case of a short lower extremity, the scoliosis will be a necessary compensation to keep the head level.

BOX 17-16

A primary scoliosis is known as an **idiopathic scoliosis**, which means that its origin is unknown. Idiopathic scolioses usually strike teenage girls and can be very severe. Care by an orthopedist is usually necessary for these individuals. However, a secondary scoliosis, usually the result of some type of asymmetry in the height of the lower extremities, is often very treatable by conservative care, as long as the primary cause is found and corrected. Keep in mind that if one lower extremity is shorter than the other, the pelvis will be unlevel, causing the spine to be tilted to one side and resulting in the head not being level. In a case like this, a secondary scoliosis is a compensation and necessary as part of the righting reflex to bring the head back to level. One additional note about a scoliosis is that it is not a pure frontal plane postural distortion; a rotational component also exists in the transverse plane. This is due to the coupling of lateral flexion and rotation at the facet joints (see Sections 7.6, 7.7, and 7.9).

Dropped Arch:

- A **dropped arch** is a frontal plane postural distortion of the foot in which the medial longitudinal arch of the foot is lessened or lost entirely; a dropped arch is known as a *flatfoot*. Some people have a rigid flatfoot in which the arch is never present; this is usually a structural problem of the bones of the feet. Other people have a supple flatfoot in which the arch is lost only on weight bearing; this is actually a hyperpronation problem of the subtalar joint of the foot and is due primarily to lax ligaments (and may be further aggravated by weak intrinsic and extrinsic foot muscles). Whether a person has a rigid or supple flatfoot, when a foot does not have its arch, certain musculoskeletal consequences occur (see Figures 17-4 and 17-5).
- Much of the shock absorption capability of the foot is dependent on the presence of the arch of the foot. When the arch is lost, shock absorption is decreased and the foot and the entire body are subjected to greater physical stress each time the foot strikes the ground.
- Further, collapsing the arch stretches the soft tissues on the plantar side of the foot, especially the plantar fascia. This results in greater tension being placed on the plantar fascia and may cause plantar fasciitis, as well as a heel spur where the plantar fascia attaches to the underside of the calcaneus.
- Loss of the arch also causes a collapse of the foot into pronation each time the foot strikes the ground. This results in a medial rotation of the tibia and femur on the foot, a rotation of the pelvis on the thigh, and may even create a rotational force on the spine.
- Additionally, loss of the arch increases a genu valgum force on the knee, resulting in excessive stress on the knee joint.
- As bad as all this is, if just one foot drops an arch, the situation may actually be worse, because it causes a drop in height of that side's lower extremity, which results in a dropped pelvis, seen as a low iliac crest height. If the spine does not compensate for the dropped pelvis, the person will have a low shoulder girdle on that side (see Figure 17-4). If the person's spine does compensate for the dropped pelvis, the person will have a compensatory scoliosis (see Figure 17-5). In fact, a great number of scolioses are secondary scolioses that are compensating for an asymmetrically short lower extremity, usually known in lay terms as a **short leg**.

BOX 17-17

A short leg can be caused by a number of things. There may be an actual difference in the height of the tibia and/or the femur. Another cause is a dropped arch in the foot or an excessive genu valgum of the knee joint. Sometimes a short leg can even be caused by tight hip joint abductor musculature. When hip abductor musculature is chronically tight, it pulls down on that side of the pelvis, creating a lower iliac crest height on that side, which appears as a short leg. Regardless of the cause, an asymmetric short leg/unlevel pelvis causes an unlevel sacral base on which the spine sits. This then causes the spine to curve scoliotically as a compensation to bring the head to a level posture!

17.7 LIMITATIONS OF STANDING IDEAL PLUMB LINE POSTURE

- Although use of a plumb line can be very helpful when analyzing a client's posture, plumb line postural analysis has certain limitations:

Transverse Plane Postural Distortions:

- As mentioned in Section 17.2, plumb line postural analyses give us a way to look for postural distortions within the frontal and sagittal planes; however, a vertical plumb line cannot be used to check for rotational distortions that occur within the transverse plane.

BOX 17-18

A plumb line cannot be used to analyze rotational postural distortions in the transverse plane, because the transverse plane is horizontal. Because a plumb line is a vertical line, it is used to analyze distortions within the two vertical planes (i.e., the frontal and sagittal planes). Without the aid of a visual plumb line, transverse plane distortions are easy to miss and must be more carefully looked for than frontal and sagittal plane distortions.

- To see a rotation of a body part, a superior view is best (Figure 17-7a). Unfortunately, viewing a client from above is logistically difficult. For this reason, transverse plane postural distortions must usually be seen and assessed from anterior, posterior, and/or lateral views, but the plumb line is not very helpful in assisting this examination (Figure 17-7b).

Standing Posture Only:

- Plumb line posture is only useful for examining our client's standing posture. If the client does not spend much of the day standing, analyzing standing posture may be largely irrelevant to his or her health. In this case it would be better to analyze the postures that the client more frequently assumes.

Questionable Importance of Static Postural Analysis:

- Static posture is just one piece of the puzzle in assessing a client's health. Many other pieces exist. Static postural analysis is an analysis of structure. Although structure does certainly affect function, the relationship is not always direct and immediate. The human body has a great deal of ability to deal with deviations from "ideal" posture, and deviations from ideal do not necessarily reflect in signs and symptoms on the part of the client. Certainly poor posture creates stresses on tissues of the body that predispose us to problems; however, these problems may not come out for a very long time, or they may never manifest. Be careful to not make too strong of a relationship between every little postural distortion and the client's presenting problem(s). Keep in mind that ideal posture is just that, ideal. Not everyone must have the same exact ideal posture; the human body comes in many shapes and forms, and it is important to not try to force every body into one standardized ideal!

BOX 17-19

What may be of much greater importance is not someone's static posture but what might be called his or her **dynamic posture**, or acture. **Acture** is a term used to describe the fluidity of someone's movement patterns. Some people when standing still may have a static posture that is less than desirable, but when they move, their movements may be clean, efficient, graceful, and healthy. In this regard, the dynamic aspect of acture may be as important, if not more important than the static aspect of posture.

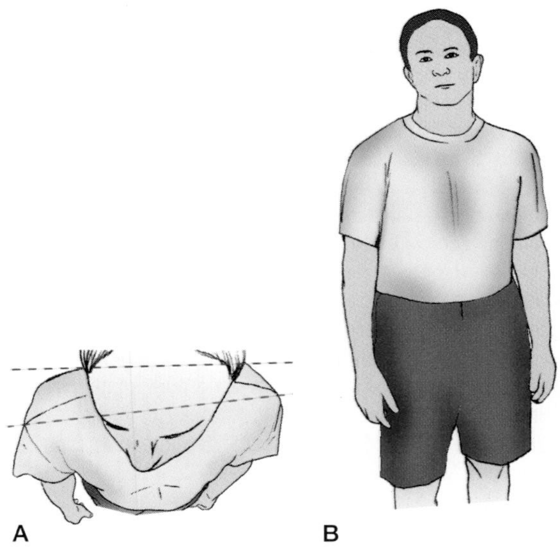

Figure 17-7 Individual with a mild/moderate scoliosis. A scoliosis is largely a rotational postural distortion in the transverse plane. The best view for any transverse plane postural assessment is superior. *A,* Superior view. Reader should note how clearly the asymmetry of the posture of the upper trunk can be seen. *B,* Anterior view, which is the more common view that we have when trying to assess transverse plane postural distortions. This perspective is not as ideal, but subtle visual clues are present. The orientation of the trunk should be noted; it is not facing perfectly anterior. In addition, the asymmetry of the arms by the sides of the body should be noted; the right hand is held further from the body than is the left hand.

☐ 17.8 EXERCISE (OVERVIEW)

- **Exercise** can be defined as performing active or passive movements for the purpose of maintaining or restoring health to the body.
- Two general types of exercise exist: (1) strengthening exercises and (2) stretching exercises.
  - **Strengthening exercises** are designed to increase the force that a muscle can generate when it contracts.
  - **Stretching exercises** are designed to increase the ability of the soft tissues of the body (including muscles) to stretch (i.e., lengthen).
- To optimize musculoskeletal health, it is important to balance our exercise regimen with both strengthening and stretching exercises.
  - Strengthening exercises create strong muscles that can more efficiently create movement of the body. Strong muscles also help to stabilize the joints of the body, decreasing the risk of injury.
  - Stretching exercises create flexible muscles (and other soft tissues) that are better able to allow for mobility of the body without injury.

☐ 17.9 STRENGTHENING EXERCISES

- Strengthening exercises are designed to increase the force that a muscle can generate when it contracts.

BOX 17-20

Stress was defined earlier in the chapter as the body's response to a stressor; and a stressor was defined as anything that asked the body to change. In this regard, strengthening exercises are stressors to the body, because they require that the body changes by growing the muscles stronger. If the proper amount of exercise is done (i.e., we place the proper amount of stress on the body), we will grow stronger and healthier. However, if excessive exercise is done, we will place an excessive amount of stress on the tissues of the body and injury might result. Whenever considering the appropriate amount of exercise to recommend to a client, especially a client who is rehabilitating from an injury, trainers should always keep in mind the ability of the tissues of the client's body to accept the level of stress that the exercises would create. Expanding the scope of stressors, all forms of bodywork can be seen to actually be stressors as well, because they ask the client's body to change and grow healthier in some manner. In this regard, stress can be very healthy. However, any change, even a good change, is a stress to the body; and too much change translates to too much stress for the client's tissues to handle. Therefore massage therapists and bodyworkers should always carefully consider the appropriateness of the massage and bodywork treatment that is performed on the client!

- Two components to **strength** exist: (1) power and (2) endurance.
  - **Power** is defined as being able to generate a maximal force for short period of time.
  - **Endurance** is defined as being able to generate a low level force for an extended period of time.
  - Power/endurance examples: Lifting 100 lb once is a display of power; lifting 1 lb 100 times is a display of endurance. Running 200 meters very quickly is an example of power; running 2000 meters slowly is an example of endurance. The well-known children's story about the tortoise and the hare exemplifies the conceptual difference between power and endurance.
- When strengthening exercises are done, they are often divided into aerobic or anaerobic exercises. The terms *aerobic* and *anaerobic* refer to the manner in which glucose is broken down to create energy for the muscles to use. (Note: For information on aerobic and anaerobic exercise and their relationship to muscle tissue, see Section 10.7.)
  - An **anaerobic exercise** is an exercise that is performed for a short period of time, with maximal exertion of the muscles. Anaerobic exercises increase the power component of strength.
  - An **aerobic exercise** is an exercise that is performed for a sustained period of time, with less than maximal exertion of the muscles. Aerobic exercises increase the endurance component of strength.
- The manner in which strengthening exercises are done can also be divided into three categories based on the type of muscular contraction that is occurring: (1) concentric contraction exercises, (2) eccentric contraction exercises, and (3) isometric contraction exercises.
- Studies have found that of the three types of contractions, eccentric contractions can generate the most force and can generate this force with the least energy output (least energy output means that an eccentric contraction burns fewer calories than a concentric or an isometric contraction for the same force output). Concentric contractions have been found to produce the lowest force, and isometric contractions are in the middle.
  - Much of the advantage that an eccentric contraction has is likely because of the increased passive tension of the sarcomere/muscle when it is stretched. (Note:

For more information on the tension [i.e., force output of a muscle], see Section 15.5.)

- An application of this knowledge might be to begin a rehabilitation program for a client or an exercise program for an unconditioned individual with eccentric contractions, because these would be the least effortful and stressful. Once the client can comfortably and successfully perform the eccentric contractions, the program can change to include isometric and then concentric contractions.

Strengthening Training Modalities and Approaches:

- Strength training can be achieved a number of ways (Figure 17-8). One approach is to simply engage in a sport or activity. Another approach is to perform a workout routine.
  - Examples of sports/activities that could be engaged in are tennis, basketball, swimming, running, and dancing. Each of these provides movement patterns

A

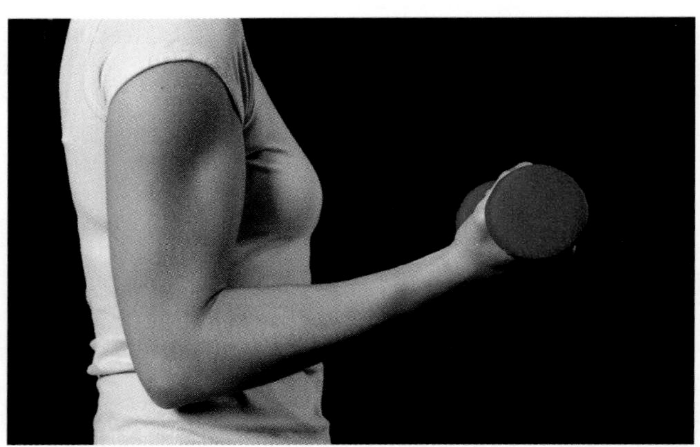

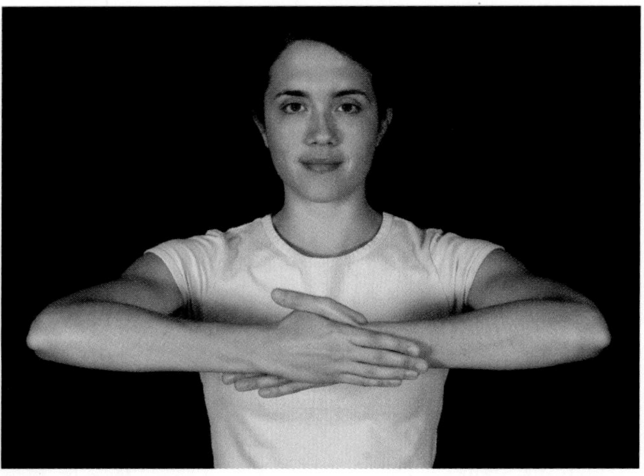

B

C

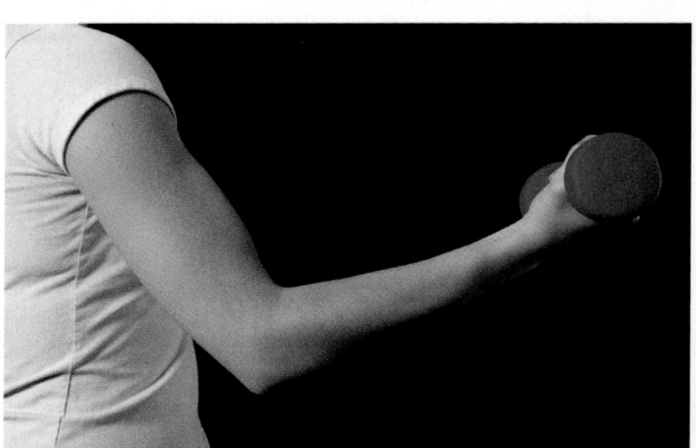

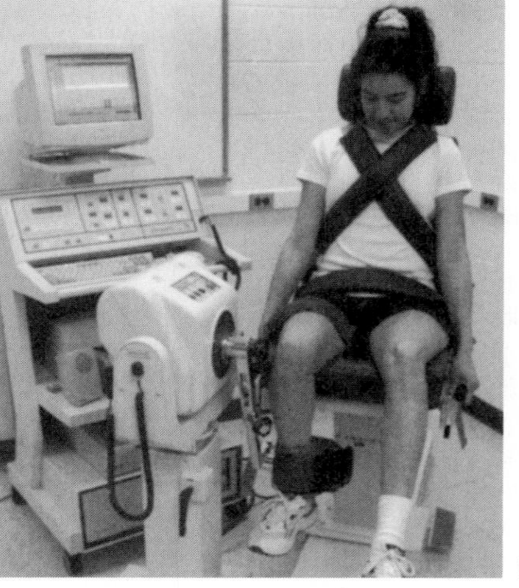

D

E

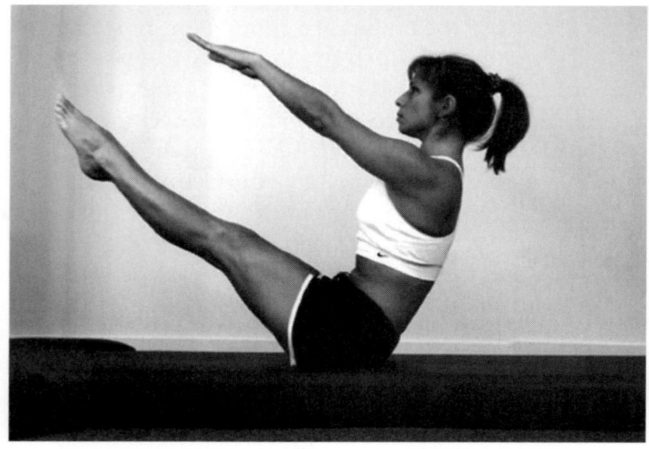

Figure 17-8 Four exercise modalities/approaches. *A,* Example of an isotonic exercise; it is a bicep curl (lifting a free weight). *B,* Example of an isometric exercise. *C,* Example of an exercise that is isotonic at one joint and isometric at another; it is a bicep curl with the arm flexed at the shoulder joint. The forearm moves through an isotonic range of motion at the elbow joint while the arm is stabilized (i.e., fixed) at the shoulder joint by an isometric contraction. *D,* Example of a variable resistance exercise; an individual is using an isokinetic machine to offer resistance to flexion of the right leg at the knee joint. *E,* Example of a core stabilization exercise for the abdominal musculature of the trunk. The individual began in a supine position, then concentrically contracted her abdominal musculature to move to this position, then isometrically holds this position for a count of three, then eccentrically contracts her abdominal musculature to return to a supine position in a controlled manner (*A, B, C, E* courtesy Joseph E. Muscolino; *D* courtesy of Biodex Medical Systems.)

that will certainly strengthen muscles of the body. When assessing the value of these sports/activities, it should be kept in mind that not every sport/activity will symmetrically strengthen all parts of the body. Every sport/activity has pros and cons; no single one is perfect. For this reason, the optimal approach might be to combine the sports/activities that are done. For example, one sport/activity could be done every Monday, Wednesday, and Friday; another could be done every Tuesday, Thursday, and Saturday. Mixing exercise routines has quite a few advantages.

❑ The alternative is to perform a workout routine that is comprised of a number of specific strengthening exercises, each one geared toward a specific muscle or muscle group. A workout routine may involve floor exercises such as push-ups and abdominal crunches, or it may involve the use of an additional resistance force such as weights, an exercise machine, or resistance tubing. (Note: Resistance tubing exercises with a tube or theraband have the advantage of being low tech, inexpensive, and extremely easy to do.) (For more on resistance tubing exercises, see Section 12.1, Figure 12-4b.)

Training Modalities

❑ A number of terms are used to describe the manner in which a strengthening exercise is done; these are called *training modalities*. Each one has advantages and disadvantages.

Isotonic Exercises:

❑ An **isotonic exercise** is the most commonly done exercise modality. It is defined as a muscle contracting and moving a constant weight through a range of motion. A typical example of an isotonic contraction would be to lift a free weight (see Figure 17-8a and c).

BOX 17-21

The term *isotonic* literally means *same tone* (*iso* means *same*). However, this term is a bit of a misnomer, because neither the tone of the muscle during the range of motion of the exercise nor the resistance force due to the free weight being moved stays the same during an isotonic exercise. Both these forces constantly change because of the constantly shifting leverage forces as the joint angle changes with the different positions of the range of motion of the exercise (the leverage forces are changing because the lever/moment arms of the muscle and resistance are constantly changing). For this reason, many trainers have dropped use of the term *isotonic*. However, given that it is still used by many people in the health and exercise field, being aware of and comfortable with this term is still important.

❑ Isotonic contractions can use concentric or eccentric contractions. Isotonic contractions may also be done closed-chain or open-chain. A closed-chain exercise is performed with the distal link of the chain of kinematic elements (i.e., body parts) fixed. Fixing the distal body part usually means having the foot on the ground or the hand either on the ground or perhaps grasping a fixed object.

❑ The advantages of an isotonic exercise is that it is low tech and easy to perform, and it perhaps best simulates real-world conditions.

❑ The disadvantage of an isotonic contraction is that it does not maximally exercise a muscle through every aspect of its range of motion. Because a muscle can generate different tension forces depending on the phase of the range of motion of the joint, lifting a constant weight must be adapted to the weakest point in the range of motion to prevent the client from being injured. This means that a greater weight could have been lifted during the stronger phases of the joint range of motion to maximally exercise the muscle.

Isometric Exercises:

❑ An **isometric exercise** modality uses an isometric muscle contraction. The muscle contracts against a force while the joint is in one position. The force is immovable so that the muscle's contractions cannot succeed in concentrically contracting (and the force does not move the muscle into an eccentric contraction by overcoming the force of the muscle's contraction) (see Figure 17-8b and c).

❑ The advantage of an isometric contraction is that it is relatively low tech and it also affords the opportunity of maximally exercising the muscle at whatever joint position is chosen.

❑ The disadvantages of an isometric contraction are that only one joint position is exercised in comparison to the full range of motion of the joint, and isometric contractions do not well simulate real-world conditions.

Variable Resistance Exercises:

❑ A **variable resistance exercise** modality requires the use of a machine that gives variable resistance to the muscle. Isokinetic and Nautilus machines are examples of variable resistance exercise machines (see Figure 17-8, *D*). **Isokinetic exercise** machines have the added aspect of keeping the speed of the joint movement constant for the entire range of the muscle's contraction.

❑ The advantage of a variable resistance exercise is that it allows for maximal exercise of a muscle at every phase of its range of motion.

❑ The disadvantages of variable resistance exercises are that they are high tech, requiring the use of somewhat expensive machines, and they do not well simulate real-world conditions.

Core Stabilization Exercises:

❑ **Core stabilization exercise** is an ideologic approach to exercise that may use many of the various exercise modalities covered previously. The focus of core stabilization exercises is to preferentially strengthen the muscles of the core of the body. The core is usually defined as the most or more proximal part of the body (i.e., the trunk, pelvis, and neck). The concept behind core stabilization is that the distal end of an attachment can better and more efficiently move if the proximal (i.e., core) end is stronger and thereby better fixed. By strengthening the spinal musculature, core stabilization also looks to create a healthier spine (see Figure 17-8, *E*). (Note: For more on core stabilization, see Section 13.6.)

Effect of Strengthening Exercises:

- The effect of strengthening exercises is to strengthen the musculature of the body (i.e., to increase the tension force that a muscle can generate without injury). Two stages to improving the performance of a muscle exist:
  - The 1st stage of an exercise program improves the strength performance of musculature by improving its neural control. Although neural control can continuously be improved and refined into the future, the increased efficiency of neural control is especially evident in the 1st month of a new exercise program and accounts for the majority of the increase in strength of musculature during that time.
  - The 2nd stage of an exercise program improves the strength performance by causing **muscle hypertrophy** (i.e., an increase in the mass of the muscle). Hypertrophy of a muscle does not involve the creation of new muscle fibers (i.e., cells). Rather, muscle hypertrophy is due to an increase in the size of the muscle fibers because of an increase in the size of the myofibrils. This increase occurs because of an increase in the amount of contractile proteins (i.e., sarcomeres within the myofibrils). The net result of increased numbers of sarcomeres is that more myosin-actin cross-bridges are present to increase the pulling force, and hence the strength of the muscle. It is the increased muscle mass of the second stage of an exercise program that accounts for the majority of the increased strength of a muscle after the first month.

BOX 17-22

Increase in mass of muscle tissue as a result of exercise is due to the addition of new sarcomeres within the myofibrils of the muscle fibers. It has been found that the newly added sarcomeres may be added to the width of the myofibrils, increasing the girth or bulk of the muscle; or they may be added to ends of the myofibrils, increasing the length of the muscle. It appears that the key determinant of how new sarcomeres are added is the type of movements performed when exercising. If an exercise program involves lengthening movements, such as those performed when dancing, or doing yoga or Pilates, sarcomeres tend to be added lengthwise. If the exercise program involves lifting free weights or primarily involves isometric contractions, sarcomeres tend to be added widthwise.

Choosing the Right Strengthening Exercise:

- When it comes to which strengthening exercise modality/approach to choose, the best exercise regimen will probably vary from individual to individual based on many factors. Following are a few of the questions that might be asked when trying to determine which approach would be best for a client. What is the purpose of the exercise program? Is the person training to achieve a particular goal? Is it a rehabilitation program focused on improving the health of a specific muscle or joint motion?

BOX 17-23

Asking a client what the purpose of their exercise regimen is might sound like a silly question. Most of us in the heath field assume that exercise is done to be healthier. However, many people do not exercise to be healthy; rather they exercise to *exorcise* their demons. Exercise may create an outlet for psychologic and emotional stress. In this regard, the optimal physical health of their bodies is not the primary focus or concern—they exercise to clear their heads. Others exercise to attain a certain goal, like being able to run a marathon or being able to lift a certain amount of weight. Again, these people are more focused on an extrinsic achievement than they are on the intrinsic health of the body. When counseling a client regarding exercise, the client's purpose for exercising must be considered and kept in mind.

- As explained previously, each exercise modality has advantages and disadvantages. Studies have not shown appreciable differences among the various strengthening modalities with regard to increasing muscle strength. Recently, more and more rehabilitation experts are leaning toward those exercises that are most easily performed by the individual client (usually low tech) and those exercises that best simulate the needs that the client has in his or her daily life.
  - However, when it comes to the best strengthening exercise for an individual, perhaps the most important question that can be asked is: What do you like to do? Many trainers, therapists, and physicians try in vain to get a client to embrace an exercise program that the client does not find enjoyable. If it is not enjoyable, the odds are that the client will discontinue the exercise program as soon as the trainer/therapist is gone and the first excuse to stop arises.
- It was stated at the beginning of this section on exercise that two aspects to exercise exist: (1) strengthening exercise and (2) stretching exercises. If optimal health is the goal, then whatever exercise regimen is chosen should also include stretching exercises.

17.10 STRETCHING EXERCISES

- Many types of stretching exercises can be done. In recent years, stretching has become very controversial; it seems that no consensus exists on exactly how and when stretching should be done. Following are the major categories of stretching:

Passive Static Stretching:

- **Passive static stretching** is the classic stretching that has been done for many decades. A body part is passively moved to a position of stretch where it is statically held for a period of time, usually 10-30 seconds. This is usually repeated three times for each stretch (i.e., three repetitions, or **reps**). A passive static stretch may be done by a therapist performing the stretch on the (passive) client. A passive static stretch may also be done by the client himself or herself, in which case the client uses another part of the body to move the body part that is being stretched. For example, the client may use the right hand to pull the head/neck into right lateral flexion to stretch the left lateral flexor muscles of the head/neck.

BOX 17-24

A number of years ago, people who did static stretching usually bounced at the end of the stretching in an effort to increase the magnitude of the stretch; this style of stretching is called **ballistic stretching**. It is universally agreed that ballistic stretching is an unhealthy way to stretch, because it stimulates the muscle spindle reflex (see Section 16.6). Because the muscle spindle reflex triggers the muscle to contract, bouncing defeats the purpose of the stretch and may even cause injury because the person is bouncing and trying to lengthen the muscle at the same time that the muscle is being stimulated to contract. However, it should be added that the muscle spindle reflex is particularly sensitive to the speed of lengthening. Therefore if the "bouncing" is done in a very gentle and slow manner, it may not stimulate the muscle spindle reflex and may be safe to do. A number of dancers and gymnasts still use a very prudent and gentle bounce in their static stretching.

Active Static Stretching:

- **Active static stretching** is similar to passive static stretching in that a body part is moved to a position of stretch where it is statically held for a period of time, typically 10-30 seconds; this procedure is usually repeated three times. The difference is that with active static stretching, the client actively uses the muscles of the region being stretched to move the body part to the position of stretch.
  - With both passive and active static stretching, in recent years more and more people have been advocating changing the manner in which they are done (from three reps held for 10-30 seconds, to approximately 10 reps, each one held for 2-3 seconds). The advantage to holding the stretch for less time and increasing the number of reps is that circulation and nutrient flow to the tissues are better promoted by increasing the movement aspect of the stretch; a greater warm up of the tissues is also achieved with greater movement. In effect, by decreasing the time that the stretch is statically held, the static aspect of the stretch is minimized in favor of more movement.

Dynamic Stretching (Mobilization):

- **Dynamic stretching**, also known as **mobilization**, seeks to greatly decrease or entirely eliminate the static aspect of the stretch and replace it with constant excursion of the joints through ranges of motion. The number of reps for each particular movement is approximately 10. Essentially, dynamic stretching is simply movement, but it is done with the intention of creating the movements that are appropriate to stretch certain target soft tissues. Remember, with every joint movement, whatever tissues are on the other side of the joint (including muscular antagonists) will be lengthened and stretched. The rationale for dynamic stretching is that it achieves stretching but with greatly improved circulation and warming of the tissues of the body.

Agonist Contract Stretching:

- **Agonist contract (AC) stretching** is a type of stretching that uses reciprocal inhibition, which is a neurologic reflex. (For more information on reciprocal inhibition, see Section 16.3.) The method of AC stretching is to actively create a joint action in the body. The mover that creates this joint action is the agonist, and it has contracted (hence the name). The result of this agonist contraction is to cause a reflex inhibition (i.e., relaxation) of the target muscle that we want to relax (i.e., the muscle that is antagonistic to the joint action and is located on the other side of the joint). At the end of the active joint movement of AC stretching, an additional force of passive stretch is usually added to the motion. This may be added by the client or a therapist/trainer.
  - For example, if the target musculature to be stretched is the extensor musculature of the shoulder joint, the client would actively move the arm into flexion at the shoulder joint. This would trigger the extensor musculature to be inhibited by reciprocal inhibition. At the end of the active range of arm flexion, the arm could be moved further into flexion, increasing the stretch of the extensors.

Active Isolated Stretching:

❑ **Active isolated stretching (AIS)** is a specific technique of stretching developed by Aaron Mattes. It incorporates two aspects: (1) the agonist contract method of stretching is done to benefit from the neurologic reflex, reciprocal inhibition, and (2) multiple reps (approximately 10) of stretches are done, each one held only 2-3 seconds. Further, Mattes uses a particular regimen of breathing: inhale and relax before the active motion; exhale on exertion to create the active joint motion.

Contract-Relax Stretching:

❑ **Contract-relax (CR) stretching** is also known as **postisometric relaxation (PIR) stretching** and is also often called **proprioceptive neuromuscular facilitation (PNF) stretching**. CR stretching uses the proprioceptive neurologic reflex of the Golgi tendon organ reflex. (Note: See Section 16.7 for more information on the Golgi tendon organ reflex and CR stretching.) The method of CR stretching is to stretch the target muscle as far as is comfortable for the client, have the client actively isometrically contract the target muscle against your resistance, and directly after the isometric contraction, have the client relax and the therapist/trainer stretches the target muscle further. The usual method of CR stretching is to have the client hold the breath in during the isometric contraction for a count of approximately 5-10 seconds; usually three reps are done.

❑ For example, if the target musculature to stretch is the extensor musculature of the hip joint, the client's thigh is passively brought as far as comfortable into flexion. The client is then asked to isometrically contract the extensors of the thigh at the hip joint against the resistance of the therapist (usually for approximately 5-10 seconds). The client is then instructed to relax the extensor musculature and the therapist moves the client's thigh further into flexion, increasing the stretch of the extensors.

Contract-Relax Agonist Contract:

❑ **Contract-relax agonist contract (CRAC)** is a combination of CR and AC stretching methods, performed sequentially—CR then AC. The premise is to use the Golgi tendon organ reflex to relax the target muscle during the CR phase, and then use reciprocal inhibition to relax the target muscle during the AC phase.

17.11 STAGES OF AN EXERCISE ROUTINE

Stages of an Exercise Routine:

- It has been conventional wisdom for decades that one should stretch before engaging in a strengthening exercise. The premise has always been that stretching makes the tissues more flexible so that there will be less chance of injury during the strengthening exercise. However, that conventional wisdom has recently been called into question.
- Recent studies have shown that little or no benefit exists to stretching before strengthening exercise; some even assert that it is detrimental to performance to stretch before this type of exercise. The reasoning is as follows:
  - When the tissues of the body are cold, the stretch will not will not be effective; tissues stretch best when they are warmed up. Thus stretching beforehand will be ineffective at best.
  - Further, because stretching causes a neural inhibition to muscle contraction by resetting the muscle spindle reflex sensitivity, stretching may actually cause the muscles to be slower to contract, both lessening the intensity of the performance of the strengthening exercise and possibly making the joints more vulnerable to sprain by decreasing the stabilization forces to the joint.
- As a result of this reasoning, conventional wisdom has changed to recommend that stretching is done after the strengthening exercise routine; it is at this point that the tissues of the body are well warmed up and will efficiently receive the benefit of the stretch!
- However, this still leaves the question of what can and should be done before the strengthening phase to help prevent muscular strains caused by forceful contractions of muscles that are not warmed up, as well as ligamentous sprains of joints that are not warmed up. In this regard, current wisdom states that mobilization (also known as *dynamic stretching*) should be done before engaging in strengthening exercises. In particular, the mobilization motions should include whatever joint motions will be done during the strength training. Further, the motions should begin with low-force, short range-of-motion movements. They should gradually progress to increasingly more forceful and greater range-of-motion movements.
- For example, if a person is about to play tennis, the person would begin the mobilization by performing forehand, backhand, and serving motions without a racquet in the hand. These motions will begin with a short arc to the range of motion and will gradually be repeated with increasingly larger arcs until the full range of motion required during the game is achieved. Once this is done, the person may repeat the process, but this time with a racquet in the hand to add the resistance force of the weight of the racquet. Once this is accomplished, the entire process may again be repeated by actually hitting a tennis ball with the opponent, but playing in midcourt so that only gentle muscular forces are needed. Then the two players move back to the baseline and begin gently rallying full court. From here, the pace and force of the hitting gradually increases until the game is at full force. This entire process might require 10-15 minutes.

  Mobilization has many advantages:
- It increases circulation, improving nutrient delivery and waste removal to the tissues.
- It warms up the tissues as a result of the active movements.
- It grooves the neural pathways necessary for the motions that will occur during the strengthening phase of the exercise program.
- It serves to stretch the soft tissues (including the muscles), because for every joint motion performed, the soft tissues on the other side of the joint are stretched.
- In reality, saying that stretching should only be done after the strengthening phase of an exercise routine is a bit fallacious, because mobilization is actually a form of stretching; it is dynamic stretching. What is true is that passive static stretching should only be done after the tissues are warmed up by the strengthening phase of an exercise routine.

BOX 17-25

Given that static stretching is not very effective unless the tissues being stretched are warmed up, it is now recommended that static stretching be done only after the strengthening phase of an exercise routine. This way, the tissues will be warmed and ready to efficiently receive and respond to the stretch. However, if a person would like to stretch but is not doing strengthening exercises, static stretching can still be done if the client begins by warming the tissues that will be stretched by some other means. Methods of warming the tissues include application of a hot pack on the region, a hot shower or bath, or perhaps best, dynamic stretching (i.e., mobilization) movements.

Following is the recommended order for the four stages of an exercise routine:

1. Mobilization (i.e., dynamic stretching)
2. Strengthening exercises
3. Stretching exercises
4. Rest and recuperation

17.12 GAIT CYCLE

- **Gait** is defined as the manner of walking.
- The **gait cycle** is defined as the cyclic pattern of engagement of muscles and joints of the body when walking.
- Walking requires a very complex coordination of muscle contractions. Although most adults take the ability to walk for granted, children need years to learn how to walk in a coordinated fashion. With advancing years, people are often challenged once again by the demands of walking.

BOX 17-26

It is estimated that an individual does not develop a mature gait pattern until approximately the age of 7 years.

- Whether our clients are children, adults, or senior citizens, athletes or nonathletes, understanding the demands of gait can be extremely valuable for therapists and trainers, given the effects that gait can have on musculoskeletal health.

Gait Cycle Specifics:

- When we walk, our gait has a repetitive or cyclic pattern. We step forward with our right foot, then our left foot, then our right foot again, then our left foot again, and so forth. Whether we walk 50 feet or 50 miles, this cyclic pattern is the same. The term *gait cycle* is used to describe this cyclic pattern of gait.
- Figure 17-9 illustrates one cycle of the gait cycle. We see that it begins when one heel strikes the ground and ends when the same side heel strikes the ground again.
- The term **stride** is used to define one cycle of the gait cycle.
  - One stride consists of two steps: (1) a left step and (2) a right step.
  - Technically the **step** of one foot begins when the heel of the other foot strikes the ground and ends when its heel strikes the ground. Each step makes up 50% of the gait cycle (or stride). In other words, two steps occur in one stride (Box 17-27).

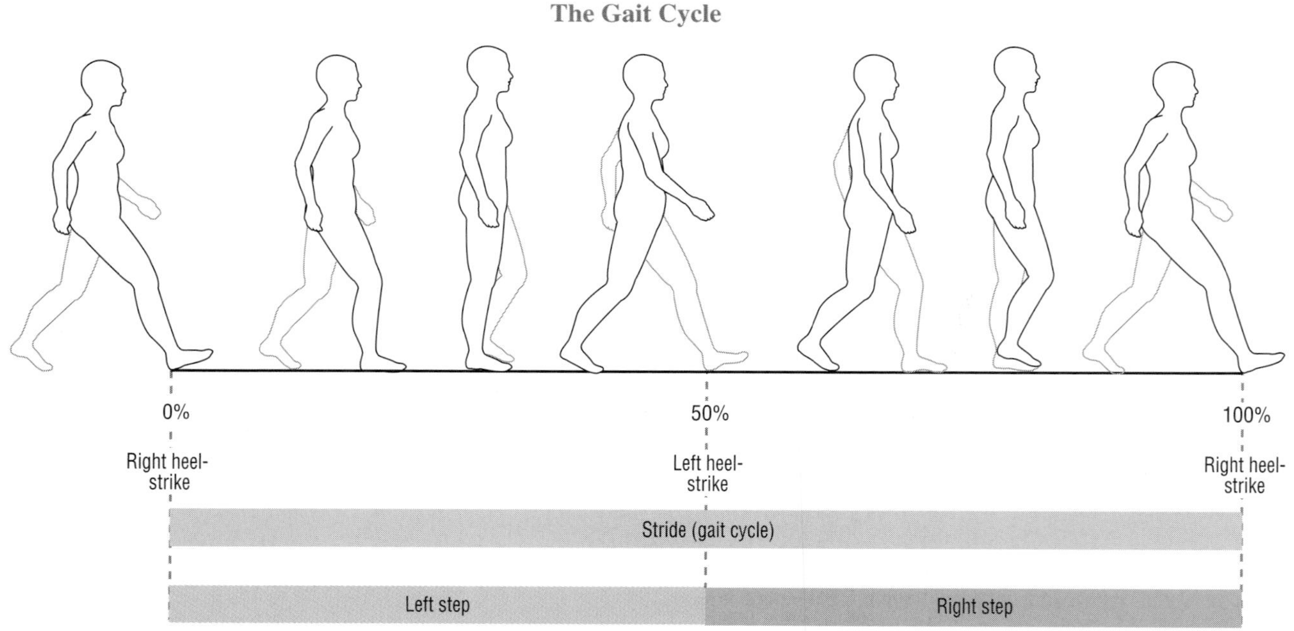

Figure 17-9 Gait cycle. The gait cycle begins with one heel-strike and ends with the same side heel-strike. One gait cycle is comprised of one stride, which in turn in composed of two steps. (Modified from Neumann DA: *Kinesiology of the musculoskeletal system: foundations for physical rehabilitation.* St Louis, 2002, Mosby.)

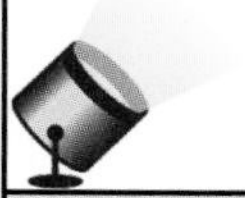

BOX 17-27 SPOTLIGHT ON FOOT FACTS

A number of additional terms are often used when describing a step of the gait cycle:

Step length is defined as the length between two consecutive heel strikes (i.e., the length of a step). Average step length of an adult is approximately 28 inches (72 cm).

Step width is the width (i.e., lateral distance) between the centers of two consecutive heel strikes. Average step width of an adult is approximately 3 inches (7-9 cm).

Step angulation is the angle created between the direction in which one is moving and the long axis of the foot. A step angulation of approximately 7-10 degrees is considered normal.

Additionally, the normal pace of walking is approximately 100 steps per minute (approximately $2^1/_2$ miles per hour [4 kilometers per hour]); and on average, each foot strikes the ground between 2000 and 10,000 times daily!

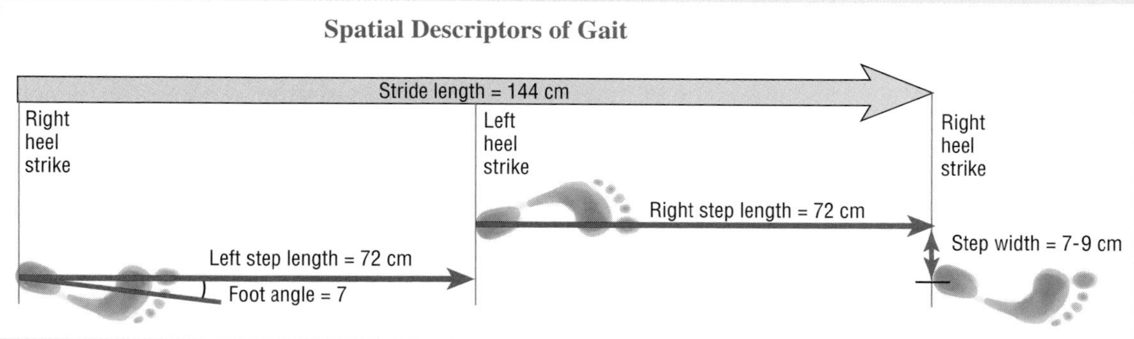

Modified from Neumann DA: *Kinesiology of the musculoskeletal system: foundations for physical rehabilitation.* St Louis, 2002, Mosby.

Gait Cycle Phases and Landmarks:

- The gait cycle has two main phases (Figure 17-10): (1) the stance phase and (2) the swing phase. These phases are correlated with the major landmarks of the gait cycle.
  - **Stance phase** begins at heel-strike and ends at toe-off.
  - **Swing phase** begins at toe-off and ends at heel-strike.

Stance Phase:

- Stance phase contains the following five landmarks of the gait cycle:

BOX 17-28

The order of landmarks of the stance phase of the gait cycle are classically considered to be heel-strike, foot-flat, midstance, heel-off, and toe-off, in that order. However, some people do not walk in that pattern. Some people reach out and begin stance phase with their toes contacting the ground before their heels.

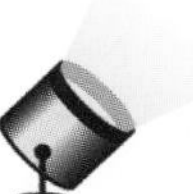

BOX 17-29 SPOTLIGHT ON THE FUNCTION OF THE FOOT DURING THE GAIT CYCLE

When walking, the foot must be supple and flexible during the early stages of the stance cycle to adapt to the uneven surfaces of the ground. This requires the foot to be in its open-packed position, which is pronation (primarily composed of eversion). Pronation allows the arches to collapse, thus allowing the foot to adapt to the contour of the ground. However, during the later stages of the stance cycle when toeing-off (i.e., pushing off) the ground, the foot must be stiff and stable to propel the body forward. This requires the foot to be in its closed-packed position, which is supination (primarily composed of inversion). Supination holds the arches high and creates a more rigid, stable foot for propulsion. The ability of the foot to change from being supple (able to pronate) to rigid (held in supination) is created by the laxity/tautness of the plantar fascia of the foot. When the plantar fascia is taut, the arches are supported and the foot becomes somewhat rigid; when the plantar fascia is lax, the arches are more mobile and the foot becomes supple. The ability of the plantar fascia to change from being lax to taut is created by the windlass mechanism (see Section 8-17). During the early stages of the stance cycle when the foot is in anatomic position, the plantar fascia is lax, resulting in a supple foot. However, during the later stages of the stance cycle when extension occurs at the metatarsophalangeal (MTP) joints, because of the windlass mechanism, the plantar fascia is pulled taut around these joints. The resulting tension in the plantar fascia is then transferred to the arches of the foot, causing them to rise, creating a rigid foot for propulsion. Thus the foot shifts between being supple and flexible during the early stance cycle to adapt to the ground, and stable and rigid during the late stance cycle for propulsion.

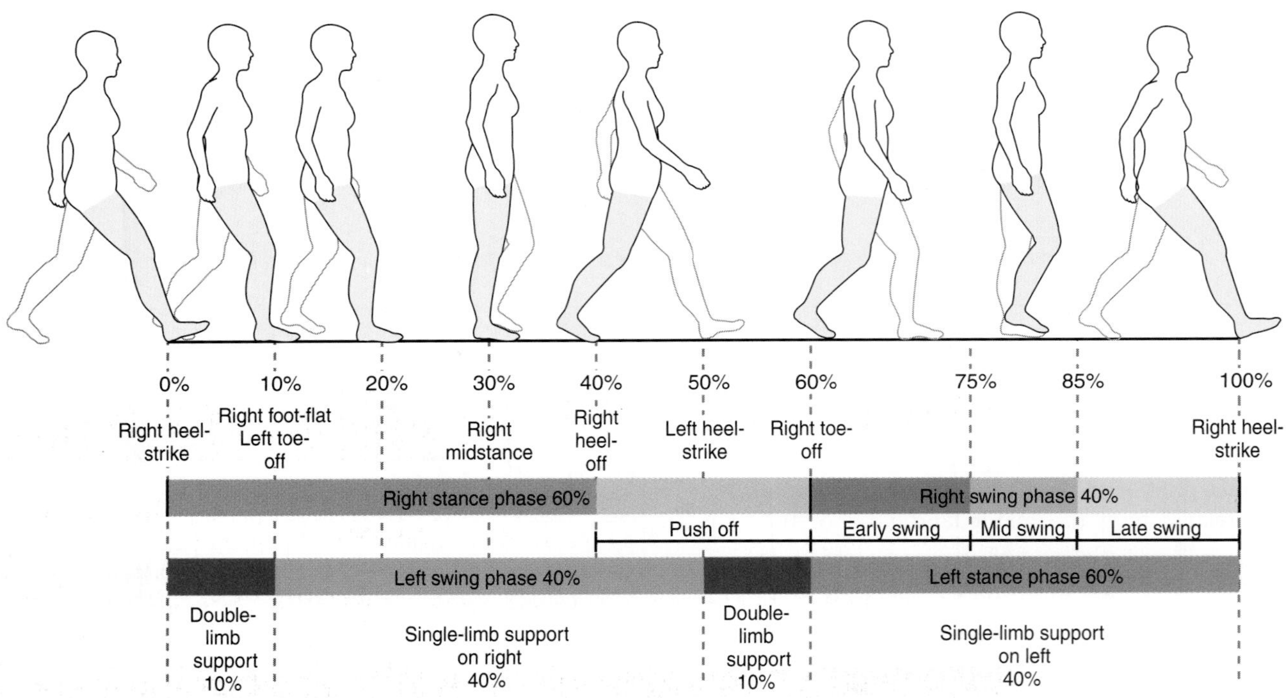

Figure 17-10 Phases and landmarks of the gait cycle. The gait cycle can be divided into two main phases: (1) the stance phase and (2) the swing phase. The stance phase is defined as when the foot is on the ground and accounts for 60% of the gait cycle for each foot; the swing phase is defined as when the foot is swinging in the air and accounts for 40% of the gait cycle for each foot. The period of double-limb support in which both feet are on the ground should be noted; walking is defined by the presence of double-limb support. The major landmarks of stance phase are heel-strike, foot-flat, midstance, heel-off, and toe-off. The swing phase is often divided into an early swing, midswing, and late swing. (Modified from Neumann DA: *Kinesiology of the musculoskeletal system: foundations for physical rehabilitation.* St Louis, 2002, Mosby.)

1. **Heel-strike** is defined as the moment that a person's heel strikes (i.e., makes contact with, the ground).
   - ❑ Heel-strike is the landmark that begins stance phase (and ends swing phase).
2. **Foot-flat** is defined as the moment that the entire plantar surface of the foot comes into contact with the ground (i.e., the foot is flat).
3. **Midstance** is the midpoint of stance phase and occurs when the weight of the body is directly over the lower extremity.
   - ❑ Midstance occurs when the greater trochanter is directly above the middle of the foot.
4. **Heel-off** is defined as the moment that the heel leaves the ground.
5. **Toe-off** is defined as the moment that a person's toes push off and leave the ground.
   - ❑ Toe-off is the landmark that ends stance phase (and begins swing phase).

Swing Phase:

- ❑ Swing phase begins with toe-off and ends with heel-strike.
- ❑ Swing phase is often subdivided into three approximately equal sections: (1) **early swing**, (2) **midswing**, and (3) **late swing**.
- ❑ When analyzing gait, our first assumption might be that stance phase and swing phase each account for 50% of the gait cycle; however, this is not true. Stance phase of any one foot actually accounts for 60% of the gait cycle, with the swing phase of that foot accounting for the other 40%. The reason for this is that a period of **double-limb support** exists in which both feet are in contact with the ground (see Figure 17-10).

BOX 17-30

It is not the speed of movement that distinguishes walking from running but the presence of double-limb support. By definition, walking has double-limb support and running does not. Interestingly, as a person speeds the pace of walking, the period of double-limb support grows increasingly smaller and smaller. At the moment that double-limb support disappears, by definition, we are running.

- ❑ As therapists and trainers, knowledge of the gait cycle is important because it allows us to understand the demands placed on the musculature, joints, and other soft tissues of the lower extremity when walking.
  - ❑ Lower extremity muscle contraction can generally be stated to occur during the gait cycle for three conceptual reasons: (1) muscles concentrically contract to create the motion needed during the gait cycle; (2) muscles eccentrically contract to decelerate the momentum motion of the gait cycle; and (3) muscles isometrically contract to stabilize and prevent motion of a body part.
  - ❑ During the early to middle stages of the stance phase, muscles of the lower extremity are primarily eccentrically contracting to slow the momentum of the body's movement. Further, during the early to middle stages, joints of the foot must be sufficiently supple to both adapt to the uneven surfaces of the ground and to absorb the stresses of the foot striking the ground.
  - ❑ During the middle to late stages of the stance phase, muscles of the lower extremity are primarily concentrically contracting to create the propulsion force of the body's movement. Further, during the middle to late stages, the joints of the foot must be sufficiently rigid to be able to allow the foot to act as a rigid lever for propulsion of the body forward.

☐ 17.13 MUSCULAR ACTIVITY DURING THE GAIT CYCLE

- ❑ The patterns of muscular coordination that occur during the gait cycle can be quite complex. Although the entire body is involved in the gait cycle, we will limit our discussion to the functional muscle groups of the lower extremity.
- ❑ Understanding these conceptual roles can be very important when working with clients who are experiencing lower extremity problems, because improper mechanics during the gait cycle often lead to functional problems throughout the body. The best way to understand and assess the cause of these improper mechanics is to have a clear understanding of the proper mechanics of gait. Once a clear assessment is made, appropriate treatment can be given.

Following are the three major conceptual roles of the musculature of the lower extremity during the gait cycle:

1. Muscles may contract concentrically to create (i.e., accelerate) a movement of the lower extremity.
2. Muscles may contract eccentrically to slow down (i.e., decelerate) a movement of the lower extremity.
3. Muscles may contract isometrically to stabilize (stop movement of) a body part.

Following is a survey of the major role(s) of the individual functional muscle groups of the lower extremity during the gait cycle. The role of the contraction of each of the major muscles of the lower extremity within the gait cycle has been determined by electromyography (EMG). (For each of these functional groups, please refer to Figure 17-11.)

BOX 17-31

Electromyography (EMG) is an assessment tool used to determine when a muscle is contracting. Because the contraction of a muscle involves a depolarization of the muscle's membrane, electricity is generated whenever a muscle contracts. That electricity can be measured by EMG. Two methods of EMG exist: one is to place surface electrodes on the skin that measure the electrical signal created by the muscles beneath them; for superficial muscles this method works fine. However, for deeper muscles, needle electrodes must be inserted into the musculature to elicit accurate results. With either method, the protocol of EMG is to put electrodes in place and then ask the person to carry out a specific movement pattern; based on the results of the EMG, it can be determined not only which muscles contracted during the movement pattern but also exactly when and how strongly each of the muscles contracted during the movement pattern. Although analysis of a muscle's potential actions is possible based on an understanding of a muscle's line of pull relative the joint it crosses, it does not tell us exactly which one of a number of possible muscles that have a particular joint action is recruited by the nervous system to contract during specific movement patterns. That information can be provided by EMG. For this reason, EMG is considered to be the most accurate means to determine the roles of muscles in movement patterns.

Hip Joint Flexor Muscles:

❑ Hip joint flexors have two roles during the gait cycle:

1. The primary role of hip joint flexors is to contract concentrically to create the forward swing of the lower extremity (i.e., flexion of the thigh at the hip joint) during the early aspect of the swing phase.

BOX 17-32

The swing phase of walking is characterized by flexion of the thigh at the hip joint. Interestingly, contraction of the hip flexor muscle group is necessary only during the 1st half of the swing phase. This is because the 2nd half of the swing phase is completed by momentum (i.e., swing phase is a ballistic motion).

2. Hip joint flexors contract eccentrically to decelerate the extension of the thigh at the hip joint that is occurring just before toe-off of the stance phase.

❑ Major hip joint flexors are the iliopsoas, sartorius, and rectus femoris.

Hip Joint Extensor Muscles:

❑ Hip joint extensors have two roles during the gait cycle:

1. Hip joint extensors contract eccentrically to decelerate the forward-swinging limb at the late aspect of the swing phase (i.e., their force of extension on the thigh at the hip joint slows down flexion of the thigh at the hip joint, which occurs during the swing phase).
2. Hip joint extensors isometrically contract forcefully on heel-strike of the stance phase to stabilize the pelvis from anteriorly tilting at the hip joint. This contraction is necessary to help prevent the pelvis and upper body from being thrown forward because of momentum when the lower extremity's forward movement is stopped by striking the ground.

❑ Major hip joint extensors are the hamstrings (i.e., biceps femoris, semitendinosus, and semimembranosus) and the gluteus maximus.

Hip Joint Abductor Muscles:

❑ The role of the hip joint abductors during the gait cycle is primarily important with regard to their action on the pelvis, not the thigh.

❑ The major function of the hip joint abductors is to contract, creating a force of depression on the pelvis during the stance phase of gait (Box 17-33, Note 1). They are particularly active during the 1st half of the stance phase, from heel-strike to midstance. By creating a force of depression on the pelvis on the stance (i.e., support) limb side, they stabilize the pelvis (and upper body), stopping it from depressing to the other side (i.e., the swing-limb side) (Box 17-33, Note 2). Without this stabilization, the pelvis would fall toward the swing-limb side, because when the body is in single-limb support, the center of weight of the body is not balanced over the support limb but rather located over thin air, toward the swing-limb side.

❑ Major hip joint abductors are the gluteus medius and gluteus minimus. The tensor fasciae latae and sartorius are also active as hip joint abductors.

BOX 17-33

Note 1: Depression of the pelvis at the hip joint is the reverse action of abduction of the thigh at the hip joint. In other words, all thigh abductor musculature can either abduct the thigh or depress the same side pelvis at the hip joint. This scenario illustrates the importance of understanding the concept of reverse actions. During the gait cycle, we are in stance phase (i.e., closed chain with the distal attachments of muscles fixed) 60% of the time. Therefore lower limb reverse actions actually occur more frequently than what are considered to be lower limb regular actions. (For more details on the concept of reverse actions, see Section 5.29.)

Note 2: As stabilizers (i.e., fixators) of the pelvis, the hip abductors are usually considered to contract isometrically. Actually, the pelvis is permitted to drop slightly toward the swing-limb side; therefore the hip abductor musculature's contraction is slightly eccentric.

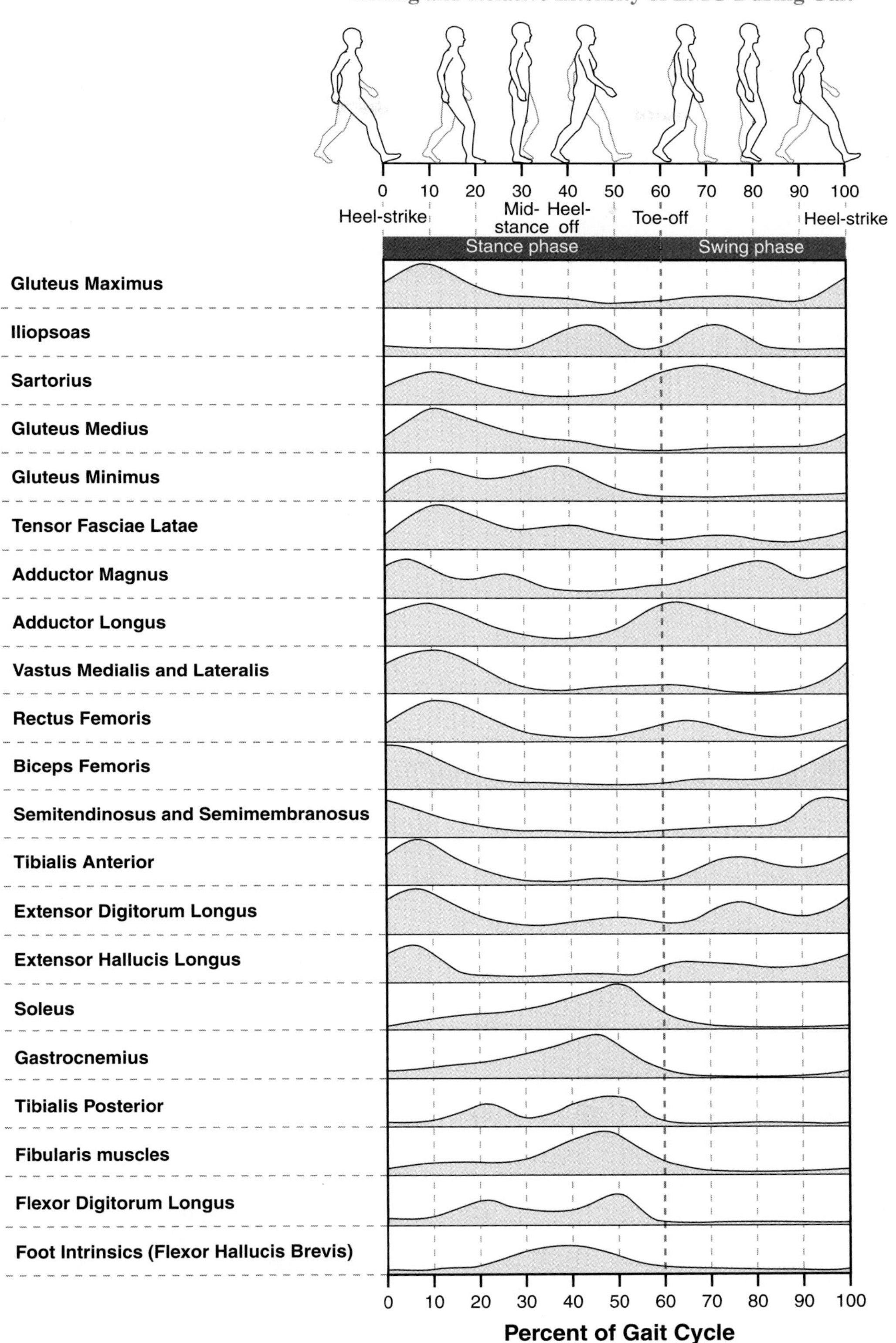

Figure 17-11 Intensity of the contractions of the major muscles of the lower extremity correlated with the phases and landmarks of the gait cycle. (Note: All references are for the right side.) (Modified from Neumann DA: *Kinesiology of the musculoskeletal system: foundations for physical rehabilitation.* St Louis, 2002, Mosby.)

Hip Joint Adductor Muscles:

- Hip joint adductors have two roles during the gait cycle:
  1. Hip joint adductors contract at heel-strike. It is believed that this contraction aids the hip joint extensors' stabilization of the hip joint as the force of hitting the ground travels up through the lower extremity.
  2. Hip joint adductors contract again just after toe-off. This contraction most likely aids in flexion of the thigh at the hip joint.

BOX 17-34

Generally the adductor muscle group has the ability to extend the thigh when it is flexed and flex the thigh when it is extended. Many muscles change their actions when their line of pull relative to the joint changes with a change in joint position. This is an example of why muscles' *anatomic actions* should not be memorized. (See Section 11.10 for an explanation of *anatomic actions*.) A muscle's action should be understood to be a function of its line of pull relative the joint it crosses; if the joint position changes, the action of the muscle can change (see Section 11.10)!

- Major hip joint adductors are the adductors longus, brevis, and magnus, as well as the pectineus and gracilis.

Hip Joint Medial Rotator Muscles:

- Hip joint medial rotators are active during the stance phase of gait.
- During stance phase, the thigh is relatively fixed (because the foot is fixed to the floor) and the pelvis is mobile. Therefore the medial rotators of the hip joint perform their reverse action of ipsilateral rotation of the pelvis at the hip joint, pulling the entire pelvis forward. (Note: For the relationship between medial rotators of the thigh at the hip joint and ipsilateral rotators of the pelvis at the hip joint, see Section 8.7.) Ipsilateral rotation of the pelvis helps to advance the swing-limb forward.
- Major hip joint medial rotators are the tensor fasciae latae and the anterior fibers of the gluteus medius and minimus.

Hip Joint Lateral Rotator Muscles:

- Hip joint lateral rotators are primarily active during the stance phase of gait.
- Hip joint lateral rotators are believed to be important toward controlling the hip joint medial rotators' action on the pelvis (i.e., the hip joint lateral rotator muscles' action of contralateral rotation of the pelvis controls the ipsilateral rotation of the pelvis of the medial rotator muscles).

BOX 17-35

The reverse action of the lateral rotator muscles of the hip joint is contralateral rotation of the pelvis at the hip joint (see Section 8.7). Contralateral rotation of the pelvis is extremely important when **planting and cutting** in sports. Planting and cutting is done when a person plants a foot on the ground and then cuts (i.e., changes the direction that he or she is running by turning the body to orient to the opposite side). For example, you plant your right foot and then turn to the left (see figure).

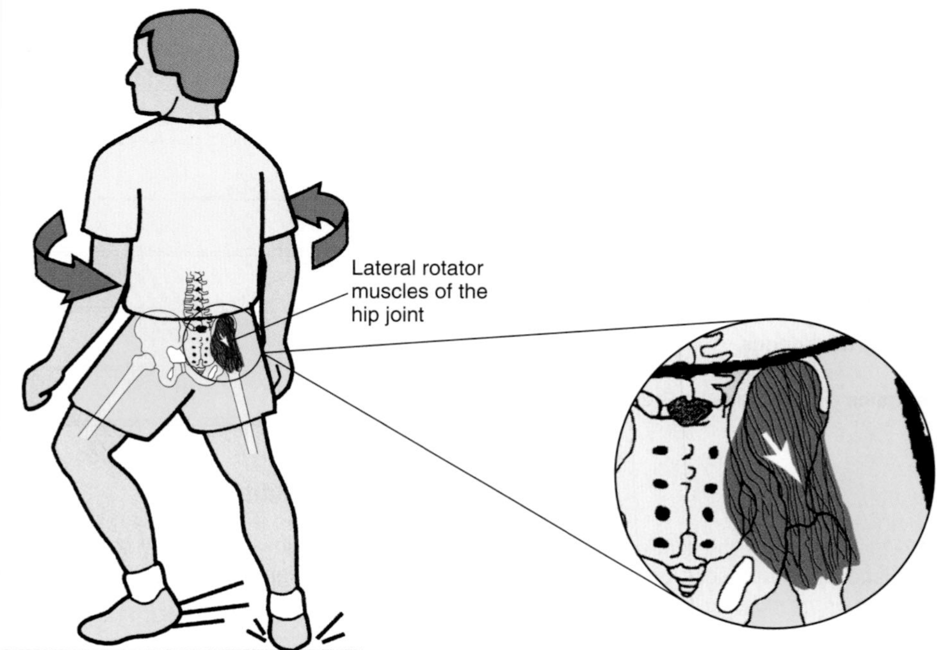

Modified from Neumann DA: *Kinesiology of the musculoskeletal system: foundations for physical rehabilitation.* St Louis, 2002, Mosby.

- Major hip joint lateral rotators are the gluteus maximus, the posterior fibers of the gluteus medius and minimus, and the deep lateral rotators of the thigh (piriformis, superior and inferior gemelli, obturators internus and externus, and quadratus femoris).

Knee Joint Extensor Muscles:

- Knee joint extensors have two roles during the gait cycle:
  1. Knee joint extensors contract concentrically at the end of swing phase to extend the leg at the knee joint and reach out with the leg in preparation for heel-strike.
  2. Knee joint extensors contract even more powerfully during the 1st half of the stance phase from heel-strike to midstance, to eccentrically contract and decelerate the knee joint flexion that occurs early in stance phase just after heel-strike and to then concentrically contract to create extension of the knee joint as we approach midstance.
- Major knee joint extensors are the quadriceps femoris group (i.e., vastus lateralis, vastus medialis, vastus intermedius, and the rectus femoris [which is also a hip joint flexor]).

Knee Joint Flexor Muscles:

- Knee joint flexors have three roles during the gait cycle:
  1. Knee joint flexors contract eccentrically to decelerate knee joint extension just before heel-strike.
  2. Knee joint flexors contract just after heel-strike. This may occur to stabilize the knee joint in the early stage of the stance phase.

BOX 17-36

Interpreting the role of the knee joint flexor musculature in the gait cycle can be difficult, because the major knee joint flexors, the hamstrings, are also hip joint extensors.

  3. Knee joint flexors contract during the swing phase to keep the foot from dragging on the ground.
- Major knee joint flexors are the hamstring muscles (i.e., biceps femoris, semitendinosus, and semimembranosus) and the gastrocnemius.

Ankle Joint Dorsiflexor Muscles:

- Ankle joint dorsiflexors have two roles during the gait cycle:
  1. Ankle joint dorsiflexors eccentrically contract to decelerate plantarflexion of the foot at the ankle joint during stance phase between heel-strike and foot-flat. This allows the foot to be lowered to the ground in a controlled and graceful manner as the body weight transfers over the stance limb.

BOX 17-37

If the foot is not brought to the ground in a controlled and graceful manner at the beginning of the stance phase, it is called **foot slap**, named for the characteristic slapping noise that the foot makes as it impacts the ground. Foot slap is usually caused by nerve compression on the nerve segments of the deep fibular nerve (a branch of the sciatic nerve) that provides motor innervation to the muscles of the anterior compartment of the leg (i.e., the dorsiflexors of the foot at the ankle joint).

  2. Ankle joint dorsiflexors contract concentrically during the swing phase of the gait cycle. This is necessary to create dorsiflexion of the foot at the ankle joint to keep the toes from scraping on the ground as the swing limb is brought forward.
- Major ankle joint dorsiflexors are the muscles of the anterior compartment of the leg (i.e., tibialis anterior, extensor digitorum longus, extensor hallucis longus, fibularis tertius).

Ankle Joint Plantarflexor Muscles:

- Ankle joint plantarflexors have two roles during the gait cycle:
  1. Ankle joint plantarflexors eccentrically contract during most of the stance phase to decelerate dorsiflexion of the ankle joint. However, because the foot is fixed to the floor, this force of plantarflexion is necessary to decelerate the reverse action of the leg moving anteriorly toward the foot (i.e., dorsiflexion or extension of the leg at the ankle joint). Without this plantarflexion force, the leg would collapse anteriorly at the ankle joint.
  2. Ankle joint plantarflexors contract more forcefully in a concentric manner at heel-off during the late stage of the stance phase to help push the foot off the floor.
- Major ankle joint plantarflexors are the gastrocnemius and soleus.

Subtalar Joint Supinator Muscles:

- Subtalar joint supinators have two roles during the gait cycle:
  1. Subtalar joint supinators contract eccentrically during the stance phase from heel-strike to foot-flat to decelerate pronation of the foot at the subtalar joint. During this phase of the gait cycle, pronation of the foot at the subtalar joint is a passive process caused by the body weight moving over the arch of the foot.

2. Subtalar joint supinators then concentrically contract between foot-flat and toe-off to supinate the foot at the subtalar joint.

- Major subtalar joint supinators are the tibialis posterior, tibialis anterior, flexor digitorum longus, flexor hallucis longus, and the intrinsic muscles of the foot.

BOX 17-38

A person with an excessively pronated foot will often overwork the foot supinators, trying to counter the tendency to overly pronate when weight bearing. As a result, pain may develop in the supinator muscles, especially the tibialis posterior and/or tibialis anterior. This condition is often called **shin splints**.

As a group, intrinsic muscles of the foot are credited with supporting the arch structure of the foot. Because excessive pronation is a collapse of the medial longitudinal arch of the foot, intrinsic muscles of the foot are considered to be supinators and active in preventing excessive pronation of the foot. However, when shoes are worn all day, much of the need for intrinsic foot muscles to contract is lost and these muscles often weaken. Weakness of the intrinsic muscles of the foot may add to the propensity of a person to develop the postural distortion pattern of excessive pronation.

Subtalar Joint Pronator Muscles:

- Subtalar joint pronators are active during the later stance phase of the gait cycle, from foot-flat to toe-off. They are believed to cocontract at this point along with the subtalar joint supinators to help stabilize the foot and make it more rigid as it readies to push off the ground for propulsion.
- Major subtalar joint pronators are the fibularis longus and brevis.

REVIEW QUESTIONS

evolve Answers to the following review questions appear on the Evolve website accompanying this book.

1. Define good posture and bad posture.

2. What is the definition of a stressor?

3. A posterior view plumb line analysis is best for assessing a postural distortion in what plane?

4. List the landmarks used when doing a lateral view plumb line analysis of posture.

5. Give an example of a frontal plane postural distortion and a sagittal plane postural distortion.

6. Explain how the concept of center of weight is important to posture.

7. Define the term *secondary postural distortion,* and give an example of a secondary postural distortion.

8. Give two examples of why a client might have a high right shoulder.

9. List three general principles of compensation within the body.

10. Give one example of an agonist/antagonist pair.

11. What are the effects of a protracted head on the neck musculature?

12. Explain how the spine might compensate for a low iliac crest height.

13. Define and give one example of adaptive shortening.

14. List the two major types of exercises.

15. What is the recommended order for the four stages of a healthy exercise routine?

16. What neurologic reflex is used during CR stretching?

17. What neurologic reflex is used during AC stretching?

18. What are the two main phases of the gait cycle?

19. Define and describe double-limb support.

20. What is the major role of the hip joint abductors during the gait cycle?

NOTES

APPENDIX
Attachments and Actions of Muscles

MUSCLES OF THE AXIAL BODY

MUSCLES OF THE HEAD

MUSCLES OF THE SCALP

Occipitofrontalis (of the Epicranius)

ATTACHMENTS

- ❑ OCCIPITALIS:
  - ❑ Occipital Bone and the Temporal Bone
    - ❒ the lateral ⅔ of the highest nuchal line of the occipital bone and the mastoid area of the temporal bone

to the

  - ❒ Galea Aponeurotica
- ❑ FRONTALIS:
  - ❒ Galea Aponeurotica

to the

  - ❒ Fascia and Skin Superior to the Eye and the Nose

ACTIONS

- ❒ 1. **Draws the Scalp Posteriorly (Occipitalis)**
- ❒ 2. **Draws the Scalp Anteriorly (Frontalis)**
- ❒ 3. Elevates the Eyebrow (Frontalis)

INNERVATION

- ❒ The Facial Nerve (CN VII)
- ❒ occipitalis: posterior auricular branch of the facial nerve
- ❒ frontalis: temporal branches of the facial nerve

Temporoparietalis (of the Epicranius)

ATTACHMENTS

- ❑ Fascia Superior to the Ear

to the

- ❑ Lateral Border of the Galea Aponeurotica

ACTIONS

- ❒ 1. **Elevates the Ear**
- ❒ 2. Tightens the Scalp

INNERVATION

- ❒ The Facial Nerve (CN VII)
- ❒ temporal branch

Auricularis Anterior, Superior, and Posterior

ATTACHMENTS

- ❑ AURICULARIS ANTERIOR: Galea Aponeurotica
  - ❒ the lateral margin

to the

- ❑ Anterior Ear
  - ❒ the spine of the helix
- ❑ AURICULARIS SUPERIOR: Galea Aponeurotica
  - ❒ the lateral margin

to the

- ❑ Superior Ear
  - ❒ the superior aspect of the cranial surface
- ❑ AURICULARIS POSTERIOR: Temporal Bone
  - ❒ the mastoid area of the temporal bone

to the

- ❑ Posterior Ear
  - ❒ the ponticulus of the eminentia conchae

ACTIONS

- ❒ 1. **Draws the Ear Anteriorly (Auricularis Anterior)**
- ❒ 2. **Elevates the Ear (Auricularis Superior)**
- ❒ 3. **Draws the Ear Posteriorly (Auricularis Posterior)**
- ❒ 4. Tightens and Moves the Scalp (Auricularis Anterior and Superior)

INNERVATION

- ❒ The Facial Nerve (CN VII)
- ❒ Auricularis Anterior and Superior: Temporal Branches
- ❒ Auricularis Posterior: Posterior Auricular Branch

MUSCLES OF FACIAL EXPRESSION

Orbicularis Oculi

ATTACHMENTS

- ❑ Medial Side of the Eye
  - ❒ ORBITAL PART: the nasal part of the frontal bone, the frontal process of the maxilla, and the medial palpebral ligament
  - ❒ PALPEBRAL PART: the medial palpebral ligament
  - ❒ LACRIMAL PART: the lacrimal bone

to the

- ❑ Medial Side of the Eye (returns to the same attachment, encircling the eye)
  - ❒ ORBITAL PART: returns to the same attachment (these fibers encircle the eye)
  - ❒ PALPEBRAL PART: the lateral palpebral ligament (these fibers run through the connective tissue of the eyelid)
  - ❒ LACRIMAL PART: the medial palpebral raphe (these fibers are deeper in the eye socket)

ACTIONS

- ❒ 1. **Closes and Squints the Eye (Orbital Part)**
- ❒ 2. Depresses the Upper Eyelid (Palpebral Part)
- ❒ 3. Elevates the Lower Eyelid (Palpebral Part)
- ❒ 4. Assists in Tear Transport and Drainage (Lacrimal Part)

INNERVATION
- ❐ The Facial Nerve (CN VII)
- ❐ temporal and zygomatic branches

Levator Palpebrae Superioris

ATTACHMENTS
- ❑ Sphenoid Bone
  - ❐ the anterior surface of the lesser wing of the sphenoid

to the
- ❑ Upper Eyelid
  - ❐ the fibrous tissue and the skin of the upper eyelid

ACTION
- ❐ **Elevates the Upper Eyelid**

INNERVATION
- ❐ The Oculomotor Nerve (CN III)

Corrugator Supercilii

ATTACHMENTS
- ❑ Inferior Frontal Bone
  - ❐ the medial end of the superciliary arch of the frontal bone

to the
- ❑ Skin Deep to the Medial Portion of the Eyebrow

ACTION
- ❐ **Draws the Eyebrow Inferiorly and Medially**

INNERVATION
- ❐ The Facial Nerve (CN VII)
- ❐ temporal branch

Procerus

ATTACHMENTS
- ❑ Fascia Over the Nasal Bone

to the
- ❑ Skin Between the Eyebrows

ACTIONS
- ❐ 1. **Draws Down the Medial Eyebrow**
- ❐ 2. Wrinkles the Skin of the Nose

INNERVATION
- ❐ The Facial Nerve (CN VII)
- ❐ superior buccal branches

Nasalis

ATTACHMENTS
- ❑ Maxilla
  - ❐ TRANSVERSE PART: the maxilla, lateral to the nose
  - ❐ ALAR PART: the maxilla, inferior and medial to the attachment of the transverse part of the nasalis

to the
- ❑ Cartilage of the Nose and the Opposite Side Nasalis Muscle
  - ❐ TRANSVERSE PART: the opposite side nasalis over the upper cartilage of the nose
  - ❐ ALAR PART: the alar cartilage of the nose

ACTION
- ❐ **Flares the Nostril**

INNERVATION
- ❐ The Facial Nerve (CN VII)
- ❐ superior buccal branches

Depressor Septi Nasi

ATTACHMENTS
- ❑ Maxilla
  - ❐ the incisive fossa of the maxilla

to the
- ❑ Cartilage of the Nose
  - ❐ the septum and the alar cartilage of the nose

ACTION
- ❐ **Constricts the Nostril**

INNERVATION
- ❐ The Facial Nerve (CN VII)
- ❐ superior buccal branches

Levator Labii Superioris Alaeque Nasi

ATTACHMENTS
- ❑ Maxilla
  - ❐ the frontal process of the maxilla near the nasal bone

to the
- ❑ Upper Lip and the Nose
  - ❐ LATERAL SLIP: the muscular substance of the lateral part of the upper lip
  - ❐ MEDIAL SLIP: the alar cartilage and the skin of the nose

ACTIONS
- ❐ 1. **Elevates the Upper Lip**
- ❐ 2. **Flares the Nostril**
- ❐ 3. Everts the Upper Lip

INNERVATION
- ❐ The Facial Nerve (CN VII)
- ❐ buccal branches

Levator Labii Superioris

ATTACHMENTS
- ❑ Maxilla
  - ❐ at the inferior orbital margin of the maxilla

to the
- ❑ Upper Lip
  - ❐ the muscular substance of the lateral part of the upper lip

ACTIONS
- ❐ 1. Elevates the Upper Lip
- ❐ 2. Everts the Upper Lip

INNERVATION
- ❐ The Facial Nerve (CN VII)
- ❐ buccal branches

Zygomaticus Minor

ATTACHMENTS
- ❑ Zygomatic Bone
  - ❐ near the zygomaticomaxillary suture

to the
- ❑ Upper Lip

- ❐ the muscular substance of the lateral part of the upper lip

ACTIONS
- ❐ 1. **Elevates the Upper Lip**
- ❐ 2. Everts the Upper Lip

INNERVATION
- ❐ The Facial Nerve (CN VII)
- ❐ buccal branches

Zygomaticus Major

ATTACHMENTS
- ❐ Zygomatic Bone
  - ❐ near the zygomaticotemporal suture

to the
- ❐ Angle of the Mouth
  - ❐ the modiolus, just lateral to the angle of the mouth

ACTIONS
- ❐ 1. **Elevates the Angle of the Mouth**
- ❐ 2. Draws Laterally the Angle of the Mouth

INNERVATION
- ❐ The Facial Nerve (CN VII)
- ❐ buccal branches

Levator Anguli Oris

ATTACHMENTS
- ❐ Maxilla
  - ❐ the canine fossa of the maxilla (just inferior to the infraorbital foramen)

to the
- ❐ Angle of the Mouth
  - ❐ the modiolus, just lateral to the angle of the mouth

ACTION
- ❐ **Elevates the Angle of the Mouth**

INNERVATION
- ❐ The Facial Nerve (CN VII)
- ❐ buccal branches

Risorius

ATTACHMENTS
- ❐ Fascia Superficial to the Masseter

to the
- ❐ Angle of the Mouth
  - ❐ the modiolus, just lateral to the angle of the mouth

ACTION
- ❐ **Draws Laterally the Angle of the Mouth**

INNERVATION
- ❐ The Facial Nerve (CN VII)
- ❐ buccal branches

Depressor Anguli Oris

ATTACHMENTS
- ❐ Mandible
  - ❐ the oblique line of the mandible, inferior to the mental foramen

to the
- ❐ Angle of the Mouth
  - ❐ the modiolus, just lateral to the angle of the mouth

ACTIONS
- ❐ 1. **Depresses the Angle of the Mouth**
- ❐ 2. Draws Laterally the Angle of the Mouth

INNERVATION
- ❐ The Facial Nerve (CN VII)
- ❐ mandibular branch

Depressor Labii Inferioris

ATTACHMENTS
- ❐ Mandible
  - ❐ the oblique line of the mandible, between the symphysis menti and the mental foramen

to the
- ❐ Lower Lip
  - ❐ the midline of the lower lip

ACTIONS
- ❐ 1. **Depresses the Lower Lip**
- ❐ 2. **Draws Laterally the Lower Lip**
- ❐ 3. **Everts the Lower Lip**

INNERVATION
- ❐ The Facial Nerve (CN VII)
- ❐ mandibular branch

Mentalis

ATTACHMENTS
- ❐ Mandible
  - ❐ the incisive fossa of the mandible

to the
- ❐ Skin of the Chin

ACTIONS
- ❐ 1. **Elevates the Lower Lip**
- ❐ 2. **Everts and Protracts the Lower Lip**
- ❐ 3. Wrinkles the Skin of the Chin

INNERVATION
- ❐ The Facial Nerve (CN VII)
- ❐ mandibular branch

Buccinator

ATTACHMENTS
- ❐ Maxilla and the Mandible
  - ❐ the external surfaces of the alveolar processes of the mandible and the maxilla (opposite the molars), and the pterygomandibular raphe

to the
- ❐ Lips
  - ❐ deeper into the musculature of the lips and the modiolus, just lateral to the angle of the mouth

ACTION
- ❐ **Compresses the Cheek (Against the Teeth)**

INNERVATION
- ❐ The Facial Nerve (CN VII)
- ❐ buccal branches

Orbicularis Oris

ATTACHMENTS
- ❐ Orbicularis oris is a muscle that, in its entirety, surrounds the mouth.

- In more detail, there are four parts to the orbicularis oris: two on the left (upper and lower) and two on the right (upper and lower). Therefore there is one part in each of the four quadrants. Each of these four parts of the orbicularis oris anchors to the modiolus on that side. From there, the fibers traverse through the tissue of the upper or the lower lips. At the midline, the fibers on each side interlace with each other, thereby attaching into each other.

ACTIONS

- 1. **Closes the Mouth**
- 2. **Protracts the Lips**

INNERVATION

- The Facial Nerve (CN VII)
- buccal and mandibular branches

MUSCLES OF MASTICATION

Temporalis

ATTACHMENTS

- Temporal Fossa
  - the entire temporal fossa except the portion on the zygomatic bone

to the

- Coronoid Process and the Ramus of the Mandible
  - the anterior border, apex, posterior border, and the internal surface of the coronoid process of the mandible, as well as the anterior border of the ramus of the mandible

ACTIONS

- 1. **Elevates the Mandible at the Temporomandibular Joint**
- 2. Retracts the Mandible at the Temporomandibular Joint

INNERVATION

- The Trigeminal Nerve (CN V)
- deep temporal branches of the anterior trunk of the mandibular division of the trigeminal nerve

Masseter

ATTACHMENTS

- Inferior Margins of Both the Zygomatic Bone and the Zygomatic Arch of the Temporal Bone
  - SUPERFICIAL LAYER: the inferior margins of the zygomatic bone and the zygomatic arch
  - DEEP LAYER: the inferior margin and the deep surface of the zygomatic arch

to the

- Angle, Ramus, and Coronoid Process of the Mandible
  - SUPERFICIAL LAYER: the angle and the inferior ½ of the external surface of the ramus of the mandible
  - DEEP LAYER: the external surface of the coronoid process, and the superior ½ of the external surface of the ramus of the mandible

ACTIONS

- 1. **Elevates the Mandible at the Temporomandibular Joint**
- 2. Protracts the Mandible at the Temporomandibular Joint
- 3. Retracts the Mandible at the Temporomandibular Joint

INNERVATION

- The Trigeminal Nerve (CN V)
  - anterior trunk of the mandibular division of the trigeminal nerve

Lateral Pterygoid

ATTACHMENTS

- Entire Muscle: Sphenoid Bone
  - SUPERIOR HEAD: the greater wing of the sphenoid
  - INFERIOR HEAD: the lateral surface of the lateral pterygoid plate of the pterygoid process of the sphenoid

to the

- Mandible and the Temporomandibular Joint (TMJ)
  - SUPERIOR HEAD: the capsule and articular disc of the temporomandibular joint
  - INFERIOR HEAD: the neck of the mandible

ACTIONS

- 1. **Protracts the Mandible at the Temporomandibular Joint**
- 2. Contralaterally Deviates the Mandible at the Temporomandibular Joint

INNERVATION

- The Trigeminal Nerve (CN V)
- lateral pterygoid nerve from the anterior trunk of the mandibular division of the trigeminal nerve

Medial Pterygoid

ATTACHMENTS

- Entire Muscle: Sphenoid Bone
  - DEEP HEAD: the medial surface of the lateral pterygoid plate of the pterygoid process of the sphenoid, the palatine bone, and the tuberosity of the maxilla
  - SUPERFICIAL HEAD: the palatine bone and the maxilla

to the

- Internal Surface of the Mandible
  - at the angle and the inferior border of the ramus of the mandible

ACTIONS

- 1. **Elevates the Mandible at the Temporomandibular Joint**
- 2. Protracts the Mandible at the Temporomandibular Joint
- 3. Contralaterally Deviates the Mandible at the Temporomandibular Joint

INNERVATION

- The Trigeminal Nerve (CN V)
- medial pterygoid nerve from the mandibular division of the trigeminal nerve

MUSCLES OF THE NECK

POSTERIOR NECK

Trapezius (The "Trap")

ATTACHMENTS

- ENTIRE MUSCLE: Occiput, Nuchal Ligament, and SPs of C7-T12
  - ENTIRE MUSCLE: external occipital protuberance and the medial ⅓ of the superior nuchal line of the occiput
  - UPPER: the external occipital protuberance, the medial ⅓ of the superior nuchal line of the occiput, the nuchal ligament, and the SP of C7
  - MIDDLE: the SPs of T1-T5
  - LOWER: the SPs of T6-T12

to the

- ENTIRE MUSCLE: Lateral Clavicle, Acromion Process, and the Spine of the Scapula
  - ENTIRE MUSCLE: lateral ⅓ of the clavicle
  - UPPER: lateral ⅓ of the clavicle and the acromion process of the scapula
  - MIDDLE: acromion process and spine of the scapula
  - LOWER: the tubercle at the root of the spine of the scapula

ACTIONS

1. **Laterally Flexes the Neck and the Head at the Spinal Joints (upper)**
2. **Extends the Neck and the Head at the Spinal Joints (upper)**
3. **Contralaterally Rotates the Neck and the Head at the Spinal Joints (upper)**
4. **Elevates the Scapula at the Scapulocostal Joint (upper)**
5. **Retracts (Adducts) the Scapula at the Scapulocostal Joint (entire muscle)**
6. **Depresses the Scapula at the Scapulocostal Joint (lower)**
7. Upwardly Rotates the Scapula at the Scapulocostal Joint (upper and lower)
8. Extends the Trunk at the Spinal Joints (middle and lower)

INNERVATION

- Spinal Accessory Nerve (CN XI)
- and C3, C4

Splenius Capitis

ATTACHMENTS

- Nuchal Ligament and the SPs of C7-T4
  - the nuchal ligament from the level of C3-C6

to the

- Mastoid Process of the Temporal Bone and the Occipital Bone
  - the lateral ⅓ of the superior nuchal line of the occiput

ACTIONS

1. **Extends the Head and the Neck at the Spinal Joints**
2. Laterally Flexes the Head and the Neck at the Spinal Joints
3. Ipsilaterally Rotates the Head and the Neck at the Spinal Joints

INNERVATION

- Cervical Spinal Nerves
- dorsal rami of the middle cervical spinal nerves

Splenius Cervicis

ATTACHMENTS

- SPs of T3-T6

to the

- TPs of C1-C3
  - the posterior tubercles of the TPs

ACTIONS

1. **Extends the Neck at the Spinal Joints**
2. **Laterally Flexes the Neck at the Spinal Joints**
3. **Ipsilaterally Rotates the Neck at the Spinal Joints**

INNERVATION

- Cervical Spinal Nerves
- dorsal rami of the lower cervical spinal nerves

Levator Scapulae

ATTACHMENTS

- TPs of C1-C4
  - the posterior tubercles of the TPs of C3 and C4

to the

- Medial Border of the Scapula, from the Superior Angle to the Root of the Spine of the Scapula

ACTIONS

1. **Elevates the Scapula at the Scapulocostal Joint**
2. **Extends the Neck at the Spinal Joints**
3. **Laterally Flexes the Neck at the Spinal Joints**
4. Ipsilaterally Rotates the Neck at the Spinal Joints
5. Downwardly Rotates the Scapula at the Scapulocostal Joint
6. Retracts (Adducts) the Scapula at the Scapulocostal Joint

INNERVATION

- Dorsal Scapular Nerve
- C3, 4, 5

Suboccipitals

Rectus Capitis Posterior Major (of Suboccipital Group)

ATTACHMENTS

- The Axis (C2)
  - the SP

to the

- Occiput
  - the lateral ½ of the inferior nuchal line

ACTIONS
- ❒ 1. **Extends the Head at the Atlanto-Occipital Joint**
- ❒ 2. Laterally Flexes the Head at the Atlanto-Occipital Joint
- ❒ 3. Ipsilaterally Rotates the Head at the Atlanto-Occipital Joint
- ❒ 4. Extends and Ipsilaterally Rotates the Atlas at the Atlantoaxial Joint

INNERVATION
- ❒ The Suboccipital Nerve
- ❒ dorsal ramus of C1

Rectus Capitis Posterior Minor (of Suboccipital Group)

ATTACHMENTS
- ❑ The Atlas (C1)
  - ❒ the posterior tubercle

to the
- ❑ Occiput
  - ❒ the medial ½ of the inferior nuchal line

ACTION
- ❒ **Extends the Head at the Atlanto-Occipital Joint**

INNERVATION
- ❒ The Suboccipital Nerve
- ❒ dorsal ramus of C1

Obliquus Capitis Inferior (of Suboccipital Group)

ATTACHMENTS
- ❑ The Axis (C2)
  - ❒ the SP

to the
- ❑ Atlas (C1)
  - ❒ the TP

ACTION
- ❒ **Ipsilaterally Rotates the Atlas at the Atlantoaxial Joint**

INNERVATION
- ❒ The Suboccipital Nerve
- ❒ dorsal ramus of C1

Obliquus Capitis Superior (of Suboccipital Group)

ATTACHMENTS
- ❑ The Atlas (C1)
  - ❒ the TP

to the
- ❑ Occiput
  - ❒ between the superior and inferior nuchal lines

ACTIONS
- ❒ 1. **Extends the Head at the Atlanto-Occipital Joint**
- ❒ 2. Laterally Flexes the Head at the Atlanto-Occipital Joint

INNERVATION
- ❒ The Suboccipital Nerve
- ❒ dorsal ramus of C1

ANTERIOR NECK

Platysma

ATTACHMENTS
- ❑ Subcutaneous Fascia of the Superior Chest
  - ❒ the pectoral and deltoid fascia

to the
- ❑ Mandible and the Subcutaneous Fascia of the Lower Face

ACTIONS
- ❒ 1. **Draws Up the Skin of the Superior Chest and Neck, Creating Ridges of Skin of the Neck**
- ❒ 2. Depresses and Draws the Lower Lip Laterally
- ❒ 3. Depresses the Mandible at the Temporomandibular Joint

INNERVATION
- ❒ Facial Nerve (CN VII)
- ❒ cervical branch

Sternocleidomastoid (SCM)

ATTACHMENTS
- ❑ STERNAL HEAD: Manubrium of the Sternum
  - ❒ the anterior superior surface
- ❑ CLAVICULAR HEAD: Medial Clavicle
  - ❒ the medial ⅓

to the
- ❑ Mastoid Process of the Temporal Bone
  - ❒ and the lateral ½ of the superior nuchal line of the occipital bone

ACTIONS
- ❒ 1. **Flexes the Neck at the Spinal Joints**
- ❒ 2. **Laterally Flexes the Neck and the Head at the Spinal Joints**
- ❒ 3. **Contralaterally Rotates the Neck and the Head at the Spinal Joints**
- ❒ 4. Extends the Head at the Atlanto-Occipital Joint
- ❒ 5. Elevates the Sternum and the Clavicle

INNERVATION
- ❒ Spinal Accessory Nerve (CN XI)
- ❒ and C2, 3

Hyoids

- ❑ The hyoids are a group of eight muscles that are superficial in the anterior neck.

Sternohyoid (of Hyoid Group)

ATTACHMENTS
- ❑ Sternum
  - ❒ the posterior surface of both the manubrium of the sternum and the medial clavicle

to the
- ❑ Hyoid
  - ❒ the inferior surface of the body of the hyoid

ACTION
- ❒ **Depresses the Hyoid**

INNERVATION
- The Cervical Plexus
- ansa cervicalis (C1, 3)

Sternothyroid (of Hyoid Group)

ATTACHMENTS
- Sternum
  - the posterior surface of both the manubrium of the sternum and the cartilage of the 1st rib

to the
- Thyroid Cartilage
  - the lamina of the thyroid cartilage

ACTION
- **Depresses the Thyroid Cartilage**

INNERVATION
- The Cervical Plexus
- ansa cervicalis (C1, 3)

Thyrohyoid (of Hyoid Group)

ATTACHMENTS
- Thyroid Cartilage
  - the lamina of the thyroid cartilage

to the
- Hyoid
  - the inferior surface of the greater cornu of the hyoid

ACTIONS
- 1. **Depresses the Hyoid**
- 2. Elevates the Thyroid Cartilage

INNERVATION
- The Hypoglossal Nerve (CN XII)
- a branch of C1 through the hypoglossal nerve

Omohyoid (of Hyoid Group)

ATTACHMENTS
- INFERIOR BELLY:
- Scapula
  - the superior border

to the
- Clavicle
  - bound to the clavicle at its central tendon
- SUPERIOR BELLY:
- Clavicle
  - bound to the clavicle at its central tendon

to the
- Hyoid
  - the inferior surface of the body of the hyoid

ACTION
- **Depresses the Hyoid**

INNERVATION
- The Cervical Plexus
- ansa cervicalis (C1-3)

Digastric (of Hyoid Group)

ATTACHMENTS
- POSTERIOR BELLY:
- Temporal Bone
  - the mastoid notch of the temporal bone

to the
- Hyoid
  - the central tendon is bound to the hyoid bone at the body and the greater cornu
- ANTERIOR BELLY:
- Mandible
  - the inner surface of the inferior border (the digastric fossa)

to the
- Hyoid
  - the central tendon is bound to the hyoid bone at the body and the greater cornu

ACTIONS
- 1. **Elevates the Hyoid**
- 2. Depresses the Mandible at the Temporomandibular Joint
- 3. Retracts the Mandible at the Temporomandibular Joint

INNERVATION
- The Trigeminal (CN V) and the Facial Nerve (CN VII)
- anterior belly: mylohyoid branch of the inferior alveolar nerve of posterior trunk of the mandibular division of the trigeminal nerve (CN V)
- posterior belly: facial nerve (CN VII)

Stylohyoid (of Hyoid Group)

ATTACHMENTS
- Styloid Process of the Temporal Bone
  - the posterior surface

to the
- Hyoid
  - at the junction of the body and the greater cornu of the hyoid bone

ACTION
- **Elevates the Hyoid**

INNERVATION
- The Facial Nerve (CN VII)
- the stylohyoid branch

Mylohyoid (of Hyoid Group)

ATTACHMENTS
- Inner Surface of the Mandible
  - the mylohyoid line of the mandible (from the symphysis menti to the molars)

to the
- Hyoid
  - the anterior surface of the body of the hyoid

ACTIONS
- 1. **Elevates the Hyoid**
- 2. Depresses the Mandible at the Temporomandibular Joint

INNERVATION
- The Trigeminal Nerve (CN V)
- the mylohyoid branch of the inferior alveolar nerve of the posterior trunk of the mandibular division of the trigeminal nerve (CN V)

Geniohyoid (of Hyoid Group)

ATTACHMENTS

- Inner Surface of the Mandible
  - the inferior mental spine of the mandible

to the

- Hyoid
  - the anterior surface of the body of the hyoid

ACTIONS

- 1. **Elevates the Hyoid**
- 2. Depresses the Mandible at the Temporomandibular Joint

INNERVATION

- The Hypoglossal Nerve (CN XII)
- a branch of C1 through the hypoglossal nerve

Scalenes

- The scalenes are a group of muscles that are found in the anterolateral neck.

Anterior Scalene (of Scalene Group)

ATTACHMENTS

- TPs of the Cervical Spine
  - the anterior tubercles of C3-6

to the

- 1st Rib
  - the scalene tubercle on the inner border

ACTIONS

- 1. **Flexes the Neck at the Spinal Joints**
- 2. **Laterally Flexes the Neck at the Spinal Joints**
- 3. **Elevates the 1st Rib at the Sternocostal and Costospinal Joints**
- 4. Contralaterally Rotates the Neck at the Spinal Joints

INNERVATION

- Cervical Spinal Nerves
- ventral rami; C4-6

Middle Scalene (of Scalene Group)

ATTACHMENTS

- TPs of the Cervical Spine
  - the posterior tubercles of C2-7

to the

- 1st Rib
  - the superior surface

ACTIONS

- 1. **Laterally Flexes the Neck at the Spinal Joints**
- 2. **Flexes the Neck at the Spinal Joints**
- 3. **Elevates the 1st Rib at the Sternocostal and Costospinal Joints**

INNERVATION

- Cervical Spinal Nerves
- ventral rami; C3-8

Posterior Scalene (of Scalene Group)

ATTACHMENTS

- TPs of the Cervical Spine
  - the posterior tubercles of C5-7

to the

- 2nd Rib
  - the external surface

ACTIONS

- 1. **Laterally Flexes the Neck at the Spinal Joints**
- 2. **Elevates the 2nd Rib at the Sternocostal and Costospinal Joints**

INNERVATION

- Cervical Spinal Nerves
- ventral rami; C6-8

Longus Colli (of Prevertebral Group)

ATTACHMENTS

- Entire Muscle: C3-T3 Vertebrae
  - the TPs and anterior bodies
  - SUPERIOR OBLIQUE PART: C3-5
    - the TPs of C3-5
  - INFERIOR OBLIQUE PART: T1-3
    - the anterior bodies of T1-3
  - VERTICAL PART:C5-T3
    - the anterior bodies of C5-T3

to the

- Entire Muscle: C1-6 Vertebrae
  - the TPs and anterior bodies; and the anterior arch of the atlas
  - SUPERIOR OBLIQUE PART: C1
    - the anterior arch of the atlas
  - INFERIOR OBLIQUE PART: C5-6
    - the TPs of C5-6
  - VERTICAL PART: C2-4
    - the anterior bodies of C2-4

ACTIONS

- 1. **Flexes the Neck at the Spinal Joints**
- 2. Laterally Flexes the Neck at the Spinal Joints
- 3. Contralaterally Rotates the Neck at the Spinal Joints

INNERVATION

- Cervical Spinal Nerves
- ventral rami; C2-6

Longus Capitis (of Prevertebral Group)

ATTACHMENTS

- TPs of the Cervical Spine
  - the anterior tubercles of C3-5

to the

- Occiput
  - the inferior surface of the basilar part of the occiput (just anterior to the foramen magnum)

ACTIONS

- 1. **Flexes the Head and the Neck at the Spinal Joints**
- 2. **Laterally Flexes the Head and the Neck at the Spinal Joints**

INNERVATION

- Cervical Spinal Nerves
- ventral rami; C1-3

Rectus Capitis Anterior (of Prevertebral Group)

ATTACHMENTS
- The Atlas (C1)
  - the anterior surface of the base of the TP

to the
- Occiput
  - the inferior surface of the basilar part of the occiput (just anterior to the foramen magnum)

ACTION
- **Flexes the Head at the Atlanto-Occipital Joint**

INNERVATION
- Cervical Spinal Nerves
- ventral rami; C1-2

Rectus Capitis Lateralis (of Prevertebral Group)

ATTACHMENTS
- The Atlas (C1)
  - the superior surface of the TP

to the
- Occiput
  - the inferior surface of the jugular process of the occiput

ACTION
- **Laterally Flexes the Head at the Atlanto-Occipital Joint**

INNERVATION
- Cervical Spinal Nerves
- ventral rami; C1-2

MUSCLES OF THE TRUNK

POSTERIOR TRUNK

Latissimus Dorsi (The "Lat")

ATTACHMENTS
- SPs of T7-L5, Posterior Sacrum, and the Posterior Iliac Crest
  - all via the thoracolumbar fascia
  - and the lowest three to four ribs and the inferior angle of the scapula

to the
- Medial Lip of the Bicipital Groove of the Humerus

ACTIONS
- 1. **Medially Rotates the Arm at the Shoulder Joint**
- 2. **Adducts the Arm at the Shoulder Joint**
- 3. **Extends the Arm at the Shoulder Joint**
- 4. **Anteriorly Tilts the Pelvis at the Lumbosacral Joint**
- 5. Elevates the Pelvis at the Lumbosacral Joint
- 6. Depresses the Scapula at the Scapulocostal Joint
- 7. Laterally Deviates the Trunk at the Scapulocostal Joint
- 8. Elevates the Trunk at the Scapulocostal Joint
- 9. Contralaterally Rotates the Trunk at the Scapulocostal Joint

INNERVATION
- The Thoracodorsal Nerve
- C6, 7, 8

Rhomboids Major and Minor

ATTACHMENTS
- THE RHOMBOIDS: SPs of C7-T5
  - MINOR: SPs of C7-T1
    - and the inferior nuchal ligament
  - MAJOR: SPs of T2-T5

to the
- THE RHOMBOIDS: Medial Border of the Scapula from the Root of the Spine of the Scapula to the Inferior Angle of the Scapula
  - MINOR: At the Root of the Spine of the Scapula
  - MAJOR: Between the Root of the Spine of the Scapula and the Inferior Angle of the Scapula

ACTIONS
- 1. **Retracts (Adducts) the Scapula at the Scapulocostal Joint**
- 2. **Elevates the Scapula at the Scapulocostal Joint**
- 3. Downwardly Rotates the Scapula at the Scapulocostal Joint
- 4. Contralaterally Rotates the Trunk at the Spinal Joints

INNERVATION
- The Dorsal Scapular Nerve
- C4, 5

Serratus Anterior

ATTACHMENTS
- Ribs #1-9
  - anterolaterally

to the
- Anterior Surface of the Entire Medial Border of the Scapula

ACTIONS
- 1. **Protracts (Abducts) the Scapula at the Scapulocostal Joint**
- 2. **Upwardly Rotates the Scapula at the Scapulocostal Joint**
- 3. Elevates the Scapula at the Scapulocostal Joint
- 4. Depresses the Scapula at the Scapulocostal Joint

INNERVATION
- The Long Thoracic Nerve
- C5, 6, 7

Serratus Posterior Superior

ATTACHMENTS
- SPs of C7-T3
  - and the lower nuchal ligament

to the
- Ribs #2-5
  - the superior borders and the external surfaces

ACTION

- **Elevates Ribs #2-5 at the Sternocostal and Costospinal Joints**

INNERVATION

- Intercostal Nerves
- intercostal nerves #2-5

Serratus Posterior Inferior

ATTACHMENTS

- SPs of T11-L2

to the

- Ribs #9-12
  - the inferior borders and the external surfaces

ACTION

- **Depresses Ribs #9-12 at the Sternocostal and Costospinal Joints**

INNERVATION

- Subcostal Nerve and Intercostal Nerves
- intercostal nerves #9-11

Erector Spinae Group

ATTACHMENTS

- Pelvis

to the

- Spine, Ribcage, and the Head

ACTIONS

- 1. **Extends the Trunk and the Neck and the Head at the Spinal Joints**
- 2. **Laterally Flexes the Trunk and the Neck and the Head at the Spinal Joints**
- 3. **Ipsilaterally Rotates the Trunk and the Neck and the Head at the Spinal Joints**
- 4. **Anteriorly Tilts the Pelvis at the Lumbosacral Joint**
- 5. Elevates the Pelvis at the Lumbosacral Joint
- 6. Contralaterally Rotates the Pelvis at the Lumbosacral Joint

INNERVATION

- Spinal Nerves
- dorsal rami of cervical, thoracic, and lumbar spinal nerves

Iliocostalis (of Erector Spinae Group)

ATTACHMENTS

- ENTIRE ILIOCOSTALIS: Sacrum, Iliac Crest, and Ribs #3-12
  - ILIOCOSTALIS LUMBORUM: Medial Iliac Crest and the Medial and Lateral Sacral Crests
  - ILIOCOSTALIS THORACIS: Angles of Ribs #7-12
  - ILIOCOSTALIS CERVICIS: Angles of Ribs #3-6

to the

- ENTIRE ILIOCOSTALIS: Ribs #1-12 and TPs of C4-7
  - ILIOCOSTALIS LUMBORUM: Angles of Ribs #7-12
  - ILIOCOSTALIS THORACIS: Angles of Ribs #1-6 and the TP of C7
  - ILIOCOSTALIS CERVICIS: TPs of C4-6

ACTIONS

- 1. **Extends the Trunk and the Neck at the Spinal Joints**
- 2. **Laterally Flexes the Trunk and the Neck at the Spinal Joints**
- 3. **Ipsilaterally Rotates the Trunk and the Neck at the Spinal Joints**
- 4. **Anteriorly Tilts the Pelvis at the Lumbosacral Joint**
- 5. Elevates the Pelvis at the Lumbosacral Joint
- 6. Contralaterally Rotates the Pelvis at the Lumbosacral Joint

INNERVATION

- Spinal Nerves
- dorsal rami of the lower cervical and the thoracic and upper lumbar spinal nerves

Longissimus (of Erector Spinae Group)

ATTACHMENTS

- ENTIRE LONGISSIMUS: Sacrum, Iliac Crest, TPs of L1-5 and T1-5, and the Articular Processes of C5-7
  - LONGISSIMUS THORACIS: Medial Iliac Crest, Posterior Sacrum, and the TPs of L1-5
  - LONGISSIMUS CERVICIS: TPs of the Upper Five Thoracic Vertebrae
  - LONGISSIMUS CAPITIS: TPs of the Upper Five Thoracic Vertebrae and the Articular Processes of the Lower Three Cervical Vertebrae

to the

- ENTIRE LONGISSIMUS: Ribs #4-12, TPs of T1-12 and C2-6, and the Mastoid Process of the Temporal Bone
  - LONGISSIMUS THORACIS: TPs of all the Thoracic Vertebrae and the Lower Nine Ribs (between the tubercles and the angles)
  - LONGISSIMUS CERVICIS: TPs of C2-6 (posterior tubercles)
  - LONGISSIMUS CAPITIS: Mastoid Process of the Temporal Bone

ACTIONS

- 1. **Extends the Trunk and the Neck and the Head at the Spinal Joints**
- 2. **Laterally Flexes the Trunk and the Neck and the Head at the Spinal Joints**
- 3. **Ipsilaterally Rotates the Trunk and the Neck and the Head at the Spinal Joints**
- 4. **Anteriorly Tilts the Pelvis at the Lumbosacral Joint**
- 5. Elevates the Pelvis at the Lumbosacral Joint
- 6. Contralaterally Rotates the Pelvis at the Lumbosacral Joint

INNERVATION

- Spinal Nerves
- dorsal rami of the lower cervical and the thoracic and lumbar spinal nerves

Spinalis (of Erector Spinae Group)

ATTACHMENTS

- ENTIRE SPINALIS: SPs of T11-L2 and C7, and the Nuchal Ligament
  - SPINALIS THORACIS: SPs of T11-L2
  - SPINALIS CERVICIS: Inferior Nuchal Ligament and the SP of C7
  - SPINALIS CAPITIS: Usually Considered to Be the Medial Part of the Semispinalis Capitis

to the

- ENTIRE SPINALIS: SPs of T5-12 and C2
  - SPINALIS THORACIS: SPs of T4-8
  - SPINALIS CERVICIS: SP of C2
  - SPINALIS CAPITIS: Usually Considered to Be the Medial Part of the Semispinalis Capitis

ACTIONS

1. **Extends the Trunk and the Neck and the Head at the Spinal Joints**
2. **Laterally Flexes the Trunk and the Neck and the Head at the Spinal Joints**
3. **Ipsilaterally Rotates the Trunk and the Neck and the Head at the Spinal Joints**

INNERVATION

- Spinal Nerves
- dorsal rami of the lower cervical and the thoracic spinal nerves

Transversospinalis Group

ATTACHMENTS

- Pelvis

to the

- Spine and the Head

ACTIONS

1. **Extends the Trunk and the Neck and the Head at the Spinal Joints**
2. **Laterally Flexes the Trunk and the Neck and the Head at the Spinal Joints**
3. **Contralaterally Rotates the Trunk and the Neck at the Spinal Joints**
4. **Anteriorly Tilts the Pelvis at the Lumbosacral Joint**
5. Elevates the Pelvis at the Lumbosacral Joint
6. Ipsilaterally Rotates the Pelvis at the Lumbosacral Joint

INNERVATION

- Spinal Nerves
- dorsal rami of cervical, thoracic, and lumbar spinal nerves

Semispinalis (of Transversospinalis Group)

ATTACHMENTS

- ENTIRE SEMISPINALIS: TPs of C7-T10 and the Articular Processes of C4-6
  - SEMISPINALIS THORACIS: TPs of T6-10
  - SEMISPINALIS CERVICIS: TPs of T1-5
  - SEMISPINALIS CAPITIS: TPs of C7-T6 and the Articular Processes of C4-6

to the

- ENTIRE SEMISPINALIS: SPs of C2-T4 and the Occipital Bone
  - SEMISPINALIS THORACIS: SPs of C6-T4
  - SEMISPINALIS CERVICIS: SPs of C2-5
  - SEMISPINALIS CAPITIS: Occipital Bone Between the Superior and Inferior Nuchal Lines

ACTIONS

1. **Extends the Trunk and the Neck and the Head at the Spinal Joints**
2. **Laterally Flexes the Trunk and the Neck and the Head at the Spinal Joints**
3. **Contralaterally Rotates the Trunk and the Neck at the Spinal Joints**

INNERVATION

- Spinal Nerves
- dorsal rami of cervical and thoracic spinal nerves

Multifidus (of Transversospinalis Group)

ATTACHMENTS

- Posterior Sacrum, Posterior Superior Iliac Spine (PSIS), Posterior Sacroiliac Ligament, and L5-C4 Vertebrae
  - LUMBAR REGION: All Mamillary Processes (not TPs)
  - Thoracic Region: All TPs
  - CERVICAL REGION: The Articular Processes of C4-7 (not TPs)

to the

- SPs of Vertebrae 2-4 Segmental Levels Superior to the Inferior Attachment

ACTIONS

1. **Extends the Trunk and the Neck at the Spinal Joints**
2. **Laterally Flexes the Trunk and the Neck at the Spinal Joints**
3. **Contralaterally Rotates the Trunk and the Neck at the Spinal Joints**
4. **Anteriorly Tilts the Pelvis at the Lumbosacral Joint**
5. Elevates the Pelvis at the Lumbosacral Joint
6. Ipsilaterally Rotates the Pelvis at the Lumbosacral Joint

INNERVATION

- Spinal Nerves
- dorsal rami of cervical, thoracic, and lumbar spinal nerves

Rotatores (of Transversospinalis Group)

ATTACHMENTS

- TP (inferiorly)

to the

- Lamina (superiorly)
  - of the vertebrae one to two levels superior

ACTIONS
- ❒ 1. **Contralaterally Rotates the Trunk and the Neck at the Spinal Joints**
- ❒ 2. **Extends the Trunk and the Neck at the Spinal Joints**

INNERVATION
- ❒ Spinal Nerves
- ❒ dorsal rami of cervical, thoracic, and lumbar spinal nerves

Quadratus Lumborum (QL)

ATTACHMENTS
- ❑ 12th Rib and the TPs of L1-4
  - ❒ the medial ½ of the inferior border of the 12th rib

to the
- ❑ **Posterior Iliac Crest**
  - ❒ the posteromedial iliac crest and the iliolumbar ligament

ACTIONS
- ❒ 1. **Elevates the Pelvis at the Lumbosacral Joint**
- ❒ 2. **Anteriorly Tilts the Pelvis at the Lumbosacral Joint**
- ❒ 3. **Laterally Flexes the Trunk at the Spinal Joints**
- ❒ 4. **Extends the Trunk at the Spinal Joints**
- ❒ 5. Depresses the 12th Rib at the Costospinal Joints

INNERVATION
- ❒ Lumbar Plexus
- ❒ T12, L1, 2, 3

Interspinales

ATTACHMENTS
- ❑ From an SP

to the
- ❑ SP directly superior
  - ❒ CERVICAL REGION: There are six pairs of interspinales located between T1-C2
  - ❒ THORACIC REGION: There are two pairs of interspinales located between T2-1 and T12-11
  - ❒ LUMBAR REGION: There are four pairs of interspinales located between L5-1

ACTION
- ❒ **Extends the Neck and the Trunk at the Spinal Joints**

INNERVATION
- ❒ Spinal Nerves
- ❒ dorsal rami

Intertransversarii

ATTACHMENTS
- ❑ From a TP

to the
- ❑ TP directly superior
  - ❒ CERVICAL REGION: There are seven pairs of intertransversarii muscles (anterior and posterior sets) located between C1 and T1 on each side of the body.
  - ❒ THORACIC REGION: There are three intertransversarii muscles between T10 and L1 on each side of the body.
  - ❒ LUMBAR REGION: There are four pairs of intertransversarii muscles (medial and lateral sets) located between L1 and L5 on each side of the body.

ACTION
- ❒ **Laterally Flexes the Neck and the Trunk at the Spinal Joints**

INNERVATION
- ❒ Spinal Nerves
- ❒ dorsal and ventral rami

Levatores Costarum

ATTACHMENTS
- ❑ TPs of C7-T11
  - ❒ the tips of the TPs

to the
- ❑ Ribs #1-12 (inferiorly)
  - ❒ the external surfaces of the ribs, between the tubercle and the angle

ACTIONS
- ❒ 1. **Elevates the Ribs at the Sternocostal and Costospinal Joints**
- ❒ 2. Extends the Trunk at the Spinal Joints
- ❒ 3. Laterally Flexes the Trunk at the Spinal Joints
- ❒ 4. Contralaterally Rotates the Trunk at the Spinal Joints

INNERVATION
- ❒ Spinal Nerves
- ❒ dorsal rami

Subcostales

ATTACHMENTS
- ❑ Ribs #10-12
  - ❒ the internal surface of the ribs, near the angle

to the
- ❑ Ribs #8-10
  - ❒ the internal surface of the ribs, near the angle

ACTION
- ❒ **Depresses Ribs #8-10 at the Sternocostal and Costospinal Joints**

INNERVATION
- ❒ Intercostal Nerves
- ❒ #8-11

ANTERIOR TRUNK

Pectoralis Major

ATTACHMENTS
- ❑ Medial Clavicle, Sternum, and the Costal Cartilages of Ribs #1-7
  - ❒ the medial ½ of the clavicle, and the aponeurosis of the external abdominal oblique

to the
- ❑ Lateral Lip of the Bicipital Groove of the Humerus

ACTIONS
- ❒ 1. **Adducts the Arm at the Shoulder Joint**
- ❒ 2. **Medially Rotates the Arm at the Shoulder Joint**
- ❒ 3. **Flexes the Arm at the Shoulder Joint (clavicu-**

lar head)

- ❐ 4. Extends the Arm at the Shoulder Joint (sternocostal head)
- ❐ 5. Abducts the Arm at the Shoulder Joint (clavicular head, above 90 degrees)
- ❐ 6. Depresses the Scapula at the Scapulocostal Joint
- ❐ 7. Protracts (Abducts) the Scapula at the Scapulocostal Joint
- ❐ 8. Elevates the Trunk at the Scapulocostal Joint
- ❐ 9. Laterally Deviates the Trunk at the Scapulocostal Joint
- ❐ 10. Ipsilaterally Rotates the Trunk at the Scapulocostal Joint

INNERVATION

- ❐ The Medial and Lateral Pectoral Nerves
- ❐ C5, 6, 7, 8, T1

Pectoralis Minor

ATTACHMENTS

- ❐ Ribs #3-5

to the

- ❐ Coracoid Process of the Scapula
  - ❐ the medial aspect

ACTIONS

- ❐ 1. **Protracts (Abducts) the Scapula at the Scapulocostal Joint**
- ❐ 2. **Depresses the Scapula at the Scapulocostal Joint**
- ❐ 3. **Elevates Ribs #3-5 at the Sternocostal and Costospinal Joints**
- ❐ 4. Downwardly Rotates the Scapula at the Scapulocostal Joint

INNERVATION

- ❐ The Medial and Lateral Pectoral Nerves
- ❐ C5, 6, 7, 8, T1

Subclavius

ATTACHMENTS

- ❐ 1st Rib
  - ❐ at the junction with its costal cartilage

to the

- ❐ Clavicle
  - ❐ the middle ⅓ of the inferior surface

ACTIONS

- ❐ 1. **Depresses the Clavicle at the Sternoclavicular Joint**
- ❐ 2. **Elevates the 1st Rib at the Sternocostal and Costospinal Joints**
- ❐ 3. Protracts the Clavicle at the Sternoclavicular Joint
- ❐ 4. Downwardly Rotates the Clavicle at the Sternoclavicular Joint

INNERVATION

- ❐ A Nerve from the Brachial Plexus
- ❐ C5, 6

External Intercostals

ATTACHMENTS

- ❐ In the Intercostal Spaces of Ribs #1-12
  - ❐ Each external intercostal attaches from the inferior border of one rib to the superior border of the rib directly inferior.

ACTIONS

- ❐ 1. **Elevates Ribs #2-12 at the Sternocostal and Costospinal Joints**
- ❐ 2. Depresses Ribs #1-11 at the Sternocostal and Costospinal Joints

INNERVATION

- ❐ Intercostal Nerves

Internal Intercostals

ATTACHMENTS

- ❐ In the Intercostal Spaces of Ribs #1-12
  - ❐ Each internal intercostal attaches from the superior border of one rib and its costal cartilage to the inferior border of the rib and its costal cartilage that is directly superior.

ACTIONS

- ❐ 1. **Depresses Ribs #1-11 at the Sternocostal and Costospinal Joints**
- ❐ 2. Elevates Ribs #2-12 at the Sternocostal and Costospinal Joints

INNERVATION

- ❐ Intercostal Nerves

Transversus Thoracis

ATTACHMENTS

- ❐ Internal Surfaces of the Sternum, Xiphoid Process, and the Adjacent Costal Cartilages
  - ❐ the inferior ⅓ of the sternum, and the costal cartilages of ribs #4-7

to the

- ❐ Internal Surface of Costal Cartilages #2-6

ACTION

- ❐ **Depresses Ribs #2-6 at the Sternocostal and Costospinal Joints**

INNVERVATION

- ❐ Intercostal Nerves

Muscles of the Anterior Abdominal Wall

Rectus Abdominis (of the Anterior Abdominal Wall)

ATTACHMENTS

- ❐ Pubis
  - ❐ the crest and symphysis of the pubis

to the

- ❐ Xiphoid Process and the Cartilage of Ribs #5-7

ACTIONS

- ❐ 1. **Flexes the Trunk at the Spinal Joints**
- ❐ 2. **Posteriorly Tilts the Pelvis at the Lumbosacral Joint**
- ❐ 3. Laterally Flexes the Trunk at the Spinal Joints
- ❐ 4. Compresses the Abdominal Contents

INNERVATION

- ❐ Intercostal Nerves
- ❐ ventral rami of T5-12

External Abdominal Oblique (of the Anterior Abdominal Wall)

ATTACHMENTS

- Anterior Iliac Crest, Pubic Bone, and the Abdominal Aponeurosis
  - the pubic crest and tubercle

to the

- Lower 8 Ribs (Ribs #5-12)
  - the inferior border of the ribs

ACTIONS

- 1. **Flexes the Trunk at the Spinal Joints**
- 2. **Laterally Flexes the Trunk at the Spinal Joints**
- 3. **Contralaterally Rotates the Trunk at the Spinal Joints**
- 4. **Posteriorly Tilts the Pelvis at the Lumbosacral Joint**
- 5. Elevates the Pelvis at the Lumbosacral Joint
- 6. Ipsilaterally Rotates the Pelvis at the Lumbosacral Joint
- 7. Compresses the Abdominal Contents

INNERVATION

- Intercostal Nerves
- ventral rami of T7-12

Internal Abdominal Oblique (of the Anterior Abdominal Wall)

ATTACHMENTS

- Inguinal Ligament, Iliac Crest, and the Thoracolumbar Fascia
  - the lateral ⅔ of the inguinal ligament

to the

- Lower Three Ribs (#10-12) and the Abdominal Aponeurosis

ACTIONS

- 1. **Flexes the Trunk at the Spinal Joints**
- 2. **Laterally Flexes the Trunk at the Spinal Joints**
- 3. **Ipsilaterally Rotates the Trunk at the Spinal Joints**
- 4. **Posteriorly Tilts the Pelvis at the Lumbosacral Joint**
- 5. Elevates the Pelvis at the Lumbosacral Joint
- 6. Contralaterally Rotates the Pelvis at the Lumbosacral Joint
- 7. Compresses the Abdominal Contents

INNERVATION

- Intercostal Nerves
- ventral rami of T7-L1

Transversus Abdominis (of the Anterior Abdominal Wall)

ATTACHMENTS

- Inguinal Ligament, Iliac Crest, Thoracolumbar Fascia, and the Lower Costal Cartilages
  - the lateral ⅓ of the inguinal ligament; the lower six costal cartilages (of ribs #7-12)

to the

- Abdominal Aponeurosis

ACTION

- Compresses the Abdominal Contents

INNERVATION

- Intercostal Nerves
- ventral rami of T7-L1

Diaphragm

ATTACHMENTS

- ENTIRE MUSCLE: Internal Surfaces of the Ribcage and Sternum, and the Spine
  - STERNAL PART: Internal Surface of the Xiphoid Process of the Sternum
  - COSTAL PART: Internal Surface of the Lower Six Ribs (Ribs #7-12) and their Costal Cartilages
  - LUMBAR PART: L1-L3
- The lumbar attachments consist of two aponeuroses, called the medial and lateral arcuate ligaments, and two tendons, called the right and left crura.

to the

- Central Tendon of the Diaphragm

ACTION

- Increases the Volume of the Thoracic Cavity (Inspiration)

INNERVATION

- The Phrenic Nerve
- C3-5

MUSCLES OF THE LOWER EXTREMITY

MUSCLES OF THE PELVIS

ANTERIOR PELVIS

Psoas Major (of the Iliopsoas)

ATTACHMENTS

- Anterolateral Lumbar Spine
  - anterolaterally on the bodies of T12-L5 and the intervertebral discs between, and anteriorly on the TPs of L1-L5

to the

- Lesser Trochanter of the Femur

ACTIONS

- 1. **Flexes the Thigh at the Hip Joint**
- 2. **Laterally Rotates the Thigh at the Hip Joint**
- 3. **Flexes the Trunk at the Spinal Joints**
- 4. **Laterally Flexes the Trunk at the Spinal Joints**
- 5. **Anteriorly Tilts the Pelvis at the Hip Joint**
- 6. Contralaterally Rotates the Trunk at the Spinal Joints
- 7. Contralaterally Rotates the Pelvis at the Hip Joint

INNERVATION

- Lumbar Plexus
- L1, 2, 3

Iliacus (of the Iliopsoas)

ATTACHMENTS

❑ Internal Ilium
  ❐ the upper ⅔ of the iliac fossa, and the anterior inferior iliac spine (AIIS) and the sacral ala

to the

❑ Lesser Trochanter of the Femur

ACTIONS

❐ 1. **Flexes the Thigh at the Hip Joint**
❐ 2. **Laterally Rotates the Thigh at the Hip Joint**
❐ 3. **Anteriorly Tilts the Pelvis at the Hip Joint**
❐ 4. Contralaterally Rotates the Pelvis at the Hip Joint

INNERVATION

❐ The Femoral Nerve
❐ L2, 3

Psoas Minor

ATTACHMENTS

❑ Anterolateral Bodies of T12 and L1
  ❐ the anterolateral bodies of T12-L1 and the disc between

to the

❑ Pubis
  ❐ the pectineal line of the pubis and the iliopectineal eminence (of the ilium and the pubis)

ACTIONS

❐ 1. **Flexes the Trunk at the Spinal Joints**
❐ 2. **Posteriorly Tilts the Pelvis at the Lumbosacral Joint**

INNERVATION

❐ L1 Spinal Nerve
❐ a branch from L1

POSTERIOR PELVIS (BUTTOCKS)

Gluteus Maximus

ATTACHMENTS

❑ Posterior Iliac Crest, the Posterolateral Sacrum, and the Coccyx
  ❐ and the sacrotuberous ligament, the thoracolumbar fascia, and the fascia over the gluteus medius

to the

❑ Iliotibial Band (ITB) and the Gluteal Tuberosity of the Femur

ACTIONS

❐ 1. **Extends the Thigh at the Hip Joint**
❐ 2. **Laterally Rotates the Thigh at the Hip Joint**
❐ 3. **Abducts the Thigh at the Hip Joint (upper ⅓)**
❐ 4. **Adducts the Thigh at the Hip Joint (lower ⅔)**
❐ 5. **Posteriorly Tilts the Pelvis at the Hip Joint**
❐ 6. Contralaterally Rotates the Pelvis at the Hip Joint
❐ 7. Extends the Leg at the Knee Joint

INNERVATION

❐ The Inferior Gluteal Nerve
❐ L5, S1, 2

Gluteus Medius

ATTACHMENTS

❑ External Ilium
  ❐ inferior to the iliac crest and between the anterior and posterior gluteal lines

to the

❑ Greater Trochanter of the Femur
  ❐ the lateral surface

ACTIONS

❐ 1. **Abducts the Thigh at the Hip Joint (entire muscle)**
❐ 2. **Flexes the Thigh at the Hip Joint (anterior fibers)**
❐ 3. **Medially Rotates the Thigh at the Hip Joint (anterior fibers)**
❐ 4. **Extends the Thigh at the Hip Joint (posterior fibers)**
❐ 5. **Laterally Rotates the Thigh at the Hip Joint (posterior fibers)**
❐ 6. **Posteriorly Tilts the Pelvis at the Hip Joint (posterior fibers)**
❐ 7. **Anteriorly Tilts the Pelvis at the Hip Joint (anterior fibers)**
❐ 8. Depresses (Laterally Tilts) the Pelvis at the Hip Joint (entire muscle)
❐ 9. Ipsilaterally Rotates the Pelvis at the Hip Joint (anterior fibers)
❐ 10. Contralaterally Rotates the Pelvis at the Hip Joint (posterior fibers)

INNERVATION

❐ The Superior Gluteal Nerve
❐ L4, 5, S1

Gluteus Minimus

ATTACHMENTS

❑ External Ilium
  ❐ between the anterior and inferior gluteal lines

to the

❑ Greater Trochanter of the Femur
  ❐ the anterior surface

ACTIONS

❐ 1. **Abducts the Thigh at the Hip Joint (entire muscle)**
❐ 2. **Flexes the Thigh at the Hip Joint (anterior fibers)**
❐ 3. **Medially Rotates the Thigh at the Hip Joint (anterior fibers)**
❐ 4. **Extends the Thigh at the Hip Joint (posterior fibers)**
❐ 5. **Laterally Rotates the Thigh at the Hip Joint (posterior fibers)**
❐ 6. **Posteriorly Tilts the Pelvis at the Hip Joint (posterior fibers)**
❐ 7. **Anteriorly Tilts the Pelvis at the Hip Joint (anterior fibers)**
❐ 8. Depresses (Laterally Tilts) the Pelvis at the Hip Joint (entire muscle)

- 9. Ipsilaterally Rotates the Pelvis at the Hip Joint (anterior fibers)
- 10. Contralaterally Rotates the Pelvis at the Hip Joint (posterior fibers)

INNERVATION
- The Superior Gluteal Nerve
- **L4, 5,** S1

Deep Lateral Rotators of the Thigh

Piriformis (of the Deep Lateral Rotators of the Thigh)

ATTACHMENTS
- Anterior Sacrum
  - and the anterior surface of the sacrotuberous ligament

to the
- Greater Trochanter of the Femur
  - the superomedial surface

ACTIONS
- 1. **Laterally Rotates the Thigh at the Hip Joint**
- 2. Abducts the Thigh at the Hip Joint (if the thigh is flexed)
- 3. Medially Rotates the Thigh at the Hip Joint (if the thigh is flexed)
- 4. Contralaterally Rotates the Pelvis at the Hip Joint

INNERVATION
- Nerve to Piriformis (of the Lumbosacral Plexus)
- L5, S1, 2

Superior Gemellus (of the Deep Lateral Rotators of the Thigh)

ATTACHMENTS
- Ischial Spine

to the
- Greater Trochanter of the Femur
  - the medial surface

ACTIONS
- 1. **Laterally Rotates the Thigh at the Hip Joint**
- 2. Abducts the Thigh at the Hip Joint (if the thigh is flexed)
- 3. Contralaterally Rotates the Pelvis at the Hip Joint

INNERVATION
- Nerve to Obturator Internus (of the Lumbosacral Plexus)
- L5, S1

Obturator Internus (of the Deep Lateral Rotators of the Thigh)

ATTACHMENTS
- Internal Surface of the Pelvic Bone Surrounding the Obturator Foramen
  - the internal surfaces of: the margin of the obturator foramen, the obturator membrane, the ischium, the pubis, and the ilium

to the
- Greater Trochanter of the Femur
  - the medial surface

ACTIONS
- 1. **Laterally Rotates the Thigh at the Hip Joint**
- 2. Abducts the Thigh at the Hip Joint (if the thigh is flexed)
- 3. Contralaterally Rotates the Pelvis at the Hip Joint

INNERVATION
- Nerve to Obturator Internus (of the Lumbosacral Plexus)
- L5, S1

Inferior Gemellus (of the Deep Lateral Rotators of the Thigh)

ATTACHMENTS
- Ischial Tuberosity
  - the superior aspect

to the
- Greater Trochanter of the Femur
  - the medial surface

ACTIONS
- 1. **Laterally Rotates the Thigh at the Hip Joint**
- 2. Abducts the Thigh at the Hip Joint (if the thigh is flexed)
- 3. Contralaterally Rotates the Pelvis at the Hip Joint

INNERVATION
- Nerve to Quadratus Femoris (of the Lumbosacral Plexus)
- L5, S1

Obturator Externus (of the Deep Lateral Rotators of the Thigh)

ATTACHMENTS
- External Surface of the Pelvic Bone Surrounding the Obturator Foramen
  - the external surfaces of: the margin of the obturator foramen on the ischium and the pubis, and the obturator membrane

to the
- Trochanteric Fossa of the Femur

ACTIONS
- 1. **Laterally Rotates the Thigh at the Hip Joint**
- 2. Contralaterally Rotates the Pelvis at the Hip Joint

INNERVATION
- The Obturator Nerve
- L3, **4**

Quadratus Femoris (of the Deep Lateral Rotators of the Thigh)

ATTACHMENTS
- Ischial Tuberosity
  - the lateral border

to the
- Intertrochanteric Crest of the Femur
  - and inferior to the intertrochanteric crest of the femur

ACTIONS
- 1. **Laterally Rotates the Thigh at the Hip Joint**
- 2. Adducts the Thigh at the Hip Joint
- 3. Contralaterally Rotates the Pelvis at the Hip Joint

INNERVATION
- Nerve to Quadratus Femoris (of the Lumbosacral Plexus)
- L5, S1

MUSCLES OF THE THIGH

ANTERIOR THIGH

Tensor Fasciae Latae (TFL)

ATTACHMENTS
- Anterior Superior Iliac Spine (ASIS)
  - and the anterior iliac crest

to the
- Iliotibial Band (ITB)
  - ⅓ of the way down the thigh

ACTIONS
- 1. **Flexes the Thigh at the Hip Joint**
- 2. **Abducts the Thigh at the Hip Joint**
- 3. **Medially Rotates the Thigh at the Hip Joint**
- 4. **Anteriorly Tilts the Pelvis at the Hip Joint**
- 5. Depresses (Laterally Tilts) the Pelvis at the Hip Joint
- 6. Ipsilaterally Rotates the Pelvis at the Hip Joint
- 7. Extends the Leg at the Knee Joint

INNERVATION
- The Superior Gluteal Nerve
- **L4, 5,** S1

Sartorius

ATTACHMENTS
- Anterior Superior Iliac Spine (ASIS)

to the
- Pes Anserine Tendon (at the Proximal Anteromedial Tibia)

ACTIONS
- 1. **Flexes the Thigh at the Hip Joint**
- 2. **Abducts the Thigh at the Hip Joint**
- 3. **Laterally Rotates the Thigh at the Hip Joint**
- 4. **Flexes the Leg at the Knee Joint**
- 5. **Anteriorly Tilts the Pelvis at the Hip Joint**
- 6. Medially Rotates the Leg at the Knee Joint
- 7. Depresses (Laterally Tilts) the Pelvis at the Hip Joint
- 8. Contralaterally Rotates the Pelvis at the Hip Joint

INNERVATION
- The Femoral Nerve
- L2, 3

Quadriceps Femoris Group ("Quads")

Rectus Femoris (of Quadriceps Femoris Group)

ATTACHMENTS
- Anterior Inferior Iliac Spine (AIIS)
  - and just superior to the brim of the acetabulum

to the
- Tibial Tuberosity
  - via the patella and the patellar ligament

ACTIONS
- 1. **Extends the Leg at the Knee Joint**
- 2. **Flexes the Thigh at the Hip Joint**
- 3. **Anteriorly Tilts the Pelvis at the Hip Joint**

INNERVATION
- The Femoral Nerve
- L2, **3, 4**

Vastus Lateralis (of Quadriceps Femoris Group)

ATTACHMENTS
- Linea Aspera of the Femur
  - the lateral lip of the linea aspera of the femur, and the anterior intertrochanteric line and gluteal tuberosity of the femur

to the
- Tibial Tuberosity
  - via the patella and the patellar ligament

ACTION
- **Extends the Leg at the Knee Joint**

INNERVATION
- The Femoral Nerve
- L2, **3, 4**

Vastus Medialis (of Quadriceps Femoris Group)

ATTACHMENTS
- Linea Aspera of the Femur
  - the medial lip of the linea aspera, and the intertrochanteric line and the medial supracondylar line of the femur

to the
- Tibial Tuberosity
  - via the patella and the patellar ligament

ACTION
- **Extends the Leg at the Knee Joint**

INNERVATION
- The Femoral Nerve
- L2, **3, 4**

Vastus Intermedius (of Quadriceps Femoris Group)

ATTACHMENTS
- Anterior Shaft and Linea Aspera of the Femur
  - the anterior and lateral surfaces of the femur and the lateral lip of the linea aspera

to the
- Tibial Tuberosity
  - via the patella and the patellar ligament

ACTION
- **Extends the Leg at the Knee Joint**

INNERVATION
- The Femoral Nerve
- L2, **3, 4**

Articularis Genus

ATTACHMENTS

- Anterior Distal Femoral Shaft

to the

- Joint Capsule of the Knee Joint

ACTION

- **Tenses and Pulls the Joint Capsule of the Knee Joint Proximally**

INNERVATION

- The Femoral Nerve
- L2, **3, 4**

MEDIAL THIGH

Pectineus (of Adductor Group)

ATTACHMENTS

- Pubis
  - the pectineal line on the superior pubic ramus

to the

- Proximal Posterior Shaft of the Femur
  - the pectineal line of the femur

ACTIONS

- 1. **Adducts the Thigh at the Hip Joint**
- 2. **Flexes the Thigh at the Hip Joint**
- 3. **Anteriorly Tilts the Pelvis at the Hip Joint**
- 4. Elevates the Pelvis at the Hip Joint

INNERVATION

- The Femoral Nerve
- **L2**, 3

Adductor Longus (of Adductor Group)

ATTACHMENTS

- Pubis
  - the anterior body

to the

- Linea Aspera of the Femur
  - the middle ⅓ at the medial lip

ACTIONS

- 1. **Adducts the Thigh at the Hip Joint**
- 2. **Flexes the Thigh at the Hip Joint**
- 3. **Anteriorly Tilts the Pelvis at the Hip Joint**
- 4. Elevates the Pelvis at the Hip Joint

INNERVATION

- The Obturator Nerve
- **L2, 3,** 4

Gracilis (of Adductor Group)

ATTACHMENTS

- Pubis
  - the anterior body and the inferior ramus

to the

- Pes Anserine Tendon (at the Proximal Anteromedial Tibia)

ACTIONS

- 1. **Adducts the Thigh at the Hip Joint**
- 2. **Flexes the Thigh at the Hip Joint**
- 3. **Flexes the Leg at the Knee Joint**
- 4. **Anteriorly Tilts the Pelvis at the Hip Joint**
- 5. Medially Rotates the Leg at the Knee Joint
- 6. Elevates the Pelvis at the Hip Joint

INNERVATION

- The Obturator Nerve
- L2, 3

Adductor Brevis (of Adductor Group)

ATTACHMENTS

- Pubis
  - the inferior ramus

to the

- Linea Aspera of the Femur
  - the proximal ⅓

ACTIONS

- 1. **Adducts the Thigh at the Hip Joint**
- 2. **Flexes the Thigh at the Hip Joint**
- 3. **Anteriorly Tilts the Pelvis at the Hip Joint**
- 4. Elevates the Pelvis at the Hip Joint

INNERVATION

- The Obturator Nerve
- L2, 3

Adductor Magnus (of Adductor Group)

ATTACHMENTS

- Pubis and Ischium
- ANTERIOR HEAD: inferior pubic ramus and the ramus of the ischium
- POSTERIOR HEAD: ischial tuberosity

to the

- Linea Aspera of the Femur
  - and the gluteal tuberosity, medial supracondylar line, and adductor tubercle of the femur

ACTIONS

- 1. **Adducts the Thigh at the Hip Joint**
- 2. **Extends the Thigh at the Hip Joint**
- 3. **Posteriorly Tilts the Pelvis at the Hip Joint**
- 4. Elevates the Pelvis at the Hip Joint

INNERVATION

- The Obturator Nerve and the Sciatic Nerve
- the obturator nerve innervates the anterior head
- the tibial branch of the sciatic nerve innervates the posterior head
- L2, 3, 4

POSTERIOR THIGH

Hamstring Group

Biceps Femoris (of Hamstring Group)

ATTACHMENTS

- LONG HEAD: Ischial Tuberosity
  - and the sacrotuberous ligament
  - SHORT HEAD: Linea Aspera
  - and the lateral supracondylar line of the femur

to the

- Head of the Fibula
  - and the lateral tibial condyle

ACTIONS
- ❒ 1. **Flexes the Leg at the Knee Joint (entire muscle)**
- ❒ 2. **Extends the Thigh at the Hip Joint (long head)**
- ❒ 3. **Posteriorly Tilts the Pelvis at the Hip Joint (long head)**
- ❒ 4. Laterally Rotates the Leg at the Knee Joint (entire muscle)
- ❒ 5. Adducts the Thigh at the Hip Joint (long head)
- ❒ 6. Laterally Rotates the Thigh at the Hip Joint (long head)

INNERVATION
- ❒ The Sciatic Nerve
- ❒ the tibial nerve and the common fibular nerve; L5, **S1**, 2

Semitendinosus (of Hamstring Group)

ATTACHMENTS
- ❑ Ischial Tuberosity

to the
- ❑ Pes Anserine Tendon (at the Proximal Anteromedial Tibia)

ACTIONS
- ❒ 1. **Flexes the Leg at the Knee Joint**
- ❒ 2. **Extends the Thigh at the Hip Joint**
- ❒ 3. **Posteriorly Tilts the Pelvis at the Hip Joint**
- ❒ 4. Medially Rotates the Leg at the Knee Joint
- ❒ 5. Medially Rotates the Thigh at the Hip Joint

INNERVATION
- ❒ The Sciatic Nerve
- ❒ the tibial nerve; L5, **S1**, 2

Semimembranosus (of Hamstring Group)

ATTACHMENTS
- ❑ Ischial Tuberosity

to the
- ❑ Medial Condyle of the Tibia
  - ❒ the posterior surface

ACTIONS
- ❒ 1. **Flexes the Leg at the Knee Joint**
- ❒ 2. **Extends the Thigh at the Hip Joint**
- ❒ 3. **Posteriorly Tilts the Pelvis at the Hip Joint**
- ❒ 4. Medially Rotates the Leg at the Knee Joint
- ❒ 5. Medially Rotates the Thigh at the Hip Joint

INNERVATION
- ❒ The Sciatic Nerve
- ❒ the tibial nerve; L5, **S1**, 2

MUSCLES OF THE LEG

ANTERIOR COMPARTMENT

Tibialis Anterior

ATTACHMENTS
- ❑ Proximal Anterior Tibia
  - ❒ the lateral tibial condyle, the proximal ⅔ of the anterior tibia, and the proximal ⅔ of the interosseus membrane

to the
- ❑ Medial Foot
  - ❒ the 1st cuneiform and 1st metatarsal

ACTIONS
- ❒ 1. **Dorsiflexes the Foot at the Ankle Joint**
- ❒ 2. **Inverts the Foot at the Tarsal Joints**

INNERVATION
- ❒ The Deep Fibular Nerve
- ❒ **L4**, 5

Extensor Digitorum Longus

ATTACHMENTS
- ❑ Proximal Anterior Fibula
  - ❒ the proximal ⅔ of the fibula, the proximal ⅓ of the interosseus membrane, and the lateral tibial condyle

to the
- ❑ Dorsal Surface of Toes #2-5
  - ❒ via its dorsal digital expansion onto the dorsal surface of the middle and distal phalanges

ACTIONS
- ❒ 1. **Extends Toes #2-5 at the Metatarsophalangeal (MTP) Joint and the Interphalangeal (IP) Joints**
- ❒ 2. **Dorsiflexes the Foot at the Ankle Joint**
- ❒ 3. **Everts the Foot at the Tarsal Joints**

INNERVATION
- ❒ The Deep Fibular Nerve
- ❒ L5, S1

Extensor Hallucis Longus

ATTACHMENTS
- ❑ Middle Anterior Fibula
  - ❒ the middle ⅓ of the anterior fibula and the middle ⅓ of the interosseus membrane

to the
- ❑ Dorsal Surface of the Big Toe (Toe #1)
  - ❒ the distal phalanx

ACTIONS
- ❒ 1. **Extends the Big Toe (Toe #1) at the Metatarsophalangeal Joint and the Interphalangeal (IP) Joint**
- ❒ 2. **Dorsiflexes the Foot at the Ankle Joint**
- ❒ 3. Inverts the Foot at the Tarsal Joints

INNERVATION
- ❒ The Deep Fibular Nerve
- ❒ **L5**, S1

Fibularis Tertius

ATTACHMENTS
- ❑ Distal Anterior Fibula
  - ❒ the distal ⅓ of the anterior fibula and the distal ⅓ of the interosseus membrane

to the
- ❑ 5th Metatarsal
  - ❒ the dorsal surface of the base of the 5th metatarsal

ACTIONS
- ❒ 1. **Dorsiflexes the Foot at the Ankle Joint**
- ❒ 2. **Everts the Foot at the Tarsal Joints**

INNERVATION
- The Deep Fibular Nerve
- L5, S1

LATERAL COMPARTMENT

Fibularis Longus

ATTACHMENTS
- Proximal Lateral Fibula
  - the head of the fibula and the proximal ½ of the lateral fibula

to the
- Medial Foot
  - the 1st cuneiform and 1st metatarsal

ACTIONS
- 1. **Everts the Foot at the Tarsal Joints**
- 2. **Plantarflexes the Foot at the Ankle Joint**

INNERVATION
- The Superficial Fibular Nerve
- L5, S1

Fibularis Brevis

ATTACHMENTS
- Distal Lateral Fibula
  - the distal ½ of the lateral fibula

to the
- Lateral Foot
  - the lateral side of the base of the 5th metatarsal

ACTIONS
- 1. **Everts the Foot at the Tarsal Joints**
- 2. **Plantarflexes the Foot at the Ankle Joint**

INNERVATION
- The Superficial Fibular Nerve
- L5, S1

SUPERFICIAL POSTERIOR COMPARTMENT

Gastrocnemius ("Gastrocs") (of the Triceps Surae)

ATTACHMENTS
- Medial and Lateral Femoral Condyles
  - and the distal posteromedial femur and the distal posterolateral femur

to the
- Calcaneus via the Calcaneal Tendon
  - the posterior surface

ACTIONS
- 1. **Plantarflexes the Foot at the Ankle Joint**
- 2. **Flexes the Leg at the Knee Joint**
- 3. Inverts the Foot at the Tarsal Joints

INNERVATION
- The Tibial Nerve
- S1, 2

Soleus (of the Triceps Surae)

ATTACHMENTS
- Posterior Tibia and Fibula
  - the soleal line of the tibia and the head and proximal ⅓ of the fibula

to the
- Calcaneus via the Calcaneal Tendon
  - the posterior surface

ACTIONS
- 1. **Plantarflexes the Foot at the Ankle Joint**
- 2. Inverts the Foot at the Tarsal Joints

INNERVATION
- The Tibial Nerve
- S1, 2

Plantaris

ATTACHMENTS
- Distal Posterolateral Femur
  - the lateral condyle and the distal lateral supracondylar line of the femur

to the
- Calcaneus
  - the posterior surface

ACTIONS
- 1. **Plantarflexes the Foot at the Ankle Joint**
- 2. **Flexes the Leg at the Knee Joint**

INNERVATION
- The Tibial Nerve
- S1, 2

DEEP POSTERIOR COMPARTMENT

Popliteus

ATTACHMENTS
- Distal Posterolateral Femur
  - the lateral surface of the lateral condyle of the femur

to the
- Proximal Posterior Tibia
  - the medial side

ACTIONS
- 1. **Medially Rotates the Leg at the Knee Joint**
- 2. **Flexes the Leg at the Knee Joint**
- 3. Laterally Rotates the Thigh at the Knee Joint

INNERVATION
- The Tibial Nerve
- L4, 5, S1

Tibialis Posterior ("Tom" of "Tom, Dick, and Harry" Muscles)

ATTACHMENTS
- Proximal Posterior Tibia and Fibula
  - the proximal ⅔ of: the posterior tibia, fibula, and interosseus membrane

to the
- Plantar Surface of the Foot

❒ metatarsals #2-4 and all the tarsal bones except the talus

ACTIONS

❒ 1. **Plantarflexes the Foot at the Ankle Joint**

❒ 2. **Inverts the Foot at the Tarsal Joints**

INNERVATION

❒ The Tibial Nerve

❒ L4, 5

Flexor Digitorum Longus ("Dick" of "Tom, Dick, and Harry" Muscles)

ATTACHMENTS

❑ Middle Posterior Tibia

❒ the middle ⅓ of the posterior tibia

to the

❑ Plantar Surface of Toes #2-5

❒ the distal phalanges

ACTIONS

❒ 1. **Flexes Toes #2-5 at the Metatarsophalangeal Joint and the Interphalangeal Joints**

❒ 2. **Plantarflexes the Foot at the Ankle Joint**

❒ 3. **Inverts the Foot at the Tarsal Joints**

INNERVATION

❒ The Tibial Nerve

❒ L5, S1, 2

Flexor Hallucis Longus ("Harry" of "Tom, Dick, and Harry" Muscles)

ATTACHMENTS

❑ Distal Posterior Fibula

❒ the distal ⅔ of the posterior fibula and the distal ⅔ of the interosseus membrane

to the

❑ Plantar Surface of the Big Toe (Toe #1)

❒ the distal phalanx

ACTIONS

❒ 1. **Flexes the Big Toe (Toe #1) at the Metatarsophalangeal Joint and the Interphalangeal Joint**

❒ 2. **Plantarflexes the Foot at the Ankle Joint**

❒ 3. **Inverts the Foot at the Tarsal Joints**

INNERVATION

❒ The Tibial Nerve

❒ L5, **S1, 2**

INTRINSIC MUSCLES OF THE FOOT

DORSAL SURFACE

Extensor Digitorum Brevis

ATTACHMENTS

❑ Dorsal Surface of the Calcaneus

to the

❑ Toes #2-4

❒ the lateral side of the distal tendons of the extensor digitorum longus muscle of toes #2-4 (via the dorsal digital expansion into the middle and distal phalanges)

ACTION

❒ **Extends Toes #2-4 at the Metatarsophalangeal and Proximal and Distal Interphalangeal Joints**

INNERVATION

❒ **The Deep Fibular Nerve**

❒ L5, S1

Extensor Hallucis Brevis

ATTACHMENTS

❑ Dorsal Surface of the Calcaneus

to the

❑ Dorsal Surface of the Big Toe (Toe #1)

❒ the base of the proximal phalanx of the big toe

ACTION

❒ **Extends the Big Toe (Toe #1) at the Metatarsophalangeal Joint**

INNERVATION

❒ **The Deep Fibular Nerve**

❒ L5, S1

PLANTAR SURFACE—LAYER I

Abductor Hallucis

ATTACHMENTS

❑ Tuberosity of the Calcaneus

❒ and the flexor retinaculum and plantar fascia

to the

❑ Big Toe (Toe #1)

❒ the medial plantar side of the base of the proximal phalanx

ACTIONS

❒ 1. **Abducts the Big Toe (Toe #1) at the Metatarsophalangeal Joint**

❒ 2. Flexes the Big Toe (Toe #1) at the Metatarsophalangeal Joint

INNERVATION

❒ The Medial Plantar Nerve

❒ S1, 2

Abductor Digiti Minimi Pedis

ATTACHMENTS

❑ Tuberosity of the Calcaneus

❒ and the plantar fascia

to the

❑ Little Toe (Toe #5)

❒ the lateral plantar side of the base of the proximal phalanx

ACTIONS

❒ 1. **Abducts the Little Toe (Toe #5) at the Metatarsophalangeal Joint**

❒ 2. Flexes the Little Toe (Toe #5) at the Metatarsophalangeal Joint

INNERVATION
- The Lateral Plantar Nerve
- S2, 3

Flexor Digitorum Brevis

ATTACHMENTS
- Tuberosity of the Calcaneus
  - and the plantar fascia

to the
- Toes #2-5
  - the medial and lateral sides of the middle phalanges

ACTION
- **Flexes Toes #2-5 at the Metatarsophalangeal and Proximal Interphalangeal Joints**

INNERVATION
- The Medial Plantar Nerve
- S1, 2

PLANTAR SURFACE—LAYER II

Quadratus Plantae

ATTACHMENTS
- The Calcaneus
  - the medial and lateral sides

to the
- Distal Tendon of the Flexor Digitorum Longus Muscle
  - the lateral margin

ACTION
- **Flexes Toes #2-5 at the Metatarsophalangeal and the Proximal and Distal Interphalangeal Joints**

INNERVATION
- The Lateral Plantar Nerve
- S2, 3

Lumbricals Pedis

- (There are four lumbrical pedis muscles, named #1, #2, #3, and #4.)

ATTACHMENTS
- The Distal Tendons of the Flexor Digitorum Longus
- **#1:** medial border of the tendon to toe #2
- **#2:** adjacent sides of the tendons to toes #2 and #3
- **#3:** adjacent sides of the tendons to toes #3 and #4
- **#4:** adjacent sides of the tendons to toes #4 and #5

to the
- Distal Tendons of the Extensor Digitorum Longus
  - the medial side of the tendons merging into the dorsal digital expansion of toes #2-5

ACTIONS
- 1. **Extends Toes #2-5 at the Proximal and Distal Interphalangeal Joints**
- 2. **Flexes Toes #2-5 at the Metatarsophalangeal Joint**

INNERVATION
- The Medial and Lateral Plantar Nerves
- S1, 2, 3
- medial plantar nerve to lumbrical pedis #1
- lateral plantar nerve to lumbricals pedis #2-4

PLANTAR SURFACE—LAYER III

Flexor Hallucis Brevis

ATTACHMENTS
- Cuboid and the 3rd Cuneiform

to the
- Big Toe (Toe #1)
  - the medial and lateral sides of the plantar surface of the base of the proximal phalanx

ACTION
- **Flexes the Big Toe (Toe #1) at the Metatarsophalangeal Joint**

INNERVATION
- The Medial Plantar Nerve
- S1, 2

Flexor Digiti Minimi Pedis

ATTACHMENTS
- 5th Metatarsal
  - the plantar surface of the base of the 5th metatarsal and the distal tendon of the fibularis longus

to the
- Little Toe (Toe #5)
  - the plantar surface of the proximal phalanx

ACTION
- **Flexes the Little Toe (Toe #5) at the Metatarsophalangeal Joint**

INNERVATION
- The Lateral Plantar Nerve
- S2, 3

Adductor Hallucis

ATTACHMENTS
- Metatarsals
- OBLIQUE HEAD: from the base of metatarsals #2-4 and the distal tendon of the fibularis longus
- TRANSVERSE HEAD: arises from the plantar metatarsophalangeal ligaments #3, 4, and 5

to the
- Big Toe (Toe #1)
  - the lateral side of the base of the proximal phalanx

ACTIONS
- 1. **Adducts the Big Toe (Toe #1) at the Metatarsophalangeal Joint**
- 2. Flexes the Big Toe (Toe #1) at the Metatarsophalangeal Joint

INNERVATION
- The Lateral Plantar Nerve
- S2, 3

PLANTAR SURFACE—LAYER IV

Plantar Interossei

ATTACHMENTS
- Metatarsals

- ❒ the medial side ("2nd Toe Side") of metatarsals #3-5:
  - ❒ **#1:** attaches onto metatarsal #3
  - ❒ **#2:** attaches onto metatarsal #4
  - ❒ **#3:** attaches onto metatarsal #5

to the

- ❑ Sides of the Phalanges and the Distal Tendons of the Extensor Digitorum Longus
  - ❒ the base of the proximal phalanges (on the "2nd Toe Side") and the dorsal digital expansion of toes #3-5:
    - ❒ **#1:** attaches to toe #3
    - ❒ **#2:** attaches to toe #4
    - ❒ **#3:** attaches to toe #5

ACTIONS

- ❒ 1. **Adducts Toes #3-5 at the Metatarsophalangeal Joint**
- ❒ 2. Flexes Toes #3-5 at the Metatarsophalangeal Joint
- ❒ 3. Extends Toes #3-5 at the Proximal and Distal Interphalangeal Joints

INNERVATION

- ❒ The Lateral Plantar Nerve
- ❒ S2, 3

Dorsal Interossei Pedis

- ❑ (There are four dorsal interossei pedis muscles, named #1, #2, #3 and #4.)

ATTACHMENTS

- ❑ Metatarsals
  - ❒ each one arises from the adjacent sides of two metatarsals:
    - ❒ **#1:** attaches onto metatarsals #1 and #2
    - ❒ **#2:** attaches onto metatarsals #2 and #3
    - ❒ **#3:** attaches onto metatarsals #3 and #4
    - ❒ **#4:** attaches onto metatarsals #4 and #5

to the

- ❑ Sides of the Phalanges and the Distal Tendons of the Extensor Digitorum Longus
  - ❒ the bases of the proximal phalanges (on the sides away from the center of the 2nd toe) and the dorsal digital expansion:
    - ❒ **#1:** attaches to the medial side of toe #2
    - ❒ **#2:** attaches to the lateral side of toe #2
    - ❒ **#3:** attaches to the lateral side of toe #3
    - ❒ **#4:** attaches to the lateral side of toe #4

ACTIONS

- ❒ 1. **Abducts Toes #2-4 at the Metatarsophalangeal Joint**
- ❒ 2. Flexes Toes #2-4 at the Metatarsophalangeal Joint
- ❒ 3. Extends Toes #2-4 at the Proximal and Distal Interphalangeal Joints

INNERVATION

- ❒ The Lateral Plantar Nerve
- ❒ S2, 3

MUSCLES OF THE UPPER EXTREMITY

MUSCLES OF THE SCAPULA/ARM

SCAPULAR MUSCLES

Supraspinatus (of Rotator Cuff Group)

ATTACHMENTS

- ❑ Supraspinous Fossa of the Scapula
  - ❒ the medial ⅔

to the

- ❑ Greater Tubercle of the Humerus
  - ❒ the superior facet

ACTION

- ❒ **Abducts the Arm at the Shoulder Joint**

INNERVATION

- ❒ The Suprascapular Nerve
- ❒ C5, 6

Infraspinatus (of Rotator Cuff Group)

ATTACHMENTS

- ❑ Infraspinous Fossa of the Scapula
  - ❒ the medial ⅔

to the

- ❑ Greater Tubercle of the Humerus
  - ❒ the middle facet

ACTION

- ❒ **Laterally Rotates the Arm at the Shoulder Joint**

INNERVATION

- ❒ The Suprascapular Nerve
- ❒ C5, 6

Teres Minor (of Rotator Cuff Group)

ATTACHMENTS

- ❑ Superior Lateral Border of the Scapula
  - ❒ the superior ⅔ of the dorsal surface

to the

- ❑ Greater Tubercle of the Humerus
  - ❒ the inferior facet

ACTIONS

- ❒ 1. **Laterally Rotates the Arm at the Shoulder Joint**
- ❒ 2. Adducts the Arm at the Shoulder Joint

INNERVATION

- ❒ The Axillary Nerve
- ❒ C5, 6

Subscapularis (of Rotator Cuff Group)

ATTACHMENTS

- ❑ Subscapular Fossa of the Scapula

to the

- ❑ Lesser Tubercle of the Humerus

ACTION

❒ **Medially Rotates the Arm at the Shoulder Joint**

INNERVATION

❒ The Upper and Lower Subscapular Nerves

❒ C5, **6**

Teres Major

ATTACHMENTS

❑ Inferior Lateral Border of the Scapula

 ❒ the inferior ⅓ of the dorsal surface

to the

❑ Medial Lip of the Bicipital Groove of the Humerus

ACTIONS

❒ 1. **Medially Rotates the Arm at the Shoulder Joint**

❒ 2. **Adducts the Arm at the Shoulder Joint**

❒ 3. **Extends the Arm at the Shoulder Joint**

❒ 4. Upwardly Rotates the Scapula at the Scapulocostal Joint

INNERVATION

❒ The Lower Subscapular Nerve

❒ C5, **6**, 7

ARM MUSCLES

Deltoid

ATTACHMENTS

❑ Lateral Clavicle, Acromion Process, and the Spine of the Scapula

 ❒ the lateral ⅓ of the clavicle

to the

❑ Deltoid Tuberosity of the Humerus

ACTIONS

❒ 1. **Abducts the Arm at the Shoulder Joint (entire muscle)**

❒ 2. **Flexes the Arm at the Shoulder Joint (anterior deltoid)**

❒ 3. **Extends the Arm at the Shoulder Joint (posterior deltoid)**

❒ 4. **Medially Rotates the Arm at the Shoulder Joint (anterior deltoid)**

❒ 5. **Laterally Rotates the Arm at the Shoulder Joint (posterior deltoid)**

❒ 6. Downwardly Rotates the Scapula at the Scapulocostal Joint (entire muscle)

❒ 7. Ipsilaterally Rotates the Trunk at the Shoulder Joint (anterior deltoid)

❒ 8. Contralaterally Rotates the Trunk at the Shoulder Joint (posterior deltoid)

INNERVATION

❒ The Axillary Nerve

❒ **C5**, 6

Coracobrachialis

ATTACHMENTS

❑ Coracoid Process of the Scapula

 ❒ the apex

to the

❑ Medial Shaft of the Humerus

 ❒ the middle ⅓

ACTIONS

❒ 1. **Flexes the Arm at the Shoulder Joint**

❒ 2. **Adducts the Arm at the Shoulder Joint**

INNERVATION

❒ The Musculocutaneous Nerve

❒ C5, 6, 7

Biceps Brachii

ATTACHMENTS

❑ LONG HEAD: Supraglenoid Tubercle of the Scapula

❑ SHORT HEAD: Coracoid Process of the Scapula

 ❒ the apex

to the

❑ Radial Tuberosity

 ❒ and the bicipital aponeurosis into deep fascia overlying the common flexor tendon

ACTIONS

❒ 1. **Flexes the Forearm at the Elbow Joint (entire muscle)**

❒ 2. **Supinates the Forearm at the Radioulnar Joints (entire muscle)**

❒ 3. **Flexes the Arm at the Shoulder Joint (entire muscle)**

❒ 4. Abducts the Arm at the Shoulder Joint (long head)

❒ 5. Adducts the Arm at the Shoulder Joint (short head)

INNERVATION

❒ The Musculocutaneous Nerve

❒ C5, 6

Brachialis

ATTACHMENTS

❑ Distal ½ of the Anterior Shaft of the Humerus

to the

❑ Ulnar Tuberosity

 ❒ and the coronoid process of the ulna

ACTION

❒ **Flexes the Forearm at the Elbow Joint**

INNERVATION

❒ The Musculocutaneous Nerve

❒ C5, **6**, 7

Triceps Brachii

ATTACHMENTS

❑ LONG HEAD: Infraglenoid Tubercle of the Scapula

❒ LATERAL HEAD: Posterior Shaft of the Humerus

 ❒ the proximal ½

❒ MEDIAL HEAD: Posterior Shaft of the Humerus

 ❒ the distal ½

to the

❑ Olecranon Process of the Ulna

ACTIONS

❒ 1. **Extends the Forearm at the Elbow Joint (entire muscle)**
❒ 2. Adducts the Arm at the Shoulder Joint (long head)
❒ 3. Extends the Arm at the Shoulder Joint (long head)

INNERVATION

❒ The Radial Nerve
❒ C6, 7, 8

MUSCLES OF THE FOREARM

ANTERIOR FOREARM—SUPERFICIAL

Pronator Teres

ATTACHMENTS

❑ HUMERAL HEAD: Medial Epicondyle of the Humerus (via the Common Flexor Tendon)
  ❒ and the medial supracondylar ridge of the humerus
❑ ULNAR HEAD: Coronoid Process of the Ulna
  ❒ the medial surface

to the

❑ Lateral Radius
  ❒ the middle ⅓

ACTIONS

❒ 1. **Pronates the Forearm at the Radioulnar Joints**
❒ 2. **Flexes the Forearm at the Elbow Joint**

INNERVATION

❒ The Median Nerve
❒ C6, 7

Flexor Carpi Radialis (of Wrist Flexor Group)

ATTACHMENTS

❑ Medial Epicondyle of the Humerus (via the Common Flexor Tendon)

to the

❑ Radial Hand on the Anterior Side
  ❒ the anterior side of the bases of the 2nd and 3rd metacarpals

ACTIONS

❒ 1. **Flexes the Hand at the Wrist Joint**
❒ 2. **Radially Deviates (Abducts) the Hand at the Wrist Joint**
❒ 3. Flexes the Forearm at the Elbow Joint
❒ 4. Pronates the Forearm at the Radioulnar Joint

INNERVATION

❒ The Median Nerve
❒ C6, 7

Palmaris Longus (of Wrist Flexor Group)

ATTACHMENTS

❑ Medial Epicondyle of the Humerus (via the Common Flexor Tendon)

to the

❑ Palm of the Hand
  ❒ the palmar aponeurosis and the flexor retinaculum

ACTIONS

❒ 1. **Flexes the Hand at the Wrist Joint**
❒ 2. Flexes the Forearm at the Elbow Joint
❒ 3. Pronates the Forearm at the Radioulnar Joint
❒ 4. Wrinkles the Skin of the Palm

INNERVATION

❒ The Median Nerve
❒ C7, 8

Flexor Carpi Ulnaris (of Wrist Flexor Group)

ATTACHMENTS

❑ Medial Epicondyle of the Humerus (via the Common Flexor Tendon) and the Ulna
  ❒ the medial margin of the olecranon and the posterior proximal ⅔ of the ulna

to the

❑ Ulnar Hand on the Anterior Side
  ❒ the pisiform, the hook of the hamate, and the base of the 5th metacarpal

ACTIONS

❒ 1. **Flexes the Hand at the Wrist Joint**
❒ 2. **Ulnar Deviates (Adducts) the Hand at the Wrist Joint**
❒ 3. Flexes the Forearm at the Elbow Joint

INNERVATION

❒ The Ulnar Nerve
❒ C7, 8

Brachioradialis (of Radial Group)

ATTACHMENTS

❑ Lateral Supracondylar Ridge of the Humerus
  ❒ the proximal ⅔

to the

❑ Styloid Process of the Radius
  ❒ the lateral side

ACTIONS

❒ 1. **Flexes the Forearm at the Elbow Joint**
❒ 2. Supinates the Forearm at the Radioulnar Joints
❒ 3. Pronates the Forearm at the Radioulnar Joints

INNERVATION

❒ The Radial Nerve
❒ C5, 6

ANTERIOR FOREARM—INTERMEDIATE

Flexor Digitorum Superficialis

ATTACHMENTS

❑ Medial Epicondyle of the Humerus (via the Common Flexor Tendon) and the Anterior Ulna, and the Radius
  ❒ HUMEROULNAR HEAD: medial epicondyle of the humerus (via the common flexor tendon) and the coronoid process of the ulna

- ❒ RADIAL HEAD: proximal ½ of the anterior shaft of the radius (starting just distal to the radial tuberosity)

to the

- ❑ Anterior Surfaces of Fingers #2-5
  - ❒ the four tendons each divide into two slips that attach onto the sides of the anterior surfaces of the middle phalanges

ACTIONS

- ❒ 1. **Flexes Fingers #2-5 at the Metacarpophalangeal and Proximal Interphalangeal Joints**
- ❒ 2. **Flexes the Hand at the Wrist Joint**
- ❒ 3. Flexes the Forearm at the Elbow Joint

INNERVATION

- ❒ The Median Nerve
- ❒ C7, **8**, T1

ANTERIOR FOREARM—DEEP

Flexor Digitorum Profundus

ATTACHMENTS

- ❑ Medial and Anterior Ulna
  - ❒ the proximal ½ (starting distal to the ulnar tuberosity) and the interosseus membrane

to the

- ❑ Anterior Surfaces of Fingers #2-5
  - ❒ the distal phalanges

ACTIONS

- ❒ 1. **Flexes Fingers #2-5 at the Metacarpophalangeal and Proximal and Distal Interphalangeal Joints**
- ❒ 2. **Flexes the Hand at the Wrist Joint**

INNERVATION

- ❒ The Median and the Ulnar Nerves
- ❒ C8, T1
- ❒ the anterior interosseus branch of the median nerve

Flexor Pollicis Longus

ATTACHMENTS

- ❑ Anterior Surface of the Radius
  - ❒ and the interosseus membrane, the medial epicondyle of the humerus, and the coronoid process of the ulna

to the

- ❑ Thumb
  - ❒ the anterior aspect of the base of the distal phalanx

ACTIONS

- ❒ 1. **Flexes the Thumb at the Carpometacarpal, Metacarpophalangeal, and the Interphalangeal Joints**
- ❒ 2. **Flexes the Hand at the Wrist Joint**
- ❒ 3. Radially Deviates (Abducts) the Hand at the Wrist Joint
- ❒ 4. Flexes the Forearm at the Elbow Joint

INNERVATION

- ❒ The Median Nerve
- ❒ the anterior interosseus branch of the median nerve; C7, **8**

Pronator Quadratus

ATTACHMENTS

- ❑ Anterior Distal Ulna
  - ❒ the distal ¼

to the

- ❑ Anterior Distal Radius
  - ❒ the distal ¼

ACTION

- ❒ **Pronates the Forearm at the Radioulnar Joints**

INNERVATION

- ❒ The Median Nerve
- ❒ anterior interosseus nerve, C7, **8**

POSTERIOR FOREARM—SUPERFICIAL

Anconeus

ATTACHMENTS

- ❑ Lateral Epicondyle of the Humerus

to the

- ❑ Posterior Ulna
  - ❒ the lateral side of the olecranon process of the ulna and the proximal ¼ of the posterior ulna

ACTION

- ❒ **Extends the Forearm at the Elbow Joint**

INNERVATION

- ❒ The Radial Nerve
- ❒ C6, 7, 8

Extensor Carpi Radialis Longus (of Wrist Extensor Group and Radial Group)

ATTACHMENTS

- ❑ Lateral Supracondylar Ridge of the Humerus
  - ❒ the distal ⅓

to the

- ❑ Radial Hand on the Posterior Side
  - ❒ the posterior side of the base of the 2nd metacarpal

ACTIONS

- ❒ 1. **Extends the Hand at the Wrist Joint**
- ❒ 2. **Radially Deviates (Abducts) the Hand at the Wrist Joint**
- ❒ 3. Flexes the Forearm at the Elbow Joint
- ❒ 4. Pronates the Forearm at the Radioulnar Joints

INNERVATION

- ❒ The Radial Nerve
- ❒ C5, **6**

Extensor Carpi Radialis Brevis (of Wrist Extensor Group and Radial Group)

ATTACHMENTS

- ❑ Lateral Epicondyle of the Humerus (via the Common Extensor Tendon)

to the

- ❑ Radial Hand on the Posterior Side
  - ❒ the posterior side of the base of the 3rd metacarpal

ACTIONS

- ❒ 1. **Extends the Hand at the Wrist Joint**

- ❒ 2. **Radially Deviates (Abducts) the Hand at the Wrist Joint**
- ❒ 3. Flexes the Forearm at the Elbow Joint

INNERVATION
- ❒ The Radial Nerve
- ❒ posterior interosseus nerve, C7, 8

Extensor Digitorum

ATTACHMENTS
- ❒ Lateral Epicondyle of the Humerus (via the Common Extensor Tendon)

to the
- ❒ Phalanges of Fingers #2-5
  - ❒ via its dorsal digital expansion onto the posterior surface of the middle and distal phalanges

ACTIONS
- ❒ 1. **Extends Fingers #2-5 at the Metacarpophalangeal and Proximal and Distal Interphalangeal Joints**
- ❒ 2. **Extends the Hand at the Wrist Joint**
- ❒ 3. Medially Rotates the Little Finger (Finger #5) at the Carpometacarpal Joint
- ❒ 4. Extends the Forearm at the Elbow Joint

INNERVATION
- ❒ The Radial Nerve
- ❒ posterior interosseus nerve, C7, 8

Extensor Digiti Minimi

ATTACHMENTS
- ❒ Lateral Epicondyle of the Humerus (via the Common Extensor Tendon)

to the
- ❒ Phalanges of the Little Finger (Finger #5)
  - ❒ attaches into the ulnar side of the tendon of the extensor digitorum muscle (to attach onto the posterior surface of the middle and distal phalanges of the little finger via the dorsal digital expansion)

ACTIONS
- ❒ 1. **Extends the Little Finger (Finger #5) at the Metacarpophalangeal and Proximal and Distal Interphalangeal Joints**
- ❒ 2. **Extends the Hand at the Wrist Joint**
- ❒ 3. Medially Rotates the Little Finger (Finger #5) at the Carpometacarpal Joint
- ❒ 4. Extends the Forearm at the Elbow Joint

INNERVATION
- ❒ The Radial Nerve
- ❒ posterior interosseus nerve; C7, 8

Extensor Carpi Ulnaris (of Wrist Extensor Group)

ATTACHMENTS
- ❒ Lateral Epicondyle of the Humerus (via the Common Extensor Tendon) and the Ulna
  - ❒ the posterior middle ⅓ of the ulna

to the
- ❒ Ulnar Hand on the Posterior Side
  - ❒ the posterior side of the base of the 5th metacarpal

ACTIONS
- ❒ 1. **Extends the Hand at the Wrist Joint**
- ❒ 2. **Ulnar Deviates (Adducts) the Hand at the Wrist Joint**
- ❒ 3. Extends the Forearm at the Elbow Joint

INNERVATION
- ❒ The Radial Nerve
- ❒ posterior interosseus nerve, C7, 8

POSTERIOR FOREARM—DEEP

Supinator

ATTACHMENTS
- ❒ Lateral Epicondyle of the Humerus and the Proximal Ulna
  - ❒ the supinator crest of the ulna

to the
- ❒ Proximal Radius
  - ❒ the proximal ⅓ of the posterior, lateral and anterior sides

ACTION
- ❒ **Supinates the Forearm at the Radioulnar Joints**

INNERVATION
- ❒ The Radial Nerve
- ❒ C6, 7

Abductor Pollicis Longus (of Deep Distal Four Group)

ATTACHMENTS
- ❒ Posterior Radius and Ulna
  - ❒ approximately the middle ⅓ of the radius, ulna, and interosseus membrane

to the
- ❒ Thumb
  - ❒ the lateral side of the base of the 1st metacarpal

ACTIONS
- ❒ 1. **Abducts the Thumb at the Carpometacarpal Joint**
- ❒ 2. Extends the Thumb at the Carpometacarpal Joint
- ❒ 3. Laterally Rotates the Thumb at the Carpometacarpal Joint
- ❒ 4. Radially Deviates (Abducts) the Hand at the Wrist Joint
- ❒ 5. Flexes the Hand at the Wrist Joint
- ❒ 6. Supinates the Forearm at the Radioulnar Joints

INNERVATION
- ❒ The Radial Nerve
- ❒ posterior interosseus nerve, C7, 8

Extensor Pollicis Brevis (of Deep Distal Four Group)

ATTACHMENTS
- ❒ Posterior Radius
  - ❒ the distal ⅓ and the adjacent interosseus membrane

to the
- ❒ Thumb
  - ❒ the posterolateral base of the proximal phalanx

ACTIONS

- ❒ 1. **Extends the Thumb at the Carpometacarpal and Metacarpophalangeal Joints**
- ❒ 2. Abducts the Thumb at the Carpometacarpal Joint
- ❒ 3. Laterally Rotates the Thumb at the Carpometacarpal Joint
- ❒ 4. Radially Deviates (Abducts) the Hand at the Wrist Joint

INNERVATION

- ❒ The Radial Nerve
- ❒ the posterior interosseus nerve, **C7**, 8

Extensor Pollicis Longus (of Deep Distal Four Group)

ATTACHMENTS

- ❑ Posterior Ulna
  - ❒ the middle ⅓ and the interosseus membrane

to the

- ❑ Thumb
  - ❒ via its dorsal digital expansion onto the posterior surface of the distal phalanx of the thumb

ACTIONS

- ❒ 1. **Extends the Thumb at the Carpometacarpal, Metacarpophalangeal, and Interphalangeal Joints**
- ❒ 2. Laterally Rotates the Thumb at the Carpometacarpal Joint
- ❒ 3. Extends the Hand at the Wrist Joint
- ❒ 4. Radially Deviates (Abducts) the Hand at the Wrist Joint
- ❒ 5. Supinates the Forearm at the Radioulnar Joints

INNERVATION

- ❒ The Radial Nerve
- ❒ posterior interosseus nerve, **C7**, 8

Extensor Indicis (of Deep Distal Four Group)

ATTACHMENTS

- ❑ Posterior Ulna
  - ❒ the distal ⅓ and the interosseus membrane

to the

- ❑ Index Finger (Finger #2)
  - ❒ attaches into the ulnar side of the tendon of the extensor digitorum muscle (to attach onto the posterior surface of the middle and distal phalanges of the index finger via the dorsal digital expansion)

ACTIONS

- ❒ 1. **Extends the Index Finger (Finger #2) at the Metacarpophalangeal and Proximal and Distal Interphalangeal Joints**
- ❒ 2. **Extends the Hand at the Wrist Joint**
- ❒ 3. Adducts the Index Finger (Finger #2) at the Metacarpophalangeal Joint
- ❒ 4. Supinates the Forearm at the Radioulnar Joints

INNERVATION

- ❒ The Radial Nerve
- ❒ posterior interosseus nerve, C7, 8

INTRINSIC MUSCLES OF THE HAND

SUPERFICIAL FASCIAL MUSCLE

Palmaris Brevis

ATTACHMENTS

- ❑ The Flexor Retinaculum and the Palmar Aponeurosis

to the

- ❑ Dermis of the Ulnar (Medial) Border of the Hand

ACTION

- ❒ **Wrinkles the Skin of the Palm**

INNERVATION

- ❒ The Ulnar Nerve
- ❒ C8, T1

MUSCLES OF THE THENAR EMINENCE

Abductor Pollicis Brevis

ATTACHMENTS

- ❑ The Flexor Retinaculum and the Carpals
  - ❒ the tubercle of the scaphoid and the tubercle of the trapezium

to the

- ❑ Proximal Phalanx of the Thumb
  - ❒ the radial (lateral) side of the base of the proximal phalanx and the dorsal digital expansion

ACTIONS

- ❒ 1. **Abducts the Thumb at the Carpometacarpal Joint**
- ❒ 2. Flexes the Thumb at the Metacarpophalangeal Joint
- ❒ 3. Extends the Thumb at the Carpometacarpal and Interphalangeal Joints

INNERVATION

- ❒ The Median Nerve
- ❒ C8, **T1**

Flexor Pollicis Brevis

ATTACHMENTS

- ❑ The Flexor Retinaculum and the Carpals
  - ❒ the trapezium

to the

- ❑ Proximal Phalanx of the Thumb
  - ❒ the radial (lateral) side of the base of the proximal phalanx of the thumb

ACTIONS

- ❒ 1. **Flexes the Thumb at the Carpometacarpal and the Metacarpophalangeal Joints**
- ❒ 2. Abducts the Thumb at the Carpometacarpal Joint

INNERVATION

- The Median and Ulnar Nerves
- C8, **T1:** (superficial head: the median nerve; deep head: the ulnar nerve)

Opponens Pollicis

ATTACHMENTS

- The Flexor Retinaculum and the Carpals
  - the tubercle of the trapezium

to the

- 1st Metacarpal (of the Thumb)
  - the anterior surface and lateral border

ACTIONS

- 1. **Opposes the Thumb at the Carpometacarpal Joint**
- 2. Flexes the Thumb at the Carpometacarpal Joint
- 3. Medially Rotates the Thumb at the Carpometacarpal Joint
- 4. Abducts the Thumb at the Carpometacarpal Joint

INNERVATION

- The Median and Ulnar Nerves
- C8, **T1**

MUSCLES OF HYPOTHENAR EMINENCE

Abductor Digiti Minimi Manus

ATTACHMENTS

- The Carpals
  - the pisiform and the tendon of the flexor carpi ulnaris

to the

- Proximal Phalanx of the Little Finger (Finger #5)
  - the ulnar (medial) side of the base of the proximal phalanx and the dorsal digital expansion

ACTIONS

- 1. **Abducts the Little Finger (Finger #5) at the Carpometacarpal and Metacarpophalangeal Joints**
- 2. Extends the Little Finger (Finger #5) at the Proximal and Distal **Interphalangeal Joints**

INNERVATION

- The Ulnar Nerve
- C8, **T1**

Flexor Digiti Minimi Manus

ATTACHMENTS

- The Flexor Retinaculum and the Carpals
  - the hook of the hamate

to the

- Proximal Phalanx of the Little Finger (Finger #5)
  - the ulnar (medial) side of the base of the proximal phalanx

ACTION

- **Flexes the Little Finger (Finger #5) at the Metacarpophalangeal Joint**

INNERVATION

- The Ulnar Nerve
- C8, **T1**

Opponens Digiti Minimi

ATTACHMENTS

- The Flexor Retinaculum and the Carpals
  - the hook of the hamate

to the

- 5th Metacarpal (of the Little Finger)
  - the anterior surface and the medial (ulnar) border of the 5th metacarpal

ACTIONS

- 1. **Opposes the Little Finger (Finger #5) at the Carpometacarpal Joint**
- 2. Flexes the Little Finger (Finger #5) at the Carpometacarpal Joint
- 3. Adducts the Little Finger (Finger #5) at the Carpometacarpal Joint
- 4. Laterally Rotates the Little Finger (Finger #5) at the Carpometacarpal Joint

INNERVATION

- The Ulnar Nerve
- C8, **T1**

MUSCLES OF THE CENTRAL COMPARTMENT

Adductor Pollicis

ATTACHMENTS

- 3rd Metacarpal
  - OBLIQUE HEAD: the anterior bases of the 2nd and 3rd metacarpals and the capitate
  - TRANSVERSE HEAD: the distal ⅔ of the anterior surface of the 3rd metacarpal

to the

- Thumb
  - OBLIQUE HEAD: the medial side of the base of the proximal phalanx and the dorsal digital expansion
  - TRANSVERSE HEAD: the medial side of the base of the proximal phalanx

ACTIONS

- 1. **Adducts the Thumb at the Carpometacarpal Joint**
- 2. Flexes the Thumb at the Carpometacarpal and Metacarpophalangeal Joints
- 3. Extends the Thumb at the Interphalangeal Joint

INNERVATION

- The Ulnar Nerve
- C8, T1

Lumbricals Manus

- (There are four lumbrical manus muscles, named #1, #2, #3, and #4.)

ATTACHMENTS

- The Distal Tendons of the Flexor Digitorum Profundus
  - **#1:** the radial (lateral) side of the tendon of the index finger (finger #2)
  - **#2:** the radial (lateral) side of the tendon of the middle finger (finger #3)
  - **#3:** the ulnar (medial) side of the tendon of the middle finger (finger #3) and the radial (lateral) side of the tendon of the ring finger (finger #4)
  - **#4:** the ulnar (medial) side of the tendon of the ring finger (finger #4) and the radial (lateral) side of the tendon of the little finger (finger #5)

to the

- Distal Tendons of the Extensor Digitorum (the Dorsal Digital Expansion)
  - the radial (lateral) side of the tendons merging into the dorsal digital expansion
  - **#1:** into the tendon of the index finger (finger #2)
  - **#2:** into the tendon of the middle finger (finger #3)
  - **#3:** into the tendon of the ring finger (finger #4)
  - **#4:** into the tendon of the little finger (finger #5)

ACTIONS

- 1. **Extends Fingers #2-5 at the Proximal and Distal Interphalangeal Joints**
- 2. **Flexes Fingers #2-5 at the Metacarpophalangeal Joint**

INNERVATION

- The Median and Ulnar Nerves
- C8, **T1** (1st and 2nd lumbricals manus: the median nerve; 3rd and 4th lumbricals manus: the ulnar nerve)

Palmar Interossei

- (There are three palmar interossei, named #1, #2, and #3.)

ATTACHMENTS

- The Metacarpal of Fingers #2, #4, and #5
  - the anterior side and on the "middle finger side" of the metacarpals:
    - **#1:** attaches to the metacarpal of the index finger (finger #2)
    - **#2:** attaches to the metacarpal of the ring finger (finger #4)
    - **#3:** attaches to the metacarpal of the little finger (finger #5)

to the

- Proximal Phalanx of Fingers #2, #4, and #5 on the "Middle Finger Side"
  - the base of the proximal phalanx and the dorsal digital expansion:
    - **#1:** attaches to the index finger (finger #2)
    - **#2:** attaches to the ring finger (finger #4)
    - **#3:** attaches to the little finger (finger #5)

ACTIONS

- 1. **Adducts Fingers #2, #4, and #5 at the Metacarpophalangeal Joint**
- 2. Flexes Fingers #2, #4, and #5 at the Metacarpophalangeal Joint
- 3. Extends Fingers #2, #4, and #5 at the Interphalangeal Joints

INNERVATION

- The Ulnar Nerve
- C8, **T1**; deep branch of the ulnar nerve

Dorsal Interossei Manus

- (There are four dorsal interossei manus muscles, named #1, #2, #3, and #4.)

ATTACHMENTS

- The Metacarpal of Fingers #1-5
  - each one arises from the adjacent sides of two metacarpals:
    - **#1:** attaches onto the metacarpal of the thumb and index finger (fingers #1 and #2)
    - **#2:** attaches onto the metacarpal of the index and middle fingers (fingers #2 and #3)
    - **#3:** attaches onto the metacarpal of the middle and ring fingers (fingers #3 and #4)
    - **#4:** attaches onto the metacarpal of the ring and little fingers (fingers #4 and #5)

to the

- Proximal Phalanx of Fingers #2, #3, and #4 on the Side Away From the Center of the Middle Finger
  - the base of the proximal phalanx and the dorsal digital expansion:
    - **#1:** attaches to the lateral side of the index finger (finger #2)
    - **#2:** attaches to the lateral side of the middle finger (finger #3)
    - **#3:** attaches to the medial side of the middle finger (finger #3)
    - **#4:** attaches to the medial side of the ring finger (finger #4)

ACTIONS

- 1. **Abducts Fingers #2, #3, and #4 at the Metacarpophalangeal Joint**
- 2. Flexes Fingers #2, #3, and #4 at the Metacarpophalangeal Joint
- 3. Extends Fingers #2, #3, and #4 at the Interphalangeal Joints

INNERVATION

- The Ulnar Nerve
- C8, **T1**; deep branch of the ulnar nerve

Bibliography

A

Abrahams PH, Marks SC Jr, Hutchings RT: *McMinn's color atlas of human anatomy*, ed 5, St. Louis, 2003, Mosby, Inc.

Alter MJ: *Science of flexibility*, ed 3, Champaign, IL, 2004, Human Kinetics.

Anderson B: *Stretching: 20th anniversary, revised edition*, Bolinas, CA, 2000, Shelter Publications, Inc.

Anderson JE: *Grant's atlas of anatomy*, ed 7, Baltimore, 1978, Williams & Wilkins.

B

Barkauskas VH, Baumann LC, Darling-Fisher CS: *Health & physical assessment*, ed 3, St. Louis, 2002, Mosby, Inc.

Bear MF, Connors BW, Paradiso MA: *Neuroscience: exploring the brain*, ed 2, Baltimore, 2001, Williams & Wilkins.

Biel A: *Trail guide to the body: how to locate muscles, bones, and more*, ed 3, Boulder, CO, 2005, Books of Discovery.

Bontrager KL: *Textbook of radiographic positioning and related anatomy*, ed 5, St. Louis, 2001, Mosby, Inc.

C

Cailliet R: *Pain series: neck and arm pain*, ed 2, Philadelphia, 1981, F.A. Davis Company.

Cailliet R: *Pain series: hand pain*, ed 3, Philadelphia, 1982, F.A. Davis Company.

Cailliet R: *Pain series: foot and ankle pain*, ed 2, Philadelphia, 1983, F.A. Davis Company.

Cailliet R: *Pain series: knee pain*, ed 2, Philadelphia, 1983, F.A. Davis Company.

Cailliet R: *Pain series: shoulder pain*, ed 2, Philadelphia, 1983, F.A. Davis Company.

Calais-Germain B: *Anatomy of movement*, Seattle, WA, 1993, Eastland Press.

Chaitow L, DeLany JW: *Clinical application of neuromuscular techniques*, vol 1, Edinburgh, 2000, Harcourt Publishers Limited.

Chaitow L, DeLany JW: *Clinical application of neuromuscular techniques*, vol 2, Edinburgh, 2002, Elsevier Science Limited.

Cipriano JJ: *Photographic manual of regional orthopaedic and neurological tests*, ed 4, Philadelphia, 2003, Williams & Wilkins.

Clark RG: *Mantar and Gatz's essentials of clinical neuroanatomy and neurophysiology*, ed 5, Philadelphia, 1975, F.A. Davis Company.

Clay JH, Pounds DM: *Basic clinical massage therapy: integrating anatomy and treatment*, Baltimore, 2003, Williams & Wilkins.

Clemente CD: *Anatomy: a regional atlas of the human body*, ed 2, Baltimore, 1981, Urban & Schwarzenberg.

Clemente CD: *Clemente anatomy: a regional atlas of the human body*, ed 4, Baltimore, 1997, Williams & Wilkins.

Cody J: *Visualizing muscles: a new ecorche approach to surface anatomy*, Lawrence, KS, University Press of Kansas.

Cohen BJ, Wood DL: *Memmler's structure and function of the human body*, ed 7, Baltimore, 2000, Williams & Wilkins.

Cramer GD, Darby SA: *Basic and clinical anatomy of the spine, spinal cord, and ANS*, St. Louis, 1995, Mosby, Inc.

D

Davies C: *The trigger point therapy workbook: your self-treatment guide for pain relief*, Oakland, CA, 2001, New Harbinger Publications, Inc.

Dimon T Jr: *Anatomy of the moving body: a basic course in bones, muscles, and joints*, Berkeley, CA, 2001, North Atlantic Books.

Dixon M: *Joint play the right way: for the peripheral skeleton*, Port Moody, British Columbia, 2003, Arthrokinetic Publishing.

Donnelly JE: *Living anatomy*, ed 2, Champaign, IL, 1990, Leisure Press.

Drake RL, Vogl W, Mitchell AWM: *Gray's anatomy for students*, Philadelphia, 2005, Elsevier Inc.

E

Enoka RM: *Neuromechanics of human movement*, ed 3, Champaign, IL, 2002, Human Kinetics.

F

Feher G: *Cyclopedia anatomicae: more than 1,500 illustrations for the human and animal figure for the artist*, New York, 1996, Black Dog & Leventhal Publishers, Inc.

Fritz S, Grosenbach MJ: *Mosby's essential sciences for therapeutic massage: anatomy, physiology, biomechanics, and pathology*, ed 2, St. Louis, 2004, Mosby, Inc.

Frye B: *Body mechanics for manual therapists: a functional approach to self-care*, ed 2, Stanwood, WA, 2004, Fryetag Publishing.

G

Gorman D: *The body moveable: blueprints of the human musculoskeletal system: its structure, mechanics, locomotor and postural functions*, sec 1, Guelph, Ontario, Ampersand Press.

Gosling JA, Harris PF, Whitmore I, Willan PLT: *Human anatomy: color atlas and text*, ed 4, St. Louis, 2002, Mosby, Inc.

Greene E, Goodrich-Dunn B: *The psychology of the body*, Baltimore, 2004, Williams & Wilkins.

Gunn C: *Bones and joints: a guide for students*, ed 4, Edinburgh, 2002, Churchill Livingstone.

Guyton AC, Hall JE: *Textbook of medical physiology*, ed 10, Philadelphia, 2000, WB Saunders Company.

H

Hale RB, Coyle T: *Albinus on anatomy: with 80 original Albinus plates*, New York, 1988, Dover Publications, Inc.

Hale RB, Coyle T: *Anatomy lessons from the great masters: 100 great figure drawings analyzed*, New York, 2000, Watson-Guptill Publications.

Hamill J, Knutzen KM: *Biochemical basis of human movement*, ed 2, Baltimore, 2003, Williams & Wilkins.

Hole JW Jr: *Student study art notebook: essentials of human anatomy and physiology*, ed 5, Dubuque, IA, 1995, Wm. C. Brown Publishers.

Hoppenfeld S: *Physical examination of the spine and extremities*, New York, 1976, Appleton-Century-Crofts.

J

Jarmey C: *The concise book of muscles*, Chichester, England, 2003, Lotus Publishing.

Jenkins DB: *Hollinshead's functional anantomy of the limbs and back*, ed 8, Philadelphia, 2002, WB Saunders Company.

Juhan D: *Job's body: a handbook for bodywork*, Barrytown, NY, 1987, Station Hill Press.

K

Kandel ER, Schwartz JH, Jessell TM: *Principles of neural science*, ed 4, New York, 2000, McGraw-Hill Companies.

Kapandji IA: *The physiology of the joints: upper limb*, vol 1, New York, 2002, Churchill Livingstone.

Kapandji IA: *The physiology of the joints: the trunk and the vertebral column*, vol 3, New York, 1980, Churchill Livingstone.

Kendall FP, McCreary EK, Provance PG: *Muscles testing and function*, ed 4, Baltimore, 1993, Williams & Wilkins.

Kendall HO, Kendall FP, Boynton DA: *Posture and pain*, Malabar, FL, 1981, Robert E. Krieger Publishing Co., Inc.

Konin JG, Wiksten DL, Isear JA Jr, Brader H: *Special tests for orthopedic examination*, ed 2, Thorofare, NJ, 2002, Slack Inc.

Kraftsow G: *Yoga for wellness: healing with the timeless teachings of viniyoga*, New York, 1999, Penguin Putnam Inc.

L

Liebenson C, editor: *Rehabilitation of the spine: practitioner's manual*, Baltimore, 1996, Williams & Wilkins.

Lieber RL: *Skeletal muscle structure, function, & plasticity: the physiological basis of rehabilitation*, ed 2, Baltimore, 2002, Williams & Wilkins.

Lowe W: *Functional assessment in massage therapy: a guide to orthopedic assessment of pain and injury conditions for the massage practitioner*, ed 3, Bend, OR, 1997, Orthopedic Massage Education & Research Institute.

Luttgens K, Deutsch H, Hamilton N: *Kinesiology: scientific basis of human motion*, ed 8, Dubuque, IA, 1992, Wm. C. Brown Communications, Inc.

M

Magee DJ: *Orthopedic physical assessment*, ed 4, Philadelphia, 2002, Elsevier Sciences.

Margareta N, Frankel VH: *Basic biomechanics of the musculoskeletal system*, ed 3, Baltimore, 2001, Williams & Wilkins.

Mattes AL: *Active isolated stretching*, Sarasota, FL, 1995, Aaron L. Mattes.

Mattes AL: *Active isolated stretching: the Mattes method*, Sarasota, FL, 2000, Aaron L. Mattes.

Mattes AL: *Specific stretching for everyone: adapted from active isolated stretching: the mattes method*, Sarasota, FL, 2000, Aaron L. Mattes.

McArdle WD, Katch FI, Katch VL: *Essentials of exercise physiology*, Media, PA, 1994, Lea & Febiger.

McAtee RE, Charland J: *Facilitated stretching: assisted and unassisted PNF stretching made easy*, ed 2, Champaign, IL, 1999, Human Kinetics.

McMinn RMH, Hutchings RT: *Color atlas of human anatomy*, Chicago, 1981, Year Book Medical Publishers, Inc.

Melzack R, Wall PD: *The challenge of pain: a modern medical classic*, ed 2, London, England, 1996, Penguin Books.

Mense S, Simons DG, Hoheisel U, Quenzer B: Lesions of rat skeletal muscle after local block of acetylcholinesterase and neuromuscular stimulation, *J Appl Physiol* 94:2494–2501, 2003.

Muscolino JE: *The muscular system manual: the skeletal muscles of the human body*, ed 2, St. Louis, 2005, Elsevier Inc.

Muscolino JE: The shoulder joint complex, *American Massage Therapy Association Message Therapy Journal* 43(1):66–73, Spring 2004.

Muscolino JE, Cipriani, S: Pilates and the 'powerhouse' I, *Journal of Bodywork and Movement Therapies: Practical Issues in Musculoskeletal Function, Treatment and Rehabilitation* 8(1):15–24, 2004.

Muscolino JE, Cipriani, S: Pilates and the 'powerhouse' II, *Journal of Bodywork and Movement Therapies: Practical Issues in Musculoskeletal Function, Treatment and Rehabilitation* 8(2):122–130, 2004.

Myers TW: *Anatomy trains: myofascial meridians for manual and movement therapists*, Edinburgh, 2002, Elsevier Science Limited.

N

Nelson DL, Cox MM: *Lehninger principles of biochemistry*, ed 3, New York, 2000, Worth Publishers.

Netter FH: *The CIBA collection of medical illustrations: musculoskeletal system-anatomy, physiology and metabolic disorders*, vol 8, part 1, Ardsley, NJ, 1987, Ciba-Geigy Corp.

Netter FH: *Atlas of human anatomy*, ed 3, Teterboro, NJ, 2003, Icon Learning Systems.

Neumann DA: *Kinesiology of the musculoskeletal system: foundations for physical rehabilitation*, St. Louis, 2002, Mosby, Inc.

Norkin CC, Levangie P: *Joint structure & function: a comprehensive analysis*, ed 2, Philadelphia, 1992, F.A. Davis Company.

Norkin CC, Levangie P: *Joint structure & function: a comprehensive analysis*, ed 3, Philadelphia, 2001, F.A. Davis Company.

Norkin CC, White DJ: *Measurement of joint motion: a guide to goniometry*, ed 3, Philadelphia, 2003, F.A. Davis Company.

O

Oatis CA: *Kinesiology: the mechanics & pathomechanics of human movement*, Philadelphia, 2004, Williams & Wilkins.

Olson TR: *A.D.A.M.: student atlas of anatomy*, Baltimore, 1996, Williams & Wilkins.

Ombregt L, Bisschop P: *Atlas of orthopedic examination of the peripheral joints*, Edinburgh, 1999, Hartcourt Brace and Company Limited.

P

Pansky B, Allen DJ: *Review of neuroscience*, New York, 1980, Macmillan Publishing Co., Inc.

Palastanga N, Field D, Soams R: *Anatomy and human movement*, ed 4, Oxford, 2002, Butterworth-Heinemann.

Peterson DH, Bergmann TF: *Chiropractic technique: principles and procedures*, ed 2, St. Louis, 2002, Mosby, Inc.

Poole RM: *The incredible machine*, Washington, D.C., 1986, National Geographic Society.

Porth CM: *Pathophysiology, concepts of altered health states*, ed. 3, Philadelphia, 1990, J.B. Lippincott Company

R

Reese NB, Bandy WD: *Joint range of motion and muscle length testing*, Philadelphia, 2002, W.B. Saunders Company.

Rigutti A: *Atlante di anatomia*, Florence, Italy, 2000, Giunti Gruppo Editoriale.

Rohen JW, Yokochi C, Lutjen-Drecoll E: *Color atlas of anatomy: a photographic study of the human body*, ed 5, Baltimore, 2002, Williams & Wilkins.

S

Saidoff DC, McDonough AL: *Critical pathways in therapeutic intervention: upper extremity*, St. Louis, 1997, Mosby, Inc.

Saidoff DC, McDonough AL: *Critical pathways in therapeutic intervention: extremities and spine*, St. Louis, 2002, Mosby, Inc.

Schuenke M, Schulte E, Schumacher U: *Thieme atlas of anatomy: general anatomy and musculoskeletal system*, New York, 2006, Georg Thieme Verlag.

Shier D, Butler J, Lewis R: *Hole's essentials of human anatomy and physiology*, ed 6, Boston, 1998, McGraw-Hill.

Simons DG, Travell JG, Simons LS: *Myofascial pain and dysfunction: the trigger point manual*, ed 2, Baltimore, 1999, Williams & Wilkins.

Smith LK, Weiss EL, Lehmkuhl LD: *Brunnstrom's clinical kinesiology*, ed 5, Philadelphia, 1996, F.A. Davis Company.

Stone RJ, Stone JA: *Atlas of skeletal muscles*, ed 4, New York, 2003, McGraw-Hill Companies, Inc.

T

Thibodeau GA, Patton KT: *Anatomy & physiology*, ed 5, St. Louis, 2003, Mosby, Inc.

Travell JG, Simons DG: *Myofascial pain and dysfunction: the trigger point manual*, vol 2, Baltimore, Williams & Wilkins.

V

Van De Graaff KM, Crawley JL: *A photographic atlas for the anatomy & physiology laboratory*, ed 5, Englewood, CO, 2003, Morton Publishing Co.

W

Walther DS: *Applied kinesiology: basic procedures and muscle testing*, vol 1, Pueblo, CO, 1981, Systems DC.

Warfel JH: *The head, neck, and trunk: muscles and motor points*, ed 4, Philadelphia, 1978, Lea & Febiger.

Warfel JH: *The extremities*, ed 4, Philadelphia, 1981, Lea & Febiger.

Watkins J: *Structure and function of the musculoskeletal system*, Champaign, IL, 1999, Human Kinetics.

Weir J, Abrahams P: *An atlas of radiological anatomy*, Chicago, 1978, Year Book Medical Publishers Inc.

Wharton J, Wharton P: *The Wharton's stretch book: featuring the breakthrough method of active-isolated stretching*, New York, 1996, Three Rivers Press.

White, TD: *Human osteology*, ed 2, San Diego, 2000, Academic Press.

Woodburne RT, Burkel WE: *Essentials of human anatomy*, ed 9, New York, 1994, Oxford University Press.

Y

Yessis M: *Kinesiology of exercise: a safe and effective way to improve bodybuilding and athletic performance*, Lincolnwood, IL, 1992, Masters Press.

Index

f = figure; b = box; t = table

D

G

Q

R

S

T

U